MANAGEMENT OF COMMON ORTHOPAEDIC DISORDERS

Physical Therapy Principles and Methods

MANAGEMENT OF COMMON ORTHOPAEDIC DISORDERS

Physical Therapy Principles and Methods

FIFTH EDITION

Betsy Myers, DHS, MPT, CSCS, CLT, CWS (Retired)
Board-Certified Clinical Specialist in Orthopaedics
Emergency Medical Responder
Associate Professor
Director, UTC Pro Bono Student-Faculty Physical Therapy Clinic
Department of Physical Therapy
University of Tennessee at Chattanooga
Chattanooga, Tennessee

June Hanks, PT, PhD, DPT, CWS, CLT
Associate Professor
Director of Anatomy Lab
Department of Physical Therapy
University of Tennessee at Chattanooga
Chattanooga, Tennessee

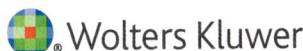

Wolters Kluwer

Philadelphia · Baltimore · New York · London
Buenos Aires · Hong Kong · Sydney · Tokyo

Acquisitions Editor: Matt Hauber
Development Editor: Greg Nicholl (freelance), Amy Millholen
Editorial Assistant: Parisa Saranj
Marketing Manager: Phyllis Hitner
Production Project Manager: Bridgett Dougherty
Design Coordinator: Stephen Druding
Art Director: Jennifer Clements
Manufacturing Coordinator: Margie Orzech
Prepress Vendor: S4Carlisle Publishing Services

Fifth Edition

Copyright © 2023 Wolters Kluwer.

Copyright © 2006 Lippincott Williams & Wilkins. Copyright © 1996, 1990 J. B. Lippincott. Copyright © 1983 Harper & Row. All rights reserved. This book is protected by copyright. No part of this book may be reproduced or transmitted in any form or by any means, including as photocopies or scanned-in or other electronic copies, or utilized by any information storage and retrieval system without written permission from the copyright owner, except for brief quotations embodied in critical articles and reviews. Materials appearing in this book prepared by individuals as part of their official duties as U.S. government employees are not covered by the above-mentioned copyright. To request permission, please contact Wolters Kluwer at Two Commerce Square, 2001 Market Street, Philadelphia, PA 19103, via email at permissions@lww.com, or via our website at shop.lww.com (products and services).

9 8 7 6 5 4 3 2 1

Printed in Mexico

Library of Congress Cataloging-in-Publication Data
ISBN-13: 978-1-975158-96-5
ISBN-10: 1-975158-96-2

Library of Congress Control Number: 2021950783

This work is provided "as is," and the publisher disclaims any and all warranties, express or implied, including any warranties as to accuracy, comprehensiveness, or currency of the content of this work.

This work is no substitute for individual patient assessment based upon healthcare professionals' examination of each patient and consideration of, among other things, age, weight, gender, current or prior medical conditions, medication history, laboratory data and other factors unique to the patient. The publisher does not provide medical advice or guidance and this work is merely a reference tool. Healthcare professionals, and not the publisher, are solely responsible for the use of this work including all medical judgments and for any resulting diagnosis and treatments.

Given continuous, rapid advances in medical science and health information, independent professional verification of medical diagnoses, indications, appropriate pharmaceutical selections and dosages, and treatment options should be made and healthcare professionals should consult a variety of sources. When prescribing medication, healthcare professionals are advised to consult the product information sheet (the manufacturer's package insert) accompanying each drug to verify, among other things, conditions of use, warnings and side effects and identify any changes in dosage schedule or contraindications, particularly if the medication to be administered is new, infrequently used or has a narrow therapeutic range. To the maximum extent permitted under applicable law, no responsibility is assumed by the publisher for any injury and/or damage to persons or property, as a matter of products liability, negligence law or otherwise, or from any reference to or use by any person of this work.

shop.lww.com

PREFACE

Much has changed since 1983 when Darlene Hertling and Randolph Kessler, MD, published the first edition of *Management of Common Musculoskeletal Disorders: Physical Therapy Principles and Methods*, originally designed with the student and entry-level physical therapist. Neuromusculoskeletal clinicians now require doctoral preparation and must have excellent skills in differential diagnosis. This completely updated fifth edition of *Management of Common Orthopaedic Disorders: Physical Therapy Principles and Methods*, is designed to prepare healthcare professionals to provide safe, effective, and holistic care for individuals with orthopaedic conditions. This book is appropriate for physical therapists, occupational therapists physician assistants, nurse practitioners, and athletic trainers along with students in these professions. In keeping with prior editions, we provide concise, user-friendly, and clinically relevant information that is supported by current research.

ORGANIZATION

The book begins with foundational science information encompassing the cellular components of body structures, tissue behavior and healing, arthrology, and gait. Next, clinical foundational chapters detail the patient history and basic physical examination. After providing this key framework, the text flows into joint-specific chapters, starting with the lower quarter to emphasize the influence of the kinetic chain.

For each joint complex, critical anatomy and biomechanics are presented. The book describes specific health history, demographic and symptom investigation, review of systems information, and potential outcome measures. The physical examination for each joint complex includes triage, systems review, quarter screen, clearing examination, and joint-specific examination. Common and potentially concerning pathologies are presented including information regarding pathophysiology, key history and physical examination findings, differential diagnosis, rehabilitation focus, and expected outcomes based on current evidence and clinical practice guidelines.

Emphasis is placed on the importance of a thorough patient history and examination of the related kinetic chain to rule out sources of patient symptoms, identify relevant deviations and impairments, identify factors that might alter rehabilitation, and expedite referral or consultation when needed. Joint-specific chapters conclude with a small case study to highlight vital concepts.

Chapter 19 presents a comprehensive introduction to pain management for the rehabilitation professional including a description of pain types, psychosocial considerations, pain screening and assessment, and interventions.

The book culminates with three detailed case studies in Chapter 20 to reinforce all aspects of the book. Beyond merely providing a sample patient intake form, each case highlights clinician interpretation of the information provided by the patient, suggests clarifying questions and additional information needed, and postulates preliminary diagnostic hypotheses. The detailed physical examination is presented in the order an experienced clinician might follow, demonstrating the clinical reasoning process in order to reach a diagnosis. Each case concludes with a prognosis and possible plan of care.

Finally, the appendices contain a glossary of key terms from the book; an integrated kinematic table of normal joint ranges, arthrokinematics motions, and the open-packed positions to use as a starting point for joint mobilizations; and a table of complete lower and upper quarter motor and sensory information including myotomes, dermatomes, and peripheral nerve innervation along with illustrative figures.

SPECIAL FEATURES

The book includes several features to assist with mastering concepts:

- Nearly 1,000 new full-color photographs and illustrations of anatomy, biomechanics, examination procedures, manual techniques, and exercises
- Tables that summarize key information
- Flow charts that emphasize processes and provide examples
- Case studies both at the end of each clinical chapter and in Chapter 20
- Kinematic summary tables for the body
- Concise presentation of peripheral and segmental innervation

CONTRIBUTORS

June Hanks, PT, PhD, DPT, CWS, CLT
Associate Professor
Director of Anatomy Lab
Department of Physical Therapy
University of Tennessee at Chattanooga
Chattanooga, Tennessee

Betsy Myers, DHS, MPT, CSCS, CLT, CWS (Retired)
Board-Certified Clinical Specialist in Orthopaedics
Emergency Medical Responder
Associate Professor
Director, UTC Pro Bono Student-Faculty Physical Therapy Clinic
Department of Physical Therapy
University of Tennessee at Chattanooga
Chattanooga, Tennessee

Gisela Sole, BScPhysio, MSc(Med)ExSci, PhD
Associate Professor
School of Physiotherapy
University of Otago
Dunedin, New Zealand

Zachary Sutton, PT, DPT, ATC, CHT
Board-Certified Clinical Specialist in Orthopaedics
McMinnville Physical Therapy, LLC
McMinnville, Tennessee

Jeremiah Tate, PT, PhD
Associate Professor
East Tennessee State University-Doctor of Physical Therapy Program
Johnson City, Tennessee

Craig A. Wassinger, PT, PhD
Associate Professor
East Tennessee State University-Doctor of Physical Therapy Program
Johnson City, Tennessee
Doctor of Physical Therapy Program
Tufts University School of Medicine
Boston, Massachusetts

ACKNOWLEDGMENTS

It takes a community! We would like to acknowledge the following individuals for their time and assistance with this fifth edition.

A special thanks to Jeremiah Tate for contributions to Chapter 3, Arthrology; Chapter 9, Ankle and Foot; and for a review of anatomy and biomechanics throughout. Thanks to Craig A. Wassinger and Gisela Sole for writing Chapter 19, Pain Management: A Mechanism-Centered Approach. Thanks to Zachary Sutton for sharing his expertise in Chapter 16, Wrist and Hand Complex. Thanks to Taylor Morgan for assisting with compilation of references and collection of articles.

We are grateful for the hard and efficient work of our University of Tennessee at Chattanooga—Doctor of Physical Therapy Department (UTC-DPT) graduate assistants and our future colleagues: Kate Carney, Mark Britt, and Anthony Errico. Your attention to detail and willingness to support this project are much appreciated.

Thank you to those serving as models for this project! Your willingness to serve as examples for exercises, mobilizations, and the like created an excellent learning resource: Becky Bandy, Kate Carney, Alan Dunlay, Anthony Errico, Krista Fumins, Rachel Grubb, Jessica Hackathorne, Ashlyn Holbrooks, Katie Johnson, Jane Keegan, Heather Marsh, Katherine Meares, Monil Patel, Stacy Takacs, Rachel Watts, and Rhonda Watts.

Thank you to Greg Nicholl, freelance development editor for Wolters Kluwer, for your guidance and patience with this project.

Wolters Kluwer would like to thank Colleen Rocus, Taka Munemoto, and Stacia Hall for their reviews during the development of this book.

June Hanks expresses deepest gratitude to her:

…parents who taught me the value of hard work and persistence.

…long-time friend Mindi whose visits and generous supply of dark chocolates literally kept me going through this project.

…hiking, pickleball, and "let's go get a burger" buddy, Wendy.

…colleague, writing partner and encourager Betsy, who had the vision, dedication, and patience to make this project a reality.

…tail-wagging companions Berkley and Benjamen who make my heart sing.

…dear twin sister, Joan, who started this life journey with me and has been my soulmate throughout…. Love forever!!!

Betsy Myers would like to thank:

…Stacy and Lexi, whose patience and support sustained me throughout this labor of love. It's time for our next adventure!

…June, your knowledge of anatomy is amazing, your editing skills are unmatched, and your track changes comments always made me smile. Thank you for taking the challenge! Ochan! Sante! Onè Respè!

…Hey, Pops, yes—it's finished!

CONTENTS

Preface v
Contributors vi
Acknowledgments vii

PART I
FOUNDATIONAL SCIENCES 1

1 Connective Tissue..2
June Hanks and Betsy Myers
- Connective Tissue Overview 2
- Connective Tissue Components 3
- Specific Connective Tissue Structures 9
- Chapter Summary 14

2 Tissue Behavior, Healing, and Repair...15
June Hanks
- Tissue Behavior 15
- Tissue Injury 17
- Tissue Healing 18
- Healing of Specific Tissues 21
- Chapter Summary 33

3 Arthrology...36
June Hanks and Jeremiah Tate
- Characteristics of Synovial Joints 36
- Joint Motion 38
- Joint Motion Assessment 43
- Chapter Summary 47

4 Spine Osteology and Arthrology...48
June Hanks
- Osteology 48
- Intervertebral Disc 55
- Facet Joints and Movement 58
- Spinal Cord Segment and Spinal Nerve 60
- Contents of Vertebral Canal 64
- Movement of the Vertebral Column 64
- Ligaments of Vertebral Column 64
- Regional Characteristics for Vertebrae, Ligaments, and Discs 68
- Sacroiliac Joint 74
- Muscles 75
- Palpation 90
- Kinematics 90
- Common Pathologies of the Vertebral Column 96
- Chapter Summary 101

5 Gait and Footwear 107
June Hanks and Betsy Myers
- Gait 107
- Standardized Assessments of Balance and Gait 113
- Footwear 114
- Foot Orthotics 117
- Chapter Summary 118

PART II
BASIC HISTORY AND PHYSICAL EXAMINATION 121

6 Patient History 122
Betsy Myers
- History 122
- Health History and General Demographics 125
- Symptom Investigation 129
- Review of Systems 141
- Chapter Summary 144

7 The Physical Examination 146
Betsy Myers
- Introduction to the Basic Physical Examination 146
- Systems Review 148
- Quarter Screen 149
- Clearing Examination 149
- Joint-Specific Examination 149
- Clinical Decision-Making 166
- Prognosis and Plan of Care 170
- Integrated Approach to Treatment 170
- Chapter Summary 172

PART III
LOWER QUARTER 175

8 Lower Quarter Screen 176
Betsy Myers
- Purpose of the Lower Quarter Screen 176
- General Rules for Lower Quarter Screening 177
- Components of the Lower Quarter Screen 177
- Chapter Summary 183

9 Ankle and Foot 185
Betsy Myers, June Hanks, and Jeremiah Tate
- Functional Anatomy of Joints 185
- Biomechanics of Ankle–Foot Complex 197
- Arches of the Foot 203
- Introduction to the Examination of the Ankle and Foot 204
- Patient History: Ankle and Foot Joint 204
- Physical Examination of the Ankle and Foot 205
- Common Foot Pathologies 224
- Common Ankle Pathologies 233
- Differential Diagnosis 245
- Additional Joint Mobilization Treatment Techniques 246
- Additional Therapeutic Exercises 248
- Chapter Summary 251

10 Knee 260
Betsy Myers and June Hanks
- Functional Anatomy 260
- Biomechanics 265
- Muscles About the Knee and Patellofemoral Joint 268
- Palpation 271
- Introduction to the Examination of the Knee 274
- History: Knee Joint 274
- Physical Examination of the Knee 275
- Common Knee Pathologies 290
- Differential Diagnosis 311
- Additional Joint Mobilization Techniques 311
- Additional Therapeutic Exercises 316
- Chapter Summary 320

11 Hip 330
Betsy Myers and June Hanks
- Functional Anatomy 330
- Biomechanics 338
- Introduction to the Examination of the Hip 341
- Patient History: Hip Joint 341
- Physical Examination: Hip Joint 342
- Common Hip Pathologies 352
- Differential Diagnosis 363
- Additional Joint Mobilization Treatment Techniques 363
- Additional Therapeutic Exercises 367
- Chapter Summary 370

12 Lumbar Spine and Sacroiliac Joint 375
Betsy Myers and June Hanks
- Introduction to the Examination of Lumbar Spine and Sacroiliac Joint 375
- Patient History: Lumbar Spine and Sacroiliac Joint 375
- Physical Examination: Lumbar Spine and Sacroiliac Joint 381
- Diagnosis of Lumbar Spine and Sacroiliac Joint Pathology 393
- Nonspecific Low Back Pain 394
- Pathoanatomic Classifications of Low Back Pain 404
- Chapter Summary 420

PART IV
UPPER QUARTER 427

13 Upper Quarter Screen 428
Betsy Myers
- Purpose of the Upper Quarter Screen 428
- General Rules for Upper Quarter Screening 428
- Components of the Upper Quarter Screen 428
- Chapter Summary 434

14 Shoulder Complex 435
Betsy Myers and June Hanks
- Functional Anatomy 435
- Joints of the Shoulder Complex 438
- Muscles 447
- Palpation 453

- Introduction to the Examination of the Shoulder Complex   455
- Patient History: Shoulder Complex   455
- Physical Examination: Shoulder Complex   458
- Common Shoulder Pathologies   474
- Differential Diagnosis   495
- Additional Joint Mobilization Techniques   496
- Additional Therapeutic Exercises   499
- Chapter Summary   504

15 Elbow Complex 513
Betsy Myers and June Hanks
- Functional Anatomy   513
- Arthrokinematics   526
- Palpation   527
- Introduction to the Examination of the Elbow   528
- Patient History: Elbow Complex   529
- Physical Examination: Elbow Complex   530
- Common Elbow Pathologies   540
- Differential Diagnosis   554
- Additional Joint Mobilization Treatment Techniques   554
- Additional Therapeutic Exercises   556
- Chapter Summary   561

16 Wrist and Hand Complex 566
Betsy Myers, June Hanks, and Zachary Sutton
- Functional Anatomy   566
- Osteology   566
- Joints of the Wrist and Hand Complex   571
- Ligaments of the Wrist and Hand Complex   577
- Muscles of the Wrist and Hand Complex   579
- Specific Anatomic Regions of the Wrist and Hand Complex   590
- Nerves Supplying the Wrist and Hand   592
- Palpation of the Wrist and Hand   596
- Introduction to the Examination of the Wrist and Hand Complex   597
- Patient History: Wrist and Hand Complex   597
- Physical Examination: Wrist and Hand   598
- Common Wrist and Hand Pathologies   613
- Differential Diagnosis   630
- Additional Joint Mobilization Treatment Techniques   630
- Additional Therapeutic Interventions   632
- Chapter Summary   636

17 Cervical and Thoracic Spine 641
Betsy Myers and June Hanks
- Introduction to the Examination of Cervical and Thoracic Spine   641
- Patient History   641
- Physical Examination: Cervical and Thoracic Spine   646
- Palpation   661
- Diagnosis of Cervical and Thoracic Spine Pathology   664
- Nonspecific Neck Pain   664
- Pathoanatomic Causes of Neck Pain and Cervical Syndromes   665
- Thoracic Pathologies   672
- Additional Exercises and Manual Therapy for the Cervicothoracic Region   681
- Chapter Summary   689

18 Temporomandibular Joint 695
Betsy Myers and June Hanks
- Functional Anatomy 695
- Joint Structure and Ligaments 698
- Muscles 700
- Arthrokinematics 702
- Palpation 703
- Introduction to the Examination of Temporomandibular Joint 706
- Patient History: Temporomandibular Joint 706
- Physical Examination: Temporomandibular Joint Complex 707
- Common Temporomandibular Joint Pathologies 714
- Interventions for Temporomandibular Dysfunction 716
- Expected Outcomes 721
- Chapter Summary 721

PART V
PAIN MANAGEMENT 725

19 Pain Management: A Mechanism-Centered Approach 726
Craig A. Wassinger and Gisela Sole
- Pain Science Definitions and Epidemiology 726
- Anatomy and Physiology 726
- Biopsychosocial Model and the Pain Neuromatrix Theory 727
- Pain Types 728
- Psychosocial Considerations in Pain 729
- Initial Pain Assessment Considerations 731
- Interventions 733
- Chapter Summary 739

PART VI
APPLIED CLINICAL REASONING 745

20 Case Studies 746
Betsy Myers
- Introduction to Case Studies 746
- Chapter Summary 761

Appendix A: Glossary 763
Appendix B: Osteokinematic and Arthrokinematic Motions 766
Appendix C: Peripheral and Segmental Nerve Innervation 768
Index 771

PART I

Foundational Sciences

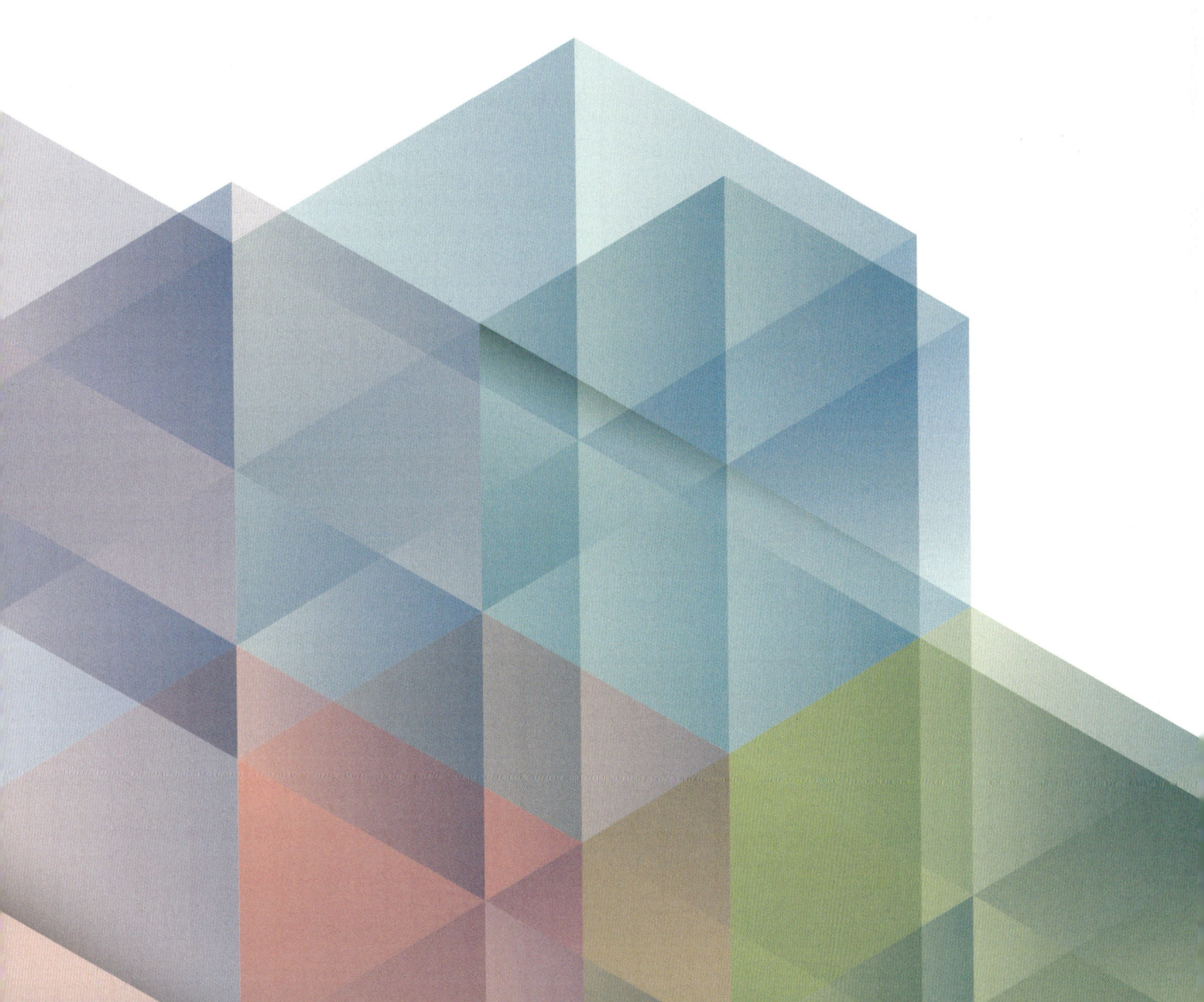

1 | Connective Tissue

June Hanks and Betsy Myers

CHAPTER OBJECTIVES

After reading this chapter, you will be able to:
1. Describe the composition of connective tissue.
2. Differentiate between loose and dense connective tissue.
3. Describe the function of fixed and transient connective tissue cells.
4. Describe the biosynthesis of the collagen molecule and the formation of collagen fibrils and fibers.
5. Differentiate among collagen types.
6. Describe the function of proteoglycans and glycosaminoglycans in the extracellular matrix.
7. Differentiate among fibrocartilage, elastic cartilage, and articular cartilage.
8. Describe the formation of bone.
9. Describe the composition of ligament, tendon, and fascia.

CONNECTIVE TISSUE OVERVIEW

The human body is composed of four major tissue types: epithelial tissue, muscle tissue, nervous tissue, and connective tissue. Connective tissue provides a framework that supports, connects, and binds together various body structures. In addition, connective tissue facilitates the exchange of nutrients between tissues and the blood, plays a role in immune system function, and assists in tissue repair.

Connective tissue consists of cells and an extracellular matrix (ECM) (Fig. 1-1). While epithelial, muscle, and nerve tissue consist mostly of cells, connective tissue consists of fewer cells and a large ECM. The ECM is composed of protein fibers (collagen, elastic, and reticular) and a gel-like substance, called *ground substance*, between the cells and fibers. Collagen proteins construct the collagen and reticular fibers; elastic fibers are formed from elastic proteins. The ground substance contains glycoproteins, proteoglycans (PGs), and glycosaminoglycans (GAGs).

Connective tissue can be described as connective tissue proper and specific connective tissue. The connective tissue discussed in this chapter is included in Figure 1-2. Common characteristics and differences in relative composition and function of connective tissue proper are presented in Table 1-1.

Loose and dense connective tissues are considered "connective tissue proper" and are distinguished by relative proportions of fibers and ground substance. Loose connective tissue has an open, spacious semiliquid composition with few fibers and an abundant amount of ground substance. Collagen and elastic fibers in loose connective tissue are arranged in an unorganized manner, forming a nonpatterned meshwork, making the tissue only slightly resistant to stress. Loose connective tissue is abundant throughout the

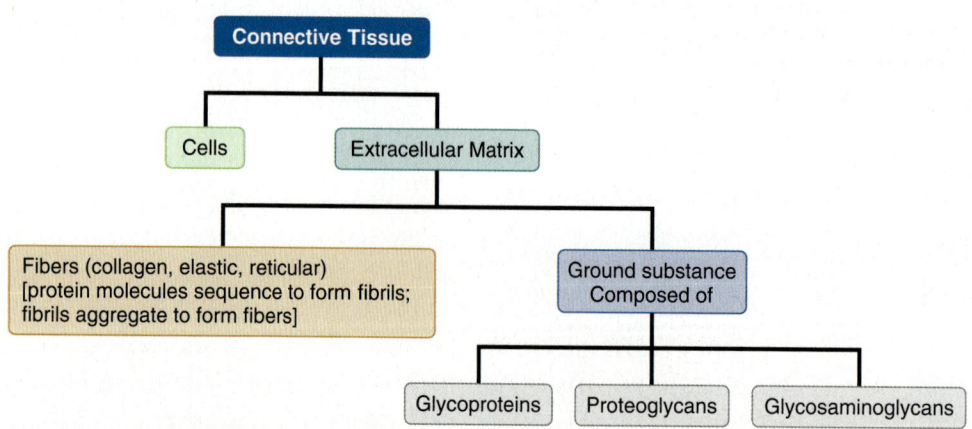

FIGURE 1-1 Connective tissue composition.

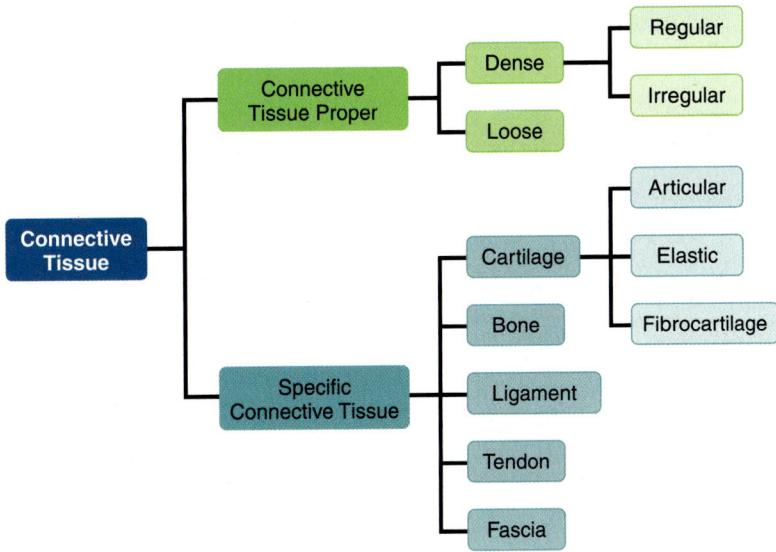

FIGURE 1-2 Proper and specific connective tissue.

TABLE 1-1			
COMPOSITION, LOCATION, AND FUNCTION OF CONNECTIVE TISSUE PROPER			
		Dense	
	Loose	*Irregular*	*Regular*
Cells	Fibroblasts, adipocytes, some macrophages with other WBC	Predominately fibroblasts	Predominately fibroblasts
Fibers	Predominately collagen; some elastin and reticulin	Collagen, elastin, reticulin	Collagen, elastin, reticulin
Relative composition	Fewer fibers; more ECM	Less ECM; more cells and fibers	Less ECM; more cells and fibers
Arrangement of fibers	Random distribution	Bundled; arranged in various directions	Bundled; arranged in uniform, parallel fashion
Primary location	Beneath epithelia; surrounding organs; lining body surfaces	Skin dermis; capsule of organs	Tendons, ligaments
Primary function	Protect, suspend, support	Protect; resist tension in multiple directions	Resist tension in direction of fiber orientation

ECM, extracellular matrix; *WBC*, white blood cell.
Modified from Cui D, Daley W, Fratkin JD, et al. *Atlas of Histology with Function and Clinical Correlations*. Lippincott Williams & Wilkins; 2011; and Gartner LP. *BRS Cell Biology and Histology*. 8th ed. Wolters Kluwer; 2019.

body, forming the tissue around vessels and organs and under the skin. Dense connective tissue has more cells (primarily fibroblasts) and fibers (primarily collagen) and less ground substance than loose connective tissue. The collagen fibers are arranged in bundles that allow for withstanding stress. In dense irregular connective tissue, the fiber bundles are arranged in various directions, allowing the tissue to withstand stresses in multiple directions. The deeper layers of the skin and the submucosa of several hollow organs are composed of dense irregular connective tissue. Tendons, ligaments, and aponeuroses are composed primarily of dense regular connective tissue that contains fibers arranged in orderly, parallel bundles affording the ability to resist tension primarily in the direction of their fiber orientation.

Specialized connective tissue includes cartilage, bone, blood, adipose, hematopoietic tissue, and lymphatic tissue. This chapter includes a discussion of cartilage, bone, ligament, tendon, and fascia.

CONNECTIVE TISSUE COMPONENTS

Cells

Embryonic mesenchymal cells differentiate into the specialized cells of connective tissue (Table 1-2). Some of the connective tissue cells are fixed cells that are formed in and remain within the connective tissue. Other cells, called *transient or wandering cells*, originate from hematopoietic stem cells, develop in bone marrow, and migrate into connective tissue from the blood (Fig. 1-3). The primary function of the cells is to

TABLE 1-2
CELLS OF CONNECTIVE TISSUE

Cells	Type	Function
Fibroblasts	Fixed	Secrete the ECM components of most tissues, primarily collagen and elastin
Chondroblasts	Fixed	Secrete the ECM components of cartilage
Osteoblasts	Fixed	Secrete the ECM components of bone
Myofibroblasts	Fixed	Secrete ECM components and have a contractile function
Adipocytes	Fixed	Lipid-storing cells that store energy, cushion and pad
Mast cells	Fixed	Develop in bone marrow; differentiate in connective tissue; distributed primarily in skin and skin appendages; secrete mediators of inflammation
Macrophages	Fixed and transient	Phagocytic cells derived from monocytes; important in immune response reactions
Lymphoid cells	Transient	Function in immune process
Plasma cells	Transient	Manufacture immunoglobulins (antibodies)
Neutrophils	Transient	Phagocytose and kill bacteria
Eosinophils	Transient	Kill parasites; phagocytose antibody-antigen complexes
Basophils	Transient	Initiate and control inflammatory processes

ECM, extracellular matrix.
Adapted from Stevens A, Lowe J. *Human Histology*. 3rd ed. Mosby/Elsevier; 2005; and Pawlina W, Ross MH. *Histology: A Text and Atlas with Correlated Cell and Molecular Biology*. 8th ed. Wolters Kluwer; 2020.

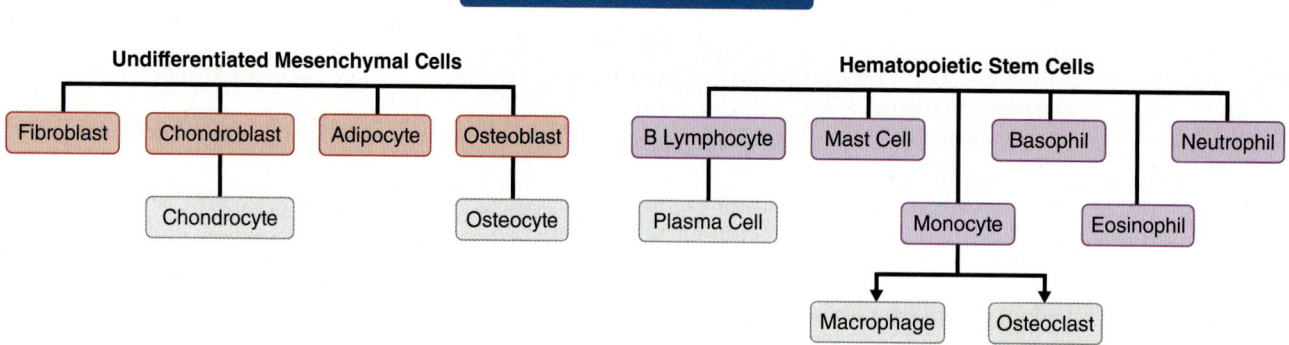

FIGURE 1-3 Origin of connective tissue cells.

secrete and maintain the ECM. The most abundant cell in connective tissue is the fibroblast that is responsible for the secretion of the ECM in most tissues. The ECM provides the supportive structural framework, communication system, and metabolic regulatory function for the cells.

Fibers

The primary types of connective tissue fibers are collagen, elastic, and reticular fibers. The amount and type of fibers dominating a particular connective tissue are dependent on structural and functional needs.

Collagen Fibers The most abundant structural protein in connective tissue is collagen.[1-3] There are at least 28 different types of collagen, with each type composed of distinctive combinations of amino acids forming chains, called *polypeptide chains* (also called α-chains).[3] The α-chains configure to form the procollagen molecule. The procollagen molecule is shortened to form the collagen molecule (formerly called *tropocollagen*). Collagen fibrils assemble to form collagen fibers.[1] The collagen fibers bundle together to form larger bundles that eventually form connective tissue structures. See Figure 1-4 for an example of the formation of tendon.

The biosynthesis of collagen fibers involves multiple intracellular and extracellular events. In the rough endoplasmic reticulum of connective tissue cells (primarily fibroblasts), amino acids assemble to form sequenced long polypeptide chains (α-chains) of a characteristic glycine-X-Y pattern, where every third amino acid of the sequence is glycine and X and Y can be any amino acid but are often proline and hydroxyproline.[4] Three polypeptide chains (α-chains) coil about a central axis in a right-handed triple-helix manner,[3] forming the procollagen molecule. Through hydrogen, covalent,

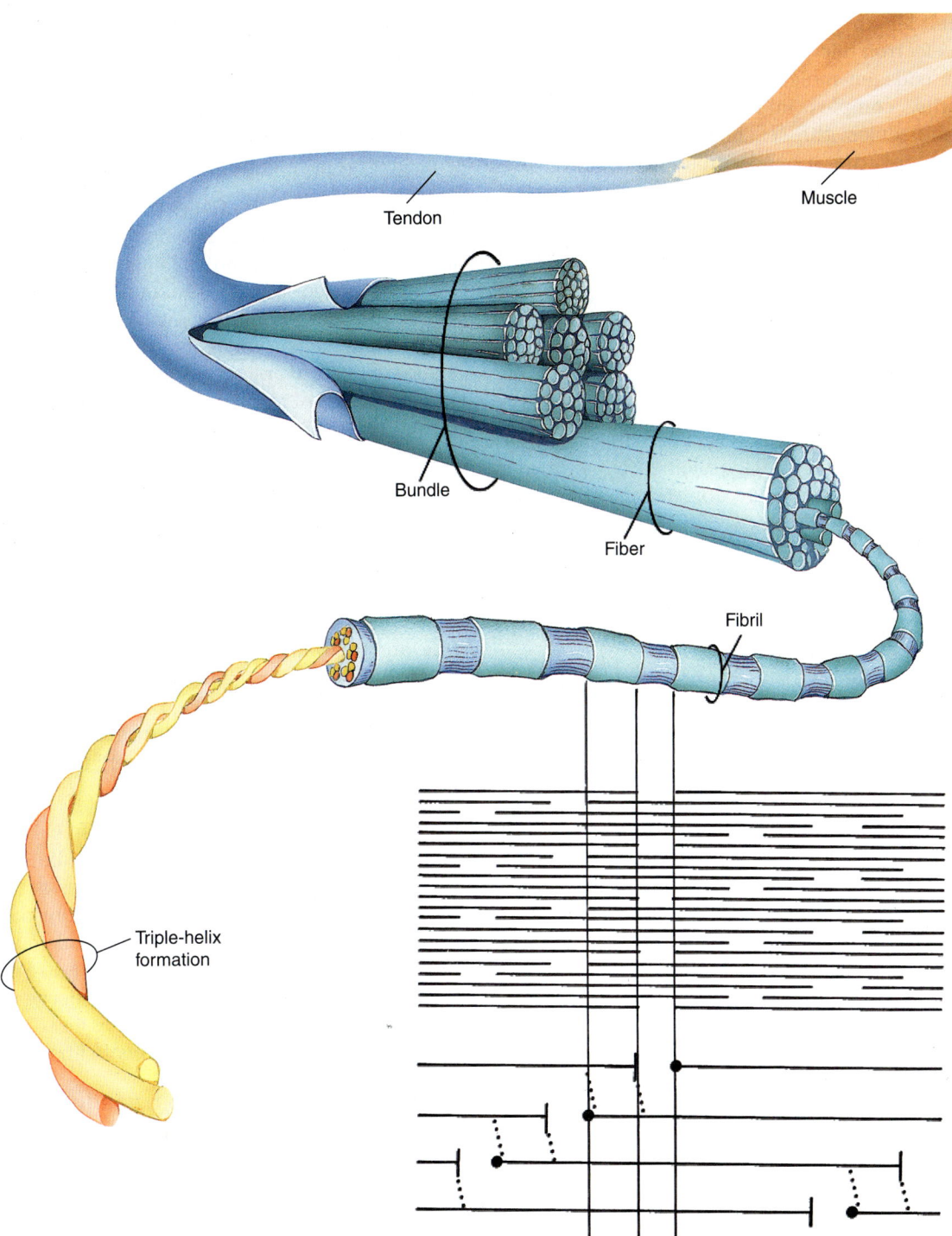

FIGURE 1-4 Example of the assembly of collagen fibers forming the collagen bundles of tendon. Note the staggered self-assembly of the chains forming the procollagen molecule. The procollagen molecule shortens to form the triple-helix collagen molecule. The collagen molecules gather to form collagen fibrils that continue to assemble forming collagen fibers. (Gartner LP. *Color Atlas and Text of Histology.* 7th ed. Wolters Kluwer; 2018: Figure 3-1.)

hydrophobic, and hydrophilic interactions, the specific α-chains fit tightly together. Upon or during secretion into the ECM, the nonhelical ends of the procollagen molecules are shortened owing to the cleavage of N- and C-terminal propeptides by extracellular peptidases (enzymes). This slightly shortened structure is now called the *collagen* molecule. The adjacent collagen molecules are displaced from one another about one-quarter step of their length, giving a striated appearance when viewed in electron micrographs.

As the collagen molecules assemble to form collagen fibrils, complex interactions occur between collagen molecules, the cell membrane surface, and components of the ground substance. Short segments at the ends of the α-chains that are not part of the glycine-X-Y repeating sequence (and thus are not triple-helical) form side chains that are modified and covalently cross-linked with components in adjacent molecules. The cross-links stabilize the collagen molecules, increasing the strength of the fibril. Various types of collagen fibrils bind together to form unique collagen fibril types. For example, in the formation of tendon, shorter type VI collagen fibrils bind to type I fibrils, forming thicker fibrils (Fig. 1-5A). In the formation of cartilage, type II fibrils are joined by short and flexible type IX fibrils with the nonhelical ends of the type IX fibrils and attached GAGs (such as chondroitin sulfate) protruding out from the type II fibril, helping to anchor the fibril to components of the ECM that will attach to the GAG (Fig. 1-5B).

The various collagen molecules are defined by the composition of the α-chains forming the procollagen molecules. The α-chains may be formed by three identical chains (homotrimers) as in collagen types II, III, VII, VIII, X, and others may be formed by two or more different chains (heterotrimers) as in collagen types I, IV, V, VI, IX, and XI. Roman numerals are assigned to categorize collagen types (called *collagens*) based on when they are discovered. The majority of collagens are fibril-forming collagens. Less abundant, but important, collagen types include fibril-associated collagens (that link fibril-forming collagens to one another or ECM components); sheet-forming and anchoring collagens (that form networks and connections in basal laminae), and transmembrane collagens (that function as adhesion receptors). See Table 1-3 for examples of collagen types, location, and function.

Elastic Fibers Elastic fibers (composed of elastin) are present in both loose and dense connective tissues, are less abundant than collagen fibers, and possess different properties. Elastin molecules are produced by fibroblasts, chondrocytes, smooth muscle, and endothelial cells. The elastin molecules have α-like chains, similar to collagen molecules, but the chains are single and do not form a triple helix. When stretched, the elastin molecule uncoils, then recoils when the stretch force is removed. The chains cross-link and form thin, flexible, rubber-like elastic fibers that branch out in multiple directions. The elastic fibers slide across each other as they move from a stretched to recoiled state. Elastic fibers interweave with collagen fibers to limit distensibility of tissue and prevent tearing. Elastic fibers are found in skin, joint structures, the tracheobronchial tree, and the walls of arteries. Structures that need more extensibility have a greater percentage of elastic than collagen fibers. For example, the aorta and ligamentum nuchae have a high percentage of elastic fibers, whereas the Achilles tendon has a relatively low percentage of elastic fibers.[5]

Reticular Fibers Reticular fibers (also called *reticulin*) may be produced by several cells, including specialized reticular cells and fibroblasts. Reticular fibers are composed of type III collagen.[6,7] Typically, the reticular fibrils are thin, branch out, and cross-link in a mesh-like pattern, providing support for cells in loose connective tissue such as around adipocytes, nerve cells, and muscle cells. Reticular fibers possess less tensile strength than do collagen and elastin fibers.

Ground Substance of Extracellular Matrix

The ground substance (also called the *interfibrillar component*) of the ECM is amorphous and contains water and a variety of specialized proteins: GAGs, PGs, and multiadhesive glycoproteins. The GAGs consist of polysaccharides with repeating disaccharide (double sugar) units and attached sulfate and carboxyl groups. The nature, linkage, and sulfation of the sugar groups distinguish the GAGs into types (Table 1-4). GAGs bind to a protein core to form PGs. An individual PG molecule may have multiple attached GAGs that stick out from the protein core, giving the appearance of a bottle brush (Fig. 1-6). The GAGs attract large amounts of water, forming a gel-like composition within the ECM. The rigidity of the GAGs contributes to the structural framework within the ECM.

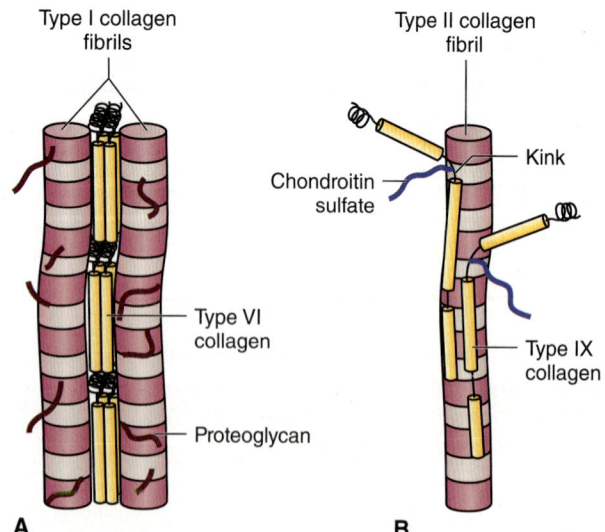

FIGURE 1-5 Binding of multiple collagen types. **A.** In tendon formation, type VI collagen molecules bind to type I fibrils forming a thicker fiber. **B.** Type IX collagen molecules bind to type II fibrils of cartilage.

TABLE 1-3
EXAMPLES OF COLLAGEN TYPES, LOCATION, AND FUNCTION

Type	Composition	Location	Function
Fibril-forming collagens			
I	$[α1(I)]_2\, α2(I)$	Connective tissue of skin, bone, tendon, ligaments, dentin, sclera, fascia, and organ capsules (accounts for 90% of body collagen)	Provides resistance to force, tension, and stretch
II	$[α1(II)]_3$	Cartilage (hyaline and elastic), notochord, and intervertebral disc	Provides resistance to intermittent pressure
III	$[α1(III)]_3$	Prominent in loose connective tissue and organs (uterus, liver, spleen, kidney, lung, etc.), smooth muscle, endoneurium, blood vessels, and fetal skin	Forms reticular fibers; arranged in a loose meshwork of thin fibers that provides a supportive scaffolding for the specialized cells of various organs and blood vessels
V	$[α1(V)]_2\, α2(V)$ or $α1(V)\, α2(V)\, α3(V)$	Distributed uniformly throughout connective tissue stroma; may be related to reticular network; localized in reticular fibers of the splenic red pulp	Localized at the surface of type I collagen fibrils along with types XII and XIV collagen to modulate biomedical properties of the fibril
Fibril-associated collagens			
VI	$[α1(VI)]_2\, α2(VI)$ or $α1(VI)\, α2(VI)\, α3(VI)$	Forms part of the cartilage matrix immediately surrounding the chondrocytes	Attaches the chondrocyte to the matrix; covalently bound to type I collagen fibrils
IX	$α1(IX)\, α2(IX)\, α3(IX)$	Found in cartilage associated with type II collagen fibrils	Stabilizes network of cartilage type II collagen fibers by interaction with proteoglycan molecules at their intersections
Sheet-forming and anchoring collagens			
IV	$[α1(IV)]_2\, α2(IV)$ or $α3(IV)\, α4(IV)\, α5(IV)$ or $[α5(IV)]_2\, α6(IV)$	Basal laminae of epithelia, kidney glomeruli, and lens capsule	Provides support and contributes to filtration-barrier functions
VII	$[α1(VII)]_3$	Present in anchoring fibrils of skin, eye, uterus, esophagus	Secures basal lamina to connective tissue fibers
Transmembrane collagen			
XIII	$[α1(XIII)]_3$	Present in bone, cartilage, intestine, skin, placenta, and striated muscles	Associated with the basal lamina along with type VII collagen

Adapted from Pawlina W, Ross MH. *Histology: A Text and Atlas with Correlated Cell and Molecular Biology*. 8th ed. Wolters Kluwer; 2020; and Liu SH, Yang RS, Shaikh R, Lane JM. Collagen in tendon, ligament and bone healing: a current review. *Clin Orthop Relat Res*. 1995;318:265–278.

TABLE 1-4
EXAMPLES OF GLYCOSAMINOGLYCANS

Name	Location	Function
Hyaluronan	Synovial fluid, vitreous humor, ECM of connective tissues	Lubricant and shock absorber
Chondroitin 4-sulfate	Cartilage, bone, heart valves	Chondroitin sulfates and hyaluronan are fundamental components of the aggrecan PG found in articular cartilage. Aggrecan confers on articular cartilage shock-absorbing properties.
Chondroitin 6-sulfate	Skin, blood vessels, heart valves	
Dermatan sulfate		Dermatan sulfates have been implicated in cardiovascular disease, tumorigenesis, infection, wound repair, fibrosis, and as a modulator in cell behavior.
Keratan sulfate	Bone, cartilage, cornea	Keratan sulfates function in cellular recognition of protein ligands, axonal guidance, cell motility, corneal transparency, and embryo implantation.
Heparan sulfate	Basal lamina, normal component of cell surface	Facilitates interaction with fibroblast growth factor (FGF) and its receptor
Heparin	Limited to granules of mast cells and basophils	Functions as an anticoagulant; facilitates interactions with FGF and its receptor

ECM, extracellular matrix; *PGs*, proteoglycans.
Modified from Pawlina W, Ross MH. *Histology: A Text and Atlas with Correlated Cell and Molecular Biology*. 8th ed. Wolters Kluwer; 2020; and Gartner LP. *BRS Cell Biology and Histology*. 8th ed. Wolters Kluwer; 2019.

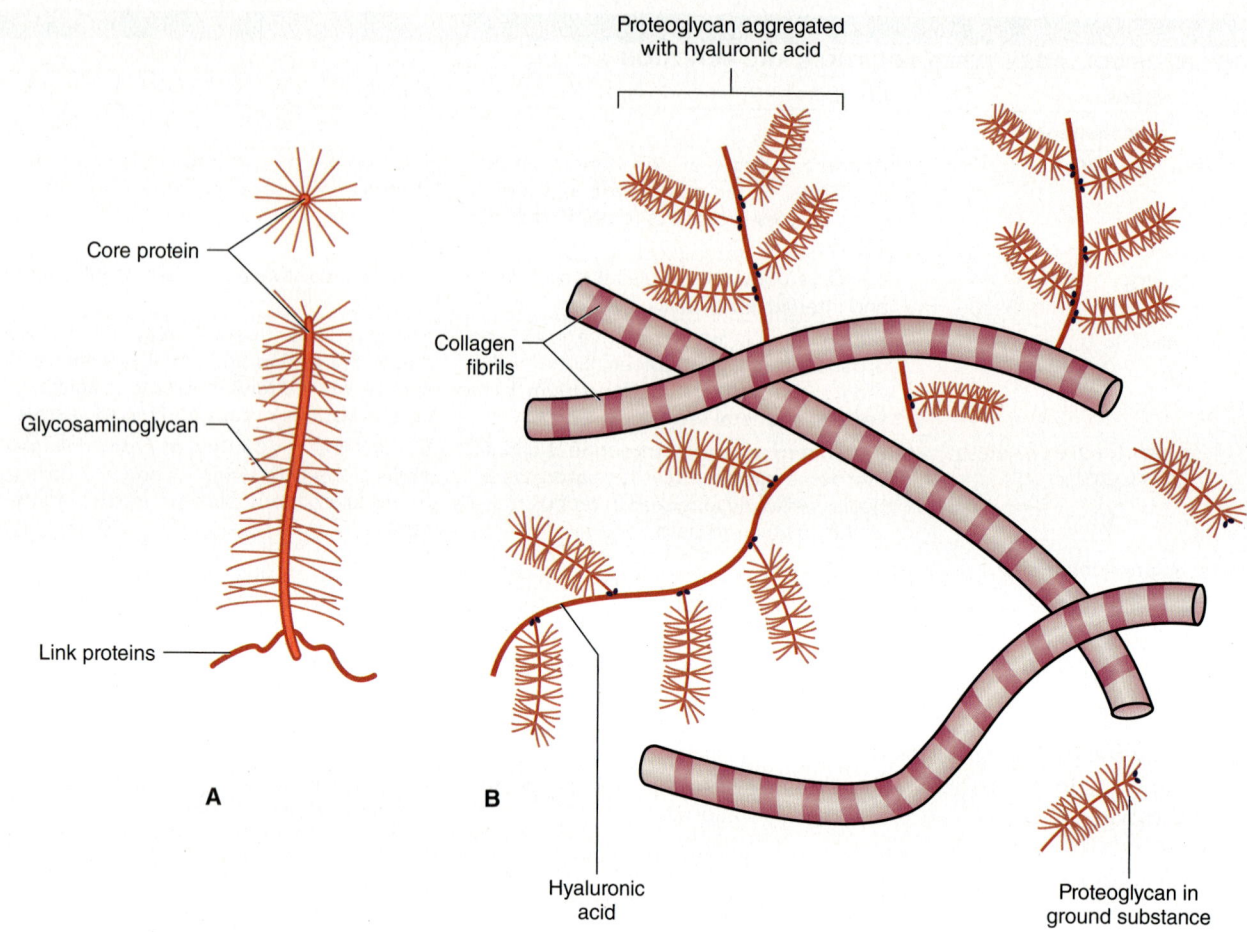

FIGURE 1-6 ECM components. **A.** Two views of a proteoglycan molecule. **B.** Various ECM molecules. *ECM,* extracellular matrix.

The GAG hyaluronan is distinctive in that it is long and rigid, does not contain sulfate, exists as a free carbohydrate chain, and is composed of many more sugars than other GAGs. Hyaluronan does not bind to protein; therefore, it does not form PGs. However, PGs indirectly bind to hyaluronan, forming giant macromolecules that attract water. These macromolecules are exceptionally abundant in the ECM of cartilage and contribute to its flexible, shock-absorbing, compression-resistant characteristic. In addition, hyaluronan binds certain growth factors to enhance or inhibit the movement of macromolecules, microorganisms, and cells within the ECM.

The number and type of GAGs attached to the protein core of PGs vary significantly, leading to great diversity among PGs (Table 1-5). Each type of connective tissue structure contains a unique composition of PGs. The PGs regulate collagen fibril formation and the

TABLE 1-5		
PROTEOGLYCANS		
Name	Location	Function
Aggrecan	Cartilage, chondrocytes	Hydrates ECM of cartilage
Decorin	Connective tissue, fibroblasts, cartilage, and bone	Functions in collagen fibril formation; by attaching to neighboring collagen molecules, helps to orient fibers; regulates thickness of the fibril and interacts with transforming growth factor β (TGF-β)
Versican	Fibroblasts, skin, smooth muscle, brain, and mesangial cells of the kidney	Possesses EGF-like domains on the core protein; participates in cell-to-cell and cell-to-ECM interactions; binds to fibulin-1
Syndecan	Embryonic epithelia, mesenchymal cells, developing lymphatic tissue cells, lymphocytes, and plasma cells	The extracellular domain binds to collagens, heparin, tenascin, and fibronectin; intracellular domain binds to cytoskeleton via actin

ECM, extracellular matrix; *EGF,* epidermal growth factor.
Modified from Pawlina W, Ross MH. *Histology: A Text and Atlas with Correlated Cell and Molecular Biology.* 8th ed. Wolters Kluwer; 2020.

binding of smaller collagen molecules into larger molecules (process of polymerization). Examples of PGs include aggrecan, decorin, versican, and syndecan. The various PGs play a role in the function and maintenance of connective tissue, contributing to the stability of the tissue by resisting compressive, tensile, and shear forces and by regulating cellular growth, differentiation, and migration. Connective tissues such as tendons and ligaments must resist tension and contain relatively small concentrations of PGs. Articular cartilage, which must resist compressive forces, contains a high concentration of PGs.

Multiadhesive glycoproteins are proteins with an attached carbohydrate molecule. Examples include fibronectin, laminin, tenascin, and osteopontin (Table 1-6). The multiadhesive glycoproteins have multiple binding sites for collagens, PGs, and GAGs and play a significant role in stabilizing the ECM. In addition, multiadhesive glycoproteins regulate and modulate the proliferation, differentiation, movement, and migration of cells within the ECM.

SPECIFIC CONNECTIVE TISSUE STRUCTURES

Connective tissue within the human body occurs in many different forms with diverse physical properties. The main types of connective tissue include cartilage, bone, ligaments, tendon, and fascia.

Cartilage

Cartilage is an avascular form of connective tissue composed of cells (immature chondroblasts and mature chondrocytes) and an expansive ECM, which is firm yet pliable. The cartilage cells produce the collagen, GAGs, PGs, and hyaluronan that are secreted into the ECM and contribute to the production and maintenance of the ECM. The supply of nutrients and removal of wastes occur through diffusion. Types of cartilage include fibrocartilage, elastic cartilage, and articular (hyaline) cartilage (Table 1-7). All types of cartilage contain type II collagen and large amounts of aggregating PGs. The large ratio of aggregating PGs to collagen allows for diffusion of substances from the blood of surrounding tissues into the chondrocytes. The significant hydration of the aggregating PGs facilitates resistance to compression forces.

Fibrocartilage contains type I and type II collagen fibers and occurs primarily in joints where little motion occurs, such as intervertebral discs and articular discs. The numerous fibers reinforce each other, making the structure ideal for bearing large stresses in multiple directions. Fibrocartilage is relatively avascular and aneural.

Elastic cartilage, sometimes called *elastic* fibrocartilage, is similar in composition to other types of cartilage but has more elastin fibers and is less prone to degeneration.[8] Elastic cartilage provides strength and elasticity and is found in structures such as the external ear and epiglottis.

Articular cartilage provides a smooth, resilient, low-friction, lubrication surface to the ends of bones in synovial joints. The articular cartilage is capable of bearing weight and distributing compressive forces over a large surface area. Articular cartilage is also capable of maintaining the force distribution properties over a person's lifetime, although the limited repair mechanisms may lead to degeneration if the tissue is injured. As with other connective tissue, articular cartilage has a small cellular and larger ground substance composition. The ECM of articular cartilage contains three types of GAGs: hyaluronan, chondroitin sulfate, and keratan sulfate. The PG aggrecan (containing chondroitin and keratan sulfate GAG chains) joins with hyaluronan,

TABLE 1-6		
MULTIADHESIVE GLYCOPROTEINS		
Name	Location	Function
Fibronectin	Present in the ECM of many tissues	Responsible for cell adhesion and mediates migration; possesses binding sites for integrins, type IV collagen, heparin, and fibrin
Laminin	Present in basal laminae of all epithelial cells and external laminae of muscle cells, adipocytes, and Schwann cells	Anchors cell surfaces to the basal lamina; possesses binding sites for collagen type IV, heparan sulfate, heparin, entactin, laminin, and integrin receptors on the cell surface
Tenascin	Giant protein formed from six chains connected by disulfide bonds	Embryonic mesenchyme, perichondrium, periosteum, musculotendinous junctions, wounds, tumors
Osteopontin	Bone	Binds to osteoclasts; possesses binding sites for calcium, hydroxyapatite, and integrin receptors on the osteoclast membrane

ECM, extracellular matrix.
Modified from Pawlina W, Ross MH. Histology: *A Text and Atlas with Correlated Cell and Molecular Biology.* 8th ed. Wolters Kluwer; 2020; and Gartner LP. *BRS Cell Biology and Histology.* 8th ed. Wolters Kluwer; 2019.

TABLE 1-7			
TYPES OF CARTILAGE			
	Fibrocartilage	*Elastic Cartilage*	*Articular Cartilage*
Characteristic	Types I and II collagen fibers; the matrix material of hyaline cartilage	Type II collagen fibers and elastin fibers; matrix material of hyaline cartilage	Matrix-containing type II collagen fibers, glycosaminoglycans, proteoglycans, and multiadhesive glycoproteins
Location	Intervertebral discs, pubic symphysis, articular discs (sternoclavicular and temporomandibular joints), knee menisci, triangular fibrocartilage complex, and insertion of tendons	External ear, external acoustic meatus, auditory (eustachian) tube, and cartilages of larynx (epiglottis, corniculate, and cuneiform cartilages)	Fetal skeletal tissue, epiphyseal plates, articular surface of synovial joints, costal cartilages of rib cage, cartilages of nasal cavity, larynx (thyroid, cricoid, and arytenoids), rings of trachea, and plates in bronchi
Function	Resists deformation under stress	Provides flexible support for soft tissues	Resists compression; provides cushioning, smooth, and low-friction surface for joints; provides structural support in respiratory system (larynx, trachea, and bronchi); forms foundation for the development of fetal skeleton and further endochondral bone formation and bone growth
Repair	Very limited capability; commonly forms scar, resulting in fibrocartilage formation		

Modified from Cui D, Daley W, Fratkin JD, et al. *Atlas of Histology with Function and Clinical Correlations*. Lippincott Williams & Wilkins; 2011; and Pawlina W, Ross MH. *Histology: A Text and Atlas with Correlated Cell and Molecular Biology*. 8th ed. Wolters Kluwer; 2020.

forming larger structures that attract and bind large amounts of water. Collagen fibers (primarily type II) are interspersed throughout the ECM and a hoop-like meshwork of collagen is formed at the joint surface. The collagen network helps to contain the water and PG molecules, contributing to resistance to compressive forces.

Bone

Bone is a dynamic, metabolically active, and rigid connective tissue that, along with cartilage, makes up the skeleton. Bone formation (called *ossification*) begins in the embryonic stage of development and continues through late adolescence. The bones continue to remodel throughout life. There are two types of bone: compact bone and spongy bone. Compact (cortical) bone surrounds spongy bone. Blood vessels supply compact bone with oxygen and nutrients through channels called *Haversian canals*. The framework of spongy bone is organized into a three-dimensional lattice-type network of bony columns called *trabeculae*, which are arranged along lines of stress. The spongy bone is porous and highly vascularized. Bone marrow and hematopoietic stem cells occupy the spaces in spongy bone (Fig. 1-7).

Bones develop from fibrous membranes and hyaline cartilage through two different ossification processes: intramembranous and endochondral. Both ossification processes involve mesenchymal cells, osteoblasts, osteoid formation, and mineralization. The processes of ossification are described in the subsequent section.

In intramembranous ossification, bone is formed from connective tissue membranes. Embryonic mesenchymal cells differentiate into capillaries and osteoblasts. Early osteoblasts cluster together to form ossification centers. The osteoblasts secrete osteoid (an unmineralized matrix) that will harden (calcify) as mineral salts are deposited onto it. Osteoblasts become entrapped in the matrix and become osteocytes. The process includes the formation of trabeculae. Osteoblasts on the outside of spongy bone form a thin connective tissue covering called *periosteum*. Compact bone usually replaces the outer layer of spongy bone, while the center of the bone remains spongy. Blood and lymphatic vessels grow into the newly formed bone and develop red bone marrow. The clavicles and bones of the skull are formed through intramembranous ossification. In fetal development, the membrane-filled spaces (fontanels) between the skull bones allow for easier passage through the birth canal. From infancy through adolescence, the fontanels change to sutures through intramembranous ossification.

The majority of bones of the skeleton, including long bones, are formed through endochondral ossification in which cartilage is replaced by bone. In this process, mesenchymal cells differentiate into chondroblasts, which secrete a cartilage matrix. The peripheral surface, called *perichondrium*, forms the shape of the future bone. A primary ossification center is formed at the central portion of the developing bone, which lengthens and widens. The chondrocytes within the growing matrix become larger. Osteogenic cells differentiate into osteoblasts, which deposit more matrix

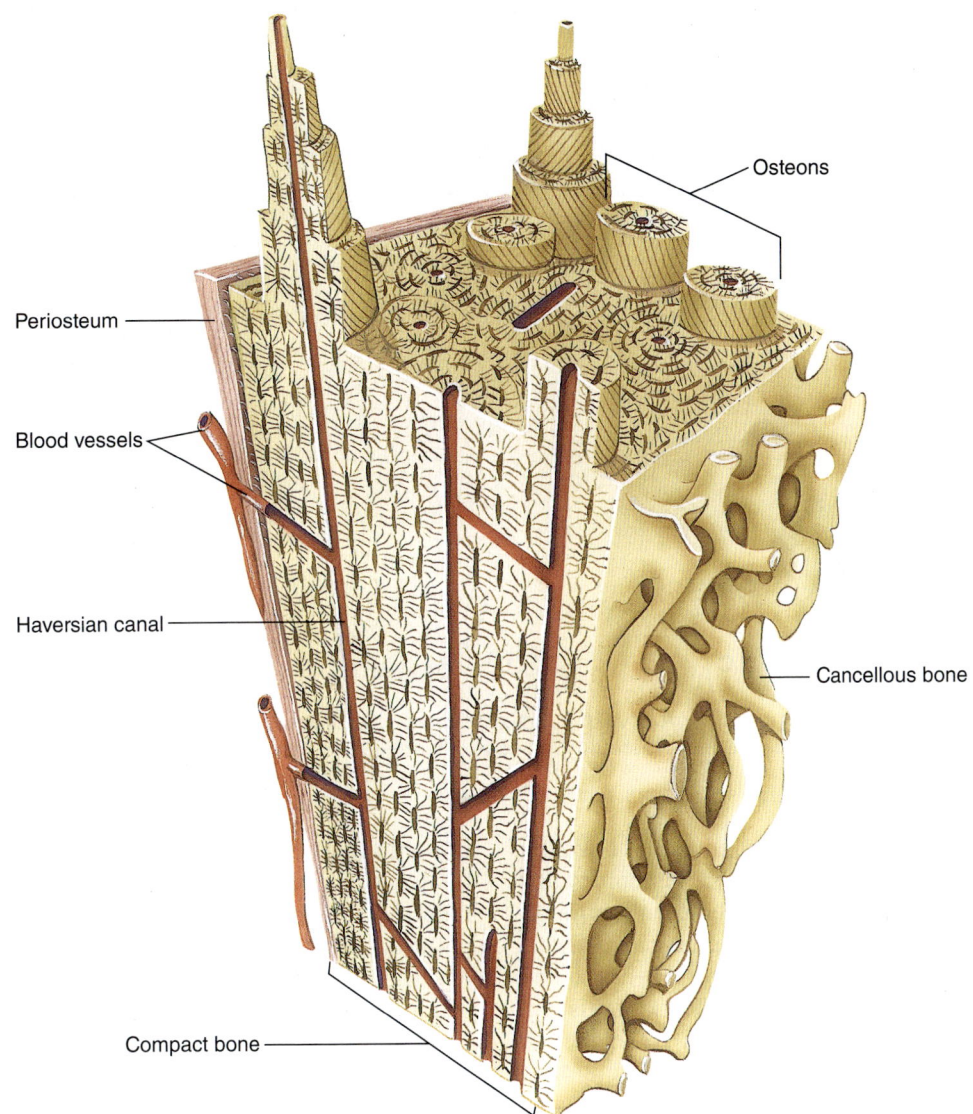

FIGURE 1-7 Section of compact bone. Blood vessels from the periosteum enter the bones through nutrient canals or smaller Volkmann canals. The osteon is composed of concentric lamellae of bone. (Gartner LP. *Color Atlas and Text of Histology.* 7th ed. Wolters Kluwer; 2018: Figure 4-1.)

under the perichondrium, forming a thin shell of compact bone known as the *bone collar*. The penetration of blood vessels into the perichondrium stimulates bone formation, transforming the perichondrium to periosteum. The bone collar deprives nutrients to the cartilage on the interior of the forming bone, causing the cartilage to disintegrate. Capillaries grow into the disintegrating cartilage and are replaced by bone.

Osteoblasts create the spongy bone trabeculae. A medullary cavity is formed at the core of the structure and is filled with capillaries and red bone marrow. Ossification continues forming the long midsection of the bone (the diaphysis). Blood vessels enter the cartilaginous epiphyses near the ends of the bones (the epiphysis), forming secondary ossification centers. Ossification proceeds outward, and the interior of the epiphysis remains spongy. By the time of full fetal skeleton formation, cartilage remains at the joint surface as articular cartilage and between the epiphysis and diastasis as the epiphyseal plate. During development, cartilage is transformed to bone on the diaphysis side of the epiphyseal plate and the bone lengthens (Fig. 1-8).

Bony remodeling occurs throughout life as a function of the ossification process of osteoblasts and the resorption process of osteoclasts.[9] In the remodeling process, old or damaged bone is resorbed and replaced by new bone. The signaling processes for osteoclast activation and reversal are unclear. Following activation, the osteoclasts resorb minerals and free

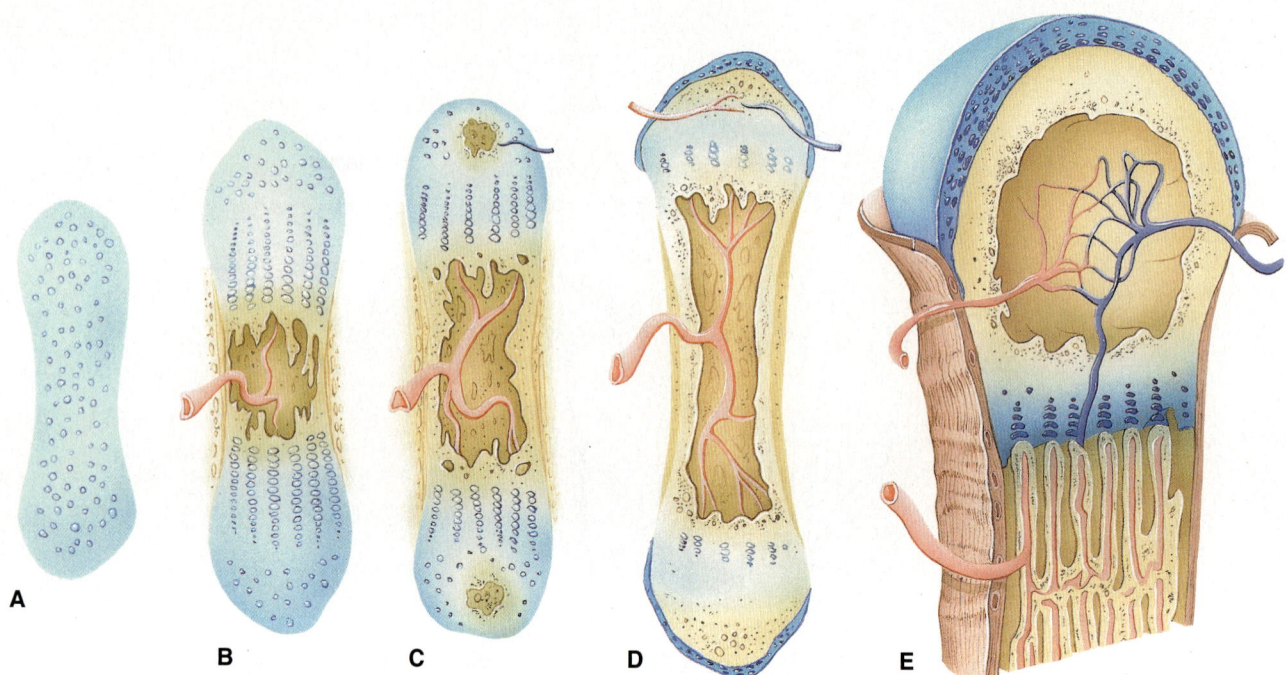

FIGURE 1-8 Endochondral bone formation. **A.** Hyaline cartilage model. **B.** Diaphysis perichondrium vascularization. **C.** Subperiosteal bone collar. **D** and **E.** Subperiosteal bone collar. (Gartner LP. *Color Atlas and Text of Histology.* 7th ed. Wolters Kluwer; 2018: Figure 4-2.)

collagen fragments, degrading any remaining collagen fragments. Osteoblasts will secrete osteoid composed of primarily type I collagen. The osteoid will mineralize, incorporating calcium and phosphate along with other minerals into the collagen matrix (Fig. 1-9). The osteoblasts will then die through cell apoptosis, incorporate into the matrix and become osteocytes, or become bone lining cells that help degrade collagen fragments.[10]

Individuals with metabolic or genetic bone diseases will demonstrate an imbalance in bone ossification and resorption. An accelerated rate of bone loss occurs in osteoporosis and hyperthyroidism. In the genetic diseases of osteopetrosis[11,12] and osteogenesis imperfecta,[12] a disruption in the metabolic turnover among osteoclasts and osteoblasts results in brittle bones that tend to fracture easily.

Ligaments

Ligaments are dense regular connective tissue that connect bones across joints. Ligaments contribute to joint function by increasing joint stability, preventing excessive motion, acting as a check or guide to direct motion, and providing proprioceptive input. Ligaments are generally named by their bony insertions (e.g., coracoacromial ligament), shape (e.g., trapezoid ligament), or relative position to each other (anterior and posterior cruciate ligaments of the knee). Ligaments may blend with the joint capsule, appearing as a thickening of the capsule, such as ligaments of the shoulder joint (e.g., glenohumeral ligaments) and hip joint (ischiofemoral, iliofemoral, pubofemoral ligaments). Ligaments may be intra-articular (such as the anterior and posterior cruciate ligaments of the knee and the interosseous talocalcaeal ligaments) or extra-articular (such as the medial and lateral collateral ligaments of the knee) (Fig. 1-10). The ECM of ligaments is composed primarily of type I collagen and water. The fibers of ligaments run primarily in the same direction but less regularly than in tendons. Some ligaments have primarily one bundle of collagen fibers running mostly straight and parallel, resisting forces in one plane, whereas others may have multiple fiber bundles oriented in varied directions, providing resistance to tension in multiple directions.

Tendons

Tendons are dense regular connective tissue that attach muscle to bone and are typically named by the muscle they attach to bone (e.g., supraspinatus tendon, flexor digitorum longus tendon). Tendons create joint motion by transferring force from muscle to bone. The composition of tendon is similar to that of ligament (i.e., composed of water, protein molecules, and collagen fibers [primarily type I]). The strength of tendons is attributed to the parallel and staggered arrangement of collagen fibers within its structure. In tendons, collagen fibers are bundled together forming primary bundles, which are then grouped together to form secondary fiber bundles.[13] These secondary

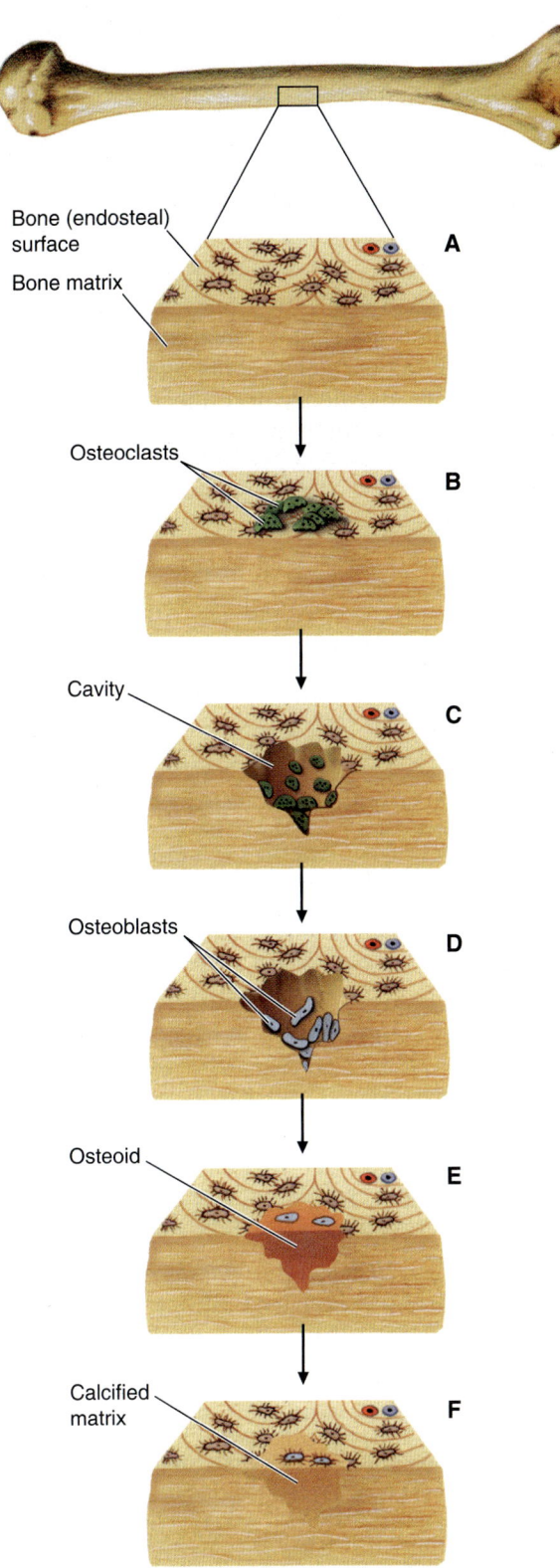

FIGURE 1-9 Bone remodeling stages. **A.** Resting cell surface. **B.** Activated osteoclasts dissolve bone. **C.** Osteoclasts produce a cavity in bone matrix. **D.** Osteoblasts are present. **E.** Osteoblasts secrete osteoid. **F.** Bone matrix is calcified. (Plowman S. *Exercise Physiology for Health Fitness and Performance.* 5th ed. Wolters Kluwer; 2017: Figure 16.3.)

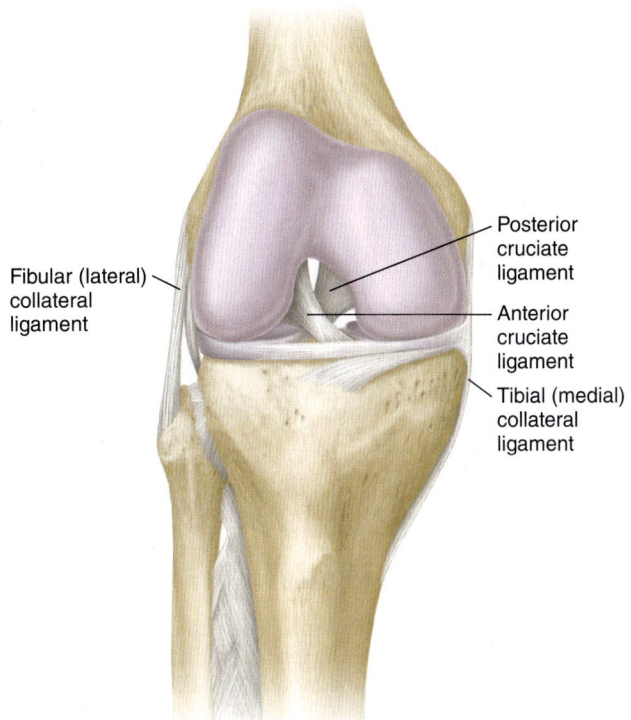

FIGURE 1-10 Ligaments of the knee (anterior view). Intra-articular ligaments are the anterior and posterior cruciate ligaments. Extra-articular ligaments include the medial and lateral collateral ligaments. (Gest TR. *Lippincott Atlas of Anatomy.* 2nd ed. Wolters Kluwer; 2020: Plate 3-59A.)

bundles group together to form tertiary fiber bundles, which, in turn, bind to form the tendon unit (see Fig. 1-4). The primary, secondary, and tertiary bundles are surrounded by connective tissue called the *endotenon*, which facilitates the gliding of bundles among themselves during movement. Continuous with and surrounding the endotenon is the epitenon that forms a sheath around the tendon unit. Surrounding the entire tendon is a peritendinous sheath, the paratenon, which allows the tendon to move against adjacent structures.[14] The tendon is attached to bone by collagen fibers that continue to the bone matrix (Fig. 1-11). It is important to note that the collagen fiber bundles are aligned in the direction of the mechanical load, which adds to the strength of the tendon. The vascular supply to tendon occurs through various surrounding tissues, such as the paratenon, and at the musculotendinous and osteotendinous junctions.[15] Some tendons, such as the biceps, supraspinatus, and Achilles, have a particularly limited blood supply. Tendons deform less than ligaments and, therefore, are able to transmit forces directly from muscle to bone. The attachment of tendon to bone (entheses) includes both fibrocartilaginous and fibrous attachments.[16,17]

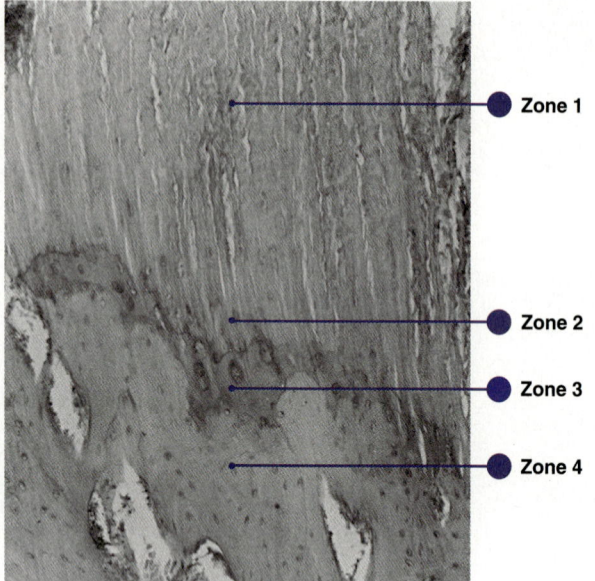

FIGURE 1-11 Electron micrograph of canine patellar tendon insertion demonstrating four zones. Zone 1, collagen fibers; Zone 2, fibrocartilage (unmineralized); Zone 3, fibrocartilage (mineralized); Zone 4, bone. (Cooper RR, Misol S. Tendon and ligament insertion. A light and electron microscopic study. *J Bone Joint Surg Am.* 1970;52(1):1-20. Copyright © 1970 by The Journal of Bone and Joint Surgery, Incorporated.)

Fascia

Fascia is composed of dense and loose connective tissue with varied organizational structure and thickness.[18] Fascia is described as superficial, deep, and visceral.[19] Superficial fascia, just deep to the dermis, forms a layer of aerolar connective tissue with a significant fat composition. The superficial fascia provides for thermoregulation, lymphatic flow, venous/arterial protection, and nerve pathways to periphery. Deep fascia covers most of the body and runs parallel and deep to the skin surface. Deep fascia may provide attachment for underlying muscles, but in most places, the muscles glide freely beneath the fascia. Extensions of deep fascia, called *investing fascia*, may envelop deeper structures such as muscles and neurovascular bundles and may form distinct fascial compartments, such as the anterior, lateral, and posterior compartments of the leg. The deep fascia attaches firmly to bone, forming an unyielding tissue around the muscles, limiting the outward expansion of muscles during contraction, and aiding venous return. In the case of repetitive microtrauma with tears to the periosteum and fleshy attachments of muscle to fascia (such as may occur with overexertion by untrained individuals), the painful condition of shin splints may develop, such as may occur with sudden overuse of the anterior compartment muscles of the leg. Significant swelling within a compartment may result in compromised blood flow throughout the compartment and subsequent ischemia and necrosis of tissue. Around certain joints, such as the ankle and wrist, thickenings of deep fascia form retinacula to hold tendons in place where they cross a joint, preventing bowstringing of tendons across the joint.

CHAPTER SUMMARY

This chapter includes an overview of cells and the ECM composing connective tissue. The fibers of the ECM include collagen, elastic, and reticular fibers. Ground substance is composed of glycoproteins, PGs, and GAGs. Fibers and ground substance form connective tissue structures, such as cartilage, bone, ligament, tendon, and fascia. A basic knowledge of connective tissue composition facilitates comprehension of the varied characteristics of these connective tissue structures.

REFERENCES

1. Lodish H, Berk A, Kaiser C, et al. *Molecular Cell Biology.* 8th ed. W. H. Freeman; 2016.
2. Kadler K, Holmes D, Trotter J, Chapman J. Collagen fibril formation. *Biochem J.* 1996;316(1):1–11.
3. Shoulders M, Raines R. Collagen structure and stability. *Annu Rev Biochem.* 2009;78:929–958. doi:10.1146/annurev.biochem.77.032207.120833
4. Glelse K, Poschl E, Aigner T. Collagens—structure, function, and biosynthesis. *Adv Drug Deliv Rev.* 2003;55(12):1531–1546.
5. Levangie P, Norkin C. *Joint Structure and Function: A Comprehensive Analysis.* 5th ed. F.A. Davis; 2011.
6. Cui D, Daley W, Fratkin J, et al. *Atlas of Histology: With Function and Clinical Correlations.* Lippincott Williams & Wilkins; 2011.
7. Pawlina W, Ross M. *Histology: A Text and Atlas with Correlated Cell and Molecular Biology.* 8th ed. Wolters Kluwer; 2020.
8. Gartner L. *BRS Cell Biology and Histology.* 8th ed. Wolters Kluwer; 2019.
9. Eriksen E. Normal and pathological remodeling of human trabecular bone: three dimensional reconstruction of the remodeling sequence in normals and in metabolic bone disease. *Endocr Rev.* 1986;7(4):379–408.
10. Newman C, Allen M. Bone remodeling. In: Mooren FC, ed. *Encyclopedia of Exercise Medicine in Health and Disease.* Springer; 2012.
11. Palagano E, Menale C, Sobacchi C, Villa A. Genetics of osteopetrosis. *Curr Osteoporos Rep.* 2018;16(1):13–25. doi:10.1007/s11914-018-0415-2
12. Balemans W, Van Wesenbeeck L, Van Hul W. A clinical and molecular overview of the human osteopetroses. *Calcif Tissue Int.* 2005;77(1):263–264.
13. Sharma P, Maffulli N. Tendon injury and tendinopathy: healing and repair. *J Bone Joint Surg Am.* 2005;87(1):187–202.
14. Allen K, Feria-Arias E, Kreulen C, Giza E. Biologics in the foot and ankle. In: Canata GL, d'Hooghe P, Hunt KJ, Kerkhoffs G, Longo U, eds. *Sports Injuries of the Foot and Ankle.* Springer; 2019.
15. Tempfer H, Traweger A. Tendon vasculature in health and disease. *Front Physiol.* 2015;6:330. doi:10.3389/fphys.2015.00330
16. Benjamen M, Toumi H, Ralphs J, et al. Where tendons and ligaments meet bone: attachment sites ('entheses') in relation to exercise and/or mechanical load. *J Anat.* 2006;208(4):471–490.
17. Benjamin M, Moriggl B, Brenner E, et al. The "enthesis organ" concept: why enthesopathies may not present as focal insertional disorders. *Arthritis Rheum.* 2004;50(10):3306–3313. doi:10.1002/art.20566
18. Benjamen M. The fascia of the limbs and back—a review. *J Anat.* 2009;214(1):1–18.
19. Gatt A, Agarwal S, Zito P. *Anatomy Fascia Layers.* StatPearls [Internet]. StatPearls Publishing; 2020.

2 | Tissue Behavior, Healing, and Repair

June Hanks

CHAPTER OBJECTIVES

After reading this chapter, you will be able to:
1. Describe tissue behavior relative to composition and response to various stresses.
2. Discuss tissue adaptations that facilitate resistance to injury and failure.
3. Discuss predisposing factors to tissue injury.
4. Describe similarities among repair processes of tissues in response to injury.
5. Discuss unique healing properties and challenges to healing in bone and nerve tissue.
6. Describe bone fracture types and methods of immobilization to promote healing.

The tissues of the body are designed to respond without injury to various internal and external forces. High forces or low repetitive forces may lead to tissue damage, leading to predictable events to promote repair and healing. The ability of specific tissues to adapt, repair, and heal varies among tissues. This chapter discusses the major body tissue response to stress, repair mechanisms, and intervention options to facilitate repair and healing.

TISSUE BEHAVIOR

The response of major body tissues to an imposed load depends on the tissue composition and health as well as factors related to the load, such as the amount, direction, and rate of loading. Within limits, healthy tissues can resist and adapt to imposed forces without failure. The German anatomist and surgeon Julius Wolff describes bone and American orthopaedist Henry Gasset Davis, and later Harold Frost, describe soft-tissue adaptations relative to stress responses.[1,2] These descriptions are referred to as "laws," stating that tissues respond and adapt to stress and heal according to the manner in which the mechanical stress is applied.[3,4] In Figure 2-1, Wolff law is depicted through bone response to axial loading of the tibia, creating a bending stress. Such stress will bend the bone, stimulating an increased thickness in the direction of the load. For example, the bone and connective tissues in an elite tennis players' dominate arm adaptively thicken and strengthen to allow for greater resistance to imposed demands. The mechanisms for adaptive change in response to stress to connective tissue are depicted in Figure 2-2, where insufficient and excessive loading is applied to connective tissue. An example is the strengthening of muscles, ligaments,

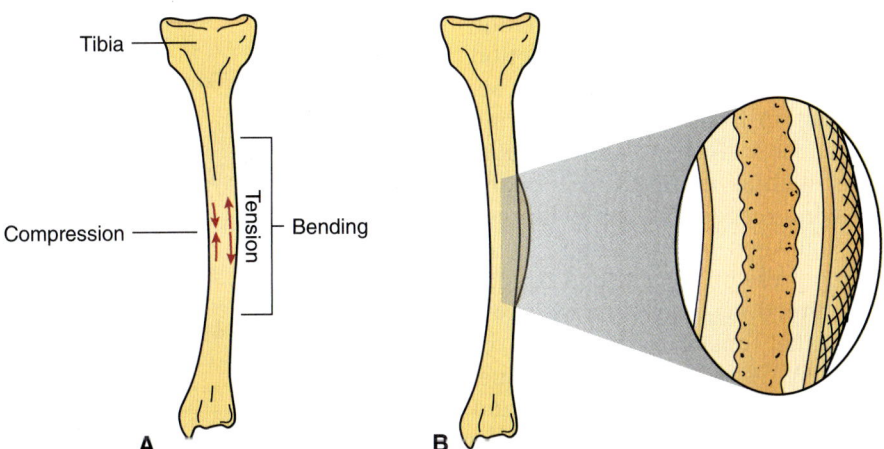

FIGURE 2-1 Depiction of Wolff law relative to bone adaptations to stress. **A.** Bending stress to bone **B.** Close up of increased thickness in response to bending stress. (Adapted from Anderson MK, Parr GP. *Foundations of Athletic Training: Prevention, Assessment, and Management.* 5th ed. Lippincott Williams & Wilkins; 2013: Figure 6.4A.)

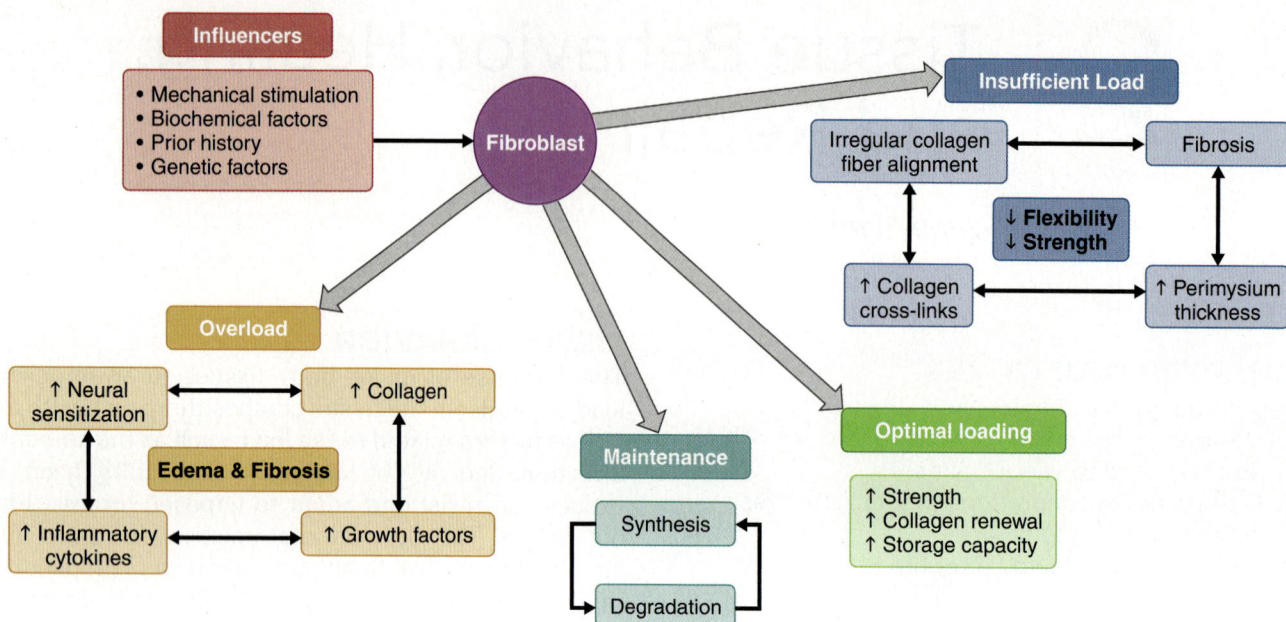

FIGURE 2-2 Response of connective tissue to excessive, optimal, and insufficient loading.

and tendons in the legs and ankles of an avid hiker, with the amount of strengthening being relative to the duration, magnitude, and rate of forces applied to the tissues. Likewise, a decrease in stress, as occurs with prolonged immobilization, results in weakened tissue that may not be able to withstand normal stress without injury and may contribute to the development of knee osteoarthrosis/osteoarthritis (OA).[5]

The composition of tissue changes with disuse, disease, age, and exposure to repeated trauma making the tissue more susceptible to injury. Some tissues may be able to adapt to a low stress over a short period of time, but eventually begin to fail with repetitive loading. A high degree of stress or rate of loading may lead to immediate failure. Stresses to tissue include compression, tension, shear, friction, and distraction (Fig. 2-3). The tissues are loaded during simple activities, such as standing up from a chair, removing laundry from the dryer, or walking to the mailbox, and complex activities such as cutting wood, hiking on a rocky path, or playing soccer. The applied forces (stresses) can be distinguished by their tendency to deform the tissues. Compression forces load tissues in equal and opposite directions, causing a widening and shortening of the tissue. Tension forces produce a narrowing and lengthening (elongation) of the tissue. With shear loading, stresses are applied in parallel and opposite directions that are not in line with each other. Torsional loading causes a structure to twist about its axis. Bending forces combine compression and tension loading. Although possible to occur separately, tissue forces most commonly occur in a combined manner. For example, during walking, the stresses to the tibia are more compressive during heel strike, tensile during stance, and torsional during the transition from stance to push-off.[6] The combined loading deforms the tissues in varying amounts and directions.

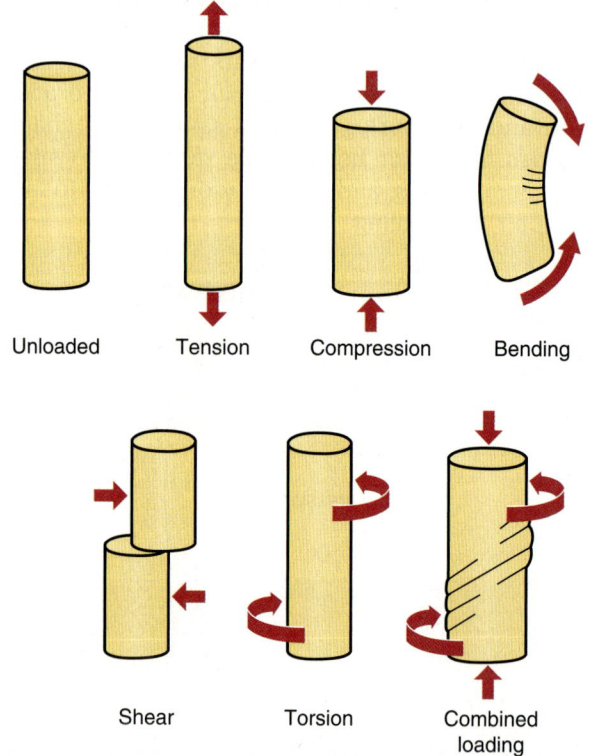

FIGURE 2-3 Various loading modes to tissues. (Adapted from Nordin M, Frankel VH. *Basic Biomechanics of the Musculoskeletal System*. 5th ed. Wolters Kluwer; 2022: Figure 2-17.)

Tissue Composition

The relative composition of biologic tissues must be appreciated to understand the response to stress. Comparison to nonbiologic materials aids understanding of the impact of loading. For example, steel is a relatively solid material and responds to stress with the same mechanical behavior, regardless of the direction of applied force. The dynamic body tissues are composed of solid and semisolid components and demonstrate varied responses, dependent on the direction, speed, and size of the applied stresses. Many tissues change/adapt their composition and their ability to function in response to the varied parameters of applied forces.[3,4] For example, tensile forces may promote an increase in type I collagen in tendons and ligaments. Tendons may respond to compression forces by increasing the amount and type of glycosaminoglycans to contribute to structural support. Joint capsules respond to focal stress by thickening to form capsular ligaments.[7] Elongation of a ligament will promote tissue changes to allow resistance necessary to maintain joint stability. This adaptive behavior demonstrates the strong association between structure, composition, and function.

Tissue Properties

The mechanical properties of tissue include stiffness, elasticity, extensibility, flexibility, and hydration. These properties allow for needed responses to stress to promote function without tissue injury. Examples include compression of the calcaneus during walking, torsion to the knee ligaments during a tennis backhand, and the pull of the Achilles tendon on the calcaneus during push-off at the start of a sprint. The sensitivity to loading direction, portion of the tissue being stressed, type and rate of load application, and the environmental conditions varies by tissue and injury.[8] Light weight bearing may be necessary to stimulate bone repair processes and prevent fracture-related disuse atrophy in some cases, whereas other fractures require non–weight bearing for a period of time for healing to occur. Adaptations to tissue demands are depicted in Figure 2-4.

As a tensile load is applied, elongation of the tissue will occur. With release of the load, the tissue will return to its prestressed dimension. With progressively increased load, the tissue will elongate (yield) even more until reaching its highest stress point. The application of a load beyond this stress point results in microfailure of the tissue, such that the tissue is not able to return to its original length with removal of the stress. Each tissue has its own maximal stress point, which may itself change owing to the direction, type and rate of load application, and environmental conditions. For example, a warmed muscle is more likely to deform than a cold one. Therefore, before stretching, the muscle should be actively warmed through gentle activity or passively warmed with application of some form of heat to obtain the best results.

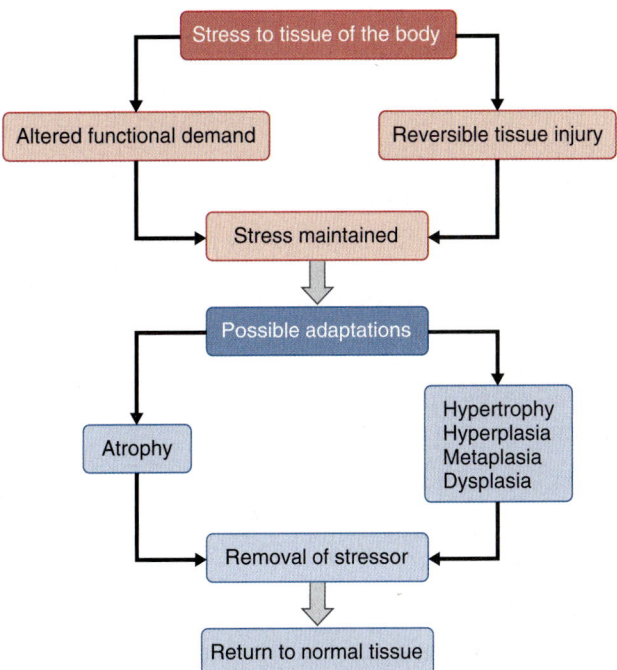

FIGURE 2-4 Adaptations of tissues to stress.

TISSUE INJURY

Applied force exceeding the maximal stress tolerance of a tissue may lead to partial or complete tissue failure. Tissue injury occurs with an interruption in continuity to any portion of a tissue, ranging from an intentional injury, as occurs with a surgical incision, to an unintentional disruption, as with an ankle ligament tear when landing on the side of the foot following a jump. The detachment of a ligament or tendon at the bony attachment is called an *avulsion*, whereas a partial or complete separation of the ligament or tendon elsewhere along its course is called a *rupture*. A fracture is failure of bony tissue. The skin over the knee may tear from a fall onto the sidewalk. With enough force, such a fall may cause a fracture of the patella. Examples of injuries relative to involved tissue include:

- Tendon/ligament: sprain, rupture, or avulsion
- Muscle: strain or tear
- Bone: fracture, dislocation, and subluxation
- Skin: abrasion, tear, or ulceration

Injury to one structure will impact the integrity of related structures and their ability to maintain normal function. For example, dislocation of the glenohumeral joint may significantly stretch or disrupt the joint capsule, rupture surrounding ligaments, and tear muscles.

Except for teeth, all tissue within the body can repair following injury. A dynamic and complex repair process begins immediately following injury to reestablish tissue continuity. The cellular and extracellular makeup, vascularity, and hydration, along with external factors such as imposed stress impact the healing rate and completeness.

Primary Tissue Injury

In most contexts, the initial injury to tissue is termed "primary injury" and is commonly the result of mechanical injury to the tissue. The natural progression of healing is acute, subacute, and chronic, described as the natural progression to healing (Fig. 2-5). If the natural progression to healing does not occur, chronic inflammation/proliferation may result.

Secondary Tissue Injury

An untreated or poorly treated primary injury may lead to a redistribution of mechanical load in the tissues, causing a "secondary injury." For example, a developed compensatory walking strategy resulting from ambulation on an unstable ankle joint may lead to undue stress on the knee meniscus or other joint structures. A loss of ankle dorsiflexion following a fracture can lead to knee hyperextension and posterior knee joint capsule elongation. Excessive motion associated with hypermobility of the glenohumeral joint may lead to faulty joint mechanics, with resultant microtrauma to joint cartilage, ligaments, and tendons. The use of an arm sling following a proximal humeral fracture may lead to a secondary elbow flexion contracture, if the elbow is not moved for an extended period of time. An imbalance of muscle strength about the hip joint may lead to excessive stress to the hip joint capsule, articular cartilage, and labrum as well as abnormal mechanics, leading to injury of the joints above and below the hip.

TISSUE HEALING

Injury to soft tissue from microtrauma, macrotrauma, or disease results in near-immediate initiation of the healing process, which is generally subdivided into three phases: inflammatory, proliferative, and remodeling. The phases of tissue healing overlap, with each phase demonstrating characteristic cellular events and clinical manifestations. Figure 2-6 graphically depicts phases of wound healing, and Table 2-1 describes predominant events, time frames, therapeutic goals, and potential interventions. The general phases of tissue healing are discussed here, with healing of specific structures discussed later in this chapter.

Inflammatory Phase

The body reacts to initial injury by an immediate attempt to minimize damage and restore homeostasis. When capillary blood flow is disrupted, platelets initiate clot formation. The capillaries initially vasoconstrict to limit blood loss and then vasodilate to allow macrophages and fibroblasts to enter the wounded area. Mediators of this vasodilation include histamine, released by mast cells, and prostaglandins, produced by resident cells at the site of injury.[9-11] The local vasodilation is promoted by products from the cascades of the inflammatory process: the complement cascade that activates circulating inactive proteins after injury; and the kinin cascade that transforms inactive enzymes, such as kallikrein, to its active form; and bradykinin that promotes vasodilation and vessel wall permeability. Fluid leaks out of vessels made more

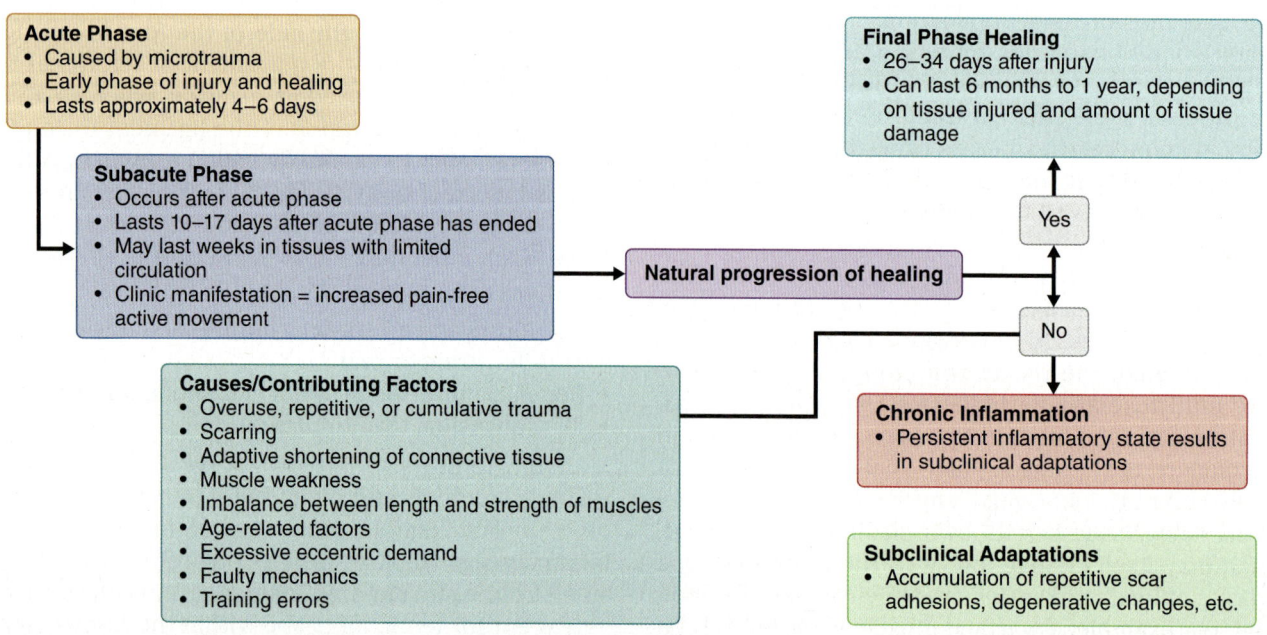

FIGURE 2-5 Progression toward healing with primary injury.

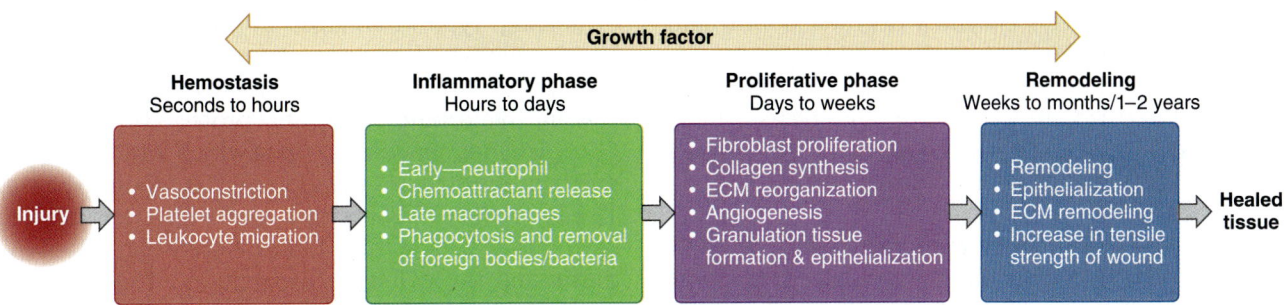

FIGURE 2-6 Phases of tissue healing with major events and approximate time frames. *ECM*, extracellular matrix.

TABLE 2-1
PHASES OF HEALING IN THE MAJORITY OF INJURED BODY TISSUES

Phase	General Time Frames*	Cellular Events	Clinical Manifestations	Therapeutic Goals	Potential Interventions
Inflammatory	• 4–6 days	Vascular • Vasoconstriction followed by vasodilation Cellular • Phagocytosis of cellular debris • Migration of pro-inflammatory cells	• Swelling, redness, heat, impaired/lost function • Pain at rest or with active motion or with stress to injured tissue	• Minimize pain and swelling • Control inflammation • Restore full, passive ROM • Prevent atrophy • Maintain soft tissue joint integrity	• Protection • Controlled rest • Cryotherapy • Compression • Elevation
Proliferative	• 6–24 days	• Angiogenesis • Granulation tissue formation • Fibroblast proliferation with collagen synthesis • Increased macrophage and mast cell activities	• Reduction in swelling, redness, heat, pain • Improvement in function	• Protect forming collagen • Direct forming collagen fibers to orient parallel to the lines of force they must withstand through controlled motion • Prevent cross-linking of collagen fibers and scar contracture	• Controlled early motion
Remodeling	• 21 days to 2 years	• Conversion of granulation tissue to collagen-filled scar • Synthesis, degradation of collagen	• Further reduction and eventual elimination of swelling, redness, heat, pain • Improved ability to tolerate tissue stress	• Promote pain-free and full function	• Controlled stress (active/resistive ROM) • Stretching • Functional activity challenges
Chronic inflammation/proliferation	• Varies	• Continued release of inflammatory products and local proliferation of mononuclear cells • Ongoing fibrocyte production of collagen	• Ongoing signs and symptoms of inflammation • Fibrosis of tissue and surrounding structures	• Reduce contributing factors	

ROM, range of motion.
*Time frames for normal phases of healing vary slightly among tissues.

permeable through the cascade processes and will enter the interstitial space, contributing to characteristic swelling in the area of injury. Neutrophils and monocytes are attracted to the area and, along with tissue macrophages (mature monocytes), act to digest and clean cellular debris and promote the activity of the fibroblasts. Neutrophils and macrophages synthesize enzymes, such as matrix metalloproteinases (MMPs) and collagenases. The enzymes degrade debris and participate in cellular proliferation, migration, angiogenesis, and cellular **apoptosis**.[9] Growth factors, such as platelet-derived growth factor and transforming growth factor-α, are released to assist in the production of biologic mediators that direct the reconstruction process.

The local inflammatory response is amplified by the release of pro-inflammatory cytokines, such as tumor necrosis factor-α and various interleukins (IL), such as IL-1 and IL-6. Chemotactic agents (e.g., neutrophils, bacterial toxins, dead and dying cells) direct the migration of cells to the site of injury. The migration of fibroblasts to the area sets the stage for the proliferative phase of healing. The magnitude of the inflammatory response depends on the injured tissue's composition and vascularity as well as the size and type of injury.[12] The inflammatory phase of healing is characterized by edema (swelling), redness, heat, and impaired or lost function. Factors contributing to the characteristic clinical manifestations are shown in Figure 2-7.

Proliferation Phase The proliferative phase begins within a few days of injury (Fig. 2-6) and is characterized by the following:

- Capillary ingrowth
- Granulation tissue formation
- Fibroblast proliferation with collagen synthesis
- Increased macrophage and mast cell activities

Local tissue ischemia and chemical mediators promote the growth of new capillaries into the area of injury. The granulation tissue is a latticework composed of new blood vessels, fibroblasts, macrophages, and loose connective tissue.[9] Functioning capillaries provide nutrition to the area and remove waste products and cellular debris. Macrophages and neutrophils promote the migration and proliferation of fibroblasts[13] that synthesize a new extracellular matrix (ECM), mainly in the form of collagen. In the early phases of healing, type III collagen is prevalent, whereas in later stages, the stronger type I collagen predominates.[10,14,15] Other components of the ECM are water, elastin, hyaluronic acids, and proteoglycans.[16,17] The ECM provides scaffolding along which additional fibroblasts and other cells migrate to the wounded area.[18] The provisional ECM is replaced with a stronger collagenous matrix as fibroblasts increase collagen synthesis and the collagen fibers bundle together in an increasingly organized manner.[10,15] As more fibroblasts are drawn into the area, new collagen, elastin, and proteoglycan molecules are synthesized, producing the initial scar tissue.[19] Some of the fibroblasts acquire contractile properties, transforming into myofibroblasts that facilitate wound contraction, thus reducing the size of the defect.[13] The proliferative process is complete when the wound is completely resurfaced.

Remodeling Phase The remodeling phase of wound healing (see Fig. 2-6) involves conversion of the granulation tissue into a collagen-filled scar. Remodeling involves the reduction of fibroblast and capillary density and the reorganization of collagen. During this phase, collagen continues to be formed, whereas older collagen is degraded by MMPs. The process of remodeling can take 1 to 2 years following wound closure. Even then, the tensile strength of the scar tissue is at most 80% of the original tissue strength.[20] The healing tissue requires controlled stress to promote collagen deposition and prevent too much contraction and adhesion among the immature collagen fibers and surrounding tissues, leading to hypomobility. The newly healed area must be protected from excessive stress that could lead to disruption.

Closed and Open Wound Healing

Closed wounding occurs when there is no disruption to the skin, whereas open wounding involves a disruption to the epidermis with possible extension to the dermis and/or deeper tissues. The normal wound healing process for closed and open wounds involves the

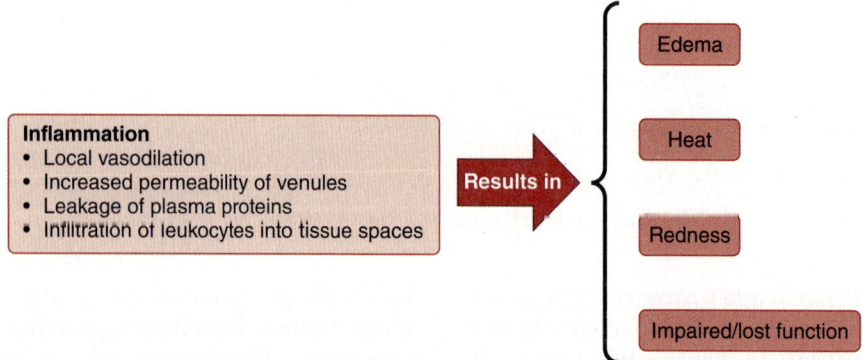

FIGURE 2-7 Events and clinical manifestations of inflammation.

inflammatory, proliferation, and remodeling phases to repair the damaged tissue.

An open wound that allows for the physical approximation of wound edges, such as a wound caused by a surgical incision, may heal by primary closure (also called *primary intention*). In such a case, there is a small tissue deficit and minimal distance that cells must travel to mitigate healing. The wound edges are held together by adhesives, sutures, or staples.[21] When the tissue defect is large and wound edges cannot be approximated, healing occurs by secondary healing (or secondary intention). This process takes more time, as the wound void must be filled by granulation tissue that is converted to scar tissue composed of collagen deposited in oriented bundles rather than the basketweave orientation of normal collagen deposition. Wound contraction and epithelialization must occur to a greater extent with secondary healing to approximate would edges.[22] In some cases, wounds heal through delayed primary closure in which the wound is left open for a few days to allow for cleansing before a primary closure procedure.[23]

Abnormalities in Wound Healing

Ideally, wounds progress through the overlapping phases of healing in a timely manner. An alteration in any stage may lead to a chronic wound or excessive scar formation. Contributing factors to chronic wounds are a self-perpetuating inflammatory phase, cellular senescence (a state of cellular arrest in which metabolically active cells fail to proliferate),[24] bacterial infection, reduced oxygenation, and a lack of nutrition.[21] Chronically inflamed wounds demonstrate excessive and prolonged inflammation due to a variety of factors, ranging from injury characteristics, such as severity and nature of wound edges (frayed versus smooth).

Factors Affecting Healing

Factors impacting wound healing are depicted in Figure 2-8. These factors may be intrinsic (within the person) or extrinsic. Local factors such as a foreign body in the wounded area or repetitive microtrauma to the healing tissues may slow progress.[25] Macrophages and other pro-inflammatory cells may fail to respond to signals from cytokines and apoptotic cells that normally bring a resolution of inflammation.[26] The chronically inflamed wound fails to progress to the proliferative phase, and the tissues may become fibrotic.[27] Systemic factors such as abnormalities in circulation, diabetes, or systemic infection may impede healing. A patient's failure to avoid positions that could create microtrauma or macrotrauma to the healing tissue may delay or prevent repair and healing. A delay in healing may create physical and psychological stress for the patient due to prolonged pain, loss of function, and the inability to perform meaningful activities.

HEALING OF SPECIFIC TISSUES

The varying composition of tissues leads to distinctive adaptations and repair processes among the major body tissues. These unique characteristics are discussed in this section.

Tendon

The healing of tendon and ligament is similar because of their comparable composition. Both structures are composed primarily of water (70–80%). The ECM of tendons and ligaments is made up of proteoglycans and other cells and about 20% type I collagen and a minor amount of elastin fibers. Tendons and ligaments have a small vascular and sensory supply. The structures adapt to functional demands through dynamic alterations in ECM composition and biomechanical properties.[28]

Tendon Injury Tendon injury occurs when the stress of mechanical loading exceeds the ability of the tissue to resist. Tendons can biomechanically adapt to repetitive loading changes. Tendon collagen fibers are more parallel, and less realignment occurs during initial loading than with ligament collagen fibers. The collagen structure of tendon allows it to resist tensile stress in the direction of the fiber orientation. The musculotendinous junction is the weakest point of the muscle-tendon unit and is the most common site of strain injuries.[29,30]

Tendons vary in compliance throughout the body. The stiffness of the digit flexors and extensors requires little change in length when muscle forces are applied in order to produce movement of associated bones. The Achilles tendon is more elastic, stretching during the latter phase of stance and releasing stored energy as the calf muscles contract producing plantarflexion. Healthy tendons tolerate repetitive light load deformation. Tensile and compression

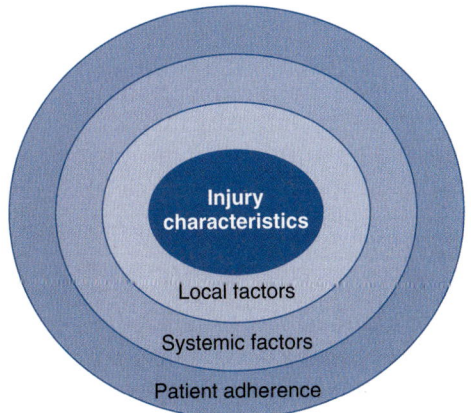

FIGURE 2-8 Factors affecting healing.

stresses are resisted according to collagen fiber orientation and proteoglycan content, respectively. As load conditions change, the tendons structurally or compositionally change in response. An abnormal load (insufficient or excessive stress) may contribute to tendinopathy.[31]

Tendinopathy, a clinical syndrome characterized by pain, diffuse or localized swelling, and impaired function,[32] may occur with overuse of a tendon. Tendon overuse injuries account for a large number of musculoskeletal injuries in sport and general practice. Most tendon trauma occurs from sudden or repetitive loading or unloading. The highly cellular and poorly vascularized and innervated composition makes the tendon highly vulnerable to injury. Although inflammation is not the hallmark of tendinopathy,[33] the inflammatory process may be demonstrated near the bony insertion and associated bursae where blood supply is greatest. The recommended term to describe tendon pathology is *tendinopathy*, rather than tendinitis.

Factors contributing to tendinopathy include age, high body mass index, biomechanical abnormalities, muscle imbalance, overuse, excessive compression, steroid use, and improper training. Tendons with insufficient blood supply, tensile strength, and flexibility are at high risk.[34] Pathologic processes associated with tendinopathy are tendinosis and peritendinitis.

- Tendinosis is characterized by intratendinous degenerative changes, such as collagen disorganization and fiber separation with blood vessel and nerve ingrowth. Tendinosis is subcategorized by location as insertional or noninsertional and may progress to a partial or complete tear if subjected to high mechanical loading.
- Peritendinitis involves inflammation of the paratenon, the thin membrane surrounding the tendon. Localized swelling and inflammatory cell infiltration occur due to repetitive loading of the structure.

Tendinitis, a less common condition, is associated with more inflammation than tendinosis. With acute injury to the tendon, the inflammatory phase of wound healing begins immediately with stabilization of bleeding through clot formation. The wounded area progresses into the inflammatory, proliferative, and remodeling phases of healing, with the repair phase (formation of a scar) predominating. This scar tissue is weaker than the original connective tissue and possesses greater amounts of minor collagens, such as types III, V, and VI rather than the type I collagen that predominates in healthy tendon. The collagen fibers demonstrate varying diameters with longitudinal splitting, partial disintegration, and the interspersion of lipid cells throughout. The ECM is not fully restored, resulting in the release of cytokines that contribute to the degenerative process.[35]

Tendons most vulnerable to injury are those that transmit large loads under eccentric conditions and those subjected to combined loading, such as the Achilles and patellar tendons in the lower extremity[36] and the supraspinatus and extensor carpi radialis brevis tendons in the upper extremity. While sporting activities are commonly associated with tendon injury, occupations that require sudden overload, repetitive overload, or rapid unloading of tendons show a high prevalence of tendinopathy. Examples include construction, meat processing, and assembly line work. Tendinopathies tend to be higher among persons with diabetes and atherosclerosis and with the use of some drugs, such as cortisone, and statins.[37]

Injury to the tendon is typically classified as acute or chronic.

- Acute:
  - Time and mechanism of injury is known
  - Includes tendon rupture and partial tendon tears
- Chronic
  - Not typically associated with known onset
  - Caused by repetitive overload
  - High amount of disorganized, immature collagen
  - Painful response to resistance of involved musculotendinous structure

Tendon Treatment to Promote Healing Poor healing of tendinopathies is due to the low oxygen content, limited vascularization, and the presence of adhesions in the involved tissue. Healing requires the formation of new, properly aligned collagen with cross-linking among fibers. The judicious application of interventions to promote tendon healing requires:

- Warm-up through active, non-to-very minimally painful exercise or local heat producing modality, such as moist heat or ultrasound
- Stretching to promote extensibility of tissues at attachment site and the antagonists before and after eccentric exercise
- Eccentric contractions of involved tendinous structure at a speed and intensity that allows completion of 20 repetitions or so before the onset of pain, with progression of speed or load when 30 repetitions or so can be completed with low/tolerable pain during the exercise.
- Cryotherapy

Failure to improve may be due to incorrect loading or speed of eccentric contractions, unrecognized external factors, nonadherence to intervention program, or incorrect diagnosis.

Ligament

The normal stabilizing function of ligaments is disrupted with ligamentous injury, leading to altered kinematics of joints. With aging, ligaments lose strength, stiffness, and viscosity. With hormonal changes, such as those occurring with pregnancy and during the menstrual cycle, ligaments may become more lax.[38] While movement promotes normal ligament behavior,[39] immobilization results in a loss of strength and stiffness.[40,41]

Ligament Injury An external load to a ligament requires deformation of the ligament to absorb the energy. A load surpassing the elastic (recovery) limit of the ligament will lead to failure and imposition of stress on other structures and ligaments to withstand the load. If the load exceeds the elastic limit of the associated structures, these structures may also fail.[42] Isolated ligament injury seldom occurs.

Ligament injury is characterized by point tenderness, joint effusion, and an identifiable mechanism of injury. Stress testing with forces applied perpendicular to the normal plane of joint motion can help differentiate the severity of ligamentous injury (e.g., varus or valgus stress testing of the elbow). The severity of ligament injury is communicated through a three-level grading system (mild, moderate, complete disruption). Patient pain and guarding again potential pain may limit clinical examination, requiring the use of magnetic resonance imaging (MRI) or other tests to diagnose injury and determine severity.

Ligament Healing Healing follows the same process as other vascularized tissue, with passage through the overlapping phases of healing. Uniquely, the intra-articular ligaments, such as the cruciate ligaments of the knee, are less vascularized than extra-articular ligaments and, therefore, exhibit less of an inflammatory response. Several months are required for the collagen and water content to return to normal levels during the remodeling phase of ligamentous healing.[43] Although the tissue may mature, the healed ligament never attains full restoration of biomechanical properties, such as tensile strength.

Ligament Treatment to Promote Healing As with tendons, strength in the direction of applied forces can be restored to the healing ligament. To facilitate scar proliferation and remodeling, periods of mobilization within a predefined range should be applied. For example, modulated low, cyclical loading may facilitate cellular migration without disrupting healing.[44] The application of ice following injury reduces bleeding, swelling, and inflammation.[45]

Ligaments may require surgical repair. The surgical approximation of torn ligament ends demonstrate more of a regeneration process and less scar formation than unrepaired ligaments.[46] However, strength advantages from surgically repaired ligaments may not be maintained.[47] The use of growth factors and gene therapy are currently being explored to improve ligament repair.

Articular Cartilage

Articular cartilage is avascular and aneural with a low metabolic rate and, therefore, has limited ability to heal following injury. Composed of water, chondrocytes, and ECM, articular cartilage changes with age, becoming less hydrated and more stiff with increased forces to underlying subchondral bone. Articular cartilage is divided into zones, with a subchondral plate separating the subchondral vascular spaces from the main matrix. Throughout the articular space, the thickness of articular cartilage varies.[48] Nutrition occurs by diffusion from synovial fluid in the joint space. A supply of nutrients is required for chondrocytes to develop, maintain, and repair the ECM. With an appropriate level of force, the structure and function of articular cartilage can be maintained throughout the lifetime. Intermittent pressure promotes healthy cartilage, whereas shear forces, prolonged static loading or a lack of loading, as occur with immobilization, alter metabolism in the cartilage and facilitate degenerative changes.[49] The viscoelasticity of articular cartilage results in time-dependent deformation when subjected to constant loading.[50]

Joints such as the knee, wrist, temporomandibular, acromioclavicular, and sternoclavicular joints have a meniscus, a form of fibrocartilage that is critical to maintaining the health and function of the joint. The meniscus helps with joint alignment and load dispersion during movement.

Articular Cartilage Injury Owing to the avascular nature of articular cartilage, a typical inflammatory response to injury is not possible. The normal cellular and extracellular synthesis and degradation is imbalanced, leading to reduced proteoglycan production and concentration.[48] With additional changes including the increase in MMPs concentration and chondrocyte apoptosis, the metabolic capacity is impaired, leading to a reduction in the ability to withstand mechanical stresses,[51] with a progressive cartilage loss, subchondral bone remodeling, osteophyte formation, and synovial inflammation. Additional factors contributing to articular cartilage changes include abnormal force transmission due to developmental aberrations, joint surface incongruity, joint instability, and disease processes, such as rheumatoid arthritis and various other forms of arthritis.

Injury to the articular cartilage is categorized by type as follows:

- Type 1: superficial, involving chondrocyte damage and ECM changes
- Type 2: partial thickness, involving chondral fractures or fissuring without penetration of subchondral bone and therefore, no provocation of an inflammatory response
- Type 3: full thickness, involving disruption into subchondral bone and the production of a significant inflammatory process

The clinical signs and symptoms of articular cartilage damage include impairment in mobility, muscle performance, and balance with consequent activity limitations. The patient may experience significant pain or little to no pain. There may be a temporary improvement in function without an improvement in tissue quality. Generally, the extent of functional loss depends on the extensiveness of articular damage, comorbidities, and combinations of other articular disorders.

Articular Cartilage Healing The repair capacity of articular cartilage is extremely limited with prospects for healing dependent on lesion depth. Without injury to subchondral bone, damaged articular cartilage becomes necrotic and progresses to degeneration.[52] The blood supply of bone may promote healing of full-thickness articular cartilage injury. The repair process results in fibrous, fibrocartilaginous, or hyaline-like cartilaginous repair, depending on the age, location, and size of the lesion.[53,54] The biochemical and biomechanical nature of newly repaired cartilage differs from normal and is of inferior tissue quality that is unable to withstand normal stresses. Degenerative changes such as fibrillation, fissuring, or frank destruction occur over time, depending on tissue loading.[55,56]

Damage to the meniscus of a joint leads to impaired mechanics. The ability of the meniscus to heal depends on the location of damage, as only the outermost portion is vascularized. The combination of articular cartilage and meniscus damage leads to a rapid deterioration of joint function.

Articular Cartilage Treatment The management of damaged articular cartilage includes conservative measures to delay major surgical intervention. Such treatment includes pain control through pharmacologic means, such as nonsteroidal anti-inflammatories, opioid and nonopioid analgesics, and intra-articular injections. The injections are most often corticosteroids, though intra-articular viscosupplementation is increasingly used. Research is progressing on the use of stem cells.[57] Other conservative measures include modalities, patient education, joint motion, strengthening exercise to improve muscular force to unload the articular surface, and low-impact aerobic exercise.

Patient symptoms, comorbidities, and expectations, along with clinical and radiographic findings, contribute to decisions for surgical interventions. For example, older patients with bicompartmental damage of the knee articular cartilage may experience better outcomes with a total knee arthroplasty, whereas a younger person with unicompartmental involvement may progress well with a high tibial osteotomy or unicompartmental arthroplasty.

Muscle

Each of the more than 430 skeletal muscles in the body possess viscoelastic properties that allow for loading and deformation to provide movement and the attainment of postures essential for normal daily function. Factors influencing muscle performance include age, temperature, and immobilization or disuse. With aging, the cross-sectional area of muscle decreases due to a reduction in the number of muscle fibers. With higher temperatures, muscle demonstrates greater elasticity and decreased stiffness, allowing greater deformation at a given load. Immobilization or disuse results in muscle atrophy due to imbalances between protein synthesis and degradation, with greater impact to type I fibers.[58] The structural and metabolic changes in muscle can be seen within 2 hours of immobilization.[59] Effects of immobilization include a reduction in cross-sectional area and reduced glycosaminoglycan levels at the musculotendinous junction.[60]

Muscle Injury Most muscle injuries occur due to excessive strain (distraction strain) or contusion, such as from a direct blow.[61] Contusion injury results in intramuscular or intermuscular hematoma, resulting in pain and loss of function. Other causes of injury are laceration, thermal stress, and myotoxic agents such as snake, bee, or bug venom, or some drugs. Muscle injury may be classified by various grading systems,[62] such as the British Athletics Muscle Injury Classification.[63]

Factors contributing to muscle injury include inadequate:

- Warm-up
- Flexibility
- Strength or endurance
- Synergistic muscle contraction
- Rehabilitation following previous injury

Muscle Healing The regenerative capacity of muscle is significant due to the rich vascularization and follows an orchestrated series of events throughout destruction, repair, and remodeling stages (Fig. 2-9). Critical to healing is the controlled motion and stress during the postacute time period to allow appropriate scar formation, muscle regeneration, orientation of collagen fibers, and restoration of tensile properties. Initially after injury, type III collagen predominates over type I collagen. Over time and with controlled mobility, type I collagen increases, and the proportion of collagen types normalize with type I exceeding type III.

Muscle Injury Treatment Complete restoration of the functional capacity of injured muscle is possible with proper management. Appropriate interventions depend on the healing stage. Inflammation and edema may decrease with elevation, compression, cryotherapy, electrical stimulation, and gentle range of motion (ROM) exercise. As healing occurs, interventions include:

- Pain-free passive ROM with minimal tissue stress
- Active-assisted ROM
- Active ROM
- Submaximal isometrics in protective ranges, then multiple angles throughout range
- Maximal isometrics at multiple angles throughout range
- Progressive resisted exercise

Bone

Bone is composed of organic, mineral, and fluid elements. Bone quality is influenced by multiple factors including:

- Diet
- Hormones
- Biomechanics

The mineral content of bone contributes stiffness and distinguishes it from other connective tissues. The collagen orientation influences the mechanical behavior in the bone layers (lamellae). The bone bends (elastic deformation) without sustaining permanent deformation. When loads are repetitively applied over a short period, the bone may change in composition (plastic deformation), such that the force will shorten and elongate with compression and tension forces, respectively. Repeated or sustained loads exceeding the capacity of deformation result in microarchitectural damage. The behavioral response of trabecular bone to stress differs according to the direction of stress in various portions of the same bone.

Bone Injury Bone injury ranges from deterioration of structure, such as occurs in osteopenia or osteoporosis, to fracture. Fracture types are described in Table 2-2 and depicted in Figure 2-10. A stress fracture is commonly encountered by clinicians who treat athletes,[64,65] with tibial stress fractures being the most common.[66] Stress fractures can be challenging to diagnose and require a detailed clinical examination that integrates patient history, contributing risk factors, and, often, confirmation with imaging (scintigraphy or MRI).[66] A premature return to full activity can complicate healing and result in delayed union or nonunion.[67,68] Some reports indicate that pain from a stress fracture may be elicited with application of ultrasound or a vibrating tuning fork over the fracture site and thus help with diagnosis. However,

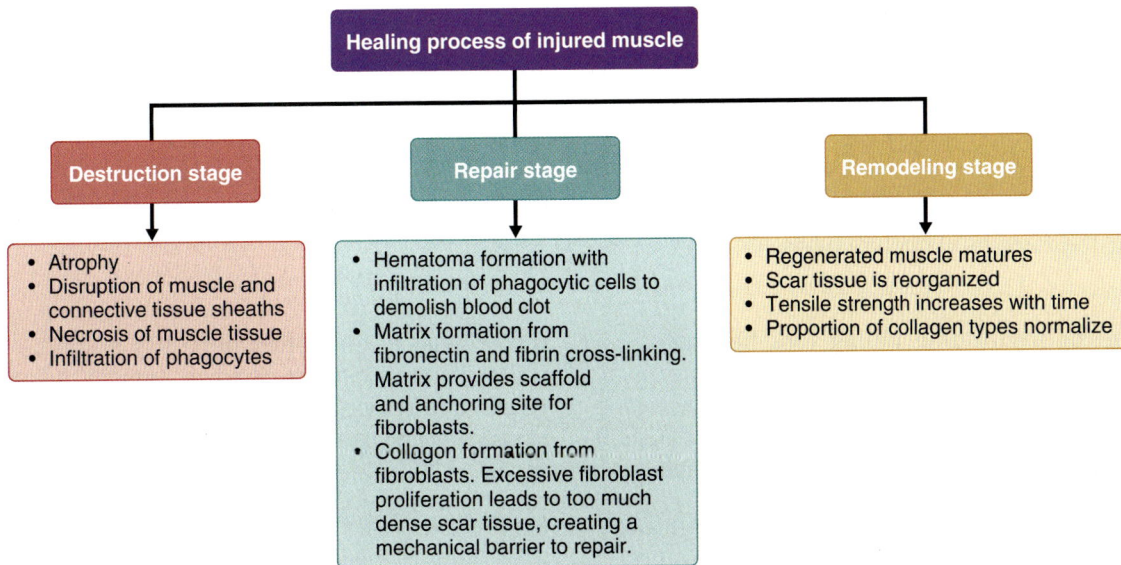

FIGURE 2-9 Healing process of injured muscle.

TABLE 2-2
FRACTURE TYPES

Fracture	Description
Avulsion	Injury to bone where tendon or ligament pulls off a piece of bone
Closed	Fractured bone does not extend through the skin, but may be seen under the skin
Comminuted	Fracture with more than two fragments of bone that have broken off; highly unstable with multiple bone fragments
Complete	Bone completely fractured through its width
Complex	Fracture that severely damages surrounding soft tissue
Compound (open)	Bone and bone fragments penetrate internal soft tissue and break through the skin; have high risk of infection
Compression	Occurs when bone is compressed beyond tolerance limit; generally occurs in vertebral bodies as result of flexion injury or without trauma in patients with osteoporosis; may occur on calcaneus when person falls from a height and lands on heel
Epiphyseal	Fracture of epiphysis and physis (growth plate)
Greenstick	Incomplete fracture only on one side of the bone; usually "bent" and fractured on the outside of the bend; considered a stable fracture; healing is quick if bone is kept rigid; common in children
Hairline	Incomplete fracture with no significant bony displacement; crack only extends into outer layer of bone; considered a stable fracture; aka fissure fracture
Impaction	Occurs when one bony fragment is driven into another; common in tibial plateau fractures
Oblique	Extends at an angle to the axis of the bone
Pathologic	Occurs when bone breaks due to weakness from a disease process, such as tumor, infection, osteoporosis, osteopenia, and some congenital bone disorders
Spiral	Extends through bone in spiral manner; unstable; may be mistakenly diagnosed as oblique fracture; resembles corkscrew running parallel to axis of bone
Stress	Extends through all or part of bone; common in spine and lower extremity (fibula, tibia, metatarsals); occurs in all age groups; not necessarily associated with history of increased activity

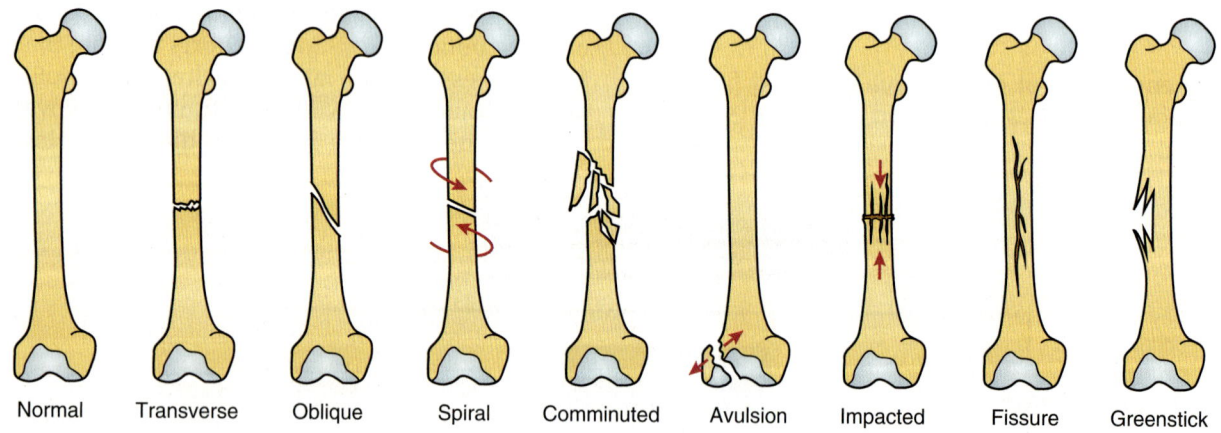

FIGURE 2-10 Examples of fracture types.

ultrasound or a vibrating tuning fork has not been supported as isolated diagnostic tests.[66] A pathologic fracture may be seen in the clinic with presenting signs and symptoms of back pain. A common cause of pathologic fracture is osteoporosis or osteopenia.

Bone Healing Normal bone healing follows an ordered set of events. Unlike other tissues, bone healing occurs through repair by the original tissue rather than scar tissue formation,[69] with strength equal or stronger than the original tissue. Intact bone has a unique capacity for regeneration and follows typical inflammation, repair, and remodeling processes.[70] Fracture healing is classically discussed in terms of primary and secondary repair.

- Primary fracture healing involves a direct attempt of bone cortex to reestablish itself after interruption (gapping) where bone on opposing sides of the gap must unite.

- Secondary fracture healing involves the formation of a callus due to responses in periosteum and surrounding soft tissues. Most fractures heal by secondary repair.

The process of fracture healing through intramembranous and/or endochondral ossification involves four distinct phases (Fig. 2-11)[70,71]:

- Hematoma formation (inflammation or granulation) phase
- Soft callus formation (reparative or revascularization) phase
- Hard callus formation (maturing or modeling) phase
- Remodeling phase

In the hematoma formation phase, the area to be healed fills with a blood clot with an inflammatory response that includes an increase in blood flow, release of growth factors, migration of neutrophils and monocytes, and phagocytosis of cellular debris. Hallmarks of the soft callus phase include the formation of cartilage and other connective tissue along with angiogenesis from preexisting vessels. Influenced by subtle differences in oxygen tension, the mechanical environment, and signals from growth factors, the periosteum starts to form bone within a few millimeters of the fracture site. Cartilage starts to form over the fracture site that initiates the calcification process. As healing progresses into the hard callus phase, the osteoblasts quickly form woven bone (lamellar bone) to bridge the gap of the fracture site, but the layers are arranged randomly and are weak. The cartilaginous layer becomes calcified and infiltrated with ingrowing blood vessels. This "clinical union" is evident on imaging, and the fracture is considered healed when the fracture line is no longer visible. During the remodeling phase, the callus is remodeled, with bone replacing cartilage and

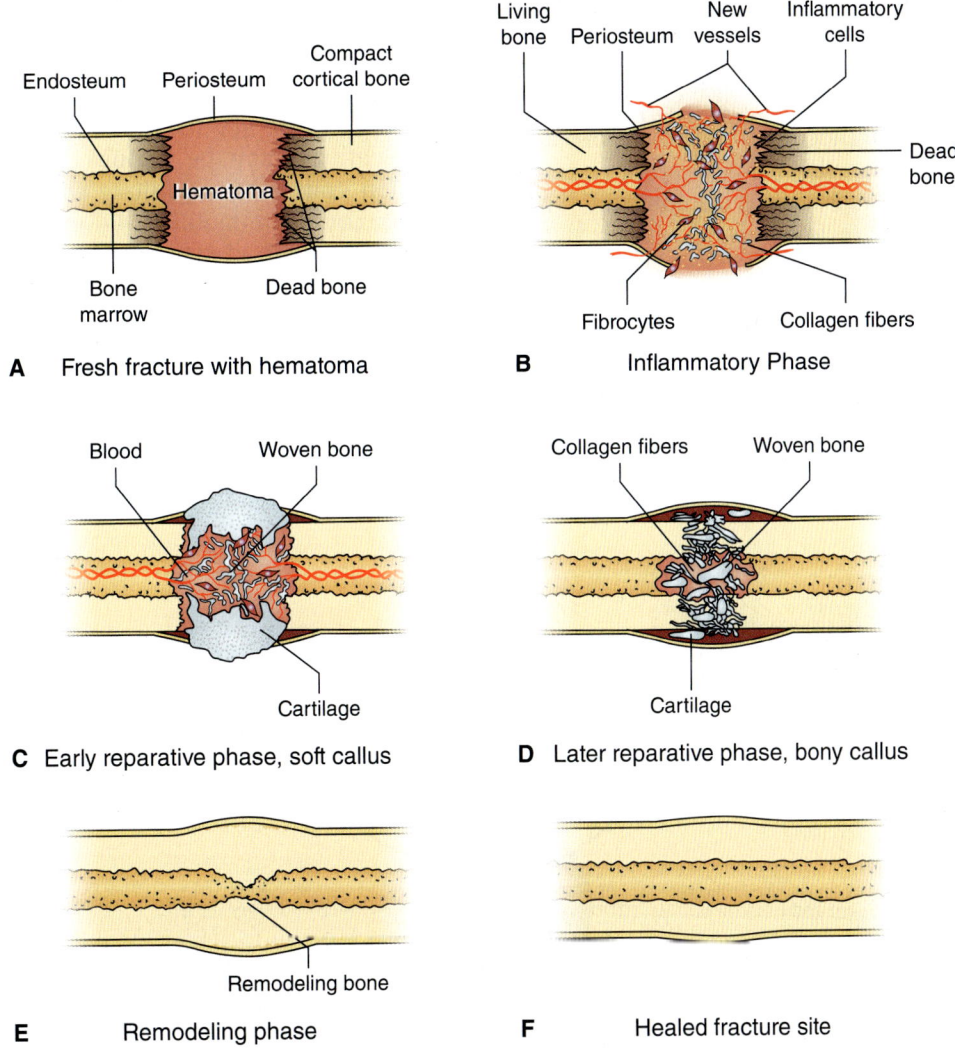

FIGURE 2-11 Phases of bone healing. (Adapted from McConnell TH, Paulson VA, Valasek MA. *The Nature of Disease: Pathology for the Health Professions*. 2nd ed. Wolters Kluwer Health; 2014: Figure 18.11.)

compact bone replacing cancellous bone. Stronger lamellar bone is remodeled through osteoclast bone resorption and osteoblast bone formation.

With rigid fixation, such as surgical internal fixation, the fracture gap is reduced and realigned and repair occurs through normal cortical bony remodeling.[72] Intramedullary nailing and functional bracing for fracture healing promotes external callus formation, with new bone formation arising from the periosteum and surrounding tissues to the fracture site. With cast immobilization, an endosteal callus bridges the gap in the bone.

Factors influencing bone healing are angiogenesis and movement at the fracture site. For capillary ingrowth to properly occur, the vascularized tissue on either side of the fracture gap must be sufficiently immobilized to allow the new capillaries to migrate and survive. While small degrees of micromotion may stimulate blood flow at the fracture site and promote the formation of the periosteal callus, too much motion prevents blood vessel bridging. Bone remodels along lines of stress[73] and is constantly undergoing remodeling as osteoclasts resorb lamellar bone and osteoblasts replace it with more dense osteonal bone.

Bone healing may be impaired by osteoporosis due to many factors, including decreased sensitivity of osteoblasts to mechanical signaling, such as strain, stretching, and vibration.[74,75] Angiogenesis is impeded,[76,77] and the quantity of estrogen receptors is decreased.

Bone Healing Treatment The management of major fractures requires a multiprofessional team to achieve strong bony union and avoid functional loss. The medical team decides on the immobilization approach (surgery versus casting, skeletal traction, splinting or bracing) (Fig. 2-12). During casting, the clinician may guide the patient through submaximal isometric exercises within the cast to minimize atrophy of muscles surrounding the fracture site. The nonimmobilized joints may be exercised as long as the fractured bones are not stressed. Once clinical union has been verified, ROM exercise involving structures crossing the fracture site can be initiated, with progression toward active resisted exercise and functional activity.

Bones that fail to heal may benefit from modalities, such as pulsed electromagnetic fields, low-intensity pulsed ultrasound,[78] and extracorporeal shockwave therapy.[79] Bone tissue engineering including the implantation of scaffolding promotes adhesion, growth, and differentiation of bone-forming cells.[80,81]

Nonoperative treatment for fractures may be utilized for patients with nondisplaced fractures without high risk of displacement, displaced fractures after acceptable alignment and stability have been achieved with closed reduction, and for patients unable to undergo anesthesia and surgery.[82] Surgical options are described in Table 2-3. The advantage of many types of surgery is early mobilization.

Postsurgical Complications While surgical intervention for fracture fixation has many advantages, complications may be serious. Figure 2-13 depicts common complications, along with contributing factors. Prolonged immobilization may be necessary for the overall health of the patient. However, undesirable consequences include:

- Cartilage degeneration
- Decreased mechanical and structural properties of ligaments
- Decreased bone density
- Weakness or atrophy of muscles

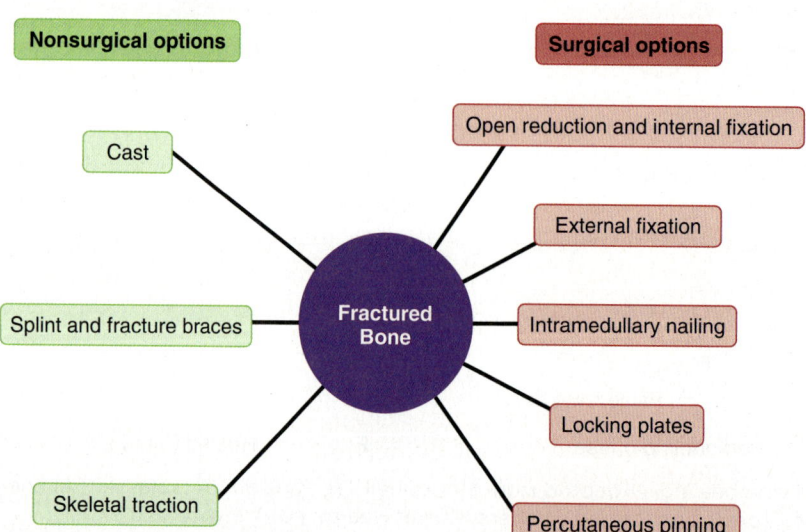

FIGURE 2-12 Nonsurgical and surgical immobilization options for fractured bone.

TABLE 2-3	
TYPES OF SURGERY FOR FRACTURE FIXATION	
Open reduction with internal fixation	Incision used to access and realign bone; bone fragments are stabilized with pins, plates, screws, or a combination of this hardware entirely within body.
External fixation	Metal rods are screwed into bone and exit body to be attached to stabilizing structure on outside body.
Intramedullary nailing	Metal rod is inserted into the medullary cavity of a bone and across the fracture to stabilize bone.
Locking plates	Metal plate with threaded screw holds and screw whose head is locked into the plate with a locknut by screwing in a threaded chamber on plate or through an adapted ring.
Closed reduction percutaneous pinning	Following closed reduction through traction, adduction, and either internal or external rotation to bring both the bony fragments into alignment, a terminally threaded pin or K-wire is placed to stabilize the bones, greater and the lesser tuberosities into alignment.

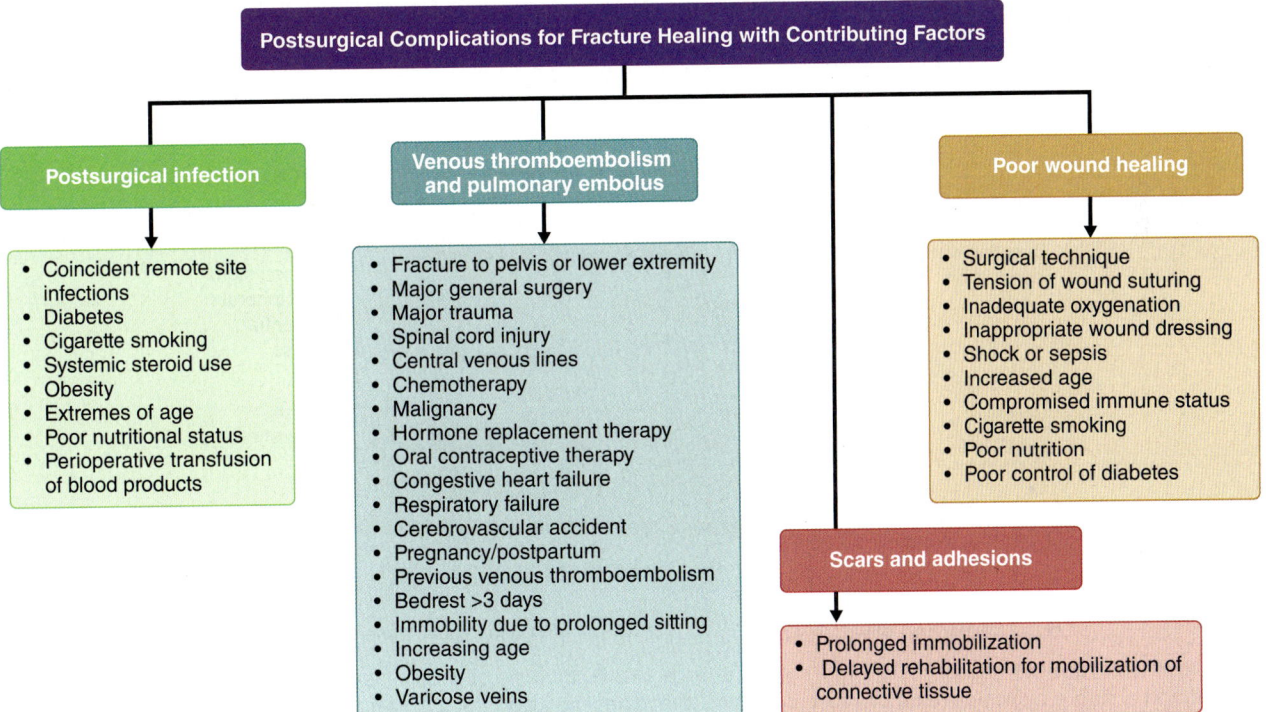

FIGURE 2-13 Potential postsurgical complications with fracture management.

Nerve

The structural division of the nervous system is the central nervous system (CNS) and the peripheral nervous system (PNS). Functionally, the nervous system can be divided into somatic and visceral parts. The CNS is composed of the brain and spinal cord, which develop from the neural tube in the embryo. The PNS is composed of all nervous structures outside the CNS and consists of the spinal and cranial nerves, visceral nerves, and plexuses and the enteric system.

The neuron (nerve cell) is the basic working unit that transmits information to other nerve cells, muscle, or gland cells. The three basic types of neurons are motor (efferent), sensory (afferent), and interneurons. In general, all motor fibers pass into the anterior (ventral) portion of the spinal cord, whereas all sensory fibers pass into the posterior aspect. Somatic motor fibers carry information away from the CNS to skeletal muscles, extending from cell bodies in the spinal cord to the muscle cells they innervate. The length of the motor nerve fibers depends on the distance from the spinal cord to the muscle. The somatic sensory afferents or general somatic afferents, together called *somatic sensory neurons*, carry information from the PNS to the CNS. Modalities transmitted by these nerves include proprioception, temperature, pain, touch, and proprioception. Interneurons transfer signals between motor and sensory neurons and also communicates with each other with circuits of varying complexity.

The neuron (Fig. 2-14) is the functional unit of the nerve and has components that resemble a tree and its branches:

- Dendrite (branches): receives information from other nerve cells or environment
- Axon (roots): conducts information and nutrition to nerve cells and tissues the nerve innervate; may

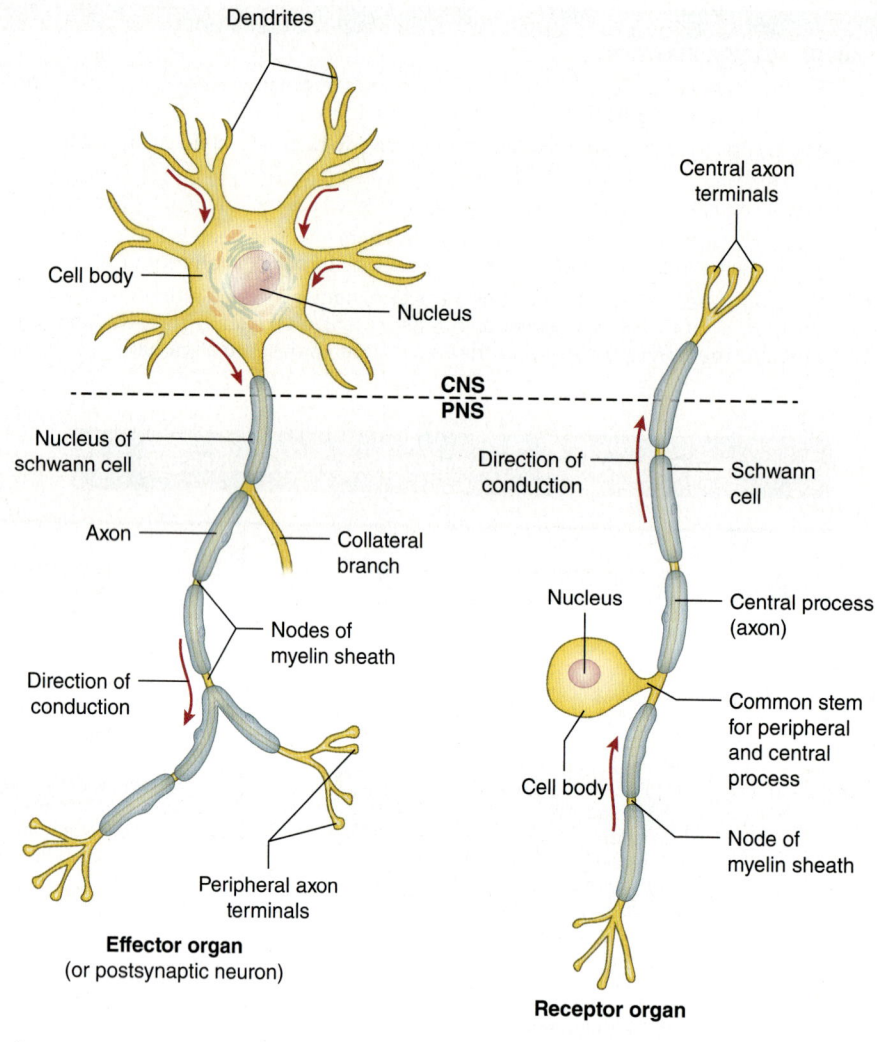

FIGURE 2-14 Anatomy of neuron. The majority of neurons are: **A.** Multipolar motor neurons, which have two or more dendrites and a single axon with one or more collateral branches; cell body is within the central nervous system (CNS) **B.** Pseudounipolar sensory neurons, which have a short common process extending from the cell body that separates into a peripheral process that conducts impulses from the receptor organ toward the cell body (located outside the CNS in sensory ganglia) and a central process that continues into the CNS. (Adapted from Dalley AF, Agur AMR. *Moore's Clinically Oriented Anatomy*. 8th ed. Wolters Kluwer; 2018:Figure 1.28.)

be covered with myelin, which increases velocity of transmission
- Cell body (trunk): contains cell nucleus; performs integrative functions
- Axon terminal (root end): transmission site for messengers (action potentials) of the nerve cell

Input received by the dendrite is transmitted along the axon as an electrical impulse toward the axon terminus. The axon may have several side branches, called *collaterals*. Within the cell body, proteins are produced and transported throughout the axon and dendrites. Communication along neurons occurs through synapses, which are contact points between axon terminals, on one side, and dendrites or cell bodies, on the other. Electrical signals from the axon convert into chemical signals via the release of neurotransmitters at the synapse and are then quickly converted back into electricity as information moves among neurons. Some axons are covered with myelin, a fatty substance that acts as insulation to the axon, allowing the axon to transmit signals over long distances.

A nerve (Fig. 2-15) is an enclosed, cable-like bundle of axons in the PNS. The nerve is like a structured highway that supports neuron function, transmitting electrochemical impulses along each axon. The axons are sometimes referred to as *fibers*. Each axon is surrounded by a connective tissue layer called the *endoneurium*. The inner portion of the endoneurium consists of a material called the *glycocalyx* and a mesh of collagen. The endoneurium prevents certain molecules from crossing from the blood into the

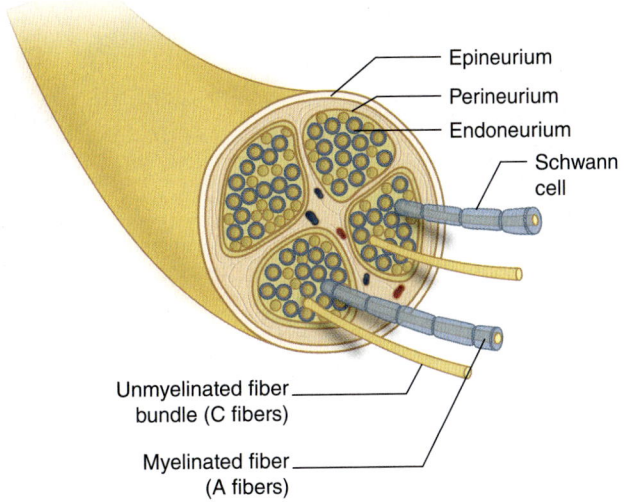

FIGURE 2-15 Anatomy of peripheral nerve. (Adapted from Golan DE, Tashjian AH, Armstron EJ, Armstrong AW. *Principles of Pharmacology: The Pathophysiologic Basis of Drug Therapy*. 3rd ed. Lippincott Williams & Wilkins; 2012: Figure 11-6.)

endoneurial fluid, a liquid within the endoneurium. With nerve irritation, the endoneurial fluid may increase and is visible on magnetic resonance neurography. Axons are bundled together into groups called *fascicles*, with each fascicle wrapped in a connective tissue layer called the *perineurium*. The connective tissue layer surrounding the entire nerve is the epineurium.[83] Blood vessels are bundled within the nerve to provide nutrients to the embedded and metabolically demanding neurons. Analogous structures in the CNS are known as *tracts*. The endoneurium is similar to the blood-brain barrier in the CNS.

The motor, sensory, and interneurons are demonstrated in the reflex arc (Fig. 2-16). For example, with a strike of the patellar tendon when the leg is relaxed, the sensory neuron receives the information of the force of the strike and quickly relays the information along the neuron to the spinal cord where the interneuron determines whether the stimulus warrants a response. If so, the motor neuron returns the impulse to the muscle of the leg, causing the lower leg to react.

Nerve/Neuron Injury The communication along neurons cannot occur if axons are damaged or broken. The nerve can be damaged by compression, stretching (traction), bruising (contusion), ischemia, electrical injury, or by laceration or tear. Nerve injury symptoms include numbness, tingling, burning, motor loss, chronic pain, or a combination of deficits. Signs of nerve injury are muscle atrophy, skin color changes, and changes to the amount of sweat produced in the injured area.

The Seddon Classification System of nerve injury[84] includes three categories, whereas the Sunderland Classification System[85] describes five categories (Table 2-4). The Sunderland grade IV and V nerve injuries require surgical intervention for potential recovery. Many nerve lesions are of mixed pathology.

Nerve Healing The generally accepted mechanisms of nerve injury repair are remyelination, collateral sprouting, and regrowth.[86,87] In the remyelination process, the Schwann cells must de-differentiate to make possible the proliferation necessary to generate new myelin. This process could take up to 3 months. Collateral sprouting may occur with partial axon lesions and may take up to 6 months to heal. Outgrowths from intact axon endings from nonmyelinated portions of the axon may occur, but the process places more fibers under the control of the remaining axons, therefore increasing the number of muscle fibers dependent on one nerve fiber and thereby decreasing motor specificity.[88] The axon regrowth rate is approximately 1 mm per day for complete lesions, with the rate dependent on the age of the patient, site of injury, mechanism of injury, and proximity of injury to the nerve cell body.[88] A faster regrowth rate may occur with proximal limb injury and injury in younger patients.[88,89]

Although nerve endogenous repair is possible following injury, the time frame is limited to approximately 12 to 18 months due to neuromuscular junction endplate changes and muscle fibrosis that occurs following injury.[83] Fibrosis extraneurally and intraneurally affects potential for repair. Extraneural fibrosis causes tethering or compression and decreases conduction velocity along the nerve. Intraneural fibrosis occurs within the internal substance of the nerve and may alter the microvasculature, impede axonal

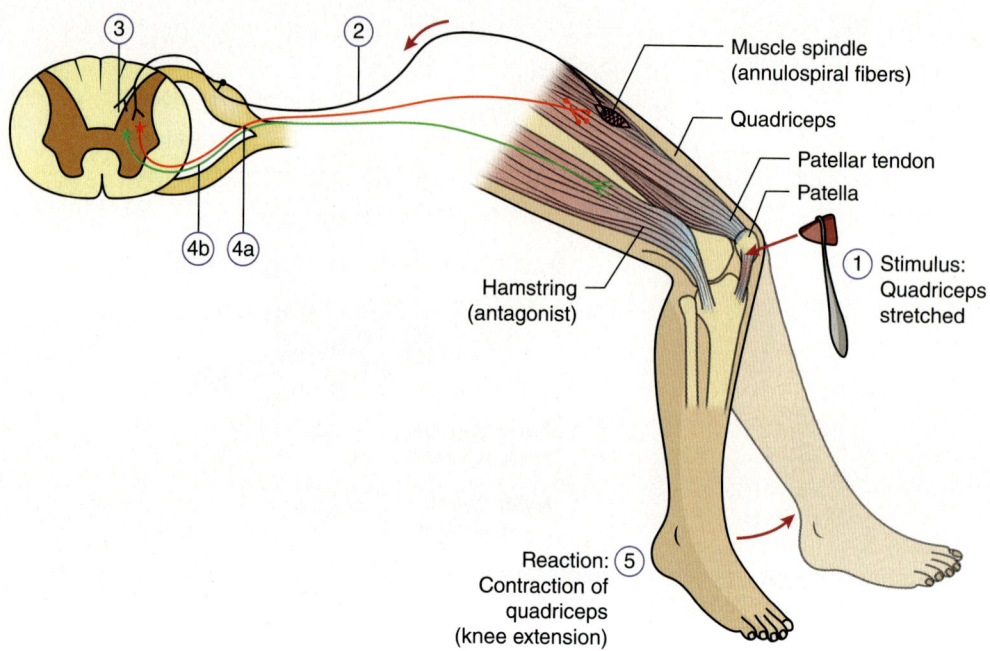

FIGURE 2-16 Example of reflex arc. *(1)* Stimulus: a relaxed quadriceps is stretched *(2)* Impulse is relayed to spinal cord along afferent neuron that bifurcates and synapses with *(3)* interneuron and *(4a)* alpha motor neuron. The alpha motor neuron stimulation leads to contraction of quadriceps (agonist). The efferent fiber *(4b)* that synapses with the interneuron leads to relaxation of hamstring (antagonist) with *(5)* resultant knee extension. (Adapted from Plowman SA, Smith DL. *Exercise Physiology for Health, Fitness, and Performance.* 5th ed. Wolters Kluwer; 2017: Figure 20.9.)

TABLE 2-4
PERIPHERAL NERVE INJURY GRADING SYSTEM

Seddon Classification	Sunderland Classification	Injury	Recovery Potential
Neuropraxia (conduction block)	Grade I	Focal demyelination without any axonal degradation; secondary to mild injury such as ischemia, compression, or toxins	Full (1 day to 3 months)
Axonotmesis	Grade II	Damage to axons; endoneurium, perineurium, and epineurium intact	Full (2-4 months)
	Grade III	Damage to axons and endoneurium; perineurium and epineurium intact	Partial (12 months)
	Grade IV	Damage to axons, endoneurium and perineurium; epineurium intact	Surgery required for recovery
Neurotmesis	Grade V	The axon, myelin sheath, and stroma are all irreversibly damaged; follows severe lesions such as laceration, percussion, or neurotoxins	Surgery required for recovery

Adapted from Sunderland S. A classification of peripheral nerve injuries producing loss of function. *Brain*. 1951;74(4):491–516; Sullivan R, Dailey T, Duncan K, Abel N, Borlongan C. Peripheral nerve injury: stem cell therapy and peripheral nerve transfer. *Int J Mol Sci*. 2016;17(12):2101; Wang M, Rivlin M, Graham J, Beredjiklian P. Peripheral nerve injury, scarring, and recovery. *Connect Tissue Res*. 2019;60(1):3–9; Tetteh ES, Bajaj S, Ghodadra NS. Basic science and surgical treatment options for articular cartilage injuries of the knee. *J Orthop Sports Phys Ther*. 2012;42(3):243–253.

migration, and impair nerve regeneration.[90,91] The degree of recovery is inversely proportional to the extent of the damage.

Nerve Treatment Paramount to treatment of nerve injury is the removal of causative factors. Compression and traction forces must be relieved. The nerve must be allowed to rest in a position of minimal to no stress. Electrical stimulation may promote reinnervation, facilitate remyelination, benefit nerve injury–induced muscle atrophy, and improve muscle function.[92] New cell-based therapies and photobiomodulation with low laser therapy may impact DNA and RNA synthesis and promote cell proliferation and protein synthesis,[93] although not exact mechanisms are not fully elucidated.

Surgical repair to nerves includes direct repair of transected nerves, segmental grafting of nerve defects with autograft nerve harvested from an uninjured host donor site, or the use of processed cadaveric allograft nerves. Despite meticulous surgical technique, incomplete neural recovery occurs frequently. Even with approximation of the ends of damaged nerves or the interposition of a graft, suboptimal recovery is common.[86,87,94]

CHAPTER SUMMARY

The healing of tissues involves an orchestrated series of events that includes inflammation, proliferation, and remodeling. The time and potential for repair differ among tissues. The cellular and extracellular composition of a tissue influences mechanical behavior, response to loading beyond the capacity of the tissue, and healing through scar tissue formation or repair by the original tissue. Factors impacting healing and functional outcomes include vascularity, oxygenation, hydration, controlled motion, and loading. Healing may be impeded by insufficient or excessive loading, cigarette smoking, the use of certain pharmacologic agents such as steroids, and comorbidities such as diabetes and cardiovascular disease. Astute timing and intensity of interventions are required for acquisition of strength, flexibility, and return to function following injury.

REFERENCES

1. Frost H. Wolff's Law and bone's structural adaptations to mechanical usage: an overview for clinicians. *Angle Orthod.* 1994;64(3):175–188.
2. Frost H. A 2003 update of bone physiology and Wolff's Law for clinicians. *Angle Orthod.* 2004;74(1):3–15.
3. Milz S, Benjamin M, Putz R. Molecular parameters indicating adaptation to mechanical stress in fibrous connective tissue. *Adv Anat Embryol Cell Biol.* 2005;178:1–71.
4. Petersen W, Hohmann G, Pufe T, et al. Structure of the human tibialis posterior tendon. *Arch Orthop Trauma Surg.* 2004;124(4):237–242.
5. Teichtahl A, Wluka A, Wijethilake P, Wang Y, Ghasem-Zadeh A, Cicuttini F. Wolff's law in action: a mechanism for early knee osteoarthritis. *Arthritis Res Ther.* 2015;17(1):207.
6. Lanyon L, WGJ H, Goodship A, Shah J. Bone deformation recorded in vivo from strain gauges attached to the human tibial shaft. *Acta Orthop Scand.* 1975;46(2):256–268.
7. Ralphs J, Benjamin M. The joint capsule: structure, composition, ageing and disease. *J Anat.* 1994;184(Pt 3):503–509.
8. Voleti P, Buckley M, Soslowsky L. Tendon healing: repair and regeneration. *Annu Rev Biomed Eng.* 2012;14:47–71.
9. Rodrigues M, Kosaric N, Bonham C, Gurtner G. Wound healing: a cellular perspective. *Physiol Rev.* 2019;99(1):665–706.
10. Komi D, Khomtchouk K, Santa Maria P. A review of the contribution of mast cells in wound healing: involved molecular and cellular mechanisms. *Clin Rev Allergy Immunol.* 2020;58(3):298–312.
11. Duchesne E, Dufresne S, Dumont N. Impact of inflammation and anti-inflammatory modalities on skeletal muscle healing: from fundamental research to the clinic. *Phys Ther.* 2017;97(8):807–817.
12. Kellett J. Acute soft tissue injuries: a review of the literature. *Med Sci Sports Exerc.* 1986;18(5):489–500.
13. Hinz B. The role of myofibroblasts in wound healing. *Curr Res Transl Med.* 2016;64(4):171–177.
14. O'Toole E. Extracellular matrix and keratinocyte migration. *Clin Exp Dermatol.* 2001;26(6):525–530.
15. Schultz G, Davidson J, Kirsner R, Bornstein P, Herman I. Dynamic reciprocity in the wound microenvironment. *Wound Repair Regen.* 2011;19(2):134–148.
16. Lee H, Jang Y. Recent understandings of biology, prophylaxis and treatment strategies for hypertrophic scars and keloids. *Int J Mol Sci.* 2018;19(3):711.
17. Werner S, Krieg T, Smola H. Keratinocyte-fibroblast interactions in wound healing. *J Investig Dermatol.* 2007;127(5):998–1008.
18. Stunova A, Vistejnova L. Dermal fibroblasts—a heterogeneous population with regulatory function in wound healing. *Cytokine Growth Factor Rev.* 2018;39:137–150.
19. Ayello E. Time heals all wounds. *Nursing.* 2004;34(4):36–41.
20. Goodman C, Fuller K. *Pathology: Implications for the Physical Therapist.* 5th ed. Elsevier; 2021.
21. Velnar T, Bailey T, Smrkolj V. The wound healing process: an overview of the cellular and molecular mechanisms. *J Int Med Res.* 2009;37(5):1528–1542.
22. Bainbridge P. Wound healing and the role of fibroblasts. *J Wound Care.* 2013;22(8):407–411.
23. Bhaumik S, Kirubakaran R, Chaudhuri S. Primary closure versus delayed or no closure for traumatic wounds due to mammalian bite. *Cochrane Database Syst Rev.* 2019;12(2):CD011822.
24. Calcinotto A, Kohli J, Zagato E, Pellegrini L, Demaria M, Alimonti A. Cellular senescence: aging, cancer, and injury. *Physiol Rev.* 2019;99(2):1047–1078.
25. Zhao R, Liang H, Clarke E, Jackson C, Xue M. Inflammation in chronic wounds. *Int J Mol Sci.* 2016;17(12):2085.
26. Kim S, Nair M. Macrophages in wound healing: activation and plasticity. *Immunol Cell Biol.* 2019;97(3):258–267.
27. Ridiandries A, Tan J, Bursill C. The role of chemokines in wound healing. *Int J Mol Sci.* 2018;19(10):3217.
28. Leong N, Kator J, Clemens T, James A, Enamoto-Iwamoto M, Jiang J. Tendon and ligament healing and current approaches to tendon and ligament regeneration. *J Orthop Res.* 2020;38(1):7–12.
29. Rehorn M, Blemker S. The effects of aponeurosis geometry on strain injury susceptibility explored with a ED muscle model. *J Biomech.* 2010;43(13):2574–2581.
30. Teitz C, Garrett W Jr, Miniaci A, Lee M, Mann R. Tendon problems in athletic individuals. *J Bone Joint Surg Am.* 1997;79:138–152.
31. McCarthy M, JA H. The mature athlete: aging tendon and ligament. *Sports Health.* 2014;6(1):41–48.
32. Khan K, Maffulli N. Tendinopathy: an Achilles' heel for athletes and clinicians. *Clin J Sport Med.* 1998;8(3):151–154.
33. Figueroa D, Figueroa F, Calvo R. Patellar tendinopathy: diagnosis and treatment. *J Am Acad Orthop Surg.* 2016;24(12):e184–e192.
34. Okewunmi J, Guzman J, Vulcano E. Achilles tendinosis injuries—tendinosis to rupture (getting the athlete back to play). *Clin Sports Med.* 2020;39(4):877–891.
35. Singh A, Calafi A, Diefenbach C, Kreulen C, Giza E. Noninsertional tendinopathy of the Achilles. *Foot Ankle Clin.* 2017;22(4):745–760.
36. Jayaseelan D, Moats N, Ricardo C. Rehabilitation of proximal hamstring tendinopathy utilizing eccentric training,

lumbopelvic stabilization, and trigger point dry needling: 2 case reports. *J Orthop Sports Phys Ther*. 2014;44(3):198–205.
37. Almekinders L, Temple J. Etiology, diagnosis and treatment of tendonitis: an analysis of the literature. *Med Sci Sports Exerc*. 1998;30:1183–1190.
38. Ruedl G, Ploner P, Linortner I, et al. Are oral contraceptive use and menstrual cycle phase related to anterior cruciate ligament injury risk in female recreational skiers? *Knee Surg Sports Tramatol Arthrosc*. 2009;17:1065–1069.
39. Abramowitch S, Woo S. An improved method to analyze the stress relaxation of ligaments following a finite ramp time based on the quasi-linear viscoelastic theory. *J Biomech Eng*. 2004;126:92–97.
40. Akeson W, Amiel D, Abel M. Effects of immobilization on joints. *Clin Orthop*. 1987;219:28–37.
41. Yasuda K, Hayashi K. Changes in biomechanical properties of tendons and ligaments from joint disuse. *Osteoarthr Cartil*. 1999;7:122–129.
42. Hildebrand K, Hart D, Rattner J. Ligament injuries: pathophysiology, healing and treatment considerations. In: Magee D, Zachezewski J, Quillen W, eds. *Scientific Foundations and Principles of Practice in Musculoskeletal Rehabilitation*. WB Saunders; 2007:23–46.
43. Steenfos H. Growth factors in wound healing. *Scand J Plast Hand Surg*. 1994;28:95–105.
44. Goodship A, Birch H, Wilson A. The pathobiology and repair of tendon and ligament injury. *Vet Clin North Am Equine Pract*. 1994;10:323–349.
45. Bleakley C, McDonough S, MacAuley D. The use of ice in the treatment of acute soft-tissue injury: a systematic review of randomized controlled trials. *Am J Sports Med*. 2004;32:251–261.
46. Richter M, Bosch J, Wippermann B, Hofmann A, Krettek C. Comparison of surgical repair or reconstruction of the cruciate ligaments versus nonsurgical treatment in patients with traumatic knee dislocations. *Am J Sports Med*. 2002;30:718–727.
47. Prentice W. Understanding and managing the healing process through rehabilitation. In: Voight M, Hoogenboom B, Prentice W, eds. *Musculoskeletal Interventions: Techniques for Therapeutic Exercise*. McGraw-Hill; 2007:19–46.
48. Tetteh E, Bajaj S, Ghodadra N. Basic science and surgical treatment options for articular cartilage injuries of the knee. *J Orthop Sports Phys Ther*. 2012;42:243–253.
49. Tozrzilli P, Grodzinsky A, Borerelli J Jr, Helfet D. Effect of impact load on articular cartilage: cell metabolism and viability, and matrix water content. *J Biomech Eng*. 1999;121:433–441.
50. Woo S, Lee T, Gomez M, Sato S, Field F. Temperature dependent behavior of the canine medial collateral ligament. *J Biomech Eng*. 1987;109(1):68–71.
51. Bijlsma J, Berenbaum F, Lafeber F. Osteoarthritis: an update with relevance for clinical practice. *Lancet*. 2011;377:2115–2126.
52. Wakitani S, Goto T, Pineda S, et al. Mesenchymal cell-based repair of large, full-thickness defects of articular cartilage. *J Bone Joint Surg Am*. 1994;76:579–592.
53. Fuller J, Ghadially R. Ultrastructural observations on surgically produced partial-thickness defects in articular cartilage. *Clin Orthop Relat Res*. 1972;86:193–205.
54. Ghadially F, Thomas I, Oryschak A, Lalonde J. Long-term results of superficial defects in articular cartilage: a scanning electron-microscope study. *J Pathol*. 1977;212:213–217.
55. Coletti J Jr, Akeson W, Woo S. A comparison of the physical behavior of normal articular cartilage and the arthroplasty surface. *J Bone Joint Surg Am*. 1972;54(1):147–160.
56. Furukawa T, Eyre D, Koide S, Glimcher M. Biochemical studies on repair cartilage resurfacing experimental defects in the rabbit knee. *J Bone Joint Surg Am*. 1980;62(1):79–89.
57. Wolfstadt J, Cole B, Viswanathan S, Chahal J. Current concepts: the role of mesenchymal stem cells in the management of knee osteoarthritis. *Sports Health*. 2015;7:38–44.
58. Hortobagyi T, Dempsey L, Fraser D, et al. Changes in muscle strength, muscle fibre size and myofibrillar gene expression after immobilization and retraining in humans. *J Physiol*. 2000;524(Part1):293–304.
59. Leivo I, Kauhanen S, Michelsson J. Abnormal mitochondria and sarcoplasmic changes in rabbit skeletal muscle induced by immobilization. *APMIS*. 1998;106:1113–1123.
60. Kannus P, Jozsa L, Kvist M, et al. The effect of immobilization on myotendinous junction: an ultrastructural, histochemical and immunohistochemical study. *Acta Physiol Scand*. 1992;144:387–394.
61. Jarvinen T, Kaariainen M, Jarvinen M, et al. Muscle strain injuries. *Curr Opin Rheumatol*. 2000;12:155–161.
62. Mueller-Wohlfahrt H, Haensel L, Mithoefer K, et al. Terminology and classification of muscle injuries in sport: the Munich consensus statement. *Br J Sports Med*. 2013;47(6):342–350.
63. Macdonald B, McAleer S, Kelly S, Chakraverty R, Johnston M, Pollock N. Hamstring rehabilitation in elite track and field athletes: applying the British Athletics Muscle Injury Classification in clinical practice. *Br J Sports Med*. 2019;53(23):1464–1473.
64. Lehman T, Belanger M, Pascale M. Bilateral proximal third fibular stress fractures in an adolescent female track athlete. *Orthopedics*. 2002;25(3):329–332.
65. Tuan K, Wu S, Sennett B. Stress fractures in athletes: risk factors, diagnosis, and management. *Orthopedics*. 2004;27(6):583–591.
66. Schneiders A, Sullivan S, Hendrick P, et al. The ability of clinical tests to diagnose stress fractures: a systematic review and meta-analysis. *J Orthop Sports Phys Ther*. 2012;42:760–771.
67. Boden B, Osbahr D. High-risk stress fractures: evaluation and treatment. *J Am Acad Orthop Surg*. 2000;8:344–353.
68. Behrens S, Deren M, Matson A, Fadale PD, Monchik KO. Stress fractures of the pelvis and legs in athletes: a review. *Sports Health*. 2013;5:165–174.
69. Lisowska B, Kosson D, Domaracka K. Positives and negatives of nonsteroidal anti-inflammatory drugs in bone healing: the effects of these drugs on bone repair. *Drug Des Devel Ther*. 2018;12:1809–1814.
70. Cheung W, Miclau T, Chow S, Yang F, Alt V. Fracture healing in osteoporotic bone. *Injury*. 2016;47(Suppl 2):S21–S26.
71. Thompson Z, Miclau T, Hu D, Helms J. A model for intramembranous ossification during fracture healing. *J Orthop Res*. 2002;20:1091–1098.
72. Marsh D, Li G. The biology of fracture healing: optimising outcome. *Br Med Bull*. 1999;46:856–869.
73. Monteleone G. Stress fractures in the athlete. *Orthop Clin North Am*. 1995;26:423–432.
74. Neidlinger-Wilke C, Stalla I, Claes L, Brand R, Hoellen I, Rubenacker S. Human osteoblasts from younger normal and osteoporotic donors show differences in proliferation and TGF beta-release in response to cyclic strain. *J Biomech*. 1995;28:1411–1418.
75. Shiels M, Mastro A, Gay C. The effect of donor age on the sensitivity of osteoblasts to the proliferative effects of TGF(beta) and 1,25(OH)(2) vitamin D(3). *Life Sci*. 2002;70(25):2967–2975.
76. Rivard A, Fabre J, Silver M, et al. Age-dependent impairment of angiogenesis. *Circulation*. 1999;99:111–120.

77. Cheung W, Sun M, Zheng Y, et al. Stimulated angiogenesis for fracture healing augmented by low-magnitude, high-frequency vibration in a rat model-evaluation of pulsed-wave Doppler, 3-D power Doppler ultrasonography and micro-CT microangiography. *Ultrasound Med Biol.* 2012;38(12):2120–2129.
78. Camal Ruggieri I, Cícero A, Issa J, Feldman S. Bone fracture healing: perspectives according to molecular basis. *J Bone Miner Metab.* 2021;39(3):311–331.
79. Haffner N, Antonic V, Smolen D, et al. Extracorporeal shockwave therapy (ESWT) ameliorates healing of tibial fracture non-union unresponsive to conventional therapy. *Injury.* 2016;47(7):1506–1513.
80. Ryu S, Lee C, Park J, et al. Three-dimensional scaffolds of carbonized polyacrylonitrile for bone tissue regeneration. *Angew Chem Int Ed Engl.* 2014;53(35):9213–9217.
81. Wang S, Li R, Xu Y, et al. Fabrication and application of a 3D-printed poly-ε-caprolactone cage scaffold for bone tissue engineering. *Biomed Res Int.* 2020;2020:2087475.
82. Patel S, Kick B, Busconi B. Fracture management. In: Magee D, Zachazewski J, Quillen W, eds. *Scientific Foundations and Principles of Practice in Musculoskeletal Rehabilitation.* WB Saunders; 2007:607–632.
83. Wang M, Rivlin M, Graham J, Beredjiklian P. Peripheral nerve injury, scarring, and recovery. *Connect Tissue Res.* 2019;60(1):3–9.
84. Seddon HJ. Three types of nerve injury. *Brain.* 1948;66:237–288.
85. Sunderland S. A classification of peripheral nerve injuries producing loss of function. *Brain.* 1951;74(4):491–516.
86. Sulaiman O, Gordon T. Effects of short and long-term Schwann cell denervation on peripheral nerve regeneration, myelination, and size. *Glia.* 2000;32(3):234–246.
87. Campbell W. Evaluation and management of peripheral nerve injury. *Clin Neurophysiol.* 2008;119(9):1951–1965.
88. Miller R. AAEE minimonograph #28: injury to peripheral motor nerves. *Muscle Nerve.* 1987;10(8):698–710.
89. Sunderland S. The anatomy and physiology of nerve injury. *Muscle Nerve.* 1990;13(9):771–784.
90. Atkins S, Smith K, Loescher A, et al. Scarring impedes regeneration at sites of peripheral nerve repair. *Neuroreport.* 2006;17(12):1245–1249.
91. Sunderland S. The function of nerve fibers whose structure has been disorganized. *Anat Rec.* 1951;109(3):503–513.
92. Modrak M, Talukder M, Gurgenashvili K, Noble M, Elfar J. Peripheral nerve injury and myelination: potential therapeutic strategies. *J Neurosci Res.* 2020;98(5):780–795.
93. de Oliveira R, de Andrade Salgado D, Trevelin L, et al. Benefits of laser phototherapy on nerve repair. *Lasers Med Sci.* 2015;30(4):1395–1406.
94. Evans G. Peripheral nerve injury: a review and approach to tissue engineered constructs. *Anat Rec.* 2001;263(4):396–404.

3 | Arthrology

June Hanks and Jeremiah Tate

CHAPTER OBJECTIVES
After reading this chapter, you will be able to:
1. Describe the characteristics of a synovial joint.
2. Discuss the innervation, nutrition, and lubrication of a synovial joint.
3. Differentiate osteokinematic and arthrokinematic movements.
4. Discuss the convex-concave pattern of movement.
5. Differentiate open-packed and close-packed joint positions.
6. Describe active, passive, and accessory joint motion.
7. Discuss the purpose, indications, contraindications, and guidelines for joint mobilization.

Arthrology is the study of types, structures, and functions of joints. A joint is formed when two bones articulate with each other. Joints are traditionally classified as fibrous, cartilaginous, and synovial by the type of tissue uniting the bones. The fibrous and cartilaginous joints are considered solid joints because the adjacent bones are held together by fibrous connective tissue or cartilage; there is no joint cavity. Little to no movement occurs at solid joints.[1] This chapter focuses on synovial joints because they are more numerous and freely moving than the other types of joints.

CHARACTERISTICS OF SYNOVIAL JOINTS
The characteristic features of synovial joints include the presence of the following:
- Joint capsule consisting of an inner synovial membrane and outer fibrous portion
- Synovial fluid produced by the inner synovial membrane of the joint capsule
- Articular cartilage (typically hyaline cartilage) covering the ends of opposing bones

The joint capsule is a double-layered collagenous structure that surrounds the joint and connects the ends of joint segments. The inner, thin, highly vascular portion of the joint capsule produces fluid into the joint cavity that nourishes and lubricates the joint surfaces. The outer fibrous portion is thicker and composed primarily of dense irregular connective tissue. Thickenings of the outer portion of the capsule may form ligaments that help reinforce the joint. These ligaments are called *intracapsular* ligaments, whereas ligaments not blended with the joint capsule are called *extracapsular* ligaments.[1,2] The articular cartilage provides stability, lubrication, and protection of the joint edges while distributing loads across the joint surface.[3] Accessory structures associated with some synovial joints include articular discs (usually composed of fibrocartilage), fat pads, bursae, sesamoid bones, and tendons.[1] Refer to Figure 3-1 for a depiction of a typical synovial joint with accessory features.

The stability of the synovial joint is provided by the shape of the articulating surfaces, the surrounding capsule, ligaments and tendons, and a negative intra-articular pressure (vacuum) within the joint. The relative contributions of these components vary by joint. For example, the hip joint, one of the most stable joints in the body, has a high-degree bony congruency along with strong capsular and ligamentous support. A significant amount of stability of the hip is derived from the vacuum effect within the joint cavity.

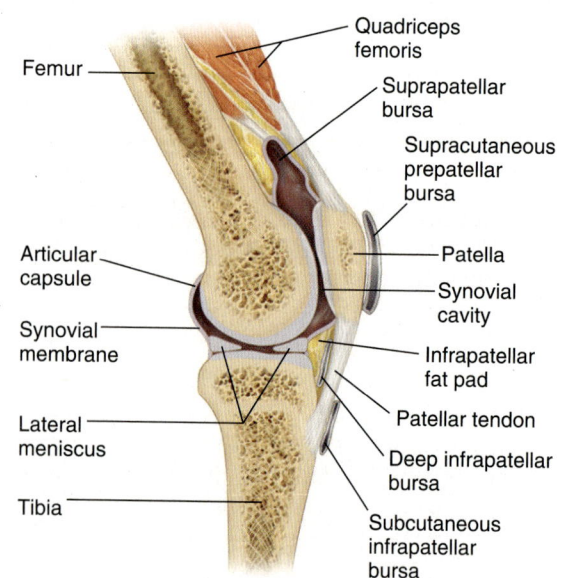

FIGURE 3-1 Typical synovial joint with major features. (Modified from Wingerd BD. *The Human Body: Concepts of Anatomy and Physiology*. 3rd ed. Lippincott Williams & Wilkins; 2014: Figure 4.19.)

In contrast, the glenohumeral joint is much more reliant on the joint capsule and surrounding musculature than on its bony structure.

Neurology

The fibrous layer of the joint capsule has limited blood supply but is richly innervated by articular branches of nerves supplying muscles passing across and acting on the joint.[1,2] Each joint is supplied by more than one nerve, with much overlap in the distribution to the joint. The joint receptors, located in the capsules, ligaments, and tendons around the joint, respond to mechanical deformation and mediate signals related to multiple modalities (proprioception, pain, and temperature) to the central nervous system where sensory input is integrated relative to static joint position, joint movement, velocity of movement, and the force of muscular contraction. The neural-mediated response coordinates muscle activity around the joint to achieve the required stability and mobility. The joint receptors can be differentiated structurally and functionally as presented in Table 3-1. Most of these receptors emit a "resting" action potential, providing an ongoing sense of joint position in space. The receptors are stimulated when deformed by forces acting on the joint. The threshold for stimulation and the speed of adaptation to movement vary among the receptors, allowing continual appraisal of joint position and movement.[4]

The function of the joint receptors should be considered in joint mobilization and other interventions involving joint movement. For example, sudden joint movements stimulate type III receptors and may result in reflex muscle contractions. Manipulations must be performed with a high velocity so that the maneuver is completed before a reflex muscular response elicited by type III receptors can act to interfere with the movement. In addition, manipulation must be performed through a very low amplitude to minimize the number of type III receptors stimulated. Gradual initiation of movement tends to stimulate the type II receptor, which effects a small facilitative muscular response. Passive and active mobilization techniques are best performed rhythmically, without sudden changes in speed or direction of movement. Pain should be avoided with joint mobilization because pain can elicit a reflex muscle response.

In synovial joints, the major pain-sensitive structures are the fibrous capsule, ligaments, and periosteum.

TABLE 3-1
DIFFERENTIATION OF JOINT RECEPTORS

Type (Function)	Location	Appearance	Conduction Speed	Stimulus	Behavior
I (Postural)	Fibrous layer of capsule, ligaments. Higher density in proximal joints	Encapsulated endings, similar to Ruffini corpuscle	Relatively slow	Change of mechanical stress to joint capsule; more active with traction than oscillating movements	Slow adapting, postural kinetic awareness (tonic stabilizers); stimulated by oscillations at end ROM (joint play or manipulation)
II (Dynamic)	Capsule, ligaments, fat pads. Higher density in distal joints	Encapsulated, similar to Pacinian corpuscle	Medium speed	Sudden changes in joint motion; may be more active with oscillation techniques than traction	Fast adapting, movement sensation (phasic movers); silent at rest, fire as movement begins; proprioceptive; stimulated by all motion, especially oscillations at mid-ROM
III (Inhibitive)	Ligaments and superficial layers of capsule (not found in longitudinal ligaments of spine)	Thinly encapsulated; similar to Golgi end organ	Fast	Stretch on end range; more active with fast manipulation techniques	Defensive receptor (provides reflex inhibition of muscle)—proprioceptive
IV (Nociceptive)	Nearly all tissues, except articular cartilage, intra-articular fibrocartilage, and synovium	Free nerve endings and plexus	Slow	Significant mechanical deformation or tension; direct mechanical or chemical irritation	Nociceptive protection (helps produce muscle guarding); stimulated by excessive pressure or tissue damage

ROM, range of motion.
Adapted from Newton RA. Joint receptor contributions to reflexive and kinesthetic responses. *Phys Ther*. 1982;62(1):22–29; Lundy-Ekman L. *Neuroscience: Fundamentals for Rehabilitation*. 4th ed. Elsevier/Saunders; 2013; and Zimny ML, Wink CS. Neuroreceptors in the tissues of the knee joint. *J Electromyogr Kinesiol*. 1991;1(3):148-157.

Articular cartilage, fibrocartilage, synovium, and compact bone are essentially aneural. Clinically, this implies that pathologic conditions affecting joint biomechanics, such as undue compression of articular cartilage, may go unnoticed in the initial stages and be recognized only when there is abnormal stress to the joint capsule or other pain-sensitive structures. This finding suggests that patients may not seek care until the condition has progressed considerably.

Nutrition and Lubrication

Joints receive nutrition from nearby vasculature and the synovial fluid within the joint cavity. Articular and fibrocartilage are avascular and rely on diffusion for nutrition.[5] The margins of associated joint structures receive some nutrients from adjacent highly vascularized structures, such as the synovium, periosteum, and peripheral capsular attachments. The more centrally located cartilaginous areas, which often comprise the primary articulating surfaces, depend on diffusion and imbibition of synovial fluid for nutrition. This arrangement means that nutrients must first pass from the capillary bed of the synovium and then diffuse through the superficial matrix of the cartilaginous surface to reach the wall of the chondrocyte. Such an exchange of nutrients and waste products at joint surfaces requires intermittent compression (approximation) and distraction (separation) of joint surfaces. The intermittent compression and distraction occur normally during weight bearing in the lower extremities and spine, intermittent contraction of muscles crossing a joint, and twisting and untwisting of the joint capsule with movement. Because joint immobilization compromises nutrition, the period of immobilization should be limited to only what is necessary for adequate healing.

Synovial fluid not only contributes to joint nutrition but also serves as a lubricant to reduce wear on joint surfaces from friction. Although appearing smooth on gross examination, articular cartilage is actually relatively rough and porous microscopically. The heavy and varied loads sustained at the joint surface require multiple lubrication processes that can be explained, in part, using the basic engineering concepts of boundary and fluid-film lubrication. In boundary lubrication, the lubricant is adsorbed (i.e., molecules are loosely held) to the surface of the contacting materials, reducing the roughness of the surfaces by filling in irregularities. With fluid-film lubrication, a separation of the joint surfaces occurs, with the load supported by the pressure developed in the fluid film.

The load-bearing surface in joints is not rigid, but relatively soft, creating a type of "elastohydrodynamic" lubrication where the pressure generated in the fluid film deforms the load-bearing surfaces, thus increasing the surface area and leading to less escape of the lubricant from between the surfaces and generating a longer-lasting lubricant film. In this case, the pressure on the articulation is lower and more sustainable. The synovial joint contact surfaces sustain various loads occurring at multiple speeds and with differing durations. Considering these varied demands in normal function, it is likely that joint lubrication involves a number of mechanisms, dependent on the loading condition at the joint.

Joint Surface Shape

The articular surfaces of synovial joints are traditionally described by similarity to geometric shapes (e.g., flat, ellipsoid, spherical). See Table 3-2 for examples. While the simplicity of this approach has value, it must be appreciated that no articular surface is a true geometric form; joint surfaces are neither spheres, ovals, ellipses, nor are they true parts of these. A more accurate description is a variation of two basic shapes: ovoid or sellar (Fig. 3-2).[6] The simple ovoid shows different curvatures of ovoid profiles in opposing planes at right angles to each other. Some joint surfaces, rather than representing a simple ovoid, might be considered a complex ovoid, or sellar (saddle-shaped), surface. A sellar surface is convex in one cross-sectional plane and concave in the plane perpendicular to it. As such, any articular surface can be considered as being part of an ovoid surface. The simple and complex ovoid articular surfaces demonstrate varying amounts of curvature and asymmetry. The joint surfaces may be nearly flat to nearly spherical, with the majority showing intermediate curvature and great variation in radius along the surface.[6]

JOINT MOTION

Kinematics describes the motion of a body or segments of a body without reference to the forces that cause the motion. Translation and rotation are the two basic

TABLE 3-2

TRADITIONAL ANATOMICAL CLASSIFICATION OF SYNOVIAL JOINTS

Type	Examples
Flat (planar)	Acromioclavicular
Hinge (ginglymi)	Elbow
Pivot (trochoid)	Atlantoaxial
	Proximal radioulnar
Bicondylar (largely uniaxial)	Knee
	Temporomandibular
Ellipsoid (biaxial)	Metacarpophalangeal
Saddle (sellar)	Carpometacarpal
	Sternoclavicular
Ball and socket (spheroid)	Hip
	Shoulder

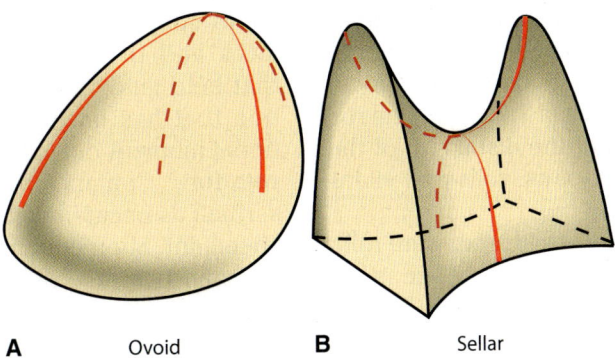

FIGURE 3-2 Ovoid **(A)** and sellar **(B)** shapes.

types of motion. *Translation* is a linear or curvilinear motion where all parts of a body or segment of a joint move parallel to and in the same direction as the other parts. With translation, all points of a body move the same distance in the same amount of time. *Rotation* refers to a circular motion about a pivot point such that different points of the same body do not move through the same distance in a given amount of time.

Definitions of joint movement require description of **osteokinematics** (rotary movement of the bony segment in space during physiologic joint motion) and **arthrokinematics** (movement between the two adjacent articular surfaces). The osteokinematic (physiologic) movement can be voluntarily generated, whereas arthrokinematic (also called *accessory*) movements typically cannot be voluntarily isolated. The amount of joint motion is guided by bony structure and constraints imposed by capsular, ligamentous, muscular, and other soft-tissue structures.

Osteokinematics

Osteokinematic movement of a joint is traditionally described in a coordinate system of planes and axes, without differentiation as to whether the described axis is the mechanical axis (as defined earlier) or the long axis of the moving bone. In this tradition, described planes and axes of movements correspond to the sagittal, frontal, or transverse plane; the plane and axis maintain a perpendicular relationship throughout the movement (Fig. 3-3). The terms *flexion* and *extension* describe angular movements between the segments articulating bone within the sagittal plane about a mediolateral axis, whereas *abduction* and *adduction* occur within the frontal plane about an anteroposterior axis. Internal and external rotation are rotational movements commonly described relative to either a vertical or longitudinal axis of the moving bone (which, depending on positioning, may coincide with the mechanical axis). The term *vertical* is typically used to describe the trunk axis in an upright position. Otherwise, the term *longitudinal* is used when referring to rotational movement.

Arthrokinematics

Arthrokinematic movements naturally occur at joint surfaces and include rolls, slides, and spins. A spin typically occurs at the joint surface as a consequence of the roll and slide, resulting from the incongruency of joint surfaces. Exceptions are the proximal radioulnar joint and the atlantoaxial joint, which spin around a true longitudinal axis. It should be noted that the term *slide*

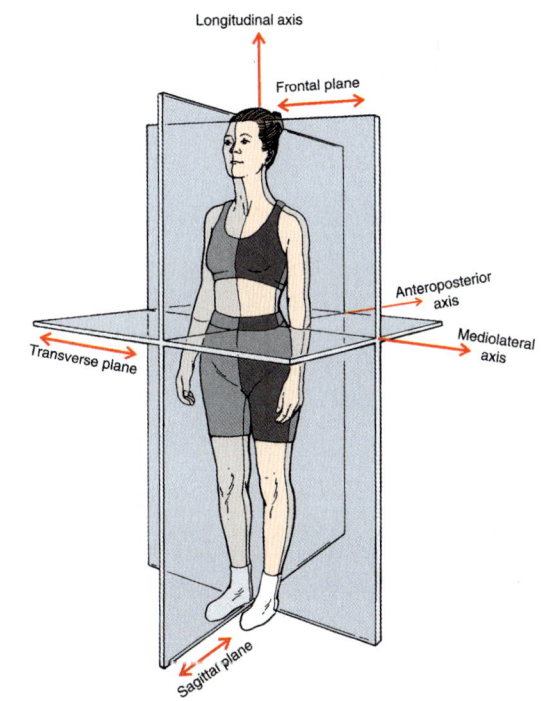

FIGURE 3-3 Cardinal planes (sagittal, frontal, transverse) and axes (mediolateral, anteroposterior, longitudinal). (Hamill J, Knutzen KM, Derrick TR. *Biomechanical Basis of Human Movement.* 5th ed. Wolters Kluwer; 2022: Figure 1-15.)

can also be referred to as glide when describing joint arthrokinematics. The term *glide* is commonly used to describe the slide motion applied in joint mobilization. Definitions and analogies are given in Table 3-3. The roll always occurs in the direction of the distal end of the moving bone. In most synovial joints, rolls and slides occur simultaneously (Fig. 3-4).

If roll occurred in the absence of slide (i.e., pure roll), the moving bone would tend to dislocate before much movement could occur at the joint surface (Fig. 3-5A). If slide took place in the absence of roll (i.e., pure slide), the joint surfaces would become impinged and full movement would not occur (Fig. 3-5B).

The concurrent movements of roll and slide allow for economy of articular cartilage with respect to the size of the joint surface necessary for movement. These concurrent movements also prevent undue wearing of isolated points on joint surfaces, which would occur if, for example, only slide took place.

Conjunct Rotation

Most motions around a joint do not occur in straight planes or along straight lines but rather the segments of bones move in space in curved paths owing to the ovoid shape and arrangement of articular joint surfaces and the capsular and ligamentous structures that help guide the movement. A special type of motion that has been described as an obligatory rotational moment occurring about two bones is **conjunct rotation**.[7] Conjunct rotation has been primarily described as occurring at the shoulder complex and the knee joint. Shoulder conjunct rotation is described by Codman paradox, demonstrated by the following sequential motions at the shoulder joint:

1. Stand with arms at the side, palms facing toward the body and thumbs extended (i.e., the thumb is pointing forward).
2. Flex the arm to 90° at the shoulder so that the thumb is pointed up.
3. Horizontally extend the arm to a position of 90° of abduction at the glenohumeral joint. The thumb is pointing upward.
4. Without rotating your arm, return the arm to your side. Note that the thumb is now pointing away from the thigh.

During this succession of three straight plane movements with return to the start position, the

TABLE 3-3				
ARTHROKINEMATIC MOVEMENTS AT JOINT (ROLL, SLIDE, SPIN) WITH TIRE ANALOGY				
Movement	Definition	Joint Example	Analogy	Tire Example
Roll	Multiple points on rotating surface contact multiple points on the opposing surface		Tire rolling down the road	
Slide	A single point on one surface contacts multiple points on the opposing surface		Nonrotating tire sliding on ice	
Spin	Single point on one surface rotates on a single point of an opposing surface		Rotating tire spinning in mud	

of a cycle of movements. Conjunction rotation of the knee is typically used to describe the external rotation of the tibia that occurs during terminal knee extension, which is also referred to as the *screw-home mechanism*.

Instant Center of Rotation

The human joint axis is complex owing to the incongruity of joint surfaces and the arthrokinematics movements of roll, slide, and spin. Unlike a door hinge whose center axis remains stationary, the center axis of a human joint moves along a curvilinear path with joint movement. This shifting in space of the center axis of rotation is called the **instant center of rotation**. Joints that demonstrate a combination of rotation and slide demonstrate a variable instant center of rotation. In some joints, such as the knee, movement of the instantaneous center of rotation is large (Fig. 3-6), whereas in most joints, the movement is relatively small. An example of the clinical relevance of the instant center of rotation is related to the complex hinge design of a functional knee brace to improve the brace's fit and overall function during high-level activity. However, simple brace designs used postoperatively (e.g., ROM knee brace) may only include a simple hinge design because these

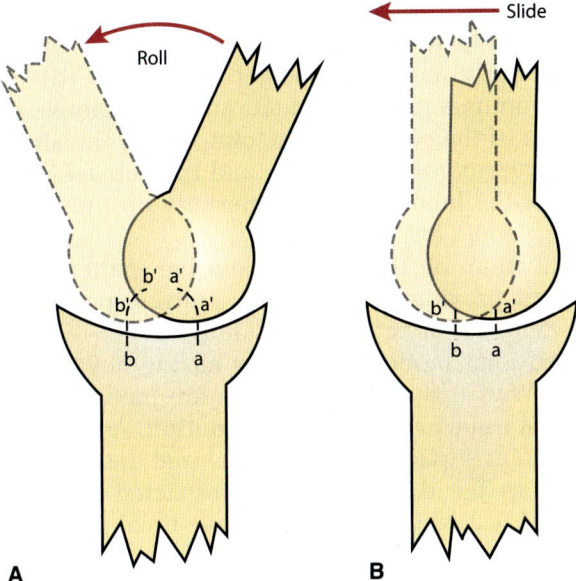

FIGURE 3-4 Arthrokinematic movements of the knee showing roll (**A**) and slide (**B**). The letters indicate points on the opposing joint surfaces contacting each other. Points a and b are on the stationary surface, and a' and b' are on the moving joint surface. During roll (**A**), points a and b contact multiple points on the moving joint surface. During slide (**B**), points a and b contact one point on the moving surface.

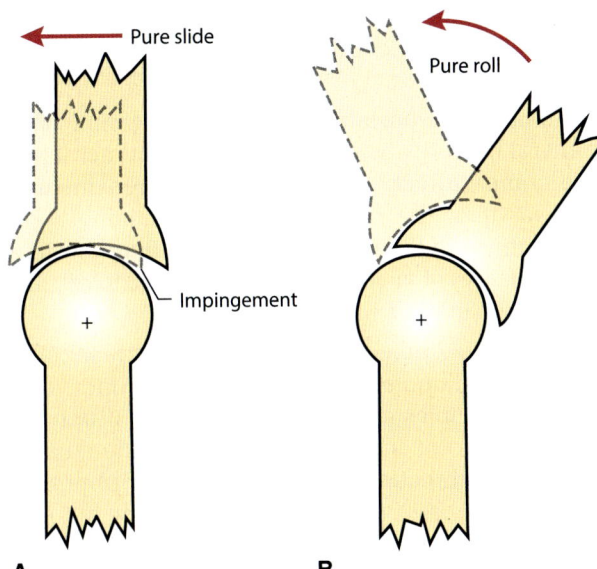

FIGURE 3-5 Example of joint movement in the absence of kinematic movement. **A.** Impingement occurs if slide occurred in the absence of roll. **B.** Dislocation occurs with roll in the absence of slide.

arm rotated externally 90°. In this case, the mechanical axis follows a path on the joint surface, tracing a triangle in space. With some movements, the conjunct rotation traces an arc or a chord or combination of both in space, from the start to completion

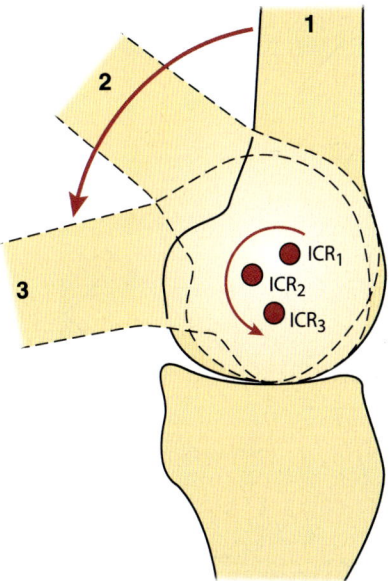

FIGURE 3-6 Instant center of rotation (ICR) of knee joint. The ICR varies by joint position. (Adapted from Oatis CA. *Kinesiology: The Mechanics and Pathomechanics of Human Movement*. 3rd ed. Wolters Kluwer; 2017: Figure 7.5B.)

types of braces are typically reserved for the first rehabilitation phase following surgery.

Convex-Concave Pattern of Movement

Most joint motions require a combination of arthrokinematic movements. The roll of a joint surface always occurs in the same direction as the moving bone. However, the shape of joint surfaces influences the direction of joint slide. The relationship between roll and slide describes a naturally occurring pattern of movement at the joint surface that minimizes the migration of the center of the convex member in the direction of the roll.[8] The roll-slide pattern is often referred to as the convex-concave "rule," stating that if a concave surface moves on a convex surface, roll and slide must occur in the same direction; if a convex joint surface moves on a concave surface, roll and slide must occur in opposite directions.[9] Consider active knee extension in the open kinetic chain. As the tibia rolls on the stationary femur (i.e., the shaft of the tibia moves anteriorly), the concave joint surface of the tibia slides anteriorly (Fig. 3-7A). In the closed kinetic chain, as an individual moves from sitting to standing, the tibia is relatively stationary. The convex surface of the femur rolls anteriorly and slides posteriorly (Fig. 3-7B) to maintain optimal joint alignment. Another example is abduction of the glenohumeral joint, where the shaft of the humerus rolls superiorly and the convex joint surface of the humerus slides inferiorly on the fixed concave glenoid fossa.

Application of the **convex-concave pattern of movement** provides a reasonable starting point for determining the direction of a slide (glide) to restore restricted joint motion, especially among novice clinicians.[8] With this approach, joints are mobilized to facilitate normal **arthrokinematic motion**. As such, a concave joint surface would be mobilized in the same direction as the direction of the restricted primary movement (e.g., the relatively concave tibial condylar surface would be mobilized anteriorly for restricted knee extension and posteriorly for restricted knee flexion). Similarly, a bone with a convex joint surface would be mobilized in the direction opposite to the restricted movement (e.g., the convex scaphoid would be mobilized with a dorsal glide on the radius for restricted wrist flexion and in a palmar direction for restricted wrist extension).

Some kinematic studies of the glenohumeral joint appear to conflict with the expected arthrokinematics based on convex-concave joint surface shapes.[10-13] However, apparent contradictions may be explained by considering[8]:

- The small net translation (slide) of the center of the humeral head relative to the size of the humeral head
- The comparatively large amount of osteokinematic movement of the humerus while remaining within the confines of the relatively small glenoid fossa
- The portion of a joint capsule, if restricted, that most likely limits a motion of interest

While the example here references movement of the convex-shaped humerus on the relatively concave glenoid, the principles can be extrapolated to other similarly shaped joint surfaces. Clinical decision-making regarding the direction of manual gliding mobilization should not be restricted solely to joint shape but must also consider tension in the surrounding tissues (e.g., joint capsule, musculature).

Close-Packed Position

Owing to their ovoid shapes, most joint surfaces vary in congruency throughout a movement. The position of greatest relative congruency between articulating surfaces is the **close-packed position** of a joint, which usually occurs somewhere near or at the end range of motion (ROM). Movement to achieve maximum joint surface congruency involves conjunct rotation that

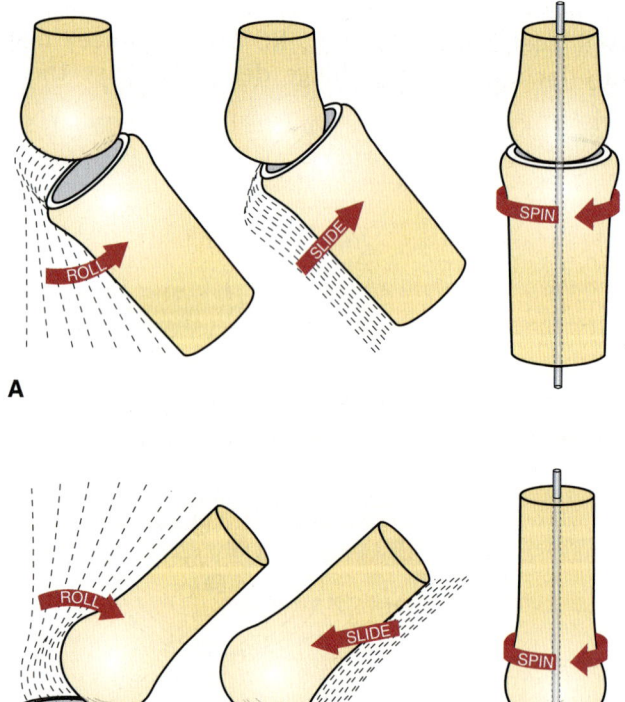

FIGURE 3-7 Joint surface movement. **A.** Concave-on-convex arthrokinematics. **B.** Convex-on-concave arthrokinematics. (Adapted from Neumann DA. *Kinesiology of the Musculoskeletal System: Foundations for Rehabilitation.* 3rd ed. Elsevier; 2017: Figure 1-8.)

serves to tighten and twist the joint capsule and ligaments. As the opposing joint surfaces are moved toward/away from maximum approximation, alternating compression and distraction of the joint surfaces occur. In the close-packed position, joint surface sliding is maximally restricted, and the application of traction and distraction forces results in minimal separation of joint spaces, adding to stability in this position. The combined effect of joint congruity (maximum contact area) and capsuloligamentous tightness provides stability and minimal joint volume in this position. Examples of close-packed positions for a joint include full (hyperextension) extension of the knee and distal radiocarpal joint and maximal abduction and external rotation of shoulder joint. See Tables 7-11 and 7-12 in Chapter 7, The Physical Examination, for close-packed positions of selected joints.

Clinical implications of the intrinsic stability of a joint in the close-packed position can be seen with injury, as most fractures and dislocations occur with the joint in this position. In a fall on an outstretched hand, the major joints of the upper extremity are in or near or in the position of maximum congruency; forces sustained beyond this position may result in fracture or dislocation (e.g., Colles fracture at the wrist, posterior dislocation at the elbow, anterior dislocation of the shoulder).

Open-Packed Position

In any position other than close-packed, the joint capsule and major supporting ligaments are less taut; thus, a joint has some "play." Normal movement between the ovoid-shaped joint surfaces requires some laxity in the surrounding capsule and ligaments. The position in which laxity of the joint capsule and surrounding ligaments allows for the least congruency is called the **open-packed (or loose-packed) position**. In the major joints of the lower extremity, open-packed positions are biased toward flexion. Generally, the joint is least congruent and thus has most "joint play" near the mid-range position. Such a position is commonly assumed by a patient with a traumatic injury to the joint to avoid approximation of joint surfaces in other positions. Adaptive shortening may occur when the joint remains in an open-packed position for an extended period of time. In such a case, treatment should be focused on regaining the full close-packed position. Open-packed position is also ideal for initial early treatment procedures to restore joint motion.

Accessory Movements

Arthrokinematic movements of joints may be referred to as *accessory joint movement* (or *component movement*). For full active or passive ROM at a joint, **accessory motions** must occur. Stated another way, normal accessory joint movement is necessary for normal osteokinematic movement. For example, for normal active elevation of the shoulder to occur, the humeral head rolls superiorly and slides inferiorly on the glenoid fossa. Another example is knee extension in non–weight bearing in which the tibia rolls in the same direction as the tibial swing and slides anteriorly. As the close-packed position of the knee is approached near full extension, the tibia must externally rotate (i.e., spin) for the complete motion to occur. If the accessory movement does not or cannot occur, it does so at the expense of the capsule or ligaments, which must be abnormally stretched, or of the articular cartilage, which must be abnormally compressed.

The more intimate the anatomic and functional relation between the joint capsule and the major supporting ligaments, the more likely it is that the close-packed position will be the most restricted position of the joint (i.e., capsular pattern of restriction). In joints where the major ligaments blend with the joint capsule (e.g., hip and shoulder), movements toward the close-packed position are often the first to be lost. In the knee, the ligaments are more easily distinguished from the joint capsule and flexion may be the most limited in a capsular restriction, whereas knee extension constitutes the close-packed position.

JOINT MOTION ASSESSMENT

Active motion at a joint occurs when muscles surrounding a joint contract and produce the joint movement. Assessment of active motion provides information regarding a person's willingness to move, coordination, muscle strength, and overall ROM. Active motion may be limited by pain due to contraction or stretching of muscles and fascia or due to stretching or compression of ligaments or joint capsule. If an individual is unable to actively move a joint easily, painlessly, and in a coordinated manner through the complete motion available for that joint, an investigation should be pursued to clarify the problem. Passive movement at a joint is performed without activation of muscles. Normally, passive motion is greater than active motion. Testing of passive motion provides information about articular surfaces and associated structures within and surrounding the joint. Active and passive physiologic motion should be examined for range (amount of motion), quality of movement, and symptom response. The physiologic movements may be used to mobilize both contractile and noncontractile tissues.

The anatomic limit of joint movement is the limit imposed by anatomic structures; the forcing of movement beyond this barrier may produce tissue injury, such as sprain, strain, dislocation, or fracture. The discrete, short-range movement of a joint at the end of passive motion is called *passive overpressure*. In normal joints, the sense of resistance to further motion felt by the clinician providing the passive overpressure is termed "end feel." Each joint has an expected normal end feel because of the bony configuration and surrounding structures. See Chapter 7, The Physical Examination, for descriptions of normal and pathologic end feels.

Hypermobility and Hypomobility

Thorough assessment of joint movement includes examination of physiologic movement (active and passive) and accessory (joint-play) movement. A joint with excessive range of movement but with adequate muscle control is considered hypermobile,[14-16] whereas such a joint without adequate protective muscular control is unstable.[16] Generalized joint hypermobility is present when the majority of synovial joints in an individual are hypermobile taking into consideration age, sex, and ethnic background.[14,15,17,18] Hypermobility is more common in females and among individuals with Asian and African ethnic backgrounds.[18-20]

Joint hypermobility may also be a clinical manifestation of a number of connective tissue diseases, such as Ehlers-Danlos syndrome or Marfan syndrome.

Hypermobility may be inherited[21] or acquired through years of consistent participation in activities requiring extremes of motion, such as gymnastics or ballet. Hypermobility may be asymptomatic and pose no problems, but in some individuals, the condition may lead to a variety of soft-tissue injuries, joint dysfunction, and pain.[15]

Joint assessment may reveal a loss of joint mobility (hypomobility). The loss of **osteokinematic motion**, such as decreased wrist extension or ankle dorsiflexion, is called *osteokinematic* (or *physiologic*) *hypomobility*. The loss of normal roll, slide, and spin that should occur along with osteokinematic movement is called *arthrokinematic* (or *accessory*) *hypomobility*. There may be a subjective report of stiffness or pain, especially when the hypomobile joint is forcibly moved. A restriction in movement at one joint may create a hypermobility at the adjacent joints to allow full range of mobility in a general area. Manual therapy for hypomobility includes soft-tissue therapies involving manual contacts, pressures, or movements focused to a particular area. Such techniques include, but are not limited to, massage, soft-tissue mobilization, acupressure, trigger point therapy, relaxation exercises, active or passive stretching of shortened muscles and associated tissues, and joint mobilization or manipulation. Postural correction and exercise to maintain improved body mechanics and joint mobility may be utilized to treat hypomobility.

Any tissue (connective, muscle, epithelial, and neural) crossing the joint may impact full motion. For example, a lack of flexibility (decreased muscle length) in the latissimus dorsi may limit full shoulder flexion and external rotation. Injury to the axillary epithelium from a thermal burn to the region can lead to significant limitation in glenohumeral movement, if joint motion is not consistently addressed during healing. In addition, neural tissues may become restricted in mobility as a result of injury (e.g., compression, post-surgical) or immobilization. For example, upper limb neural tension tests involve placing multiple joints in specific positions to sequentially stress nerves as they course through tissues and across joints. Neural mobilization may be necessary to restore the dynamic balance between relative movement of neural tissues and surrounding tissue interfaces.

Joint Mobilization

The purpose of passive **joint mobilization** is to increase joint ROM, decrease pain, promote muscle relaxation, and improve muscle performance. The term "mobilization" is most commonly used to denote a movement within the range of a joint that does not involve a high-velocity thrust movement. Defined in this manner, the joint mobilization is a passive slow movement that may be applied with a sustained stretch or with an oscillatory motion: a gentle, coaxing, repetitive, rhythmic movement. The mobilization is performed over a wide range of movements (referred to as *grades*) and at a speed that can be resisted by the patient.[16] The passive stretch or oscillatory movements are intended to reduce pain or joint restriction. The term "manipulation" describes a passive high-velocity movement of small amplitude that occurs near the joint's anatomic limit of motion and without guarding by the patient. A manipulation is within the joint's anatomic limit and is performed at a high speed. In this text, the term "joint mobilization" refers to both joint mobilization and joint manipulation.

To determine the need for joint mobilization, the clinician evaluates joint accessory mobility including distraction, compression, and gliding movements at the joint surface to assess the amount of movement available and the symptom response. Joint accessory motion is assessed, and joint mobilization forces are applied relative to the treatment plane, described as a plane perpendicular to a line running from the axis of rotation to the deepest portion of the concave articular surface. In a mobilization maneuver, the treatment plane remains with the concave articular surface, regardless of whether the moving aspect of the joint is concave or convex.[9]

The direction of movement during treatment is either perpendicular or parallel to the treatment plane. Gliding mobilizations are applied parallel to the treatment plane and are usually performed in the direction in which the joint mobility test has shown that the glide is actually restricted. Gliding mobilization in the direction opposite, the restriction should be considered if the mobilization in the direction of the restriction produces pain or if treatment in that direction is ineffective. Joint distraction techniques are applied perpendicular to the treatment plane; the entire bone is moved so that the joint surfaces are separated.

Indications and Contraindications for Joint Mobilization Indication for joint mobilization includes joint restriction due to loss of accessory joint motion that causes pain or restriction during normal physiologic movement. There are numerous causes of loss of accessory motions, including capsuloligamentous tightening or adherence; internal derangement resulting from a cartilaginous loose body or meniscus displacement; reflex muscle guarding; and bony blockage resulting from hypertrophic degenerative changes. The loss of accessory motion due to capsular or ligamentous tightness or adherence is a primary indication. Other causes of joint dysfunction are relative contraindications.

Absolute contraindications for joint mobilization include the following:

- Any undiagnosed lesion
- Joint ankylosis
- Close-packed position

Absolute contraindications for spinal joint mobilization include the following:

- Cauda equina lesions producing disturbance of bladder or bowel function if the lumbar spine is being treated
- Where the integrity of ligaments may be affected by the use of steroids, traumatized upper cervical ligaments, Down syndrome, rheumatoid collagen necrosis of the vertebral ligaments, particularly if the cervical spine is being treated
- Any indication of vertebrobasilar insufficiency in the cervical spine if the cervical spine is being treated; and active inflammatory and infective arthritis

Relative contraindications for joint mobilization include the following:

- Joint effusions from trauma or disease
- Arthrosis (e.g., degenerative joint disease) if acute or causing a bony block to movement to be restored
- Rheumatoid arthritis
- Metabolic bone disease, such as osteoporosis, Paget disease, and tuberculosis
- Internal derangement
- General debilitation (e.g., influenza, chronic disease)
- Hypermobility—patients with hypermobility may benefit from gentle joint-play techniques if kept within the limits of motion. Patients with potential necrosis of the ligaments or capsule should not be mobilized

- Pregnancy, if the lumbar spine or pelvis is being treated
- Spinal cord involvement or suspected aneurysm in the area being treated

Relative contraindications for spinal mobilization include the following:

- Spondylolisthesis or severe scoliosis in the area being treated
- Where there are symptoms derived from severe radicular involvement

General Guidelines for Joint Mobilization Generally, the rate, rhythm, and intensity of mobilization must be adjusted according to how the patient presents (e.g., pain versus stiffness) and according to the response of the patient to the applied technique. In the application of manual therapy techniques, the following points should be considered:

- Room setup:
  - The temperature of the room should be comfortable and free of distracting noises.
- Position of the patient:
  - The patient must be relaxed and in a position in which the joint under treatment is accessible with full range of movement unrestricted.
  - All other joints should be in a resting, well-supported position.
- Position of structure to be treated:
  - During an assessment mobilization, the joint should be tested in the open-packed position if the patient is capable of attaining that position.
  - Typically, the open-packed position is used when the patient has an acute condition; this "resting" position of the patient may be the position that the injured joint adopts rather than the classic resting position for a normal joint.
  - As treatment progresses, the joint may be positioned at or near the end of the available range before application of the mobilization force so that the restricting tissue is in its most stretched position. In some cases, the position to use is the one in which the joint is least painful.
- Position of the clinician:
  - The clinician should be relaxed and positioned relative to the patient to allow for proper body mechanics as well as close body contact with the patient for optimal control and direction of forces during the mobilization.
  - Ideally, the force will be directed with gravity assistance, especially when treating larger joints.
- Clinician hand placement and stabilization:
  - Hand placement is critical for establishing appropriate stabilization and for the transmission of force in the intended direction. The stabilizing hand and mobilizing hand should be positioned as

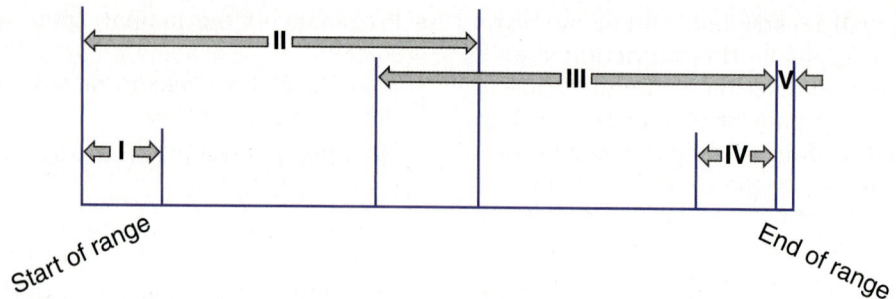

FIGURE 3-8 Grades of mobilization.

close to the joint surface as possible to allow force application as intended.
- A larger contact surface with the hands is preferred, as this position is typically more comfortable to the patient. Though this may vary, typically, the proximal bone is stabilized with the clinician's hands, a belt, the treatment surface, or an assistant, and the distal bone is mobilized.
- The grip must be firm, yet painless and reassuring with fingertips free to palpate tissues being treated.
- Application of forces:
  - The arms and body of the clinician are used to impart the passive movement to the joint, with the hands of the clinician used to sense and feel the movement rather than directly producing the movement.
- Force type and direction:
  - Distraction, or separation of joint surfaces, occurs with movement at a right angle to and away from the treatment plane.
  - Gliding occurs with movement parallel to the treatment plane. Gliding movements are typically performed with a slight amount of distraction.
- Amount of force:
  - The amount of force used depends on the intent of the manual procedure and other factors such as the following:
    - Age, sex, and general health status of the patient
    - Barrier to motion
    - Type and severity of movement disorder
- Ongoing assessment:
  - Each technique may be an assessment technique and treatment technique; therefore, the clinician continually re-assesses during treatment.

Joint Mobilization Technique Joint mobilization directed toward limited accessory joint movements within or at the limit of joint motion may be necessary to restore normal joint function. The anatomic limit to the joint motion is specific to each joint and is determined by the shape of joint surfaces and the surrounding capsules and ligaments. The passive mobilization techniques are typically graded on a scale that reflects the speed of movement and the degree of stretch imparted to tissues. In the system promoted by Maitland,[16] there are five grades of movement (Fig. 3-8). The joint movements are performed at varying speeds and amplitudes (portions of the joint-play movement). The grades are as follows:

- Grade I: slow, small-amplitude movement performed at the beginning of range; movement takes place within the joint; used to reduce pain.
- Grade II: slow, large-amplitude movement that does not move into resistance or the limit of the available range; used to reduce pain.
- Grade III: slow, large-amplitude movement that reaches the limit of the available range; used to increase mobility.
- Grade IV: slow, small-amplitude movement performed into resistance, up to the limit of available range; used to increase mobility.
- Grade V: fast, small-amplitude, high-velocity movement, usually performed at the end of the available range; also called *thrust* technique or manipulation.

The criteria for selection of speed and grade to be used for mobilization include (1) the degree of pain or protective muscle spasm during the passive joint-play movement (irritability) (Table 3-4) and (2) the degree of restriction of joint-play movement. Joints may also be stretched with a stationary hold at the end of a limited range or may be moved toward and away from the limit of motion with slow, oscillating movements or sharp, staccato-type movements. The slow, smooth oscillatory movements may be best suited for grades I and II to treat more irritable, painful conditions, whereas quick, staccato-type movements are useful in

TABLE 3-4

GRADES BASED ON DURATION, TYPE, AND IRRITABILITY OF SYMPTOMS

Duration of Symptoms	Grades
Acute	Grades I and II indicated
Subacute	Grades II and III indicated
	Grade V moderately indicated
Chronic	Grades III and IV indicated
	Grade V strongly indicated

treating stiff joints using grades III and IV. Grade IV and V maneuvers are used to stretch or break down adhesions. The skill and experience of the clinician and the clinical presentation of the patient should guide the grades used. Grades I to IV should be utilized before consideration of a grade V maneuver.

The duration of joint mobilization in a treatment session is determined by the treatment goals, the patient's symptoms, and the movement signs during and after the technique. Generally, within a given session, techniques to reduce pain with movement are performed for a short duration (1–2 minutes, once or twice), whereas techniques to reduce joint stiffness are performed for a longer duration and more frequently with gentle techniques interspersed to minimize soreness.[16]

During a treatment session, graded mobilization may be used in combination with osteokinematic motions. For example, in treating joint stiffness with wrist extension, grades III and IV mobilization may be used with active and passive wrist extension. It should be noted that the primary goal of joint mobilization is to restore normal joint mechanics to allow full, pain-free use of the joint. Forcing osteokinematic movement on a joint with an accessory movement restriction risks damage to the joint by compressing isolated portions of articular cartilage and may increase pain and muscle guarding by overstretching portions of the surrounding joint capsule and ligaments. Targeted and appropriately applied specific passive mobilization provides a safer, more efficient, and less painful method of increasing motion in joints. For example, if glenohumeral inferior slide is limited or absent with glenohumeral elevation, the superior portion of the joint capsule and surrounding structures may be impinged and the condition worsened with repeated shoulder elevation. In this case, treatment directed toward the limited accessory motion should improve the pain-free range of physiologic motion.

CHAPTER SUMMARY
Joint mobility is a component of the overall patient examination (see Chapter 7, The Physical Examination). The effective application of joint mobilization techniques in the management of musculoskeletal disorders requires proficiency in evaluating accessory joint movements, correlating findings with knowledge of normal accessory movements at the joint, and taking into account other presenting signs and symptoms in the examination. The patient's symptom response and joint mobility should be assessed throughout and at the end of each treatment as well as over time following each treatment session.

REFERENCES
1. Drake RL, Vogl AW, Mitchell AWM. *Gray's Anatomy for Students.* 3rd ed. Churchill Livingstone/Elsevier; 2015.
2. Oatis CA. *Kinesiology: The Mechanics and Pathomechanics of Human Movement.* 3rd ed. Wolters Kluwer; 2017.
3. Hamill J, Knutzen KM, Derrick TR. *Biomechanical Basis of Human Movement.* 5th ed. Wolters Kluwer; 2022.
4. Lundy-Ekman L. *Neuroscience: Fundamentals for Rehabilitation.* 4th ed. Elsevier/Saunders; 2013.
5. Pawlina W, Ross MH. *Histology: A Text and Atlas with Correlated Cell and Molecular Biology.* 8th ed. Wolters Kluwer; 2020.
6. Williams P, Warwick R, Myson M, Bannister L, eds. *Gray's Anatomy.* 37th ed. Churchill Livingstone; 1989.
7. Straiton J, Todd B, Venner R. Radiographic assessment of knee joint rotation. *J Anat.* 1987;155:189–193.
8. Neumann D. The convex-concave rules of arthrokinematics: flawed or perhaps just misinterpreted? *J Orthop Sports Phys Ther.* 2012;42(2):53–55.
9. Kaltenborn F. *Manual Mobilization of the Joints, Volume I: The Extremities.* 7th ed. Norli; 2011.
10. Matsuki K, Matsuki K, Yamaguchi S, et al. Dynamic in vivo glenohumeral kinematics during scapular plane abduction in healthy shoulders. *J Orthop Sports Phys Ther.* 2012;42(2):96–104.
11. Harryman D 2nd, Sidles J, Clark J, McQuade K, Gibb T, Matsen F 3rd. Translation of the humeral head on the glenoid with passive glenohumeral motion. *J Bone Joint Surg Am.* 1990;72(9):1334–1343.
12. Howell S, Galinat B, Renzi A, Marone P. Normal and abnormal mechanics of the glenohumeral joint in the horizontal plane. *J Bone Joint Surg Am.* 1988;70(2):227–232.
13. Johnson A, Godges J, Zimmerman G, Ounanian L. The effect of anterior versus posterior glide joint mobilization on external rotation range of motion in patients with shoulder adhesive capsulitis. *J Orthop Sports Phys Ther.* 2007;37(3):88–99.
14. Hakim A, Grahame R. Joint hypermobility. *Best Pract Res Clin Rheumatol.* 2003;17(6):989–1004.
15. Simmonds J, Keer R. Hypermobility and the hypermobility syndrome. *Man Ther.* 2007;12(4):298–309.
16. Hengeveld E, Banks K. *Maitland's Peripheral Manipulation.* 4th ed. Elsevier; 2005.
17. Grahame R, Hakim AJ. Hypermobility. *Curr Opin Rheumatol.* 2008;20(1):106–110.
18. Singh H, McKay M, Baldwin J, et al. Beighton scores and cut-offs across the lifespan: cross-sectional study of an Australian population. *Rheumatology (Oxford).* 2017;56(11):1857–1864.
19. Beighton P, Solomon L, Soskolne C. Articular mobility in an African population. *Ann Rheum Dis.* 1973;32(5):413–418.
20. Wordsworth P, Ogilvie D, Smith R, Sykes B. Joint mobility with particular reference to racial variation and inherited connective tissue disorders. *Br J Rheumatol.* 1987;26(1):9–12.
21. Child A. Joint hypermobility syndrome: inherited disorder of collagen synthesis. *J Rheumatol.* 1986;13(2):239–243.

4 | Spine Osteology and Arthrology

June Hanks

CHAPTER OBJECTIVES

After reading this chapter, you will be able to:
1. Differentiate between the appendicular and axial skeleton.
2. Describe the osteology and associated connective tissue in the vertebral column regions.
3. Describe the components of the intervertebral disc and the response to loading.
4. Discuss the impact of facet joint orientation on movement.
5. Describe the musculature that moves and stabilizes the vertebral column.
6. Discuss the kinematics of vertebral column and sacroiliac joint.
7. Describe common pathologies affecting the spinal column.

The skeleton has two components: appendicular and axial. The appendicular skeleton consists of bones of the extremities, and the axial skeleton consists of bones of the vertebral column, ribs, sternum, and cranium. The component parts of the appendicular skeleton are discussed in chapters throughout this text. The cranium is described in Chapter 18, Temporomandibular Joint. The focus of this chapter is the osteology, articular movement, stability, and associated muscles of the vertebral column and sacroiliac joint (SIJ).

OSTEOLOGY

The vertebral column is 72 to 75 cm (~2 feet, 5 inches) long. There are 33 vertebrae: 7 cervical, 12 thoracic, 5 lumbar, 5 sacral, 4 coccygeal (Fig. 4-1). An intervertebral disc (IVD) lies between each of the vertebrae from the first and second cervical to the fifth lumbar vertebra and top of the sacrum. One-fourth of the length of

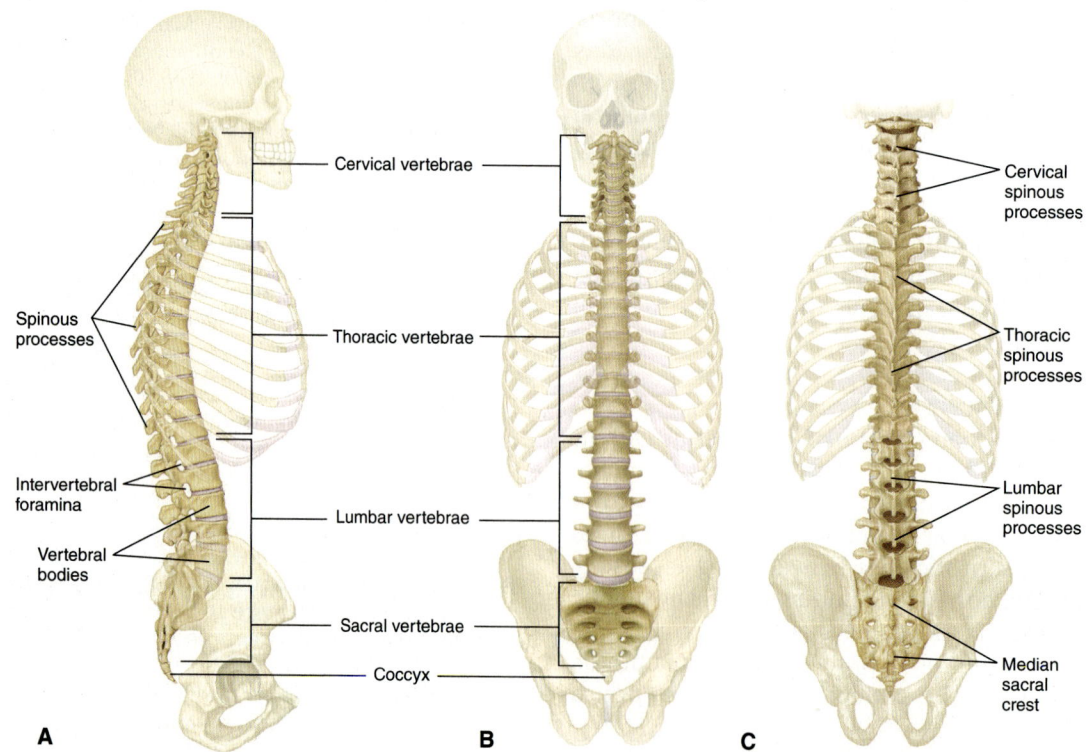

FIGURE 4-1 Vertebral column showing cervical, thoracic, lumbar, sacral and coccygeal levels from **(A)** Sagittal view, **(B)** anterior view, and **(C)** posterior view. (Modified from Pansky B, Gest TR. *Lippincott's Concise Illustrated Anatomy: Back, Upper Limb & Lower Limb*. Vol. 1. Lippincott Williams & Wilkins; 2014:Figure 1.2B–D.)

the vertebral column is from the IVDs. The vertebral column:

- Protects spinal cord and spinal nerves
- Supports the weight of the body
- Provides partly rigid, partly flexible axis for body and pivot for head
- Plays a role in posture and locomotion

The normal curvatures of the vertebral column are named primary (kyphosis) and secondary (lordosis). In the sagittal plane, the primary curve is convex posteriorly and concave anteriorly, whereas the secondary curves are concave posteriorly and convex anteriorly. The lordotic curvatures progressively develop in the cervical and lumbar spine during normal maturation during the transition to an upright posture (Fig. 4-2). Except for a slight lordotic lumbar curvature evident on magnetic resonance imaging (MRI), the spinal curvature is all kyphotic in a newborn. As an infant begins to explore the environment from a prone position, the cervical lordotic curvature develops as a result of the pull of extensor musculature on the head and neck. The hip flexor muscles pull inferiorly on the anterior pelvis with crawling, tilting the pelvis anteriorly relative to the hips and creating a relative position of lumbar spine lordosis. In the progression to standing and walking, the lumbar lordotic curve further develops, with the line of gravity passing through or near the first or second lumbar vertebrae. The normal curvatures allow the vertebral column to sustain compressive loads because of the sharing of forces between the vertebrae by the stretched connective tissues and muscles on the convex side of the curves.

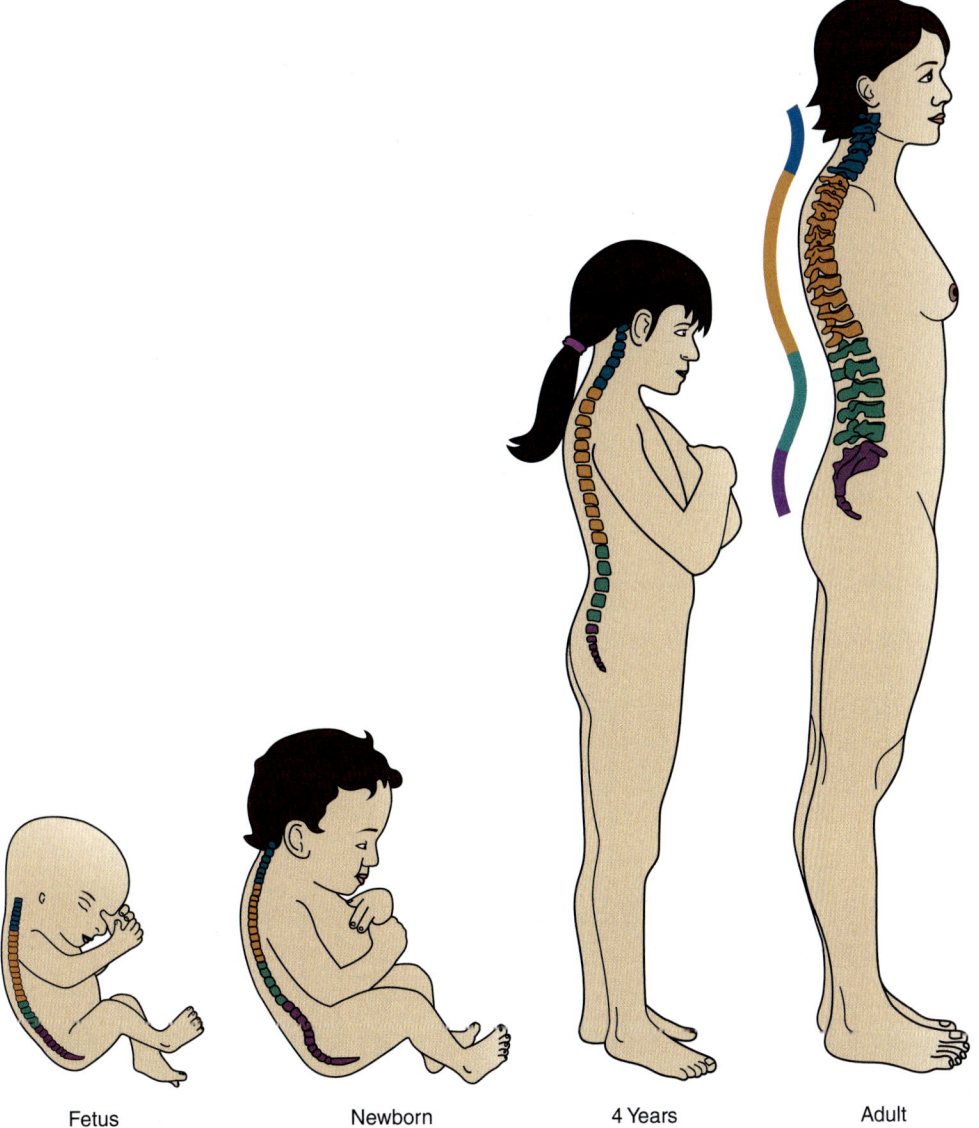

FIGURE 4-2 Curvatures of vertebral column during maturation. (Adapted from Moore KL, Dalley AF, Agur AMR. *Clinically Oriented Anatomy*. 8th ed. Wolters Kluwer; 2018; Figure 2.23.)

Normal Alignment and Curvatures

Normal alignment and common sagittal plane alignment faults are shown in Figure 4-3.

In the adult, the ideal line of gravity passing through the vertebral column in the optimal upright posture varies, but, in general, passes near the mastoid

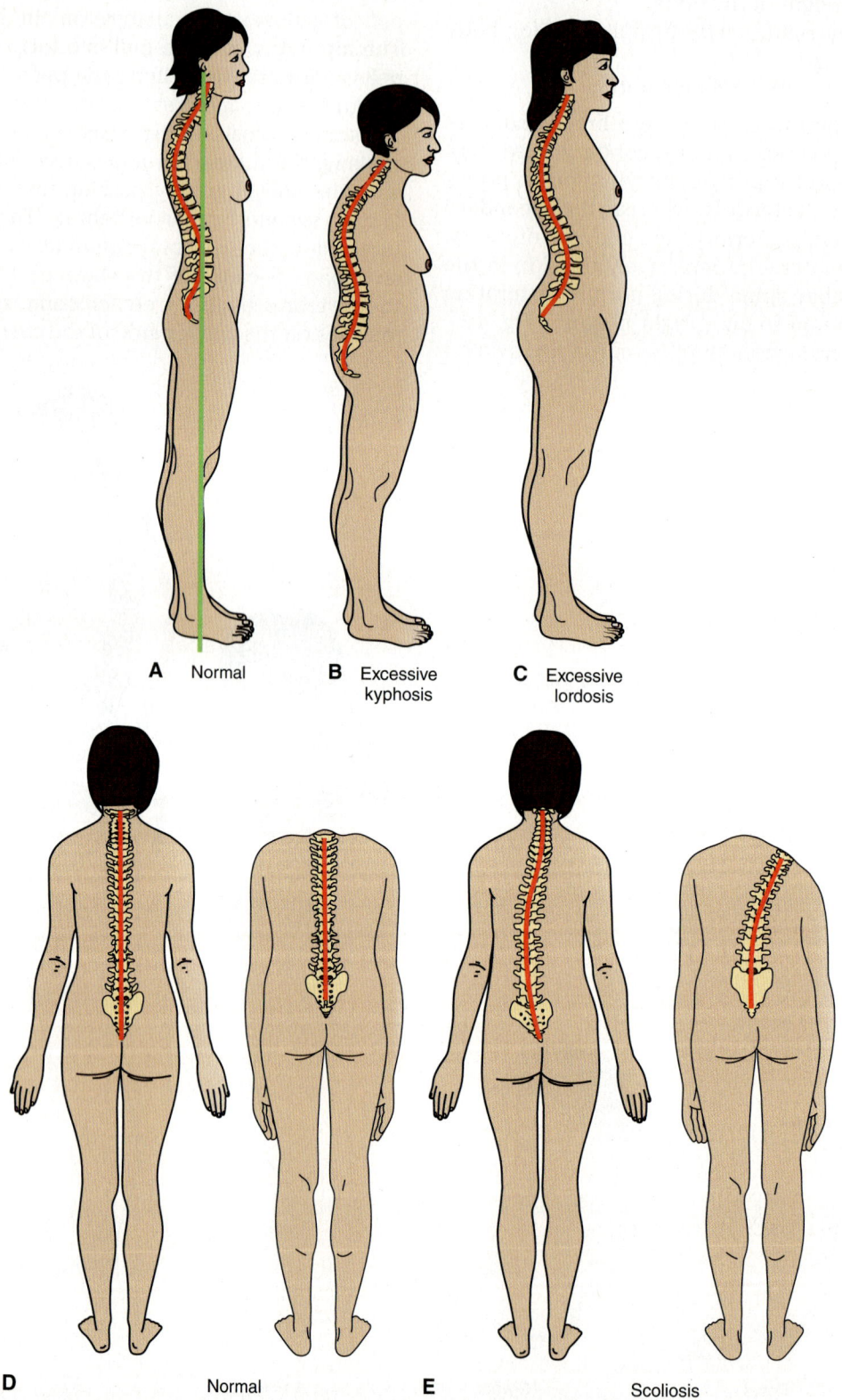

FIGURE 4-3 Alignment of vertebral column. Sagittal plane: normal alignment **(A)**, excessive kyphosis **(B)**, and excessive lordosis **(C)**. Frontal plane: normal alignment **(D)** and scoliosis **(E)**. (Adapted from Moore KL, Dalley AF, Agur AMR. *Clinically Oriented Anatomy*. 8th ed. Wolters Kluwer; 2018; Figure B2-18A-E.)

process of the temporal bone, just anterior to the second sacral vertebra, slightly posterior to the hip joint, and anterior to the knee and ankle joints (Fig. 4-3A). Normal alignment of the vertebrae can be altered by disease, trauma, chronic postural stresses, age, and reduced activity. An abnormal alignment may be an exaggeration of a normal curvature for that region of the spine (e.g., excessive thoracic kyphosis or lumbar lordosis), a lessened or reversal of the expected curvature for the region (e.g., flat or kyphotic lumbar curvature), or a scoliotic curvature.

Scoliosis is an abnormal lateral curvature of the spine, often with an accompanying rotational component, as shown in Figure 4-3E. Though scoliosis can occur in any portion of the spine, the thoracic spine is commonly affected (Fig. 4-4). In most cases, the cause of scoliosis is unknown (idiopathic scoliosis). Scoliosis may also be congenital, neuromuscular, and degenerative. (See Chapter 17, Cervical and Thoracic Spine, for more details.)

In older adults, an exaggerated kyphosis may be due to a compression fracture of the thoracic vertebral body, leading to reduced height (Fig. 4-5). The majority of spinal fractures are compression fractures, also called wedge fractures. The weight of the body above the fracture causes the anterior portion of the vertebral body to be compressed, creating a wedge-shaped appearance. Compression fractures most commonly occur in the midthoracic to mid-lumbar region and are common in younger patients with major trauma and in older patients with minor trauma. Osteoporosis, tumors, or other pathologies change and weaken the bone structure, leading to nontraumatic or low-load fracture. Osteoporotic spine fractures are associated with increased risk of additional fractures,[1-3] mortality, disability, and long-term functional deficits.[3-5] Isolated single-vertebral body fractures in the thoracic spine typically do not cause spinal instability. However, simultaneous fractures of the vertebral body and posterior portions of the vertebra or the sternum are likely to result in clinically relevant instability.[6] Burst fractures (Fig. 4-5B) occur from axial compressive forces and may result in severe vertebral body collapse, with retropulsion into the spinal canal causing spinal cord injury.

A common fracture site in the lumbar vertebrae is at the junction of the pedicle and lamina of the vertebrae, the pars interarticularis. A fractured pars interarticularis is called **spondylolysis**. The normal oblique lumbar radiograph shows a visible outline of a Scottish Terrier dog, called the "Scotty dog," with the neck of the Scotty dog representing the pars interarticularis. When the Scotty dog neck is absent, the condition is called *spondylolysis*. When fractures occur on both sides, one vertebra may translate forward over the neighboring vertebra, creating the **spondylolisthesis**. Figures 4-6A and B shows the normal pars interarticularis with the neck of the Scotty dog visible, and Figure 4-6C shows the forward slippage of the fifth lumbar vertebra on the sacrum, creating a spondylolisthesis. Spondylolysis typically occurs in childhood due to repetitive stress. The vertebrae respond by gradually adding new bone in the stressed area. However,

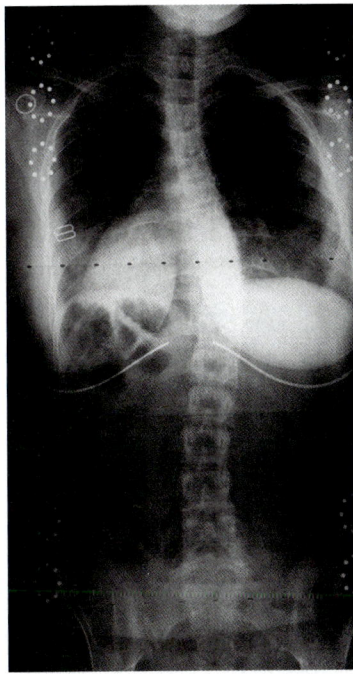

FIGURE 4-4 Radiograph, posterior-to-anterior, showing left thoracic scoliosis. (Weinstein SL, Flynn JM, Crawford HA. *Lovell and Winters's Pediatric Orthopaedics.* 8th ed. Vol 1. Wolters Kluwer; 2021; Figure 16-8.)

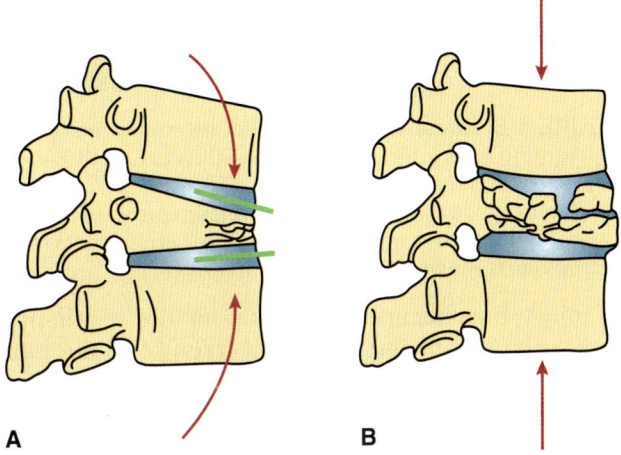

FIGURE 4-5 Sagittal view of compression fracture **(A)** and burst fracture **(B)**. (Adapted from Hickey JV, Strayer AL. *The Clinical Practice of Neurological Neurosurgical Nursing.* 8th ed. Wolters Kluwer; 2020; Figure 15-5.)

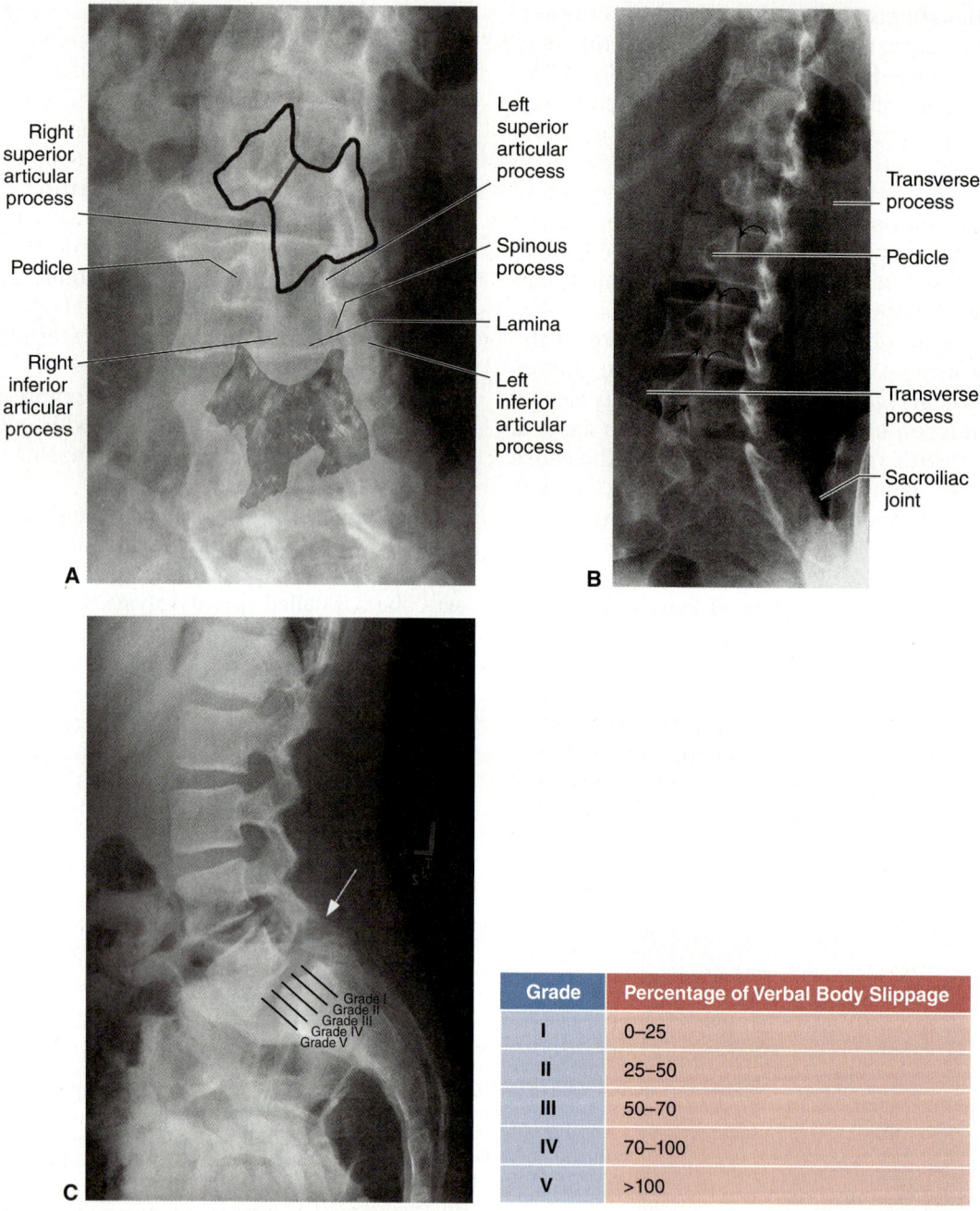

FIGURE 4-6 Lateral and lateral oblique views of vertebral column. **A.** Radiograph with outline of Scottish Terrier highlighting pars interarticularis. (Smith WL, Farrell TA. *Radiology 101: The Basics and Fundamentals of Imaging.* 4th ed. Lippincott Williams & Wilkins; 2014; Figure 9.10A.) **B.** Radiograph without outline of Scottish Terrier. (Smith WL, Farrell TA. *Radiology 101: The Basics and Fundamentals of Imaging.* 4th ed. Lippincott Williams & Wilkins; 2014; Figure 9.10B.) **C.** Spondylolisthesis, lateral view. Grade 2 anterior spondylolisthesis. (Iyer RS, Chapman T. *Pediatric Imaging: The Essentials.* Wolters Kluwer; 2016; Figure 36.10A.)

an injury that occurs too quickly for the repair process to be completed leads to a fracture of the pars interarticularis. In athletes, spondylolysis is common among gymnasts and American football linemen who repeatedly stress the lumbar spine in extension. The condition may progress to a spondylolisthesis. In contrast, degenerative spondylolisthesis may result from deterioration of the facet joints and disc with aging.

Typical Vertebrae

The vertebrae vary in size and shape throughout the spine. Table 4-1 details regional features of vertebrae. Regardless of vertebral column region, the general structure of a vertebra is the same and consists of a vertebral body, the vertebral arch, and multiple processes (Fig. 4-7). The anteriorly located vertebral body

TABLE 4-1
COMPARISONS OF VERTEBRAE BY REGION

Region	Part	Distinguishing Features	Movement Characteristics
Cervical	Vertebral body	Wider side to side than anteroposterior. Commonly form uncovertebral joints on lateral sides of C3 or C4–C6 or C7	Greater overall range of motion than other regions Within region: • Most flexion/extension occurs between occiput and C1 • Most rotation occurs between C1 and C2 • Relatively flat and horizontal orientation of facet joint allows greater movement than in other regions
	Vertebral foramen	Large and triangular	
	Transverse processes	Foramina transversaria C1–C7—passage of vertebral arteries, venous and sympathetic plexuses (C1–C6) and small vertebral veins (C7). Anterior and posterior tubercles	
	Articular processes	Superior facets directed superoposteriorly; inferior facets directed inferoanteriorly	
	Spinous processes	Short (C3–C5); bifid (C3–C6); long (C6 and C7)	
Thoracic	Vertebral body	Heart shaped; 1–2 costal facets for articulation with rib	Limited movement due to attachment of ribs
	Vertebral foramen	Circular and smaller than cervical or lumbar region	
	Transverse processes	Long and strong; length decreases T1–T12; T1–T10 have facets for articulation with tubercle of rib	
	Articular processes	Nearly vertical articular facets; superior facets oriented posterior and slightly lateral; inferior facets oriented slightly anterior and medial; planes of facets lie in an arc centered around the vertebral body	
	Spinous processes	Long with a posteroinferior slope	
Lumbar	Vertebral body	Large; kidney shaped on superior view	Sagittal orientation and shape of facet joints allow flexion and extension and limit rotation and lateral flexion
	Vertebral foramen	Triangular; smaller than in cervical region and larger than in thoracic region	
	Transverse processes	Long; accessory process on posterior surface of base of each process	
	Articular processes	Nearly vertical facets; superior facets face posteromedial; inferior facets face anterolateral	
	Spinous processes	Short and stout with posterior alignment with vertebral body	

Adapted from Moore KL, Dalley AF, Agur AMR. *Clinically Oriented Anatomy.* 8th ed. Wolters Kluwer; 2018; Tables 2.1, 2.2, and 2.3.

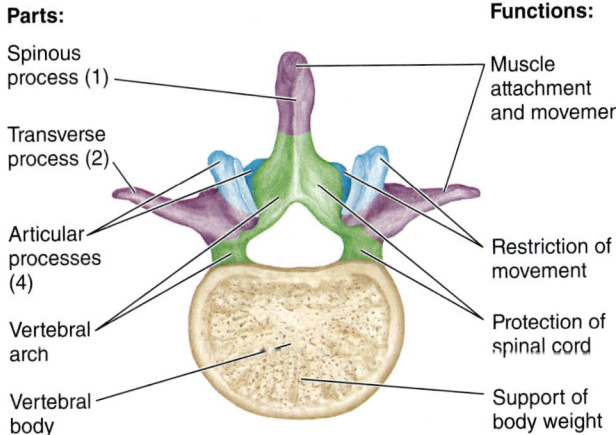

FIGURE 4-7 Major components of a typical vertebra, with function of each part identified. (Gest TR. *Lippincott Atlas of Anatomy.* 2nd ed. Wolters Kluwer; 2020; Plate 1-06D.)

is generally thicker than other parts of the vertebra and supports weight. The vertebral arch is composed of the pedicles and laminae that, together with the vertebral body, form the vertebral foramen (canal) that houses and protects the spinal cord, spinal nerve roots and the surrounding membranes, fat, and blood vessels. Bony processes that arise from the vertebral arch are as follows:

- One spinous process
- Two transverse processes
- Two superior articular processes
- Two inferior articular processes

Figure 4-8 shows a typical vertebra in each moveable spinal region. The transverse and spinous processes provide attachment sites for deep muscles. The superior and inferior articular processes restrict

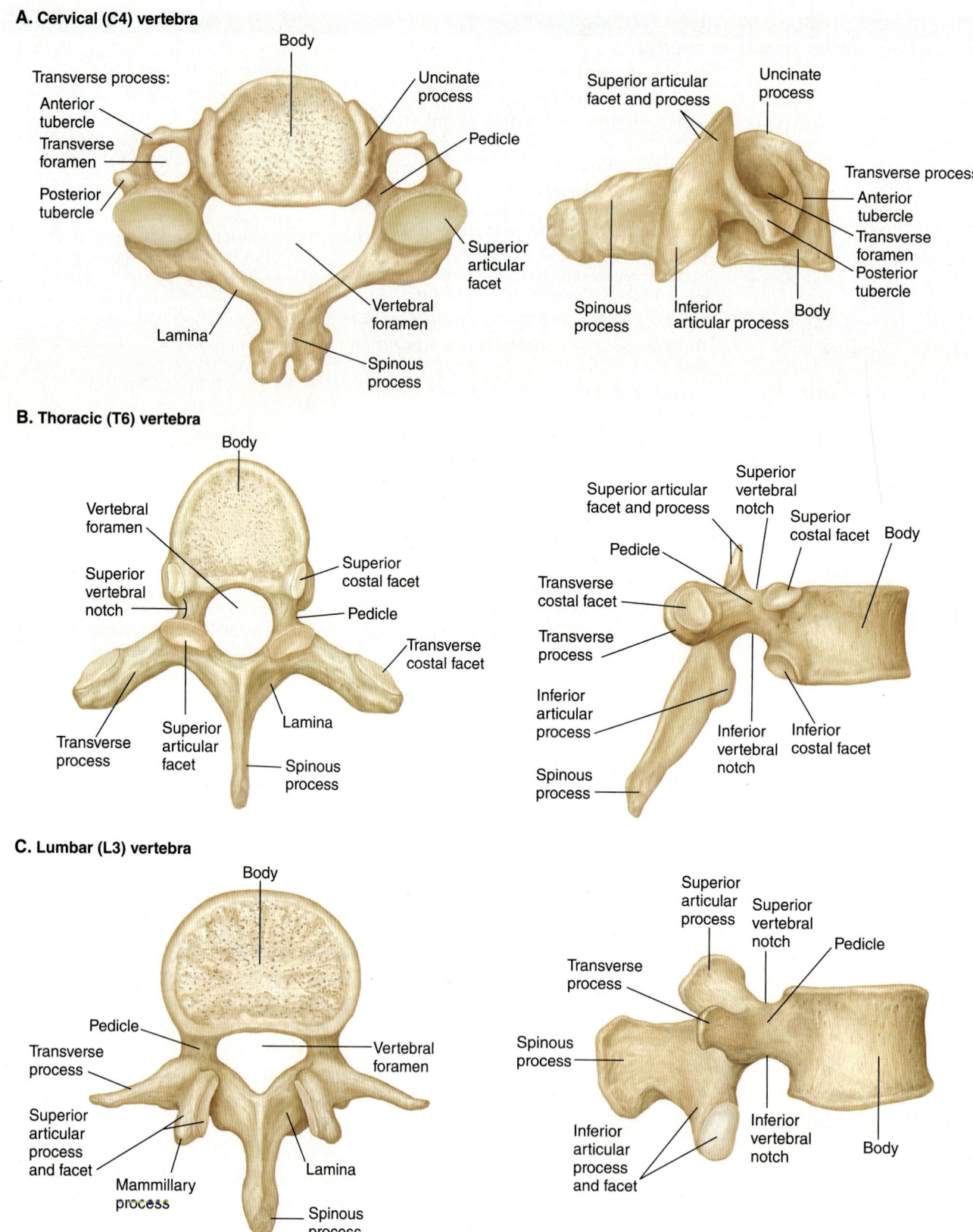

FIGURE 4-8 Typical vertebrae in vertebral column with superior view on left and lateral view on right. **A.** Cervical. **B.** Thoracic. **C.** Lumbar. (Gest TR. *Lippincott Atlas of Anatomy*. 2nd ed. Wolters Kluwer; 2020; Plates 1-04 and 1-06.)

movement. The inferior and superior pedicles of adjacent vertebrae form the IV foramen for passage of a spinal nerve and spinal (posterior root) ganglion (Fig. 4-9). The inferior and superior articular surfaces of adjacent vertebrae form the facet (zygapophyseal) joint. The superior and inferior surfaces of the vertebral body are covered with hyaline cartilage that forms vertebral end plates. Except for the epiphyseal rim (at the periphery), the bone of the vertebral body is spongy. At the epiphyseal rim, the bone smooth. This region, a secondary ossification center, provides protection to the vertebral bodies and allows diffusion of fluid between the IVD and the capillaries in the vertebral body.

INTERVERTEBRAL DISC

The IVDs between adjacent vertebral bodies consist of an outer annulus fibrosis and inner nucleus pulposus.[7] There is no disc between the C1 and C2 vertebrae. There is a disc between each of the cervical, thoracic, and lumbar vertebrae and a disc between the fifth lumbar and first sacral vertebra. Disc thickness and shape varies in each region, with the greatest thickness in the cervical and lumbar areas, the most uniform thickness in the thoracic region, and a greater thickness anteriorly than posteriorly in the cervical and lumbar regions. This variation in thickness helps produce the secondary curves of the vertebral column.

Intervertebral Disc Biomechanics

The biomechanical interaction between the annulus fibrosis and the nucleus pulposus allows for shock absorption to protect the vertebral bone from potential damage with loading from body weight, muscular activation, and lifting.[8] The annulus fibrosis is composed of multiple concentric layers of fibrocartilage that insert/attach into the annular epiphysis. The fibers in each layer are oblique in orientation, aligned approximately 65° from vertical.[9] The fibers within each adjacent layer cross obliquely in opposite directions (Fig. 4-10).[10] The fiber orientation provides significant resistance against vertical distraction, shear, and torsion stress. The annulus fibrosus is more vascularized and innervated in the peripheral portion. Overall, fibers of the annulus are thicker and more numerous anteriorly and laterally than posteriorly.

The IVD deforms in response to imparted forces, becoming broader with compression and thinner with tensile stresses (Fig. 4-11). In healthy discs, the cells in the IVD produce the proteoglycans that bind and release water, thereby generating an intradiscal osmotic pressure that maintains the biomechanical function.[11] The deformation is nonlinear and time dependent,[12] demonstrating viscoelastic properties.[13-15] The predominant load on the IVD is compression, as occurs during standing.[16]

The stresses sustained by and within the discs vary with vertebral column flexion, extension, lateral flexion, and rotation, with the nucleus serving as a semifluid fulcrum. The water content of the nucleus pulposus is high at birth and decreases with aging. The gel-like composition contributes to the flexibility and resilience of the IVD and vertebral column. Degenerated IVDs have reduced capacity to bind water owing to a reduced proteoglycan content and, therefore, are less able to resist fluid flow of the nucleus pulposus when subjected to loading.[11] The annular fibers become disorganized[17] with an altered response to compressive loads.[18-20]

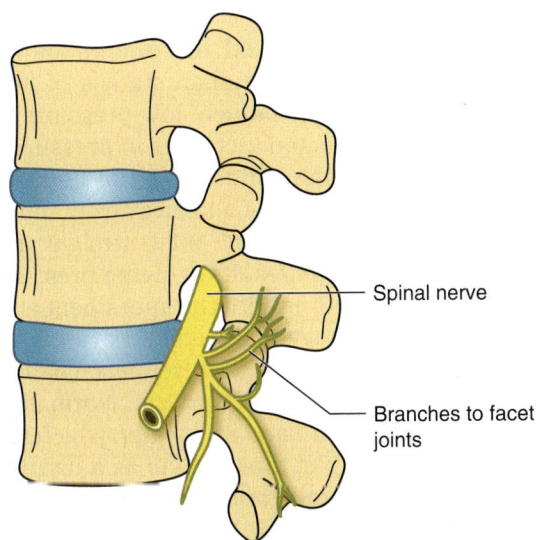

FIGURE 4-9 Spinal nerve passes through IV foramen formed by superior and inferior pedicles of adjacent vertebrae. Branches of the posterior ramus supply muscles, facet joints, and skin.

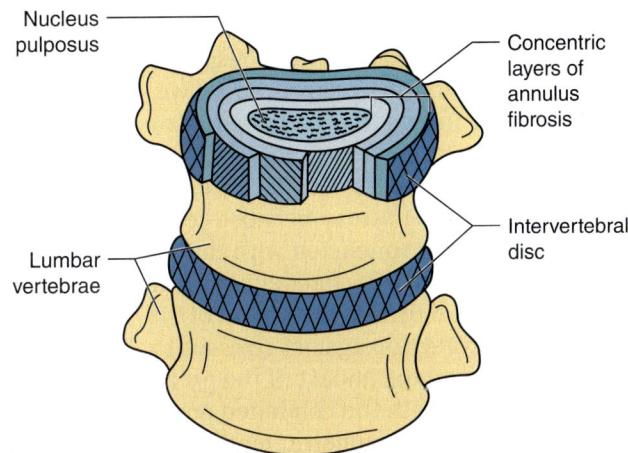

FIGURE 4-10 Intervertebral disc. (Adapted from Oatis CA. *Kinesiology: The Mechanics and Pathomechanics of Human Movement.* 3rd ed. Wolters Kluwer; 2017; Figure 34.7.)

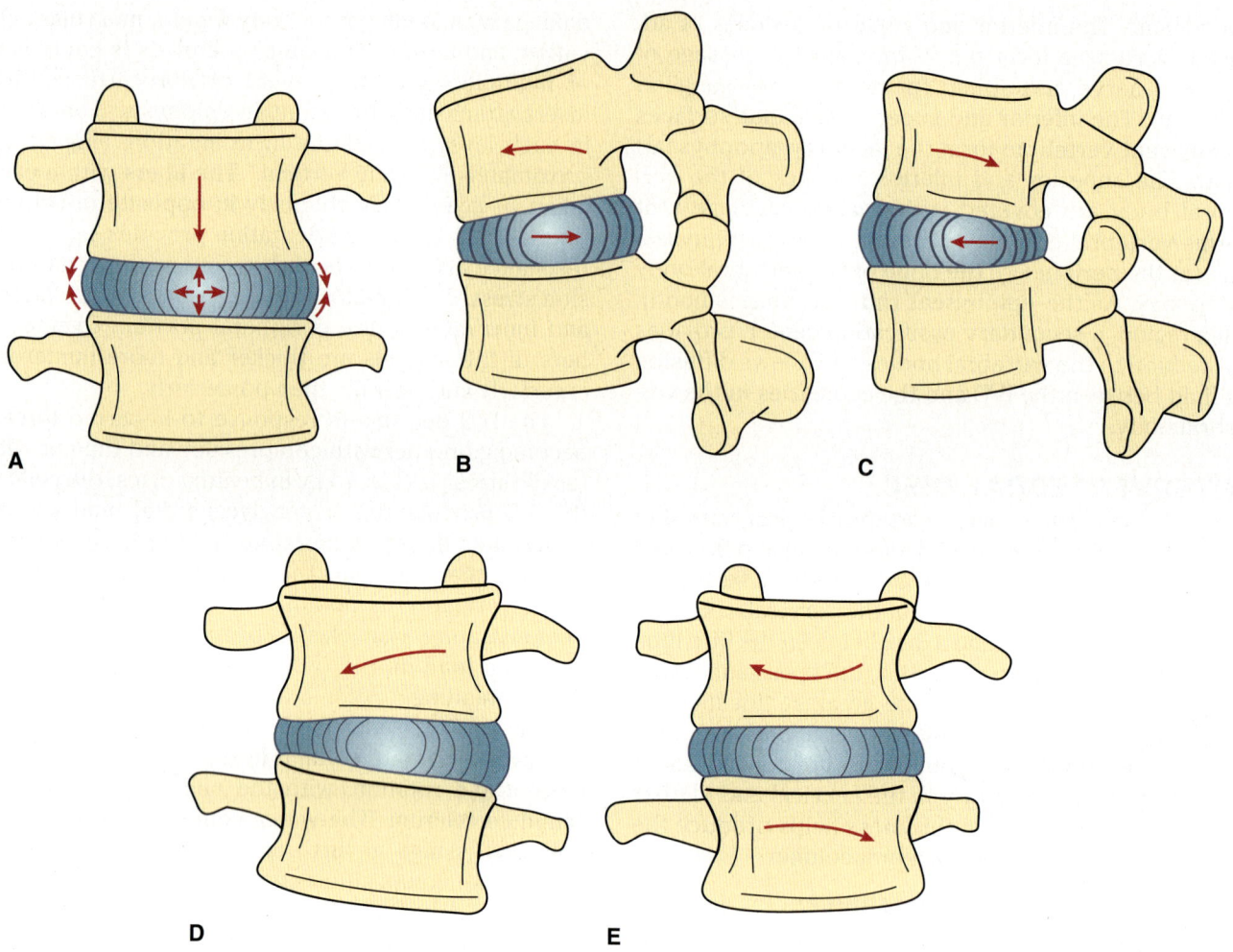

FIGURE 4-11 Disc response to compression and tension with axial compression **(A)**, spine flexion **(B)**, spine extension **(C)**, lateral flexion **(D)**, and axial rotation **(E)**.

The stress on the layers of the annulus fibrosis differs with movements of the adjacent vertebral bodies. For example, with lumbar extension, the posterior annular fibers are compressed, whereas the anterior fibers undergo a tensile stress (Fig. 4-12A). The alternating direction of collagen fibers within adjacent annular layers makes the IVD ideal for tolerating compressive loading. However, this crisscross arrangement of collagen fibers results in less resistance to rotation (torsional) stress because fewer annular fibers are subjected to tension with the rotation in one direction (Fig. 4-12B). Fortunately, in the lumbar spine, rotation is limited by the orientation of the facet joints, leading to a protection against stresses to the annulus fibrosis. However, the impact of the protective mechanism is lessened with the combined movement of flexion with rotation. Asymmetric motions are important risk factors, as more than 60% of low back injuries are associated with trunk twisting.[21]

The pressure sustained by the IVD varies with the body position. Pioneering studies by Nachemson[22] and others[23-25] have informed the understanding of loading of the IVD. In vivo human studies of lumbar IVD pressure indicate a relatively low pressure in the resting supine position and increases in pressure with weight bearing and combinations of flexion, especially when a load is held in front of and away from the body (Fig. 4-13). Lifting a load with the knees straight and sitting in a slumped posture results in higher pressures in the lumbar IVD than lifting with the knees bent and sitting erect.[22,26] The change in intradiscal pressure with positional changes suggests that frequent changes in position may help with disc nutrition. Normally, the disc contains between 70 and 88% water, which makes it nearly incompressible; thus, it acts as a distributor of force at the vertebral level. A reduction in hydration and elasticity in the IVD leads to a loss in ability to store energy, distribute stresses, and resist loads.[27]

Intervertebral Disc Nutrition

The nucleus pulposus is not vascularized and has limited healing capacity. The IVD receives nutrition

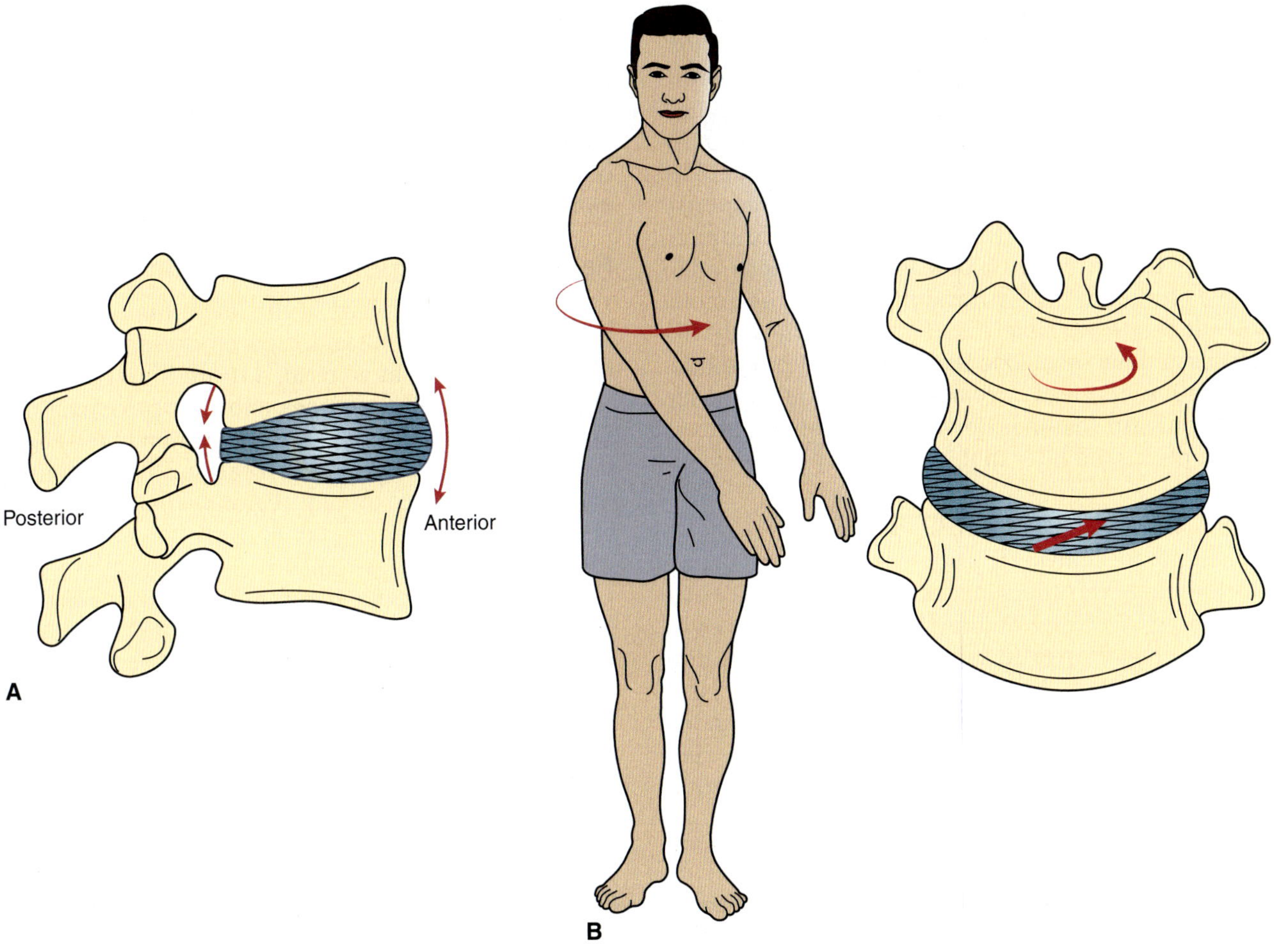

FIGURE 4-12 Stress to annular fibers of intervertebral disc with extension **(A)** and axial rotation **(B)**. (Adapted from Oatis CA. *Kinesiology: The Mechanics and Pathomechanics of Human Movement*. 3rd ed. Wolters Kluwer; 2017; Figures 32.14 and 32.15.)

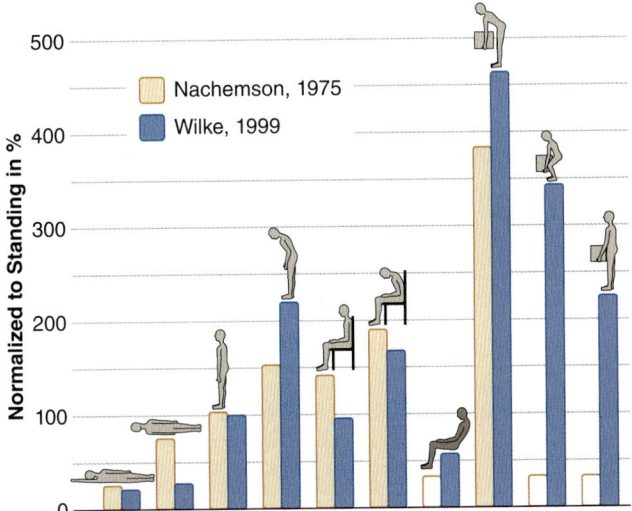

FIGURE 4-13 Pressure in the lumbar intervertebral disc. (Data from Nachemson A. Towards a better understanding of low-back pain: a review of the mechanics of the lumbar disc. *Rheumatol Rehabil*. 1975;14(3):129-143 and Wilke H, Neef P, Caimi M, Hoogland T, Claes L. New in vivo measurements of pressures in the intervertebral disc in daily life. *Spine*. 1999;24(8):755-762.)

by diffusion from blood vessels in the peripheral annulus fibrosis and the adjacent vertebral bodies.[28] Movement assists with nutrition of the IVD. The cells within the IVD must have nutrients to manufacture building blocks for proteoglycans that contribute to hydration and regulate collagen fibrillogenesis.[29] The loss of nutrient supply can occur with biomechanical changes affecting hydration, decreased oxygen due to atherosclerosis or blood disorders,[30] exposure to vibration,[31,32] or smoking.[33]

Intervertebral Disc Pathology The IVD is a common site of spinal pathology due to the varied loads sustained with positional changes, the viscoelastic properties, and variable disc hydration with time of day and loading. The position of the nucleus pulposus within the annulus fibrosis as a result of movement and sustained postures confirmed in studies using MRI technology. For example, in the lumbar spine, the nucleus pulposus tends to migrate posteriorly with flexion and anteriorly with extension,[34-38] with the extent of migration correlated with the degree of the flexion-extension angle.[34] Studies of the cervical spine indicate an overall posterior migration of the nucleus pulposus with cervical spine extension, with the degree of posterior migration varying among individuals.[39,40] These findings are challenged by Nazari and colleagues[41] who report that rather than migrate, the nucleus pulposus deforms by lengthening under various loads. The hydrostatic properties of the disc influence response to loading. The observation that the nucleus pulposus moves toward the side of least load is reported in multiple studies.[34,35,37,38,42] Possibly, differences among studies indicate variable responses both between individuals and between disc levels, along with potential degenerative changes within the disc that influence the response to loading. Herniated nucleus pulposus (HNP) is discussed later in this chapter.

FACET JOINTS AND MOVEMENT

The facet (zygapophyseal) joints are formed by the articulations between the superior and inferior articular processes of adjacent vertebrae, forming plane synovial joints. The superior articulating facet is directed dorsally to some degree, and the inferior articulating facet is directed anteriorly. The facet joints are surrounded by a thin, loose joint capsule that attaches to the margins of the articulating vertebrae. The facet joints permit gliding between the articular surfaces. Facet joints and IVD together are part of the three-part spinal motion segment. These components of the spinal motion segment allow for mobility while preventing potentially injurious movements.[43] Figure 4-14 illustrates the relative amount of movement of the cervical, thoracic, and lumbar regions in the sagittal, frontal, and horizontal planes.

Facet Joint Regional Orientation

The orientation of plane of the facet joint surfaces determines the amount and type of motion available at the IV segment.[44] In general, a more horizontal orientation of facet joint surfaces allows greater axial rotation, whereas a more vertical orientation in the sagittal or frontal plane limits axial rotation.[9] Facet joint orientation is distinct among regions when pooled data of vertebral movement at multiple levels examined within a region (Fig. 4-15).[45]

In the lower cervical spine, the superior articular processes are oriented approximately 45° to the transverse plane and, on average, 0° to the frontal plane.[6] The orientation of the facets transition from a slightly posteromedial to somewhat posterolateral orientation from C3–C7. The midthoracic superior articular processes are more vertical, oriented approximately 60°

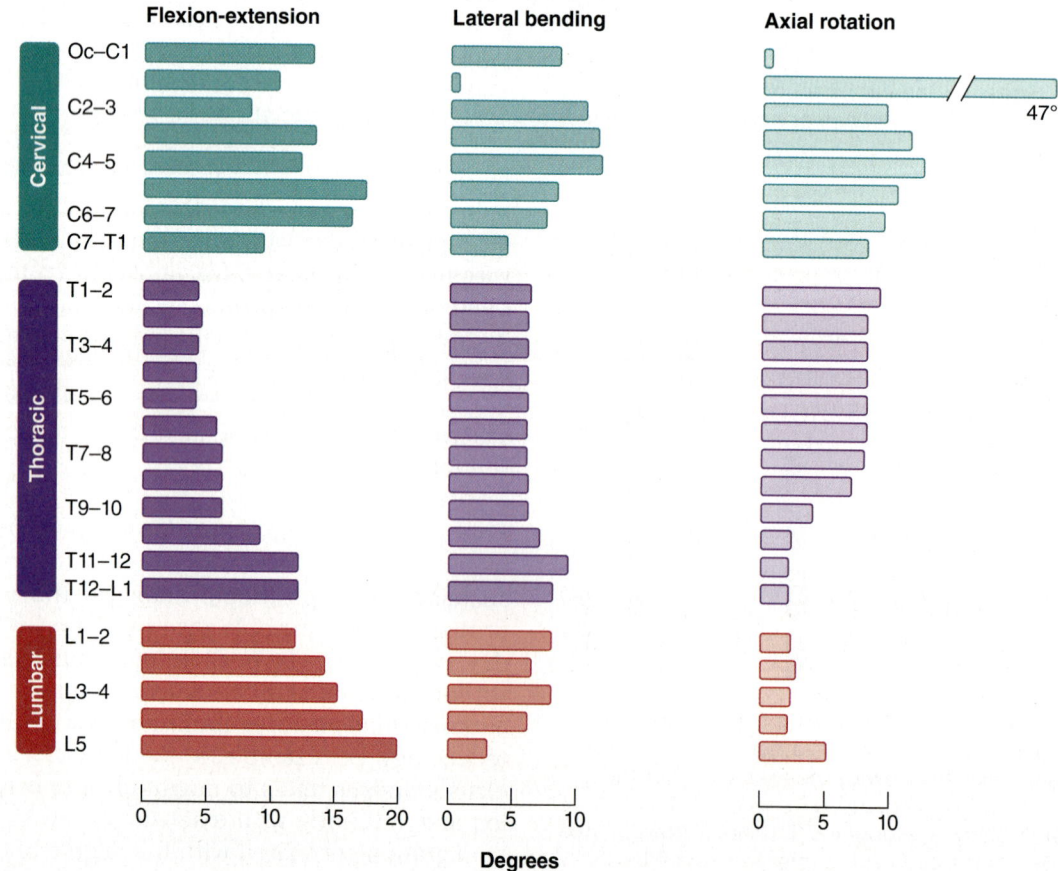

FIGURE 4-14 Summary of overall maximal range of motion allowed across three planes.

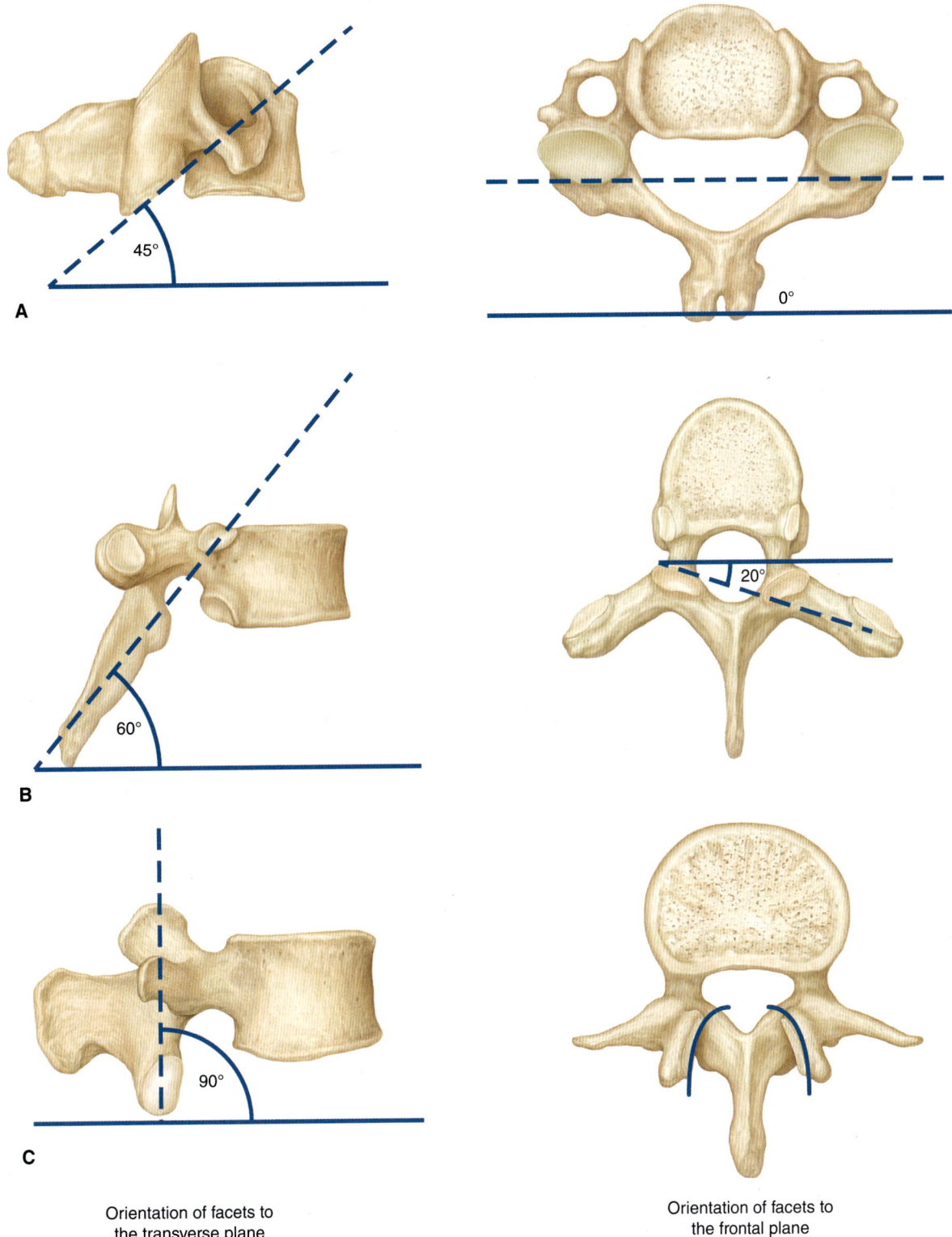

Orientation of facets to
the transverse plane

Orientation of facets to
the frontal plane

FIGURE 4-15 Facet joint orientation in sagittal (*left*) and frontal (*right*) view. **(A)** Mid-cervical vertebra. **(B)** Mid-thoracic vertebra. **(C)** Mid-lumbar vertebra. (Gest TR. *Lippincott Atlas of Anatomy*. 2nd ed. Wolters Kluwer; 2020; Plates 1-04 and 1-06.)

to the transverse plane and a 20° angle to the frontal plane. The lumbar superior articular processes are a curved posteromedial shape, oriented 90° to the horizontal plane.[6] The frontal plane orientation is such that the anterior portion faces primarily medially and the posterior aspect faces anteriorly. Moving from superior to inferior in the vertebral column, the facet joint orientation transitions suddenly, or gradually over two to three segments, to orient in the manner of the adjacent region.[44-46]

Facet Joint and Intervertebral Disc Height

The size of the IVD relative to the associated vertebral body influences the amount of movement permitted at the facet joints. The smallest disc-to-vertebral height ratio is in the thoracic region. The relatively thin IVDs limit the amount of sagittal and frontal plane motion before bony compression, a factor contributing to stability of the thoracic spine.

Facet Joint Innervation

The facet joints are innervated by articular branches from the medial branches of the spinal nerve dorsal rami (see Fig. 4-9). Each articular branch supplies two adjacent joints.

Close- and Open-Packed Position

In the spine, the position that increases the contact area of the articulating surfaces and tension in the surrounding capsular ligaments (close-packed position) is the anatomic or slightly extended position. Some of the capsular ligamentous fibers are taut with movement beyond the anatomic or slightly extended position. At C1–C2, the close-packed position is flexion. The open-packed position is moderate flexion of most of the facet joints.[9] With extension of the vertebral column, the load on the facet joints is greater than with flexion.

The close-packed position may be lost following a pathologic process, trauma, or prolonged immobilization. Inability to assume the close-packed position may lead to increased dysfunction and, as a result, a more unstable open-packed position is maintained. The open-packed versus closed-packed position must be considered during joint mobilization and manipulation. The joint to be moved is most often placed in an open-packed position. The surrounding joints may need to be placed in a close-packed position to allow a focus of mobilization or manipulative force to the target joint.

SPINAL CORD SEGMENT AND SPINAL NERVE

The spinal cord segment is the portion of the spinal cord that bears the rootlets and roots to form one bilateral pair of spinal nerves. There are 31 pairs of spinal nerves: 8 cervical, 12 thoracic, 5 lumbar, 5 sacral, and 1 coccygeal. Each spinal nerve is a mixed peripheral nerve formed by the union of the anterior (ventral) and posterior (dorsal) roots of a specific spinal cord segment (Fig. 4-16). The name of the spinal cord segment is the same as the spinal nerves arising from it. For example, the C8 spinal cord segment forms the C8 spinal nerve. The C8 spinal nerve exits the vertebral canal through the IV foramen formed by the C7 and T1 vertebrae. (See Table 4-2 and Fig. 4-17 for the level of nerve exit from the vertebral column of each of the spinal nerves.)

Just after formation and exit from the IV foramen, the spinal nerve divides into an anterior (ventral) ramus and posterior (dorsal) ramus. Some of the anterior rami join together to form a plexus (web of nerves) to supply a body region. The anterior rami of C5–T1 form the brachial plexus roots that form nerves to innervate the upper limb. The anterior rami of L1–L4, with contributions from T12, form the lumbar plexus to supply portions of the lower extremity. The sacral plexus is composed of anterior rami of spinal nerves S1–S4. The lumbosacral plexus is formed by the lumbosacral trunk (L4–L5) and sacral plexus. The branches of the lumbosacral plexus supply the posterior thigh, most of the lower leg, the entire foot, and part of the pelvis. The plexuses, nerve roots, and peripheral nerves are shown in Chapter 7, The Physical Examination, in Tables 7-10 and 7-11. The plexus formations are shown in Figure 4-18.

Along with the facet joints, innervation of the vertebral column is provided by the recurrent meningeal branches of the spinal nerves (see Fig. 4-9). These recurrent meningeal branches arise either from the

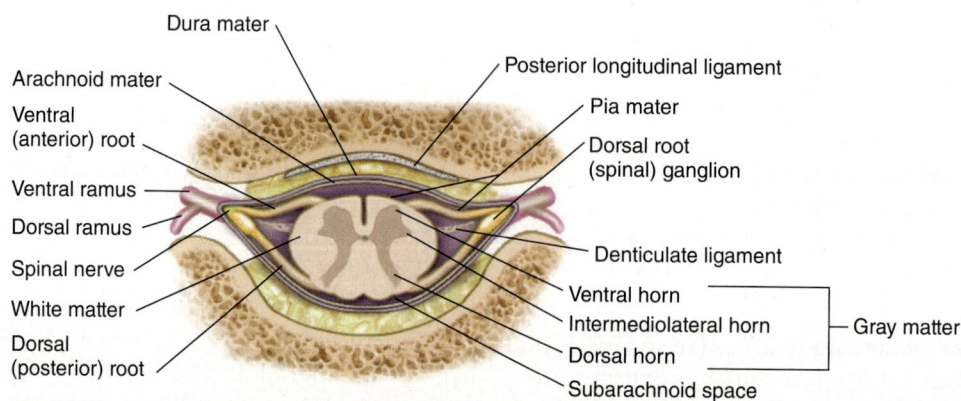

FIGURE 4-16 Formation of a spinal nerve, cross-sectional view. (Gest TR. *Lippincott Atlas of Anatomy*. 2nd ed. Wolters Kluwer; 2020; Plate 1-18.)

CHAPTER 4 | SPINE OSTEOLOGY AND ARTHROLOGY   61

TABLE 4-2		
SPINAL NERVE EXIT FROM VERTEBRAL COLUMN		
Segment Level	Nerves	Level of Nerve Exit from Vertebral Column
Cervical	C1–C8	Nerve C1 passes superior to arch of C1 vertebra Nerves C2–C7 pass through IV foramina superior to corresponding vertebrae Nerve C8 passes through IV foramen between C7 and T1 vertebrae
Thoracic	T1–T12	Nerves T1–L5 pass through IV foramina inferior to the corresponding named vertebra
Lumbar	L1–L5	
Sacral	S1–S5	Nerves S1–S4 branch into anterior and posterior rami within sacrum; anterior rami pass through anterior sacral foramina, posterior rami pass through posterior sacral foramina
Coccygeal[†]	Co1	Nerve S5 and Co1 (if present) pass through sacral hiatus

[†]Coccygeal nerves may be absent.
Adapted from Moore KL, Dalley AF, Agur AMR. *Clinically Oriented Anatomy*. 8th ed. Wolters Kluwer; 2018; Table 2.13.

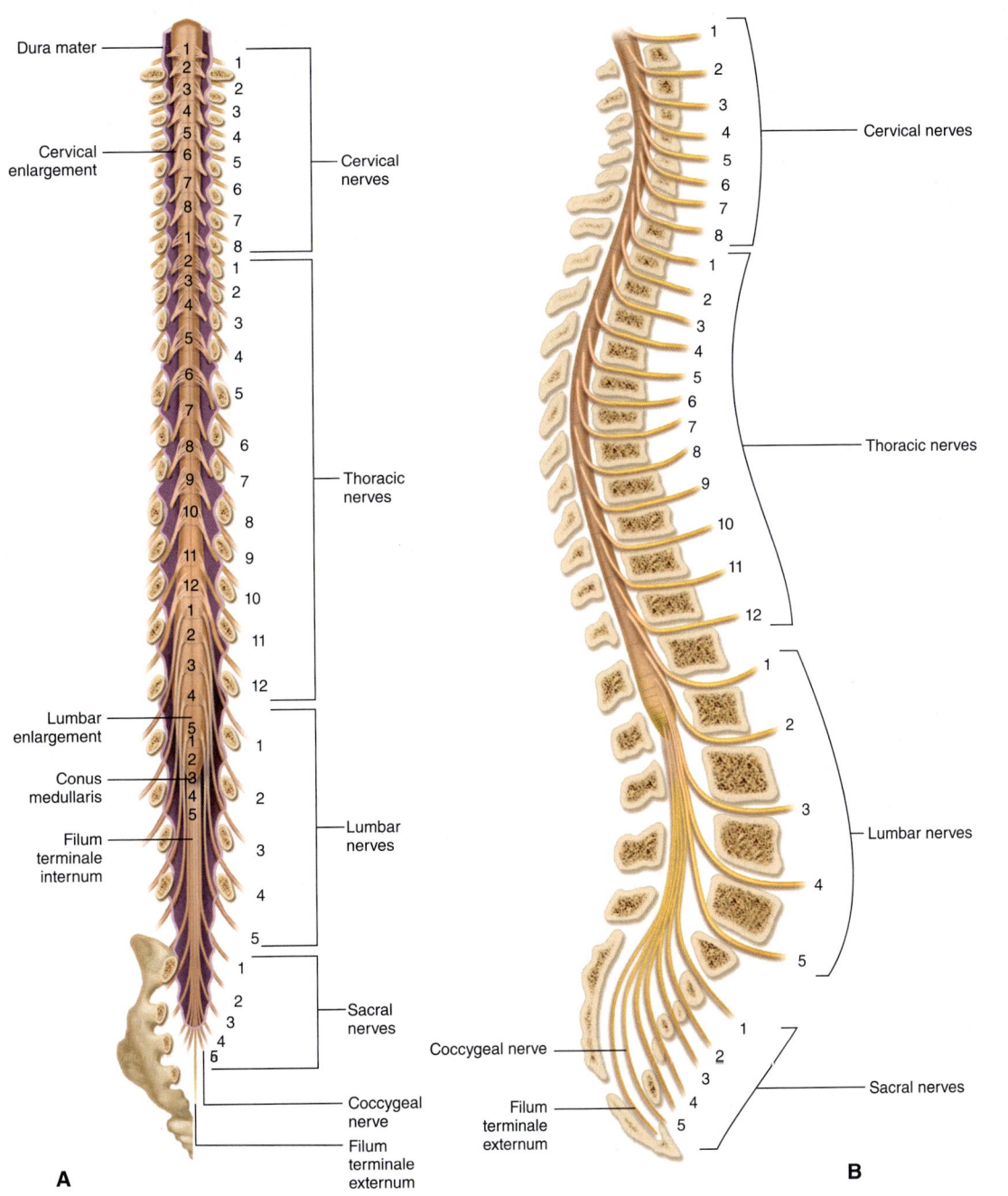

FIGURE 4-17 Vertebral column, spinal cord, spinal ganglia, and spinal nerves. **A.** Lateral view. **B.** Anterior view. (Modified from Pansky B, Gest TR. *Lippincott's Concise Illustrated Anatomy: Back, Upper Limb & Lower Limb*. Vol. 1. Lippincott Williams & Wilkins; 2014: Figure 1.16C&D.)

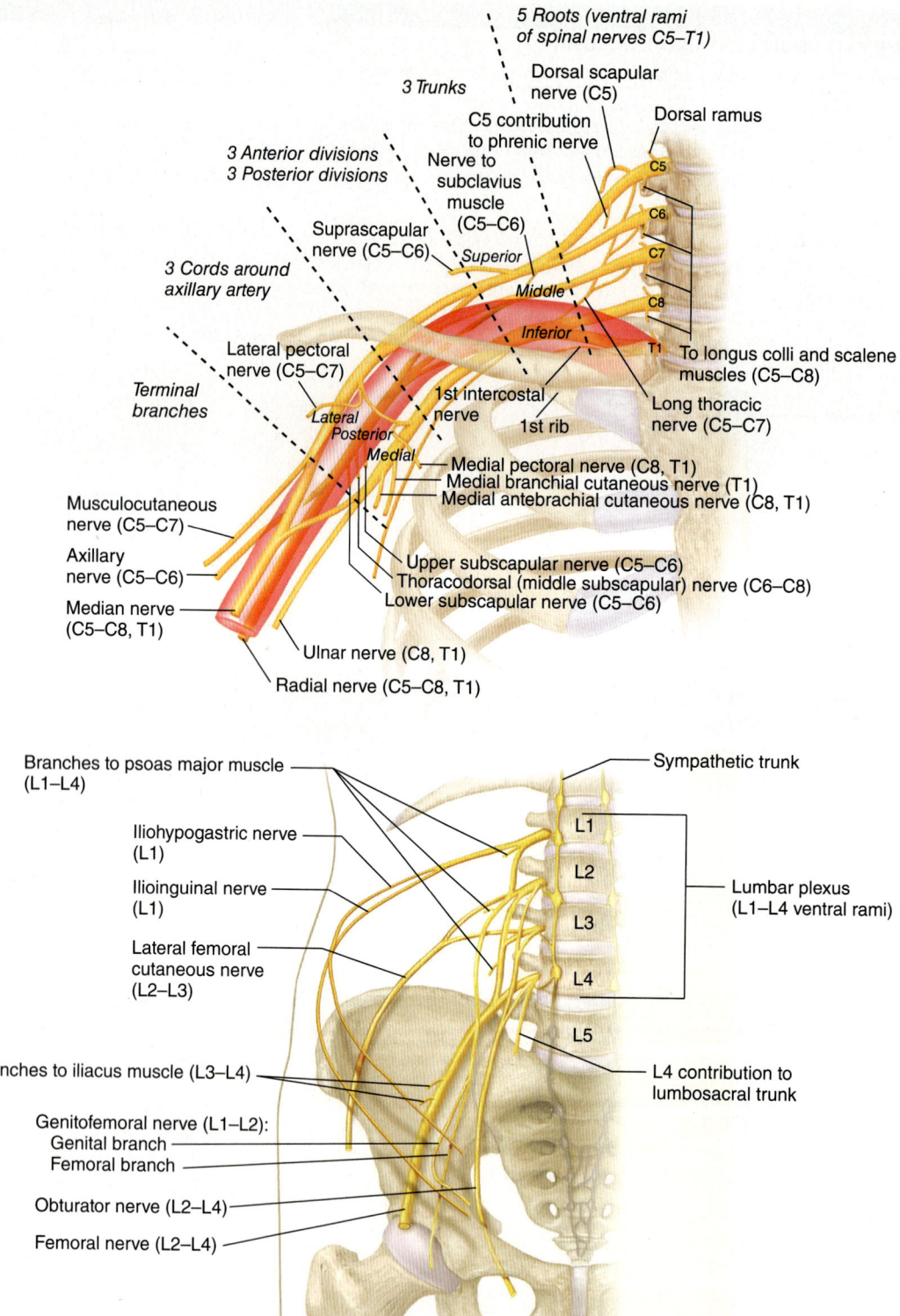

FIGURE 4-18 Plexuses formed by anterior rami of spinal nerves. **A.** Brachial plexus. **B.** Lumbar plexus. **C.** Sacral plexus, anterior view. **D.** Sacral plexus, posterior view. (Gest TR. *Lippincott Atlas of Anatomy*. 2nd ed. Wolters Kluwer; 2020; Plates 2-14, 3-14, and 3-25.)

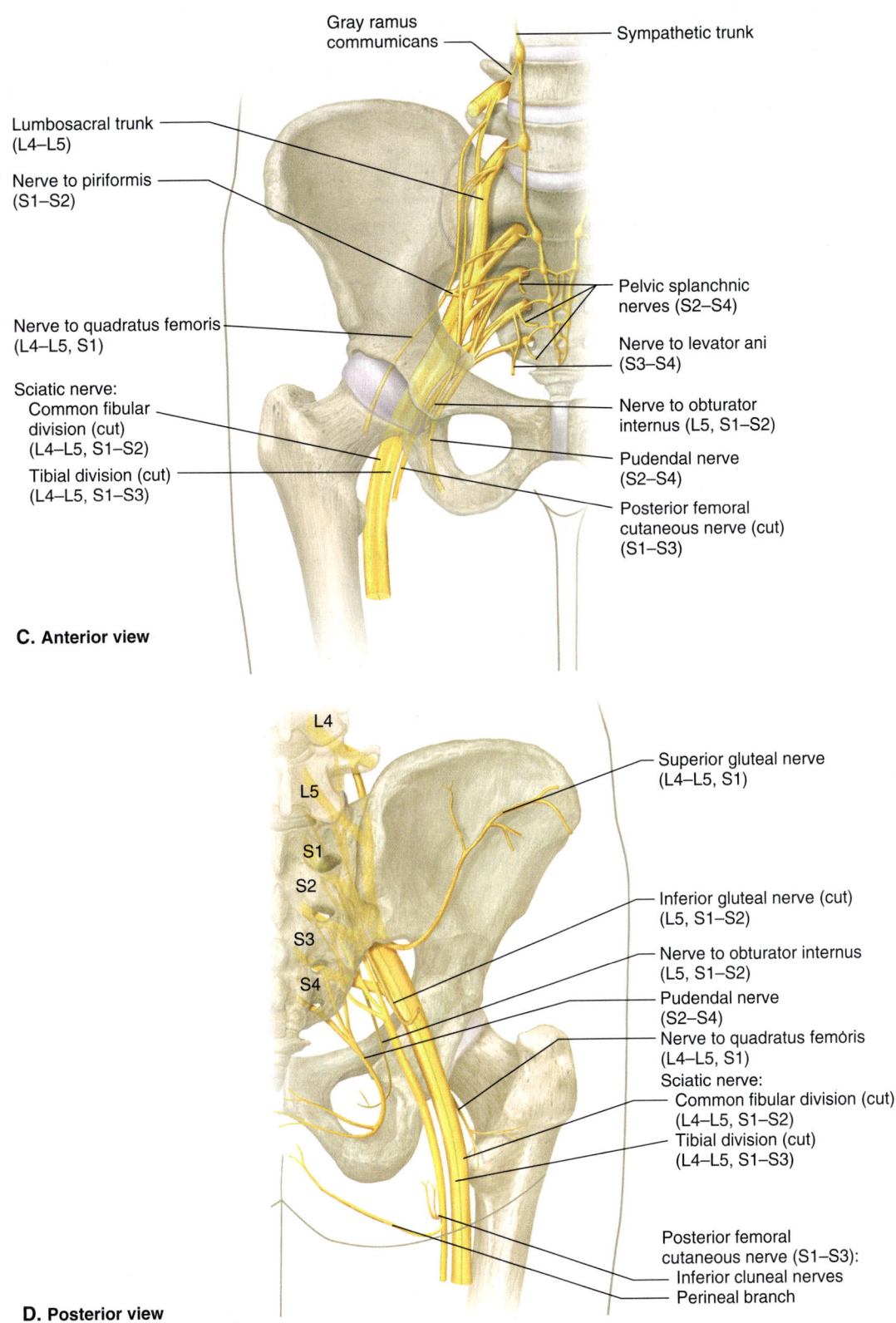

C. Anterior view

D. Posterior view

FIGURE 4-18 (continued)

spinal nerve before the division into anterior and posterior rami or from the anterior ramus immediately after it is formed. As the spinal nerve exits the IV foramen, some of the recurrent meningeal branches remain outside the IV foramen to supply the vertebral bodies, IVDs, and periosteum associated with the anterior longitudinal ligament (ALL). Some of the recurrent meningeal branches reenter the IV foramen to supply the periosteum associated with the posterior vertebral bony structures, the ligamenta flava, annuli fibrosi of the posterior and posterolateral IVDs, posterior longitudinal ligament (PLL), spinal dura mater, and blood vessels in the vertebral canal.

CONTENTS OF VERTEBRAL CANAL

The contents of the vertebral canal include the spinal cord, spinal cord nerve rootlets, spinal meninges, and neurovascular structures that supply these structures. The spinal cord occupies the superior 2/3 of the vertebral canal, beginning as a continuation of the medulla oblongata at the foramen magnum and ending as the conus medullaris. During development, the vertebral column grows faster than the spinal cord; thus, the spinal cord is shorter than the vertebral canal. At birth, the end of the spinal cord lies at approximately the L4–L5 level. As growth continues, the spinal cord further ascends such that by adulthood, the spinal cord terminates at the L2 level in most (Fig. 4-19A), but may be as high as T12 and as low as L4. There is an increasing obliquity and length of the spinal nerve roots such that the most inferior spinal nerve roots are the longest. The loose bundle of spinal nerve roots on the inferior end of the spinal cord resembles a horse's tail and is called the *cauda equina* (Latin, horse tail). From the tip of the conus medullaris, a delicate fibrous connective tissue, the filum terminale, descends along with the spinal nerves. The inferior portion of the filum terminale attaches to the dura mater and the first segment of the coccyx, forming the coccygeal ligament (Fig. 4-19B).

The spinal cord is covered by three membranous meningeal layers: the pia mater, arachnoid mater, and dura mater. The outermost layer, the dura mater, is composed primarily of fibrous tissue and is separated from the periosteum of the vertebral canal by the epidural space that contains a venous plexus and fat. The dura mater forms a long tube-like sheath, called the *spinal dural sac*, within the vertebral canal. The dural sac is continuous with the cranial dura mater superiorly and anchored to the coccyx inferiorly. Each pair of anterior and posterior rootlets extend laterally from the spinal cord and are surrounded by the dura mater as they pass to the IV foramen. The dura mater forms a sleeve, called a *dural root sheath*, around the spinal nerve roots and blends with the epineurium (outermost covering of the spinal nerves), attaching to the periosteum of the IV foramen. The dura mater is supplied by the recurrent meningeal nerves. The arachnoid mater lies against the dura mater, but is not attached to it. The innermost layer of meninges covering the spinal cord is the pia mater. The space between the arachnoid mater and the pia mater is the subarachnoid space. The cerebrospinal fluid (CSF) is contained within the subarachnoid space. The arachnoid trabeculae are thin, delicate threads of connective tissue strands passing between the arachnoid mater and the pia mater. Denticulate ligaments, composed of a fibrous sheet of pia mater, pass longitudinally along each side of the spinal cord. The denticulate ligaments and filum terminale suspend the spinal cord within the dural sac. (See Fig. 4-18 to clarify the relationship of the spinal cord, nerve rootlets, nerve roots, spinal ganglia, spinal nerves, and meninges.)

MOVEMENT OF THE VERTEBRAL COLUMN

The range of motion of the vertebral column varies by region and among individuals. The compressibility and elasticity of the IVDs contribute to mobility as well as limit mobility, if abnormal. Additional limits to mobility of the vertebral column include:

- Orientation and shape of facet joints and associated joint capsules
- Thickness of vertebral body
- Resistance of the surrounding connective tissues
- Attachment to the rib cage

Movements of the vertebral column are flexion, extension, lateral flexion, and rotation. The movements are produced by back muscles, anterior and anterolateral abdominal muscles, and gravity. The motion segment of the vertebral column is defined as two adjacent vertebrae and consists of three joints. One joint is formed between the two vertebral bodies and the intervening IVD. The other two joints are the facet joints formed by the adjacent vertebrae. Except for the C1 and C2 vertebrae that move relatively independent of other IV segments, movements occur at multiple spinal motion segments at once. Although movement at an individual IV segment is small, the cumulative movement at multiple segments produces a large range of motion overall. The attachment of ribs limits movement of the thoracic region. The overall movement is greater in the cervical region than in the lumbar region because of the IVD and vertebral body height ratio, large articular surfaces with nearly horizontal orientation, loose joint capsules, and relatively less surrounding soft tissue. (See Fig. 4-14 for a comparison of available movement throughout the vertebral column.)

LIGAMENTS OF VERTEBRAL COLUMN

The ligaments of the spine provide stability, maintain curvatures, and guide motion. The major ligaments

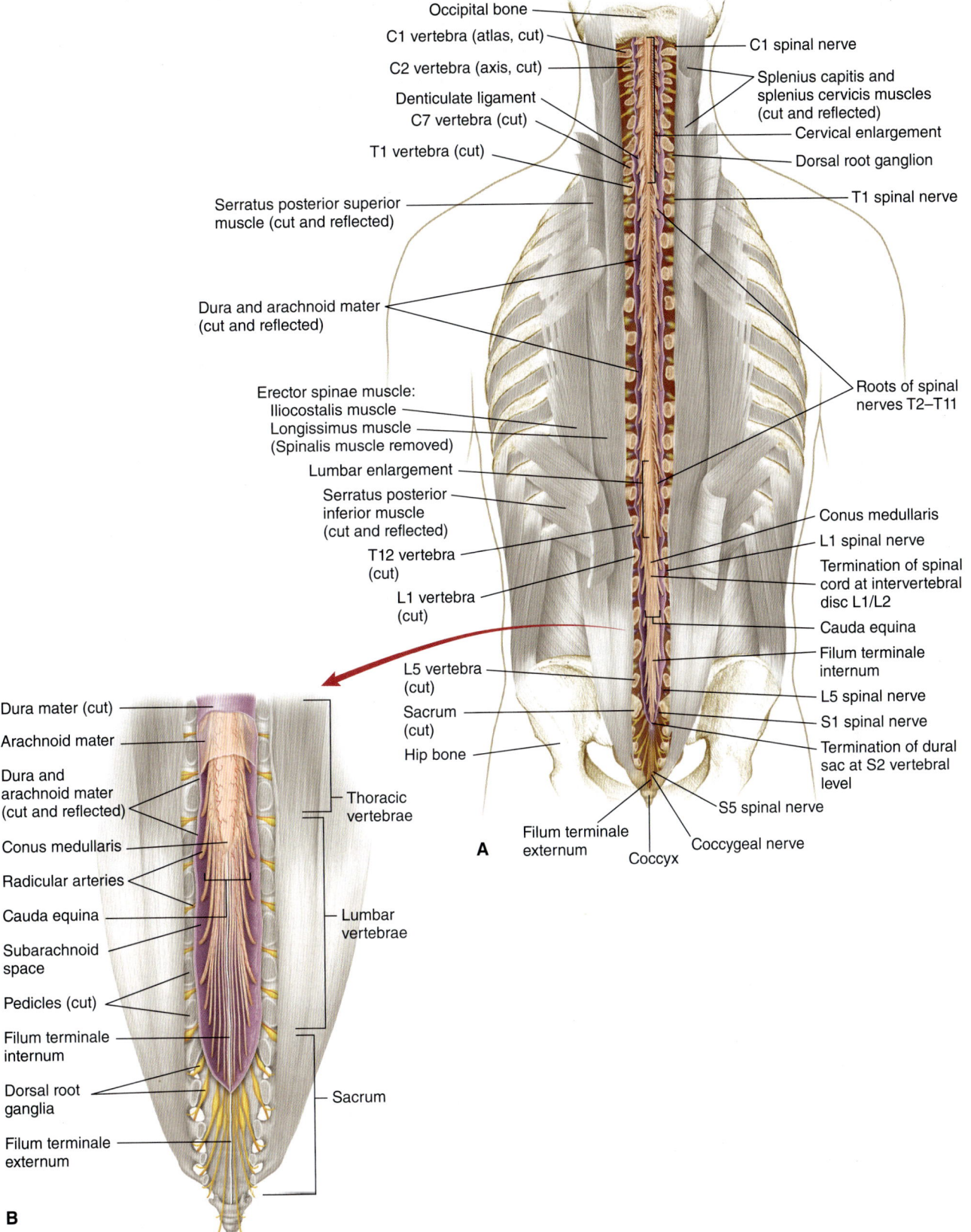

FIGURE 4-19 Spinal cord and vertebral column, posterior view. **A.** Spinal cord descent to termination at approximately L2 vertebra. **B.** Inferior portion of spinal cord and vertebral column showing conus medullaris and filum terminale. (Gest TR. *Lippincott Atlas of Anatomy*. 2nd ed. Wolters Kluwer; 2020; Plates 1-19 and 1-21.)

are summarized in Table 4-3 and depicted in Figure 4-20. The iliolumbar ligament passes between transverse processes of the L4 and L5 vertebrae to the internal lip of the adjacent iliac crest and reinforces the L5–S1 articulation.[47]

The broad ALL runs the length of the vertebral column, with the width increasing during the descent inferiorly. The ALL attaches to the basilar portion of the occipital bone and extends along the anterior vertebral column, blending with the anterior surfaces of the IVDs and ending on the pelvic surface of the sacrum. The ALL is taut in extension and helps limit the natural lordosis of the cervical and lumbar spine.

The narrow PLL runs from C2 to the sacrum within the vertebral canal, attached to the posterior aspect of the vertebral bodies. The fibers of the PLL blend with the IVD outer fibers, providing reinforcement to the IVD, particularly during vertebral column flexion. Unlike the ALL, the PLL narrows during the descent inferiorly and is thus most narrow in the lumbar region where limited support is given to prevent IVD protrusion or herniation.

The ligamentum flavum consists of approximately 80% elastin and 20% collagen. The composition allows the ligament to exert a relatively constant resistance throughout the flexion range of motion of the vertebral column. The ligamentum flavum is thickest in the lumbar region. The ligament exerts a small constant compressive force between the vertebrae.

The intertransverse ligaments pass between the adjacent transverse vertebra. The fibers of the intertransverse ligaments blend with the intertransverse muscles, particularly in the cervical and thoracic spine. In the lumbar region, the intertransverse ligaments are thin.

The interspinous ligaments pass between the adjacent spinous processes, providing resistance to flexion. The deeper fibers contain more elastin and blend with those of the ligamenta flava, whereas the more superficial fibers are more collagen rich and blend with the supraspinous ligaments and nuchal ligament.

The supraspinous ligaments attach along the tips of the spinous processes and, along with the interspinous ligaments, resist flexion by limiting separation of

TABLE 4-3

MAJOR LIGAMENTS OF THE VERTEBRAL COLUMN

Ligament	Attachments	Function	Characteristics
Anterior longitudinal	Extends along anterolateral aspects of bodies and IVDs from pelvic surface of sacrum to anterior tubercle of C1 and occipital bone	Limits hyperextension of column; maintains stability of IV joints	Continues in upper C region as anterior atlanto-occipital and atlantoaxial membrane Strong and broad
Posterior longitudinal	Runs within vertebral canal along posterior aspect of vertebral bodies and IVDs Attached to posterior edges of vertebral bodies from C2 to sacrum	Limits hyperflexion of column and herniation (posterior protrusion of disc)	Continues as tectorial membrane in upper cervical region Narrow and weak Contains many pain receptors; may hypertrophy
Ligamentum flavum	Extends vertically from lamina above to lamina below	Limits separation of vertebral lamina (stops abrupt flexion of vertebral column to minimize injury to IVDs) Strong elastic component helps to preserve normal curves of column and assist with straightening column after flexing	Continues as posterior atlanto-occipital and atlantoaxial membrane in upper cervical region Broad, yellow fibrous tissue with high elastin content
Intertransverse	Extends between adjacent transverse processes	Limits flexion; limits lateral flexion to contralateral side	Cervical region fibers are few; thoracic region fibers and local muscle intertwine; lumbar region fibers are thin and membranous
Interspinous	Extends between adjacent spinous processes	Limits flexion	Continues superiorly as Nuchal ligament (aka ligamentum nuchae) or merges with it
Supraspinous	Extends along apices of spinous process from C7 to sacrum	Limits flexion	Continues superiorly as (merges superiorly with) the nuchal ligament (aka ligamentum nuchae)
Nuchal ligament (aka ligamentum nuchae)	Extends base of skull to C7, extending posteriorly from spinous processes	Limits flexion	Provides muscle attachments to the cervical spinous processes without the necessity of long spinous processes that would impede extension of the neck

C, cervical; IVDs, intervertebral discs.
Adapted from Moore KL, Dalley AF, Agur AMR. *Clinically Oriented Anatomy.* 8th ed. Wolters Kluwer; 2018:97-125.

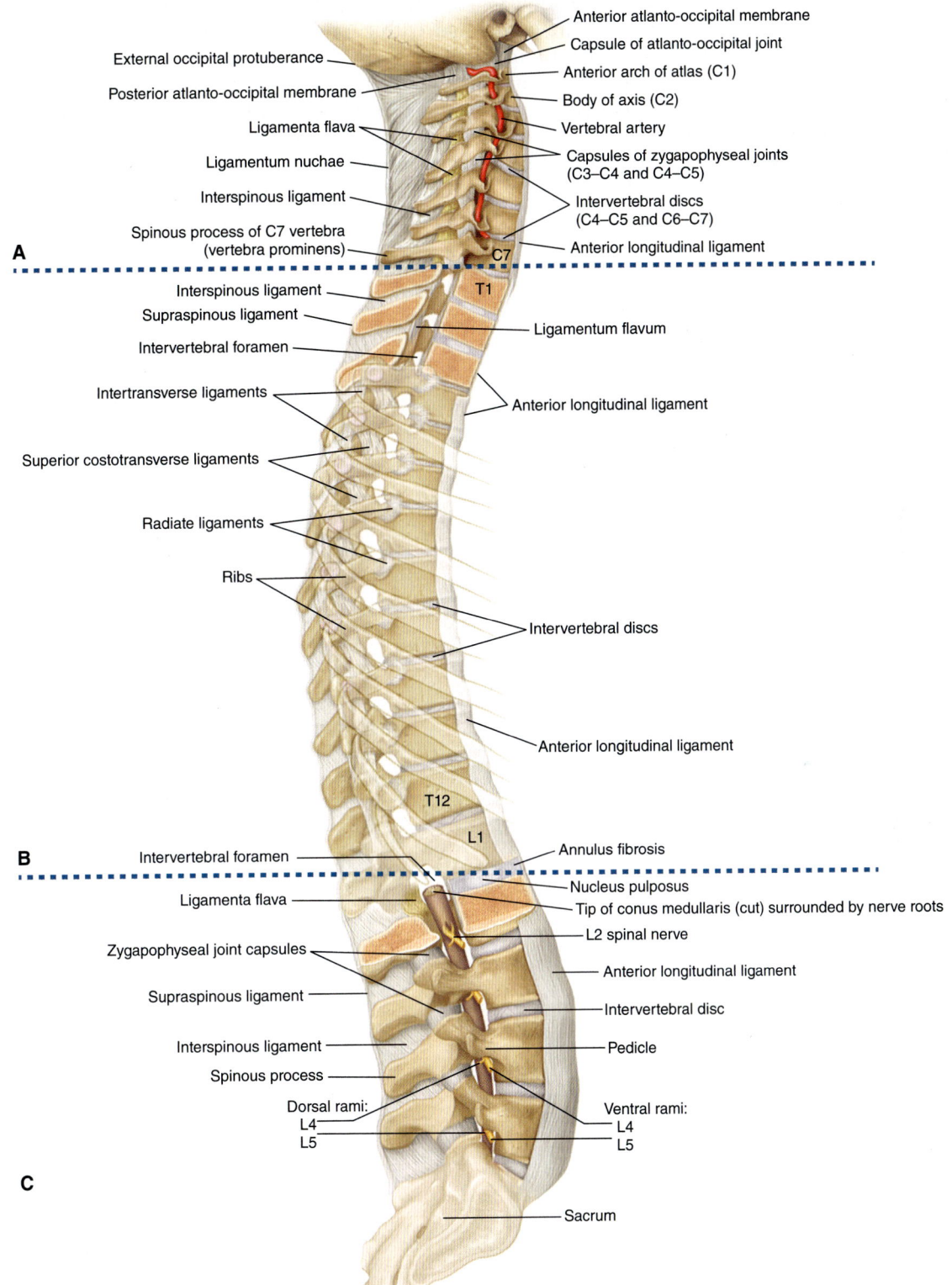

FIGURE 4-20 Major ligaments of the (A) cervical (B) thoracic (C) lumbar regions. (Gest TR. *Lippincott Atlas of Anatomy*. 2nd ed. Wolters Kluwer; 2020; Plates 1-10A, 1-11A, and 1-12A.)

the spinous processes. The supraspinous ligaments are more robust in the cervical region than in the lumbar region. Supraspinous ligament fibers blend with those of the thoracolumbar fascia. The supraspinous ligament is prone to rupture in the lumbar region at the extremes of lumbar flexion.

The nuchal ligament (aka ligamentum nuchae) is a midline ligament extending posteriorly from the tips of the spinous processes of the cervical vertebra. The nuchal ligament runs from the base of the skull to the seventh cervical vertebra.

REGIONAL CHARACTERISTICS FOR VERTEBRAE, LIGAMENTS, AND DISCS

Although portions of the vertebral column share common characteristics, each region has unique features that contribute to the function in that region and to the overall function of the spine. Figure 4-21 highlights

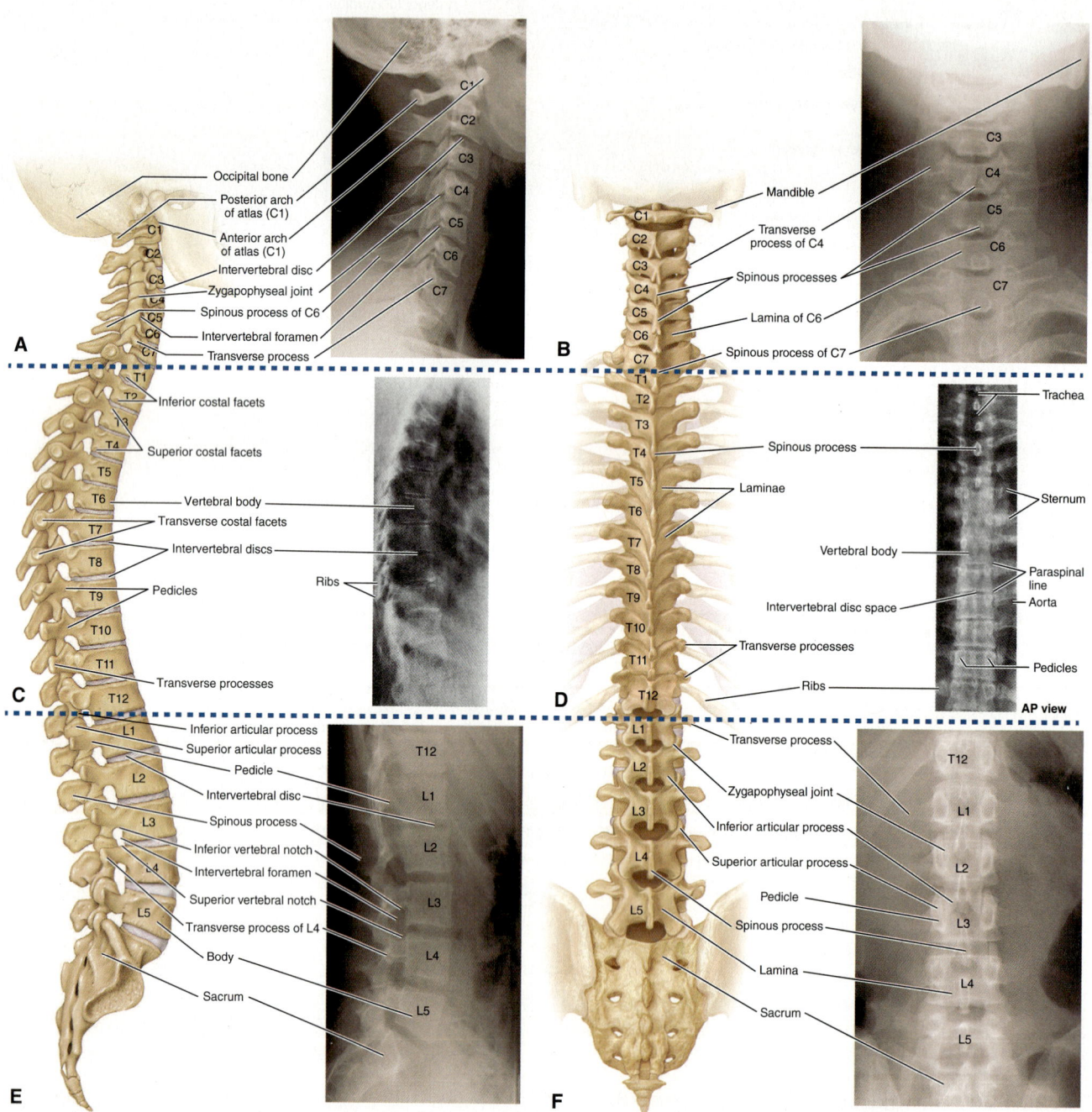

FIGURE 4-21 Osteologic features and radiographs. **A** and **B**. Cervical spine. **C** and **D**. Thoracic spine. **E** and **F**. Lumbar spine. Lateral view (**A, C,** and **E**). Posterior-anterior view (**B, D,** and **F**). (**A-B, E-F:** Modified from Gest TR. *Lippincott Atlas of Anatomy.* 2nd ed. Wolters Kluwer; 2020; Plates 1-05, 1-07, and 1-08; **C-D:** Farrell TA. *Radiology 101: The Basics and Fundamentals of Imaging.* 5th ed. Wolters Kluwer; 2020; Figure 9.6.)

CHAPTER 4 | SPINE OSTEOLOGY AND ARTHROLOGY

the cervical, thoracic, and lumbar regions of the vertebral column.

Cervical Vertebrae and Ligaments

Cervical Vertebrae The first and second cervical vertebrae have unique shapes and features and are considered atypical vertebrae. Figure 4-20A depicts the seven cervical vertebrae. A unique feature of vertebrae in this region is the transverse foramina, a foramen (hole) in the transverse processes for passage of the vertebral artery. The vertebral artery is located just anterior to the spinal nerve roots in the neck in its ascent toward the foramen magnum.

Upper Cervical Vertebrae The upper cervical spine (craniovertebral joints) includes the atlanto-occipital joints, formed by articulations between the C1 vertebra and the occiput, and the atlantoaxial joints, formed by articulations between the C1 and C2 vertebrae. The C1 vertebra is called the *atlas*, and the C2 vertebra is called the *axis*. There is no IVD in the craniovertebral joints. Figure 4-22 shows the unique osteologic features of the C1 and C2 vertebrae.

The C1 vertebra is ring shaped with no body or spinous process. The large lateral masses bear the weight of the skull. Projecting from the lateral masses are transverse processes that are more laterally positioned than other vertebrae, making the atlas the widest of the cervical vertebrae. The superior articular portion of the lateral masses bears kidney-shaped condyles that articulate with the occiput. The anterior and posterior arches of the atlas connect the lateral masses to form the complete ring of the bone. The arches bear a centrally located tubercle. The groove for the vertebral artery is located on the superior surface of the posterior arch. The vertebral artery and C1 nerve run in this groove. The atlanto-occipital joints permit nodding of the head, as in the "yes" movement

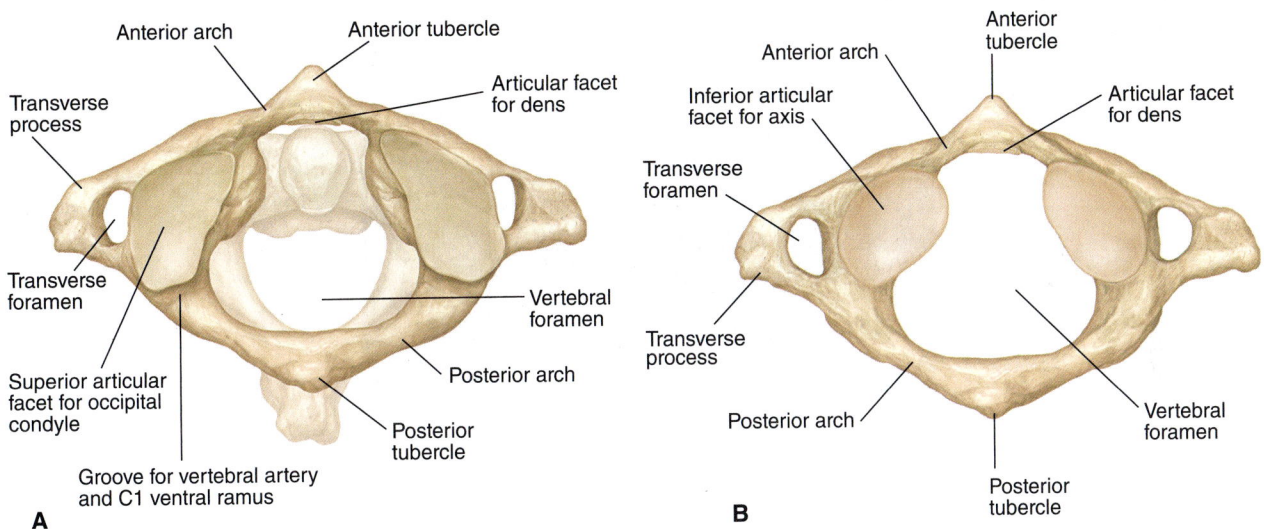

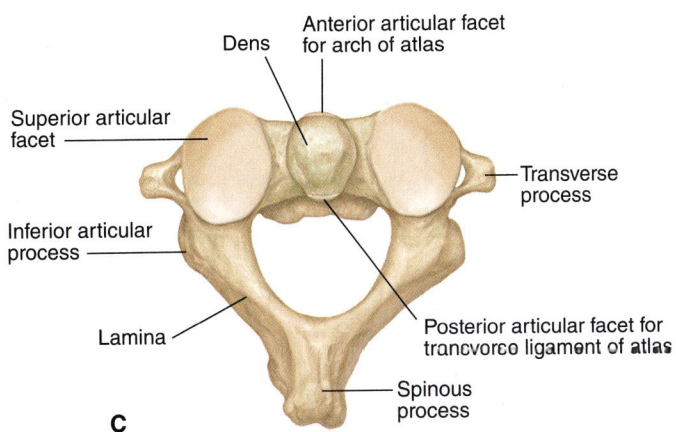

FIGURE 4-22 Articulated C1 and C2 vertebrae. **A.** C1, superior view. **B.** C1, inferior view. **C.** C2, superior view. (Gest TR. *Lippincott Atlas of Anatomy*. 2nd ed. Wolters Kluwer; 2020; Plate 1-04A-C.)

to indicate approval or agreement, with some lateral tilting/bending of the head.

The C2 vertebra is called the axis due to the large superior articular facets on which the atlas sits and rotates. The superior projection of C2 is the dens (odontoid process). The atlantoaxial joints include the two lateral atlantoaxial joints, formed by the inferior articular facets of the lateral masses of C1 and the superior articular facets of C2, and the articulation between the anterior surface of the dens with the posterior central aspect of the C1 anterior arch. The lateral atlantoaxial joints are synovial joints, and the median atlantoaxial joint is a pivot joint. The dens is held in place by the transverse ligament of the atlas that passes between the tubercles on the medial aspect of the lateral masses of C1. The transverse ligament of the atlas prevents dislocation of the axis posteriorly and the atlas anteriorly. The vertebral foramen for the spinal cord is located just posterior to the transverse ligament of the atlas. The large bifid spinous process of C2 can be palpated deep in the posterior neck. The atlantoaxial joints permit rotation of the head, as in the "no" movement, indicating disapproval. During this rotation, the occiput and C1 rotate as a unit on the C2 vertebra. To view the upper cervical vertebrae, an open mouth radiograph may be required (Fig. 4-23). In the upper cervical spine, the space available for the spinal cord is approximately two-thirds of the anteroposterior size of the vertebral canal (Fig. 4-24). The extra space in this region allows for slight slippage/displacement of the upper cervical vertebrae without impingement on the spinal cord.

Middle and Lower Cervical Vertebrae The C3–C6 vertebrae are similar in structure with small rectangular-shaped bodies that are wider side to side than anterior to posterior. Between the uncinate processes of the cervical vertebra, a synovial-like articular cavity, called the *uncovertebral joint* (aka the joint of Luschka), may form at the lateral margins (Fig. 4-25). Bone spurs

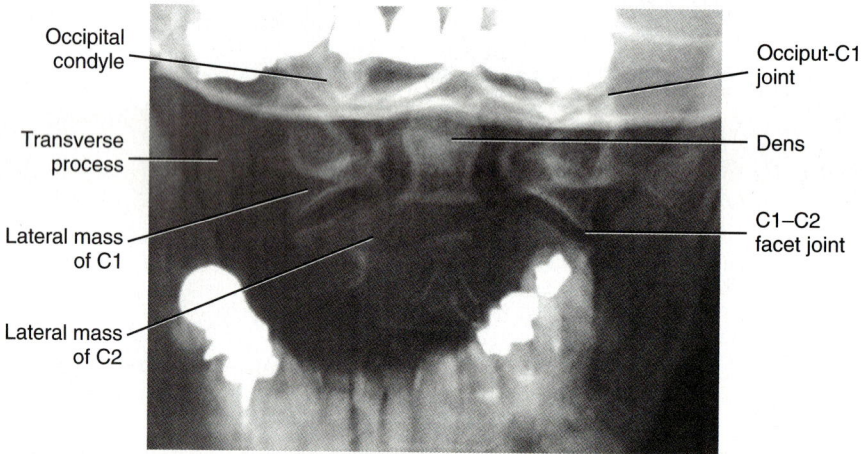

FIGURE 4-23 Anteroposterior open mouth radiograph demonstrating the occiput-C1 and the atlantoaxial articulations. (Nordin M, Frankel VH. *Basic Biomechanics of the Musculoskeletal System*. 5th ed. Wolters Kluwer; 2022; Figure 12-3.)

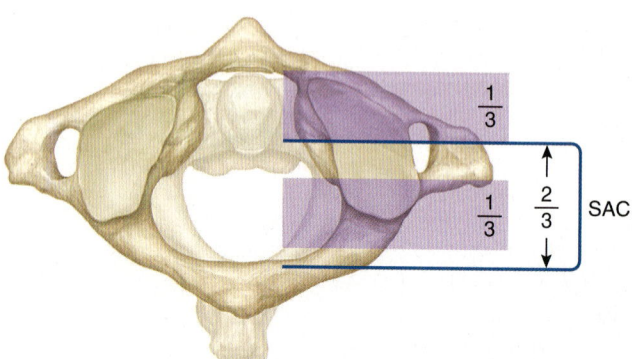

FIGURE 4-24 The upper cervical spine, superior view. The space available for the spinal cord (SAC) within the spinal canal is greater in the upper cervical region than in the mid-to-lower portions of the spine. (Adapted from Gest TR. *Lippincott Atlas of Anatomy*. 2nd ed. Wolters Kluwer; 2020; Plate 1-04 A.)

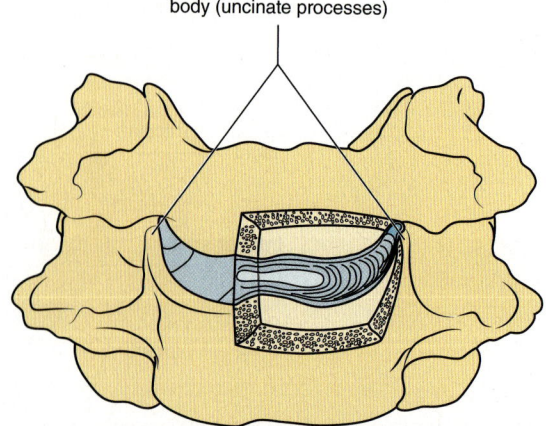

FIGURE 4-25 Middle and lower cervical vertebrae, anterior view, demonstrating uncovertebral joints. (Adapted from Moore KL, Dalley AF, Agur AMR. *Clinically Oriented Anatomy*. 8th ed. Wolters Kluwer; 2018; Figure 2.16.)

commonly occur at the uncovertebral joints. The C7 spinous process is larger than the other spinous processes in the cervical spine; thus, C7 is called the *vertebra prominens*.

Ligaments of Cervical Vertebrae

The ligaments of the upper cervical vertebrae are the anterior and posterior atlanto-occipital membranes, the cruciate ligament and the alar ligaments (Fig. 4-26). The anterior membrane's central portion is a continuation of the ALL. The anterior membrane is broad and strong, whereas the posterior membrane is broad and weak. The cruciate ligament of the atlas is formed by the transverse ligament of the atlas and vertical extensions from the transverse ligament to the occiput and C2 vertebra. This cross-shaped cruciate ligament contributes to stabilization of the dens. The alar ligaments, passing from the lateral sides of the dens superiorly to the lateral margins of the foramen magnum, form strong cords that prevent excessive rotation between the occiput and C2. The tectorial membrane, a continuation of the PLL and located just posterior to the central atlantoaxial joint complex, extends superiorly from the C2 vertebral body, through the foramen magnum, and to the floor of the occipital bone of the cranium (Fig. 4-27).

Thoracic Vertebrae

The middle thoracic vertebrae demonstrate the typical characteristics of the thoracic vertebrae, whereas the upper and lower thoracic vertebrae share features of the cervical and lumbar vertebrae, respectively.

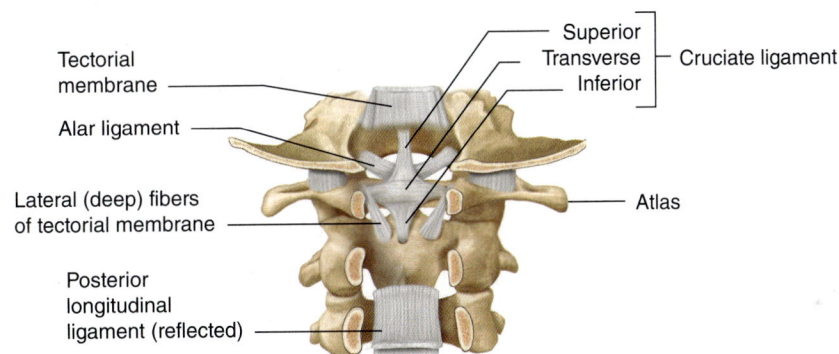

FIGURE 4-26 Upper cervical spine ligaments, posterior view. (Modified from Pansky B, Gest TR. *Lippincott's Concise Illustrated Anatomy: Back, Upper Limb & Lower Limb.* Vol. 1. Lippincott Williams & Wilkins; 2014:Figure 1.5C.)

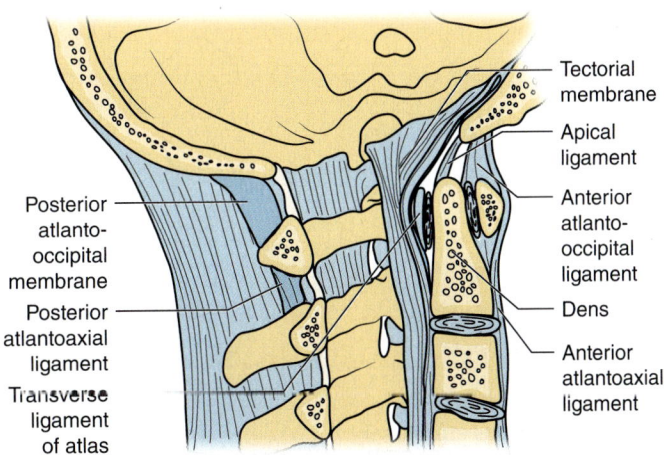

FIGURE 4-27 Medial view of right half of hemi-dissected head and upper cervical spine showing ligaments of cervical spine and ligament name changes. (Adapted from Oatis CA. *Kinesiology: The Mechanics and Pathomechanics of Human Movement.* 3rd ed. Wolters Kluwer; 2017; Figure 26.12.)

Flexion, extension, and lateral flexion are limited in the thoracic region due to the orientation of the facet joints, attachment of the ribs, and downward projection of the spinous processes. As with other regions of the vertebral column, the bony portions are sometimes considered in columns: posterior, middle, and anterior. In the thoracic region, the sternal column is added (Fig. 4-28). The posterior column is more susceptible to distraction injuries, whereas the anterior and sternal columns are more likely to fracture due to excessive flexion and compression loads.

The T1 vertebra has complete costal facets on superior edge of each side of the vertebral body for articulation with the head of rib 1 and a demifacet on inferior edge that contributes to the articular surface for the head of rib 2. The heads of ribs 2 to 11 articulate with the superior demifacet of the corresponding vertebral body, the IVD, and the inferior costal demifacet of the vertebral body above (Fig. 4-29). The T12 vertebra serves as a transitional vertebra, with the superior half bearing only one facet for articulation with ribs. Consequently, the stresses to the T12 vertebra make it prone to fracture.

Lumbar Vertebrae

The lumbar vertebral bodies are large and thick, allowing the acceptance of weight from the upper body. The vertical orientation and distinctive concave shape of the articular processes, with the posterior aspect in coronal plane and the medial/lateral aspect in sagittal plane, dictates the predominance of flexion and extension movement allowed in the region and limits rotation. The lumbar vertebral bodies are taller anteriorly than posteriorly, as are the IVDs, contributing to the normal lumbar lordosis and the lumbosacral angle (Fig. 4-30). Compared to other lumbar vertebrae, the inferior articular processes of L5 are more vertical, anterior, and lateral in orientation, allowing more rotation at the L5–S1 junction than elsewhere in the lumbar spine and limiting forward slippage of the L5 vertebra on the sacrum in standing. The transverse processes of the lumbar vertebrae bear small accessory processes for attachment of the intertransversarii muscles. The posterior portion of the superior articular facet bears small tubercles, the mammillary processes, that serve as an attachment site for the lumbar portion of the multifidi and intertransversarii muscles. The robust vertebral body of L5 is taller anteriorly

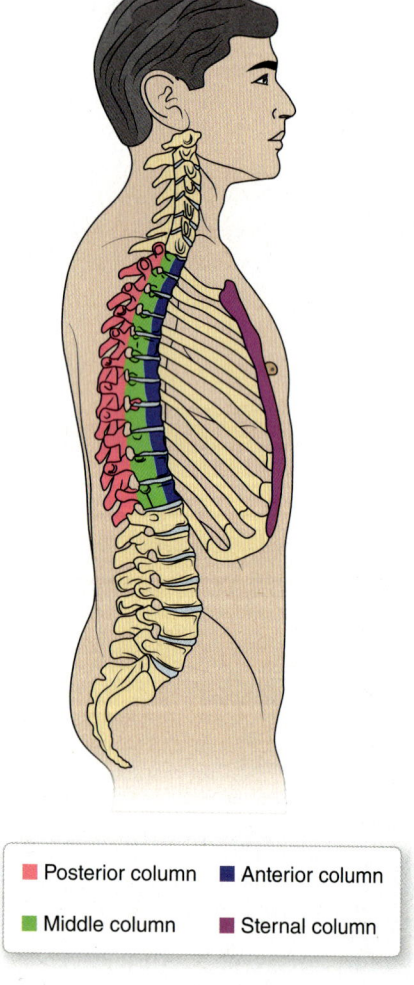

FIGURE 4-28 Vertebral columns in thoracic spine, articulated lateral view. Posterior, middle, and columns are present throughout spine. (Derived from Denis, F. The three column spine and its significance in the classification of acute thoracolumbar spinal injuries. *Spine*. 1983;8(8):817–831; and Berg EE. The sternal-rib complex: a possible fourth column in thoracic spine fractures. *Spine*. 1993;18(13):1916–1919.)

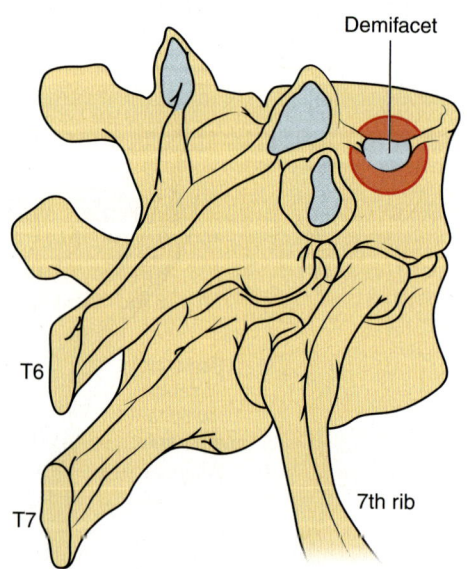

FIGURE 4-29 Demifacets on posterolateral aspect of superior and inferior surfaces of vertebral bodies. (Adapted from Oatis CA. *Kinesiology: The Mechanics and Pathomechanics of Human Movement*. 3rd ed. Wolters Kluwer; 2017; Figure 29.4.)

Sacrum

The triangularly shaped sacrum is composed of five fused vertebrae in adults. The inferior portion of the sacrum is non–weight bearing. The role of the sacrum is to transmit the weight of the trunk and upper extremities to the pelvic girdle. The vertebral canal of the vertebral column continues in the sacrum as the sacral canal, which contains the terminal portion of the cauda equina. The anterior and posterior sacral foramina provide the exit point for the anterior and posterior rami of the spinal nerves (see Fig. 4-18C, D). The anterior proximal portion of the sacrum, the sacral base, projects anteriorly as the sacral promontory. The apex is the inferior end of the sacrum, articulating with the coccyx. The pelvic surface of the sacrum is smooth and concave, forming the posterior aspect of the bony pelvis. The posterior surface is rough and bears crests: median, intermediate, and lateral. The upside-down U-shaped sacral hiatus is an opening on the inferior aspect of the sacrum that is continuous with the sacral canal. The superior lateral surfaces of the sacrum are ear shaped (C-shaped) and are called the *auricular surfaces*. The auricular surfaces on each side of the sacrum articulate with the reciprocating auricular surface of each iliac wing to form an SIJ on each side (Fig. 4-31).[49] The SIJs, fused pelvic bones (ilium, ischium, and pubis), and pubic symphysis form the pelvic ring.

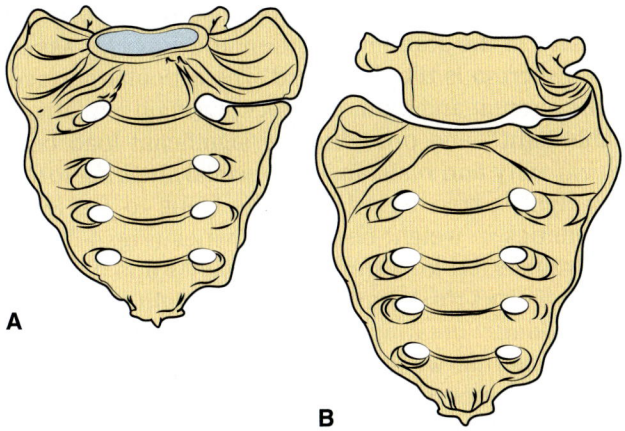

FIGURE 4-30 Sacrum, anterior view. **A.** Partial lumbarization of the first sacral vertebra. **B.** Partial sacralization of the fifth lumbar vertebra. (Adapted from Oatis CA. *Kinesiology: The Mechanics and Pathomechanics of Human Movement.* 3rd ed. Wolters Kluwer; 2017; Figure 35.8.)

and sloped, providing significant contribution to the angle between the lumbar and sacral portions of the vertebral column (see Fig. 4-21E). A common abnormality in the lumbar spine is a full or partial fusion of L5 with the sacrum (aka sacralization of the lumbar vertebra or lumbarization of the first sacral vertebra) (Fig. 4-30).[48]

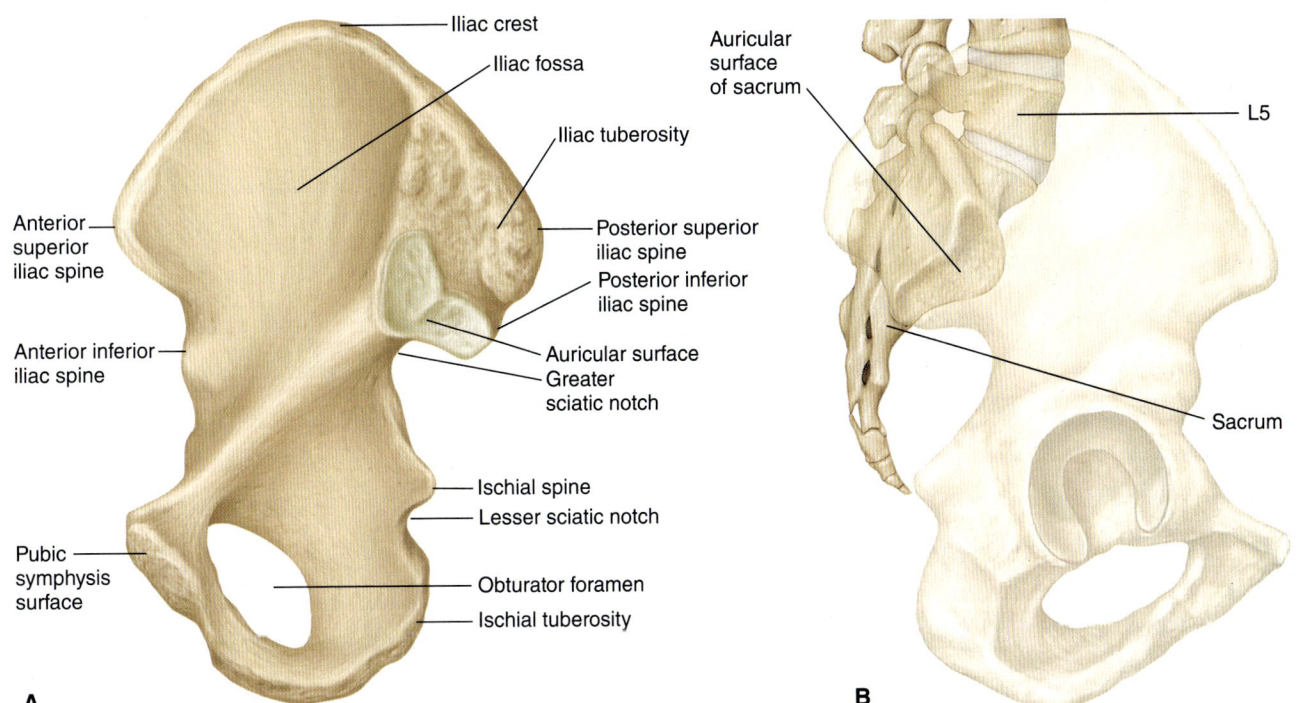

FIGURE 4-31 Sacroiliac joint formed by articulation of auricular surfaces. **A.** Ilium. (Gest TR. *Lippincott Atlas of Anatomy.* 2nd ed. Wolters Kluwer; 2020; Plate 6-03A.) **B.** Sacrum. (Modified from Gest TR. *Lippincott Atlas of Anatomy.* 2nd ed. Wolters Kluwer; 2020; Plate 1-03.)

Coccyx

The most inferior portion of the vertebral column is the coccyx, a small triangular-shaped bone formed by the fusion of one to four vertebrae. The first coccygeal vertebra, vertebra Co1, is the largest of the coccygeal vertebrae and often remains separate from the fused bones. The Co1 vertebra may fuse with the sacrum with aging. The coccyx bears no weight in standing, but flexes and bears some weight in sitting. Attaching to the coccyx are portions of the gluteus maximus (GMax), coccygeus muscles, and the median fibrous band of the pubococcygeus muscles (aka the anococcygeal ligament).

SACROILIAC JOINT

The auricular surfaces of the sacrum are composed primarily of the first two and the upper part of the third sacral vertebrae and are directed posteroinferiorly and laterally. In the standing position, the superior aspect of the sacrum is tilted forward. The articular surfaces of the sacrum and ilium interlock, forming a relatively stable joint[49] and providing for significant load bearing capacity and resistance to vertical shearing forces as weight is transferred from the trunk to the lower extremities in weight-bearing activities (Fig. 4-32).[50,51] The transferred load through the pelvis and hips may rise as high as three times the body weight during normal walking,[51] creating significant stress on the SIJ.

The sacrum wedges between the ilia and is stabilized by ligaments that prevent separation of the joint surfaces (Table 4-4). The anterior and posterior sacroiliac ligaments surround the interosseous ligament, which is the strongest of the supporting ligaments. The short and long posterior sacroiliac ligamentous fibers blend with those of the interosseous ligament. The

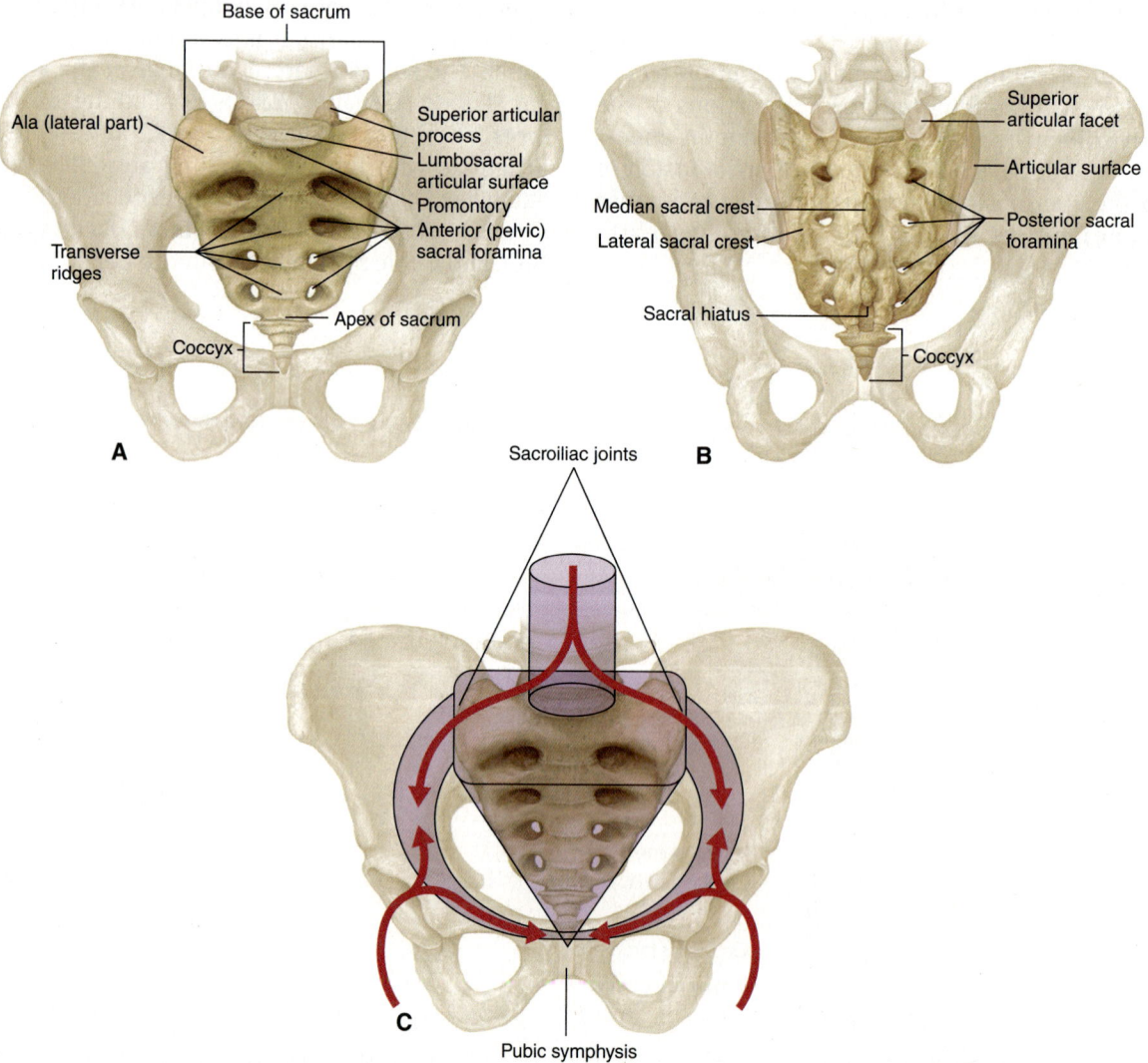

FIGURE 4-32 Sacroiliac joint as part of pelvic basin with osteologic landmarks. **A.** Anterior view. **B.** Posterior view. **C.** Transferring of load between the trunk and the lower extremities. (Modified from Gest TR. *Lippincott Atlas of Anatomy*. 2nd ed. Wolters Kluwer; 2020; Plate 1-09.)

TABLE 4-4		
LIGAMENTS STABILIZING THE SACROILIAC JOINT		
Ligament	*Location/Attachments*	*Function*
Anterior sacroiliac	Thickening of anterior portion of joint capsule	Reinforces interosseous ligament
Posterior sacroiliac	Thickening of posterior portion of joint capsule	Reinforces interosseous ligament
Short and long posterior sacroiliac	Short: Passes between the first and second tubercles on the dorsum of the sacrum to PSIS and internal lip of iliac crest Long: Passes between the third and fourth tubercles of sacrum to PSIS and internal lip of iliac crest	Reinforces interosseous ligament
Interosseous	Passes between sacral and ischial tuberosities	Stabilizes joint (primary) during weight transfers of upper body from trunk to ilia
Sacrotuberous	Passes between lateral margins of the sacrum and PSIS to ischial tuberosity	Anchors inferior end of sacrum to ischium; resists superior and posterior rotation of sacrum in forceful weight bearing
Sacroiliac	Passes between lateral margins of the sacrum to ischial spine	Anchors inferior end of sacrum to ischium; resists superior and posterior rotation of sacrum in forceful weight bearing

PSIS, posterior superior iliac spine.
Adapted from Shi D, Wang F, Wang D, Li X, Wang Q. 3-D finite element analysis of the influence of synovial condition in sacroiliac joint on the load transmission in human pelvic system. *Med Eng Phys.* 2014;36(6):745-753.

sacrotuberous and sacrospinous ligaments provide stabilizing reinforcement to the SIJ (Fig. 4-33).[52]

The SIJ capsule has characteristics of a synovial joint[49] with smooth articulating surfaces. With aging, the joint capsule becomes more fibrotic and less mobile and the smooth articulating surfaces become rough, expressing reciprocating depressions and elevations within subchondral bone and cartilage. The articulating surfaces are covered with hyaline and articular cartilage.[49,53,54] The ilium cartilage is thinner with more dense collagen bundles that extend into the subchondral bone endplate and fewer proteoglycans than sacral cartilage. The subadjacent cancellous bone of the ilium is thicker than that of the sacrum.[55,56] For reasons that are unclear, degenerative changes occur more often on the iliac side of the SIJ.[57]

Computed tomography (CT) imaging allows clear visualization of degenerative changes of the SIJ. In asymptomatic (pain-free) individuals, studies indicate increasing degeneration with aging,[58,59] with more than 85% of asymptomatic individuals demonstrating degeneration by the sixth decade and more than 90% by the eighth decade of life.[59] The image-detected degenerative changes do not correlate with pain related to the SIJ.

The sacrum moves relative to the ilium in all directions, though the magnitude is limited to approximately 3° in flexion-extension, 1.5° in axial rotation, and 0.8° in lateral bending.[56] The SIJ may cause low back pain,[60] though differentiation of pain originating from the SIJ versus related structures, such as the IVD, facet joints, or dorsal rami of spinal nerves, is difficult. Similarities exist among pain-referral patterns for lumbar disc, facet joint, and SIJ pathology.[61] Potential pain-generating sources of the SIJ are intra- and extra-articular structures, such as the SIJ capsule[62] and ligaments.[63] A composite map of the pain-referral patterns developed from sensory diagrams following injection in asymptomatic individuals implicates an area 3 × 10 cm inferior to the posterior superior iliac spine (PSIS) as the area most likely to represent SIJ pain, though radiation beyond this area may exist.[61] Confirmatory image-guided injections can aid diagnosis of SIJ-related pain.[60] (Chapter 12, Lumbar Spine and Sacroiliac Joint, explains special tests and interventions for the SIJ.)

MUSCLES

The muscles of the trunk act in the following ways: to position the spine and stabilize it, to provide the power to lift and carry objects, to produce movement against gravity, and to act as guidewires to prevent excessive movement in a direction of imbalance. The muscles of the back can be divided into extrinsic (containing one attachment outside the vertebrae and ribs) and intrinsic with multiple layers within each division, as summarized in Table 4-5 and depicted in Figures 4-34 to 4-36. The extrinsic back muscles produce and control limb movements and participate in respiration and proprioception. The intrinsic (deep) back muscles act directly on the vertebral column to produce movement and maintain static positions. Table 4-6 provides a summary of principle muscles producing movement at the intervertebral joints.

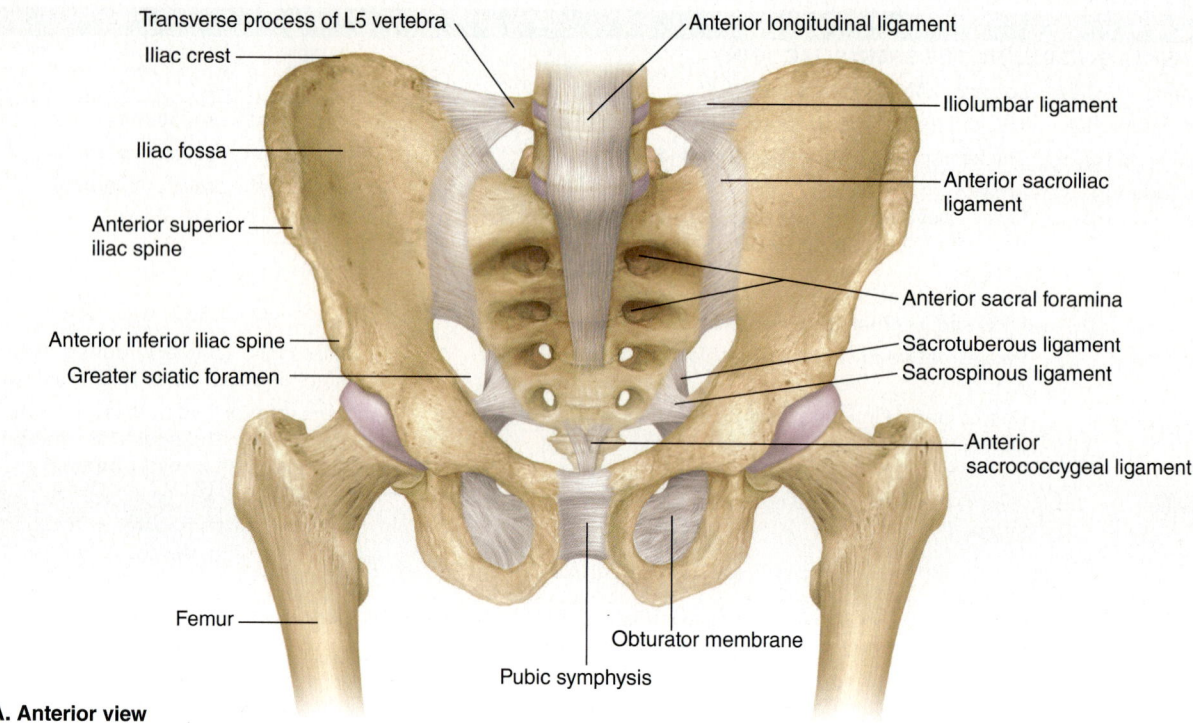

A. Anterior view

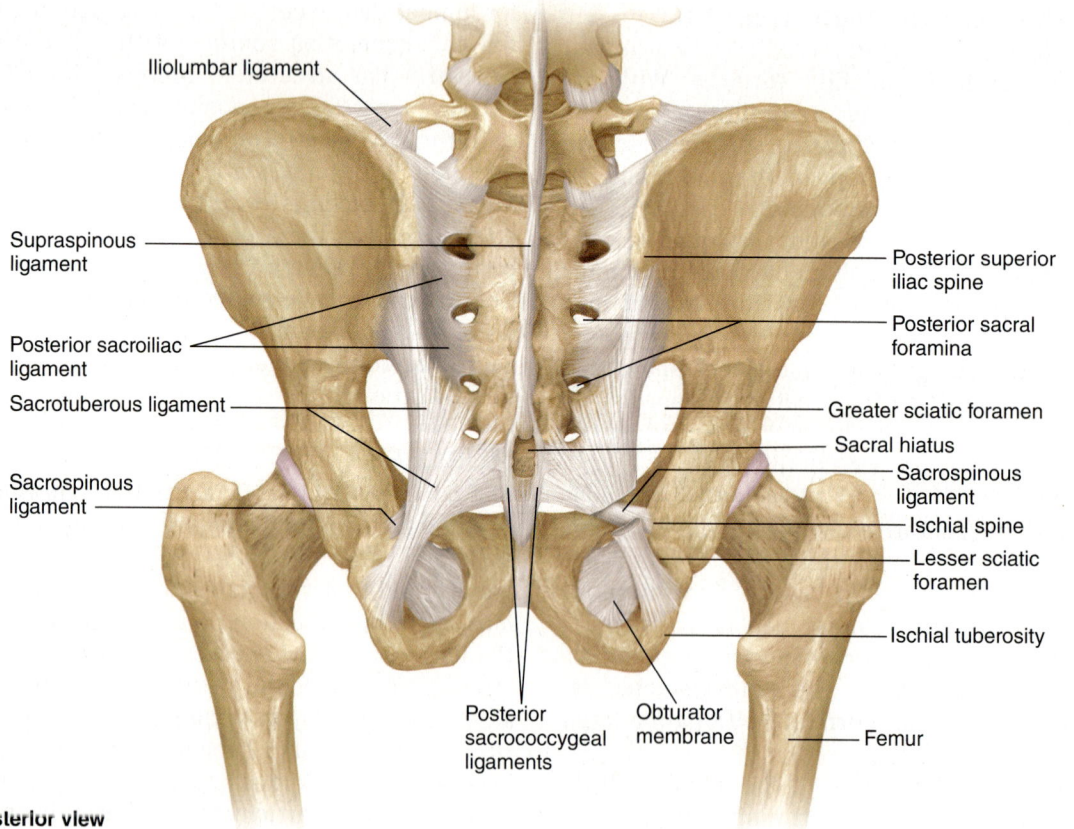

B. Posterior view

FIGURE 4-33 Stabilizing ligaments of sacroiliac joint. **A.** Anterior view. **B.** Posterior view. (Gest TR. *Lippincott Atlas of Anatomy*. 2nd ed. Wolters Kluwer; 2020; Plate 1-06.)

TABLE 4-5
EXTRINSIC AND INTRINSIC MUSCLES OF THE BACK (BY LAYER)

Extrinsic Group		
• Limb and trunk movement (global); respiration • Anchor upper limb and scapula to trunk	Superficial layer	Trapezius Latissimus dorsi Levator scapulae Rhomboid major Rhomboid minor
	Intermediate layer	Serratus posterior superior Serratus posterior inferior
Intrinsic (Deep) Group		
• Posture • Movement of trunk and head (local)	Superficial layer	Splenius (cervicis and capitus)
	Intermediate layer (erector spinae group)	Iliocostalis Longissimus Spinalis
	Major deep layer (transversospinalis group)	Semispinalis (cervicis and capitus) Multifidus Rotatores
	Minor deep layer	Interspinales Intertransversarii Levator costarum

Adapted from Moore KL, Dalley AF, Agur AMR. *Clinically Oriented Anatomy.* 8th ed. Wolters Kluwer; 2018; Tables 2.4, 2.5, and 2.6.

Extrinsic Back Muscles

The extrinsic back muscles connect the vertebral column with the scapula, clavicle, and humerus to move the scapula and produce and control the upper limb movements. For the most part, these muscles receive nerve supply from the anterior rami of the cervical spinal nerves. The trapezius is supplied by the spinal accessory nerve, cranial nerve XI. The functional role of the intermediate extrinsic back muscles, the serratus posterior superior and inferior, is debated. Based strictly on muscle attachments, these muscles have been thought to contribute to elevation and depression of the ribs, thus impacting respiration. However, cadaveric and electromyographic (EMG) studies show little evidence to support this role.[64,65]

Intrinsic Back Muscles

The intrinsic back muscles control movements of the back and help maintain posture. These muscles are encased by deep fascia and pass from the cranium to the pelvis. In the thoracic and lumbar regions, the deep fascia surrounding the intrinsic back muscles constitutes the thoracolumbar fascia. The thoracolumbar fascia has extensive attachments, including a lateral connection to the abdominal muscles, a medial attachment to spinal ligaments and facet joint capsules, and an inferior attachment to the iliolumbar ligament, the iliac crest, and the SIJ.[66] The medial portion of the thoracolumbar fascia divides into anterior, middle, and posterior layers that surround the quadratus lumborum, erector spinae, and multifidus muscles. The quadratus lumborum primarily laterally flexes the lumbar spine. During gait, the quadratus lumborum, assisted by the psoas muscle, holds the pelvis in a neutral position. The posterior superficial components of the thoracolumbar fascia provide a connection between the latissimus dorsi and the GMax, thereby contributing to the transfer of forces between the spine, pelvis, and lower limbs.[67,68]

Superficial Layer The superficial layer of intrinsic back muscles, the splenius capitis and splenius cervicis, wrap around the neck much like a bandage. The splenius muscles attach to the nuchal ligament and spinous processes of the lower cervical and first six thoracic vertebrae and extend superiorly and laterally to attach to the skull and cervical transverse processes.

Intermediate Layer Deep to the superficial layer muscles and inferiorly, the erector spinae muscle group lies in a groove between the spinous processes and angles of the ribs, a position that allows their primary action of extension of the vertebral column and head (acting bilaterally) and lateral flexion of the spine (acting unilaterally). The erector spinae muscle group is divided, from lateral to medial, into three columns of muscles: iliocostalis, longissimus, and spinalis. The three columns of muscles have a common attachment via a broad tendon to the iliac crest, sacrum, sacroiliac ligaments, sacral and inferior lumbar spinous processes, and supraspinous ligament. Further divisions of these columns are made based on the superior attachments in the lumbar, thoracic, cervical, and cranial regions.

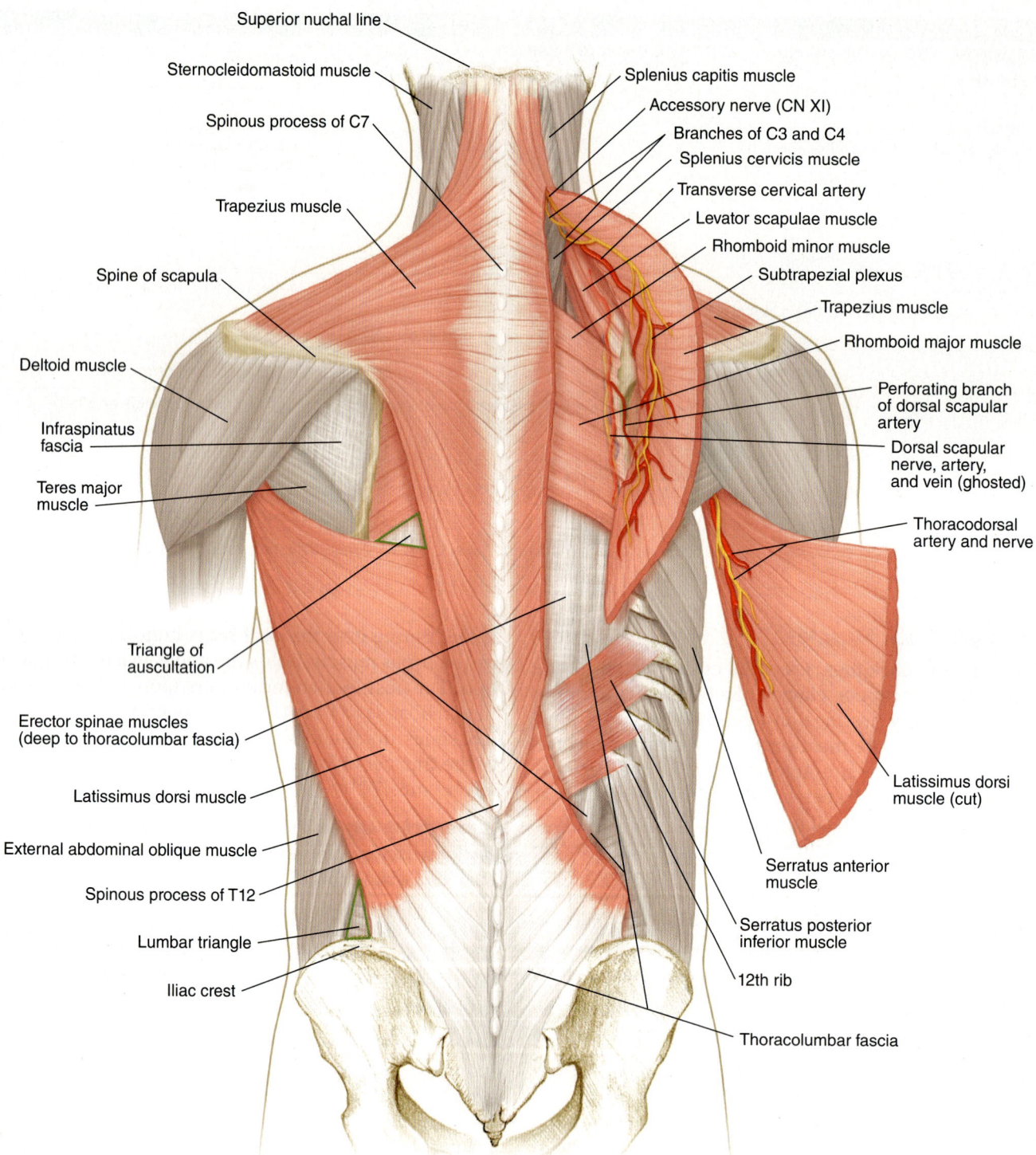

FIGURE 4-34 Extrinsic muscles of the back. *CN*, cranial nerve. (Gest TR. *Lippincott Atlas of Anatomy*. 2nd ed. Wolters Kluwer; 2020; Plate 1-14.)

Major Deep Layer The major deep layer of intrinsic back muscles is named the transversospinalis muscles owing to their attachments to the transverse process and spinous processes. From superficial to deep, the transversospinalis muscles are the semispinali, multifidi, and rotatores. The multifidi are largest in the lumbar region, where they play a major role in dynamic stabilization.[69-74] The rotatores muscles are most developed in the thoracic region.

CHAPTER 4 | SPINE OSTEOLOGY AND ARTHROLOGY

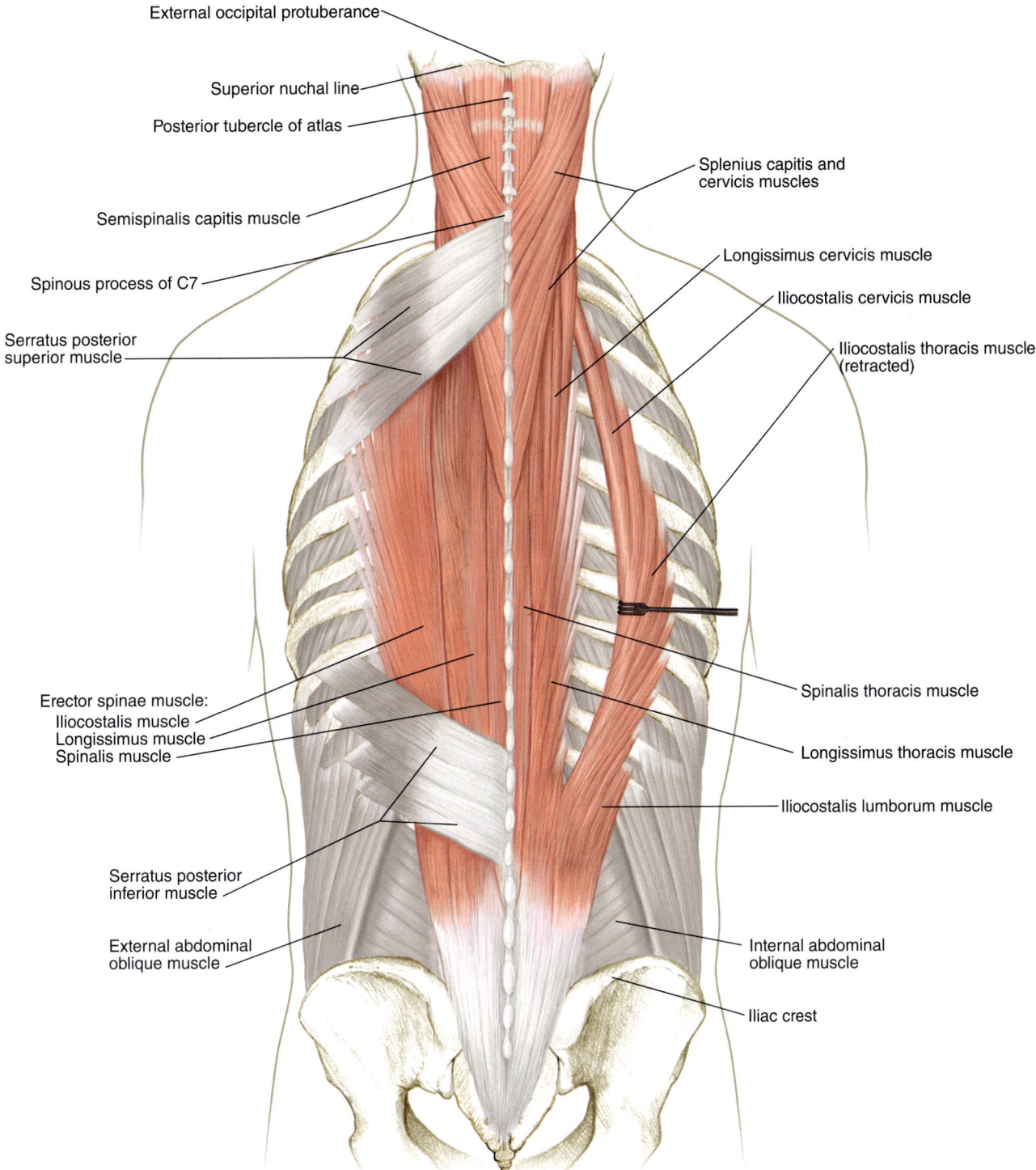

FIGURE 4-35 Intrinsic muscles, superficial and intermediate layers. (Gest TR. *Lippincott Atlas of Anatomy*. 2nd ed. Wolters Kluwer; 2020; Plate 1-15.)

Minor Deep Layer The minor deep layer of intrinsic back muscles is the interspinales (singular: interspinalis), intertransversarii, and levatores costarum. The attachments of the interspinales and intertransversarii are the spinous processes and transverse processes. The levatores costarum attaches to the transverse processes and the ribs.

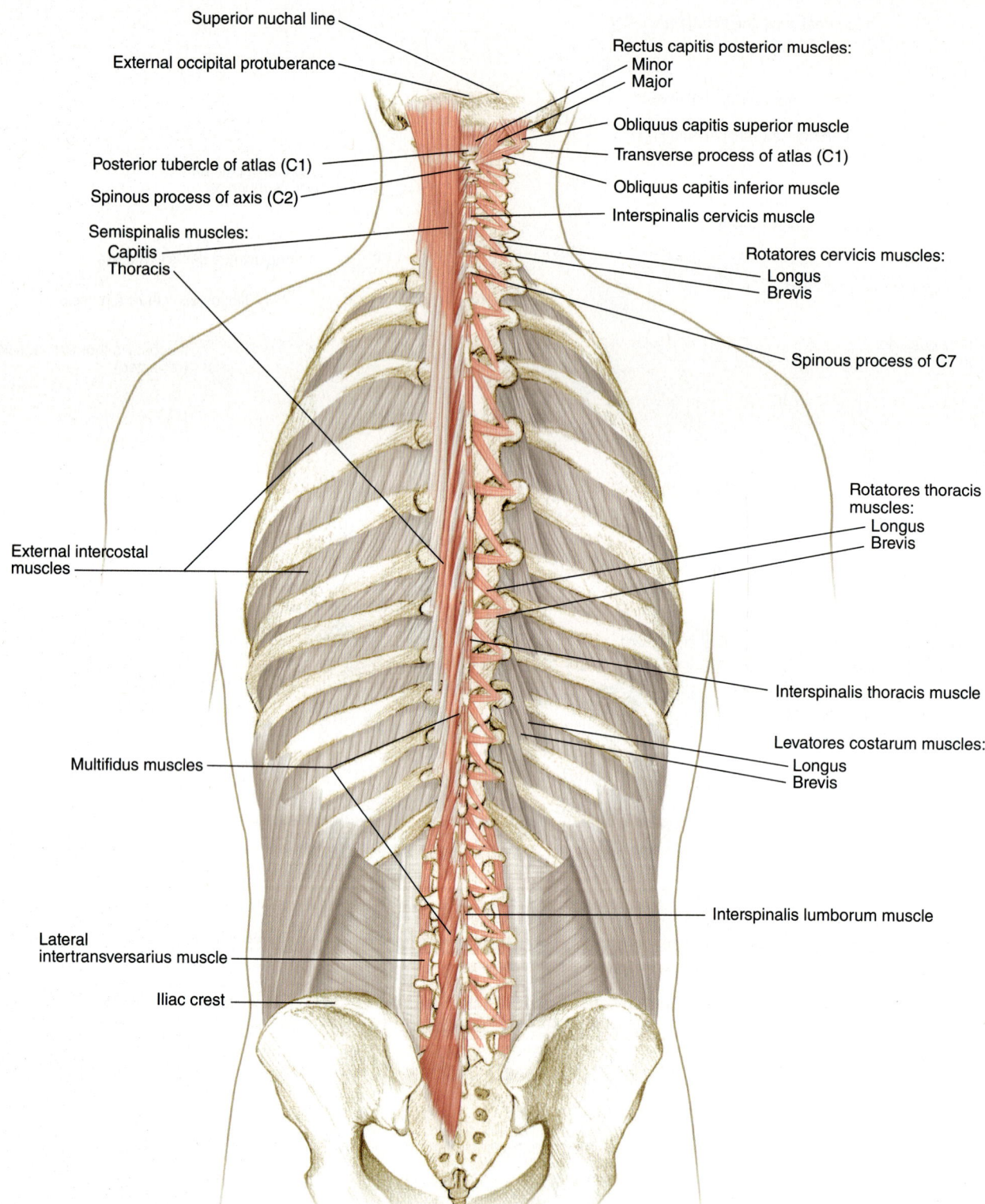

FIGURE 4-36 Intrinsic muscles, major deep and minor deep layers. (Gest TR. *Lippincott Atlas of Anatomy*. 2nd ed. Wolters Kluwer; 2020; Plate 1-16.)

Stabilizing Muscles

Several muscles work together with the back muscles to move the spine and rib cage, increase intra-abdominal pressure, and assist lumbopelvic stability (Table 4-7). As a group, the abdominal muscle fibers run in multiple directions and exert movement and stabilizing forces on the trunk (Fig. 4-37). The thoracic diaphragm is activated during trunk movement

TABLE 4-6
PRINCIPAL MUSCLES PRODUCING MOVEMENT OF INTERVERTEBRAL JOINTS

	Flexion*	Extension	Lateral Flexion*	Rotation
Movement of cervical intervertebral joints	Bilateral action of: • Longus colli • Scalene • Sternocleidomastoid	Deep neck muscles: • Semispinalis cervicis and iliocostalis cervicis • Splenius cervicis and Levator scapulae • Splenius capitis • Multifidus • Longissimus capitis • Semispinalis capitis • Trapezius	Unilateral action of: • Iliocostalis cervicis • Longissimus capitis and cervicis • Splenius capitis and cervicis • Intertransversarii • Scalenes	Unilateral action of: • Rotatores • Semispinalis capitis and cervicis • Multifidus • Splenius cervicis
Movement of thoracic and lumbar intervertebral joints	Bilateral action of: • Rectus abdominis • Psoas major	Bilateral action of: • Erector spinae • Multifidus • Semispinalis thoracis	Unilateral action of: • Iliocostalis thoracis and lumborum • Longissimus thoracis • Multifidus • External and internal oblique • Quadratus lumborum • Rhomboids • Serratus anterior	Unilateral action of: • Rotatores • Multifidus • Iliocostalis • Longissimus • External oblique acting synchronously with opposite Internal oblique • Splenius thoracis

* From the standing position, trunk flexion is the result of gravity and controlled by the erector spinae bilaterally, whereas lateral flexion is controlled by the contralateral erector spinae.
Adapted from Moore KL, Dalley AF, Agur AMR. *Clinically Oriented Anatomy*. 8th ed. Wolters Kluwer; 2018; Tables 2.7 and 2.8.

TABLE 4-7
STABILIZING MUSCLES OF THE TRUNK

Group	Muscles	Attachments	Action
Anterolateral abdominal wall	Rectus abdominis	• Pubic symphysis and pubic crest • Xiphoid process and costal cartilages 5-7	• Flexes trunk • Compresses abdominal viscera • Stabilizes and control tilt of pelvis
	External oblique	• External surfaces of lower 8 ribs • Linea alba, pubic tubercle, anterior half of iliac crest	• Flexes trunk • Compresses abdominal viscera
	Internal oblique	• Thoracolumbar fascia, anterior 2/3 iliac crest, connective tissue deep to lateral 1/3 of inguinal ligament • Inferior borders of ribs 10-12, linea alba, pecten pubis (via conjoint tendon)	
	Transversus abdominis	• Internal surfaces of costal cartilages 7-12, thoracolumbar fascia, iliac crest, connective tissue deep to lateral 1/3 of inguinal ligament • Linea alba with aponeurosis of internal oblique, pubic crest and pecten pubis via conjoint tendon	• Compresses abdominal viscera
Posterior abdominal wall	Psoas major	• Transverse processes of lumbar vertebrae and sides of bodies of T12-L5 vertebrae and intervening IVDs • Lesser trochanter of femur	• Flexes thigh (with iliacus) • Flexes vertebral column • Balances trunk
	Quadratus lumborum	• Medial half of inferior border of 12th ribs and tips of lumbar transverse processes • Iliolumbar ligament and internal lip of iliac crest	• Extends and laterally flex vertebral column • Stabilizes 12th rib during inspiration

(continued)

TABLE 4-7 (continued)
STABILIZING MUSCLES OF THE TRUNK

Group	Muscles		Attachments	Action
Pelvic floor	Coccygeus (aka ischio-coccygeus)		• Ischial spine • Inferior end of sacrum and coccyx	• Forms small part of pelvic diaphragm that supports pelvic viscera • Flexes coccyx
	Levator ani	Iliococcygeus Pubococcygeus Puborectalis	• Body of pubis; tendinous arch of obturator fascia; ischial spine • Perineal body; coccyx; anococcygeal ligament; wall of prostate or vagina, rectum and anal canal	• Forms most of the pelvic diaphragm that helps support pelvic viscera and increases abdominal pressure
	Obturator internus		• Pelvic surfaces of ilium and ischium; obturator membrane • Great trochanter of femur	• Rotates thigh laterally • Assists in holding head of femur in acetabulum • Supports floor of pelvis
	Piriformis		• Pelvic surface of S2–S4 segments; superior margin of greater sciatic notch and sacrotuberous ligament	• Rotates thigh laterally • Abducts thigh • Assists in holding head of femur in acetabulum • Supports floor of pelvis

IVD, intervertebral disc.
Adapted from Moore KL Dalley AF, Agur AMR. *Clinically Oriented Anatomy*. 8th ed. Wolters Kluwer; 2018; Tables 5.2, 5.13, and 6.2.

to impact intra-abdominal pressure and support the trunk during movement of the trunk and lower limbs.

Abdominal Muscles The stabilizing role of the abdominal muscles on the trunk (Figs. 4-38 and 4-39) is well documented.[75-77] The transversus abdominis (TrA) demonstrates continuous activation throughout trunk flexion and extension.[78] The TrA is the first trunk muscle to be activated during perturbations in standing and remains active throughout dorsal and ventral trunk loading.[78] During limb movement, the TrA is activated, regardless of limb movement or direction of forces acting on the spine.[79] The rectus abdominis, internal oblique, external oblique, and TrA muscles are activated along with the erector spinae muscles during the performance of plank exercises.[77] Weakness and lack of motor control of deep trunk muscles, such as the lumbar multifidus and TrA muscles, are common in low back pain.[80] Strengthening of deep back and abdominal muscles has been associated with improvements in pain and functional outcomes among persons with low back pain.[75,76,81-83]

Pelvic Floor Muscles The pelvic diaphragm (coccygeus and levator ani muscles and covering fascia) forms the deep layer muscles of the pelvic floor. The levator ani is composed of three muscles: the pubococcygeus, puborectalis, and iliococcygeus (Fig. 4-40). The levator ani joins the coccygeus to form a base in the pelvis to:

- Support the pelvic organs
- Increase intra-abdominal pressure

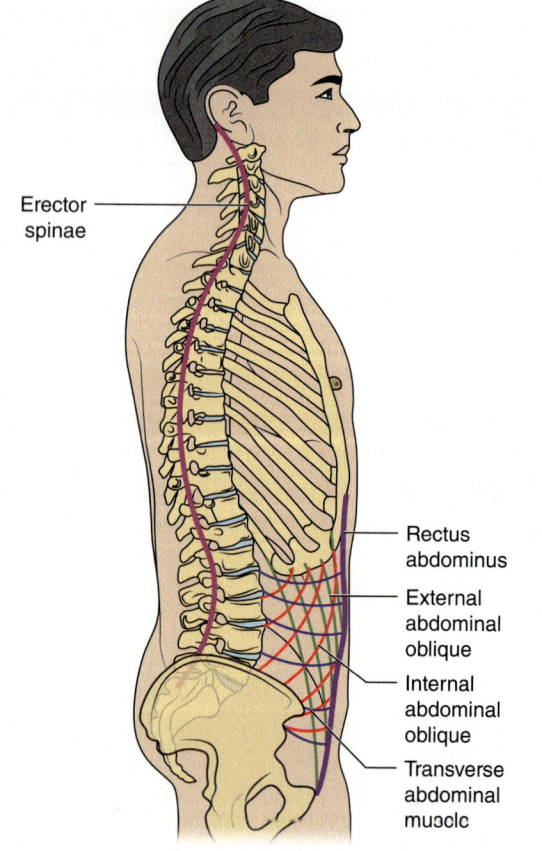

FIGURE 4-37 Erector spinae and abdominal muscles provide movement and balance to trunk. (Adapted from Nordin M, Frankel VH. *Basic Biomechanics of the Musculoskeletal System*. 5th ed. Wolters Kluwer; 2022; Figure 11-4.)

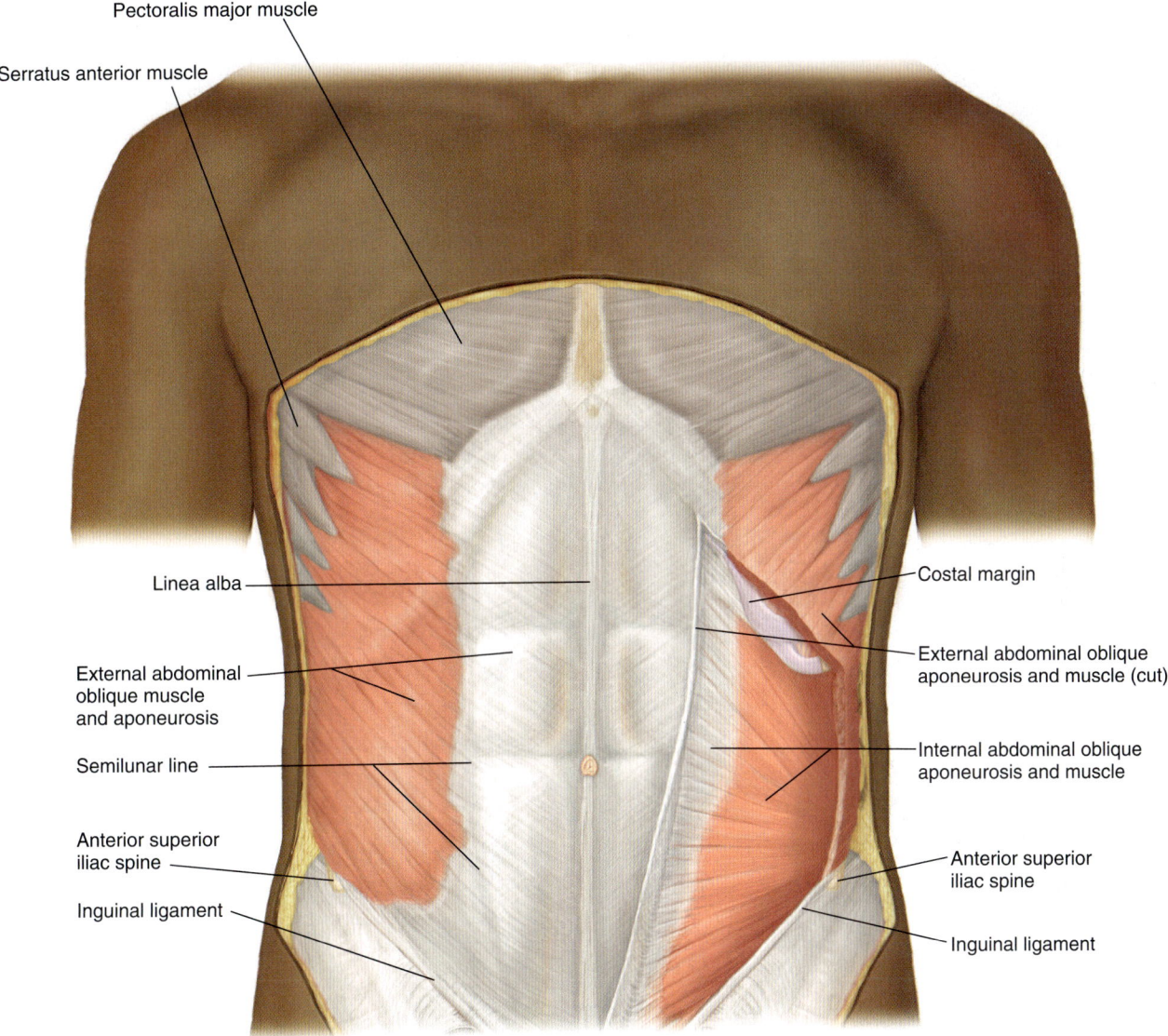

FIGURE 4-38 Abdominal muscles: rectus abdominis, external oblique, internal oblique. Note varied direction of muscle fibers among the muscles. (Gest TR. *Lippincott Atlas of Anatomy*. 2nd ed. Wolters Kluwer; 2020; Plate 5-04.)

- Inhibit bladder activity
- Support the rectum during defecation
- Assist lumbopelvic stability

The piriformis and obturator internus form the posterosuperior and lateral walls of the pelvis, respectively (Figs. 4-40 and 4-41). Posteriorly, the obturator internus becomes tendinous as the muscle turns laterally to pass through the lesser sciatic foramen to continue to the attachment on the greater trochanter of the femur. The medial surface of the obturator internus is covered by fascia that is thickened as a tendinous arch providing attachment for muscles of the pelvic floor. An inferior view of the pelvic floor is depicted in Figure 4-42. (Refer to Chapter 12, Lumbar Spine and Sacroiliac Joint, for more information about pelvic floor muscle dysfunction.)

To provide stability to the trunk, the muscles of the pelvic floor, abdominals, lumbar multifidus, and thoracoabdominal diaphragm work together synergistically. Studies using EMG and palpation indicate the abdominal muscles are recruited during contraction of the pelvic floor muscles (PFMs),[84-86] with varied contributions from individual abdominal muscles as the position of the lumbar spine changes.[87] Contracting together, the abdominals, PFMs, and diaphragm increase intra-abdominal pressure[88] and stabilize the spine. The strength and endurance of the PFMs are thus an integral part of spinal stability.

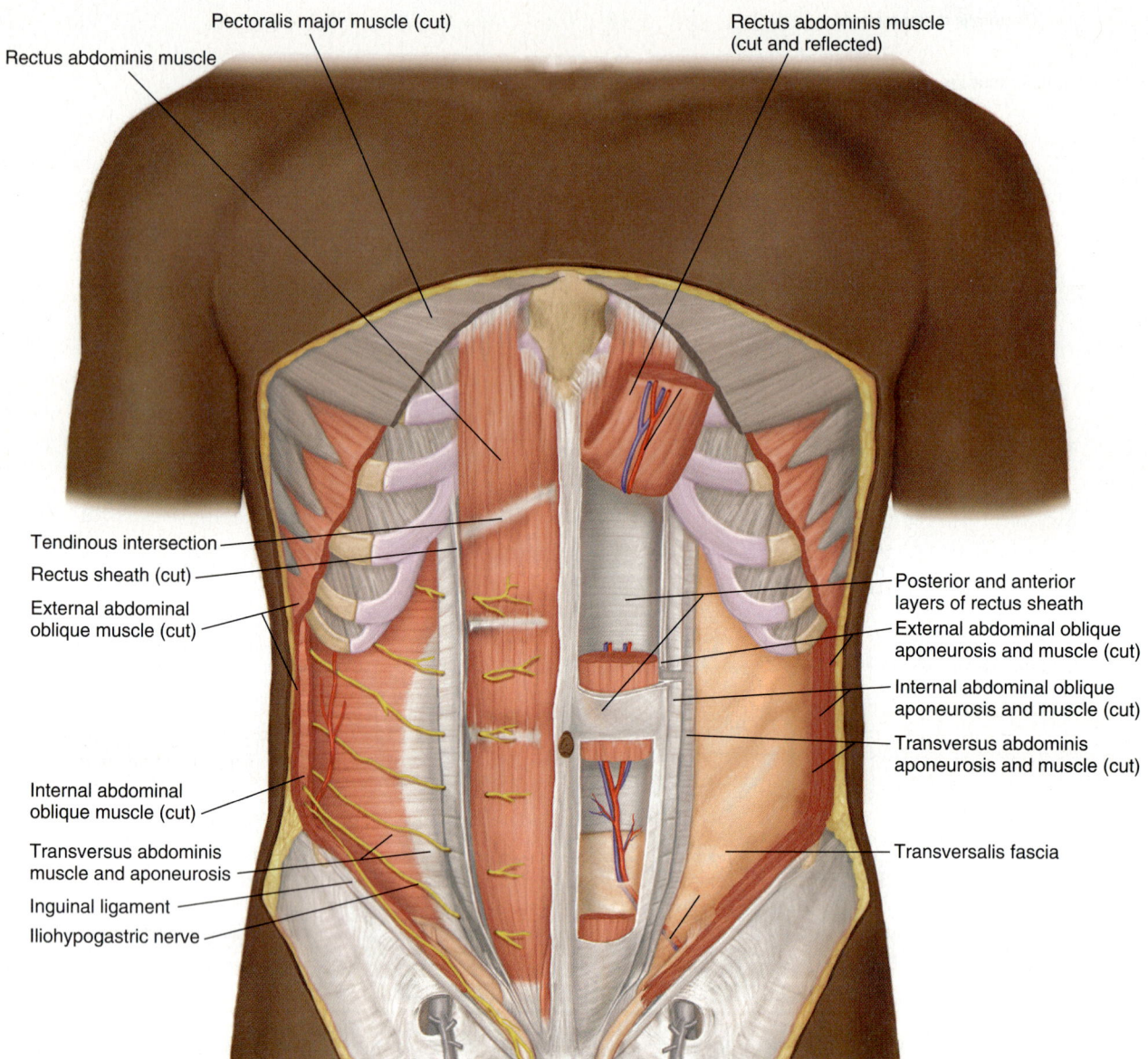

FIGURE 4-39 Abdominal muscles with rectus abdominis, external oblique, internal oblique and transversus abdominis partially dissected on the left abdomen. (Gest TR. *Lippincott Atlas of Anatomy*. 2nd ed. Wolters Kluwer; 2020; Plate 5-05.)

Gluteal Muscles Major muscle groups acting on the pelvis and lower limb influence trunk movement. The psoas major attaches proximally to the anterolateral aspect of the vertebral bodies and transverse processes and then passes distally with the iliacus to attach to the greater trochanter. Though primarily a muscle of the lower limb, the psoas major is a potential extensor of the lumbar spine and a flexor of the lumbar spine on the pelvis, depending on the relative positions and fixation of the spine, pelvis, and femur.

The GMax has bony and connective tissue attachments. The majority of the distal attachment is to the iliotibial tract, which inserts into the lateral condyle of the tibia. The rest of the GMax attaches distally to the greater tuberosity of the femur. The action of the GMax is to extend the flexed thigh, participate in lateral rotation and to steady the thigh.[89] Multiple studies of weight-lifting exercises show the greatest GMax activation with the step-up exercise and variations (lateral, diagonal, and crossover step-up).[90-92] These exercises are unilateral and require the GMax to extend the hip joint, while simultaneously working with the gluteus medius (GMe) to maintain the pelvis level and control excessive femur adduction and medial rotation. Greater muscle activation is required for the GMax and GMe when exercises are performed in the weight-bearing position.[93] The extent of GMax activation is influenced by trunk positioning. For example, a forward lunge with the trunk flexed relative to the hip and pelvis places greater demand on and activation of the GMax than with the trunk extended.[94] In relaxed standing, slight, but

CHAPTER 4 | SPINE OSTEOLOGY AND ARTHROLOGY   85

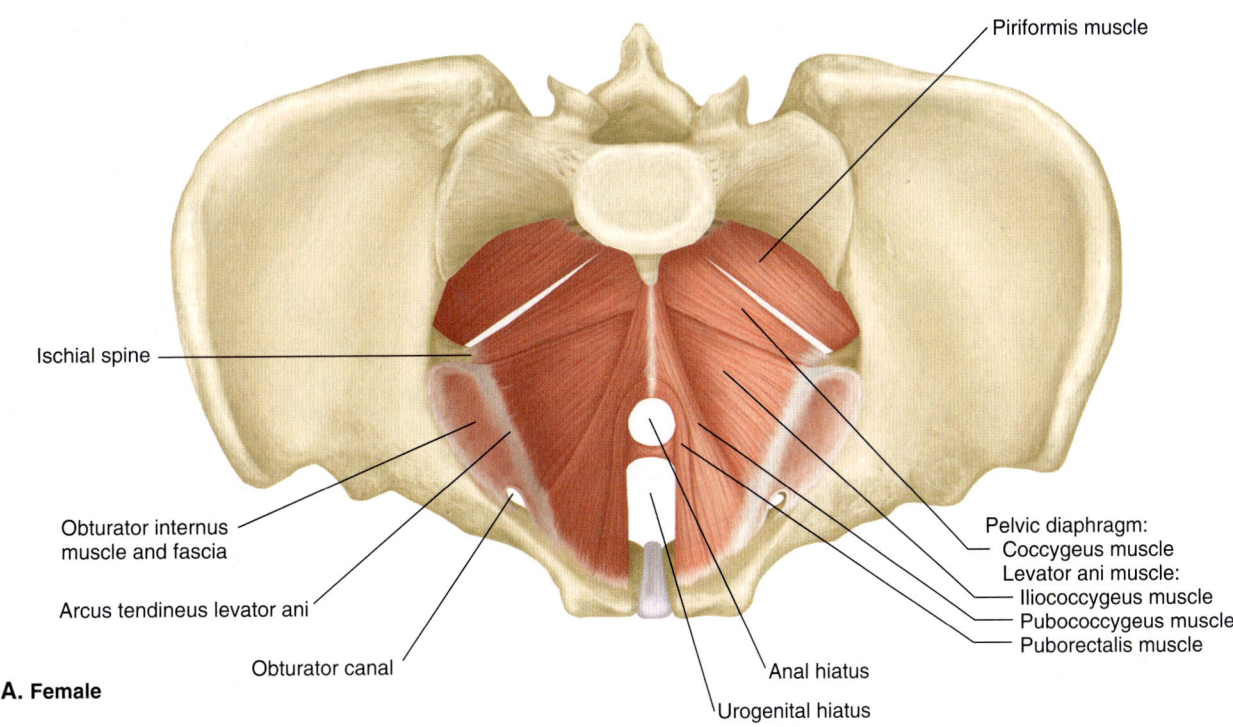

A. Female

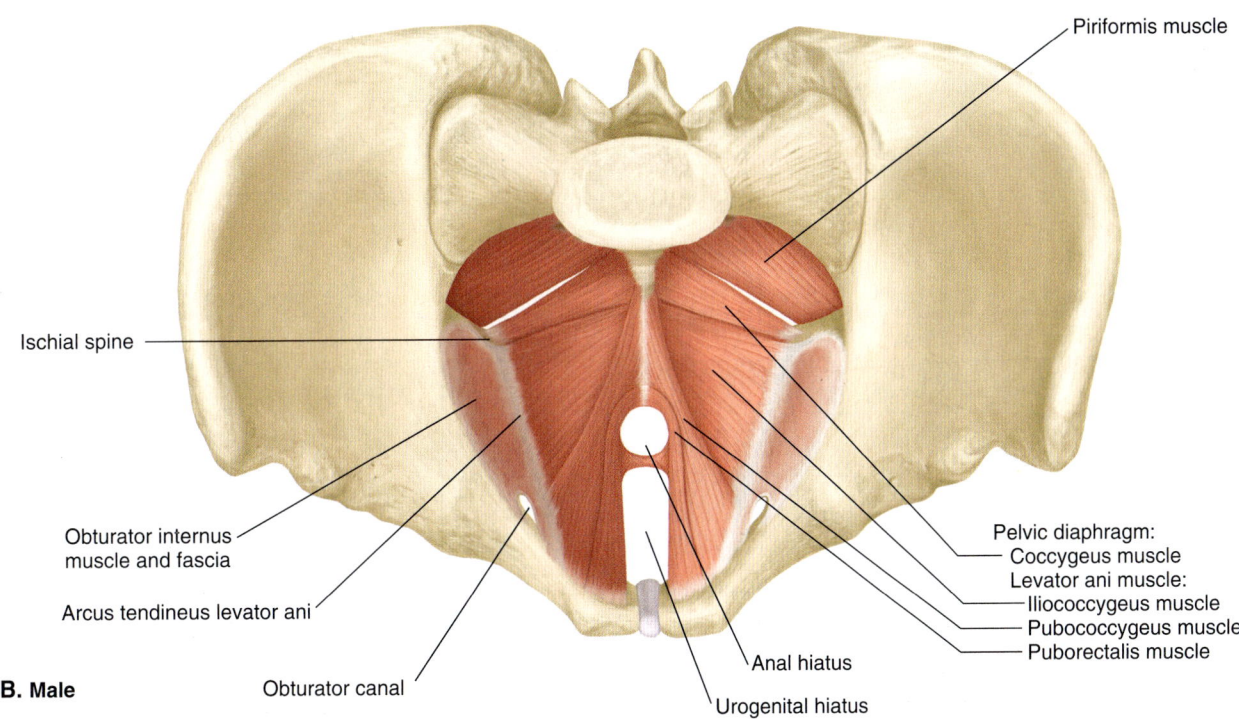

B. Male

FIGURE 4-40 Pelvic floor muscles, superior view. **A.** Female. **B.** Male. (Gest TR. *Lippincott Atlas of Anatomy*. 2nd ed. Wolters Kluwer; 2020; Plate 6-24.)

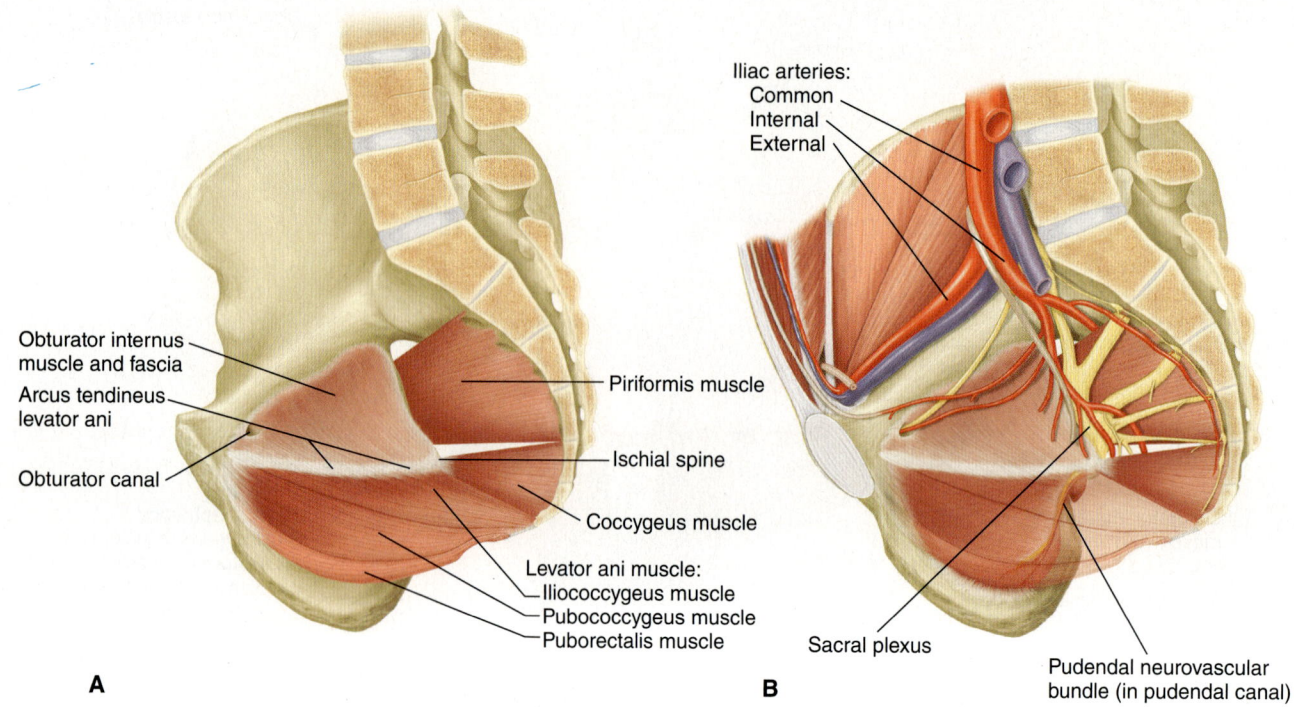
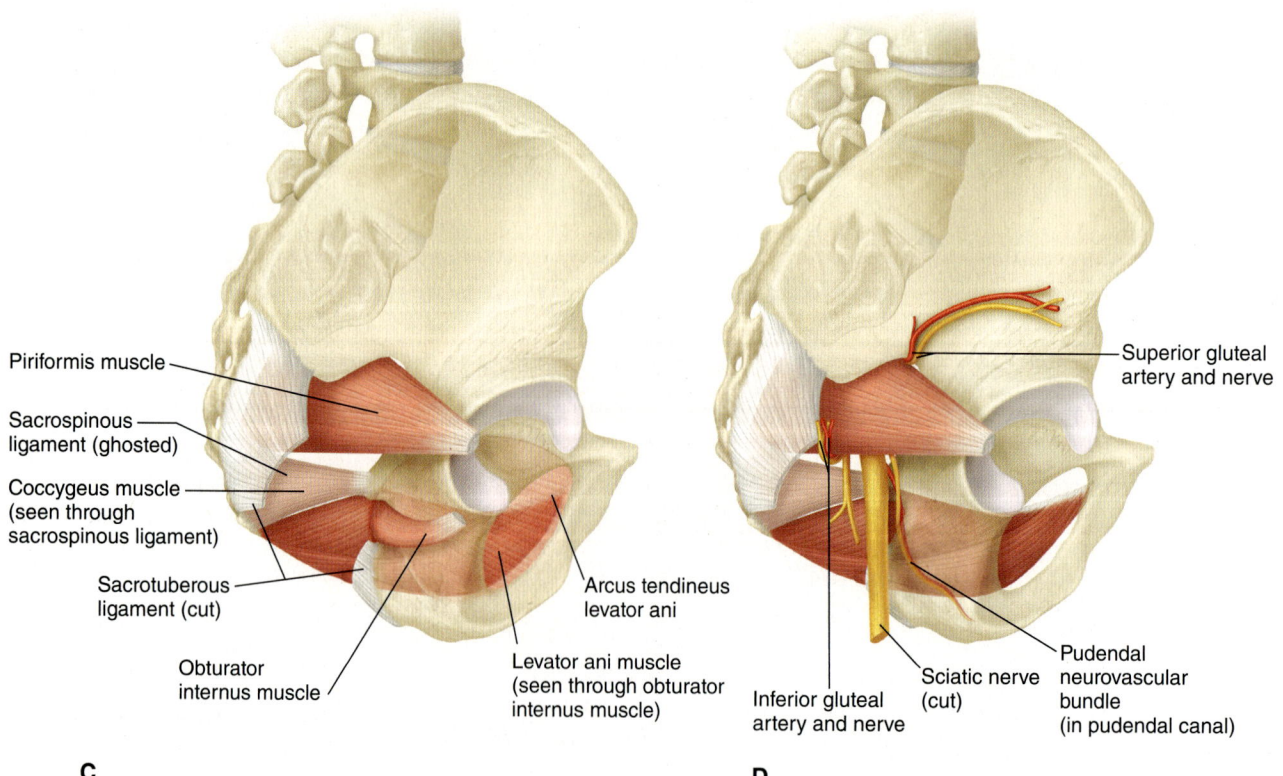

FIGURE 4-41 Pelvic floor muscles. **A** and **B**. Medial view. **C** and **D**. Lateral view. Relationships to nerves and vessels (**B** and **D**) (Gest TR. *Lippincott Atlas of Anatomy*. 2nd ed. Wolters Kluwer; 2020; Plate 6-25.)

CHAPTER 4 | SPINE OSTEOLOGY AND ARTHROLOGY 87

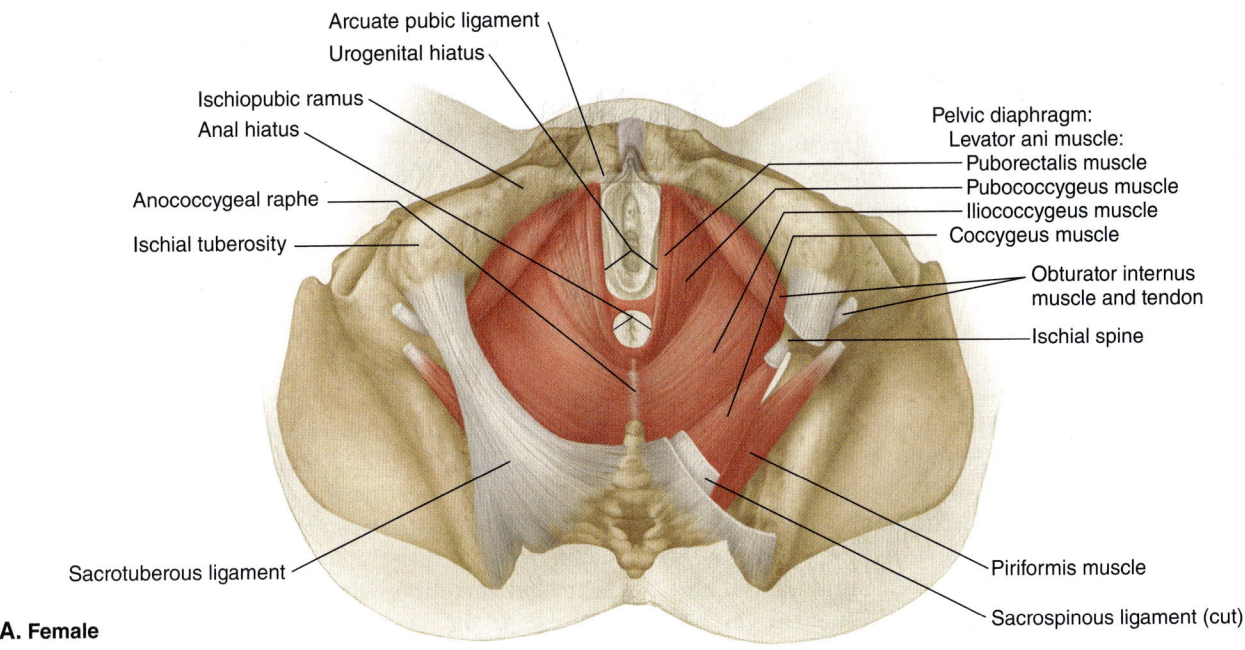

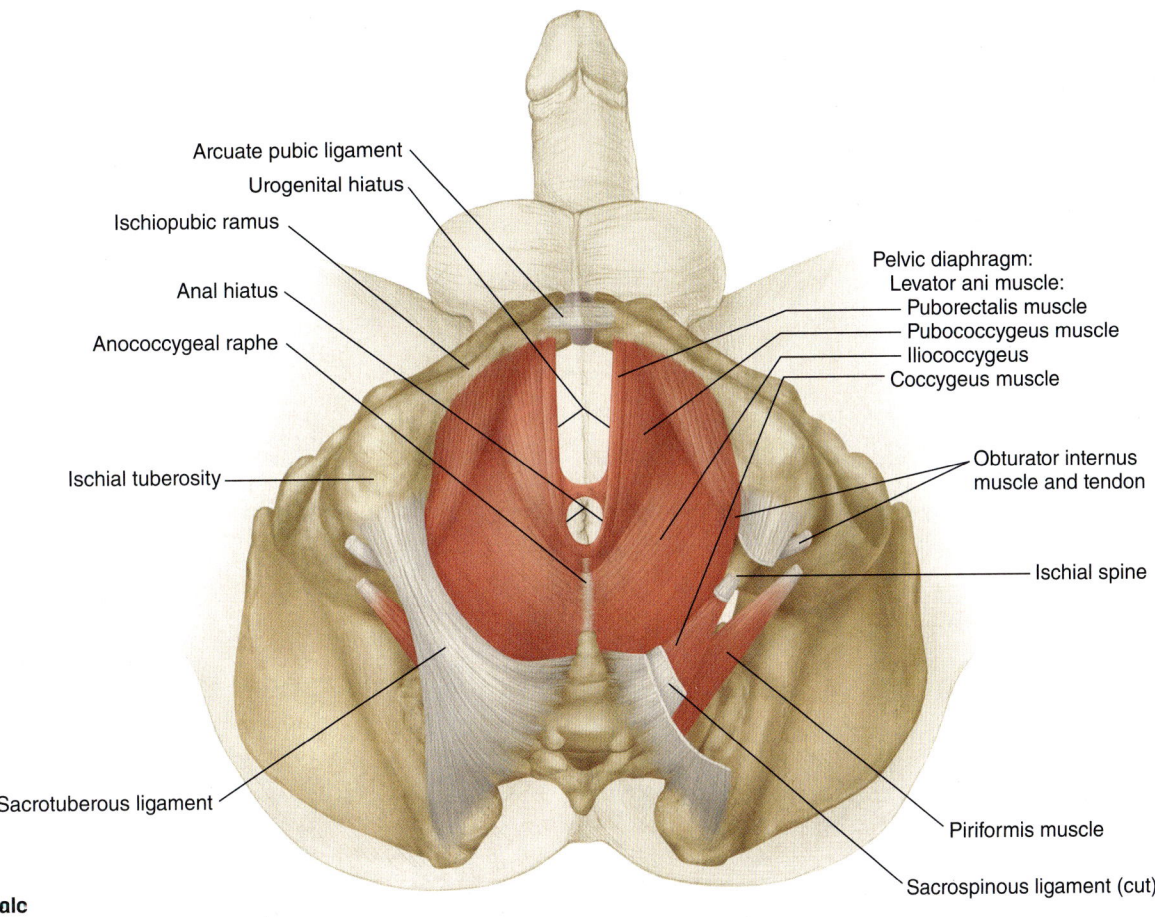

FIGURE 4-42 Pelvic floor muscles, inferior view. **A.** Female. **B.** Male. (Gest TR. *Lippincott Atlas of Anatomy*. 2nd ed. Wolters Kluwer; 2020; Plate 6-26.)

constant activity in superficial muscles of the back and abdomen is present, supporting the idea that opposing muscles act as "guy wires" on the torso.[95] While intermittent bursts of EMG activity can be seen in standing,[95,96] investigations of standing in a completely relaxed posture indicate some activity, even if slight.[95] The torso is unlikely totally balanced in upright by passive mechanisms.

Suboccipital Muscles

The muscle compartments of the suboccipital region are located just inferior to the external occipital protuberance of the occiput and deep to the trapezius, splenius, and semispinalis muscles (Fig. 4-43). The suboccipital muscle attachments include the posterior skull and the C1 and C2 vertebrae. See Table 4-8 for attachments. All of the suboccipital muscles are innervated by the posterior ramus of C1 spinal nerve, the suboccipital nerve. The suboccipital nerve emerges in the suboccipital triangle near the vertebral artery (see Fig. 4-43). The obliquus capitis inferior is the only one of these muscles with no attachment to the skull. The suboccipital muscles are primarily postural muscles,[97] with actions on the head. These small muscles are important to stabilize the upper cervical spine where, when only the larger muscles are used, focal areas of instability develop during normal motion.[98]

Anterior and Lateral Neck Muscles

In addition to the suboccipitals, muscles acting on the head and neck (Table 7-8) are located anterior, posterior, and lateral. The suprahyoid and infrahyoid muscles act mostly as accessory muscles of swallowing and mastication. Through their action as stabilizers of the hyoid bone, these muscles help improve flexion of the neck.[99-101] The action of the sternocleidomastoid (SCM) muscle on the head and neck depends on whether the muscle is acting bilaterally or unilaterally. With bilateral contraction, the SCM can act in a variety of ways: to extend the head at the C1/C2 vertebrae; flex the upper cervical vertebra so that the neck is flexed and the chin is brought to the manubrium; or extend the upper cervical vertebrae while flexing the inferior vertebrae, thus thrusting the chin forward while the head is kept level.[89] Acting unilaterally, the SCM acts to laterally flex the neck to the same side while rotating the head so that the face turns upward toward the contralateral side. Pathology of the SCM or its innervation may result in torticollis in which the cervical muscles contract or shorten

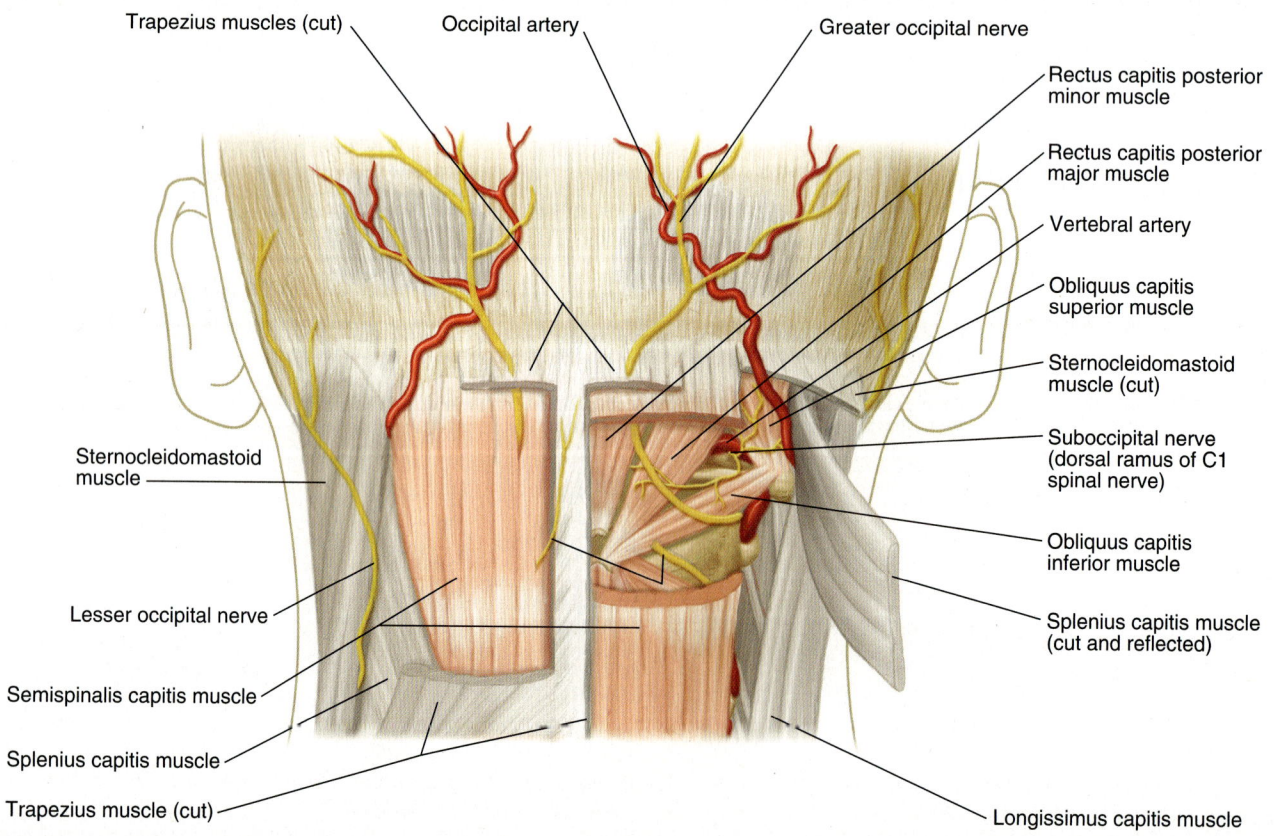

FIGURE 4-43 Suboccipital triangle. Muscles, nerves, and blood vessels. (Gest TR. *Lippincott Atlas of Anatomy*. 2nd ed. Wolters Kluwer; 2020; Plate 1-17.)

TABLE 4-8
MUSCLES ACTING ON HEAD AND NECK

Muscle Group	Muscles	Origin/Superior Attachment	Insertion/Inferior Attachment	Main Action on Vertebral Column or Scapulae
Suboccipital muscles	Rectus capitis posterior major	Spinous process C2 vertebra	Occiput: lateral part of inferior nuchal line	Bilateral contraction: extend C1/C2 Unilateral contraction: rotate C1/C2 to same side as head is rotated
	Rectus capitis posterior minor	Posterior tubercle of C1 vertebra	Occiput: medial part of inferior nuchal line	
	Obliquus capitis inferior	Posterior tubercle of C2 vertebra	Transverse process of C1 vertebra	
	Obliquus capitis superior	Transverse process of C1 vertebra	Occiput: between superior and inferior nuchal lines	Extend C1/C2
Suprahyoid muscles	Geniohyoid Stylohyoid Digastric	Mandible, temporal bone, or mandible	Hyoid	Flex neck*
Infrahyoid muscles	Sternohyoid Omohyoid Sternothyroid Thyrohyoid	Sternum, clavicle, scapula, or thyroid cartilage	Hyoid	Flex neck*
Sternoclei-domastoid		Lateral surface of mastoid process of temporal bone and lateral half of superior nuchal line	Sternal head: anterior surface of manubrium of sternum Clavicular head: superior surface of medial third of clavicle	Unilateral contraction: laterally flex neck* and rotates it so that face is turned superiorly toward opposite side Bilateral contraction: extends neck at atlanto-occipital joints; flexes cervical vertebrae so that chin approaches manubrium; extends superior cervical vertebrae so chin is thrust forward with head kept level
Trapezius		Medial third of superior nuchal line, external occipital protuberance, nuchal ligament, spinous processes C7-T12 vertebrae, and lumbar and sacral spinous processes	Lateral third of clavicle, acromion, and spine of scapula	Elevates, retracts, and rotates scapula superiorly Superior fibers: elevate scapula/shoulders Middle fibers: retract scapulae Inferior fibers: depress scapulae Superior and inferior fibers working together: rotate scapulae superiorly With shoulders fixed, bilateral contraction extends neck; unilateral contraction produces lateral flexion to same side†
Prevertebral muscles	Longus colli	Anterior tubercle C1 vertebra; bodies of C1-C3 and transverse processes of C3-C6 vertebrae	Bodies of C5-T3 vertebrae; transverse processes of C3-C5 vertebrae	Flexes neck with rotation to opposite side, if acting unilaterally*
	Longus capitis	Occipital bone	Anterior tubercles of C3-C6 transverse processes	Flexes head†
	Rectus capitis anterior	Base of cranium	Lateral mass of C1, anterior surface	
	Anterior scalene	Transverse processes C3-C6 vertebrae	First rib	
Lateral vertebral muscles	Rectus capitis lateralis	Occipital bone	Transverse process C1 vertebra	Flexes and helps stabilize head†
	Splenius capitis	Inferior half of nuchal ligament and spinous processes of T1-T6 vertebrae	Lateral portion of superior nuchal line; lateral aspect of mastoid process	Laterally flex and rotates head and neck to the same side; acting bilaterally, extends head and neck**
	Levator scapulae	Posterior tubercles of transverse processes C2-C6 vertebrae	Superior part of medial border of scapula	Downward rotation of scapula; tilts glenoid cavity inferiorly
	Middle scalene	Posterior tubercles of transverse processes C5-C7 vertebrae	Superior surface of first rib	Flexes neck laterally*; elevates first rib during forced inspiration
	Posterior scalene		External surface of second rib	Flexes neck laterally*; elevates second rib during forced inspiration

* Flex neck = anterior (or lateral) bending of C2-C7 vertebrae.
† Flex head = anterior (or lateral) bending of head relative to vertebral column at atlanto-occipital joints.
** Rotation of head occurs at atlantoaxial joints.

causing the head to tilt in the position of a unilateral contraction. The condition may occur prenatally due to intrauterine impairment of the SCM, a fibrous tissue tumor, or during birth if the infant's head is pulled and the SCM is injured.[102,103] In adults, spasmodic torticollis (cervical dystonia) may occur with characteristics of involuntary contraction of neck muscles, resulting in a disabling, abnormal head posture.[104,105] The trapezius acts on the head and neck when the shoulders are fixed. The prevertebral muscles enable fine movements of the head and neck. These muscles are richly supplied with mechanoreceptors that are largely integrated into the muscles' strong proprioceptive function and implicated in the production of dizziness in patients with dysfunction in this region.[106] The large muscles in the cervical spine region are active intermittently, primarily playing a role in torque production, whereas the deeper muscles show more continuous activity, consistent with a tonic supportive role.[97]

PALPATION

Most of the bones and many of the muscles surrounding the vertebral column can be palpated. General landmarks are helpful to guide the clinician in determining vertebral levels (Fig. 4-44). For example, the vertebral border of the scapula is approximately 2 inches (the width of three fingers) from the spinous processes of the thoracic vertebra. Horizontal lines connecting key bony landmarks provide a guide to identifying the following spinous processes:

- Root of the scapular spines (T3)
- Inferior scapular angles (T7)
- Top of the iliac crests (L4/L5 interspace)

The PSIS lies just inferior and lateral to the skin dimples near the junction of the sacrum and ilium. A horizontal line connecting the PSIS lies at the S2 spinous process.

The spinous processes of most vertebrae can be felt in the midline of the neck and back, particularly when the neck and trunk are positioned in flexion. The long spinous processes of the C6, C7, and T1 vertebrae are quite prominent. The long inferiorly sloping spinous processes of the thoracic spine can be appreciated. In relatively thin individuals, the transverse process and ribs in the thoracic region are identifiable.

With the patient sitting and leaned forward, the spinous processes of the lumbar spine can be felt. Specific guidance to palpation can be found in Chapter 12, Lumbar Spine and Sacroiliac Joint, and Chapter 17, Cervical and Thoracic Spine.

KINEMATICS

The spinal motion segment, the smallest functional unit of the spine, allows a combination of movements that are restrained by the bony structure and surrounding soft tissues.[107] In the vertebral column, the IVD and facets[108] work together to constrain spinal kinematics. Additional restraint is provided by joint capsules and ligaments. As indicated previously in this chapter, with a few exceptions, movement occurring at any isolated intervertebral joint is relatively small. However, when motion is added across all moveable segments of the vertebral column, the overall movement is quite large (see Fig. 4-14).[9]

Spinal Coupling

Classically, lateral flexion and rotation movement in the spine is considered "coupled" movement, meaning that a motion about an axis occurs concurrently with (couples with) another motion whose axis is in another plane. With coupled motions, one motion cannot occur without the other.[109] Ipsilateral coupling is when lateral flexion and rotation occur in the same direction. An example of cervical spine ipsilateral coupled movement is depicted in Figure 4-45 where left lateral flexion is accompanied by left rotation. Likewise, left rotation is accompanied by left lateral flexion. An example of contralateral coupling is left lateral flexion with right rotation and vice versa.

In the C2 through C7 vertebrae, the angle of the facet joints to the horizontal and frontal planes (see Fig. 4-15) suggests that the movements are ipsilaterally coupled in this region.[110] For example, the left superior facet joint of C3 is in the same orientation as the right inferior facet joints of all cervical vertebrae below this level. The ipsilateral coupling of movements in the mid- to lower cervical region[111] and in the majority of the thoracic spine is generally accepted.

In a critical analysis of the literature, Legaspi and Edmund[109] describe controversial coupling studies in the lumbar spine. Although many studies report coupling exists, there is little agreement on whether coupling is ipsilateral or contralateral or both, depending on the sagittal plane position of the lumbar spine.[109,111-113] The lack of consensus on the presence or direction of coupling in the lumbar spine challenges the use of the term in discussion of lumbar spine motion.

Movement and Impact on Neural Structures

Movement impacts the available free space within the vertebral canal and IV foramina. With flexion of the neck and back, the spinal cord is stretched over anteriorly located bony and ligamentous structures. Flexion increases the size of the intervertebral foramen. With an extended position, the space within the vertebral canal and foramina is more limited than in neutral.[114] With rotation, the size of the IV foramen decreases on the side of the direction of the rotation and increases on the contralateral side.[115] A reduction in the IV foramen size occurs ipsilateral to the side of lateral flexion and increases on the contralateral side. A reduction in free space within the vertebral canal or IV foramen may potentially compromise neural structures when space is limited.[114]

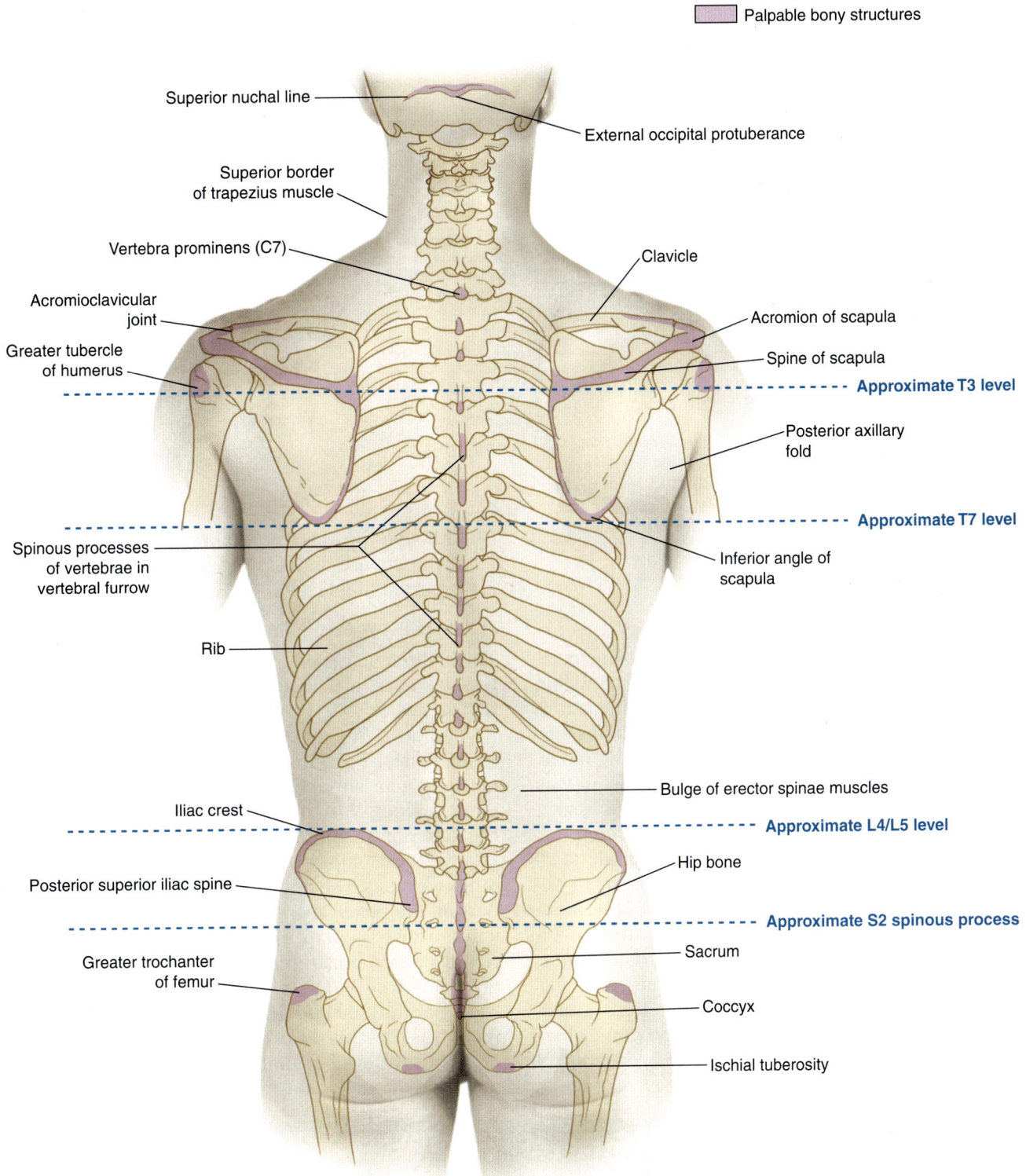

FIGURE 4-44 Major palpable bony landmarks of spine, posterior view. (Gest TR. *Lippincott Atlas of Anatomy*. 2nd ed. Wolters Kluwer; 2020; Plate 1-02.)

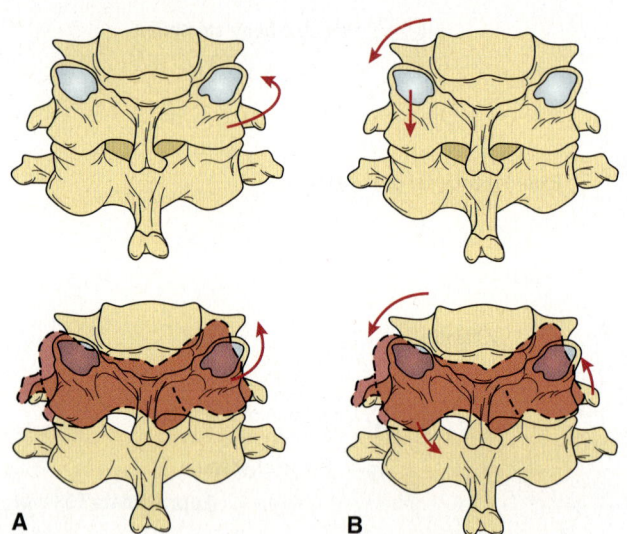

FIGURE 4-45 Example of ipsilateral coupling, posterior view. **(A)** Left rotation with left sidebending. **(B)** Left sidebending with left rotation. (Adapted from Oatis CA. *Kinesiology: The Mechanics and Pathomechanics of Human Movement.* 3rd ed. Wolters Kluwer; 2017; Figures 26.18 and 26.19.)

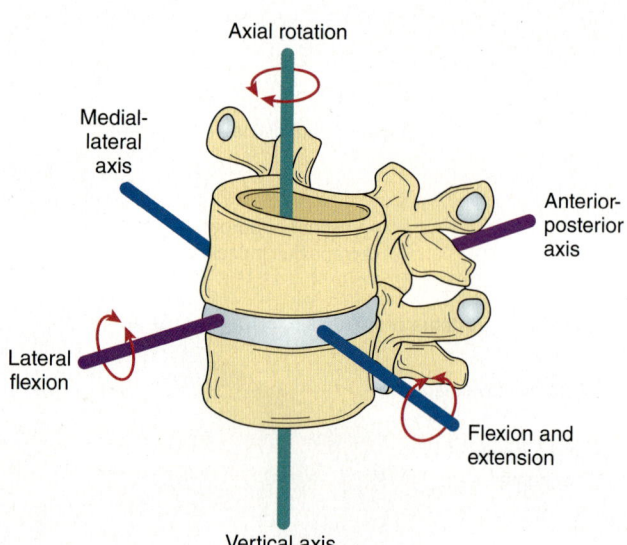

FIGURE 4-46 Osteokinematic movement of the vertebral column.

Osteokinematic Movement

As described in Chapter 3, Arthrology, osteokinematic movement is classically described as a rotation within the sagittal, frontal, or horizontal plane, with the axis of motion occurring through or near the articulating surfaces (Fig. 4-46).[116] In the spine, osteokinematic movement is considered at the "interbody joint" defined as the IVD with the adjacent vertebral bodies and associated endplates.[9] Movement in the vertebral column is described from superior to inferior, in anatomic position, with reference to the direction of movement determined by a point on the anterior side of the more superior vertebral segment. For example, with a C4–C5 right axial rotation, the C4 vertebral body rotates right, whereas the spinous process of C4 moves to the left. Varying reports exist regarding normal spinal movement because of differences in study methods and characteristics of participants, such as age and gender.[117-119]

Although the exact normal range of motion values for the spine are difficult to establish, general trends are reported (Table 4-9).

Arthrokinematic Movement

The arthrokinematics of IV motion describes the motion between articular facets.[9] The facet joints are flat or nearly flat. Terms to describe arthrokinematic motion at the facet joints include approximation (compression) of joint surfaces, separation (gapping) between joint surfaces, and sliding (gliding) between joint surfaces. With flexion, the inferior facet joints of the superior vertebra slide superiorly and anteriorly relative to the superior articular facet joints of the inferior vertebra. The opposite occurs with extension. In flexion, the posterior ligaments are taut, whereas the anterior disc is compressed. With extension, the anterior ligaments are stretched, whereas the posterior annular fibers of the IVD are compressed. With rotation, sliding at the articular surfaces occurs in the same direction as the rotation of the vertebral body. Examples of sliding at the facet joints are shown in Figure 4-47.

TABLE 4-9

GENERAL TRENDS IN REPORTED RANGE OF MOTION IN SPINAL REGION

Joint or Region	Flexion	Extension	Total Arc in Sagittal Plane	Rotation	Lateral Flexion
Atlanto-occipital joint	5°	10°	15°	Negligible	5°
Atlantoaxial joint complex	5°	10°	15°	30–40°	Negligible
Cervical (C2–C7)	35–40°	55–60°	90–100°	30–35°	30–35°
Thoracic	30–40°	15–20°	45–60°	25–35°	25–30°
Lumbar	45–55°	15–25°	60–80°	5–7°	20°

Adapted from Neumann D. *Kinesiology of the Musculoskeletal System: Foundations for Rehabilitation.* 3rd ed. Elsevier; 2017.

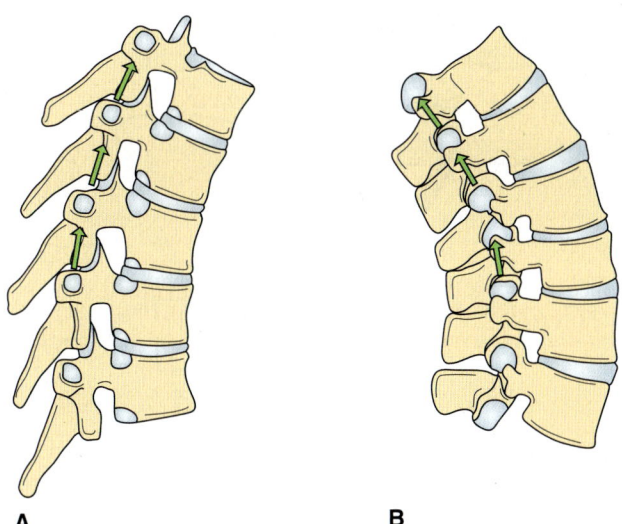

FIGURE 4-47 Examples of sliding at facet joints with flexion and extension. Flexion in thoracic spine **(A)** and extension in lumbar spine **(B)**.

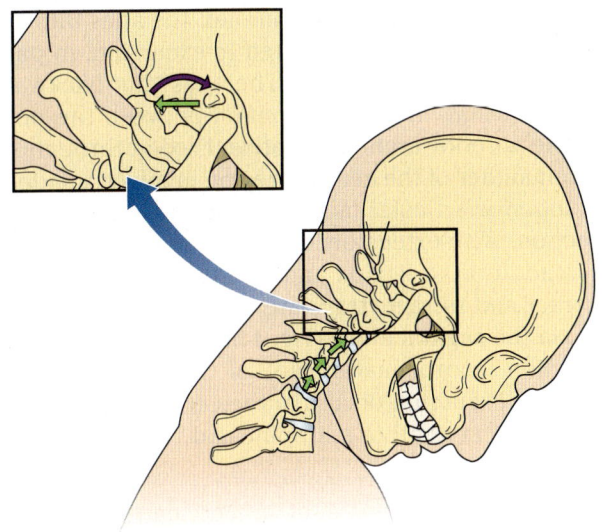

FIGURE 4-48 Sagittal plane flexion of head and neck demonstrating the roll (purple arrow) and slide (green arrow) motions of atlanto-occipital, atlantoaxial, and intracervical regions.

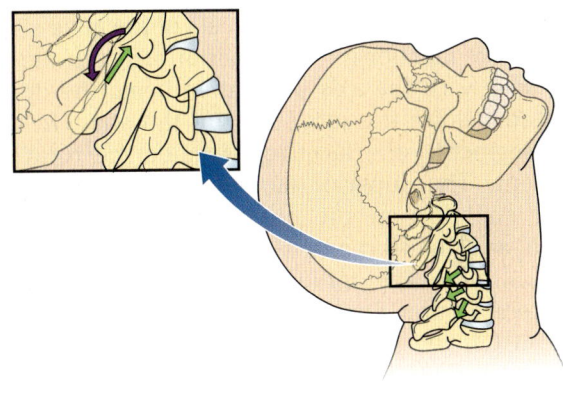

FIGURE 4-49 Sagittal plane extension of head and neck demonstrating the roll (purple arrow) and slide (green arrow) motions of atlanto-occipital, atlantoaxial, and intracervical regions.

Osteokinematic and Arthrokinematic Movement by Region

The distinctive bony features of each region of the vertebral column lead to unique available osteokinematic and arthrokinematic movements in each region.

Movement in Cervical Region The cervical region is the most mobile within the entire vertebral column. The osteokinematic movements are flexion, extension, rotation, and lateral sidebending. The atypically shaped C1 and C2 vertebrae facilitate precise positioning of the head to allow adjustments for seeing, hearing, and equilibrium.

Sagittal Plane Movement in Cervical Region The sagittal plane osteokinematic and arthrokinematic movements of the cervical region are flexion and extension at the atlanto-occipital, atlantoaxial, and intracervical (C2–C7) levels. Though variable, the amount of extension typically exceeds that of flexion by a ratio of 1.5:1. Approximately 25% of sagittal plane motion occurs at the atlanto-occipital and atlantoaxial joints, with the rest occurring throughout the remainder of the cervical spine. In addition, protraction and retraction occur. The sagittal kinematic movements of the atlanto-occipital, atlantoaxial, and C2–C7 vertebrae are depicted in Figures 4-48 and 4-49.

At the atlanto-occipital joint, the deep concavity of the atlas lateral masses limits translation of the convex occipital condyles in a lateral, anterior, and posterior direction, but permits nodding movements of the occiput on the atlas, as in an affirmative "yes" gesture. With flexion of the head on the atlas, the occipital condyles roll forward and the occipital condyles concurrently translate downward and backward.[120] Without the concurrent downward and backward slide, the occipital condyles would roll up and over the anterior wall of the socket.[121] The opposite occurs with extension of the head on the atlas. Following typical convex-on-concave rules, an expected slide opposite the direction of roll occurs.[9] The extent of the roll and slide is limited by tension in the articular capsule, the atlanto-occipital membranes, and alar ligaments.

At the atlantoaxial joint complex, the atlas tilts forward with flexion, but is limited in excursion, in part, by the transverse ligament. The atlas tilts backward with extension, limited by contact between the dens and the anterior arch of the atlas. Flexion throughout the remainder of the cervical region involves a slide of the superior articular facet in a superior and anterior direction. With extension, the opposite occurs.

In addition to flexion and extension, the head can protract and retract (translate anteriorly and posteriorly) in the sagittal plane (Fig. 4-50). With protraction/retraction, approximately 60% of the anterior/posterior head excursion occurs in the cervical spine, with 30% in the cervicothoracic spine and 10% in the lower thoracic regions.[122]

Horizontal Plane Movement in Cervical Region The movement of axial rotation in the cervical region occurs primarily at the atlantoaxial joint (Fig. 4-51), with the remainder occurring throughout the rest of the cervical spine.[110,123,124] Little rotational movement occurs at the atlanto-occipital joint due to the shape of the occipital condyles. The shape of the atlantoaxial joint complex is ideal for rotational movement. The relatively flat inferior articular facets of the atlas slide in an arc-like manner on the superior articular facets of the axis, with the axis of rotation being the dens. The head follows the movement of the atlas. In the C2–C7 segments, the facet joints guide the rotation movement. The superior facets slide anterior and slightly superior on the contralateral side to the rotation and inferior and slightly posterior on the ipsilateral side. The rotation movement is coupled with lateral flexion. For example, during right rotation of C3 on C4, the right inferior articular facet of C3 slides inferior and posterior, whereas the left inferior articular facet slides anterior and slightly superior on the corresponding superior articular facets of C4.

Frontal Plane Movement in the Cervical Region The frontal plane movement of lateral flexion occurs primarily in the C2–C7 portion of the cervical spine. Approximately 5° of lateral flexion occurs at the atlanto-occipital joint, whereas little to no lateral flexion movement occurs at the atlantoaxial joint complex. Refer to Figure 4-52. With lateral flexion, there is a small amount of rolling of the convex occipital condyles on

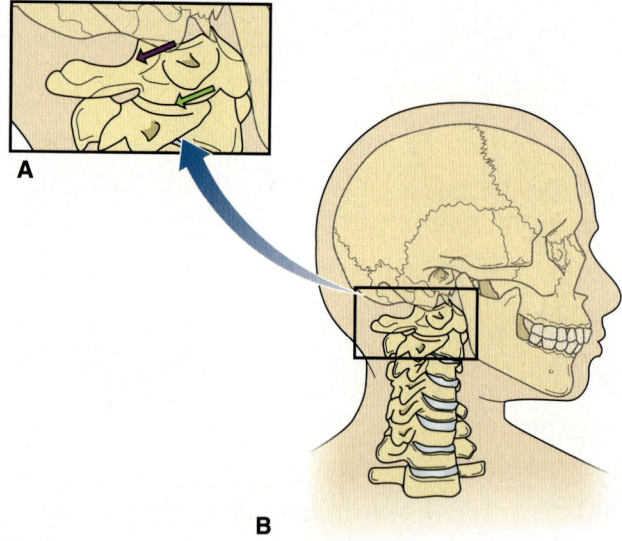

FIGURE 4-51 Cervical rotation **(A)** Close-up at atlantoaxial complex, with roll (*purple arrow*) and slide (*green arrow*). **(B)** Intracervical region (C2-C7), anterior view.

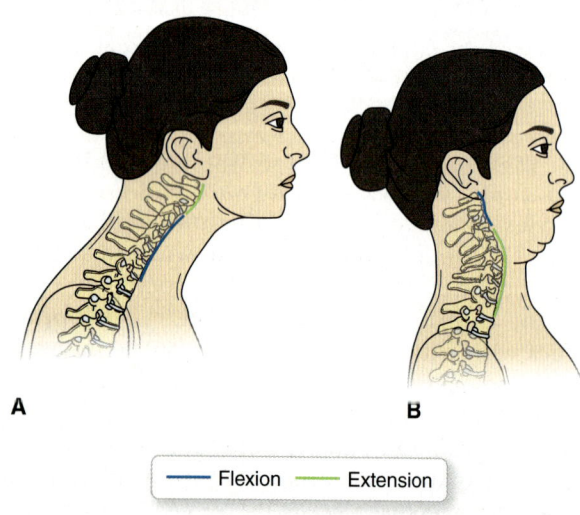

FIGURE 4-50 Cervical protraction **(A)**, retraction **(B)**.

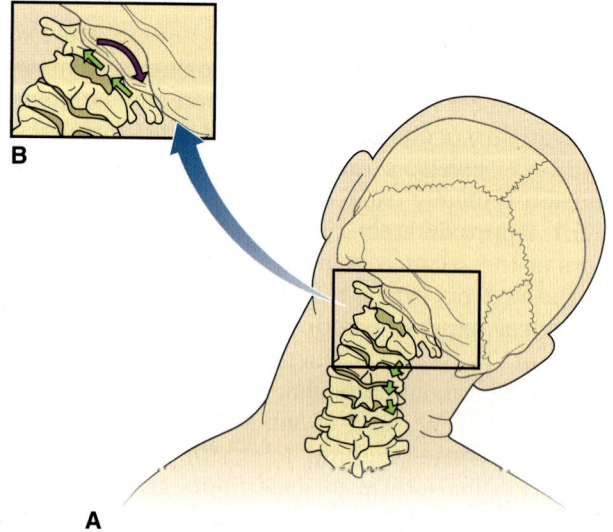

FIGURE 4-52 Cervical lateral flexion, posterior view. **A.** Intracervical region **B.** Atlanto-occipital joint, close-up with roll (*purple arrow*) and slide (*green arrow*).

the superior articular facets of the atlas. Considering a typical convex-on-concave movement pattern, the occipital condyles slide opposite the direction of the roll. With lateral flexion at C2–C7, the superior and inferior articular facets slide in the same direction as rotation. For example, with left lateral flexion of C4 on C5, the left inferior articular facet of C4 slides inferior and posterior, whereas the right inferior articular facet slides superior and anterior on the corresponding superior articular facets of C5.

Movement in Thoracic Region The attachment of the ribs to the thoracic vertebrae limits movement of the region and provides a stable base for muscle to control the cervical region, protect the organs, and support breathing. In both the thoracic and lumbar regions, movement occurs in all three planes, with the direction and extent of movement influenced by the resting posture, orientation of the facets, and height of the IVDs. The thin discs in the thoracic region contribute to the overall stability of the region. The arthrokinematic movement in the thoracic region is similar to the cervical region (Figs. 4-48, 4-49, 4-51, and 4-52), but with less excursion and slight differences due to the different vertebral shapes, rib attachments, and orientation of the facet joints. The following applies to both the midcervical and majority of the thoracic region:

- Flexion/extension: Inferior articular facet of vertebra above slides superiorly in flexion and inferiorly in extension on superior articular facet of vertebra below.
- Axial rotation: Inferior articular facets of the vertebra above slide in the same direction as the direction of rotation on the superior articular facets of the vertebra below.
- Lateral flexion: Inferior articular facet of vertebra above on ipsilateral side of the direction of lateral flexion (i.e., concave side) slides inferiorly on the superior articular facet of vertebra below. On the contralateral side, the inferior articular facet the vertebra above slides superiorly on the superior articular facet of the vertebra below.

Sagittal Plane Movement in Thoracic Region Greater flexion than extension is available in the thoracic spine (Figs. 4-47 and 4-48). The degree of flexion is limited by tension in the posterior ligaments and the facet joint capsules. Extension is limited by the broad ALL and by the potential approximation of the thoracic spinous processes. The lower thoracic facet joints have a more sagittal plane orientation than the more superior thoracic facet joints, allowing more sagittal plane motion in the inferior thoracic region.[125]

Horizontal Plane Movement in Thoracic Region Throughout the thoracic region, rotation occurs, but with less excursion in the lower segments. As previously discussed, the direction of roll and slide at the facet joints is the same as in the cervical spine. As the thoracolumbar junction is approached, the facet joints are oriented more vertically, contributing to the decreased rotation.

Frontal Plane Movement in Thoracic Region Although the facet joints in the thoracic region are primarily oriented in the frontal plane, suggesting freedom of movement with lateral flexion, the rib attachments limit motion in the frontal plane.

Movement in Lumbar Region The motion in the lumbar spine is similar to that in the thoracic spine (see Table 4-9), but distributed over fewer segments: 5 segments in the lumbar region versus 12 segments in the thoracic region. This indicates mobility is favored over stability in the lumbar region.[125] The lumbar facet joints in each motion segment are not perfectly matched in orientation to neighboring lumbar facet joints,[126] contributing to a greater available range of motion throughout the lumbar spine. The vertical orientation of the facets provides for more bony impact and greater stability during movement.[125] Motion at the L5–S1 segment differs from that of the thoracolumbar and L1–L5 motion segments and is described separately.

Sagittal Plane Movement in Lumbar Region During flexion of the lumbar spine, passive tension increases tension in the posterior connective tissues. With the lower end of the spine fixed, such as during an attempt to touch the toes when long sitting or in standing, the hamstrings are stretched and the lumbar lordosis is reversed. As shown in Figure 4-47B, flexion of the lumbar spine involves superior and anterior sliding of the inferior articular facets. With a progressive increase in flexion, the anterior portion of the disc sustains a mounting compressive load and the posterior ligaments are increasingly stretched, requiring the disc and ligaments to support more of the total spinal load. With full flexion, the facet joints and articular capsules contribute additional restraint to the forward migration of the superior vertebra.[127] While the facet joints carry little to no load in the anatomic position, with flexion beyond 7 to 8°, the load on the facet increases such that at full flexion, the load is similar to the high loads on the facet joints in extension.[128] With full flexion, the load on the contact area within an individual facet joint decreases, resulting in higher contact pressure. With trunk muscle activation in a fully flexed position, the contact pressure in the facet joints rises even more and can potentially damage the facet joint, especially if the high contact pressure must be sustained for a period of time.[9]

Flexion of the lumbar spine increases the size of the vertebral canal and IV foramina,[129] providing more space for exiting spinal nerves.[130] The flexed lumbar spine position may temporarily reduce pressure on an impinged nerve root. However, with excessive or sustained flexion, the passive flexion stiffness of the posterior lumbar tissues decrease,[12,131] and the disc loses fluid.[132] With sustained flexion, a posterior migration of the nucleus pulposus is promoted due to the increased compression of the anterior disc. The risk of low back injury is increased with such positioning.[133] While the annulus fibrosis of a healthy disc may be able to contain the nucleus pulposus, a disc with weak, cracked, or fissured annular layers may bulge or break open in a posterior or posterolateral direction, resulting in impingement on the PLL, spinal cord, or nerve root. Refer to the section on HNP later in this chapter.

With lumbar extension, the facets of the superior vertebra slide posterior and inferior (approximate) on the facets of the inferior vertebra. The forces acting on the facet joints[128] and contact pressures within the facet joints increase with extension.[134] A sustained hyperextended posture may place a damaging stress on the facet joints, contributing to low back pain. The size of the IV foramen and vertebral canal decreases with extension,[129] and the nucleus tends to deform anteriorly.[135] With lumbar flexion, the facet joints distract, and the nucleus tends to deform posteriorly.

Many functional activities require movement in the sagittal plane with interaction between the trunk and the lumbar spine and between the pelvis and the femurs (hips). Examples include bending over to pick up a sock, lifting the leg to put on a shoe, and walking up steep steps. The movement between flexion and extension in the lumbar spine should be smooth and rhythmical, with a balance between a reversal of the lumbar lordosis and pelvic rotation.

Horizontal Plane Movement in Lumbar Region Except at the lumbosacral junction, axial rotation in the lumbar spine is significantly limited because of physical restriction (approximation) at the facet joints (Fig. 4-53). The articular cartilage in the contralateral facet joint is compressed, and tension of some of the annular fibers of the IVD increases with axial rotation. Because not all annular fibers are under tension and thus resisting the deformation of the nucleus pulposus with rotation, the IVD is vulnerable to injury with rotational movement.

Front Plane Movement in Lumbar Region Lateral flexion in the lumbar spine is limited, but to a lesser extent than axial rotation. The ligaments on the side opposite the lateral flexion become taut, further restricting motion.

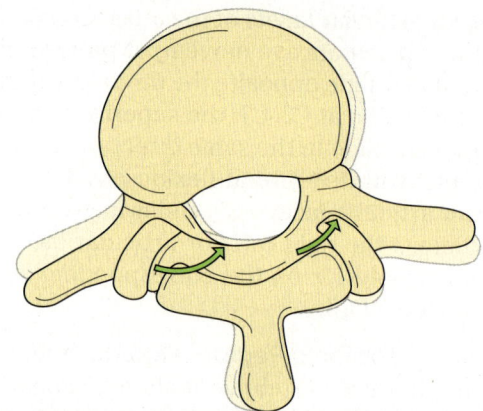

FIGURE 4-53 Horizontal plane kinematics depicted in lumbar spine, superior view.

COMMON PATHOLOGIES OF THE VERTEBRAL COLUMN

Several spinal pathologies have been discussed previously in this chapter to include osteoporosis, abnormal curvatures, abnormal alignment, torticollis, and fractures. This section discusses degenerative disc disease (DDD), HNP, and spinal stenosis. The reader is referred to Chapter 12, Lumbar Spine and Sacroiliac Joint, and Chapter 17, Cervical and Thoracic Spine, for a region-specific discussion of pathologies.

Degenerative Disc Disease

The degenerative process of the IVD, named degenerative disc disease (DDD), begins as early as adolescence, with increasing prevalence with aging.[136] Spinal imaging of persons who are asymptomatic is 50% for ages 30 to 39 and 90% ages 65 years or older.[137] The high prevalence among asymptomatic persons indicates that degenerative changes such as disc deterioration, loss of disc height, disc protrusion, and facet arthropathy are part of normal aging and not necessarily part of a pathologic condition requiring intervention. Although degenerative changes on imaging are observed in persons with chronic low back pain,[138] the degree of degeneration is not associated with the presence or intensity of low back pain or degree of disability.[139-141]

Although degenerative findings on imaging do not necessarily correlate with the severity of symptoms, the clinical presentation of DDD is often neck or back pain. With aging, the nucleus pulposus loses water content,[142] resulting in a disc height reduction and abnormal loading on the IVD, vertebral endplates, and facet joints. The relative composition of the disc changes in response to the altered loading. Macromolecules, such as proteoglycans and collagens, change in proportion throughout the extracellular matrix. An alteration in the biosynthesis of cells responsible for maintaining and repairing the disc, such as metalloproteases, collagenases, and aggrecanases, creates an imbalance between synthesis and degradation. The influx of vascular granulation and sensory nerves along with the release of cytokines and pro-inflammatory cells can result in an imbalance between degeneration and tissue healing, remodeling, and degradation.[143] Scar tissue impairs nutrition to the disc. Contributing factors to DDD,[144,145] in addition to age-related changes, include:

- Genetics
- Lifestyle (e.g., smoking, excessive alcohol consumption, physical inactivity)
- Excessive loading through sport or occupation
- Comorbidities (e.g., diabetes, obesity)
- Injury

Degenerative changes may lead to chronic instability of spinal segments, functional changes, and greater susceptibility to injury.[136] In summary, the multifactorial process of DDD includes an abnormal cell–mediated response to structural alterations and failure (Fig. 4-54),[20] with an end result of asymptomatic or symptomatic DDD. Symptomatic DDD may present as neck or back pain, with or without radiculopathy, and with varying degrees of disability.[146]

Herniated Nucleus Pulposus

The term **herniated nucleus pulposus** (aka herniated disc) typically refers to a posterior or posterolateral migration of the disc nucleus against sensitive neural tissue, such as the spinal cord, cauda equina, anterior or posterior nerve roots, or spinal nerve (Fig. 4-55). In addition, vertebral endplate fragments, cartilage, fragmented apophyseal bone, annular tissue, or any combination thereof may dislodge and press against neural structures (Fig. 4-56).[147,148] Although herniation can occur to any disc, the discs of the cervical and lumbar spine are at highest risk due to the lordotic curvature and greater mobility. The disc itself can be a pain generator[149] owing to pressure on innervated portions of the annulus fibrosus.[150] Symptomatic cervical disc herniation (CDH) and lumbar disc herniation (LDH) increase with age, with incidence higher in women than men.[151]

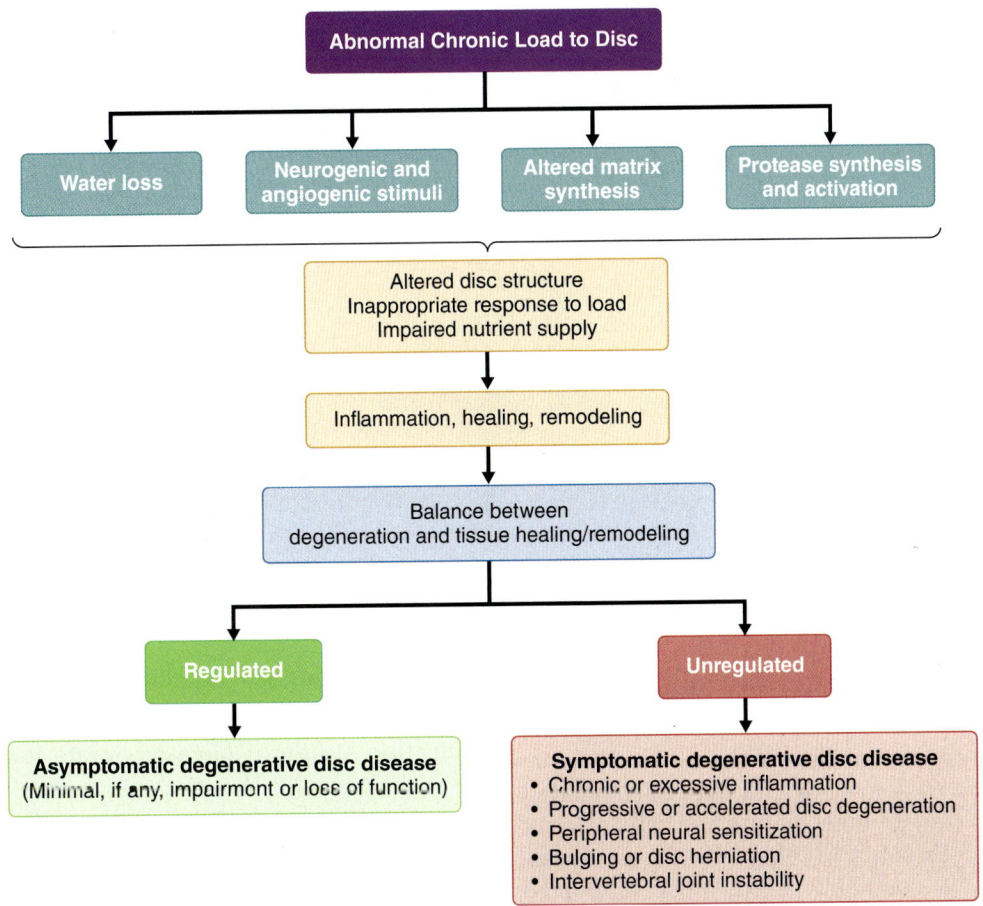

FIGURE 4-54 Degenerative disc disease process.

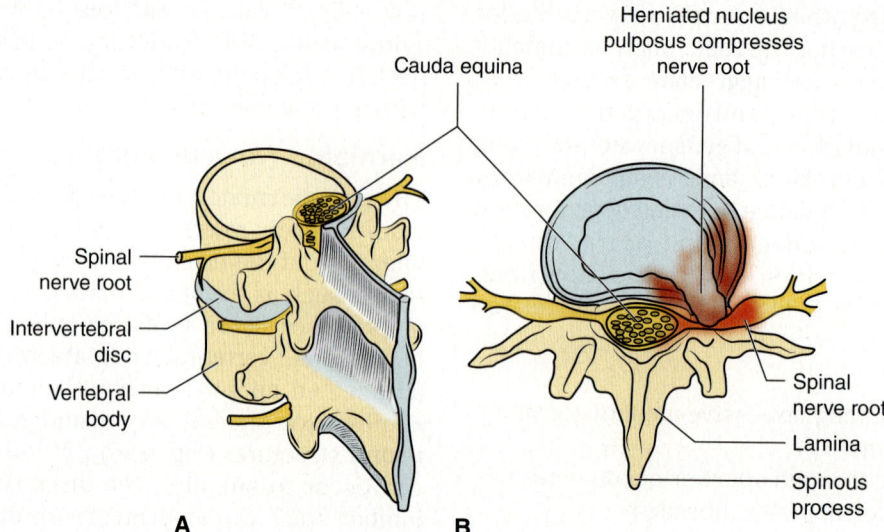

FIGURE 4-55 Intervertebral disc pathology. **A.** Normal lumbar vertebrae, intervertebral disc, and spinal nerve root. **B.** Herniated nucleus pulposus with nerve root compression. (Adapted from Pellico LH. *Focus on Adult Health Medical-Surgical Nursing*. Wolters Kluwer Health; 2013; Figure 46-7.)

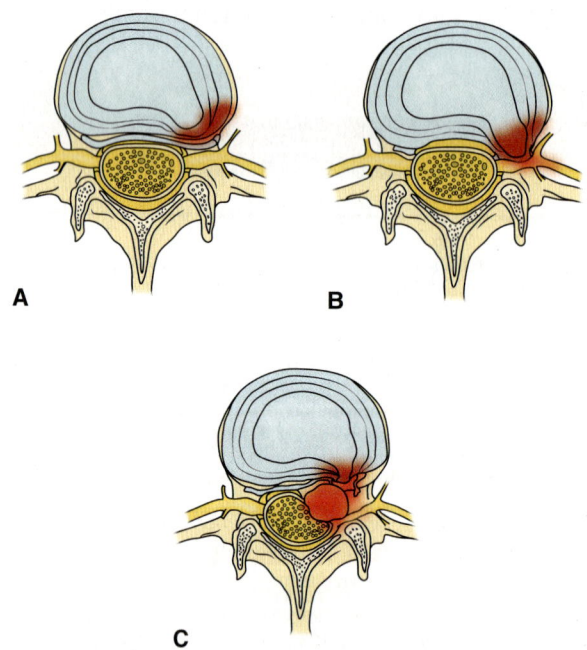

FIGURE 4-56 Superior view of disc depicting pathologic disc conditions. **A.** Bulge. **B.** Rupture/herniation. **C.** Sequestration. (Adapted from Rhee JM, Boden SD. *Operative Techniques in Spine Surgery*. 3rd ed. Wolters Kluwer; 2022; Figure 11.2.)

Classification of Herniated Nucleus Pulposus and Nerve Root Involvement

Classification systems for disc herniation and nerve root involvement evidenced on MRI have been created in an attempt to clarify nomenclature and categories of pathologic involvement.[152-156] Table 4-10 describes classification systems commonly used. Most supported nomenclatures have moderate-to-strong interobserver reliability, though the classification term "disc bulge" is a source of confusion and disagreement.[152,157] The Combined Task Force (CTF)[148,158] and Jensen's classification system[156] have moderate levels of interobserver agreement,[152] with the interobserver agreement on the CTF being slight stronger.[154] The CTF is a pathology-based system providing clarifying nomenclature and classification categories of disc herniation for use among radiologists and other healthcare providers.[148] The CTF-Version 2.0 is a simple classification

TABLE 4-10
DIAGNOSTIC SYSTEMS FOR DISC HERNIATION AND NERVE ROOT PATHOLOGY

Type	System	Terms
Disc herniation	Combined Task Force (CTF)[148]	Diagnostic categories: • Normal • Congenital/developmental variation • Degeneration • Trauma • Infection/inflammation • Neoplasia • Morphologic variant of uncertain significance Diagnostic subcategories used to characterize the interpretation: • Possible • Probable • Definite
	Jensen[156]	Categories: • Normal • Bulge • Protrusion • Extrusion
Nerve root compression	van Rijn[157]	Two grades: • Present • Not present
	Pfirrmann (Pfirrmann, 2004)	Four grades: • No compromise • Contact of disc material with nerve root • Deviation of nerve root • Compression of nerve root

Adapted from Fardon D, Williams A, Dohring E, Murtagh F, Gabriel Rothman S, Sze G. Lumbar disc nomenclature: version 2.0: recommendations of the combined task forces of the North American Spine Society, the American Society of Spine Radiology and the American Society of Neuroradiology. *Spine J.* 2014;14(11):2525-2545; Jensen MC, Brant-Zawadzki MN, Obuchowski N, Modic MT, Malkasian D, Ross JS. Magnetic resonance imaging of the lumbar spine in people without back pain. *N Engl J Med.* 1994;331(2):69-73; van Rijn J, Klemetsö N, Reitsma J, et al. Observer variation in MRI evaluation of patients suspected of lumbar disk herniation. *AJR Am J Roentgenol.* 2005;184(1):299-303; Pfirrmann CW, Dora C, Schmid MR, Zanetti M, Hodler J, Boos N. MR image-based grading of lumbar nerve root compromise due to disk herniation: reliability study with surgical correlation. *Radiology.* 2004;230(2):583-588.

of diagnostic terms, and expansion into more precise subclassifications aids the understanding of reports of imaging studies. Although the CTF focuses on the lumbar spine, the system can be extrapolated for use in the cervical and thoracic spine.[155]

Classification systems of nerve root compression include the van Rijn's classification and the Pfirrmann classification system.[152] No single classification system predominates because of the lack of a reference gold standard against which to determine accuracy of imaging findings and the paucity of the studies to determine clinical application of the systems.

The Michigan State University (MSU) classification was created to assist with surgical decision-making regarding disc herniation. The categories in the MSU classification are based on herniation size and location within the disc. Interobserver reliability was 98% using the criteria. Surgical decisions based on the use of the MSU classification, with smallest lesions excluded from surgical intervention, demonstrate good patient outcomes.[159] Figure 4-57 illustrates the basic MSU classification categories.

Cervical Disc Herniation

CDH is a common source of neck and/or arm pain. Depending on size and location, CDH may lead to cervical

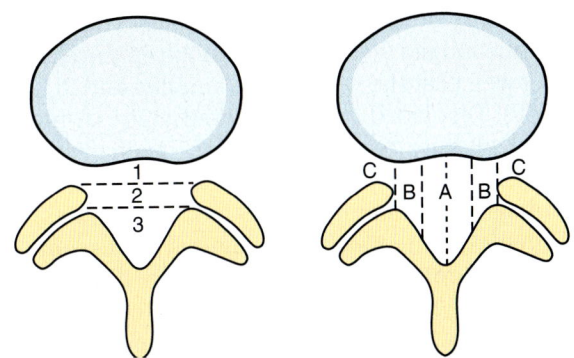

FIGURE 4-57 Michigan State University classification uses size and location of herniated disc to create categories. (Adapted from Mysliwiec L, Cholewicki J, Winkelpleck M, Eis G. MSU classification for herniated lumbar discs on MRI: toward developing objective criteria for surgical selection. *Eur Spine J.* 2010;19(7):1087-1093; Figures 1 and 2.)

radiculopathy. Symptoms include pain that follows a myotomal distribution and sensory symptoms (numbness, burning, tingling) that follow a dermatomal pattern.[160,161] The space-occupying lesion typically encroaches on the spinal nerve in or near the IV foramen. In the cervical spine, the C6 and C7 nerve roots are most commonly affected. Reduced IVD height and degenerative changes to the uncovertebral or facet joints are common factors.[162] An HNP is less the cause of radiculopathy in the cervical spine than the lumbar spine. Tumors or infection of the spine are not common, but may be a causative factor.[163] Careful history taking and physical examination should be conducted with imaging and electrophysiologic studies, as appropriate, to rule out conditions that may mimic cervical radiculopathy. These conditions include peripheral entrapment neuropathy, such as carpal tunnel syndrome; rotator cuff and shoulder disorders; and thoracic outlet syndrome.[149,162]

Thoracic Disc Herniation

Thoracic disc herniation (TDH) is rare. The estimated frequency is 1 per 1,000,000 people.[164] The incidence of asymptomatic TDH is much higher than symptomatic TDH.[165,166] Most asymptomatic thoracic herniated discs are diagnosed incidental to imaging findings. Presenting symptoms of TDH are usually nonspecific, such as pain in the chest wall, upper or lower extremity, or groin.[167] Surgery is considered when conservative treatment fails and in the presence of intractable pain, radiculopathy, or myelopathy symptoms.[168] Compared to CDH and LDH, TDHs rarely necessitate surgery.[169]

Lumbar Disc Herniation

LDH is one of the most common causes of low back pain in the general population.[147] In mild cases, the nucleus demonstrates minor displacement, yet remains contained within the concentric, layered annular fibers. In more moderate-to-severe cases, the nucleus may bulge and protrude past the vertebral body rim. In more extreme cases, the nucleus may extrude into or become lodged (sequestered) in the epidural space, moving well past the walls of the annulus and PLL (see Fig. 4-56). Displaced or sequestered material may be partially or fully resorbed through mechanisms not fully eludicated,[170] but likely involving proteoglycan and phagocytic activity. Extruded and sequestered discs demonstrate more spontaneous regression than bulging or protruding discs, and both have greater possibility of regression than bulging or protruding discs.[171] Although any level can be affected, most LDHs involve the L4–L5 or L5–S1 levels. An HNP between L5 and S1 is shown in Figure 5-58.

Treatment for Herniated Nucleus Pulposus

The first line of treatment for symptomatic HNP is conservative care that includes interventions to restore

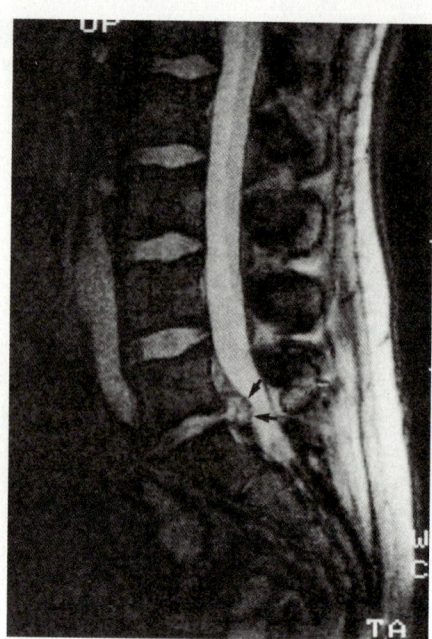

FIGURE 4-58 Magnetic resonance imaging, sagittal view, showing herniated disc (*arrows*). (Dudek RW, Louis TM. *High Yield: Gross Anatomy*. 5th ed. Lippincott Williams & Wilkins; 2015; Figure 1-4A.)

mobility and reduce peripheral symptoms, education/counseling, epidural injections, anti-inflammatory medications, and opioids. Surgery may be required when conservative treatment fails. In the cervical spine, an anterior cervical discectomy with fusion (ACDF) is a common surgical procedure for CDH. Although the ACDF is a relatively safe and effective intervention for persons who fail conservative treatment, it restricts motion at the fused segments, subjecting neighboring segments to higher stress and accelerated degeneration.[172] In the lumbar spine, common surgical procedures include laminotomy, laminectomy, discectomy, microdiscectomy, and spinal fusion. The long-term surgical success rate for LDH is lower than that for CDH.[173] A poor surgical outcome includes failure to relieve symptoms immediately after surgery or recurrence of sciatica/radiculopathy after a pain-free period.[174] Factors contributing to surgical failure include an operation performed at the wrong level, inadequate decompression, spinal instability, and failure to remove a sequestered disc fragment.[175] High-quality prognostic studies with long-term follow-up, clear definitions for inclusion, and the use of valid and reliable outcome measures for the assessment of pain, disability, and quality of life are scarce.[176]

Spinal Stenosis

Spinal stenosis is a general term that includes narrowing of the central, lateral, and foraminal openings of the vertebral column. The decreased size of the central vertebral canal can compress the spinal cord, whereas lateral and foraminal stenosis may compress nerve roots. Spinal stenosis can be congenital (developmental) or acquired or both. Degenerative spinal stenosis is the most common acquired type.[177] Degenerative changes may exacerbate congenital spinal stenosis.[178] Other types of acquired spinal stenosis include spondylitic/spondylolisthetic, iatrogenic (e.g., postlaminectomy, postfusion), post-traumatic, and metabolic (e.g., Paget disease).[177] Regardless of cause, spinal stenosis can cause pain, disability, impaired function, and reduced quality of life.[179] For a diagnosis of spinal stenosis, a sufficient degree of narrowing is required to compress neural structures and impact motor and sensory nerve function. For this reason, imaging and clinical examination findings are not always correlated.[180,181] Though clinical symptoms are not always classic, an accurate interpretation of imaging and symptoms is critical for management decisions.

Central stenosis is caused by disc protrusion, hypertrophic joints, degenerative spondylolisthesis, and ligamentum flavum buckling or hypertrophy. Figure 4-59 shows stenosis of the central canal anteriorly from bulging discs and posteriorly from hypertrophy of the ligamenta flava. The space in the vertebral canal is affected by movement. With flexion of the neck and back, the spinal cord lengthens and stretches over the bony and ligamentous structures. During extension, the posterior elements including the ligamentum flavum may fold or buckle, leading to reduced space for the spinal cord.[182]

Compromise of neural structures in the lumbar central vertebral canal may lead to neurogenic claudication. Symptoms of neurogenic claudication are pain, tingling, cramping, and weakness or heaviness in the legs. Typically, symptoms commence or are worsened with walking, standing, or hip extension and improve with trunk forward flexion, sitting, or lying supine with the hips and knees flexed. Narrowing of the cervical canal may present clinically as a myelopathy with or without radiculopathy.

Lateral stenosis may occur due to a bone spurs (osteophytes), disc degeneration, swelling of the connective tissue sheath around the spinal nerve root, or hypertrophy of ligaments or capsules. Such compression can lead to an altered transmission of sensory or motor impulses (radiculopathy), radicular "shooting" pain along the path of the corresponding dermatome, or weakness in the associated myotome, causing an increase in leg symptoms.[114] A reduction in reflexes may be found on clinical examination.

Myelopathy is an injury to the spinal cord because of severe compression. Compression of the spinal cord causes neural dysfunction, resulting in pain, loss of balance and coordination, weakness, and numbness in the related areas of compromise. Other symptoms include clumsiness, difficulty with fine motor skills, and abnormal reflexes, along with bowel and bladder dysfunction. Cervical myelopathy is more common than thoracic or lumbar myelopathy. Without treatment, permanent spinal cord and nerve damage may result. See Chapter 17, Cervical and Thoracic Spine, for more details.

CHAPTER SUMMARY

This chapter reviews the general structure of the spine and the biomechanical functions. The most important function of the spine is to protect the spinal cord and exiting nerves from potentially damaging forces or motions. The result of degeneration, disease, or injury to any portion of the vertebral column or supportive structures is instability that impacts the motion and function of the spinal motion segments. Pain, motor weakness, diminished or absent reflexes, anesthesia or paresthesia, and functional impairment may occur. The source of spinal pain is complex and not always identifiable. Diagnosis and successful interventions require an orderly evaluation, including a careful history, thorough physical examination, and diagnostic imaging or other diagnostic testing. The following chapters in this text aids the clinician to develop skill in diagnosis, treatment, and appropriate referral in the management of spinal abnormalities: Chapter 6, Patient History; Chapter 7, The Physical Examination; Chapter 8, Lower Quarter Screen; Chapter 13, Upper Quarter Screen; Chapter 17, Cervical and

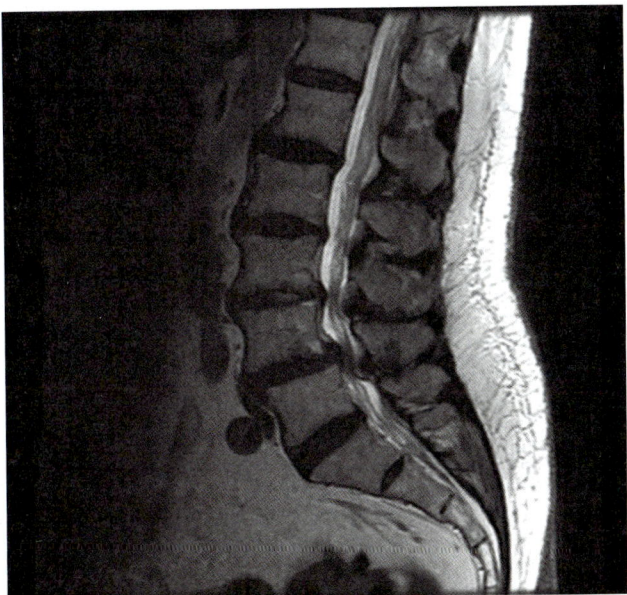

FIGURE 4-59 Magnetic resonance imaging showing spinal stenosis at L3–L5 with an L4–L5 spondylolisthesis. (Biller J. *Practical Neurology*. 5th ed. Wolters Kluwer; 2017; Figure 26.1.)

Thoracic Spine; and Chapter 19, Pain Management: A Mechanism-Centered Approach.

REFERENCES

1. Balasubramanian A, Zhang J, Chen L, et al. Risk of subsequent fracture after prior fracture among older women. *Osteoporos Int.* 2019;30(1):79–92.
2. Banefelt J, Åkesson K, Spångéus A, et al. Risk of imminent fracture following a previous fracture in a Swedish database study. *Osteoporos Int.* 2019;30(3):601–609.
3. Bliuc D, Nguyen N, Nguyen T, Eisman J, Center J. Compound risk of high mortality following osteoporotic fracture and refracture in elderly women and men. *J Bone Miner Res.* 2013;28(11):2317–2324.
4. Zeytinoglu M, Jain R, Vokes T. Vertebral fracture assessment: enhancing the diagnosis, prevention, and treatment of osteoporosis. *Bone.* 2017;104:54–65.
5. Suzuki N, Ogikubo O, Hansson T. The course of the acute vertebral body fragility fracture: its effect on pain, disability and quality of life during 12 months. *Eur Spine J.* 2008;17(10):1380–1390.
6. Nordin M, Frankel VH. *Basic Biomechanics of the Musculoskeletal System.* 5th ed. Wolters Kluwer; 2022.
7. Mitchell U, Helgeson K, Mintken P. Physiological effects of physical therapy interventions on lumbar intervertebral discs: a systematic review. *Physiother Theory Pract.* 2017;33(9):695–705.
8. Jaumard N, Welch W, Winkelstein B. Spinal facet joint biomechanics and mechanotransduction in normal, injury and degenerative conditions. *J Biomech Eng.* 2011;133(7):071010.
9. Neumann D. *Kinesology of the Musculoskeletal System: Foundations for Rehabilitation.* 3rd ed. Elsevier; 2017.
10. Heuer F, Schmidt H, Klezl Z, Claes L, Wilke H. Stepwise reduction of functional spinal structures increase range of motion and change lordosis angle. *J Biomech.* 2007;40(2):271–280.
11. Emanuel K, Vergroesen P, Peeters M, Hdsolewijn R, Kingma I, Smit T. Poroelastic behaviour of the degenerating human intervertebral disc: a ten-day study in a loaded disc culture system. *Eur Cell Mater.* 2015;29:330–340; discussion 340-1.
12. Adams M, Dolan P. Time-dependent changes in the lumbar spine's resistance to bending. *Clin Biomech (Bristol, Avon).* 1996;11(4):194–200.
13. O'Connell G, Jacobs N, Sen S, Vresilovic E, Elliott D. Axial creep loading and unloaded recovery of the human intervertebral disc and the effect of degeneration. *J Mech Behav Biomed Mater.* 2011;4(7):933–942.
14. van der Veen A, Bisschop A, Mullender M, van Dieën J. Modelling creep behaviour of the human intervertebral disc. *J Biomech.* 2013;46(12):2101–2103.
15. Boxberger J, Orlansky A, Sen S, Elliott D. Reduced nucleus pulposus glycosaminoglycan content alters intervertebral disc dynamic viscoelastic mechanics. *J Biomech.* 2009;42(12):1941–1946.
16. Smit T, Odgaard A, Schneider E. Structure and function of vertebral trabecular bone. *Spine.* 1997;22(24):2823–2833.
17. Adams M, Roughley P. What is intervertebral disc degeneration, and what causes it? *Spine.* 2006;31(18):2151–2161.
18. Hwang D, Gabai A, Yu M, Yew A, Hsieh A. Role of load history in intervertebral disc mechanics and intradiscal pressure generation. *Biomech Model Mechanobiol.* 2012;11(1–2):95–106.
19. Vergroesen P, van der Veen A, van Royen B, Kingma I, Smit T. Intradiscal pressure depends on recent loading and correlates with disc height and compressive stiffness. *Eur Spine J.* 2014;23(11):2359–2368.
20. Vergroesen P, Kingma I, Emanuel K, et al. Mechanics and biology in intervertebral disc degeneration: a vicious circle. *Osteoarthritis Cartilage.* 2015;23(7):1057–1070.
21. Kumar S, Dufresne R, Van Schoor T. Human trunk strength profile in lateral flexion and axial rotation. *Spine.* 1995;20(2):169–177.
22. Nachemson A. Towards a better understanding of low-back pain: a review of the mechanics of the lumbar disc. *Rheumatol Rehabil.* 1975;14(3):129–143.
23. Andersson G, Murphy R, Ortengren R, Nachemson A. The influence of backrest inclination and lumbar support on lumbar lordosis. *Spine.* 1979;4(1):52–58.
24. Andersson B, Ortengren R, Nachemson A, Elfström G. Lumbar disc pressure and myoelectric back muscle activity during sitting. IV. Studies on a car driver's seat. *Scand J Rehabil Med.* 1974;6(3):128–133.
25. Andersson B, Ortengren R, Nachemson A, Elfström G, Broman H. The sitting posture: an electromyographic and discometric study. *Orthop Clin North Am.* 1975;6(1):105–120.
26. Wilke H, Neef P, Caimi M, Hoogland T, Claes L. New in vivo measurements of pressures in the intervertebral disc in daily life. *Spine.* 1999;24(8):755–762.
27. Hertling D, Kessler RM. *Management of Common Musculoskeletal Disorders: Physical Therapy Principles and Methods.* 4th ed. Lippincott Williams & Wilkins; 2006.
28. Urban J, Smith S, Fairbank J. Nutrition of the intervertebral disc. *Spine.* 2004;29(23):2700–2709.
29. Yaltirik C, Timirci-Kahraman Ö, Gulec-Yilmaz S, Ozdogan S, Atalay B, Isbir T. The evaluation of proteoglycan levels and the possible role of ACAN Gene (c.6423T>C) variant in patients with lumbar disc degeneration disease. *In Vivo.* 2019;33(2):413–417.
30. Naseer Z, Bachabi M, Jones L, Sterling R, Khanuja H. Osteonecrosis in sickle cell disease. *South Med J.* 2016;109(9):525–530.
31. Hirano N, Tsuji H, Ohshima H, Kitano S, Itoh T, Sano A. Analysis of rabbit intervertebral disc physiology based on water metabolism. II. Changes in normal intervertebral discs under axial vibratory load. *Spine.* 1988;13(11):1297–1302.
32. McCann M, Patel P, Pest M, et al. Repeated exposure to high-frequency low-amplitude vibration induces degeneration of murine intervertebral discs and knee joints. *Arthritis Rheumatol.* 2015;67(8):2164–2175.
33. Jackson A, Dhawale A, Brown M. Association between intervertebral disc degeneration and cigarette smoking: clinical and experimental findings. *JBJS Rev.* 2015;3(3).
34. Fennell A, Jones A, Hukins D. Migration of the nucleus pulposus within the intervertebral disc during flexion and extension of the spine. *Spine.* 1996;21(23):2753–2757.
35. Beattie P, Brooks W, Rothstein J, et al. Effect of lordosis on the position of the nucleus pulposus in supine subjects. A study using magnetic resonance imaging. *Spine.* 1994;19(18):2096–2102.
36. Edmondston S, Song S, Bricknell R, et al. MRI evaluation of lumbar spine flexion and extension in asymptomatic individuals. *Man Ther.* 2000;5(3):158–164.
37. Fazey P, Song S, Price R, Singer K. Nucleus pulposus deformation in response to rotation at L1-2 and L4-5. *Clin Biomech (Bristol, Avon).* 2013;28(5):586–589.
38. Brault J, Driscoll D, Laakso L, Kappler R, Allin E, Glonek T. Quantification of lumbar intradiscal deformation during flexion and extension, by mathematical analysis of magnetic resonance imaging pixel intensity profiles. *Spine.* 1997;22(18):2066–2072.
39. Kim Y, Kim S, Park S, Hong S, Chung S. Effects of cervical extension on deformation of intervertebral disk and migration of nucleus pulposus. *PM R.* 2017;9(4):329–338.

40. Elmaazi A, Morse C, Lewis S, Qureshi S, McEwan I. The acute response of the nucleus pulposus of the cervical intervertebral disc to three supine postures in an asymptomatic population. *Musculoskelet Sci Pract.* 2019;44:102038.
41. Nazari J, Pope M, Graveling R. Reality about migration of the nucleus pulposus within the intervertebral disc with changing postures. *Clin Biomech (Bristol, Avon).* 2012;27(3):213–217.
42. Périé D, Sales de Gauzy J, Curnier D, Hobatho M. Intervertebral disc modeling using a MRI method: migration of the nucleus zone within scoliotic intervertebral discs. *Magn Reson Imaging.* 2001;19(9):1245–1248.
43. Inoue N, Orías A, Segami K. Biomechanics of the lumbar facet joint. *Spine Surg Relat Res.* 2020;4(1):1–7.
44. Shinohara H. Changes in the surface of the superior articular joint from the lower thoracic to the upper lumbar vertebrae. *J Anat.* 1997;190 (Pt 3):461–465.
45. Pal G, Routal R, Saggu S. The orientation of the articular facets of the zygapophyseal joints at the cervical and upper thoracic region. *J Anat.* 2001;198(Pt 4):431–441.
46. Pal G, Routal R. Mechanism of change in the orientation of the articular process of the zygapophyseal joint at the thoracolumbar junction. *J Anat.* 1999;195(Pt 2):199–209.
47. Shi D, Wang F, Wang D, Li X, Wang Q. 3-D finite element analysis of the influence of synovial condition in sacroiliac joint on the load transmission in human pelvic system. *Med Eng Phys.* 2014;36(6):745–753.
48. Drake RL, Vogl AW, Mitchell AWM. *Gray's Anatomy for Students.* 3rd ed. Churchill Livingstone/Elsevier; 2015.
49. Le Huec J, Tsoupras A, Leglise A, Heraudet P, Celarier G, Sturresson B. The sacro-iliac joint: a potentially painful enigma. Update on the diagnosis and treatment of pain from microtrauma. *Orthop Traumatol Surg Res.* 2019;105(1s):S31–S42.
50. Vleeming A, Schuenke M, Masi A, Carreiro J, Danneels L, Willard F. The sacroiliac joint: an overview of its anatomy, function and potential clinical implications. *J Anat.* 2012;221(6):537–567.
51. Casaroli G, Bassani T, Brayda-Bruno M, Luca A, Galbusera F. What do we know about the biomechanics of the sacroiliac joint and of sacropelvic fixation? A literature review. *Med Eng Phys.* 2020;76:1–12.
52. Hammer N, Höch A, Klima S, Le Joncour J, Rouquette C, Ramezani M. Effects of cutting the sacrospinous and sacrotuberous ligaments. *Clin Anat.* 2019;32(2):231–237.
53. Bowen V, Cassidy J. Macroscopic and microscopic anatomy of the sacroiliac joint from embryonic life until the eighth decade. *Spine.* 1981;6(6):620–628.
54. Forst S, Wheeler M, Fortin J, Vilensky J. The sacroiliac joint: anatomy, physiology and clinical significance. *Pain Physician.* 2006;9(1):61–67.
55. McLauchlan G, Gardner D. Sacral and iliac articular cartilage thickness and cellularity: relationship to subchondral bone end-plate thickness and cancellous bone density. *Rheumatology (Oxford).* 2002;41(4):375–380.
56. Kiapour A, Joukar A, Elgafy H, Erbulut D, Agarwal A, Goel V. Biomechanics of the sacroiliac joint: anatomy, function, biomechanics, sexual dimorphism, and causes of pain. *Int J Spine Surg.* 2020;14(Suppl 1):3–13.
57. Kampen W, Tillmann B. Age-related changes in the articular cartilage of human sacroiliac joint. *Anat Embryol (Berl).* 1998;198(6):505–513.
58. Vogler J 3rd, Brown W, Helms C, Genant H. The normal sacroiliac joint: a CT study of asymptomatic patients. *Radiology.* 1984;151(2):433–437.
59. Eno J, Boone C, Bellino M, Bishop J. The prevalence of sacroiliac joint degeneration in asymptomatic adults. *J Bone Joint Surg Am.* 2015;97(11):932–936.
60. Polly D Jr. The sacroiliac joint. *Neurosurg Clin N Am.* 2017;28(3):301–312.
61. Fortin J, Dwyer A, West S, Pier J. Sacroiliac joint: pain referral maps upon applying a new injection/arthrography technique. Part I: asymptomatic volunteers. *Spine.* 1994;19(13):1475–1482.
62. Szadek K, Hoogland P, Zuurmond W, de Lange J, Perez R. Nociceptive nerve fibers in the sacroiliac joint in humans. *Reg Anesth Pain Med.* 2008;33(1):36–43.
63. Szadek K, Hoogland P, Zuurmond W, De Lange J, Perez R. Possible nociceptive structures in the sacroiliac joint cartilage: an immunohistochemical study. *Clin Anat.* 2010;23(2):192–198.
64. Loukas M, Louis RG Jr, Wartmann C, et al. An anatomic investigation of the serratus posterior superior and serratus posterior inferior muscles. *Surg Radiol Anat.* 2008;30(2):119–123.
65. Vilensky J, Baltes M, Weikel L, Fortin J, Fourie L. Serratus posterior muscles: anatomy, clinical relevance, and function. *Clin Anat.* 2001;14(4):237–241.
66. Benjamen M. The fascia of the limbs and back—a review. *J Anat.* 2009;214(1):1–18.
67. Vleeming A, Schuenke M, Danneels L, Willard F. The functional coupling of the deep abdominal and paraspinal muscles: the effects of simulated paraspinal muscle contraction on force transfer to the middle and posterior layer of the thoracolumbar fascia. *J Anat.* 2014;225(4):447–462.
68. Vleeming A, Pool-Goudzwaard A, Stoeckart R, van Wingerden J, Snijders C. The posterior layer of the thoracolumbar fascia. Its function in load transfer from spine to legs. *Spine.* 1995;20(7):753–758.
69. Panjabi M. The stabilizing system of the spine. Part I. Function, dysfunction, adaptation, and enhancement. *J Spinal Disord.* 1992;5(4):383–389; discussion 397.
70. Panjabi M, Abumi K, Duranceau J, Oxland T. Spinal stability and intersegmental muscle forces. A biomechanical model. *Spine.* 1989;14(2):194–200.
71. Cholewicki J, McGill S. Mechanical stability of the in vivo lumbar spine: implications for injury and chronic low back pain. *Clin Biomech (Bristol, Avon).* 1996;11(1):1–15.
72. Freeman M, Woodham M, Woodham A. The role of the lumbar multifidus in chronic low back pain: a review. *PM R.* 2010;2(2):142-146; quiz 141 p following 167.
73. Kliziene I, Sipaviciene S, Klizas S, Imbrasiene D. Effects of core stability exercises on multifidus muscles in healthy women and women with chronic low-back pain. *J Back Musculoskelet Rehabil.* 2015;28(4):841–847.
74. Wilke H, Wolf S, Claes L, Arand M, Wiesend A. Stability increase of the lumbar spine with different muscle groups. A biomechanical in vitro study. *Spine.* 1995;20(2):192–198.
75. O'Sullivan P, Phyty G, Twomey L, Allison G. Evaluation of specific stabilizing exercise in the treatment of chronic low back pain with radiologic diagnosis of spondylolysis or spondylolisthesis. *Spine.* 1997;22(24):2959–2967.
76. Saragiotto B, Maher C, Yamato T, et al. Motor control exercise for chronic non-specific low-back pain. *Cochrane Database Syst Rev.* 2016; (1):CD012004.
77. Calatayud J, Casaña J, Martín F, et al. Trunk muscle activity during different variations of the supine plank exercise. *Musculoskelet Sci Pract.* 2017;28:54–58.
78. Cresswell A, Grundström H, Thorstensson A. Observations on intra-abdominal pressure and patterns of abdominal intra-muscular activity in man. *Acta Physiol Scand.* 1992;144(4):409–418.
79. Hodges P, Richardson C. Contraction of the abdominal muscles associated with movement of the lower limb. *Phys Ther.* 1997;77(2):132–142; discussion 142–4.

80. Hides J, Jull G, Richardson C. Long-term effects of specific stabilizing exercises for first-episode low back pain. *Spine*. 2001;26(11):E243–E248.
81. Cai C, Yang Y, Kong P. Comparison of lower limb and back exercises for runners with chronic low back pain. *Med Sci Sports Exerc*. 2017;49(12):2374–2384.
82. França F, Burke T, Hanada E, Marques A. Segmental stabilization and muscular strengthening in chronic low back pain: a comparative study. *Clinics (Sao Paulo)*. 2010;65(10):1013–1017.
83. França F, Burke T, Caffaro R, Ramos L, Marques A. Effects of muscular stretching and segmental stabilization on functional disability and pain in patients with chronic low back pain: a randomized, controlled trial. *J Manipulative Physiol Ther*. 2012;35(4):279–285.
84. Neumann P, Gill V. Pelvic floor and abdominal muscle interaction: EMG activity and intra-abdominal pressure. *Int Urogynecol J Pelvic Floor Dysfunct*. 2002;13(2):125–132.
85. Madill S, McLean L. Relationship between abdominal and pelvic floor muscle activation and intravaginal pressure during pelvic floor muscle contractions in healthy continent women. *Neurourol Urodyn*. 2006;25(7):722–730.
86. Sapsford R, Hodges P. Contraction of the pelvic floor muscles during abdominal maneuvers. *ACMR*. 2001;82(8):1081–1088.
87. Sapsford R, Hodges P, Richardson C, Cooper D, Markwell S, Jull G. Co-activation of the abdominal and pelvic floor muscles during voluntary exercises. *Neurourol Urodyn*. 2001;20(1):31–42.
88. Hemborg B, Moritz U, Löwing H. Intra-abdominal pressure and trunk muscle activity during lifting. IV. The causal factors of the intra-abdominal pressure rise. *Scand J Rehabil Med*. 1985;17(1):25–38.
89. Moore KL, Dalley AF, Agur AMR. *Clinically Oriented Anatomy*. 8th ed. Wolters Kluwer; 2018.
90. Simenz C, Garceau L, Lutsch B, Suchomel T, Ebben W. Electromyographical analysis of lower extremity muscle activation during variations of the loaded step-up exercise. *J Strength Cond Res*. 2012;26(12):3398–3405.
91. Neto W, Soares E, Vieira T, et al. Gluteus maximus activation during common strength and hypertrophy exercises: a systematic review. *J Sports Sci Med*. 2020;19(1):195–203.
92. Macadam P, Cronin J, Contreras B. An examination of the gluteal muscle activity associated with dynamic hip abduction and hip external rotation exercise: a systematic review. *Int J Sports Phys Ther*. 2015;10(5):573–591.
93. Reiman M, Bolgla L, Loudon J. A literature review of studies evaluating gluteus maximus and gluteus medius activation during rehabilitation exercises. *Physiother Theory Pract*. 2012;28(4):257–268.
94. Farrokhi S, Pollard CD, Souza RB, Chen YJ, Reischl S, Powers CM. Trunk position influences the kinematics, kinetics, and muscle activity of the lead lower extremity during the forward lunge exercise. *J Orthop Sports Phys Ther*. 2008;38(7):403–409.
95. Woodhull-McNeal A. Activity in torso muscles during relaxed standing. *Eur J Appl Physiol Occup Physiol*. 1986;55(4):419–424.
96. Soames R, Atha J. The role of the antigravity musculature during quiet standing in man. *Eur J Appl Physiol Occup Physiol*. 1981;47(2):159–167.
97. Conley M, Meyer R, Bloomberg J, Feeback D, Dudley G. Non-invasive analysis of human neck muscle function. *Spine*. 1995;20(23):2505–2512.
98. Winters J, Peles J. Neck muscle activity and 3-D head kinematics during quasi-static and dynamic traking movements. In: Jack MW, Woo S, eds. *Multiple Muscle Systems: Biomechanics and Movement Organization*. Springer-Verlag; 1990:461–480.
99. Khan Y, Bordoni B. Anatomy, head and neck, suprahyoid muscle. In: StatPearls. StatPearls Publishing; 2021.
100. Moroney S, Schultz A, Miller J. Analysis and measurement of neck loads. *J Orthop Res*. 1988;6(5):713–720.
101. Siegmund G, Blouin J, Brault J, Hedenstierna S, Inglis J. Electromyography of superficial and deep neck muscles during isometric, voluntary, and reflex contractions. *J Biomech Eng*. 2007;129(1):66–77.
102. Sargent B, Kaplan S, Coulter C, Baker C. Congenital muscular torticollis: bridging the gap between research and clinical practice. *Pediatrics*. 2019;144(2).
103. van Vlimmeren L, Helders P, van Adrichem L, Engelbert R. Torticollis and plagiocephaly in infancy: therapeutic strategies. *Pediatr Rehabil*. 2006;9(1):40–46.
104. Jinnah H, Berardelli A, Comella C, et al. The focal dystonias: current views and challenges for future research. *Mov Disord*. 2013;28(7):926–943.
105. De Pauw J, Van der Velden K, Meirte J, et al. The effectiveness of physiotherapy for cervical dystonia: a systematic literature review. *J Neurol*. 2014;261(10):1857–1865.
106. Kennedy C. The cervical spine. In: Hall C, Brody L, eds. *Therapeutic Exercise: Moving Toward Function*. Lippincott Williams & Wilkins; 1998:525–548.
107. Izzo R, Guarnieri G, Guglielmi G, Muto M. Biomechanics of the spine. Part I: spinal stability. *Eur J Radiol*. 2013;82(1):118–126.
108. Schmidt H, Heuer F, Claes L, Wilke H. The relation between the instantaneous center of rotation and facet joint forces—a finite element analysis. *Clin Biomech (Bristol, Avon)*. 2008;23(3):270–278.
109. Legaspi O, Edmond S. Does the evidence support the existence of lumbar spine coupled motion? A critical review of the literature. *J Orthop Sports Phys Ther*. 2007;37(4):169–178.
110. Salem W, Lenders C, Mathieu J, Hermanus N, Klein P. In vivo three-dimensional kinematics of the cervical spine during maximal axial rotation. *Man Ther*. 2013;18(4):339–344.
111. Cook C, Hegedus E, Showalter C, Sizer PS Jr. Coupling behavior of the cervical spine: a systematic review of the literature. *J Manipulative Physiol Ther*. 2006;29(7):570–575.
112. Cook C. *Orthopedic Manual Therapy an Evidence-Based Approach*. Prentice Hall; 2007.
113. Kaltenborn F. *Manual Mobilization of the Joints, Vol 2: The Spine*. 4th ed. Norli; 2003.
114. Orita S, Inage K, Eguchi Y, et al. Lumbar foraminal stenosis, the hidden stenosis including at L5/S1. *Eur J Orthop Surg Traumatol*. 2016;26(7):685–693.
115. Muhle C, Resnick D, Ahn J, Südmeyer M, Heller M. In vivo changes in the neuroforaminal size at flexion-extension and axial rotation of the cervical spine in healthy persons examined using kinematic magnetic resonance imaging. *Spine*. 2001;26(13):E287–E293.
116. Brasiliense L, Lazaro B, Reyes P, Dogan S, Theodore N, Crawford N. Biomechanical contribution of the rib cage to thoracic stability. *Spine*. 2011;36(26):E1686–E1693.
117. Edmondston S, Waller R, Vallin P, Holthe A, Noebauer A, King E. Thoracic spine extension mobility in young adults: influence of subject position and spinal curvature. *J Orthop Sports Phys Ther*. 2011;41(4):266–273.
118. Dvořák J, Vajda E, Grob D, Panjabi M. Normal motion of the lumbar spine as related to age and gender. *Eur Spine J*. 1995;4(1):18–23.
119. Yukawa Y, Kato F, Suda K, Yamagata M, Ueta T. Age-related changes in osseous anatomy, alignment, and range of motion of the cervical spine. Part I: radiographic data from

over 1,200 asymptomatic subjects. *Eur Spine J.* 2012;21(8): 1492–1498.
120. Bogduk N, Mercer S. Biomechanics of the cervical spine. I: normal kinematics. *Clin Biomech (Bristol, Avon).* 2000; 15(9):633–648.
121. Oatis CA. *Kinesiology: The Mechanics and Pathomechanics of Human Movement.* 3rd ed. Wolters Kluwer; 2017.
122. Persson P, Hirschfeld H, Nilsson-Wikmar L. Associated sagittal spinal movements in performance of head pro-and retraction in healthy women: a kinematic analysis. *Man Ther.* 2007;12(2):119–125.
123. Zhang Q, Teo E, Ng H, Lee V. Finite element analysis of moment-rotation relationships for human cervical spine. *J Biomech.* 2006;39(1):189–193.
124. Kang J, Chen G, Zhai X, He X. In vivo three-dimensional kinematics of the cervical spine during maximal active head rotation. *PLoS One.* 2019;14(4):e0215357.
125. Masharawi Y, Rothschild B, Dar G, et al. Facet orientation in the thoracolumbar spine: three-dimensional anatomic and biomechanical analysis. *Spine.* 2004;29(16):1755–1763.
126. Jiang X, Chen D, Li Z, Lou Y. Correlation between lumbar spine facet joint orientation and intervertebral disk degeneration: a positional MRI analysis. *J Neurol Surg A Cent Eur Neurosurg.* 2019;80(4):255–261.
127. Cyron B, Hutton W. The tensile strength of the capsular ligaments of the apophyseal joints. *J Anat.* 1981;132(Pt 1): 145–150.
128. Shirazi-Adl A, Drouin G. Load-bearing role of facets in a lumbar segment under sagittal plane loadings. *J Biomech.* 1987;20(6):601–613.
129. Inufusa A, An H, Lim T, Hasegawa T, Haughton V, Nowicki B. Anatomic changes of the spinal canal and intervertebral foramen associated with flexion-extension movement. *Spine.* 1996;21(21):2412–2420.
130. Scannell J, McGill S. Lumbar posture—should it, and can it, be modified? A study of passive tissue stiffness and lumbar position during activities of daily living. *Phys Ther.* 2003;83(10):907–917.
131. McGill S, Brown S. Creep response of the lumbar spine to prolonged full flexion. *Clin Biomech (Bristol, Avon).* 1992;7(1):43–46.
132. Adams M, Hutton W. The effect of posture on the fluid content of lumbar intervertebral discs. *Spine.* 1983;8(6): 665–671.
133. Beach T, Parkinson R, Stothart J, Callaghan J. Effects of prolonged sitting on the passive flexion stiffness of the in vivo lumbar spine. *Spine J.* 2005;5(2):145–154.
134. Jaumard N, Bauman J, Weisshaar C, Guarino B, Welch W, Winkelstein B. Contact pressure in the facet joint during sagittal bending of the cadaveric cervical spine. *J Biomech Eng.* 2011;133(7):071004.
135. Tsantrizos A, Ito K, Aebi M, Steffen T. Internal strains in healthy and degenerated lumbar intervertebral discs. *Spine.* 2005;30(19):2129–2137.
136. Kos N, Gradisnik L, Velnar T. A brief review of the degenerative intervertebral disc disease. *Med Arch.* 2019;73(6):421–424.
137. Brinjikji W, Luetmer P, Comstock B, et al. Systematic literature review of imaging features of spinal degeneration in asymptomatic populations. *AJNR Am J Neuroradiol.* 2015;36(4):811–816.
138. Chou D, Samartzis D, Bellabarba C, et al. Degenerative magnetic resonance imaging changes in patients with chronic low back pain: a systematic review. *Spine.* 2011;36(21 Suppl): S43–S53.
139. Takatalo J, Karppinen J, Niinimäki J, et al. Association of modic changes, Schmorl's nodes, spondylolytic defects, high-intensity zone lesions, disc herniations, and radial tears with low back symptom severity among young Finnish adults. *Spine.* 2012;37(14):1231–1239.
140. Berg L, Hellum C, Gjertsen Ø, et al. Do more MRI findings imply worse disability or more intense low back pain? A cross-sectional study of candidates for lumbar disc prosthesis. *Skeletal Radiol.* 2013;42(11):1593–1602.
141. Steffens D, Hancock M, Maher C, Williams C, Jensen T, Latimer J. Does magnetic resonance imaging predict future low back pain? A systematic review. *Eur J Pain.* 2014;18(6):755–765.
142. Antoniou J, Steffen T, Nelson F, et al. The human lumbar intervertebral disc: evidence for changes in the biosynthesis and denaturation of the extracellular matrix with growth, maturation, ageing, and degeneration. *J Clin Invest.* 1996;98(4):996–1003.
143. Risbud M, Shapiro I. Role of cytokines in intervertebral disc degeneration: pain and disc content. *Nat Rev Rheumatol.* 2014;10(1):44–56.
144. Colombini A, Lombardi G, Corsi M, Banfi G. Pathophysiology of the human intervertebral disc. *Int J Biochem Cell Biol.* 2008;40(5):837–842.
145. Khan A, Jacobsen H, Khan J, et al. Inflammatory biomarkers of low back pain and disc degeneration: a review. *Ann N Y Acad Sci.* 2017;1410(1):68–84.
146. Middendorp M, Vogl T, Kollias K, Kafchitsas K, Khan M, Maataoui A. Association between intervertebral disc degeneration and the Oswestry Disability Index. *J Back Musculoskelet Rehabil.* 2017;30(4):819–823.
147. Shan Z, Fan S, Xie Q, et al. Spontaneous resorption of lumbar disc herniation is less likely when modic changes are present. *Spine.* 2014;39(9):736–744.
148. Fardon D, Williams A, Dohring E, Murtagh F, Gabriel Rothman S, Sze G. Lumbar disc nomenclature: version 2.0: recommendations of the combined task forces of the North American Spine Society, the American Society of Spine Radiology and the American Society of Neuroradiology. *Spine J.* 2014;14(11):2525–2545.
149. Rao R. Neck pain, cervical radiculopathy, and cervical myelopathy: pathophysiology, natural history, and clinical evaluation. *J Bone Joint Surg Am.* 2002;84(10):1872–1881.
150. Bogduk N, Windsor M, Inglis A. The innervation of the cervical intervertebral discs. *Spine.* 1988;13(1):2–8.
151. Kim Y, Kang D, Lee I, Kim S. Differences in the incidence of symptomatic cervical and lumbar disc herniation according to age, sex and National Health Insurance eligibility: a pilot study on the disease's association with work. *Int J Environ Res Public Health.* 2018;15(10).
152. Li Y, Fredrickson V, Resnick D. How should we grade lumbar disc herniation and nerve root compression? A systematic review. *Clin Orthop Relat Res.* 2015;473(6):1896–1902.
153. Solgaard Sorensen J, Kjaer P, Jensen S, Andersen P. Low-field magnetic resonance imaging of the lumbar spine: reliability of qualitative evaluation of disc and muscle parameters. *Acta Radiol.* 2006;47(9):947–953.
154. Arana E, Kovacs F, Royuela A, et al. Influence of nomenclature in the interpretation of lumbar disk contour on MR imaging: a comparison of the agreement using the combined task force and the Nordic nomenclatures. *AJNR Am J Neuroradiol.* 2011;32(6):1143–1148.
155. Imaad-ur-Rehman Hamid R, Akhtar W, Shamim M, Naqi R, Siddiq H. Observer variation in MRI evaluation of patients with suspected lumbar disc herniation and nerve root compression: comparison of neuroradiologist and neurosurgeon's interpretations. *J Pak Med Assoc.* 2012;62(8): 826–829.

156. Jensen MC, Brant-Zawadzki MN, Obuchowski N, Modic MT, Malkasian D, Ross JS. Magnetic resonance imaging of the lumbar spine in people without back pain. *N Engl J Med.* 1994;331(2):69–73.
157. van Rijn J, Klemetsö N, Reitsma J, et al. Observer variation in MRI evaluation of patients suspected of lumbar disk herniation. *AJR Am J Roentgenol.* 2005;184(1):299–303.
158. Fardon D, Milette P. Nomenclature and classification of lumbar disc pathology. Recommendations of the Combined Task Forces of the North American Spine Society, American Society of Spine Radiology, and American Society of Neuroradiology. *Spine.* 2001;26(5):E93–E113.
159. Mysliwiec L, Cholewicki J, Winkelpleck M, Eis G. MSU classification for herniated lumbar discs on MRI: toward developing objective criteria for surgical selection. *Eur Spine J.* 2010;19(7):1087–1093.
160. Radhakrishnan K, Litchy W, O'Fallon W, Kurland L. Epidemiology of cervical radiculopathy. A population-based study from Rochester, Minnesota, 1976 through 1990. *Brain.* 1994;117(Pt 2):325–335.
161. Slipman C, Plastaras C, Palmitier R, Huston C, Sterenfeld E. Symptom provocation of fluoroscopically guided cervical nerve root stimulation. Are dynatomal maps identical to dermatomal maps? *Spine.* 1998;23(20):2235–2242.
162. Carette S, Fehlings M. Clinical practice. Cervical radiculopathy. *N Engl J Med.* 2005;353(4):392–399.
163. Shelerud R, Paynter K. Rarer causes of radiculopathy: spinal tumors, infections, and other unusual causes. *Phys Med Rehabil Clin N Am.* 2002;13(3):645–696.
164. Quint U, Bordon G, Preissl I, Sanner C, Rosenthal D. Thoracoscopic treatment for single level symptomatic thoracic disc herniation: a prospective followed cohort study in a group of 167 consecutive cases. *Eur Spine J.* 2012;21(4):637–645.
165. Williams M, Cherryman G, Husband J. Significance of thoracic disc herniation demonstrated by MR imaging. *J Comput Assist Tomogr.* 1989;13(2):211–214.
166. Oltulu I, Cil H, Ulu M, Deviren V. Clinical outcomes of symptomatic thoracic disk herniations treated surgically through minimally invasive lateral transthoracic approach. *Neurosurg Rev.* 2019;42(4):885–894.
167. Kato K, Yabuki S, Otani K, et al. Unusual chest wall pain caused by thoracic disc herniation in a professional baseball pitcher. *Fukushima J Med Sci.* 2016;62(1):64–67.
168. Bouthors C, Benzakour A, Court C. Surgical treatment of thoracic disc herniation: an overview. *Int Orthop.* 2019;43(4):807–816.
169. Hott J, Feiz-Erfan I, Kenny K, Dickman C. Surgical management of giant herniated thoracic discs: analysis of 20 cases. *J Neurosurg Spine.* 2005;3(3):191–197.
170. Zhong M, Liu J, Jiang H, et al. Incidence of spontaneous resorption of lumbar disc herniation: a meta-analysis. *Pain Physician.* 2017;20(1):E45–E52.
171. Chiu C, Chuang T, Chang K, Wu C, Lin P, Hsu W. The probability of spontaneous regression of lumbar herniated disc: a systematic review. *Clin Rehabil.* 2015;29(2):184–195.
172. Wigfield C, Gill S, Nelson R, Langdon I, Metcalf N, Robertson J. Influence of an artificial cervical joint compared with fusion on adjacent-level motion in the treatment of degenerative cervical disc disease. *J Neurosurg.* 2002;96(1 Suppl):17–21.
173. Dohrmann G, Mansour N. Long-term results of various operations for lumbar disc herniation: analysis of over 39,000 patients. *Med Princ Pract.* 2015;24(3):285–290.
174. Rogerson A, Aidlen J, Jenis L. Persistent radiculopathy after surgical treatment for lumbar disc herniation: causes and treatment options. *Int Orthop.* 2019;43(4):969–973.
175. Suk K, Lee H, Moon S, Kim N. Recurrent lumbar disc herniation: results of operative management. *Spine.* 2001;26(6):672–676.
176. Wong J, Côté P, Quesnele J, Stern P, Mior S. The course and prognostic factors of symptomatic cervical disc herniation with radiculopathy: a systematic review of the literature. *Spine.* 2014;14(8):1781–1789.
177. Botwin K, Gruber R. Lumbar spinal stenosis: anatomy and pathogenesis. *Phys Med Rehabil Clin N Am.* 2003;14(1):1–15, v.
178. Ciricillo SF, Weinstein P. Lumbar spinal stenosis. *West J Med.* 1993;158(2):171–177.
179. Chad D. Lumbar spinal stenosis. *Neurol Clin.* 2007;25(2):407–418.
180. Maus T. Imaging of spinal stenosis: neurogenic intermittent claudication and cervical spondylotic myelopathy. *Radiol Clin North Am.* 2012;50(4):651–679.
181. Willén J, Wessberg P, Danielsson B. Surgical results in hidden lumbar spinal stenosis detected by axial loaded computed tomography and magnetic resonance imaging: an outcome study. *Spine.* 2008;33(4):E109–E115.
182. Chen I, Vasavada A, Panjabi M. Kinematics of the cervical spine canal: changes with sagittal plane loads. *J Spinal Disord.* 1994;7(2):93–101.

5 | Gait and Footwear

June Hanks and Betsy Myers

CHAPTER OBJECTIVES
After reading this chapter, you will be able to:
1. Describe the events and periods in gait cycle phases.
2. Define temporal and distance terminology utilized in gait analysis.
3. Describe the characteristics of normal gait.
4. Discuss expected motions of the ankle, foot, knee, hip, pelvis, and trunk during gait.
5. Describe muscle activity during the gait cycle.
6. Describe the methods of gait analysis.
7. Differentiate various gait abnormalities.
8. Discuss the effect of age and gender on gait.
9. Describe utilization of assistive devices and impact on gait.
10. Describe the impact of footwear and foot orthotics on gait, balance, and joint stress.

GAIT

One of the most important normal daily activities is walking. Although gait and walking are often used interchangeably, there is a difference. *Walking* refers to a mode of locomotion, whereas *gait* describes a way or manner of walking. Normal gait is a sequence of limb motions that progresses the body forward while maintaining stability, absorbing shock, and conserving energy. The purpose of this chapter is to provide a logical description of gait that provides a foundation for analysis of normal walking and common gait deviations.

Phases of Gait Cycle

The gait cycle is measured from two consecutive initial contacts of the same foot. As shown in Figure 5-1, if the right foot is considered the reference limb, one gait cycle will start when the right foot contacts the ground and ends when the right foot contacts the ground again. The events of the gait cycle are considered in two phases: stance phase and swing phase, which occupy approximately 60 and 40% of one gait cycle, respectively. Stance phase is the period of time the reference foot is on the ground. During stance, the lower extremity accepts body weight and provides limb support. Swing phase is the period of time the reference foot is off the ground and moving forward as the body is moving forward. The phases of the gait cycle can be subdivided into events occurring sequentially in each phase, as outlined in Table 5-1.

Temporal and Distance Terminology

The timing of the gait cycle is shown in Figure 5-2. The period of time during gait when both feet are in contact with the surface is called *double support*. When walking at a normal speed, double support occurs twice in one gait cycle and takes a total of approximately 20% of the cycle. This means single-limb support during one gait cycle occupies approximately 80% of the time. These time frames vary with the speed of walking: as one walks faster, the swing phase becomes longer and the stance phase and double support phases shorter. The transition from walking to running is marked by the disappearance of the double support phase. During running, there is a period of time when neither foot is on the ground.

Terms to describe distance variables during a gait cycle are depicted in Figure 5-3. The stride length is the distance between two successive foot contacts of the same foot. The length of one stride includes all the events in one gait cycle. Step length is the distance between two successive foot contacts of opposite extremities. Because stride and step length depend directly on the length of the lower extremity, these measures must be normalized for comparison among individuals. Step width is the width of the walking base, measured as the side-to-side distance between the midpoint of the foot contacts. The degree of toe-out (or less commonly, toe-in) is measured as the angle (in degrees) formed between each foot's line of progression and a reference line on the sole of the foot, typically defined as angle between the center of the heel and approximately the second toe.

Timing variables include stance time, swing time, and single- and double-limb support time. Within a single gait cycle, the amount of time that elapses for each variable can be recorded. Another timing variable is cadence, which is the number of steps taken in a unit of time, typically steps per minute. The walking speed is the distance covered by the body in a unit of time. The term *walking speed* is preferred to *walking velocity*, unless the direction of walking is reported.

108 PART I | FOUNDATIONAL SCIENCES

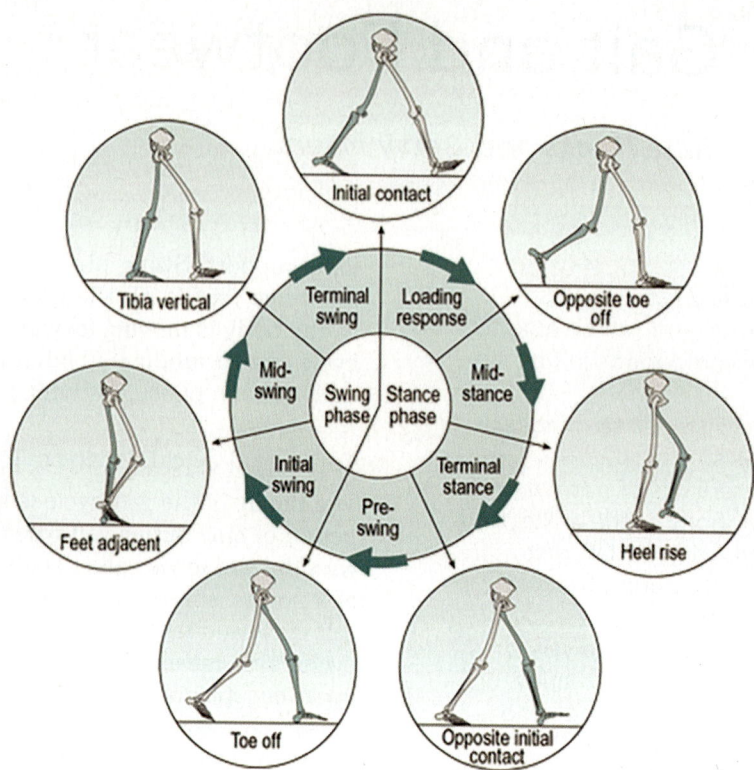

FIGURE 5-1 Phases and timing of the gait cycle, beginning with right foot initial contact. (Reprinted with permission from Levine D, Richards J, Whittle, MW. *Whittle's Gait Analysis*. 5th ed. Churchill Livingstone/Elsevier; 2012: Figure 2.1.)

TABLE 5-1		
EVENTS AND PERIODS DURING PHASES OF GAIT		
Phase of Gait	**Events**	**Periods**
Stance	• Initial contact • Opposite toe off • Heel rise • Opposite initial contact	• Loading response • Midstance • Terminal stance • Pre-swing
Swing	• Toe off • Feet adjacent • Tibia vertical	• Initial swing • Midswing • Terminal swing

The walking speed can be calculated as stride length divided by the time to complete a gait cycle using the following formula:

(speed [meter/second] = stride length [meter]/cycle time [second])

To calculate walking speed using the parameter of cadence rather than cycle time, one must consider that cadence, if recorded in steps per minute, corresponds to half-strides per 60 seconds or full strides

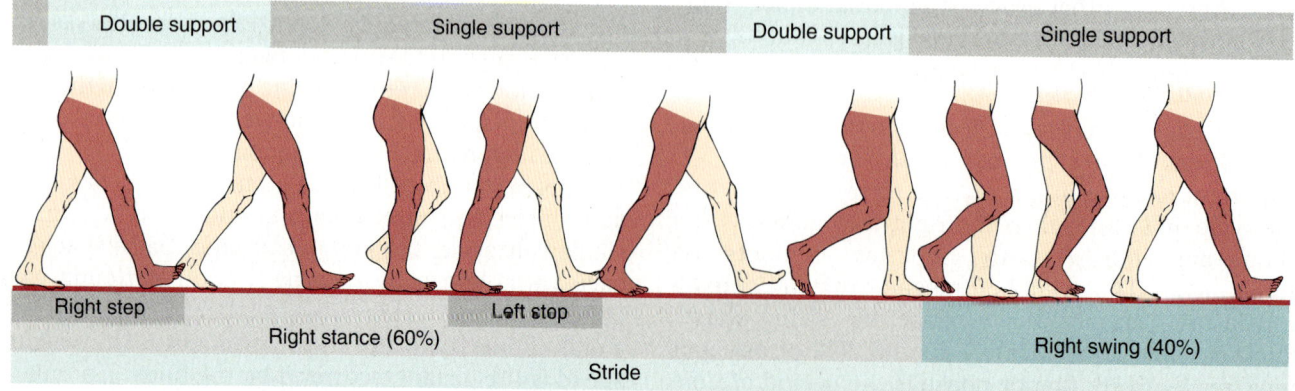

FIGURE 5-2 A single gait cycle from initial contact of one foot to the subsequent initial contact of the same foot. A gait cycle includes two periods of single-limb support and two periods of double-limb support. (Modified from Oatis CA. *Kinesiology: The Mechanics and Pathomechanics of Human Movement*. 3rd ed. Wolters Kluwer; 2017: Figure 48-1.)

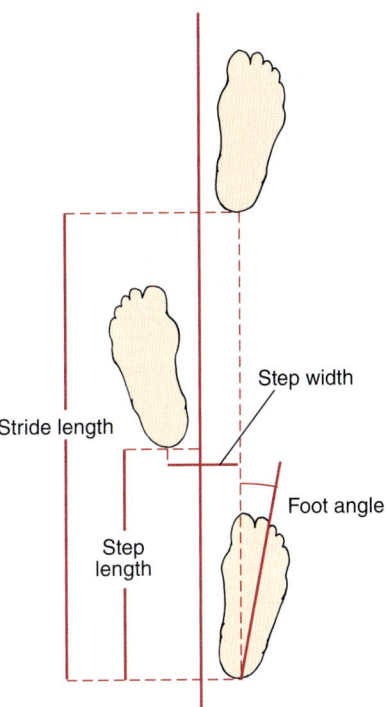

FIGURE 5-3 Distance variables in the gait cycle. (Modified from Oatis CA. *Kinesiology: The Mechanics and Pathomechanics of Human Movement.* 3rd ed. Wolters Kluwer; 2017: Figure 48-4.)

per 120 seconds. The speed can thus be calculated using the following formula:

(speed [meter/second] = stride length [meter] × cadence [step/minute/120])

Because walking speed depends on both stride length and cadence, one can alter either variable to change walking speed. Most commonly, people alter walking speed by adjusting both stride length and cadence.[1]

Characteristics of Normal Gait

Although overall motions of the trunk, pelvis, hip, knee, and ankle during walking have been reported,[2-5] intrasubject and intersubject variability exists in the specific magnitude of motion of body segments, especially with frontal and transverse plane motions.[6] The "normal" range of motion at each joint during walking, as assessed in the motion analysis laboratory, demonstrates large standard deviations; thus, reported values of peak motion at each joint must be interpreted with caution. However, the approximate joint motions as viewed from the sagittal plane during normal walking arc 20° of flexion and 20° of extension at the hip, 0 to 60° of flexion at the knee, 7° of dorsiflexion to 25° of plantarflexion at the ankle,[7] and more than 40° of 1st metatarsophalangeal (MTP) joint extension.[8] Motion at the pelvis is minimal, with a slight anterior tilt during terminal stance. The upper extremities move in a reciprocal, rhythmical pattern relative to the lower extremities.

Joint movements in the frontal plane are considerably less than those in the sagittal plane. From initial contact to late stance, the hip moves from neutral to approximately 10° of adduction, with the greatest adduction demonstrated as weight shifts toward the stance limb during single support. During swing, the hip moves into abduction and then back to the neutral position by initial contact. Knee motion in the frontal plane is very limited, with reported ranges from 2 to 10° of adduction.[6,9,10] The degree of the frontal plane components of ankle and foot inversion and eversion varies greatly among individuals during stance and swing. The rearfoot follows a pattern of inversion (consistent with supination) at initial contact, progressing to slight eversion (consistent with pronation) and returning to inversion (supination) at late stance.[11] During swing, the foot position varies, typically returning to a supinated position before initial contact. The foot follows a pattern of motion similar to the rearfoot.[12]

The lower extremity joint motions in the transverse plane are small and variable. During swing of the reference limb, the pelvis transversely rotates forward and is accompanied by slight external hip rotation until initial contact. From initial contact to late stance, the pelvis transversely rotates backward. At initial contact, the femur is in near-neutral to slight internal rotation, then gradually externally rotates during loading through late stance and part of swing, then assuming a slight external rotation until initial contact again. The transverse plane movement of the tibia is similar to that of the femur, with internal rotation after initial contact followed by a gradual external rotation by midstance that continues until midswing. The rotations of the femur and tibia contribute to the rotation at the knee, which follows a similar pattern.

As described in Chapter 9, Ankle and Foot, motions of the leg and foot are coupled. At initial contact, the rearfoot is in slight inversion (supination). As weight acceptance progresses toward midstance, the foot pronates and the tibia internally rotates,[13] providing shock absorption and accommodation of the foot to the contact surface.[14] From midstance to heel rise, the foot supinates again and maintains supination through toe off,[11] providing a rigid lever for propulsion. As the ankle and foot supinate, the tibia externally rotates.[15]

While the tibia and femur are rotating in the transverse plane, the knee is flexing and extending in the sagittal plane. The knee moves from nearly full extension at initial contact to flexion during loading to early midstance and then extends again at midstance to heel rise. As the knee flexes, the femur and tibia internally rotate, with the tibia rotating farther internally than the femur. Thus, the tibia is internally rotated relative to the femur, a position described as internal rotation of the knee. As the knee extends, the femur and tibia externally rotate, with the tibia rotating farther externally than the femur. The knee then externally rotates as it extends. The total excursion of knee rotation during gait is relatively small, ranging from 8 to 15°.[10,16]

Muscle Activity During Gait

Muscle activation patterns and periods of peak activation during the gait cycle have been demonstrated using electromyography.[17,18] The majority of muscle activity occurs during transitions between the phases of gait, as can be seen in Figure 5-4. During the loading response from initial contact to midstance, the gluteus maximus, quadriceps, and tibialis anterior muscles are most active, whereas from midstance to terminal stance, the gastrocnemius/soleus muscles demonstrate peak activity. The iliopsoas is most active during initial swing, and the hamstrings peak in activity during terminal swing.[1] It should be noted that during gait, the majority of muscles provide a burst of activity in one portion of the cycle while slowing a motion in the opposite direction in different portions of the cycle. That is, muscles accelerate limb movement in one direction and decelerate (slow) limb movement in the opposite direction. For example, ankle dorsiflexion occurs during swing phase to clear the toes; the ankle dorsiflexors are also active early in stance to lower the foot to foot flat.

Methods of Gait Analysis

Gait analysis ranges from visual observation to camera-based systems with force plates and electromyography. Elaborate and highly technologic systems yield useful objective kinetic and kinematic data, but cost limits utilization in the clinical setting. Useful data can be obtained from visual observation of a person walking from variety of angles while looking for the presence or absence of specific abnormalities.[19] Any type of gait analysis must be coupled with an assessment that synthesizes the history, physical examination, and complaints of the patient. The clinician must keep in mind that an observed abnormal gait pattern is, in effect, what remains from a patient's pathology and their attempt to compensate for it.[20] For example, a patient with weak dorsiflexors may flex the hip more on that side during swing to allow for toe clearance. An alternative explanation is that the abnormal movement pattern is used to compensate for another problem that needs to be identified.[1]

The clinician must decide whether to allow the individual being observed to walk at a self-selected pace or at a predetermined pace, such as walking in time to a metronome or a preset speed on a treadmill. Gait parameters vary significantly with changes in walking speed in persons with and without pathology.[21] Some

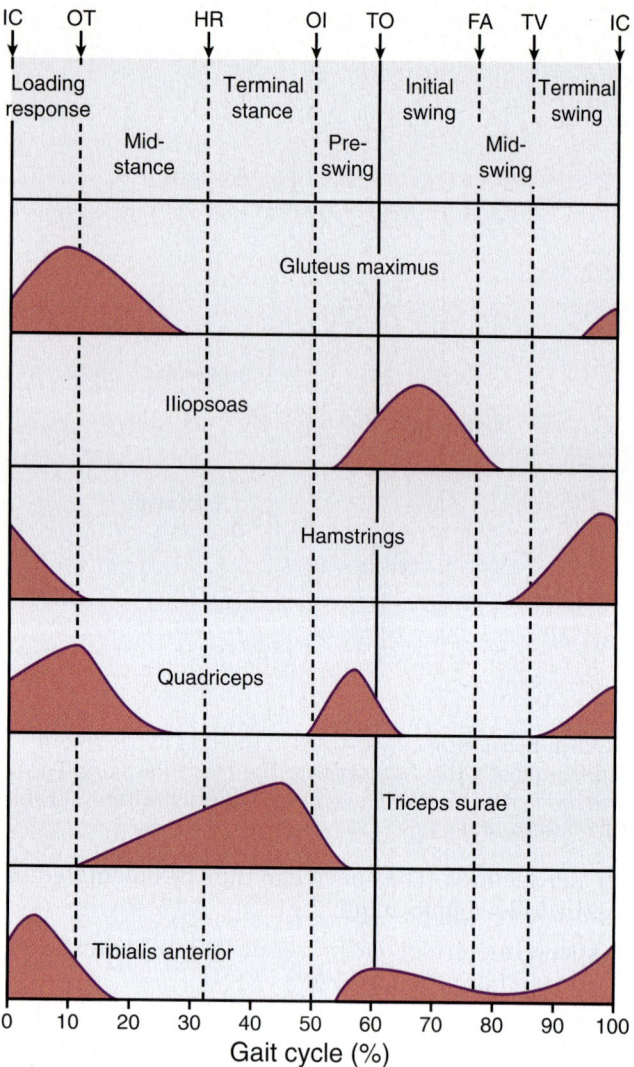

FIGURE 5-4 Muscle activity during the gait cycle. *FA*, foot adjacent; *HR*, heel rise; *IC*, initial contact; *OI*, opposite initial contact; *OT*, opposite toe off; *TO*, toe off; *TV*, tibia vertical. (Reprinted with permission from Levine D, Richards J, Whittle MW. *Whittle's Gait Analysis*. 5th ed. Churchill Livingstone/Elsevier; 2012: Figure 2.10.)

individuals find it difficult to walk naturally at externally imposed speeds, whereas others with motor control problems may be unable to walk safely or may be unable to walk at all at certain speeds.

The recommended length of walkway during visual observation is 8 m (26 feet), with a longer walkway of at least 12 m (39 feet) for fast walkers. For significant pathologic gait, a shorter walkway of 3 m (10 feet) may be sufficient.[1] The clinician should view the patient walking from a front, back, and side view. The visual analysis should be systematically approached,[19] with focus starting with the ankle and foot, and progressing proximally, or from the trunk and pelvis and moving toward the ankle and foot. The patient should be asked to walk barefoot and with footwear. When analyzing from the side, the clinician should view from both the right and left sides of the patient. The frontal plane analysis should be performed from an anterior and posterior view. Gait analysis charts, such as the one designed by the Rancho Los Amigos Medical Center (Fig. 5-5), may aid the visual analysis. In addition, normal speed and slow-motion videos are helpful, allowing repeated viewing by the clinician without undue fatigue of the patient.

Gait Abnormalities

The clinician must be careful to identify gait abnormalities in descriptive terms, avoiding pathologic terms because not all individuals with a particular pathology will necessarily demonstrate the same gait pattern.

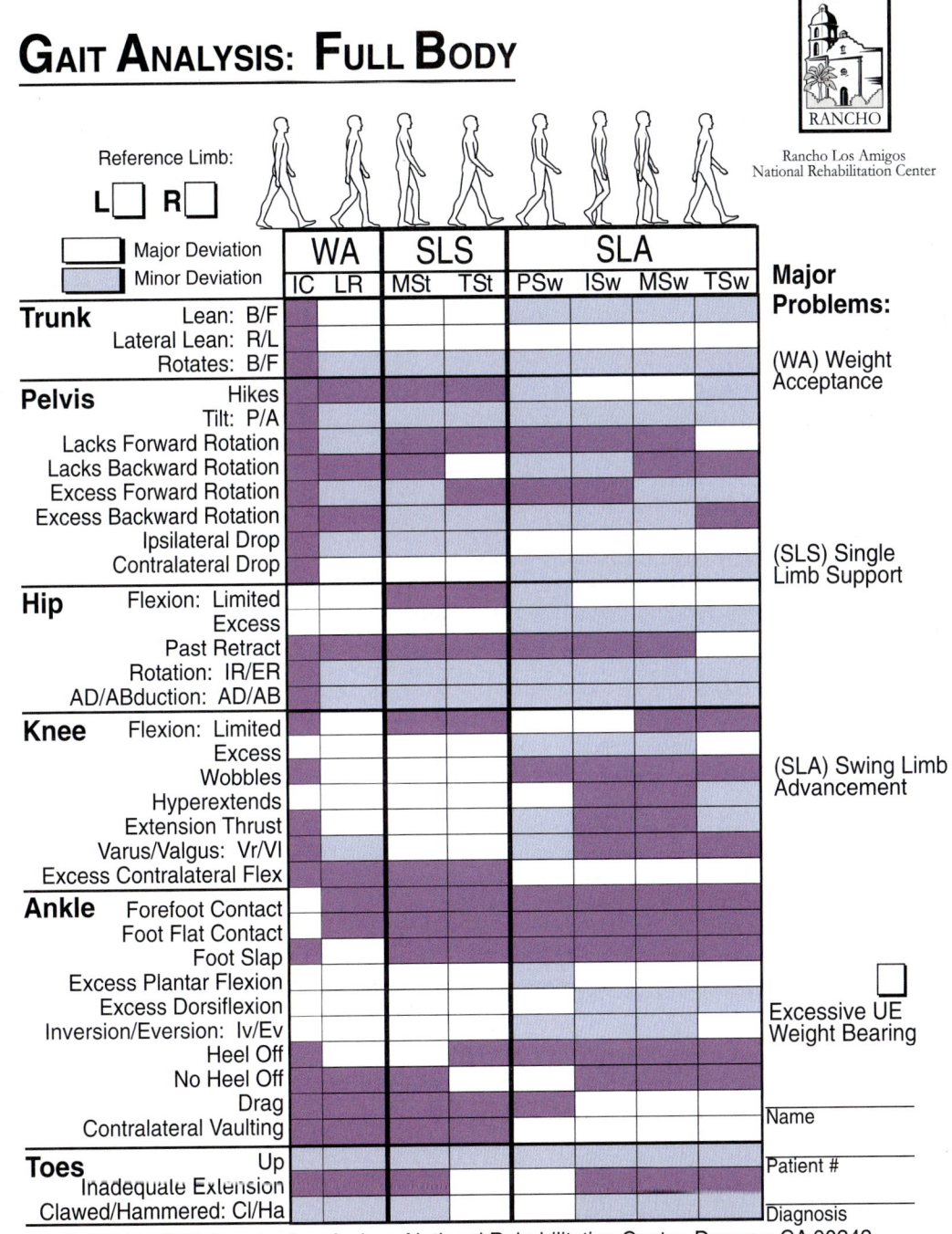

FIGURE 5-5 Rancho Los Amigos Gait Assessment Form. (Reprinted with permission from Rancho Los Amigos National Rehabilitation Center's Physical Therapy Department and Pathokinesiology Laboratory, Downey, California.)

For example, the term "parkinsonian gait" should be avoided, as gait among persons with Parkinson disease varies and changes with time and therapeutic intervention. A sample of common gait abnormalities with potential contributing factors is provided in Table 5-2.

Impact of Age on Gait

The effect of aging on gait is widely reported in the literature.[22-25] Self-selected walking speed decreases with advanced age.[26-30] Although older adults adopt a slower gait speed and higher foot clearance strategies when navigating obstacles, they are more likely to fail clearing an obstacle with their lead limb, making it difficult to recover balance.[31] Age-associated reductions in peak ankle plantarflexion power generation as well as ankle plantarflexion and hip extension range of motion have been identified at self-selected and fast walking speeds.[25] A decline in ability to dual task (e.g., talk while walking) increases the risk of falls.[32,33] Changes in gait, such as increased variability in stride length and swing time, contribute to a high incidence of falls among older adults,[34-36] along with other age-associated changes such as vision impairment, neurologic disorders, foot problems, and adverse effects from medications.[37] Walking speed is a component of many frailty assessment tools[38-41] and is considered one of the most suitable assessments in research and clinical evaluation of older adults.[41,42]

TABLE 5-2
COMMON GAIT ABNORMALITIES WITH DESCRIPTIONS AND COMMON CAUSES

Gait Abnormalities	Description	Potential Contributing Factors
Lateral trunk bending (also called compensated Trendelenburg gait)	Bending of the trunk toward the supporting limb in stance	• Painful hip • Hip abductor weakness • Abnormal hip joint • Wide walking base • Unequal leg length
Posterior trunk lean	Leaning of the trunk backward in early stance	• Weak hip extensors
Increased lumbar lordosis	Lumbar lordosis is exaggerated in midstance to late stance	• Hip flexor tightness • Weakness of muscles of anterior abdominal wall
Circumduction	Lower limb is swung out to the side and advanced during swing	• Weak hip flexors • Leg length discrepancy
Hip hiking	The pelvis is lifted on the side of the swing leg; usually seen during slow walking	• Leg length discrepancy
Steppage	Hip and knee flexion are exaggerated to lift foot higher to clear the ground	• Inadequate dorsiflexion control
Vaulting	Rising up on toes of stance-phase leg to increase ground clearance for swing-phase leg; usually seen during slow walking	• Leg length discrepancy
Excessive knee extension	Normal stance-phase flexion is minimal or lost	• Weak knee extensors
Excessive knee flexion	Stance-phase knee flexion is increased (at initial contact and/or heel rise)	• Contracture of knee flexors • Contracture of hip flexors • Spasticity of knee flexors
Inadequate dorsiflexion control	During loading at initial contact, foot is lowered abruptly (foot slap) During swing, toes are unable to clear the ground	• Weakness of ankle dorsiflexors
Insufficient push off	Inadequate push off phase with lack of heel rise; whole foot is lifted off ground at once	• Weakness of gastrocnemius/soleus or Achilles tendon pathology • Weakness of intrinsic foot muscles • Foot deformity or pain that prevents normal forefoot loading
Wide walking base	Feet are farther apart than the typical 4-6 inches during gait	• Limb deformity (e.g., abducted hip, valgus knee) • Fear of falling
Narrow walking base	Feet are closer together than normal during gait	• Limb deformity (e.g., adducted hip, varus knee)
Antalgic gait	Reduced stance time on painful limb with correspondingly longer time on pain-free limb	• Pain with weight bearing

Modified from Levine D, Richards J, Whittle, MW. *Whittle's Gait Analysis*. 5th ed. Churchill Livingstone/Elsevier; 2012; and Hoppenfeld S. *Physical Examination of the Spine and Extremities*. Appleton-Century-Croft/Prentice-Hall; 1976.

Assistive Devices and Gait

Walking with an assistive device such as a walker, crutch, or cane is sometimes necessary to reduce loading on healing tissues, reduce pain, or improve stability with walking. Assistive devices must be carefully chosen to allow for the most normal gait pattern while providing the necessary stability for safety. The cognitive attention necessary to manage the assistive device while avoiding potential environmental hazards and attending to changes in contact surface variations in evenness and friction must also be considered. A standard and wheeled walker provide an increased base of support. However, a wheeled walker allows a more normal gait pattern and requires less attention to coordinate movement and direction of the walker with components of the gait cycle than a standard walker.[43,44] A standard walker is likely easier to maneuver if non–weight bearing on one lower limb must be maintained. A straight cane has been shown to reduce pressure on the hip when used on the contralateral side[45] but does not allow unweighting of the lower extremity to the same extent as crutches or a walker.[43] The postural control required for safe crutch use is much greater than that for a walker.[46] These factors indicate that the patient's problem and recovery goal must be considered in the selection of devices to assist gait.

STANDARDIZED ASSESSMENTS OF BALANCE AND GAIT

Many standardized tests are available to assess balance and gait. The Performance-Oriented Mobility Assessment and the Dynamic Gait Index include activities to assess both balance and gait.[47,48] Standardized assessments of balance, such as the Berg Balance Scale,[49] should be utilized among patients with a history of falls, older patients, and patients with balance deficits (Table 5-3). The Functional Reach Test (Fig. 5-6) assesses the patient's limits of stability for static balance, and results can be

TABLE 5-3
STANDARDIZED GAIT AND BALANCE ASSESSMENTS

Tool	Tool Basics
Berg Balance Scale	• Assesses static and dynamic balance for lower level tasks such as transfers, turning, single leg balance, and picking up an object from the floor • Scoring: 0-56 • 14 tests scored 0-4, with lower scores indicating lower function • Normative data available based on age, diagnosis • Common cutoff score for fall risk is <45[49] • Common uses: fall risk assessment in a wide variety of orthopaedic and nonorthopaedic patient populations
Performance-Oriented Mobility Assessment (POMA)	• Gait and balance assessment for older adults that includes a balance section and gait assessment section • Scoring: 0-28 • Balance section includes tasks such as sitting and standing balance, rising/sitting, and turning • Gait assessment examines gait components including gait initiation, step length, symmetry, and continuity, path deviation, and base of support • 16 items scored 0-1 or 0-2, with lower scores indicating lower function • Fall risk: <19 high risk, 19-24 moderate risk[49]
Dynamic Gait Index (DGI)	• Gait and balance assessment that includes walking on a level surface, changing speeds, walking with head movements, turning, stepping over and around an obstacle, and steps • Scoring: 0-24 • 8 items scores 0-3, with lower scores indicating lower function • Cutoff score for increased fall risk in community-dwelling older adults: <19[47] • Minimal detectable change (for risk of falling): 3 points[48] • Common uses: fall risk in the elderly and those with neurologic dysfunction such as stroke, Parkinson disease, and multiple sclerosis
Timed Up and Go (TUG)	• Time for patient to rise from a standard arm chair, walk 3 m or 10 feet using an assistive device if needed, turn, and return to sitting. • Patients who take ≥ 12 seconds to complete the test are considered a fall risk[50]
6-Minute Walk Test	• Distance covered by a patient walking overground with or without an assistive device for 6 minutes. The patient may stop to rest as desired but cannot be paced by the examiner. • Minimal detectable change: (older adults) 48 m[51] • Common diagnoses: hip and knee osteoarthritis, hip and knee arthroplasty, variety of neurologic disease

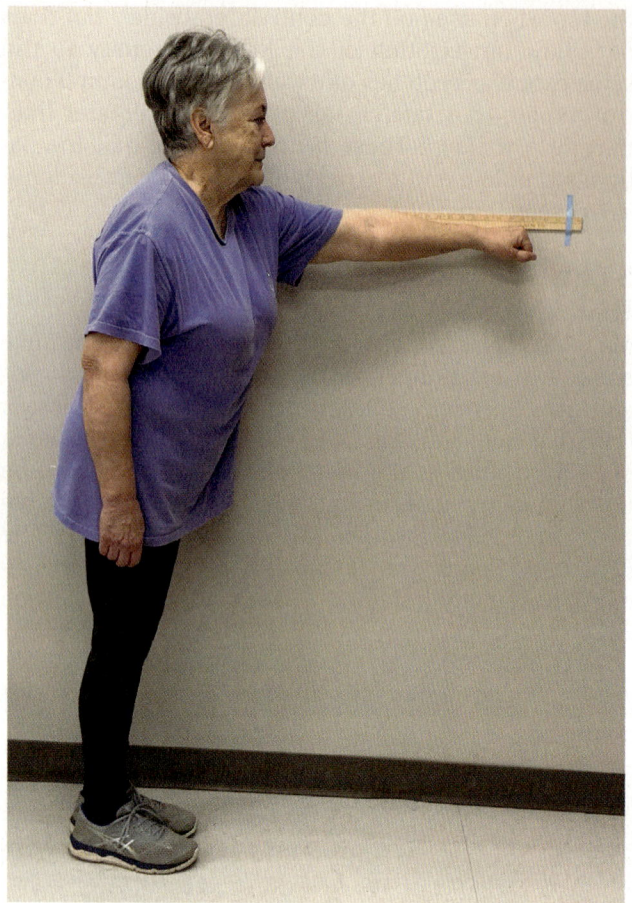

FIGURE 5-6 Functional Reach Test. The patient stands near a wall with feet together, shoulder flexed 90°, and fist closed. The patient then leans forward as far as possible without taking a step or leaning on the wall. The distance that is reached is recorded.

compared to normative values based on age, diagnosis, and living situation. Additional assessments of functional mobility include the Timed Up and Go and the 6-Minute Walk Test.[50,51]

FOOTWEAR

Footwear impacts gait, balance, and joint stress and, therefore, should be assessed in nearly all patients. Footwear and footwear modification can be an important component of injury prevention and rehabilitation. For the elderly, proper footwear selection should be part of fall prevention. Sadly, in one study,[52] 75% of patients who sustained a hip fracture in a fall were wearing footwear with at least one suboptimal feature (e.g., no attached heel). In another study, the majority of elderly reported wearing slippers in the house, and 11% wore shoes that were determined to be so old as to be "beyond repair."[53] Slippers are commonly worn because they are easy to don, soft, flexible, and comfortable. However, slippers are likely to be a fall risk because many of them lack an attached heel and do not have slip-resistant soles. There are seven main functions of footwear:

- Protect the plantar foot
- Provide traction
- Optimize alignment
- Provide foot stability
- Attenuate shock
- Provide energy return
- Offer a sense of individuality and cosmesis

There are many types of footwear, including slippers, sandals, athletic shoes, dress shoes, boots, and heels. Within each type of shoe, there are many varieties. For some examples, athletic shoes may be court shoes, walking shoes, cleats, road running shoes, trail running shoes, or racing flats. Likewise, heels may vary from a small, chunky "kitten" heel to an 8-inch, pencil-thin stiletto. Footwear can be made of a wide variety of materials—from flexible fabric, moldable leather, to stiff synthetic materials. Shoes may be open or closed toe and have a wide or small toe box. Shoes may slip on or have Velcro or lacing to make them more adjustable. Shoes may be securely attached to the foot with an enclosed heel counter or a heel strap or be loose posteriorly, like a flip flop.

Footwear Components

Figure 5-7 and Table 5-4 identify and describe important components of a typical shoe. The "last" is the mold from which a shoe is made. Shoes made from curved molds tend to provide more cushioning, whereas those made from straight molds tend to be more rigid. Similarly, slip-lasted construction design used in moccasin-type shoes is more flexible, whereas the board-lasted construction of an Oxford dress shoe is more rigid. Strobel-lasted construction designs are found in neutral running shoes, providing more flexibility than slip-lasted designs and less firmness than board-lasted designs.

The outsole primarily provides traction and can assist with shock absorption. On some running shoes, the outsole may contain a heel outflare to increase medial and lateral stability. However, this can also serve as a pivot point or fulcrum, increasing the risk of a lateral ankle sprain. The midsole is the primary shoe component to absorb shock,[54] reducing impact loading. Shoes with thicker midsoles provide more cushioning but may also decrease plantar sensation, making balance more challenging.[55] Midsoles are commonly constructed from ethylene-vinyl acetate (EVA), polyurethane (PU), air, or gel. Many shoes have midsoles of dual density[56] to absorb shock at heel strike but a more rigid medial heel and midfoot to decrease pronation. The insole, or sock liner, may be fixed or

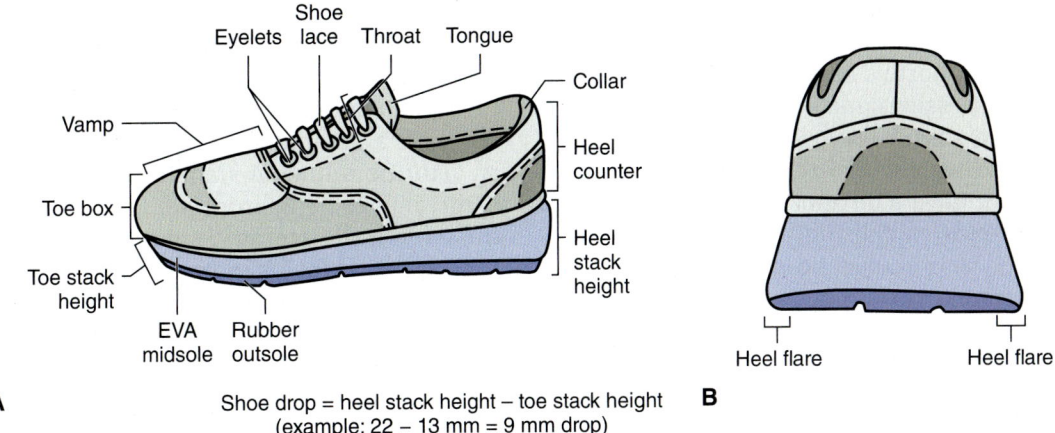

FIGURE 5-7 Components of footwear. **A.** Medial view. **B.** Posterior view.

removable. If orthotics are used, removable insoles should be taken out and the orthotic inserted.

The heel counter encircles the calcaneus. A heel counter that feels rigid when squeezed medial-laterally can help control foot pronation. The toe box should provide adequate room for the toes. A soft toe box with adequate height should be chosen to accommodate toe deformities. A narrow toe box may increase the risk for corns, blisters, and a hallux valgus deformity (bunion). Shoe drop is the difference between the heel height and the forefoot height (a 1-inch heel has a 1-inch drop). Shoes with a greater drop increase pressure on the forefoot and require more MTP extension but less dorsiflexion range for gait. Individuals who only walk in shoes with heels are likely to have a plantarflexion contracture, making ambulation without shoes problematic.

Footwear can be both a solution to and a source of foot and lower extremity pain. Individuals with standing jobs reported that wearing cushioned footwear or cushioned insoles reduced lower extremity fatigue and did so more than merely standing on a cushioned mat.[57] Footwear modification can also allow an athlete to continue to compete with less pain. For example, an athlete with a hyperextension injury to the great toe (also known as *turf toe*) can be put into a shoe with less of a break (less flexibility) at the MTP joint to decrease stress to the injured tissue. Choosing a shoe with a rocker-bottom design allows for the wearer to roll through the stance phase of gait with significantly less dorsiflexion range and MTP extension. This can be quite beneficial for an individual with ankle or great toe degenerative joint disease or an ankle fusion. In some circumstances, such as gymnastics or skating, footwear modifications are extremely limited.

Fitting Footwear

Many individuals report foot pain when wearing shoes.[58] Most likely, the shoes fit improperly[58] or are inappropriate for a given individual's foot structure and/or purpose. Poor shoe fit can increase the risk of falls, damage the integument, cause pain, and create gait deviations. Shoes should be assessed for length, width, heel fit, toe box and break, and shape. Shoe

TABLE 5-4	
KEY FOOTWEAR COMPONENTS	
Component	*Key Aspect*
Outsole	Provides traction
Midsole	Provides shock absorption
Insole	Prevents the foot from sliding within the shoe Absorbs sweat Helps control odor When new can provide a limited amount of shock absorption
Heel counter	Encircles calcaneus Rigid heel counter can help control pronation
Toe box	Provide enough depth for toes and toe deformities May be open, closed, or steel toed for some occupations
Throat	Opening for the foot
Collar	Cushioned area around the top of the shoe

rigidity should match the patient's needs. For example, the shoe of an individual should be difficult to twist if a patient needs a supportive shoe. Table 5-5 provides a basic guide for assessing shoe fit.

Clinicians can assess the outsole for signs of excessive wear and insight into the patient's gait. New shoes should not have a distinct wear pattern. Shoes with excessive wear or holes no longer provide their desired function and should be replaced. Figure 5-8 shows common wear patterns.

Running Shoes

Running is a popular fitness activity, and running-related injuries are commonly seen in outpatient clinics.

TABLE 5-5	
ASSESSING SHOE FIT	
Assessment	Method
Length	• Half inch longer than the longest toe
Shoe width	• Use the pinch test by pinching the medial and lateral vamp together. If fabric can be gathered, the shoe is too wide. • Check to see if there is any wearing in the region of a hallux valgus deformity
Heel fit	• Heel should be snug and not piston up and down during gait • Consider if the heel height is safe for the patient
Toe box	• Check to see if the patient can extend the toes slightly within the toe box and if there are any wear patterns from toe hyperextension
Toe break	• The break of the shoe should correspond with the patient's MTP
Last	• Place the bottom of the shoe against the plantar aspect of the patient's foot. The shoe shape (last) should match the shape of the patient's foot.
Rigidity	• Use the twist tests, twist the shoe front to back and rotate it across its axis • A supportive shoe will have little give, whereas a flexible shoe will be easily twisted.

MTP, metatarsophalangeal joint.

Running shoes are categorized as cushioned, stability, and motion control, making a continuum from soft to rigid (Fig. 5-9).

A cushioned shoe would be appropriate for a runner with a supinatory foot type, an older runner, or an arthritic runner. A stability, or neutral shoe, as the name implies, is appropriate for a runner with a neutral foot, or the average runner. A motion control shoe has a midsole that is more firm than a stability shoe,[56] which may reduce pronation and tibial internal rotation.[59] A motion control shoe may be appropriate for runners who overpronate. Theoretically, runners who overpronate and have conditions such as patellofemoral pain or plantar fasciopathy may benefit from a motion control shoe.[59] Various lacing strategies can also be used to help reduce pronation velocity.[55]

When choosing a running shoe, it is also important to consider shoe drop. Running shoe drop ranges from 0 to 14 mm, with the average running shoe having a drop of about 10 mm. Recall that a higher drop means less dorsiflexion range is required for normal gait. However, in terms of running, it is important to consider that a lower drop increases load on the Achilles tendon. Shoe drop should be considered when changing from one shoe model to another, as most runners can only tolerate a 2 to 4 mm decrease in drop without feeling signs of overloading of the Achilles tendon.[60] Conversely, runners with Achilles tendinopathy may benefit from the reduced loading of a shoe with a higher drop (in addition to any necessary changes in training). Minimalist shoes are ultra lightweight with very little or no shoe drop.[56] Transitioning from running in a more traditional 10-mm drop shoe into a minimalist shoe is best done by first changing to perhaps an 8-mm drop shoe for 2 to 4 months followed by a 4-mm drop shoe for another 2 to 4 months before finally trying the minimalist shoe. Minimalist shoes result in significantly greater tibial internal rotation and higher loading rates than traditional running shoes.[61] In addition, because minimalist shoes basically only protect the plantar surface of the foot, they are generally only indicated for individuals with a neutral foot and no musculoskeletal problems.

Footwear Recommendations

Table 5-6 provides some common problems that may benefit from footwear modifications. With more than

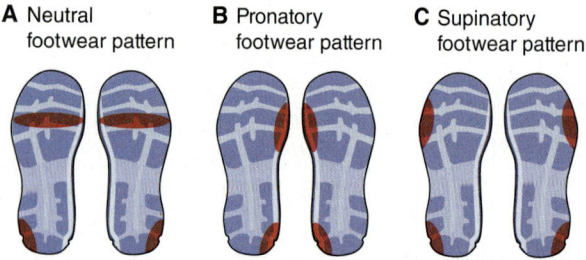

FIGURE 5-8 Common outsole wear patterns. (Adapted from Staheli LT. *Fundamentals of Pediatric Orthopedics.* 5th ed. Staheli, Inc./Wolters Kluwer; 2016; Figure 9.83.)

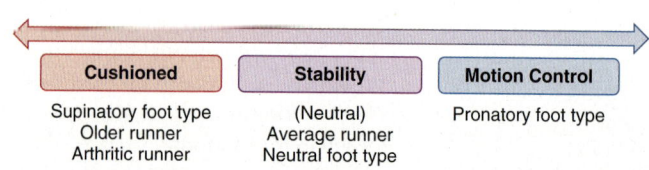

FIGURE 5-9 Continuum of running shoes.

TABLE 5-6
FOOTWEAR RECOMMENDATIONS

Problem	Example	Footwear Recommendations
Fall risk	Patient with poor balance such as elderly, post-fracture, or poststroke	• Proper length • Ensure heel does not piston • Heel counter or heel strap • Laces or Velcro to secure shoe • Outsole with traction* • Heel height < 1 inch
Decreased sensation	Patient with diabetes or peripheral neuropathy	• Full shoe (non-sandal type) with enclosed toe and hard outsole to protect against objects entering or pushing through the shoe • Soft materials with room in toe box • Low/no heel height • Wear socks
Decreased great toe extension	Patient with hallux valgus, hallux rigidus, or turf toe	• Rigid midsole • Rocker-bottom shoe
Decreased ankle dorsiflexion	Patient with ankle degenerative joint disease or after an ankle fracture	• Heel lift • Rocker-bottom shoe • Safe heel height
Increased pronation	Patient with pes planus	• Rigid heel counter • Straight-lasted shoe • Upper made of more rigid materials • No/low heel height • Motion control shoe
Lack of shock absorption	Patient with degenerative joint disease or rheumatoid arthritis who needs cushioning, patient with a supinatory foot type	• Midsole with shock-absorbing material • Shock-absorbing insert • Curve-lasted shoe • Cushioned shoe

*For some patients, such as those with Parkinson disease who walk with a shuffling gait, a shoe with minimal traction might be more appropriate.

50 brands and models of running shoes,[56] and new models coming out once or twice a year, it can be difficult for clinicians to make solid recommendations for their patients who are runners. Several running magazines publish a yearly guide to running shoes. In addition, shoe make and model information can be found online, including key details such as shoe class and shoe drop. However, finding a knowledgeable associate at a local running store can be invaluable.

FOOT ORTHOTICS

Although a thorough discussion of foot orthotics is outside the scope of this text, a brief summary is provided. There are three main functions of foot orthotics:

- Assist with weight distribution across the plantar aspect of the foot
- Provide cushioning and shock absorption
- Control foot motion

Orthotics can be excavated to make room for bony prominences. Padding can be used to cushion areas of pain.

Prefabricated Foot Orthotics

Prefabricated (off-the-shelf) foot orthotics can be expected to provide adequate cushioning by using shock-absorbing materials such as Sorbothane or gel. These may prove useful for individuals who cannot afford the most appropriate pair of shoes, a new pair of shoes, or require additional shock absorption for comfort. Some prefabricated orthotics provide a more rigid base, which may help patients with overpronation, for example, prefabricated orthotics and exercise may be beneficial for individuals who hyperpronate who have patellofemoral pain syndrome,[62] plantar fasciopathy,[63] flat feet,[64] or osteoarthritis-related lower extremity pain.[65] Orthotics that support the medial longitudinal arch appear to improve static and dynamic balance in healthy elderly adults[66] and in individuals with chronic ankle instability.[67] Clinicians may choose to try taping the patient's foot to see if this increased support provides symptom relief. If so, it is quite possible that this small intervention may be beneficial. Currently, the evidence for the use of orthotics to prevent overuse injuries is unclear.[68]

Custom Foot Orthotics

Custom orthotics are individually made from a cast or mold of a patient's feet. Custom orthotics are usually made based on the subtalar joint neutral theory (see Chapter 9, Ankle and Foot), cost between $200 and $400, and may or may not be covered by insurance.

Currently, there is limited evidence to support the use of custom orthotics for musculoskeletal conditions.[62] However, custom devices may be beneficial for individuals with hallux valgus, individuals with significant foot deformities including those due to rheumatoid arthritis,[69] and individuals with conditions that have not improved with conservative interventions, such as footwear modification, load management strategies, and exercise.

Heel Lifts and Wedges

Heel lifts and wedges may be used in most standard footwear with or without orthotics. A heel lift is a wedge that is thicker posteriorly and tapered anteriorly. A heel lift is placed in the rear of the shoe under the calcaneus. A heel lift is equivalent to increasing the drop of a shoe, thereby reducing the amount of dorsiflexion required for gait. A heel lift may be used if a patient lacks the dorsiflexion range or gastrocnemius length required for normal gait or if this motion is painful. A heel wedge also essentially lengthens the lower extremity. As such, it may be used to even out a leg length discrepancy. Because of the potential to create an ankle plantarflexion contracture long term, a full-length insert may be superior to a heel lift. Because there is limited space inside the shoe, an external shoe lift may be required if the limb length is more than 5 mm or so. External shoe lifts are both costly and effect cosmesis, which may limit patient adherence.

A medial wedge is thicker medially and tapered laterally. Placing a medial wedge under the calcaneus can reduce the amount of rearfoot pronation by acting as a sort of buttress to calcaneal eversion. This can be useful for individuals with tibialis posterior dysfunction[70] or a rigid hindfoot varus. A lateral heel wedge can be used to promote rearfoot eversion. There is some evidence that a lateral heel wedge may unload the medial compartment of the knee, reducing pain in individuals with medial compartment degenerative joint disease.[71,72] Medial and lateral forefoot wedges can compensate for forefoot varus and valgus, respectively, thereby reducing the amount of compensatory rearfoot motion.[73] Chapter 9, Ankle and Foot, contains additional details on these pathologies.

CHAPTER SUMMARY

Clinical and laboratory gait analysis informs decision-making to improve locomotion capacity in individuals of all ages, occupation, and sport. In planning interventions, the clinician should consider patient's goals, safety, efficiency, pain complaints, footwear, history of falls, and fear of falling. The use of digital video assists visual observation and allows the patient to see the impact of therapeutic interventions impacting gait.

REFERENCES

1. Levine D, Richards J, Whittle MW. *Whittle's Gait Analysis*. 5th ed. Churchill Livingstone/Elsevier; 2012.
2. Burnfield J, Shu Y, Buster T, Taylor A. Similarity of joint kinematics and muscle demands between elliptical training and walking: implications for practice. *Phys Ther.* 2010;90(2):289–305.
3. Murray M, Drought A, Kory R. Walking patterns of normal men. *J Bone Joint Surg Am.* 1964;46:335–360.
4. Murray M, Kory R, Sepic S. Walking patterns of normal women. *Arch Phys Med Rehabil.* 1970;51(11):637–650.
5. Murray M. Gait as a total pattern of movement. *Am J Phys Med.* 1967;46(1):290–333.
6. Kadaba M, Ramakrishnan H, Wootten M, Gainey J, Gorton G, Cochran G. Repeatability of kinematic, kinetic, and electromyographic data in normal adult gait. *J Orthop Res.* 1989;7(6):849–860.
7. Levangie PK, Norkin CC. *Joint Structure and Function: A Comprehensive Analysis*. 5th ed. F.A. Davis; 2011.
8. Nawoczenski D, Baumhauer J, Umberger B. Relationship between clinical measurements and motion of the first metatarsophalangeal joint during gait. *J Bone Joint Surg.* 1999;81(3):370–376.
9. Gilbert S, Chen T, Hutchinson I, et al. Dynamic contact mechanics on the tibial plateau of the human femur during activities of daily living. *J Biomech.* 2014;47(9):2006–2012.
10. Lafortune M, Cavanagh P, Sommer HR, Kalenak A. Three-dimensional kinematics of the human knee during walking. *J Biomech.* 1992;25(4):347–357.
11. Nester C. The relationship between transverse plane leg rotation and transverse plane motion at the knee and hip during normal walking. *Gait Posture.* 2000;(3):251–256.
12. Oatis CA. *Kinesiology: The Mechanics and Pathomechanics of Human Movement*. 3rd ed. Wolters Kluwer; 2017.
13. Reischl S, Powers C, Rao S, Perry J. Relationship between foot pronation and rotation of the tibia and femur during walking. *Foot Ankle Int.* 1999;20(8):513–520.
14. McPoil T, Knecht H. Biomechanics of the foot in walking: a function approach. *J Orthop Sports Phys Ther.* 1986;7(2):69–72.
15. Houglum PA, Burtoti DB. *Brunnstrom's Clinical Kinesiology*. 6th ed. F.A. Davis; 2012.
16. Kettelkamp D, Johnson R, Smidt G, Chao E, Walker M. An electrogoniometric study of knee motion in normal gait. *J Bone Joint Surg Am.* 1970;52(4):775–790.
17. Winter D, Yack H. EMG profiles during normal human walking: stride-to-stride and inter-subject variability. *Electroencephalogr Clin Neurophysiol.* 1987;67(5):402–411.
18. Shaivi R. Electromyographic patterns in adult locomotion: a comprehensive review. *J Rehabil Res Dev.* 1985;22(3):85–98.
19. Gronley J, Perry J. Gait analysis techniques. Rancho Los Amigos Hospital gait laboratory. *Phys Ther.* 1984;64(12):1831–1838.
20. Rose G. Clinical gait assessment: a personal view. *J Med Eng Technol.* 1983;7(6):273–279.
21. Zijlstra W, Rutgers A, Van Weerden T. Voluntary and involuntary adaptation of gait in Parkinson's disease. *Gait Posture.* 1998;1(7):53–63.
22. Bohannon R. Comfortable and maximum walking speed of adults aged 20–79 years: reference values and determinants. *Age Aging.* 1997;26(1):15–19.
23. Cunningham D, Rechnitzer P, Pearce M, Donner A. Determinants of self-selected walking pace across ages 19 to 66. *J Gerontol.* 1982;37(5):560–564.
24. DeVita P, Hortobagyi T. Age causes a redistribution of joint torques and powers during gait. *J Appl Physiol.* 2000;88(5):1804–1811.

25. Kerrigan D, Todd M, Della Croce U, Lipsitz L, Collins J. Biomechanical gait alterations independent of speed in the healthy elderly: evidence for specific limiting impairments. *Arch Phys Med Rehabil*. 1998;79(3):317–322. doi:10.1016/s0003-9993(98)90013-2
26. Elble R, Thomas S, Higgins C, Colliver J. Stride-dependent changes in gait of older people. *J Neurol*. 1991;238(1):1–5.
27. Hageman P, Blanke D. Comparison of gait of young women and elderly women. *Phys Ther*. 1986;66(9):1382–1387.
28. Himann J, Cunningham D, Rechnitzer P, Paterson D. Age-related changes in speed of walking. *Med Sci Sports Exerc*. 1988;20(2):161–166.
29. Hollman J, Kovash F, Kubik J, Linbo R. Age-related differences in spatiotemporal markers of gait stability during dual task walking. *Gait Posture*. 2007;26(1):113–119.
30. Murray M, Kory R, Clarkson B. Walking patterns in healthy old men. *J Gerontol*. 1969;24(2):169–178.
31. Muir B, Bodratti L, Morris C, Haddad J, van Emmerik R, Rietdyk S. Gait characteristic during inadvertent obstacle contact in young, middle-aged and older adults. *Gait Posture*. 2020;77:100–104.
32. Beauchet O, Annweiler C, Dubost V, et al. Stops walking when talking: a predictor of falls in older adults? *Eur J Neurol*. 2009;16(7):786–795.
33. Lundin-Olsson L, Nyberg L, Gustafson Y. "Stops walking when talking" as a predictor of falls in elderly people. *Lancet*. 1997;349(9052):617.
34. Verghese J, Holtzer R, Lipton R, Wang C. Quantitative gait markers and incident fall risk in older adults. *J Gerontol A Biol Sci Med Sci*. 2009;64(8):896–901.
35. Khow K, Visvanathan R. Falls in the aging population. *Clin Geriatr Med*. 2017;33(3):357–368.
36. Deandrea S, Lucenteforte E, Bravi F, Foschi R, La Vecchia R, Negri E. Risk factors for falls in community-dwelling older people: a systematic review and meta-analysis. *Epidemiology*. 2010;21(5):658–668.
37. Ambrose A, Paul G, Hausdorff J. Risk factors for falls among older adults: a review of the literature. *Maturitas*. 2013;75(1):51–61.
38. Gill T, Baker D, Gottschalk M, Peduzzi P, Allore H, Byers A. A program to prevent functional decline in physical frail, elderly persons who live at home. *N Engl J Med*. 2002;347(14):1068–1074.
39. Fried L, Tangen C, Walston J, et al; Cardiovascular Health Study Collaborative Research Group. Frailty in older adults: evidence for a phenotype. *J Gerontol A Biol Sci Med Sci*. 2001;56(3):146–156.
40. Fried L, Ferrucci L, Darer J, Williamson J, Anderson G. Untangling the concepts of disability, frailty, and comorbidity: implications for improved targeting and care. *J Gerontol A Biol Sci Med Sci*. 2004;59(3):255–263.
41. Abellan van Kan G, Rolland Y, Bergman H, Morley J, Kritchevsky S, Vellas B. Frailty assessment of older people in clinical practice. Expert opinion of a Geriatric Advisory Panel. *J Nutr Health Aging*. 2007;12(1):29–37.
42. Fritz S, Lusardi M. White paper: "Walking speed: The sixth vital sign". *J Geriatric Phys Ther*. 2009;32(2):2–9.
43. Melis E, Torres-Moreno R, Barbeaum H, Lemaire E. Analysis of assisted-gait characteristics in persons with incomplete spinal cord injury. *Spinal Cord*. 1999;37(6):430–439.
44. Kegelmeyer D, Parthasarathy S, Kostyk S, White S, Kloos A. Assistive devices alter gait patterns in Parkinson disease: advantages of the four-wheeled walker. *Gait Posture*. 2013;38(1):20–24.
45. Krebs D, Robbins C, Lavine L, Mann R. Hip biomechanics during gait. *J Orthop Sports Phys Ther*. 1998;28(1):51–59.
46. Martins M, Santos C, Costa L, Frizera A. Feature reduction and multi-classification of different assistive devices according to the gait pattern. *Disabil Rehabil Assist Technol*. 2016;11(3):202–218.
47. Shumway-Cook A, Gruber W, Baldwin M, Liao S. The effect of multidimensional exercises on balance, mobility, and fall risk in community-dwelling older adults. *Phys Ther*. 1997;77(1):46–57. doi:10.1093/ptj/77.1.46
48. Romero S, Bishop M, Velozo C, Light K. Minimum detectable change of the Berg Balance Scale and Dynamic Gait Index in older persons at risk for falling. *J Geriatr Phys Ther*. 2011;34(3):131–137. doi:10.1519/JPT.0b013e3182048006
49. Lima C, Ricci N, Nogueira E, Perracini M. The Berg Balance Scale as a clinical screening tool to predict fall risk in older adults: a systematic review. *Physiotherapy*. 2018;104(4):383–394. doi:10.1016/j.physio.2018.02.002
50. Olsson Möller U, Kristensson J, Midlöv P, Ekdahl C, Jakobsson U. Predictive validity and cut-off scores in four diagnostic tests for falls—a study in frail older people at home. *Phys Occup Ther Geriatr*. 2012;30(3):189–201. doi:10.3109/02703181.2012.694586
51. Perera S, Mody S, Woodman R, Studenski S. Meaningful change and responsiveness in common physical performance measures in older adults. *J Am Geriatr Soc*. 2006;54(5):743–749.
52. Sherrington C, Menz H. An evaluation of footwear worn at the time of fall-related hip fracture. *Age Ageing*. 2003;32(3):310–314. doi:10.1093/ageing/32.3.310
53. Menant J, Steele J, Menz H, Munro B, Lord S. Optimizing footwear for older people at risk of falls. *J Rehabil Res Dev*. 2008;45(8):1167–1181. doi:10.1682/jrrd.2007.10.0168
54. Piaolin P, Shaolan D, Zhikang W, Yifan Z, Jiahao P. Effect of running speed and midsole type on foot loading in heel–toe running. *J Appl Biomech*. 2020;36(3):134–140. doi:10.1123/jab.2019-0236
55. Xiaole S, Wing-Kai L, Xini Z, Junqing W, Weijie F. Systematic review of the role of footwear constructions in running biomechanics: implications for running-related injury and performance. *J Sports Sci Med*. 2020;19(1):20–37.
56. Ramsey C, Lamb P, Kaur M, Baxter G, Ribeiro D. How are running shoes assessed? A systematic review of characteristics and measurement tools used to describe running footwear. *J Sports Sci*. 2019;37(14):1617–1629. doi:10.1080/02640414.2019.1578449
57. Anderson J, Williams A, Nester C. A narrative review of musculoskeletal problems of the lower extremity and back associated with the interface between occupational tasks, feet, footwear and flooring. *Musculoskeletal Care*. 2017;15(4):304–315. doi:10.1002/msc.1174
58. de Castro A, Rebelatto J, Aurichio T. The relationship between wearing incorrectly sized shoes and foot dimensions, foot pain, and diabetes. *J Sport Rehabil*. 2010;19(2):214–225. doi:10.1123/jsr.19.2.214
59. Cheung R, Ng G, Chen B. Association of footwear with patellofemoral pain syndrome in runners. *Sports Med*. 2006;36(3):199–205. doi:10.2165/00007256-200636030-00002
60. Lussiana T, Fabre N, Hébert-Losier K, Mourot L. Effect of slope and footwear on running economy and kinematics. *Scand J Med Sci Sports*. 2013;23(4):e246–e253. doi:10.1111/sms.12057
61. Sinclair J, Fau-Goodwin J, Richards J, Shore H. The influence of minimalist and maximalist footwear on the kinetics and kinematics of running. *Footwear Sci*. 2016;8(1):33–39. doi:10.1080/19424280.2016.1142003
62. Willy R, Hoglund L, Barton C, et al. Patellofemoral pain. *J Orthop Sports Phys Ther*. 2019;49(9):CPG1-CPG95.

63. Schuitema D, Greve C, Postema K, Dekker R, Hijmans J. Effectiveness of mechanical treatment for plantar fasciitis: a systematic review. *J Sport Rehabil.* 2020;29(5):657–674.
64. Desmyttere G, Hajizadeh M, Bleau J, Begon M. Effect of foot orthosis design on lower limb joint kinematics and kinetics during walking in flexible pes planovalgus: a systematic review and meta-analysis. *Clin Biomech.* 2018;59:117–129.
65. Wagner A, Luna S. Effect of footwear on joint pain and function in older adults with lower extremity osteoarthritis. *J Geriatr Phys Ther.* 2018;41(2):85–101.
66. Ma C, Lam W-K, Chang B-C, Lee W. Can insoles be used to improve static and dynamic balance of community-dwelling older adults? A systematic review on recent advances and future perspectives. *J Aging Phys Act.* 2020;28(6):971–986.
67. Gabriner M, Braun B, Houston M, Hoch M. The effectiveness of foot orthotics in improving postural control in individuals with chronic ankle instability: a critically appraised topic. *J Sport Rehabil.* 2015;24(1):68–71.
68. Kelly J, Valier A. The use of orthotic insoles to prevent lower limb overuse injuries: a critically appraised topic. *J Sport Rehabil.* 2018;27(6):591–595.
69. Arias-Martín I, Reina-Bueno M, Munuera-Martínez PV. Effectiveness of custom-made foot orthoses for treating forefoot pain: a systematic review. *Int Orthop.* 2018;42(8):1865–1875.
70. Ling S, Lui T. Posterior tibial tendon dysfunction: an overview. *Open Orthop J.* 2017;11:714–723.
71. Tohyama H, Yasuda K, Kaneda K. Treatment of osteoarthritis of the knee with heel wedges. *Int Orthop.* 1991;15(1):31–33.
72. Butler R, Marchesi S, Royer T, Davis I. The effect of a subject-specific amount of lateral wedge on knee mechanics in patients with medial knee osteoarthritis. *J Orthop Res.* 2007;25(9):1121–1127.
73. Gross M. Lower quarter screening for skeletal malalignment—suggestions for orthotics and shoewear. *J Orthop Sports Phys Ther.* 1995;21(6):389–405.

PART II

Basic History and Physical Examination

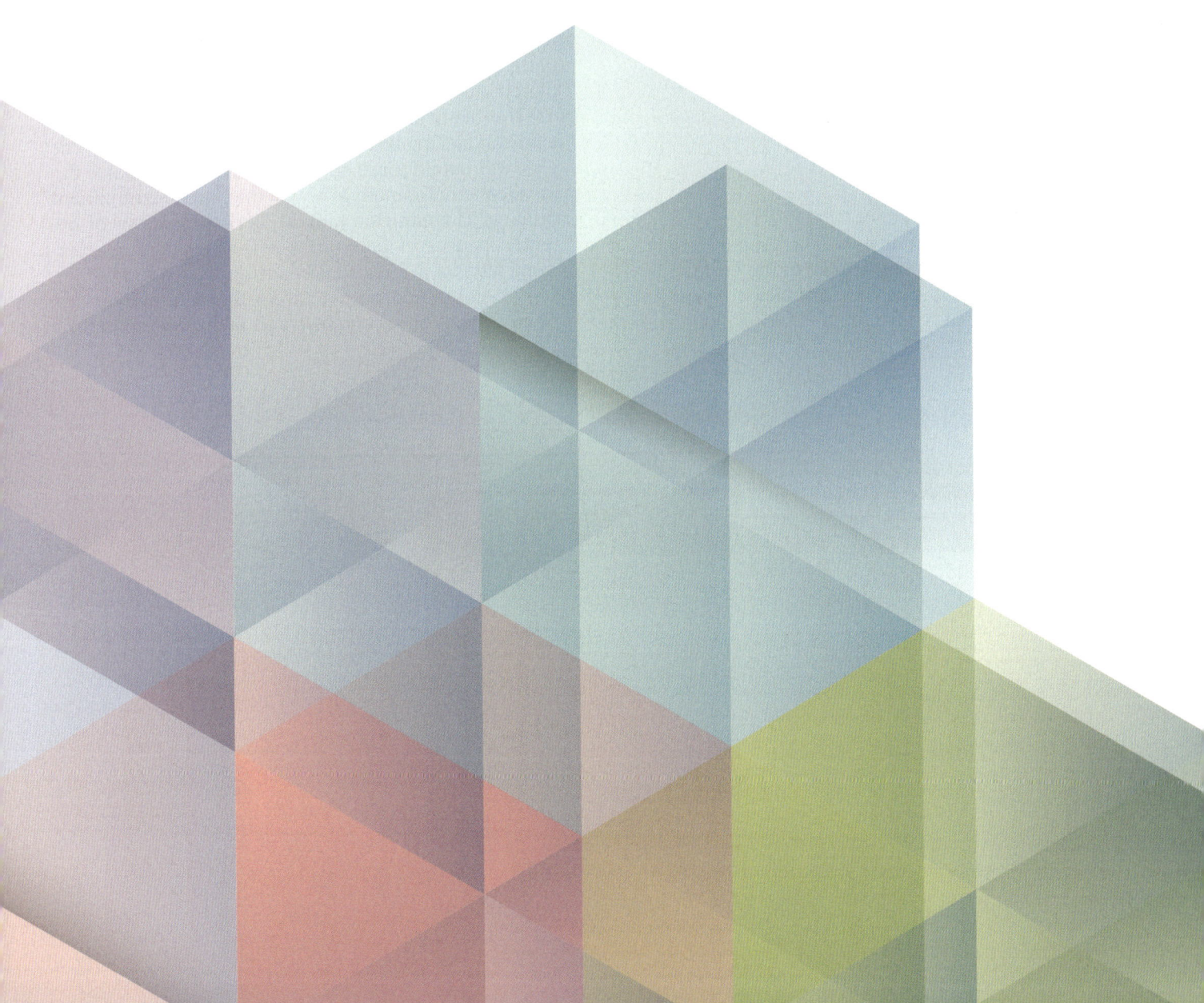

6 | Patient History
Betsy Myers

CHAPTER OBJECTIVES
After reading this chapter, you will be able to:
1. State the key elements of the patient history.
2. Describe methods to efficiently and effectively take a patient history.
3. Describe the rationale for performing a thorough patient history.
4. Describe key information to obtain from the patient regarding health history and demographics, symptom investigation, and review of systems.
5. Determine how to choose relevant systems to explore during the review of systems.

HISTORY

The evaluation consists of two main parts: the history and the physical examination. The patient history is arguably the most important part of the evaluation. The history is composed of three elements: health history and demographics, symptom investigation, and the review of systems (Fig. 6-1). Together, these three elements help to establish patient rapport, determine that it is safe to proceed to the physical examination, generate hypotheses regarding differential diagnosis to help focus the physical examination, provide context for the patient's condition, establish goals, and determine whether the patient may benefit from any referrals.

Figure 6-2 provides a sample outpatient intake form (sometimes known as a medical history form) that includes many of the key components of the history. Forms, such as these, are extremely useful in providing a broad overview of the patient, allowing for a more holistic and efficient patient encounter. Intake forms can be provided electronically or sent by mail to patients when scheduling their evaluation or be completed onsite before this first patient visit.

The history-taking process should begin with the clinician making introductions and explaining how the visit will unfold. Care should be taken to organize the physical environment in a way that maximizes patient privacy. The clinician should alert the patient of potential pauses to take notes, either by hand or electronically, as a means of ensuring best patient care. The room should be set up so that the patient can be in a position of comfort and allow eye contact. If

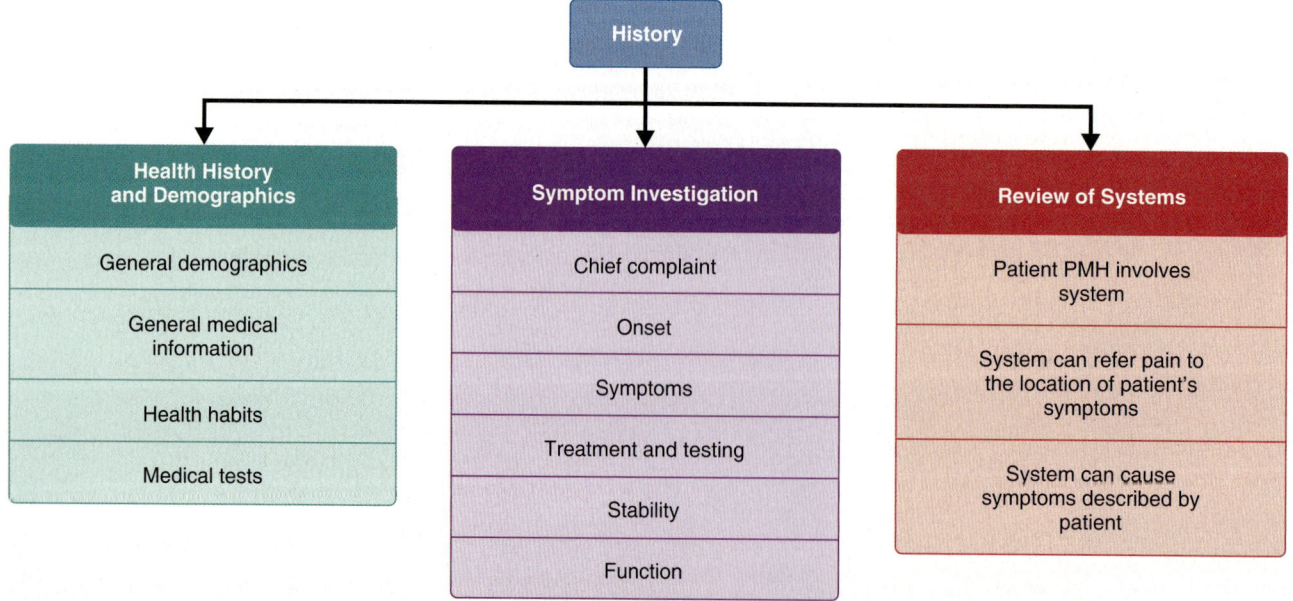

FIGURE 6-1 Key elements of the history. *PMH*, past medical history.

Intake Form

Name: _____ Date: _____ Age: ___

Gender: _____ Pronoun: _____ Race/Ethnicity: _____ Preferred language: _____

Reason for visit: _____

When did this start? _____

How did this occur? ☐ No apparent reason ☐ _____

Have you had this problem in the past? ☐ No ☐ Yes If so, please describe (how often, how long it lasted, how resolved). _____

What activities are you having difficulty performing (hobbies, sports, exercise, work): _____
_____

Describe any treatment you have tried so far to assist with this and the result (ibuprofen, ice)
_____

Describe any testing you have received for this and the result (x-ray, MRI, etc.):
_____

Mark the location of your symptom(s) on the diagrams below:

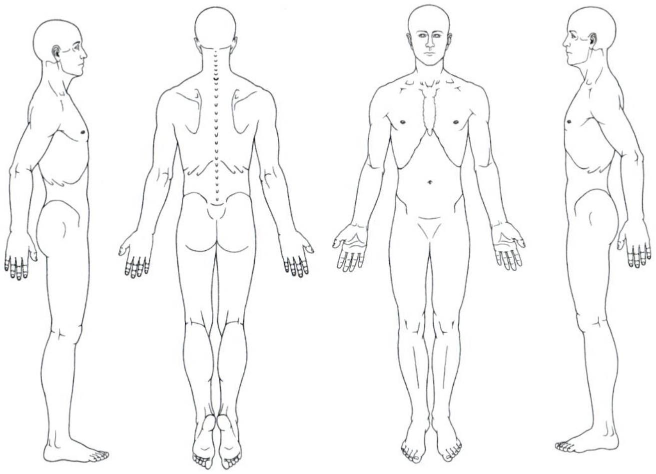

Using the following scale, 0 = No pain, 10 = Worst pain imaginable, Emergency Department necessary
  what is your pain level **right now**? ___/10
  During the last 48 hours, what was your pain: **at best** ___/10 **at worst:** ___/10

Overall are you: ☐ getting better ☐ getting worse ☐ staying the same

Describe your symptoms: ☐ pins and needles   ☐ burning   ☐ aching   ☐ dull
    ☐ sharp ☐ stabbing   ☐ throbbing   other: _____

What makes your symptoms **better**? ☐ activity ☐ rest ☐ morning ☐ end of day
    ☐ sitting ☐ walking   ☐ ice ☐ heat ☐ medications: _____ Other: _____

What makes your symptoms **worse**? ☐ activity ☐ rest ☐ morning ☐ end of day
    ☐ sitting ☐ walking   ☐ ice ☐ heat ☐ medications: _____ Other: _____

FIGURE 6-2 Intake form.

Goal(s) for therapy: _____

Mark any boxes if you have a history of, or have recently experienced, the following:

☐ High blood pressure	☐ Cancer	☐ Nail changes
☐ High cholesterol	☐ Night sweats	☐ Skin changes
☐ Heart disease	☐ Night pain	☐ Vision changes
☐ Chest pain	☐ Ulcer	☐ Easy bruising
☐ Leg cramping with walking	☐ Constipation	☐ Excessive weight gain or loss
☐ Feel a heartbeat in your abdomen	☐ Incontinence	☐ Headaches
☐ Lightheadedness	☐ Abdominal pain	☐ Arthritis
☐ Diabetes	☐ Changes in menstrual pattern	☐ Muscle weakness
☐ Stroke	☐ Numbness, tingling	☐ Fatigue
☐ Epilepsy / seizures	☐ Walking or balance difficulties	☐ Morning stiffness
☐ Asthma / breathing problems	☐ Long-term steroid use	☐ Trauma (car accident or fall)

Are you currently pregnant? ☐ No ☐ Yes
List prior surgeries: _____
List any other diagnoses or injuries: _____
List any medications/supplements you are taking: _____
List any allergies (i.e., latex, adhesives, sulfa, etc.)? _____
Occupation: _____ Currently working? ☐ No ☐ Yes
Recreational activities/sports: _____
How often do you exercise? ☐ 0 days/week   ☐ 1–4 days/week   ☐ 5–7 days/week
On average, how many minutes of moderate or strenuous exercise (e.g., at least a *brisk* walk) do you engage in per week? ____
On average, how many alcoholic drinks do you have per week? _____
Do you smoke? ☐ No ☐ Yes: ___packs/d, ___ yrs ☐ Former smoker: date quit _____packs/d, __yrs,
On average, how many hours of sleep do you get per night? _____
    Does this current problem affect your sleep? ☐ No ☐ Yes
Do you currently feel stressed? ☐ No ☐ Yes
Do you feel down, depressed, or hopeless? ☐ No ☐ Yes
Please note if you need any accommodations or have any preferences that may affect your therapy (i.e., religion, physical disability, etc.). _____

FIGURE 6-2 (*continued*)

documenting on an electronic health record, at times, it might be helpful to show the screen to the patient. For example, the patient could view the list of patient medications entered by a primary care provider.

When interviewing a patient, clinicians should use a funnel approach, starting with open-ended questions, followed by more closed-ended or specific questions, and progressing to specific yes/no questions. Rather than randomly asking a series of preset questions, clinicians should have a purpose for each question, using the patient's answer to guide the next question. This approach allows patients to tell their story in an efficient manner.

Pattern recognition for musculoskeletal pathology is important and can help clinicians be more efficient. However, each patient situation must be considered individually. For example, although it is rare that shoulder pain is caused by a Pancoast tumor, clinicians must consider this pathology within the differential diagnoses in a patient with shoulder pain who has a long history of smoking.[1] Although many times it is possible to identify a pathoanatomic cause to a patient's chief complaint, this, in itself, is insufficient for developing a plan of care. Consider two patients presenting with reports consistent with a full-thickness rotator cuff tear: each unable to raise the affected arm out to the side. The first patient is an 18-year-old who reports the injury was the result of a wrestling competition last week. The second patient is a 75-year-old who reports the problem has been long-standing but made worse when transferring his spouse from the bed to a wheelchair. Without uncovering these contextual factors during the history, an individualized plan of care cannot be created.

How questions are phrased depends on the amount and type of information available to the clinician. For example, beginning the interview by asking a patient: "What brought you in today?" would seem to be an appropriate starting point. However, if the patient has completed an intake form, such as the one in Figure 6-2, asking this question makes it clear to the patient that the clinician has not paid attention to the information already provided. In this case, the clinician should begin the interview by acknowledging having read through the patient intake information: "I see that you are having problems with your right knee that began last week after a fall. Can you tell me more about what made you fall?" The clinician should demonstrate active listening skills through the appropriate use of silence and summarizing patient information. "Let me see if I am understanding you correctly...." Clinicians should ask clarifying questions when necessary: "When you say you couldn't walk after the injury, do you mean you were unable to walk *normally* or that it was too painful to bear any weight on that leg?" Clinicians may choose to repeat or restate key pieces of information to ensure they understand the patient's narrative.

Clinicians should monitor verbal and nonverbal communication throughout the visit. This includes using patient-first language, monitoring tone, nodding or stating verbal encouragement for the patient to continue, maintaining good posture, and demonstrating appropriate body language. Talkative patients may require redirecting: "You have voiced several concerns, what is the primary concern that we should focus on today?" Emotional patients may benefit from reassurance. The clinician should show empathy for the patient's situation accordingly: "That must have been difficult to get around for a few days. I'm sorry that happened to you. Can you tell me more about how you were able to walk immediately after you injured your knee?" At times, it is necessary for clinicians to ask questions that appear unrelated or extremely personal. It is important that clinicians explain the reason for asking such personal questions and use nonjudgmental language: "Some patients with hip pain experience incontinence. Is this something you have experienced?" By developing patient rapport, providing background for questions, and gathering nonthreatening information first, the patient is more likely to provide necessary personal information such as this.

HEALTH HISTORY AND GENERAL DEMOGRAPHICS

The health history and general demographic information are obtained by reviewing the patient's medical record and, in an outpatient setting, reviewing intake forms completed by the patient or caregiver. The majority of this information can be gained before seeing the patient and then clarified or expanded upon when face-to-face with the patient. Figure 6-3 provides examples of the importance of investigating this information for each patient. The successful clinician does not attempt to treat the patient's chief complaint in isolation but instead cares for the patient as a whole.

General Demographics

Because the prevalence of many disease processes varies by age, gender, and race/ethnicity, the clinician should review the patient's general demographic information to begin to form diagnostic hypotheses (Fig. 6-4). For example, given two patients with knee pain, a 13-year-old and a 65-year-old, the younger patient is much more likely to have patellofemoral pain syndrome[2] whereas the older patient is more likely to have knee osteoarthritis.[3] In addition, rheumatoid arthritis[4] is more prevalent in females than males, whereas Dupuytren disease is more prevalent in individuals of North-Western European descent.[5]

The clinician should understand the patient's social history. Does the patient live alone? If the patient is a minor or unable to give consent, who is the primary caregiver? Can someone assist with a home exercise program, if needed? In what environment does the individual live? Are there stairs to navigate? It is important to know whether the patient is a student or currently working. What are the patient's job demands and schedule needs? Knowing a patient's occupational demands can assist with both goal planning and scheduling.

Knowledge of the patient's (and caregiver's) level of education will allow the clinician to present

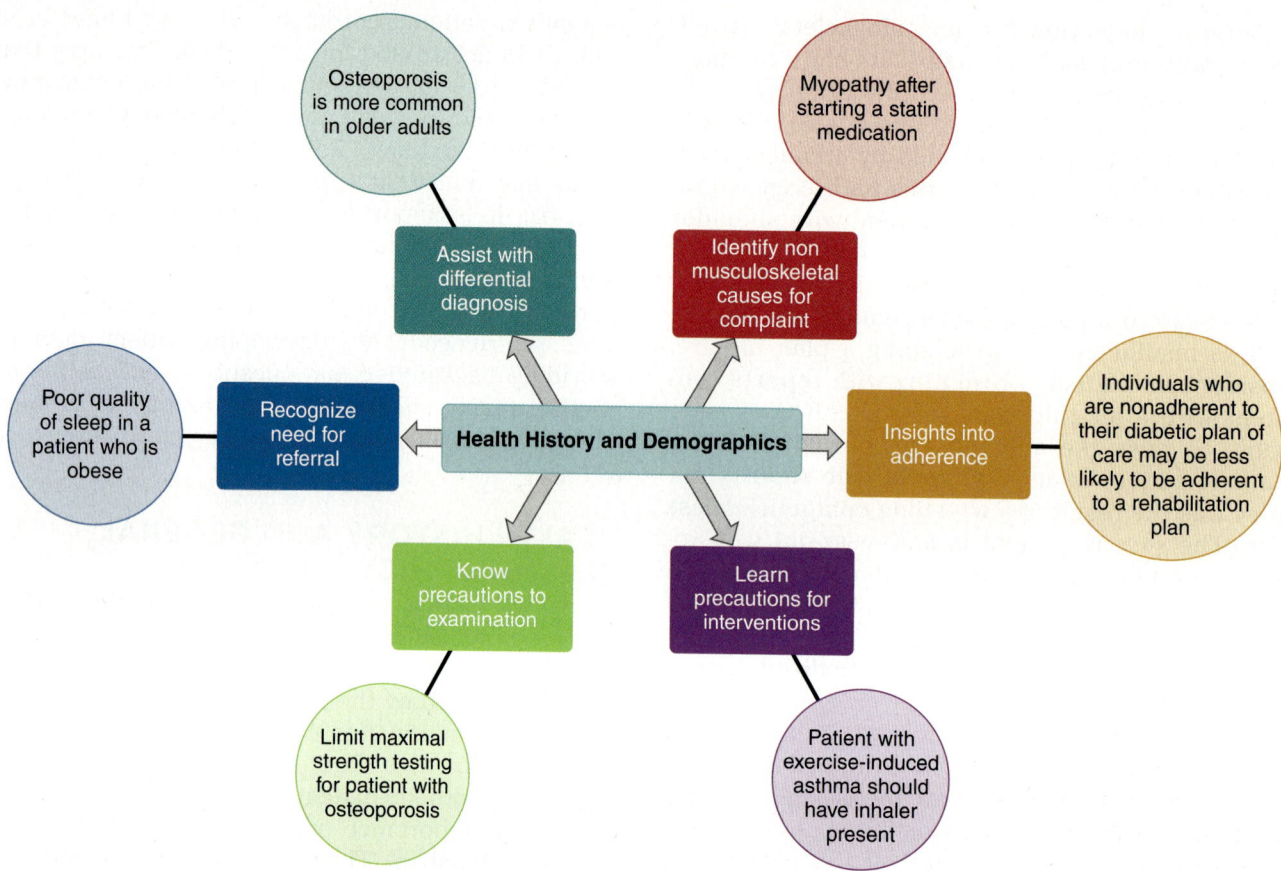

FIGURE 6-3 Importance of thoroughly investigating health history and general demographics.

information and instructions at an appropriate level to maximize learning. Determination of the preferred language is vital to accurate communication. If the clinician is not fluent in this language, a translator should be provided.

Health History

A patient's health history can be grouped into three parts: general medical information, health habits, and medical tests.

General Medical Information The clinician should understand the patient's prior illnesses, injuries, surgeries, allergies, family history, and medications. Many times, patients do not list this information because they do not think it is relevant to the reason they are coming to therapy. For example, a patient may not mention a prior lumbar surgery or diabetes because they do not think it could be related to a new onset of foot pain. The clinician should ask about the presence of allergies. This is particularly important for allergies to adhesives (commonly used for taping or electrotherapy), sulfa (commonly used in iontophoresis and topical agents for wound management), and latex (used in some equipment, such as resistance bands). Knowing a patient's family history helps identify family health risks such as cancer, high cholesterol, hypertension, coronary artery disease, asthma, obesity, autoimmune diseases, arthritis, and dementia.[6,7] The clinician should perform a complete medication reconciliation[8,9] including medications prescribed to the patient for the current condition, medications prescribed for other conditions, over-the-counter medications, herbs and supplements, and recreational or illicit drugs. Patients should be asked if they notice any side effects from their medications including the "4Ds": dizziness, drowsiness, depression, or disturbed vision.

Table 6-1 provides a framework for performing medication reconciliation. Medication use can provide insights into the patient's current condition (response to anti-inflammatory medication), undisclosed medical conditions (use of glucose-lowering medication in a patient who did not equate his "touch of sugar" with diabetes), intervention modification (need to use rate of perceived exertion rather than target heart rate for exercise intensity in a patient taking β blockers, such as atenolol), and identify potential problems, such as polypharmacy and drug interactions. Patients may take antihistamines to combat pruritus, a common

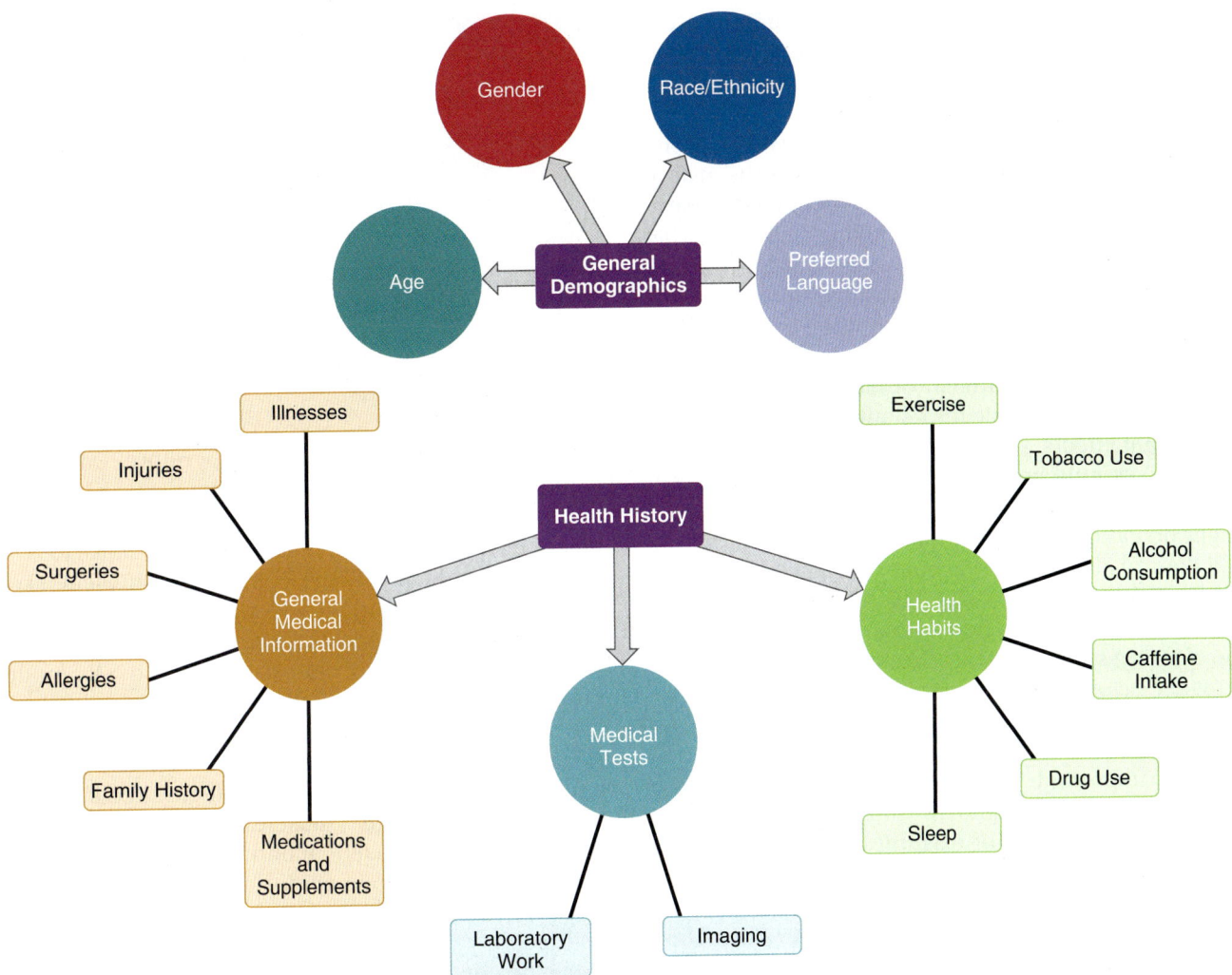

FIGURE 6-4 General demographics and health history.

TABLE 6-1
MEDICATION RECONCILIATION
Clinicians should learn the following information regarding patient medication:
• Medication name, dose, frequency • When started, when last taken, any recent changes in prescription • The patient's understanding of what the medication is for • Does the medication seem to be working? • Do the patient notice any increase in symptoms or do symptoms start after taking the medication?
Patients should be asked about the use of specific medications:
• Acetaminophen, nonsteroidal anti-inflammatories • Pain medications • Steroids • Blood pressure medication • Nitroglycerin • Cholesterol-lowering medication • Blood sugar medication • Sleep aides • Allergy medications • Mood-altering drugs • Laxatives

adverse drug reaction.[6] Medications may be used to treat the side effects of other medicines: a patient may take a proton-pump inhibitor, such as omeprazole, to treat an ulcer caused by nonsteroidal anti-inflammatory medication.

Screening for cardiac-related medications is important for many reasons. Patients prescribed nitroglycerin should have this with them during exercise. In addition, coronary artery disease is a systemic condition that increases the likelihood of the patient having peripheral arterial disease.[10] Therefore, the clinician may need to consider peripheral arterial disease as a differential diagnosis for a patient with a history of a coronary bypass surgery who reports leg pain during gait. Statin medications, antibiotics, and corticosteroid medications have been linked to tendinopathy.[11,12] Some medications may mask the signs and symptoms of disease. For examples, self-prescription of an H2 receptor blocker (e.g., cimetidine) to treat perceived gastroesophageal reflux disease may mask esophageal cancer and laxatives may mask a space-occupying tumor within the colon. It is important to identify any long-term use of corticosteroids, which produces a variety of adverse effects including osteoporosis; proximal muscle weakness; generalized tissue edema; thin, fragile skin; collagen tissue weakening; and immunosuppression.[6]

Clinicians should query their patients regarding the use of sleep aides because these increase the risk of falls and poor-quality sleep negatively impacts nearly all body systems.[13] Patients taking mood-altering drugs may benefit from a biopsychosocial approach to care or referral for nonpharmacologic interventions. Clinicians should ask patients about the use of supplements as well as prescribed medications. Consider a patient coming for treatment of fatigue who has been self-prescribing turmeric for its anti-inflammatory and antioxidant effects. On physical examination, the clinician notices mild ankle swelling. The astute clinician would recognize not only that leg edema and fatigue might be indicative of liver failure but also that herbal and dietary supplements account for roughly 9% of all cases of acute liver toxicity and turmeric, in particular, has been linked to hepatotoxicity.[14] Knowing this, the clinician should contact the patient's primary care provider before proceeding with treatment.

Health Habits Understanding a patient's health habits is important for health promotion and disease prevention, early diagnosis and reduction of the severity and duration of existing diseases, reduction of disability, and improvement in function. Clinicians should ask about the patient's frequency, intensity, time, and type (FITT) of exercise. This information opens up discussions with the patient regarding the American College of Sports Medicine's guidelines for general health and may assist with improving adherence to a long-term exercise program. This is particularly important, given the link between obesity, diabetes, and long-term disability.[15]

Identifying high-risk health behaviors can assist with generating diagnostic hypotheses and planning treatment and, therefore, should be included within the history and intake form. Individuals with anxiety or depression, post-traumatic stress disorder, attention-deficit disorder, and sleep disorders are most at risk for substance abuse, including drugs and alcohol.[8] Abuse of drugs or medications such as antidepressants can lead to physical symptoms, including tachycardia and weakness, and also alter pain perception.[8] Around 6% of the US population is estimated to have an alcohol use disorder.[16] The National Institute on Alcohol Abuse and Alcoholism notes that consuming more than 7 alcoholic drinks per week for women and 14 for men is cause for concern.[16] Clinicians should consider screening for alcohol abuse using the CAGE method (Table 6-2).[17] Smoking increases the risk of certain types of cancer, delays healing, and increases patient perception of pain.[8,18] Therefore, when encountering a patient with an insidious onset of shoulder pain who is a 50-pack-year smoker, the clinician must consider lung cancer as a potential cause for the patient's complaint. If the condition is musculoskeletal in origin, the patient will likely heal more slowly than someone with the same condition who does not smoke. Clinicians may choose to use the 5A's model (Table 6-3) to assess patient readiness to quit smoking.[19] Coffee, tea, and other caffeine-containing beverages are extremely popular worldwide. Caffeine use and withdrawal have many physiologic effects[6] including headache,[20] fatigue, muscle spasms, nervousness, palpitations, increased blood pressure, increased production of stomach acid, sleep disorders, and decreased pain threshold.[21]

Sleep is critical to many body functions, including tissue healing, pain modulation, cardiovascular health, immune function, cognition, learning, and memory.[13] Reduced quality of sleep can affect work, recreational activities, and the quality of life. The most common causes of sleep disturbances are insomnia, sleep apnea, and restless leg syndrome,[22] but musculoskeletal pain, particularly hip and shoulder pain, can also affect sleep quality.[23,24] Sleep disturbances are common in patients with depression and the elderly.[25] Because night pain and sleep disturbances may be a warning sign of undiagnosed metastatic disease,[26,27] patients should be asked about their sleep quantity and quality as well as if their current condition is impacting sleep. A positive screen may result in the need for sleep hygiene education or referral.

TABLE 6-2
CAGE METHOD OF SCREENING FOR ALCOHOL ABUSE

	Have you ever:
Cut	thought you should cut down on your drinking?
Annoyed	been annoyed by someone who criticized your drinking?
Guilty	felt guilty about your drinking?
Eye-opener	had an eye-opener?
Action	If 1 yes: discussion regarding alcohol use and follow-up later If >1 yes: intervention and referral are likely needed

TABLE 6-3
5As MODEL TO ASSESS FOR PATIENT READINESS TO QUIT SMOKING

Ask about tobacco use
Advise about tobacco cessation
Assess willingness to try quitting
Assist attempt to quit
Arrange for follow-up

Through routine assessment of patient health habits and the promotion or reinforcement of a healthy lifestyle, the clinician can assist with needed behavioral change, enhanced the quality of life, and improved outcomes.

Medical Tests Clinicians should review any laboratory or clinical tests available in the medical record. This can be useful for detecting trends in weight, blood pressure, and blood glucose, as well as assisting with referral needs. For example, a patient with low back pain who reports frequent urination might be experiencing symptoms of hyperglycemia, urinary tract infection, or benign prostatic hyperplasia. In reviewing the patient medical record, the clinician finds the patient has normal blood glucose, white blood cell count, and urinalysis as well as a referral to a urologist. This informs the clinician that the patient's report is being investigated by the patient's primary caregiver. The clinician should check the urologist's assessment once available to ensure that the patient's urinary issues are distinct from the patient's back pain.

Clinicians should ask clarifying questions regarding any items marked on the intake form to obtain further details. For example, if the patient marked a history of cancer, the clinician should inquire regarding the type of cancer, treatments received, whether the cancer is in remission, and when the patient was last seen by an oncologist. It is wise for clinicians to assess for pertinent negatives,[19] that is, to ask safety questions as patients may not report certain conditions because they do not feel they are relevant to their chief complaint. Specifically, clinicians should ensure the patient has no history of diabetes; heart problems; allergies to latex, adhesives, and sulfa; or prior surgeries or injuries in the affected quadrant. Lastly, the clinician should ask the patient's self-perception of his or her general health, as this can provide insights into the patient's self-efficacy and the patient's overall impression of his or her physical and emotional situation.

SYMPTOM INVESTIGATION

To best understand the physical, psychological, financial, and social costs of the patients' current condition, the patient's symptoms should be explored, perhaps using the mnemonic *COSTS + Function and Goals* (Chief complaint, Onset, Symptoms, Treatment and testing, Stability along with the patient's Function and Goals) (Fig. 6-5).

Clinician questioning will vary based on the information available before seeing the patient. For example, if the patient has not completed an intake form providing background information on the reason for the visit, the clinician might begin with a more broad, open-ended statement such as, "Tell me what brings you to see me today?" However, if a patient already provided this information, the question must be rephrased, noting what information the patient has already provided and requesting clarification: "I see that your right shoulder has been bothering you since playing rugby last week. Can you tell me more about that?" The specific inquiries during the initial history-taking naturally vary according to the site of the lesion, the nature of the lesion, and other factors. Questions particularly important for specific anatomic regions are discussed in the respective chapters dealing with those regions. There are, however, certain routine inquiries that should be included in virtually every case.

Chief complaint
Onset
Symptoms
Treatment and testing
Stability

+ patient
function and goals

FIGURE 6-5 COSTS + Function and Goals.

Chief Complaint

What is the patient's chief complaint? Often, pain is the primary reason patients seek therapy. However, patients may also report their main problem to be stiffness, weakness, feelings of instability, or giving way. Likewise, patients generally link their complaint with the impact on function: "I have right knee pain that limits my ability to hike." This initial information helps to focus the examination on a specific body region, the lower extremity, in this case. In contrast, the patient's chief complaint might be more global: "When I get up in the morning, my whole body is stiff." In this scenario, the clinician should consider the possibility of a more systemic problem, such as rheumatoid arthritis.[19]

It is also important to understand how the patient came to see the clinician. Did the patient's family identify a decline in the patient's status, but the patient did not agree? Was the patient referred to a facility not recognizing that, while close to the medical provider's office, both offices were 2 hours from the patient's home and less optimal than the patient's hometown clinic? Did the referring provider believe surgery was the best course of action, yet the patient wanted to pursue conservative treatment because it was not possible to take the required time off work after surgery? These initial insights into the patient's perception of the problem are critical to shaping the patient interview.

Onset

Clinicians should obtain a timeline and mechanism of onset for the patient's chief complaint (Fig. 6-6).

Timeline To help determine the stage of the patient's condition, the clinician should establish a timeline of symptoms. How long ago did the patient first notice symptoms? For traumatic injuries, the acute phase of healing predominates for the first 6 days, followed by the subacute phase from weeks 2 to 6.[28,29] Finally, the maturation and remodeling phase begins around the sixth week postinjury[28] and may last 1[30] to 2 years.[10,28,31] An acute condition will require a more gentle approach to examination and protection of injured structures, whereas a subacute condition can tolerate more intensive examination and treatment. Individuals with chronic pain may have a degree of central sensitization.[32] This type of pain appears to be due to altered central processing without overt (and current) tissue injury.[33] As such, the physical examination is less likely to be able to identify a specific anatomic lesion. Alternatively, the problem might be an acute exacerbation of a chronic condition, such as a patient with chronic low-level low back pain who now has severe pain shooting down his right leg and is unable to stand fully upright.

Mechanism of Onset Understanding how the problem occurred is quite useful in developing diagnostic hypotheses and an examination strategy.

The exact nature of the event or mechanism of injury should be determined so that correlation can be made to symptoms and signs for interpretation. Determining the direction and nature of forces producing the injury may give insight regarding which tissues may have been stressed. The clinician should establish if the onset was gradual and progressive, which might indicate a degenerative condition, or due to a traumatic event. If the onset was the result of a one-time trauma, could this trauma have reasonably been avoided? For example, when evaluating a patient who sustained a fractured radius in a fall, the clinician should consider if the fall occurred due to poor balance, poor vision in an unfamiliar situation, or just plain back luck. How much force was involved in the trauma? An 18-year-old patient who sustained a fractured vertebra in a high-speed motor vehicle accident would likely have a very different prognosis than an 82-year-old patient who sustained an insufficiency fracture from something as minor as bending over to tie her shoes.

If a patient reports a sudden onset of a red, painful, swollen joint without trauma, the clinician should suspect conditions such as septic arthritis, gout, or osteomyelitis.[19] Symptoms starting after a new job might indicate a subpar workstation, whereas symptoms starting after a new workout routine might indicate that the patient was underprepared for the new task or has an overuse injury. Recurrent problems, such as repeated ankle sprains, would seem to indicate that the cause of the condition has not been rectified.

An insidious onset unrelated to injury or unusual activity should always be viewed with suspicion

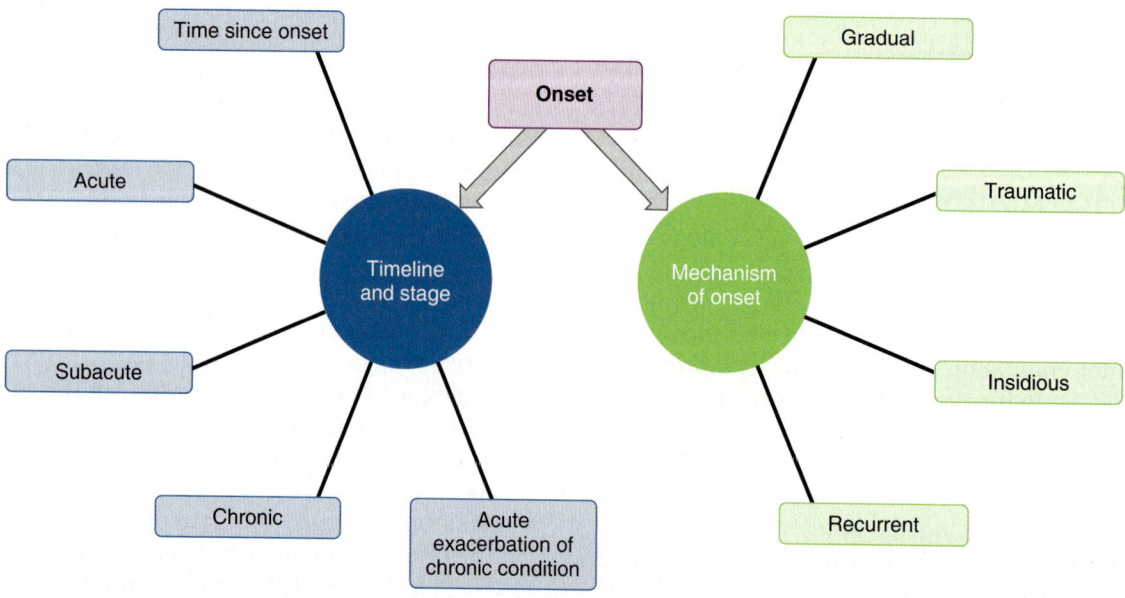

FIGURE 6-6 Key information to obtain regarding the onset of patient symptoms.

because this history is typical of a neoplasm.[19] However, degenerative lesions or lesions caused by tissue fatigue are common and may also arise in this manner. If the patient blames some injury or activity, keep in mind that he or she may or may not be correct.

Symptoms

Clinicians must gain information regarding the patient's symptoms including location, quality, severity, constancy, modifying factors, 24-hour pattern, irritability, and any associated symptoms (Fig. 6-7).

Location Symptom location should be clearly defined. It is useful to ask patients if they can point with one hand or one finger to the primary area of symptoms and then any areas to which the symptoms spread. Clinicians should consider all possible pain generators for the region of the patient's symptoms. For example, if a patient reports symptoms in the region of the hip, the clinician should not make the mistake of assuming the symptoms arise from the hip joint. Rather, the symptoms might be referred from the low back, sacroiliac joint, intestines, or bladder.[8] Likewise, unilateral paresthesia in the palmar aspect of the hand and first and second digit suggests peripheral (median) nerve involvement, whereas tingling in all four extremities suggests spinal cord involvement or some other more serious pathologic process.

Does the patient have symptoms in a small local area, multiple small regions, or more globally? Patients reporting symptoms at a single joint might be experiencing a sprain. In contrast, patients reporting multiarticular symptoms should make the clinician suspicious of a connective tissue disorder,[19] such as rheumatoid arthritis or systemic lupus erythematosus. Patients reporting more global symptoms may be experiencing central sensitization[32] or conditions such as fibromyalgia and chronic fatigue syndrome.[33]

It may be useful to ask the patient to note the area(s) of symptoms on a body diagram (Fig. 6-8). A key can be used for patients to describe the quality of symptoms. The clinician should then question the patient to determine the nature of each area of complaint and start to determine whether a relationship exists between regions. For example, symptoms from the L5 nerve root might cause local right low back pain. However, when exacerbated, the symptoms may extend from the right low back into the right lower leg. In this situation, the patient might have back symptoms without leg symptoms but would not have leg symptoms without also having back symptoms.[34]

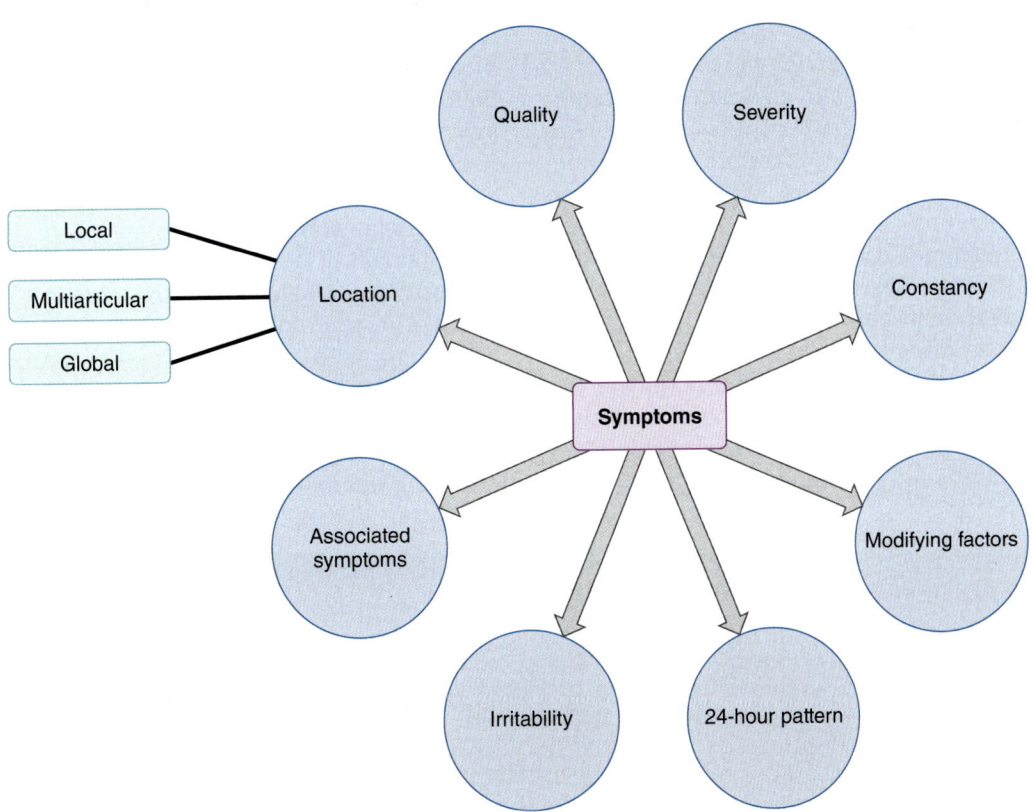

FIGURE 6-7 Key information to obtain regarding patient symptoms.

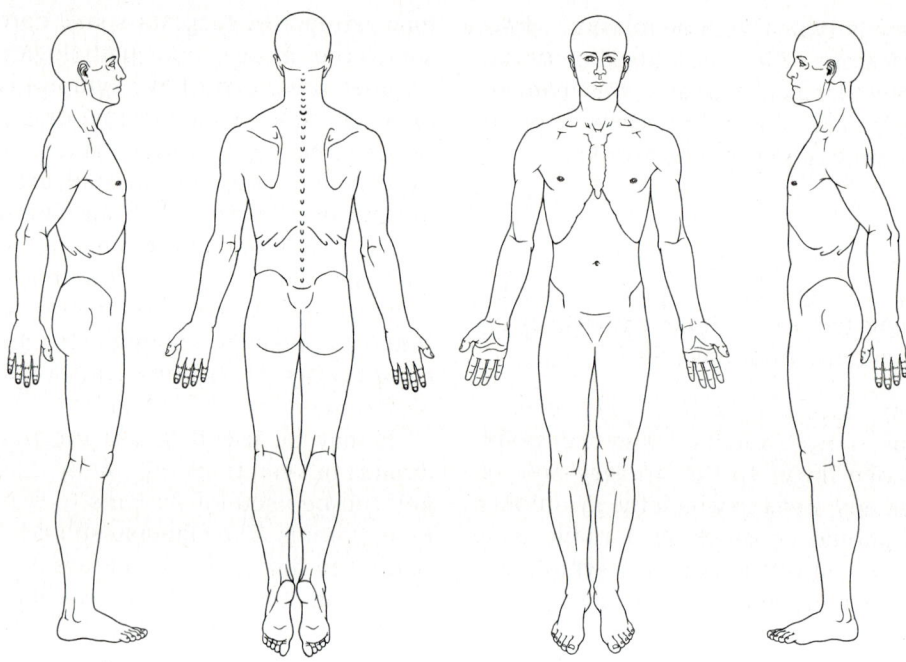

FIGURE 6-8 Body diagram.

It may also be possible that the patient has two areas of symptoms (right low back pain and right leg pain), with one having no particular influence on the other.

It is possible that the patient has two distinctly separate areas of complaint: left knee pain and right hip pain. In either case, the clinician should take care to specifically track the behavior of each region. The regions might be labeled P1 (problem 1) and P2 (problem 2) on the body diagram, and clinician documentation must clearly reflect the patterns of each problem. Given the potential for time constraints in the clinic, the clinician may ask the patient which problem he would like to focus on during the initial visit and defer thorough investigation of the remaining problem until the next session. Last, the patient may note that his right hip pain has been an ongoing, minor problem for which he does not want to seek treatment and that he would prefer to focus solely on the left knee pain. In this case, although thorough investigation of the hip pain is not required, the clinician must respect the patient's hip pain and understand how to avoid exacerbating this during the examination and plan of care.

Quality of Symptoms The clinician should ask about the characteristics of the patient's symptoms. Pain that is described as dull and aching is generally consistent with somatic pain, whereas shooting or tingling symptoms are more indicative of neurologic pain.[34] Table 6-4 provides some common descriptors for symptoms of musculoskeletal and nonmusculoskeletal sources.[8] By concentrating solely on pain, the clinician is likely to overlook some other important symptoms. The clinician should consider symptom descriptors as a component of the overall patient picture and use this information to help shape the physical examination. Reports of grinding with active range of motion are consistent with articular degeneration. However, if present, this finding may be inconsequential to the patient's current complaint. Clinicians should always ask about the presence of neurologic symptoms, including numbness or tingling sensations. If present,

TABLE 6-4				
POSSIBLE SOURCES OF PATIENT-REPORTED SYMPTOMS				
Musculoskeletal	*Neurogenic*	*Visceral*	*Vascular*	*Emotional*
Sore, hurting	Shooting, sharp	Diffuse, poorly localized	Throbbing	Miserable
Achey	Burning, hot searing	Boring, gnawing	Pounding	Exhausting
Dull	Numbness, tingling	Deep steady ache	Pulsing	Fatiguing
Heavy, deep	Electrical		Beating	Nauseating
Cramping				Frightening
Catching, grinding				
Popping, snapping				

the clinician should perform a complete upper and/or lower quarter neurologic screen. Likewise, psychological screening should be considered for patients using certain descriptors, such as miserable or frightening.

Severity It is important to clarify symptom intensity, particularly in regard to patient pain complaint. There are several options for reliably documenting pain severity (Table 6-5).[35] Tracking changes in pain intensity over time is particularly useful to determining the effectiveness of a plan of care. Although developed specifically for pain, these scales can be modified to rate the intensity of other symptoms, such as numbness or tingling.

Constancy of Symptoms Are the symptoms constant or intermittent? Pain that is inflammatory in nature may increase or decrease with activity or position change but is constantly present. In contrast, intermittent pain would indicate a mechanical cause. Patients frequently confuse consistency for constancy. For example, a patient with hallux valgus may report having constant foot pain, when really meaning the pain is consistently present during the terminal stance phase of gait on the affected side.

Modifying Factors Clinicians should ask about aggravating and relieving factors. Inflammatory conditions tend to feel better with movement, anti-inflammatory medications, or ice, whereas rest or prolonged positioning causes stiffness. Symptoms that are mechanical in nature tend to be exacerbated with specific activities that stress the involved tissue, such as weight bearing or contraction, but relieved by rest. Given the prevalence of pharmacotherapy, clinicians should explicitly ask about the use of analgesics, anti-inflammatories, muscle relaxers, steroids, and injections, and the impact on symptoms.

24-Hour Pattern The clinician should ask the patient to describe a typical day to determine the 24-hour pattern of symptoms.[36] Stiffness on first getting up in the morning that lasts less than 30 minutes is consistent with osteoarthritis,[37] whereas stiffness lasting longer than this should make the clinician consider another condition, such as rheumatoid arthritis, as a differential diagnosis.[19] Patients whose symptoms start near the end of the workday may be experiencing postural fatigue.[34] The clinician should ask if this pattern is consistently present, even on days when the patient is not working. How often do the patient's symptoms occur? Are they daily or less frequently? Each of these questions provides clues as to possible causes or perpetuating factors for the patient's chief complaint.

Irritability The clinician must determine the **irritability** of the patient's condition[38,39]: the tissue's ability to handle stress. Tissue irritability includes how easily symptoms are provoked; once provoked, how intense the symptoms are; and how long it takes for symptoms to return to baseline. Patients with low tissue irritability can be examined more vigorously, whereas patients with high tissue irritability must be cared for more cautiously. McClure and Michener[40] provided operational definitions for irritability (Table 6-6). Tissue irritability is generally related to the extent of tissue injury and stage of healing.[41] At times, a patient may not clearly fit into one category: a patient may report high disability despite having only 2/10 pain. In cases such as this, clinicians must use clinical judgment to best categorize the patient's level of irritability.

Associated Symptoms The clinician should ask if the patient has any other symptoms associated with the problem.[19] For example, when these symptoms arise, does the patient get dizzy or nauseous? Symptoms that are inconsistent with musculoskeletal dysfunction must be viewed with some suspicion and may require medical consultation or referral.

Treatment and Testing

Inquiring about previous management can assist with examination and treatment planning (Fig. 6-9). The clinician should know what treatment was performed for this or a similar condition, when treatment occurred, and what was the result. If, for example, a patient reported that anti-inflammatory medication and ice had no effect, it is quite possible that the patient does not have an inflammatory condition and, therefore, further attempts to control inflammation are unlikely to have

TABLE 6-5	
DOCUMENTING PAIN SEVERITY	
Scale	Descriptor
Numeric pain rating scale	0–10 scale with zero being no pain and 10 being the worst imaginable pain
Visual analog scale	Documenting on a 10-cm line labeled no pain on the far left and worst possible pain on the far right
Verbal pain rating scale	Pain is described as none, minimal, moderate, severe, or unbearable
Wong-Baker FACES rating scale	Patient chooses from a series of faces meant to depict varying amounts of distress. This may be most appropriate for young children, patients with communication impairments, or patients who are illiterate

TABLE 6-6			
TISSUE IRRITABILITY			
None	*Low*	*Moderate*	*High*
• Pain free • No resting or night pain • Low degree of disability	• Pain < 3/10 • No resting or night pain • May have minimal pain with over-pressure to motion • Low disability	• Pain 4–6/10 • Intermittent resting or night pain • May have end range pain	• Pain > 6/10 • Consistent resting or night pain • Generally, has pain before end range • High degree of disability

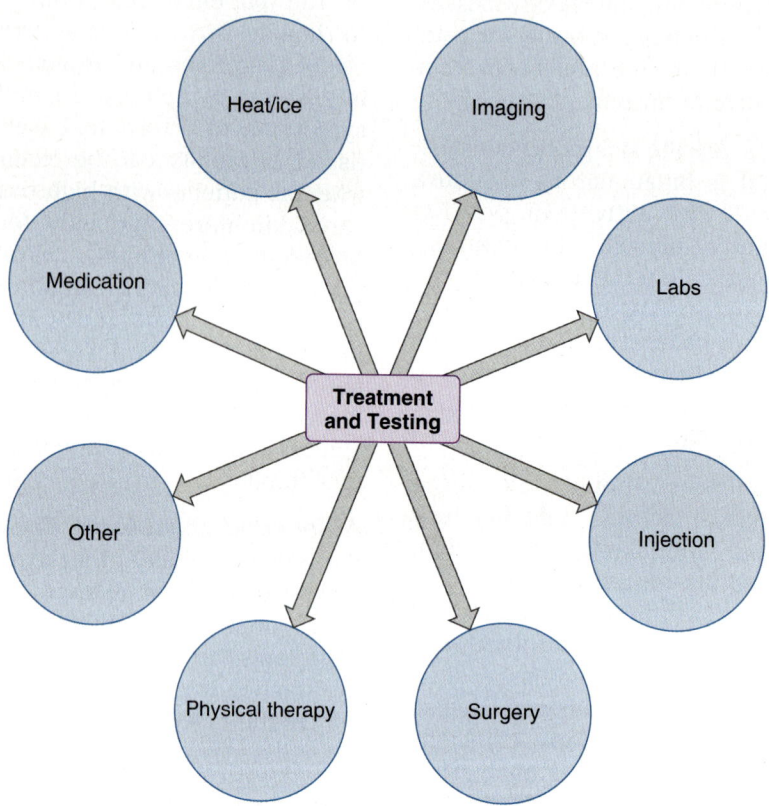

FIGURE 6-9 Key information to obtain regarding prior treatment and testing.

a positive effect. Similarly, a patient who reported only transient relief from 5 months of chiropractic manipulation is unlikely to respond well to a plan of care that focuses on manipulation. The clinician should also strive to understand the patient's judgment of the value of prior treatment. Consider a patient who comes to the clinic with right shoulder pain. The patient reported a prior history of left shoulder pain, for which therapy and medications were not beneficial, but surgery resolved the issue. The patient might be less inclined to fully engage in rehabilitation for this new right shoulder complaint unless the clinician provides substantial education and evidence-based rationale that supports a trial of conservative care.

It is wise to find out the patient's opinions on the current problem.[7] Regardless of the accuracy of the patient's insight, the patient is assured that the clinician is interested in the patient's thoughts and involving him or her in the plan of care.

Clinicians should inquire regarding tests or procedures performed for this current condition and the results.

Other Investigations Diagnostic imaging studies and other investigations can help identify structural abnormalities and can assist with ruling out serious pathologies, such as tumors. A clinician's ability to order, interpret, and be reimbursed for these studies varies by state.[42] A working knowledge of radiologic fundamentals and terminology greatly facilitates the study of the musculoskeletal system and enhances understanding of the radiologist's report. Basic proficiency in film interpretation is considered within the scope of practice.[42] Given the radiologist's advanced training, clinicians should also review the details of the radiology report before proceeding. The report will include patient information, clinical information, the part investigated, findings, impression, and any recommendations. This section provides a brief overview of key diagnostic imaging studies and electrodiagnostic testing. The reader is referred to other sources for additional details.[43–45]

Radiographs Plain film radiography (an x-ray) is the most common first-order diagnostic screening procedure in the evaluation of musculoskeletal diseases and dysfunction. X-ray films need not be taken routinely in all patients, and a particular radiologic lesion does not necessarily prove that it is the source of the patient's symptoms. They are often of most value in demonstrating that no abnormality is present in the bone or joints. At times, findings simply support a moderately firm clinical diagnosis; in other cases, however, the films may provide the only clue to a clinically obscure situation, such as a metastatic lesion.[46] If radiographs or radiograph reports interpreted by a radiologist are available, they should be reviewed. If they are not available but the examiner believes they are needed, the examiner must request them before proceeding with treatment.

Radiographs expose the patient to a small amount of radiation, are universally available, and are relatively inexpensive. Radiographs are best used to identify fractures and dislocations. More than one view of the same region may be required for full visualization. For example, both lateral and anterior views may be required to reveal a distal fibula fracture. Some fractures, such as stress fractures and scaphoid fractures, do not show up on x-ray. Lack of joint space provides an indication of degenerative joint disease.[47] Clinicians should use the mnemonic ABCS when viewing radiographs to ensure a consistent and methodical approach to image interpretation (Table 6-7). Figures 6-10 to 6-12 provide examples of common abnormal radiographic findings.

TABLE 6-7		
ABCs OF RADIOGRAPH INTERPRETATION		
	Examine	*Pathology Examples*
A: Adequacy, Architecture, Alignment	Adequacy: is the image of adequate quality and include all areas required for interpretation Architecture: number and size of bones Alignment: bone-to-bone relationship	Fracture, dislocation
B: Bones	Bone density: general and local bone density, cortical outlines	Osteoporosis, osteophytes
C: Cartilage space	Joint space width, subchondral bone density, epiphyseal plates	Degenerative joint disease
S: Soft-tissue space	Size of musculature, fat pad location	Effusion or foreign bodies

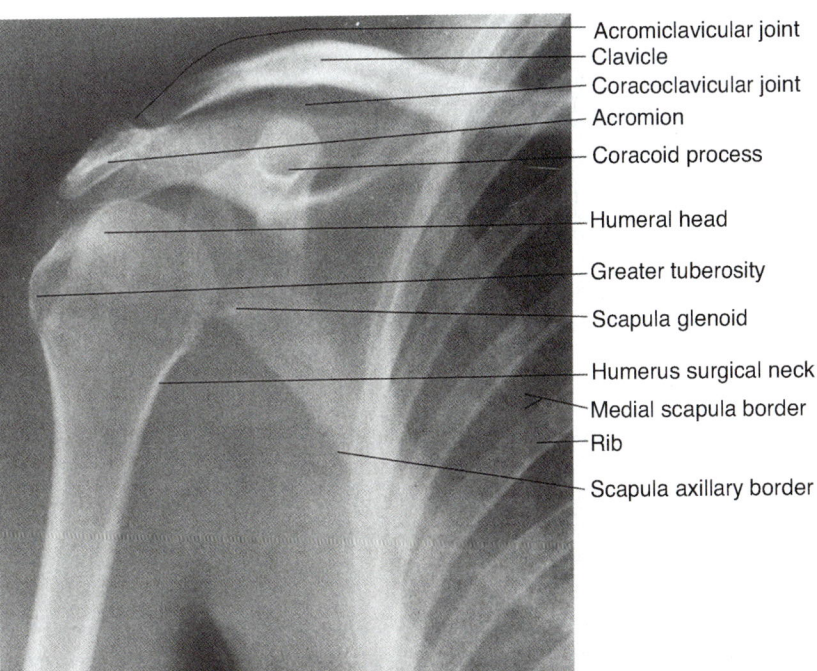

FIGURE 6-10 Right shoulder radiograph with humerus externally rotated. (Smith WL, Farrell TA. *Radiology 101: The Basics and Fundamentals of Imaging*. 4th ed. Lippincott Williams & Wilkins; 2014: Figure 6.5B.)

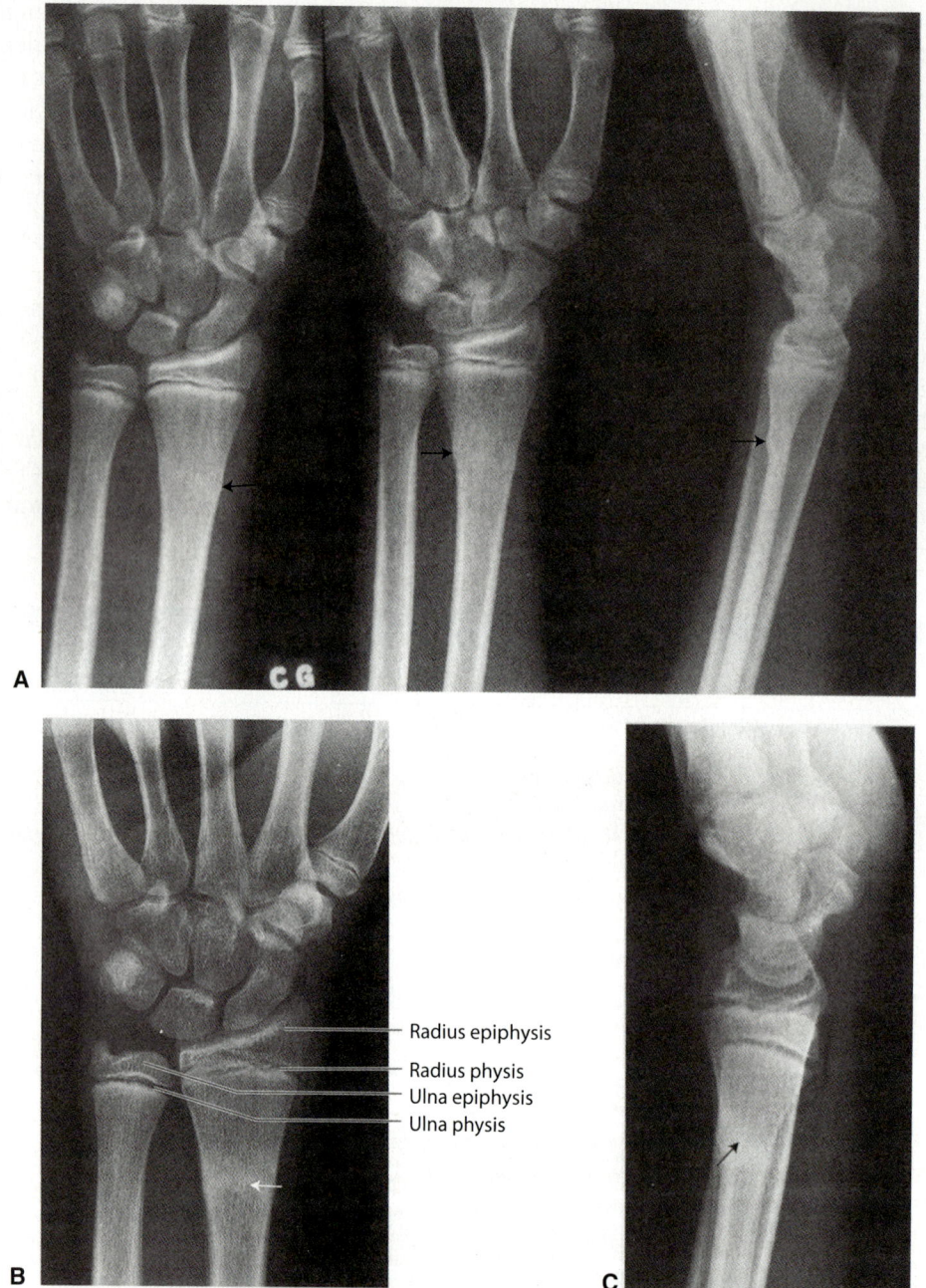

FIGURE 6-11 A. Left wrist radiographs. Nondisplaced distal left radius fracture (*arrow*). Left wrist posteroanterior **(B)** and lateral **(C)** radiographs. Six weeks after left distal radius fracture with signs of bone healing. The dense white zone (*arrows*) is the typical appearance of a healing fracture. (Smith WL, Farrell TA. *Radiology 101: The Basics and Fundamentals of Imaging*. 4th ed. Lippincott Williams & Wilkins; 2014: Figure 6.34B, C.)

Computed Tomography Computed tomography (CT scan) exposes the patient to a greater amount of radiation than a radiograph, significantly increasing its ability to detect differences in tissue contrast. For example, conventional radiographs can detect a 10% difference in x-ray attenuation, CT scans can detect differences less than 0.5%.[45] CT scans create two- and three-dimensional images of body structures that can be manipulated and viewed from any plane. CT scans are able to detect subtle and complex fractures, intra-articular abnormalities, and some bone and soft-tissue tumors (Fig. 6-13). CT scans are often used for imaging of the lungs and other organs.

Magnetic Resonance Imaging Magnetic resonance imaging (MRI) uses magnets to produce a strong electric field that forces protons to align within the field-providing images that can be viewed in multiple

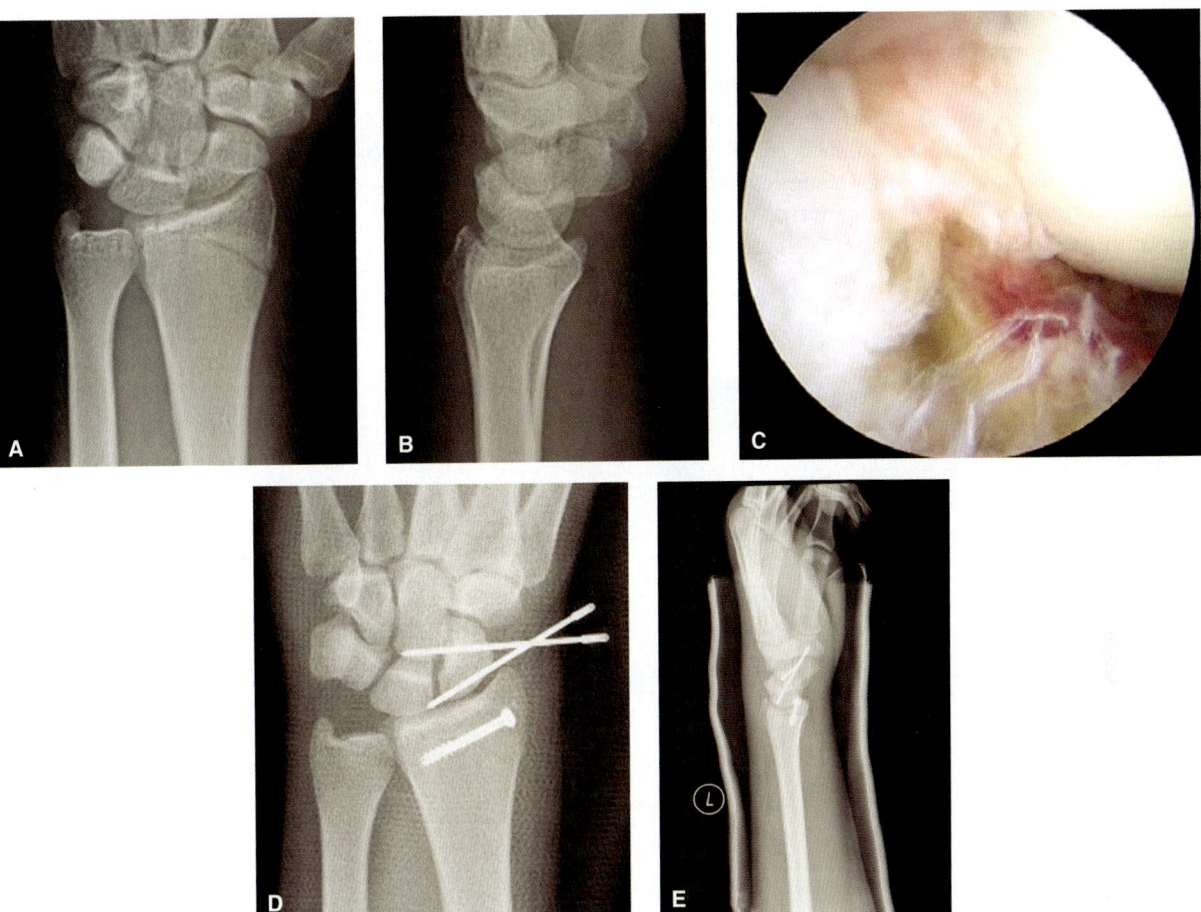

FIGURE 6-12 Anteroposterior (AP) **(A)** and lateral **(B)** radiograph showing displaced left intra-articular radial styloid fracture without apparent carpal malalignment. **C.** Arthroscopic examination revealed scapholunate interosseous ligament injury. **D.** AP radiograph demonstrates the radial styloid fracture treated with internal fixation and the intercarpal ligament injury treated with percutaneous wire placement. **E.** Lateral postoperative radiograph of the wrist. (Ricci WM, Ostrum RE. *Orthopaedic Knowledge Update: Trauma*. American Academy of Orthopedic Surgeons; 2016: Figure 26.8A-C, E, F.)

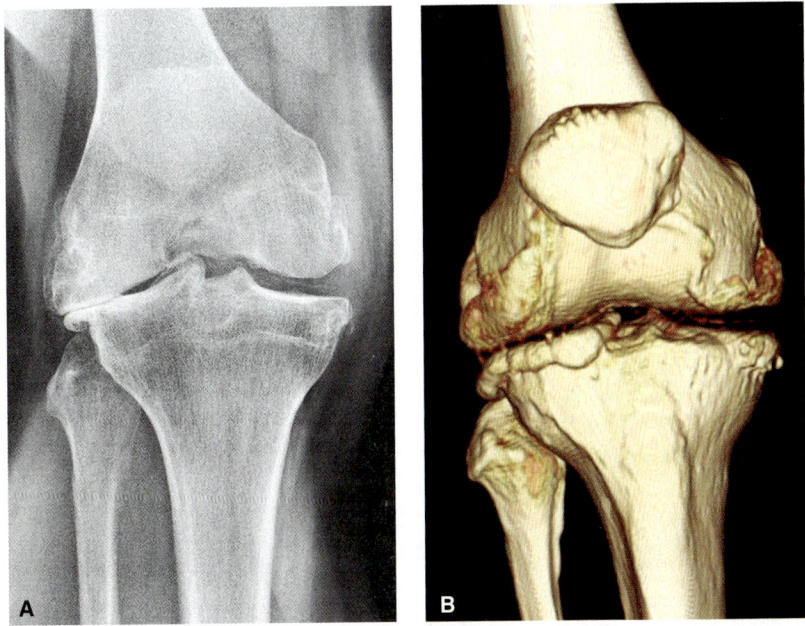

FIGURE 6-13 **A.** Radiograph of the right knee demonstrating advanced osteoarthritis. **B.** Three-dimensional reconstructed computed tomography images demonstrating advanced three-compartmental osteoarthritis. (Greenspan A, Gershwin ME. *Imaging in Rheumatology: A Clinical Approach*. Wolters Kluwer; 2018: Figure 5.40A, B.)

planes. MRIs provide excellent soft-tissue contrast and can also identify areas of inflammation. MRIs do not expose the patient to ionizing radiation. MRIs can be performed with or without the addition of a contrast dye to enhance image quality. MRIs (Fig. 6-14) are the imaging method of choice for soft-tissue lesions, such as injuries to menisci, labrum, ligament, or tendon. MRIs cost more than radiographs and may not be appropriate for individuals with implanted metal devices or claustrophobia.

Radionucleotide Bone Scan A bone scan (Fig. 6-15A) is a very sensitive nuclear imaging test that detects increased bone activity. As such, bone scans are able to identify subtle fractures, bone tumors, and bone or joint infections. However, bone scans are not very

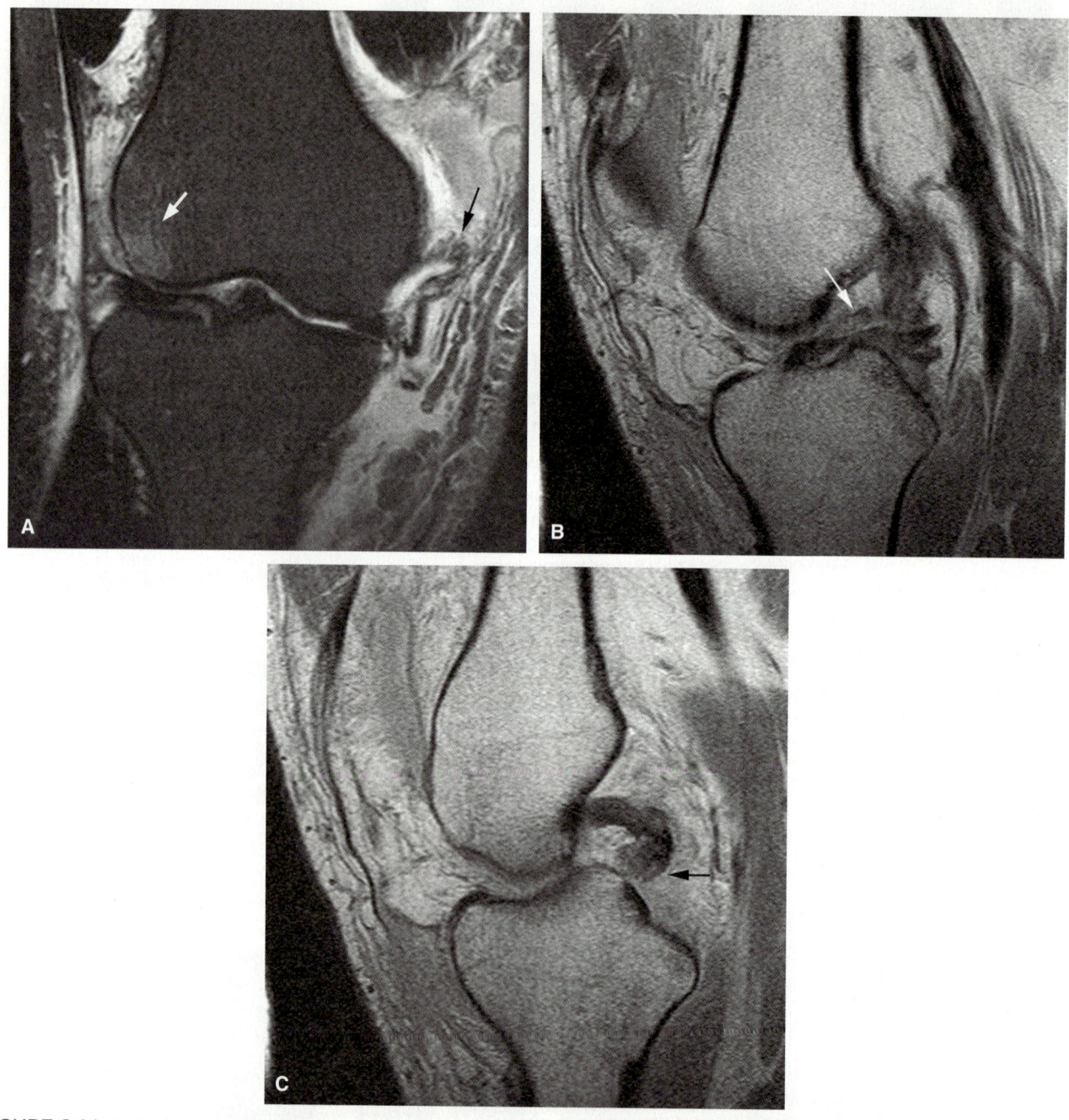

FIGURE 6-14 A. Coronal magnetic resonance imaging (MRI) showing a complete tear of the medial collateral ligament (*black arrow*) with lateral femoral condyle bone bruise (*white arrow*). B. Sagittal MRI showing tear of the anterior cruciate ligament (*white arrow*). C. Sagittal MRI showing tear of the posterior cruciate ligament (*black arrow*). (Chew FS. *Musculoskeletal Imaging: The Essentials*. Wolters Kluwer; 2019: Figure 5.34.)

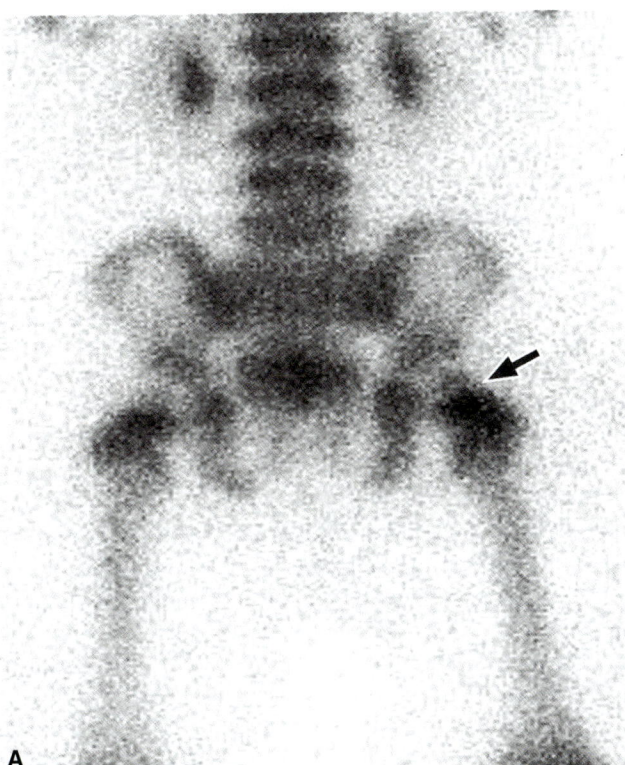
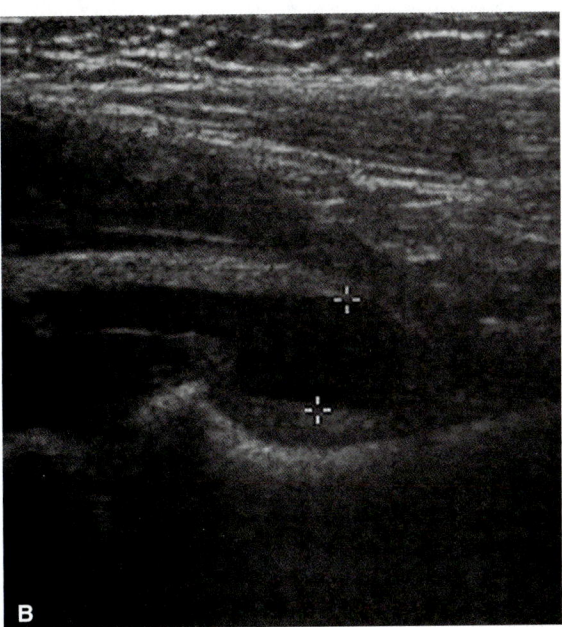

FIGURE 6-15 An infant boy presented with fever, irritability, and decreased left leg mobility. **A.** Bone scan demonstrating increased uptake in the proximal femur and left hip joint (*arrow*) suggestive of septic arthritis. **B.** Ultrasound performed on the same day showing large effusion (*calipers*) in the left hip. The hip joint was aspirated and cultured which confirmed the diagnosis. (Lee EY. *Pediatric Radiology: Practical Imaging Evaluation of Infants and Children.* Wolters Kluwer; 2018: Figure 22.6A, C.)

specific, as areas of increased uptake may also indicate degenerative conditions, such as osteoarthritis.

Ultrasound Imaging Diagnostic ultrasound imaging (Fig. 6-15B) creates images out of reflected sound waves. Diagnostic ultrasound can be useful in identifying superficial lesions in the muscle, tendon, and ligaments. This modality is low cost and does not involve radiation. However, interpretation of imaging relies heavily on operator skill.

Electrodiagnostic Testing Electromyography (EMG) and nerve condition study (NCS) are electrodiagnostic tests that measure electrical activity in the muscles and nerves. An EMG is an invasive test in which a needle (called an *electrode*) is inserted into the muscle of interest. The electrode picks up electrical signals within the muscle and displays them as wave forms. An NCS uses electrodes to measure the speed of electrical impulses over a nerve. These tests are generally performed together to help determine the presence, location, and extent of damage to the nerves and muscles. These studies are useful in diagnosing conditions such as carpal tunnel syndrome, radiculopathy, neuropathy, and certain muscular diseases.

When reviewing this information, the clinician must be aware of the diagnostic accuracy of various imaging modalities. For example, CT arthrography has a sensitivity of 0.91 and a specificity of 0.89 for detecting hip labral tears, whereas MRI has sensitivity of 0.72 and specificity of 0.76.[48] In addition, while the presence of pathology, such as joint space narrowing on a radiograph, is an indicator of osteoarthritis,[47] this pathology may not be the cause of the patient's pain complaint. Being part of an integrated electronic health record system facilitates communication among all providers. Without this access, clinicians should strive to obtain test results and other key information from the appropriate provider. This is particularly important in cases of post-operative care. It is not unheard of that a patient may come to therapy with a prescription that simply states: "Diagnosis: 2 weeks s/p rotator cuff repair, evaluate and treat." Without knowing the extent of the tear, the degree to which a repair was possible, and the patient's tissue quality, the clinician has inadequate information for the examination and cannot create an appropriate plan of care.

Stability

The clinician should establish the clinical course of the patient's condition (stability); overall is the condition improving, staying the same, or worsening (Fig. 6-16). Conditions that are improving in a timely manner

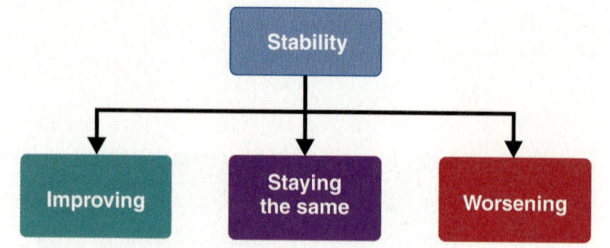

FIGURE 6-16 Key information to obtain regarding the stability of the patient's condition.

merely require support of the existing interventions, whereas conditions that are worsening require careful investigation and a change in intervention strategies.

Function

It is vital for clinicians to link the patient's chief complaint with the patient's abilities and functional limitations. The clinician should learn how this problem has affected the patient's ability to dress, groom, walk, work, assist with household chores, participate in recreational activities, and so on. Some tasks may be possible but with difficulty, pain, or modification. The clinician must know the patient's response to symptoms. Is the patient continuing to perform aggravating activities that might prolong recovery? In contrast, has the patient stopped performing a variety of activities due to fear of harm? Clinicians should be cautious in the method of asking questions regarding function. For example, asking: "What is this problem preventing you from doing?" is very different from the following series of questions: "Can you tell me what things you are having difficulty with or that you are doing differently because of this problem? What things are you avoiding as a result of this problem? Given what we've discussed so far, I'm wondering if you can tell me a little about the things that you are unable to perform due to this problem?" Functional deficits should be compared with the patient's normal occupation and daily activity level. Like pain intensity, any stated functional difficulties must be correlated with the apparent severity and extent of the problem found in the physical examination and any inconsistencies must be considered.

Clinicians should consider having the patient complete a self-reported outcome tool. Outcome tools not only assist with tracking changes in patient function over time, but also help guide the physical examination, intervention choices and exercise parameters, and assist with determining functional goals. A wide variety of reliable and valid outcome tools are available. While a complete review of outcome measures is beyond the scope of this text, the reader will find additional information on various joint-specific (e.g., Neck Disability Index or NDI), region-specific (e.g., Lower Extremity Function Scale or LEFS), and disease-specific (e.g., Western Ontario and McMaster Universities Osteoarthritis Index or WOMAC) tools within the appropriate chapters.

The Patient-Specific Functional Scale (PSFS) allows the patient to create an individualized outcome tool for comparison over time by ranking how difficult it is to perform up to five tasks on a 0 to 10 scale (Fig. 6-17). The minimum important difference on the PSFS is 1.3 points and is relatively stable across body regions.[49] Clinicians may also choose to have a patient rate the degree of change from baseline using the Global Rating

Instructions: Identify two to five activities you are having difficulty doing or are unable to perform as a result of the condition you came to therapy to address. Rate your ability to perform each task today using the following scale: 0 = unable to perform activity, 10 = able to perform activity as well as before this condition. We will use this same scale to assess how your abilities have changed during the course of rehabilitation.

Activity	Initial rating Date:	Date:	Date:	Date:
1.				
2.				
3.				
4.				
5.				

FIGURE 6-17 Patient-Specific Functional Scale. (Adapted from Stratford P, Gill C, Westaway M, Binkly J. Assessing disability and change on individual patients: a report of a patient specific measure. *Physiother Can*. 1995;47:258-263.)

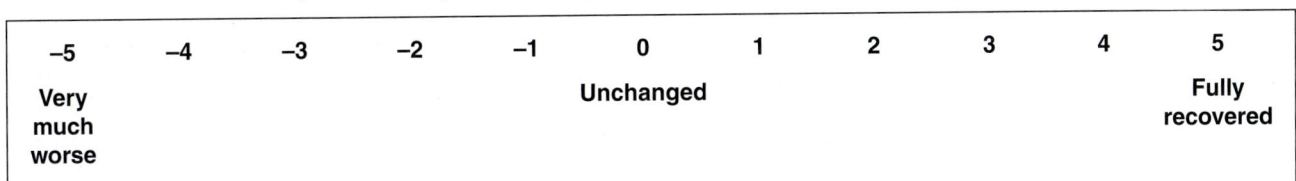

FIGURE 6-18 Global rating of change. (Adapted from Kamper SJ, Maher CG, Mackay G. Global rating of change scales: a review of strengths and weaknesses and considerations for design. *J Man Manip Ther.* 2009;17(3):163–170.)

of Change Scale (Fig. 6-18). Clinicians must complete the instruction statement to outline the desired comparison time point. For example, the patient may be asked to compare changes since the time of injury or the start of therapy. The minimum clinically important change is 2 points.[50]

Goals

The clinician should clearly identify the patient's goal(s) for rehabilitation. Once the physical examination is complete and the clinician has a better understanding of the patient's situation and diagnosis, the clinician must revisit these patient goals to create mutually agreed-upon rehabilitation goals that are specific, measurable, achievable, relevant, and time bound. These steps are vital to maximizing patient adherence and outcomes.

The clinician must determine whether a patient's stated goal is realistic. For example, a patient who has used a walker for the past 5 years may want to stop using the walker and ambulate without any assistive device. However, after thoroughly evaluating the patient, the clinician's best prognosis might be that the patient would be able to ambulate safely with a cane but not without an assistive device. In this case, the clinician must discuss the rationale for this prognosis and note that, once achieved, the patient–clinician team will reassess to see if the patient's original goal might, indeed, be possible at that time.

Some patient goals are realistic but do not require ongoing therapy to achieve. For example, consider a runner who is currently using a walking boot while recovering from an ankle fracture. The patient's stated goal is to return to marathon running. The patient need not be in therapy until completing a 26.2-mile run. Rather, the clinician must determine at what point the patient is safe to progress running mileage without clinician guidance. Should the patient be able to run just 1 mile? What type of running quality and pace are required? Should the patient be symptom-free during and after running? In this case, the clinician might recommend two goals: (1) In 12 weeks the patient is able to run 3 miles two times in a week without significant deviation, ankle pain, or ankle swelling and (2) in 12 weeks, the patient will verbalize how to safely progress running to return to marathon distances.

REVIEW OF SYSTEMS

During the **review of systems**, the clinician asks the patient questions regarding potentially relevant body systems (Table 6-8). Not all systems require screening for every patient. Figure 6-19 provides guidance to help clinicians know how to choose relevant systems to review.

The clinician must screen any system in which the patient has a positive past medical history (e.g., screen the cardiovascular system for a patient with a history of hypertension). Systems should also be screened based on symptom location to identify referred pain (Fig. 6-20). Last, systems should be screened based on the nature of reported symptoms (the nervous system should be screened if there is a report of numbness). See Table 6-4 for some common descriptors for symptoms of nonmusculoskeletal sources, including neurogenic, visceral, vascular, and emotional.

Red flags are signs and symptoms that might indicate the presence of serious or nonmusculoskeletal pathology for which referral is required. Using red flags in isolation has not been proven to be useful.[51] However, a successful strategy is systematic screening for red flags by asking patients key questions regarding the presence of certain key symptoms, followed by more specific, clarifying questions to determine whether referral or consultation is warranted.[52] To improve the clinician's ability to consistently and efficiently identify potential red flags, some key questions should be included within the intake form (see Fig. 6-2). When positive, further questioning regarding the condition is required. For example, a patient might report having significant weight loss. Although this could be a warning sign of metastatic disease, weight loss would be considered appropriate if the patient recently had bariatric surgery. Alternatively, the 10- or 23-item Optimal Screening for Prediction of Referral and Outcome (OSPRO) can be utilized.[51,52]

Psychological factors have been associated with increased pain intensity, increased utilization of medical services, and physical disability.[53–57] In addition, psychological factors may adversely affect functional

TABLE 6-8
REVIEW OF SYSTEMS

System	Sample Screening Questions
Cardiovascular	• Do your symptoms increase with exertion? • Do you experience lightheadedness? • Do you have excessive fatigue?
Pulmonary	• Do you have any shortness of breath? • Do you have a cough? Is it productive?
Eyes, ears, nose, throat	• Do you have difficulty swallowing? • Have you noticed any changes in your vision?
Gastrointestinal	• Do you have any nausea or vomiting? • Are your symptoms affected by what you eat or when? • Have you noticed any discoloration in your urine or stools?
Genitourinary/reproductive	• Do you have difficulty urinating? • Have you had any incontinence? • When was your last menstrual cycle?
Endocrine	• Do you feel excessively cold or hot? • Do you have tingling or numbness? • Do you notice that you need to urinate often?
Hematologic/lymphatic	• Do you have any "swollen glands" or areas of swelling? • Do your legs cramp when walking? • Do you bruise easily?
Neurologic	• Do you feel any weakness or tingling? • Have you had any difficulties with your memory? • Have you ever experienced a seizure or been unconscious?
Integumentary	• Do you have any rashes or open wounds? • Have you noticed any changes in your moles or freckles? • Do you have any areas of itchiness?
Psychiatric	• Do you have little interest in doing things? • Do you feel down, depressed, or hopeless? • Do you feel anxious?
Constitutional symptoms*	• Have you noticed any change in your energy level? • Have you recently had a temperature? • Do you have any night sweats?

*Although not a system, clinicians should ask about the presence of constitutional symptoms during the review of systems.

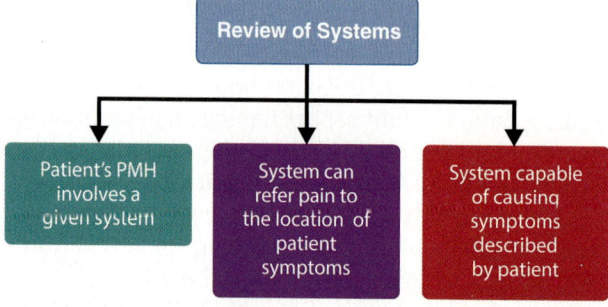

FIGURE 6-19 Clinician guide to systems capable of causing symptoms described by patient. *PMH*, past medical history.

outcomes.[55–57] **Yellow flags** are items that indicate the potential for pain-associated psychological distress and fear-avoidance beliefs.[33] The OSPRO-YF is a concise instrument that can be used in an outpatient setting to identify yellow flags.[57,58] For example, depression is the most common mental disorder, affecting roughly 7% of all adults and 13% of adolescents in the United States.[59] Although many undergo treatment, including medications and counseling, roughly 35% of adults and 60% of adolescents do not undergo any treatment.[59] Clinicians are encouraged to screen patients for depression using the first two psychiatric questions[61] provided in Table 6-8. A follow-up question "Is help needed?" is recommended if the patient responds affirmatively to either question.[60]

Clinicians should always ask about the presence of constitutional symptoms[7,61] such as malaise, fatigue, weakness, night pain, weight change (amount, time), confusion, elevated body temperature, and sweats. **Constitutional symptoms** are a nonspecific cluster of signs and symptoms that signal possible systemic disease process or pathology. When identified, constitutional symptoms require referral for further investigation. Although not the focus of this book, there are several excellent resources for clinicians to improve differential diagnosis problem-solving.[8,9,51,58]

After gathering all relevant information in the health history and demographics, symptom investigation, and review of systems, the clinician should summarize what appear to be key points for the patient. For example: "We've talked about several things so far. Let me make sure I understand. It seems that your main concerns are.... Is that correct?" Then, the clinician should ask if the patient has any additional symptoms that have not previously been mentioned and if the patient has any questions or concerns. Pausing to allow the patient a moment to reflect on what has transpired in the visit to this point may help the patient recall additional details of symptom behavior or related past medical history that provide valuable insight into the patient's condition. As a transition into the physical examination, the clinician should explain to the patient what the next phase of the evaluation entails. It is important to note, that although the formal history-taking process may have been completed, additional crucial pieces of information may come to light during the physical examination. Taking the time to perform a thorough patient history has several advantages including:

- Establishing patient rapport
- Understanding the patient's impression of the situation
- Knowing the timeline of the patient's condition
- Understanding the nature, stage, severity, and irritability of the patient's chief complaint

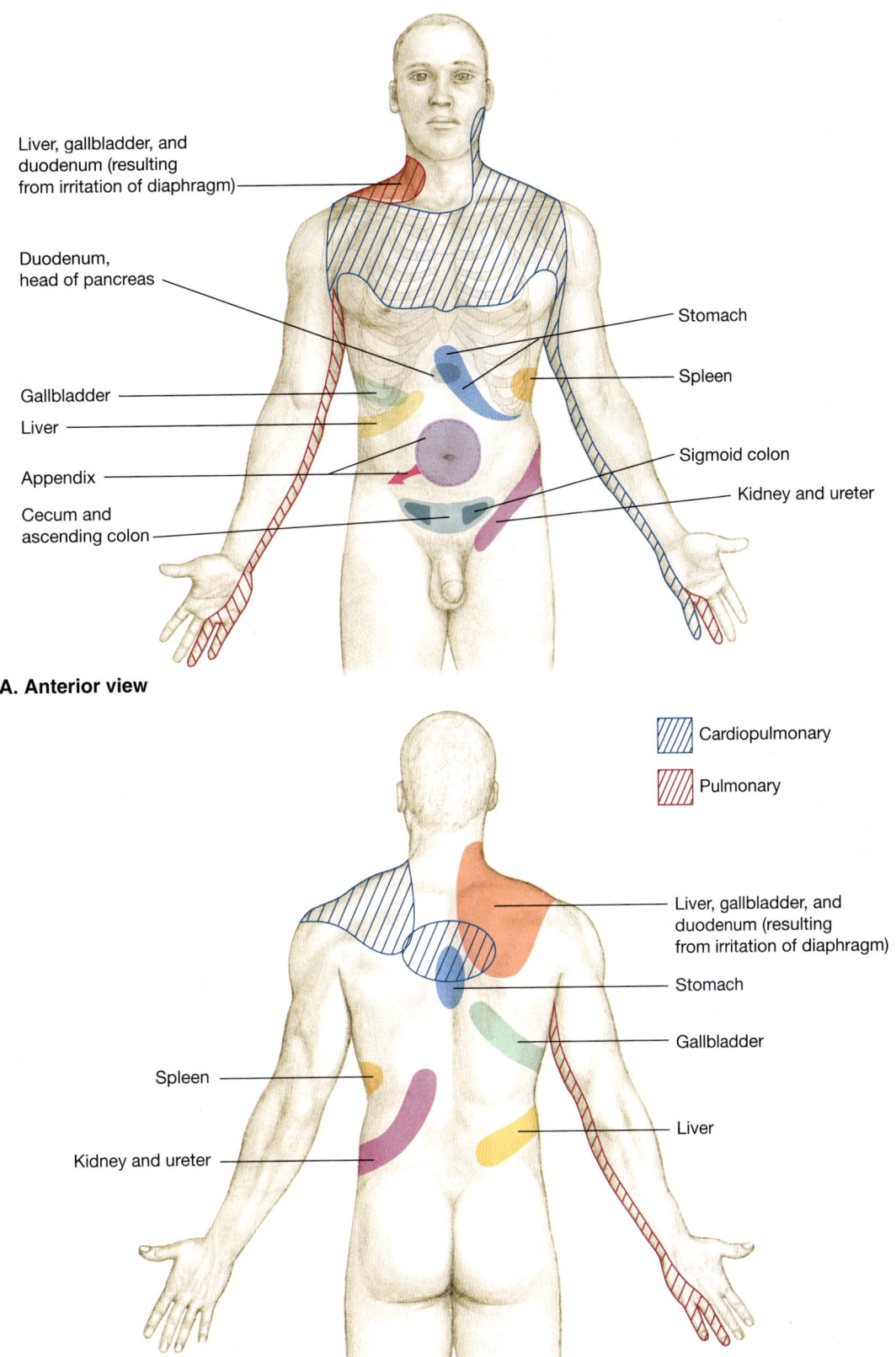

FIGURE 6-20 Common sites of viscera-referred pain. **A.** Anterior view. **B.** Posterior view. (Modified from Gest TR. *Lippincott Atlas of Anatomy*. 2nd ed. Wolters Kluwer; 2020: Plate 8-08.)

- Understanding patient functional limitations and activity restrictions
- Understanding contributing factors condition
- Generating hypotheses regarding differential diagnosis
- Determining whether it is safe to proceed to the physical examination
- Focusing the physical examination
- Identifying precautions for examination and interventions
- Identifying rehabilitation goals
- Determining whether the patient may benefit from a referral

Not only is patient rapport developed, but the skilled clinician is likely to have nearly 75% of the information required to make a final diagnosis.[62]

CHAPTER SUMMARY

The history is composed of three elements: health history and demographics, symptom investigation, and the review of systems. Clinicians should use the mnemonic COSTS + Function and Goals to investigate patient symptoms. The review of systems is a targeted screening of relevant body systems based on patient's past medical history, symptom location, and the nature of reported symptoms. The history helps establish patient rapport, provides context for the patient's condition, and assists with goal setting. Obtaining a thorough patient history helps determine whether it is safe to proceed to the physical examination and if the patient may benefit from any referrals. The history helps generate hypotheses regarding differential diagnosis and focuses the physical examination.

REFERENCES

1. Villgran V, Cheiran S. Pancoast syndrome. StatPearls. 2020. Accessed May 28, 2020. https://www.ncbi.nlm.nih.gov/books/NBK482155/?report=printable
2. Willy R, Hoglund L, Barton C, et al. Patellofemoral pain: clinical practice guidelines linked to the International Classification of Functioning, Disability and Health from the Academy of Orthopaedic Physical Therapy of the American Physical Therapy Association. *J Orthop Sports Phys Ther.* 2019;49(9):CPG1–CPG95.
3. Kolasinski SL, Neogi T, Hochberg MC, et al. 2019 American College of Rheumatology/Arthritis Foundation guideline for the management of osteoarthritis of the hand, hip, and knee. *Arthritis Rheumatol.* 2020;72(2):149–162.
4. van Vollenhoven RF. Sex differences in rheumatoid arthritis: more than meets the eye. *BMC Med.* 2009;7:12.
5. Riesmeijer S, Werker P, Nolte I. Ethnic differences in prevalence of Dupuytren disease can partly be explained by known genetic risk variants. *Eur J Hum Genet.* 2019;27(12):1876–1884.
6. Holland L Jr, Adams M, Brice J. *Core Concepts in Pharmacology.* 5th ed. Pearson; 2018.
7. Boissonault JS, Boissonault WG, Hetzel SJ. Development of a physical therapy patient-interview student assessment tool: a pilot study. *J Phys Ther Educ.* 2013;27(1):35–47.
8. Goodman CC, Heick J, Lazaro RT. *Differential Diagnosis for Physical Therapists: Screening for Referral.* 6th ed. Elsevier; 2018.
9. Boissonault WG. *Primary Care for the Physical Therapist: Examination and Triage.* 2nd ed. Elsevier/Saunders; 2011.
10. Myers BA. *Wound Management: Principles and Practice.* 4th ed. Pearson; 2020.
11. Godoy-Santos AL, Bruschini H, Cury J, et al. Fluoroquinolones and the risk of Achilles tendon disorders: update on a neglected complication. *Urology.* 2018;113(1):20–25.
12. Kirchgesner T, Larbi A, Omoumi P, et al. Drug-induced tendinopathy: from physiology to clinical applications. *Joint Bone Spine.* 2014;81(6):485–492.
13. Siengsukon C, Al-dughmi M, Stevens S. Sleep health promotion: practical information for physical therapists. *Phys Ther.* 2017;97(8):826–836.
14. Luber RP, Rentsch C, Lontos S, et al. Turmeric induced liver injury: a report of two cases. *Case Reports Hepatol.* 2019;2019:6741213.
15. Riebe D, Franklin BA, Thompson P, et al. Updating ACSM's recommendations for exercise preparticipation health screening. *Med Sci Sport Exerc.* 2015;47(11):2473–2479.
16. National Institute on Alcohol Abuse and Alcoholism. Alcohol use disorder. National Institute of Health. Accessed August 20, 2020. https://www.niaaa.nih.gov/alcohol-health/overview-alcohol-consumption/alcohol-use-disorders
17. Ewing JA. Detecting alcoholism: the CAGE questionnaire. *JAMA.* 1984;252(14):1905–1907.
18. Abate M, Vanni D, Pantalone A, Salini V. Cigarette smoking and musculoskeletal disorders. *Muscles Ligaments Tendons J.* 2013;3(2):63–69.
19. Bikley LS. *Bates' Guide to Physical Examination and History Taking.* 13th ed. Wolters Kluwer; 2021.
20. Mostofsky E, Mittleman MA, Buettner C, Li W, Bertisch SM. Prospective cohort study of caffeinated beverage intake as a potential trigger of headaches among migraineurs. *Am J Med.* 2019;132(8):984–991.
21. Juliano LM, Huntley ED, Harrell PT, Westerman AT. Development of the caffeine withdrawal symptom questionnaire: caffeine withdrawal symptoms cluster into 7 factors. *Drug Alcohol Depend.* 2012;124(3):229–234.
22. Nijs J, Mairesse O, Neu D, et al. Sleep disturbances in chronic pain: neurobiology, assessment, and treatment in physical therapist practice. *Phys Ther.* 2018;98(5):325–335.
23. Martinez R, Reddy N, Mulligan EP, Hynan LS, Wells J. Sleep quality and nocturnal pain in patients with hip osteoarthritis. *Medicine.* 2019;98(41):1–5.
24. Khazzam MS, Mulligan EP, Brunette-Christiansen M, Shirley Z. Sleep quality in patients with rotator cuff disease. *J Am Acad Orthop Surg.* 2018;26(6):215–222.
25. Becker NB, Jesus SN, João KADR, Viseu JN, Martins RIS. Depression and sleep quality in older adults: a meta-analysis. *Psychol Health Med.* 2017;22(8):889–895.
26. Bhatt P, Greenberg E, Suh B. Differential diagnosis of a pathological spine fracture. *J Orthop Sports Phys Ther.* 2018;48(7):595.
27. Downie A, Williams CM, Henschke N, et al. Red flags to screen for malignancy and fracture in patients with low back pain: systematic review. *Br Med J.* 2014;348(7942):12.
28. Kisner C. Soft tissue injury, repair, and management. In: Kisner C, Colby LA, Borstad J, eds. *Therapeutic Exercise: Foundations and Techniques.* 7th ed. F.A. Davis; 2018.
29. Enwemeka CS. Connective tissue plasticity: ultrastructural, biomechanical, and morphometric effects of physical factors on intact and regenerating tendons. *J Orthop Sports Phys Ther.* 1991;14(14):198–212.

30. Childs D. Overview of wound healing and management. *Surg Clin North Am.* 2017;97(1):189–207.
31. Lazaro R, Burke-Doe A. Injury, inflammation, healing, and repair. In: Goodman CC, Fuller KS, eds. *Pathology: Implications for the Physical Therapist.* 4th ed. Elsevier; 2015:216–261.
32. Alrwaily M, Timko M, Schneiider M, et al. Treatment-based classification system for low back pain: revision and update. *Phys Ther.* 2016;96(7):1057–1066.
33. Jones MA, Rivett DA. *Clinical Reasoning in Musculoskeletal Practice.* Elsevier; 2019.
34. McKenzie R, May S. *The Lumbar Spine: Mechanical Diagnosis and Therapy.* Vol 1. Spinal Publications; 2013.
35. Berman A, Snyder S. *Skills in Clinical Nursing.* 8th ed. Pearson; 2016.
36. Hengeveld E, Banks K. *Maitland's Vertebral Manipulation.* 8th ed. Vol 1. Churchill Livingstone/Elsevier; 2014.
37. O'Sullivan S, Schmitz T, Fulk G. *Physical Rehabilitation.* 6th ed. F.A. Davis; 2014.
38. Maitland G. *Vertebral Manipulation.* 5th ed. Butterworth Heinemann; 1986.
39. McKenzie R, May S. *The Human Extremities: Mechanical Diagnosis and Therapy.* Spinal Publications; 2017.
40. McClure P, Michener L. Staged approach for rehabilitation classification: shoulder disorders (STAR-Shoulder). *Phys Ther.* 2015;95(5):791–800.
41. Logerstedt DS, Scalzitti DA, Bennell KL, et al. Knee pain and mobility impairments: meniscal and articular cartilage lesions. Revision 2018. *J Orthop Sports Phys Ther.* 2018;48(2):A1–A50.
42. Orthopaedic Section. *Diagnostic and Procedural Imaging in Physical Therapist Practice.* American Physical Therapy Association; 2016.
43. McKinnis L. *Fundamentals for Musculoskeletal Imaging.* 2nd ed. F.A. Davis; 2005.
44. Orth D. *Essentials of Radiologic Science.* 2nd ed. Wolters Kluwer; 2017.
45. Gunderman R. *Essential Radiology: Clinical Presentation, Pathophysiology, Imaging.* 3rd ed. Thieme; 2014.
46. Traver K, Haack RM, Krause D. Ewing sarcoma of the femur. *J Orthop Sports Phys Ther.* 2018;48(7):594.
47. Cibulka M, Bloom M, Enseki KR, Macdonald C, Woehrle J, McDonough C. Hip pain and mobility deficits—hip osteoarthritis: revision 2017. Clinical practice guidelines linked to the International Classification of Functioning, Disability, and Health from the Orthopaedic Section of the American Physical Therapy Association. *J Orthop Sports Phys Ther.* 2017;47(6):A1–A37.
48. Reiman MP, Thorborg K, Goode AP, Cook CE, Weir A, Hölmich P. Diagnostic accuracy of imaging modalities and injection techniques for the diagnosis of femoroacetabular impingement/labral tear: a systematic review with meta-analysis. *Am J Sport Med.* 2017;45(11):2665–2677.
49. Abbott J, Schmitt J. Minimum important differences for the Patient-Specific Functional Scale, 4 region-specific outcome measures, and the NumericPain Rating Scale. *J Orthop Sports Phys Ther.* 2014;44(8):560–564.
50. Kamper SJ, Maher CG, Mackay G. Global rating of change scales: a review of strengths and weaknesses and considerations for design. *J Man Manip Ther.* 2009;17(3):163–170.
51. Heick J, Peterson S, Jain T. Principles of differential screening (Independent Study Course 29.3.1). Academy of Orthopaedic Physical Therapy; 2019:1–17.
52. George S, Beneciuk J, Bialosky J, et al. Development of a review-of-systems screening tool for orthopaedic physical therapists: results from the Optimal Screening for Prediction of Referral and Outcome (OSPRO) cohort. *J Orthop Sports Phys Ther.* 2015;45(7):512–526.
53. Niknejad B, Bolier R, Henderson CR, et al. Association between psychological interventions and chronic pain outcomes in older adults: a systematic review and meta-analysis. *JAMA Intern Med.* 2018;178(6):830–839.
54. Abbema R, Lakke S, Reneman M, et al. Factors associated with functional capacity test results in patients with non-specific chronic low back pain: a systematic review. *J Occup Rehabil.* 2011;21(4):455–473.
55. Perry M, Starkweather A, Baumbauer K, Young E. Factors leading to persistent postsurgical pain in adolescents undergoing spinal fusion: an integrative literature review. *J Pediatr Nurs.* 2018;38:74–80.
56. Martinez-Calderon J, Meeus M, Struyf F, Luque-Suarez A. The role of self-efficacy in pain intensity, function, psychological factors, health behaviors, and quality of life in people with rheumatoid arthritis: a systematic review. *Physiother Theory Pract.* 2020;36(1):21–37.
57. Lentz T, Beneciuk J, Bialosky J, et al. Development of a yellow flag assessment tool for orthopaedic physical therapists: results from the optimal screening for prediction of referral and outcome (OSPRO) cohort. *J Orthop Sports Phys Ther.* 2016;46(5):327–345.
58. George S, Beneciuk J, Lentz T, et al. Optimal Screening for Prediction of Referral and Outcome (OSPRO) for musculoskeletal pain conditions: results from the validation cohort. *J Orthop Sports Phys Ther.* 2018;48(6):460–475.
59. National Institute of Mental Health. Major depression. Accessed August 5, 2020. https://www.nimh.nih.gov/health/statistics/major-depression.shtml#part_155721
60. Mohd-Sidik S, Arroll B, Goodyear-Smith F, Zain AMD. Screening for depression with a brief questionnaire in a primary care setting: validation of the two questions with help question. *Int J Psychiatry Med.* 2011;41(2):143–154.
61. Enthoven W, Geuze J, Scheele J, et al. Prevalence and "red flags" regarding specified causes of back pain in older adults presenting in general practice. *Phys Ther.* 2015;96(3):305–312.
62. Peterson M, Holbrook J, Van Hales D, Smith N, Staker L. Contributions of the history, physical examination, and laboratory investigation in making medical diagnoses. *West J Med.* 1992;156(2):163–165.

7 | The Physical Examination

Betsy Myers

> **CHAPTER OBJECTIVES**
> After reading this chapter, you will be able to:
> 1. Describe the purposes of the physical examination.
> 2. State the key components of the systems review.
> 3. Describe the key components of a basic joint examination.
> 4. Describe classic physical examination findings for bone, articular cartilage, fibrocartilage, capsule, ligament, bursa, muscle, and tendon lesions.
> 5. Compare and contrast various methods of assessing muscle performance.
> 6. State key components to document when making a patient diagnosis.

INTRODUCTION TO THE BASIC PHYSICAL EXAMINATION

A comprehensive examination is *the most important step* in the management of patients with musculoskeletal disorders. The examination begins with obtaining a thorough history. Based on the history, the clinician must understand the global status of the patient and recognize the need for referrals. The clinician must clarify the nature and extent of the condition as well as the patient's functional limitations. The first decision clinicians must make is to determine whether the patient's condition appears to fall within their scope of practice. Next, it is imperative that the clinician quickly recognize any potential danger (red flag) signs and symptoms that would preclude the ability to safely proceed to the physical examination.

Clinicians should use the history to develop a basic strategy for the physical examination and have a narrow list of potential diagnoses. The physical examination is a series of tests and measures used, among other things, to confirm or refute these differential diagnoses by changing the patient's familiar symptoms. It is important for clinicians to understand that there are many purposes for performing the physical examination; arriving at a diagnosis is only one of those. The purposes of the physical examination are as follows:

- Identify the affected area or target tissue
- Determine the presence, and importance, of any red flags
- Reproduce patient symptoms
- Classify a patient into a diagnostic category
- Determine the stage of healing
- Identify secondarily involved structures
- Identify contributing factors to dysfunction or symptoms
- Identify issues that might alter rehabilitation interventions, precautions, or patient prognosis
- Expedite referral and consultation when needed
- Collect baseline information from which to judge changes over time

Clinicians must not succumb to confirmation bias by only collecting information that will rule in a suspected pathology[1] but must also perform tests that might rule out the pathology. This is particularly true when patients arrive at the clinic with a given diagnosis. The examination strategy must not be narrowed prematurely. Clinicians should cautiously avoid holding firmly to an initial hypothesis despite competing or new information uncovered during the examination.[1] Lastly, clinicians should consider at least one potential diagnosis that is possible, but less likely based on the history, that would be potentially dangerous if missed.[2] For example, a patient reporting hip and groin pain during gait may be experiencing symptoms due to musculoskeletal dysfunction of the hip, pelvis, or lumbar spine, including a strain or herniated disc. If the patient also reported a recent abdominal surgery, the clinician must also consider the potential for osteomyelitis or abscess.[3] However, if the patient exhibits pain only with activity, a pathology of the vasculature may be suspected.

Cyriax believed that all pain arises from a lesion and that treatment must reach this lesion.[4] Cyriax's hypothesis is well applied in some cases. Consider a sprinter who skipped his warm-up because he was late to practice and sustained a proximal hamstring strain. Appropriate treatment would include progressive hamstring loading[5] and manual therapy[6] to the site of lesion. However, this viewpoint is too simplistic in other scenarios. Some tissue lesions may be the result of problems in another region. For example, the knee pain of patellofemoral pain syndrome may be the result of proximal hip weakness or poor neuromuscular control.[7] Therefore, directing treatment solely toward the knee is unlikely to result in lasting benefit. Another example is a patient with low back pain and a magnetic resonance imaging (MRI)–confirmed herniated disc who continues to have back pain after the lesion was addressed via lumbar discectomy. Clearly, the removal of the presumed pain-inducing lesion did not result in the patient's desired outcome. One must also consider the complexities of chronic musculoskeletal pain, where, among other things, pain persists long after normal tissue healing time.[8]

Although it is not always possible to confirm pathology or a target tissue, clinicians must utilize strong clinical reasoning to classify a patient into a diagnostic category within their scope of practice.[9] At times, it might not be possible to identify a clear cluster, syndrome, or category to which a patient clearly fits. Impairments have a reasonable chance of being linked to patient-reported functional limitations.[10] In these situations, clinicians may direct the plan of care toward lessening symptoms and alleviating impairments, in an attempt to improve function.[9] Constant subjective and objective reassessment is used to judge the effect of the intervention strategy, and the plan of care should be modified accordingly.

Figure 7-1 describes the main components of the physical examination for musculoskeletal pathology. Like the history, the physical examination begins more broadly with the systems review before progressively fine-tuning the area of chief complaint, ultimately leading the clinician to perform a thorough investigation for joint-specific pathology. Similarly, it is important that clinicians not perform a set series of objective tests without consideration for the individual patient. Rather, clinicians must carefully consider the information received to date and assess the implications of those data points.

The reason the patient came to the clinic influences the basic physical examination. If a patient comes with a traumatic onset of symptoms, the clinician should consider if the injury could have been averted along with ways to prevent injury recurrence. For example, a patient who sustained a wrist fracture from a fall is likely to benefit from balance testing and a fall risk

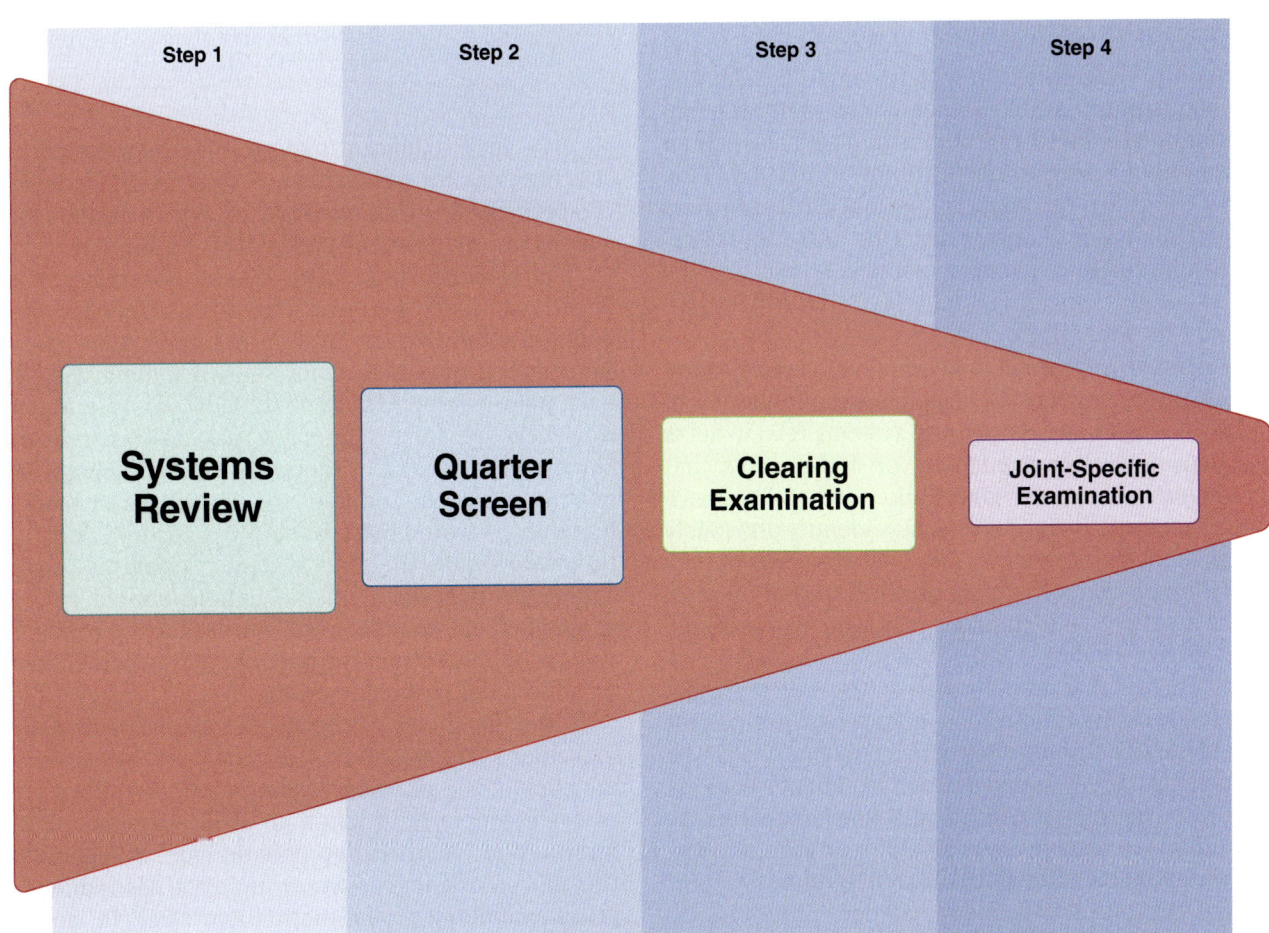

FIGURE 7-1 Funnel components of the physical examination.

assessment in addition to the examination of her upper quarter. Patients with overuse injuries would benefit from a thorough history investigating extrinsic factors, including training errors such as a novice runner beginning a marathon training program with a 10-mile run. However, the clinician must also consider the role intrinsic factors might have in perpetuating the patient's condition and examine the patient for muscle imbalances and structural malalignments, even if the patient has had a surgical procedure. Clinicians should investigate the circumstances behind the onset of symptoms and the reason leading to the decision for surgery. Did the patient sustain a direct trauma, fall, noncontact injury, or overuse injury, or does the patient have a structural malalignment that contributed to the injury? The patient who sustained a noncontact anterior cruciate ligament injury while cutting in practice would benefit from a thorough dynamic biomechanical assessment, including bilateral lower extremities and the trunk.[11] This is crucial because failure to correct deficits increases the likelihood of recurrence.[12]

There are several approaches to the patient examination, including those attributed to Cyriax,[4,13,14] Kaltenborn,[15] Maitland,[16] McKenzie,[17,18] and Sahrmann.[19] Regardless of which system is selected, the clinician must establish a sequential method to ensure that no crucial test or step is omitted, as such an omission could prevent accurate interpretation. This chapter describes the basic framework of the physical examination. Later chapters describe how this framework is adapted for each joint complex.

SYSTEMS REVIEW

The **systems review** is a limited examination of key body systems and serves several key purposes (Table 7-1). In combination with the history, the systems review helps the clinician identify risk factors or impairments that may require referral or consultation with other disciplines. For example, the clinician may identify previously undiagnosed hypertension. The systems review may identify impairments that may be addressed in therapy, such as a patient with shoulder pain who also presents with decreased balance and subsequent increased risk for falls. Factors that alter the plan of care may be identified in the systems review, such as knee pain in a patient with a history of chronic obstructive pulmonary disease. The systems review should assess the patient's communication and learning style to identify barriers to learning and methods to resolve them. Most importantly, the systems review allows the clinician to determine whether it is safe to proceed with the remainder of the physical examination. Consider a patient with reports of mild low back pain whose blood pressure is 205/110 mm Hg. This patient should be referred to a primary care provider because such significant hypertension puts the patient at a high risk for an adverse medical event, such as a cerebrovascular event, and further physical examination may further increase the patient's blood pressure.

The clinician must consider the possibility of referred pain (see Chapter 6, Patient History) and thoroughly investigate any system that may refer pain to the location of patient symptoms. A patient with low back pain may be experiencing musculoskeletal pain. However, this same complaint may also arise from a kidney infection.[20–22] Failure to perform percussion testing or ask this patient about changes in bladder function[23,24] would lead to misdiagnosis and delay appropriate treatment. Any system capable of causing symptoms described by the patient should also be screened. For example, a patient describing back pain as a throbbing or pulsing pain should be screened for an abdominal aortic aneurysm.[25]

Although the musculoskeletal system and neuromuscular systems will be the primary focus of the remainder of the physical examination, a cursory view of each system is required to avoid overlooking key information for providing holistic care. Screening for the musculoskeletal system includes assessment of gross symmetry, global motion and strength, and patient height and weight. Screening the neuromuscular system includes noting the patient's gross coordinated movements to include gait, balance, and mobility, as

TABLE 7-1
COMPONENTS OF THE SYSTEMS REVIEW

System	Components
Communication and learning preferences	Communication Affect Cognition Preferred language Preferred learning style
Cardiovascular	Heart rate Blood pressure Edema
Pulmonary	Oxygen saturation Respiratory rate
Integument	Integrity Scarring Pliability Color Nail status
Musculoskeletal	Gross symmetry Global range of motion and strength Height Weight
Neuromuscular	Gross coordinated Gross motor function
Other systems	System able to refer pain to the location of patient symptoms System capable of causing symptoms described by the patient

well as gross motor function (motor control and motor learning). Identifying that a patient reporting knee pain has a body mass index of 32.0 (class I obesity) provides the clinician with relevant and actionable information, including education regarding activity guidelines, interventions that might unload the affected joint, and possible referral to a dietician. Likewise, noting that a patient with shoulder pain requires multiple attempts to rise from a standard chair should spur the clinician to further investigate possible lower extremity strength deficits.

The clinician must use the systems review to make the following four critical decisions:

1. Is it safe to proceed with the physical examination?
2. Is the patient's complaint due to referred pain?
3. Is there a need to rule out significant local pathology before proceeding further?
4. Would the patient benefit from any referrals?

For example, if a cervical spine fracture is suspected, the clinician should move directly to applying clinical guidelines, such as the Canadian cervical spine rule.[26,27] To continue with the examination without reasonably ruling out a cervical spine fracture would be potentially catastrophic. Similarly, if a scaphoid fracture is suspected, the clinician should move directly into performing the cluster of tests to rule out a fracture,[28–30] because the result of any additional tests and measures is inconsequential if imaging or referral is required.

QUARTER SCREEN

The history provides initial guidance regarding where to begin the physical examination, but the history alone is insufficient. For example, consider a patient reporting wrist pain. Moving directly to the location of the patient's symptoms to perform wrist palpation, joint mobility assessment, and special tests would fail to detect a more proximal source of symptoms from the cervical region. **Quarter screens** help narrow the working hypotheses generated from the history to tell the clinician where to focus a more detailed joint-specific examination. The lower quarter screen is performed when a patient has symptoms in the lower body or lumbar/thoracic region, whereas the upper quarter screen is performed when a patient has symptoms in the upper body or cervical/thoracic region. Quarter screens include observation; gross assessment of structure and posture; a lower or upper quarter neurologic screen; assessment of lower or upper extremity motion, muscle length, and strength; and functional testing. The screen is organized by patient position to maximize efficiency. The purposes for the quarter screens are as follows:

- Rule out sources of patient symptoms
- Identify relevant deviation and impairments within the kinetic chain
- Identify issues that might alter rehabilitation interventions, precautions, or patient prognosis
- Expedite referral and consultation when needed.

Refer to Chapter 8, Lower Quarter Screen, and Chapter 13, Upper Quarter Screen, for complete details.

CLEARING EXAMINATION

The possibility of referred pain (see Chapter 6, Patient History) must be considered when determining the area to be singled out as the primary area of a focused examination. The history or referral from another provider or both may implicate the involved area, but other possibilities must be considered. For example, knee pain may be of local origin (at the knee) but could possibly be referred from the hip. It is not necessary to perform an in-depth examination of both the hip and the knee in every situation. Rather, a "clearing examination" is performed on the joints proximal and distal to the region of symptoms. The **clearing examination** is done by asking the patient to actively move each joint within the suspected areas and by applying passive overpressure to the extremes of each motion. If the patient's familiar pain or dysfunction is noted in a particular area, this area should be examined in depth. To build on our example, a child with an insidious onset of knee pain may, in fact, be complaining of knee pain referred from the hip region due to a slipped capital femoral epiphysis. In this case, examination of the knee itself would be unremarkable, yet a clearing examination of the hip would lead the clinician to the true source of the child's complaint.

JOINT-SPECIFIC EXAMINATION

The basic joint-specific physical examination is presented in this chapter and described in detail in later chapters. The basic aims of the joint-specific examination are to detect the level of dysfunction and reproduce the patient's symptoms by provocation of the affected joint or tissues. The main components of the joint-specific examination are as follows:

- Structure
- Range of motion (ROM)
- Muscle length
- Muscle performance
- Sensory tests
- Reflexes
- Neurodynamic tests
- Accessory motions
- Special tests
- Palpation
- Gait, transfers, mobility
- Functional testing (including balance and proprioception)

The information presented in the subsequent section is grouped conceptually. However, like the quarter screen, the clinician should organize the joint-specific examination by patient position to maximize efficiency.

Structure

The upper and lower quarter screens include a cursory view of the patient's overall structure and posture (see Tables 8-1 and 8-2 in Chapter 8, Lower Quarter Screen, and Table 13-1 in Chapter 13, Upper Quarter Screen). Once the clinician has narrowed the area of chief complaint down to a local joint complex, the clinician should inspect this local region more closely for structural abnormalities. Assessment of structural alignment is of utmost importance following the healing of fractures. A person who has sustained a Colles fracture invariably demonstrates some residual angulation dorsally and radially, resulting in a "dinner-fork" deformity. With such a deformity, restoration of full wrist flexion and ulnar deviation should not be expected.[31] Likewise, the presence of local bony hypertrophy at the margins of superficial joints is a sign of degenerative joint disease (DJD). Thus, local structural assessment becomes important for treatment planning and goal setting.

Range of Motion

ROM tests include active and passive physiologic movements of the involved joint. When properly interpreted, findings from these tests can yield very specific information relating to both the nature and extent of the pathologic process. The organization and interpretation of these tests follow a process similar to that proposed by Cyriax.[4,32]

Active Range of Motion Active range of motion (AROM) yields very general information regarding the patient's functional status, primarily demonstrating the patient's willingness and ability to use the part. Ideally, AROM should be performed against gravity. Moving a part actively through a range does not, in isolation, provide a true indication of the available ROM or the strength of a part. For example, if a patient is asked to lift an arm overhead and only lifts it to the horizontal, additional information is required to determine whether the loss of function is due to pain, weakness, or stiffness. The quantity and quality of AROM as well as any signs and symptoms should be noted and documented. In some cases, the clinician may find it useful to have the patient perform repeated active motions to determine the effect on range and symptoms.[17,18,33,34]

Quantity of Active Motion The ROM through which the patient is able to move the part should be measured by some easily reproducible method, such as a goniometer or inclinometer.

Quality of Active Motion Any motion deviations should be described. For example, a typical abnormal movement pattern for a patient with shoulder pain would be excessive scapular elevation during composite shoulder abduction rather than moving with a normal scapulohumeral rhythm.

Signs and Symptoms If pain is reported, the clinician must consider the patient's account regarding at what point in the range of movement the pain occurs as well as what factors increase or decrease the pain. Pain with movement may indicate a muscle strain. In such an instance, pain would be further increased with resisted testing of the involved muscle. Gentle overpressure to AROM should allow the clinician to move the part slightly farther than the patient is able to move actively. Sometimes, symptoms are only noted at end range, which the patient may tend to avoid by actively moving just short of this point. Production of the patient's familiar pain, as opposed to end range strain, that arises only from overpressure would indicate an injured structure is being stretched.[35]

The existence of a painful arc of movement is best detected on active, weight-bearing, or antigravity movements. A painful arc of movement, in which pain is felt throughout a small arc in the midrange of motion, suggests an irritable structure being pulled across a protuberance (such as a nerve root pulled across a disc herniation during a straight leg raise) or pinched between two structures (such as a portion of the rotator cuff tendons being compressed between the greater tubercle and the coracoacromial arch during shoulder abduction). Patients may also report sensations such as catching or clicking during active motion, which may indicate defects in the articular cartilage, labrum, or the menisci. Other sensations include a feeling of instability, indicative of capsular laxity or damage to a ligament or joint capsule.

The presence of crepitus can be appreciated audibly and by palpating over the involved area. Muscle contraction during active movement compresses the joint surfaces. Crepitus usually indicates roughening of joint surfaces. Fine crepitus at a joint suggests early wearing of articular cartilage, whereas coarser crepitus implies considerable cartilaginous degeneration. A creaking sound, not unlike that which a large tree makes when swaying in the wind, often occurs when bones articulate in the late stages of joint surface degeneration. Crepitus over a tendon indicates areas of increased friction between the tendon and its sheath because of swelling or roughening of either the tendon or the sheath.

Clicking during motion may be the result of a normal vacuum effect and is also common in hypermobile joints in which the ligamentous laxity enables a bone to click as it moves in relation to an underlying bone.[36] Clicking can also be pathologic, as in the case of a displaced temporomandibular disc.[37] Snapping may be heard or felt around joints as ligaments of tendons catch and then slip over bony prominences or scar tissue, as in snapping hip syndrome and trigger finger.

Passive Range of Motion To assess passive range of motion (PROM), the clinician moves the part through the major motions that normally occur at the joint being moved. PROM quantity, end feel, quality, and associated symptoms should be noted and documented. The relationship between PROM, AROM, and symptoms helps the clinician determine whether there is joint stiffness, muscle weakness, or pain-limiting motion (Fig. 7-2).

Quantity of Passive Motion The ROM through which the clinician is able to move the part should be measured by some easily reproducible method, such as a goniometer or inclinometer. The examiner must determine whether movement is normal, restricted (hypomobile), or greater than normal (hypermobile). For patients exhibiting hypermobility, the clinician should consider whether the hypermobility is isolated to the motion being assessed or the joint being examined, or whether the patient is globally hypermobile. The Beighton score, also known as the *modified Carter Wilkinson scale*, is a quick and easy assessment consisting of five movements (Fig. 7-3). Although there is no universally agreed-upon cutoff, a patient scoring 4 or more is considered to have generalized ligamentous laxity.[38]

If there is a loss of motion, the clinician should consider if the restriction is in a capsular or noncapsular pattern (Fig. 7-4).

A **capsular pattern of restriction** indicates the loss of mobility of the entire joint capsule.[14] Only joints that are controlled by muscles have a capsular pattern of restriction. Thus, joints such as the tibiofibular and sacroiliac do not exhibit capsular patterns. Capsular restrictions typically accompany acute trauma to a joint (effusion), or prolonged immobilization of a joint

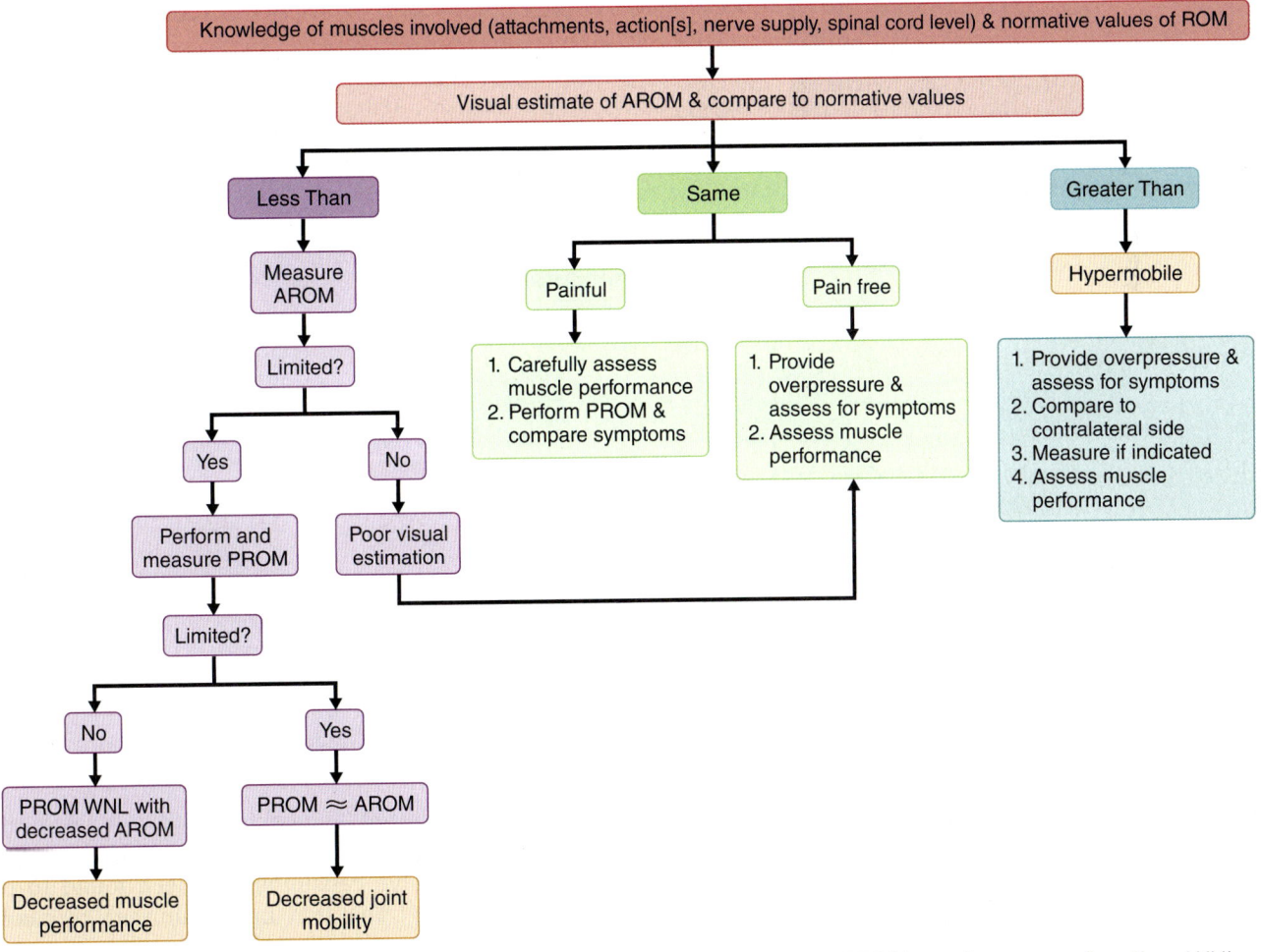

FIGURE 7-2 Range of motion (ROM) algorithm. *AROM*, active range of motion; *PROM*, passive range of motion; *WNL*, within normal limits.

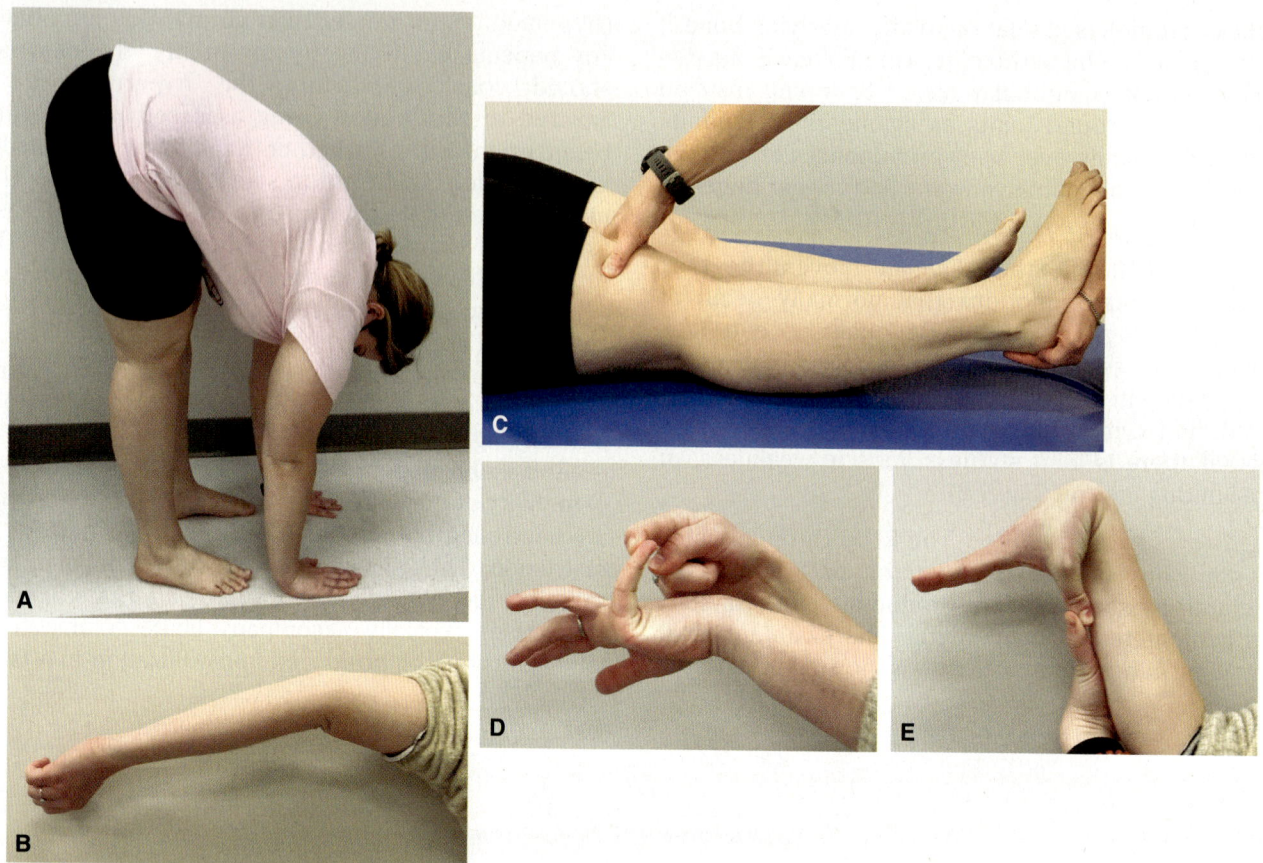

FIGURE 7-3 Beighton score for systemic hypermobility. **A.** Ability to palm the floor with knees straight. **B.** Elbow hyperextension. **C.** Knee hyperextension. **D.** 5th metacarpal hyperextension. **E.** Ventral flexion of thumb to forearm.

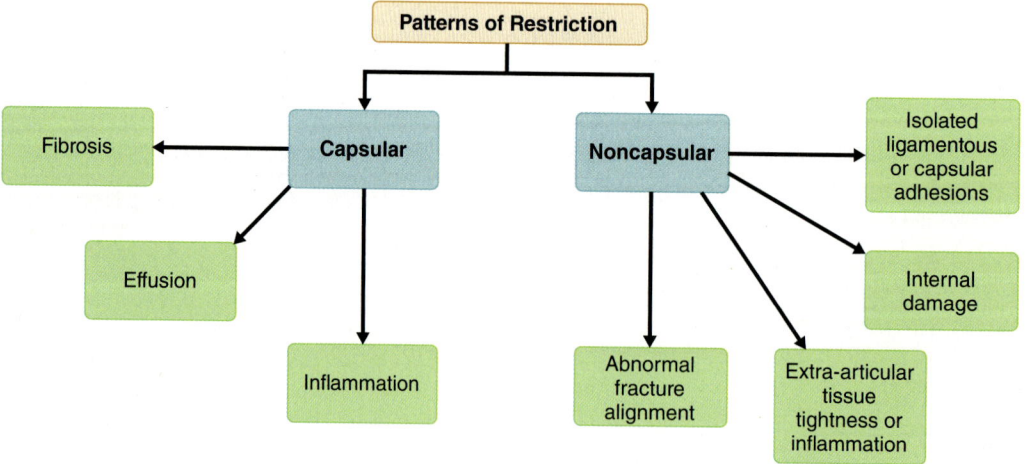

FIGURE 7-4 Patterns of joint restriction.

(fibrosis). The concept of capsular patterns of restriction is evolving. Traditionally, capsular patterns of restriction have been thought to occur in patients with arthritis or DJD. While DJD may include capsular fibrosis, inflammation, or effusion, by definition, DJD is a pathology involving articular cartilage. As such, the presence of a capsular or **noncapsular pattern of restriction** should not be used to confirm or refute the presence of DJD.[39–42] The pattern of motion loss in patients with adhesive capsulitis has been found to be highly variable.[43,44] This may be due, in part, to inconsistencies of diagnostic definitions (idiopathic adhesive capsulitis, systemic secondary adhesive capsulitis, or extrinsic secondary adhesive capsulitis)[45] as well as the

TABLE 7-2
CAPSULAR PATTERNS OF THE LOWER QUARTER

Joint(s)	Proportional Limitations
Thoracic spine	Limitation of sidebending and rotation > extension
Lumbar spine	Limitation of extension > sidebending
Sacroiliac, symphysis pubis, sacrococcygeal	Pain when joints are stressed
Hip	Limitation of flexion/internal rotation > limitation of abduction/extension; no or little limitation of remaining motions
Tibiofemoral (knee)	Flexion grossly limited; slight limitation of extension
Talocrural	Limitation of plantarflexion > dorsiflexion
Talocalcaneal (subtalar)	Limitation of inversion > eversion
Midtarsal	Limitation of supination > pronation
1st metatarsal-phalangeal	Significant limitation of extension; slight limitation of flexion
Metatarsophalangeal (II-V)	Variable; tend toward flexion restrictions
Interphalangeal	Tend toward extension limitations > flexion limitations

Adapted Kaltenborn FM, Evjenth O, Kaltenborn T, Vollowitz E. *The Spine: Basic Evaluation and Mobilization Techniques*. 2nd ed. Olaf Norlis Bokhandel Universitetsgaten; 1993; Kaltenborn FM. *Manual Mobilization of the Joints: The Extremities*. 5th ed. Olaf Norlis Bokhandel Universitetsgaten; 1999; Cyriax J. *Textbook of Orthopedic Medicine: Vol 1. Diagnosis of Soft Tissue Lesions*. 8th ed. W.B. Saunders; 1989; and Edmond S. *Manipulations and Mobilizations: Extremity and Spinal Techniques*. Mosby; 1993.

TABLE 7-3
CAPSULAR PATTERNS OF THE UPPER QUARTER

Joint(s)	Proportional Limitations
Temporomandibular	Limitation of mouth opening
OA joint	Limitation of forward bending > backward bending
AA joint	Restriction with rotation
Lower cervical spine (C3-T2)	Limitation of all motions except flexion (sidebending = rotation > backward bending)
Sternoclavicular	Limitation of full elevation; pain at extreme range of motion
Acromioclavicular	Limitation of full elevation; pain at extreme range of motion
Glenohumeral	Limitation of external rotation > abduction > internal rotation
Humeroulnar	Limitation of flexion > extension
Humeroradial	Limitation of flexion > extension
Proximal radioulnar	Limitation; pronation = supination
Distal radioulnar	Limitation; pronation = supination
Wrist	Limitation; flexion = extension
Midcarpal	Limitation equal all directions
Trapeziometacarpal	Limitation abduction > extension
Carpometacarpals II-V	Limitation of flexion > extension
Upper extremity digits	Limitation of flexion > extension

AA, atlantoaxial joint; *OA*, occipitoatlantal joint.
Adapted from Kaltenborn FM, Evjenth O, Kaltenborn T, Vollowitz E. *The Spine: Basic Evaluation and Mobilization Techniques*. 2nd ed. Olaf Norlis Bokhandel Universitetsgaten; 1993; Kaltenborn FM. *Manual Mobilization of the Joints: The Extremities*. 5th ed. Olaf Norlis Bokhandel Universitetsgaten; 1999; Cyriax J. *Textbook of Orthopedic Medicine: Vol 1. Diagnosis of Soft Tissue Lesions*. 8th ed. W.B. Saunders; 1989; and Edmond S. *Manipulations and Mobilizations: Extremity and Spinal Techniques*. Mosby; 1993.

stage when the condition is assessed. Tables 7-2 and 7-3 list the commonly accepted capsular patterns of the lower and upper quarters, respectively.

Noncapsular patterns of joint restrictions typically occur with intra-articular mechanical blocks or extra-articular lesions. A common example of an isolated ligamentous adhesion is that of adherence of the medial collateral ligament (MCL) at the knee to the medial femoral condyle during healing of a sprain. This results in restriction of knee flexion PROM with extension range being full.[46] Isolated capsular lesions can occur as a result of trauma, but also from surgical interventions for capsular laxity where only certain areas of the capsule are selectively tightened. Internal derangements include displacements of pieces of torn menisci and/or cartilaginous loose bodies. These typically produce a mechanical block to movement in a noncapsular pattern. The most common example is a "bucket-handle" tear of the medial meniscus, resulting in a block to knee extension, with flexion remaining relatively free (in the absence of significant effusion).

Abnormal fracture healing, such as a "dinner-fork" deformity of a Colles fracture, will result in a noncapsular loss of motion. Extra-articular tissue tightness, such as reduced lengthening of muscles from contracture (fibrosis) or myositis ossificans, and extra-articular inflammation, such as those accompanying acute bursitis, also result in noncapsular patterns of restriction.

Signs and Symptoms As with AROM, the patient's report of pain with PROM should be investigated. Stress on injured tissue, such as a sprained ligament, may cause pain. Patients with instability may report a sensation of sliding or giving way, and both the patient and the clinician may appreciate a "clunk" during PROM. An audible "crack" may occur when traction is applied to a joint, stretching the joint capsule and causing gas bubbles within the synovial fluid to collapse.[47] Snapping, clicks, and crepitus may also occur.

End Feel **End feel** is the quality of resistance to the movement the examiner feels when coming to the end point of a particular movement. Some end feels may be normal or pathologic, depending on the movement they accompany at a particular joint and the point in the range of movement at which they are felt.[4,14,48] Other end feels are strictly pathologic. Table 7-4 describes the various types of end feels along with examples of each. It should be noted that for end feel descriptions, intra-rater reliability is good, but inter-rater reliability may be lower.[49]

Interpretation of Symptoms with Active and Passive Range of Motion
Active and passive motion testing helps determine tissue irritability. Recall from Chapter 6, Patient History, that tissue irritability is the ability of tissue to handle stress. Patients with minimal pain with overpressure are described as having low tissue irritability, patients with pain at the end of the ROM have moderate tissue irritability, and patients with pain before end range have high tissue irritability (see Table 6-6).

It is possible to differentiate muscle strains from ligament sprains by comparing symptoms created with AROM and PROM. If a patient reports pain at end range PROM, the lesion is likely a tissue that is being stretched. If a patient reports pain with AROM, the lesion might be the contracting muscle-tendon unit or a (contractile or inert) structure on the opposite side of the joint that is being stretched.

A patient with an anterior talofibular ligament sprain would have pain with active and passive ankle inversion because these stretch the ligament. The pain would be slightly greater if the ankle is plantarflexed slightly because this lengthens the ligament to a greater extent. However, active and passive eversion would be pain free because the ligament is not stressed with these movements.

In contrast, a fibularis strain may cause pain with active eversion because of the increased tension within the contractile unit, but also with active and passive inversion, as the muscle is lengthened with movement in this direction. However, passive eversion would be pain free. It should be noted that mild strains may require a greater stress to the contractile unit, such as with resisted testing, than AROM to elicit symptoms. Likewise, a mild strain may not be sufficiently stressed to elicit symptoms when subjected to maximal tissue lengthening.

The clinician must also consider the effect of biarticular structures when there is pain at end ranges. For example, a patient with a hamstring strain may report no pain with active or passive knee extension when in the supine position but would likely report pain when knee extension is performed while seated. This is sometimes referred to as the *constant-length phenomenon*. In sitting, the hamstring is lengthened over the hip joint, but in supine, it is not. The addition of knee extension from a seated position further stretches the hamstring muscle.

Muscle Length
The purpose of assessment of muscle length (flexibility) is to determine whether the ROM occurring at a joint is limited or excessive by the intrinsic joint structures or by the muscles crossing the joint. Muscle length is tested by the clinician stabilizing one end of the

TABLE 7-4
NORMAL AND PATHOLOGIC END FEELS

End Feels	Description	Normal Example	Pathologic Example
Capsular	Firm, leathery feeling felt with a slight give	Shoulder external rotation	When this end feel occurs sooner than full range (adhesive capsulitis)
Ligamentous	Firm with little or no give	Abduction of the extended knee	
Bony	Abrupt end feel with no give	Elbow extension	When this end feel occurs sooner than full range (hypertrophic bony changes or malunion)
Soft-tissue approximation	Soft end feel	Knee flexion Hip flexion in a patient who is obese	When this end feel occurs sooner than full range (elbow flexion in an individual with elbow effusion)
Muscular	Rubbery, less firm than capsular	Straight leg raise	
Guarding	Abrupt stop to motion, may have rebound	NA	Reflexive muscle contraction trying to prevent further motion
Boggy	Soft, mushy	NA	Effusion
Internal derangement or springy	A pronounced, springy rebound at the end point of movement	NA	Mechanical block from a meniscal tear
Empty	No resistance	NA	Examiner stops motion due to patient report of extreme apprehension or pain

muscle and slowly and smoothly moving the body part to stretch the muscle. When assessing muscle length, clinicians should note the range of movement, the quality of movement, and pain complaints. Muscle tone and the quality of resistance to end range should also be noted. Hypermobility should be further examined to determine whether the excessive movement is isolated to a particular muscle group or whether the hypermobility is systemic. A hurdler may develop excessive hamstring length only on the lead leg, whereas a punter may have excessive hip flexor length. In contrast, a dancer is likely to have excessive bilateral hamstring length in addition to global hypermobility.

Muscle Performance

The relative strength, endurance, and control of muscles should be assessed. Several methods of assessing muscle performance are presented in Table 7-5.[14,32,50-54] This section provides a brief overview of the use and interpretation of this key assessment; the method(s) chosen depend on the individual patient situation. Motor control is a part of screening the neuromuscular system. Motor control is also assessed as part of the quality of movement during AROM testing and observed while a patient is performing functional tasks.

Manual Muscle Testing Manual muscle testing is the most universal method of assessing muscle strength. Close attention to substitution patterns minimizes the chance of erroneous results. Muscle weakness, if elicited, may be caused by an upper motor neuron lesion, a nerve root lesion, injury to a peripheral nerve, pathology at the neuromuscular junction, or by a lesion of the muscle, its tendons, or the bony insertions themselves. Length-tension relationships, muscle imbalance, and positional weakness must be considered when interpreting a manual muscle test.[55]

Myotomal Testing Myotomal testing is used to identify neurologic involvement by testing the strength of specific muscles that are *primarily* innervated by one spinal nerve root. Table 7-6 includes the **myotomes** for the lower quarter, and Table 7-7 includes the myotomes for the upper quarter. Strength should be assessed using traditional manual muscle testing. However, functional testing can be used for S1/2 (toe walk), L4 (heel walk), and L3 (squat).[56]

Cyriax Testing Cyriax testing,[14] also known as **isometric testing in a midrange position**, is a part of selective tissue tension testing and is designed to assess the status of the muscle-tendon unit along with its innervation. These strong isometric strength tests are performed with the joint held in a static, midrange position. Maximal contraction is not normally used because this would cause increase in the activation of synergist muscles. The use of a midrange position allows for optimal length for maximal muscle contraction. Slight changes in position may help distinguish a muscle from its synergist; for example, testing resisted elbow flexion with the forearm in a neutral, pronated, and supinated position might preferentially activate the brachioradialis, brachialis, or biceps.[50] By not allowing any joint motion, there is no change in stress applied to the surrounding capsule and ligaments and there is no change in articular surface contact. Table 7-8 lists the six possible outcomes of Cyriax testing.[14] Interpretation is based on the relationship between the patient's ability to generate force and the reported pain with testing. Like manual muscle testing, this form of assessment is commonly used but may lack reliability.[43] The clinician must also consider that muscle contraction across the joint will increase joint compressive forces, which might create pain in the presence of a fracture or local articular surface lesion.

TABLE 7-5		
MUSCLE PERFORMANCE ASSESSMENT		
Method	Purpose	Grading
Manual muscle testing (MMT)	To differentiate the strength of one muscle from other muscles by precise positioning and application of resistance	0–5 scale or handheld dynamometer
Myotomal testing	To identify neurologic involvement by testing muscles that are primarily innervated by one spinal nerve root	0–5 scale
Isometric testing in a midrange position (also known as Cyriax testing)	To identify a contractile lesion	Strong or weak, painful or painless
Fatigue testing	To identify how a muscle performs over time	Narrative documentation
Functional testing	To observe how an individual performs tasks	Narrative documentation
Isokinetic testing	To assess muscle strength, power, and/or fatigue using various speeds and contraction types	Torque, work

TABLE 7-6
LOWER EXTREMITY PERIPHERAL AND SEGMENTAL MOTOR INNERVATION

Muscles	Peripheral Nerve	Nerve Root	Myotome	Plexus
Iliopsoas	Femoral	L1-L3	L1, L2	Lumbar
Pectineus	Femoral	L2-L3		Lumbar
Sartorius	Femoral	L2-L3		Lumbar
Quadriceps femoris	Femoral	L2-L4	L3	Lumbar
Gracilis	Obturator	L2-L3		Lumbar
Adductor brevis	Obturator	L2-L4		Lumbar
Adductor longus	Obturator	L2-L4		Lumbar
Adductor magnus	Obturator, tibial division of sciatic	L2-L4		Lumbar
Obturator externus	Obturator	L3-L4		Lumbar
Tensor fasciae latae	Superior gluteal	L4-L5		Sacral
Gluteus medius	Superior gluteal	L5-S1		Sacral
Gluteus minimus	Superior gluteal	L5-S1		Sacral
Tibialis anterior	Deep fibular	L4-L5	L4	Sacral
Extensor digitorum longus	Deep fibular	L5-S1		Sacral
Extensor hallucis longus	Deep fibular	L5-S1	L5	Sacral
Extensor digitorum brevis	Deep fibular	S1-S2		Sacral
Gemellus superior	Nerve to obturator internus	L5-S1		Sacral
Obturator internus	Nerve to obturator internus	L5-S1		Sacral
Gemellus inferior	Nerve to quadratus femoris	L5-S1		Sacral
Quadratus femoris	Nerve to quadratus femoris	L5-S1		Sacral
Piriformis	Nerve to piriformis	L5-S2		Sacral
Semimembranosus	Tibial division of sciatic nerve	L5-S1	S1	Sacral
Semitendinosus	Tibial division of sciatic nerve	L5-S1	S1	Sacral
Biceps femoris	Tibia division of sciatic nerve (long head), common fibular division of sciatic nerve	L5-S2		Sacral
Gluteus maximus	Inferior gluteal	L5-S2		Sacral
Fibularis	Superficial fibular	L5-S1	S1, S2	Sacral
Tibialis posterior	Tibial	L4-L5		Sacral
Gastrocnemius	Tibial	S1-S2	S1, S2	Sacral
Soleus	Tibial	S1-S2		
Flexor digitorum longus	Tibial	S2-S3		Sacral
Flexor hallucis longus	Tibial	S2-S3		Sacral
Small muscles of foot	Lateral plantar	S1-S2		Sacral
Flexor digitorum brevis	Medial plantar	S2-S3		Sacral
Flexor hallucis brevis	Medial plantar	S2-S3		Sacral
Perineal and sphincters	Pudendal	S2-S4		Sacral

Adapted from Williams PL, Warwick R, Dyson M, Bannister LH. *Gray's Anatomy*. 37th ed. Churchill Livingstone, 1989.

Fatigue Testing Fatigue testing is used in situations where a patient can perform a task for a period of time before symptoms develop. For example, a marathoner may report knee pain occurring 10 to 12 miles into a training run. This athlete would benefit from an expansion of traditional manual muscle testing. After initial strength testing, the patient would perform a fatigue test, followed by repeat manual muscle testing. The fatigue test could be done in two ways. First, the patient could run a distance just short of the typical onset of pain. Alternatively, the patient could perform repeated resisted exercise of the muscle(s) perceived to be the culprit. A decline in strength on the affected side more than the unaffected side or the reproduction of pain would indicate that muscle fatigue is a part of the patient's pathology.

Functional Testing Functional testing involves observing the patient performing the functional task of reported difficulty. In many aspects, this can be similar to fatigue testing, in that the patient's form may decline over time with a given task. For example, a person who stocks shelves may report back pain that begins 1-hour into an 8-hour shift. Observation of the patient's form and comparison with how the form may change over time could provide valuable insights into the patient's condition.

TABLE 7-7
UPPER EXTREMITY PERIPHERAL AND SEGMENTAL MOTOR INNERVATION

Muscle	Peripheral Nerve	Nerve Root	Myotome	Plexus
Sternocleidomastoid	Accessory	CN XI		Cranial
Trapezius	Accessory	CN XI		Cranial
Cervical muscles	Cervical	C1–C4	C1	Cervical
Diaphragm	Phrenic	C3–C5		Cervical, brachial
Scaleni	Phrenic	C3–C5		Cervical, brachial
Levator scapulae	Dorsal scapular	C5 (C3–C4)		Cervical, brachial
Rhomboids	Dorsal scapular nerve	C4–C5		Cervical, brachial
Infraspinatus	Suprascapular	C4–C6		Cervical, brachial
Supraspinatus	Suprascapular	C4–C6		Cervical, brachial
Teres minor	Axillary	C4–C6		Cervical, brachial
Deltoid	Axillary	C5–C6	C5	Brachial
Biceps brachii	Musculocutaneous	C5–C6	C6	Brachial
Brachialis	Musculocutaneous	C5–C6		Brachial
Coracobrachialis	Musculocutaneous	C5–C7		Brachial
Subscapularis	Subscapular	C5–C7		Cervical, brachial
Teres major	Subscapular	C6–C7		Cervical, brachial
Latissimus dorsi	Thoracodorsal	C6–C8		Brachial
Triceps brachii	Radial	C6–C8	C7	Brachial
Anconeus	Radial	C7–T1		Brachial
Brachioradialis	Radial	C5–C7		Brachial
Extensor carpi radialis longus	Radial	C5–C8	C6	Brachial
Extensor carpi radialis brevis	Posterior interosseous	C6–C8	C6	Brachial
Supinator	Posterior interosseous	C5–C6		Brachial
Abductor pollicis longus	Posterior interosseous	C7–C8		Brachial
Extensor carpi ulnaris	Posterior interosseous	C7–C8	C6	Brachial
Extensor digiti minimi	Posterior interosseous	C7–C8		Brachial
Extensor digitorum	Posterior interosseous	C7–C8		Brachial
Extensor indicis	Posterior interosseous	C7–C8		Brachial
Extensor pollicis brevis	Posterior interosseous nerve	C7–C8		Brachial
Extensor pollicis longus	Posterior interosseous nerve	C7–C8	C8	Brachial
Flexor carpi radialis	Median	C6–C7	C7	Brachial
Pronator teres	Medial	C6–C7		Brachial
Flexor digitorum superficialis	Median	C7–T1		Brachial
Abductor pollicis brevis	Median	C8–T1		Brachial
Flexor digitorum profundus	Median, ulnar	C8–T1		Brachial
Flexor pollicis brevis	Median	C8–T1		Brachial
Flexor pollicis longus	Median	C8–T1		Brachial
Lumbricals (the two lateral)	Median	C8–T1		Brachial
Opponens pollicis	Median	C8–T1		Brachial
Flexor carpi ulnaris	Ulnar	C7–C8	C7	Brachial
Palmaris longus	Ulnar	C8–T1		Brachial
Lumbricals (the two medial)	Ulnar	C8–T1		Brachial
Abductor digiti minimi	Ulnar	C8–T1		Brachial
Adductor pollicis	Ulnar	C8–T1		Brachial
Flexor digiti minimi brevis	Ulnar	C8–T1		Brachial
Interossei	Ulnar	C8–T1	T1	Brachial
Opponens digiti minimi	Ulnar	C8–T1		Brachial

CN, cranial nerve.
Adapted from Williams PL, Warwick R, Dyson M, Bannister LH. *Gray's Anatomy*. 37th ed. Churchill Livingstone, 1989.

TABLE 7-8
CYRIAX TESTING* INTERPRETATION

Outcome	Interpretation
Strong and painless	No contractile lesion
Strong and painful	Minor contractile lesion, first-degree strain
Weak and painful	Severe contractile lesion, second-degree strain
Weak and painless	Complete rupture of muscle/tendon unit or nerve damage
Painful on repetition	Intermittent claudication, possible fatigue or minor lesion
All painful	Gross lesion, fracture, pain-associated psychological distress

*Also known as Isometric Testing in a Midrange Position

Isokinetic Testing Isokinetic testing is expensive, time-consuming, and may lack validity because tested movements are in the open kinetic chain, isolated to a single joint, and do not replicate functional speeds. However, the objectivity and reliability of isokinetic testing make this an ideal research tool.

Sensory Tests A pin, wisp of cotton, monofilament, and tuning fork may be used to clinically assess sensation. Pressure or tension on a nerve will usually result in loss of conduction along the large myelinated fibers first and the small unmyelinated fibers last. Therefore, minor deficits will often be manifested first by loss of vibration sense, with sensation to touch and noxious stimulation being reduced with more severe or long-lasting pressure.

The sensory examination is begun with a quick "scan" of skin sensation. To do this, the clinician runs a finger over the skin to be tested on both regions and asks the patient whether the areas generally feel the same and normal. When performing detailed sensory tests for light touch (with a wisp of cotton or fingertip), a particular area on the unaffected side is tested and the patient is asked if the sensation is perceived. Then, the involved side is tested. The patient is again asked if the sensation is felt, and if so, if the sensation felt the same as the unaffected side. This procedure is followed when testing each key dermatomal segment and each peripheral nerve sensory distribution (Fig. 7-5). Sensory deficits and asymmetries in perception are noted.

Pain sensation can then be tested with a pin, pinwheel, or other sharp object. Only light tapping should be used. The clinician should randomly alternate between testing with the pin (sharp) and testing light touch (dull). The timing of the stimuli should be irregular so that the patient does not know when to expect the next pinprick or touch. The patient should be asked to close their eyes and indicate if a sensation is felt or if the sensation is sharp or dull and to identify the area being assessed.

Other sensations, which can be tested if abnormalities are found, are deep pressure, two-point discrimination, vibration sense, hot or cold sensation, proprioception, and stereognosis.

Any abnormality of sensation is mapped out on a body chart. Positive finding should be reexamined regularly so that any changes in neurologic impairment can be identified and the appropriate action taken.

Reflexes

Lower motor neuron lesions, such as segmental or peripheral nerve disorders, may result in diminution of certain deep tendon reflexes, whereas more central, upper motor neuron lesions may cause hyperreflexia. The deep tendon reflexes are elicited by tapping the tendon a number of times. Incipient root involvement is missed if reflexes are tested once. Routine examinations should include tapping the tendon six successive times to uncover the fading reflex response that indicates developing root signs.[48] Commonly used deep tendon reflexes are listed in Table 7-9.

The important assessments to make when testing deep tendon reflexes are whether the responses at homologous tendons are symmetrical and whether any responses are clonic. Reflexes should be compared bilaterally and graded using either a 0 to 4+ or noting the response (Table 7-10).[57] If it is difficult to elicit a reflex, the clinician may consider having the patient perform the **Jendrassik maneuver** to reinforce the reflex.[58] To reinforce lower extremity reflexes, immediately before tapping the tendon, the clinician should ask the patient to clench his or her teeth or attempt to pull apart his or her clenched hands. The reinforcement contraction for upper extremity reflexes is for the patient to perform leg adduction. When documenting this, the clinician should note the reflex grade and that reinforcement was used.

The presence of hyporeflexia is difficult to judge because some persons normally have reflexes that are difficult to elicit. In general, if it is equally difficult to elicit responses at corresponding tendons, no significance should be attributed to the finding. However, if upper extremity responses are difficult to elicit but lower extremity responses are strong, myelopathy or some other more serious pathologic process should be considered.

Clonus is an exaggerated, rhythmic, oscillating stretch reflex. The presence of clonus suggests an upper motor lesion.[59] If noted, the clinician should check the patient's plantar reflex (Babinski reflex). The Babinski reflex test involves stroking the lateral aspect of the foot and observing the movement of the toes. A normal response is for all the toes to flex. An abnormal response is extension of the great toe and, possibly, fanning of the remaining toes. An abnormal response in a

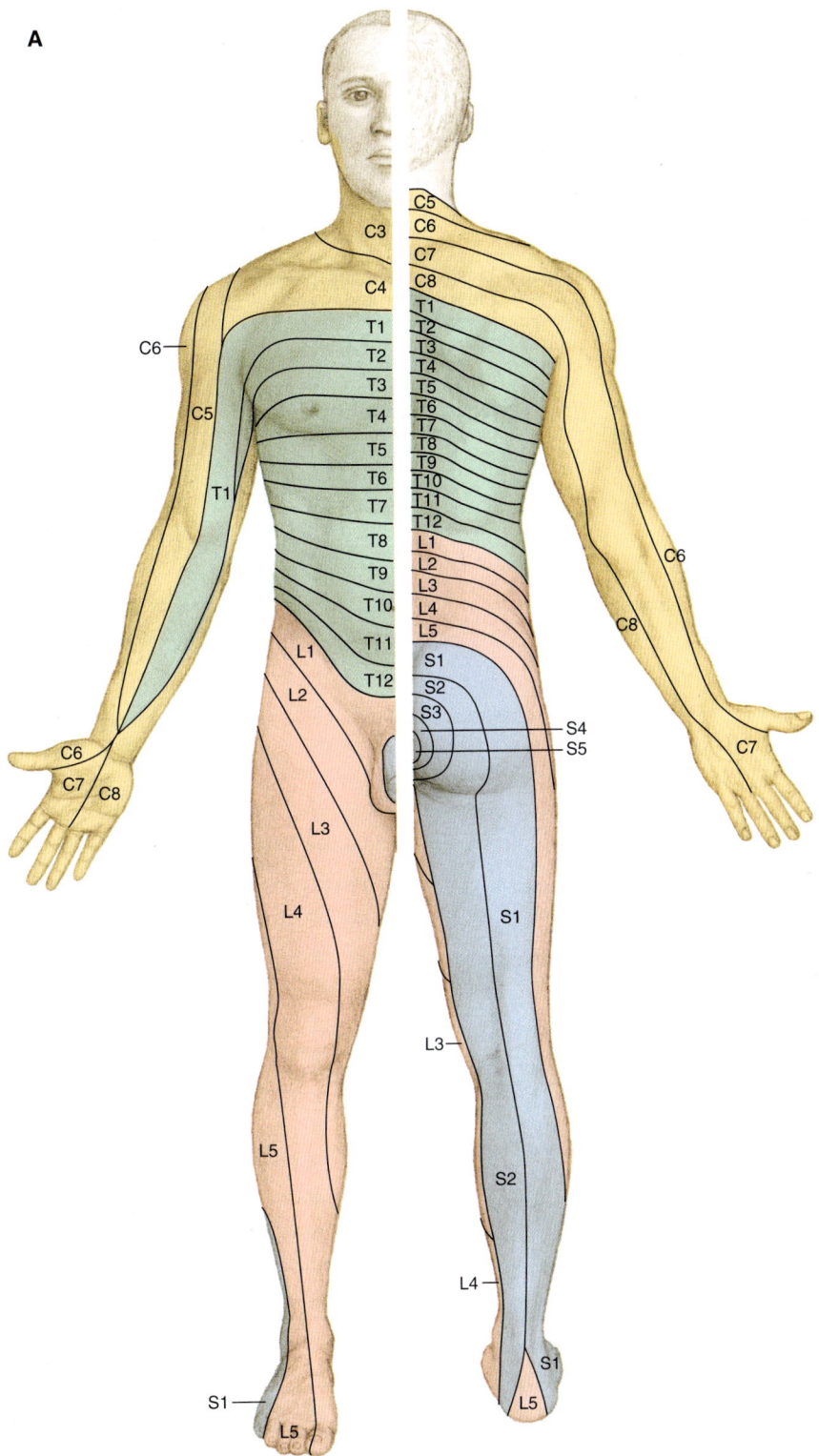

FIGURE 7-5 Peripheral sensory nerve distribution and dermatomes. Dermatomal (A) and upper extremity (B) and lower extremity (C) peripheral nerve distribution. (Modified from Gest TR. *Lippincott Atlas of Anatomy*, 2nd ed. Wolters Kluwer; 2020: Plates 2-53, 2-54, 3-69, 3-70, and 4-03.)

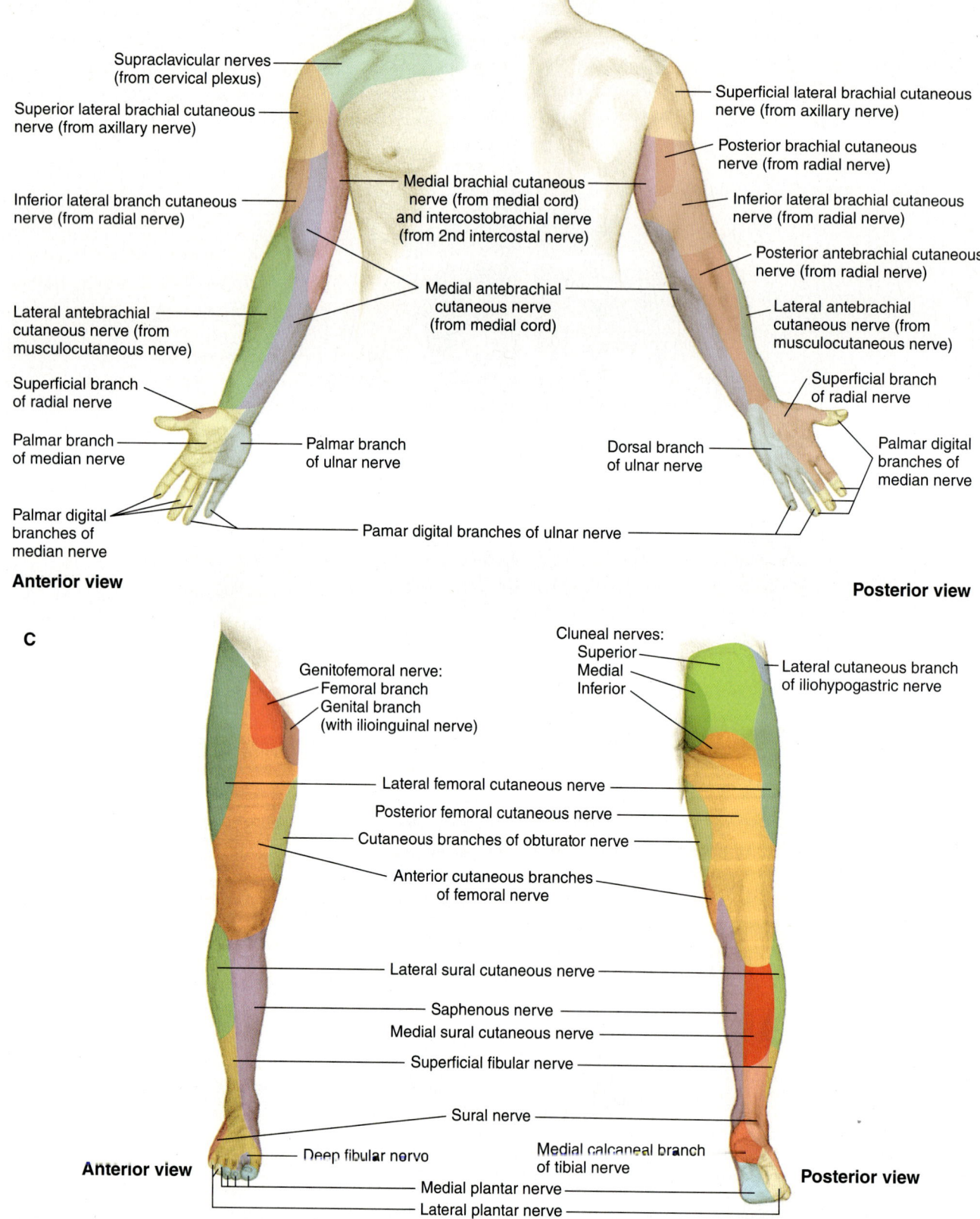

FIGURE 7-5 (continued)

TABLE 7-9
REFLEX TESTING

Spinal Nerve Root	Tendon Reflex
S1/2	Achilles
L3	Patellar
C5	Biceps
C6	Brachioradialis
C7	Triceps
Trigeminal nerve	Jaw jerk

TABLE 7-10
REFLEX GRADES

Grade	Response
0	Absent
1+	Diminished
2+	Normal
3+	Hyperreflexive
4+	Clonus

patient over 2 years of age raises the suspicion of an upper motor neuron lesion.[60] The Hoffmann test is a sensitive but nonspecific test for upper motor neuron lesion, such as cervical myelopathy.[61] It is performed with the patient in a relaxed seated position. The clinician holds the patient's middle phalanx of the 3rd digit and flicks the distal phalanx into flexion. An abnormal response is involuntary flexion of the thumb and index finger.

Neurodynamic Tests

Neurodynamic tests examine the extensibility of the nervous system because tension within the nerve and its connective tissue can be a source of symptoms. Examples of neurodynamic tests include the straight leg raise, slump test, and upper limb tension tests described in Chapter 12, Lumbar Spine and Sacroiliac Joint, and Chapter 17, Cervical and Thoracic Spine. Testing procedures follow the same format as those of joint movement. The resting symptoms are established before testing. The clinician notes the range of movement, end feel, and symptom behavior with the test movement.

Accessory Motions

AROM and PROM reflect osteokinematic movements. Moving one of the articular surfaces of a joint parallel or perpendicular to the joint line assesses arthrokinematic motions. Arthrokinematic motions are also known as *accessory motions* or *joint play*. The treatment plane is at right angles to a line drawn from the axis of rotation to the center of the concave articulating surface and lies in the concave surface. Passively moving the distal bone perpendicular to the treatment plane is called *traction* or *distraction*. When this motion is directed parallel to the axis of a distal long bone, this is called *long-axis distraction*. Traction and distraction increase the distance between joint surfaces, thus unloading the joint surfaces (Fig. 7-6A). Passively moving the distal bone parallel to the treatment plane is called a *glide* (Fig. 7-6B). The examiner may also provide a rotational mobilization, called *spin*, in which the distal bone and articular surface are rotated clockwise or counterclockwise (Fig. 7-6C).

Accessory motions should be assessed in the open-packed (or loose-packed) position. The **open-packed position** is the position in which laxity of the capsule and ligaments is greatest and there is the least bony contact (minimal congruency between the articular surfaces). Therefore, the open-packed position has the greatest amount of joint play available. Because of the lack of bony and soft-tissue support, dislocations are more likely to occur when injuries occur when the joint is in the open-packed position. If limitations in ROM or pain prevent the examiner from placing the joint in the open-packed position, the position most closely approximating the open-packed position should be used for assessment.

Passive accessory motions are designed to stress various portions of the joint capsule and major ligaments to detect the presence of painful lesions affecting these structures or loss of continuity of these structures. Traction and distraction create a global stretch of the joint capsule and surrounding tissues. Gliding provides a more local stretch to a specific region of the capsule. Spin can be used to facilitate normal arthrokinematics spin, such as conjunct rotation of the knee during terminal knee extension.

Accessory motion assessment entails determination of the amount of excursion present in a particular direction, the type of resistance felt at the end of ROM (end feel), and any symptoms created (pain, guarding, or instability). Excursion is determined by comparing the joint with the same joint on the contralateral side.[48] The examiner may also rely on prior clinical experience for determining the amount of joint mobility, particularly if the contralateral side is dysfunctional.[62] Joint mobility is evaluated by performing either a glide or traction mobilization and grading the amplitude of excursion.[15] Maitland initially described a 0 to 6 grading scale moving from fused to grossly hypermobile.[48] However, simplifying grading into three categories (hypomobile, normal, or hypermobile)[14] improves reliability and does not alter treatment.[62–66]

Joint hypomobility may be the result of tissue fibrosis and increased collagen deposition, abnormal fracture healing, or the result of protective muscle spasm and inflammation. Hypomobile joints may benefit from joint mobilizations to improve accessory motion and osteokinematic range.[15] Joint mobilizations can initially be performed in the open-packed position but may progress to near end range to provide a more aggressive and specific stretch to restricted tissues.[35,65] Joint hypermobility may be the result of a partial or complete rupture of the structure being

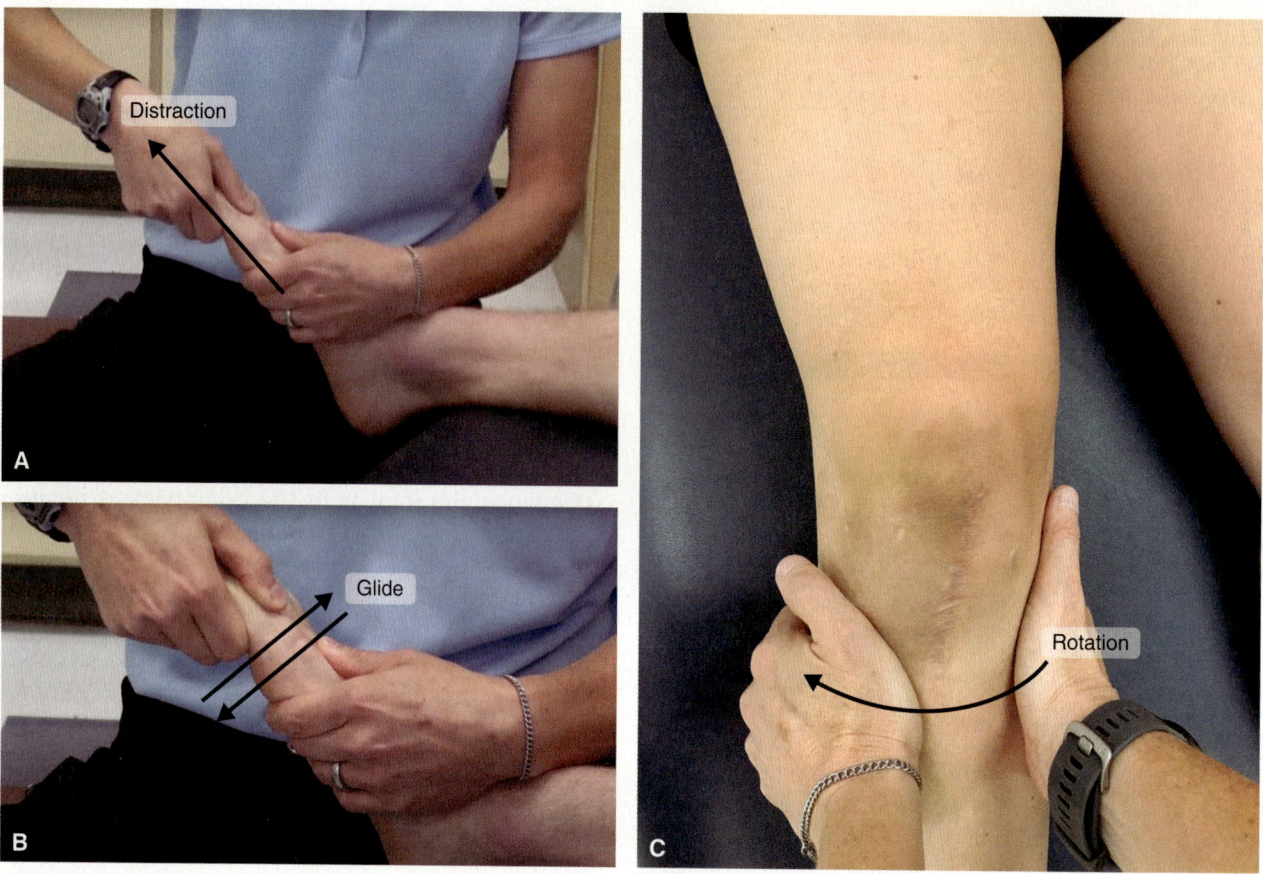

FIGURE 7-6 Accessory motion. **A.** Joint distraction. **B.** Dorsal and plantar glide. **C.** Rotational mobilization.

assessed, systemic hypermobility, or a dysplastic joint (such as hip dysplasia). Hypermobile joints may benefit from taping, bracing, or stabilization via exercises in addition to education to avoid postures or positions that increase stress to the joint or affected tissues.[15] Normal mobility implies the structures being tested are normal. The presence of pain or guarding suggests the presence of a sprain or tear of the structure being stressed. Painful joints may benefit from small-amplitude joint mobilizations in the open-packed position to modulate pain. Figure 7-7 describes the six possible findings of accessory motion testing and their

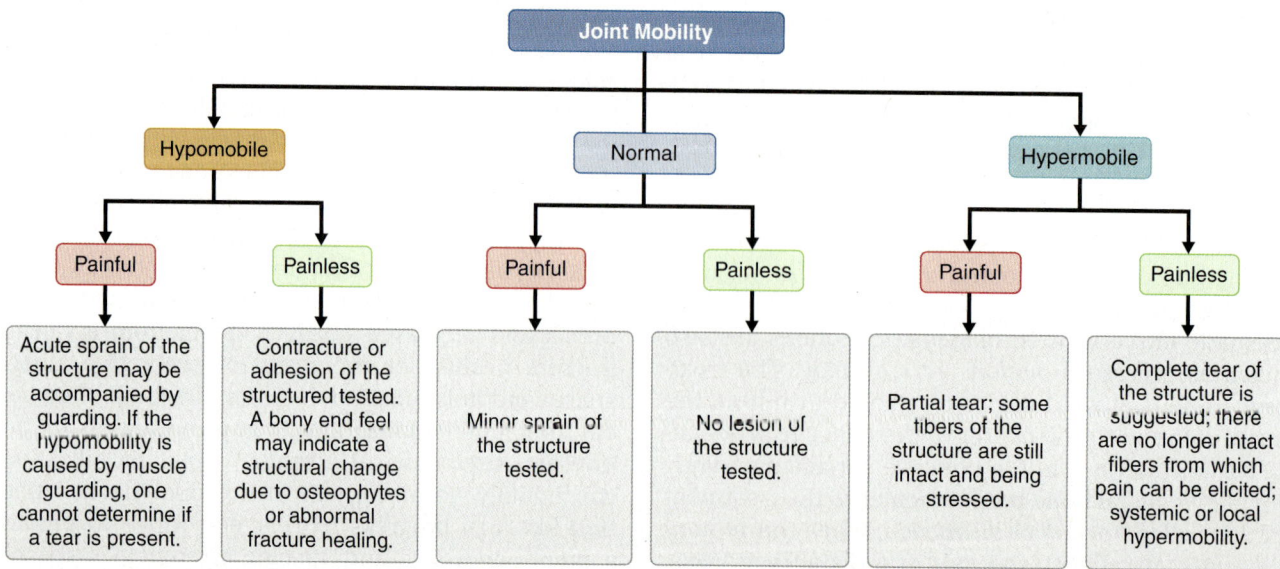

FIGURE 7-7 Interpretation of joint mobility assessment.

probable interpretation. Joint-specific chapters later in the book provide specific methods for performing joint mobilization techniques.

The close-packed position is the position of the joint in which the capsule and ligaments are most taut and there is maximal bony congruency. Therefore, the close-packed position is the position with the least amount of joint play, making fractures more likely when injuries occur when the joint is in this position. The close-packed position can be used therapeutically to block motion at a given joint. For example, the spinal segments above and below a segment to be mobilized may be "locked" into a close-packed position in order to attempt to localize the mobilizing force to a particular level.[16] Descriptions of open- and close-packed positions for various joints are provided in Tables 7-11 and 7-12.

Special Tests

Special tests are procedures that pertain to the specific anatomy and pathologic condition of the peripheral joint or spinal region being examined. These tests are structured to uncover a specific type of pathology, condition, or injury. The use of the term "special" to describe these tests may be misleading because it implies these tests have a high degree of accuracy and reliability. Although the phrase "additional tests" is more appropriate, common convention within the medical community continues to use "special test" to describe this category of tests and measures. Although each joint complex has multiple special tests, the clinician need not perform every procedure. Special tests are most helpful when the history and previous portions of the examination have led the examiner to suspect the nature of the pathology or condition. This is because some tests may create false positives. For example, the Finkelstein test for de Quervain tenosynovitis commonly produces symptoms when the pathology is not, in fact, present.[67] Special tests include tests for ligamentous laxity (e.g., Lachman test) and muscle-tendon ruptures (e.g., external rotation lag test).

Provocation tests are specific types of special tests that attempt to create or increase the patient's familiar symptoms. While active and passive motion along with overpressure, accessory motions, and resisted testing may be capable of creating the patient's familiar symptoms, some structures require additional strategies. This may include repeated active motions and sustained pressures. Should these fail to reproduce the pain, greater stress on the structures can be achieved by combined motions or by coupling movements in two or three directions (e.g., quadrant tests). The Hawkins-Kennedy test for shoulder impingement and the patellar grind test for patellofemoral pain syndrome are additional examples of provocation tests.

Because many special tests create or exacerbate symptoms, they are best reserved for later in the physical examination. This is because the clinician may not gain accurate information on assessments, such as muscle performance, if the patient's condition has been sufficiently irritated by special tests. Special tests specific to each joint complex are discussed within the appropriate chapters.

TABLE 7-11

OPEN- AND CLOSE-PACKED POSITIONS OF THE LOWER QUARTER

Open-Packed Position	Joint(s)	Close-Packed Position
Midway between flexion and extension	**Vertebral**	Maximal extension
30° flexion, 30° abduction, and slight lateral rotation	**Hip**	Ligamentous: full extension, abduction, and internal rotation Bony: 90° flexion, slight abduction, and slight external rotation
25° flexion	**Knee**	Full extension
	Ankle/Foot	
Mid-inversion/eversion and 10° plantar flexion	Talocrural	Full dorsiflexion
Midway between extremes of range of motion with 10° plantar flexion	Subtalar	Full inversion
Midway between extremes of range of motion with 10° plantar flexion	Midtarsal	Full supination
Midway between supination and pronation	Tarsometatarsal	Full supination
	Toes	
0–10° extension	Metatarsophalangeal	Full extension
Slight flexion	Interphalangeal	Full extension

Adapted from Kaltenborn FM, Evjenth O, Kaltenborn T, Vollowitz E. *The Spine: Basic Evaluation and Mobilization Techniques.* 2nd ed. Olaf Norlis Bokhandel Universitetsgaten; 1993; Kaltenborn FM. *Manual Mobilization of the Joints: The Extremities.* 5th ed. Olaf Norlis Bokhandel Universitetsgaten; 1999; and Cyriax J. *Textbook of Orthopedic Medicine: Vol 1. Diagnosis of Soft Tissue Lesions.* 8th ed. W.B. Saunders; 1989.

TABLE 7-12
OPEN- AND CLOSE-PACKED POSITIONS OF THE UPPER QUARTER

Open-packed	Joint	Close-packed
	Spine	
Midway between flexion and extension	**Vertebral**	Maximal extension
Jaw slightly open (freeway space)	**Temporomandibular**	Maximal retrusion (mouth closed with teeth clenched) or maximal anterior position (mouth maximally opened)
	Shoulder Complex	
Arm resting by side	Sternoclavicular	Shoulder maximally elevated
Arm resting by side	Acromioclavicular	Shoulder abducted 90°
55–70° abduction; 30° horizontal adduction; neutral rotation	Glenohumeral	Maximum abduction and external rotation
	Elbow/Forearm	
70° flexion and 10° supination	Humeroulnar	Full extension and supination
Full extension and supination	Humeroradial	90° flexion, 5° supination
70° flexion and 35° supination	Proximal radioulnar	5° supination, full extension
10° supination	Distal radioulnar	5° supination
	Wrist/Hand	
Neutral with slight ulnar deviation	Radio/ulnocarpal	Full extension with radial deviation
Neutral with slight flexion and ulnar deviation	Midcarpal	Full extension
Midway between flexion/extension, midflexion, and midextension	Carpometacarpal (2nd through 5th)	Full opposition
Midway between flexion/extension and between abduction/adduction	1st carpometacarpal	Full opposition
Slight flexion	1st MCP	Full extension
Slight flexion	MCP 2nd to 5th	Full flexion
10° flexion	Proximal IP	Full extension
30° flexion	Distal IP	Full extension

MCP, metacarpophalangeal; *IP*, interphalangeal.
Adapted from Blanpied P, Gross A, Elliott J, et al. Neck pain: revision 2017. Clinical practice guidelines linked to the international classification of functioning, disability and health from the orthopaedic section of the American Physical Therapy Association. *J Orthop Sports Phys Ther.* 2017;47(1):A1–A83; Davenport D, Colaco H, Kavarthapu V. Examination of the adult spine. *Br J Hosp Med.* 2015;76(12):C182–C195; and Dawson C, Mudgal CS. Staged description of the Finkelstein test. *J Hand Surg.* 2010;35(9):1513–1515.

Palpation

Relying on palpation to provide insights into a patient's condition can be grossly misleading. First, palpating the area of a patient's pain complaint fails to take into account the possibility of referred pain. Without first using the history and prior pieces of the physical examination as a guide, the clinician would be proceeding by guesswork rather than science. Second, local tenderness can be misleading, as conditions such as tendinopathy and chronic pain are known to create both local and more generalized hyperalgesia.[18,68,69] Third, some structures, such as the labrum of the shoulder or hip, are not readily assessed via palpation.

Once the region of pathology has been sufficiently narrowed via the history and preceding examination components, careful and methodical palpation can provide significant insights into physiologic and structural changes. The palpatory examination includes, but is not necessarily limited to, palpation of the myofascial structures in the form of layer palpation and palpation of the bony structures. The tissues that can be palpated include the skin, subcutaneous fascia, blood vessels, nerves, muscle sheaths, muscle bellies, musculotendinous junctions, tendons, deep fascia, ligaments, bones, and joint margins. The uninvolved side should be palpated first so that the patient has an idea of what to expect. Palpation should be organized according to layers, assessing the status of the skin, subcutaneous soft tissues, and bony structures (including tendon and ligament attachments). Significant findings are documented. For practical purposes, the palpation examination has been categorized into the assessment of skin, swelling, pulses, mobility, structure, and tenderness.

Skin Observation of the skin for structural changes, such as open wounds callus, and color changes is performed during the system review. When a scar exists, whether surgical or traumatic, the type of surgery or injury should be determined because it may have some bearing on the present problem. Blemishes such as large, brownish, pigmented areas (café au lait spots), and localized hairy regions often accompany underlying bony defects, such as spina bifida. Calluses develop with increased shear or compressive stresses; blisters occur with increased shear between the skin and the subcutaneous tissue. When an open wound is observed, the clinician should determine whether it is of traumatic origin or of insidious origin, as often accompanies diabetes. When palpating the skin, the clinician should note tissue temperature, moisture, and texture.

Temperature Palpation of skin temperature is a qualitative assessment and should be recorded as increased, normal, or decreased. An infrared thermometer can reliably measure temperature to the nearest 0.1°F. Infrared thermography is used for differential diagnosis of certain conditions, such as the diabetic neuropathic osteoarthropathy known as *Charcot foot*.[70] However, in most cases, this degree of accuracy is not required. Skin temperature will be elevated in the presence of an underlying inflammatory process or with reduced sympathetic activity.[71] A reduction in skin temperature may accompany vascular deficiency or increased sympathetic activity.[72]

Moisture and Texture Moisture and texture may be altered with changes in vascularity or changes in sympathetic activity to the part. In the presence of increased sympathetic activity, such as that which commonly occurs in the chronic stages of reflex sympathetic dystrophy, the skin will be abnormally moist and very smooth. With reduced sympathetic activity, sometimes preceding a reflex sympathetic dystrophy, the skin may be dry and scaly.

Swelling Generalized edema should be noted as part of the cardiovascular system review. Bilateral edema may be a sign of heart failure or electrolyte imbalances, whereas unilateral edema may be due to trauma, venous insufficiency, or lymphedema. Edema should be graded on a 1+ to 4+ scale based on the tissue's response to the clinician's thumb or index finger firmly pressing into the area for 5 seconds (Table 7-13).

Intra-articular swelling is called **effusion**. Effusion limits joint ROM. Effusion within the knee should make the clinician suspect an intra-articular fracture or anterior cruciate ligament rupture. Effusion can be measured using circumferential measurements or special tests, such as the ballottement or modified stroke test (see Chapter 10, Knee).

Localized swelling is common with bursitis but may also occur with an abscess. Certain disease process, such as rheumatoid arthritis, causes synovial inflammation.

Pulses Palpating for the pulse of major arteries in the region can assist in assessing the status of blood supply to the part. Although commonly thought of as pertaining only to the management of patients with open wounds, the palpation examination is a vital part of identifying pathologies such as compartment syndrome and intermittent claudication, which may be first seen in an outpatient setting. Pulses should be graded on a 0 to 3+ scale (Table 7-14).

Mobility The movement of the skin over the underlying but superficial structures should be assessed. Normal soft tissue is supple and easily moved against underlying tissue. This is especially important following healing of surgical and other traumatic wounds. Any scars present should be assessed for thickness and mobility. Scars that are not mobile and pliable can restrict motion, particularly when crossing a joint. No more pressure than what is necessary is used. A common mistake is to press harder and harder in an attempt to distinguish deep structures. The deep palpatory examination includes compression, which is palpation through layers of tissue perpendicular to the tissue, and shear. Shear is the movement of the myofascial tissues between layers, moving parallel to the tissue. Translational and longitudinal muscle play are effective assessment tools for assessing the mobility of a muscle or muscle group within a fascial sheath. Palpation may progress to probing, grasping, or displacing muscle bellies and tendons. Resistance to displacement or stretch and crepitus or "catching" should be noted. It can be most revealing to palpate the entire extent of a tendon sheath during contraction of its respective muscle. Crepitus, creaking, or vibration,

TABLE 7-13
EDEMA CLASSIFICATION

Grade	Description
1+	Barely perceptible depression
2+	Easily identifiable depression that rebounds within 15 seconds.
3+	Depression rebounds in 15–30 seconds
4+	Depression lasts for >30 seconds

Adapted from Myers BA. *Wound Management: Principles and Practice.* 4th ed. Pearson; 2020.

TABLE 7-14
PULSE EXAMINATION

Grade	Description
0	Absent pulse
1+	Decreased pulse
2+	Normal pulse that is easily palpable
3+	Bounding pulse

as if the tendon needs lubrication, may represent tenosynovitis.

Depending on the body part being tested, either the palm or the fingertips are used to detect restrictions. On broad body surfaces, the palm is firmly but lightly placed on the skin and then displaced in all directions to identify tension and resistance to gentle displacement. More vigorous displacement in the form of skin rolling (if tolerated and indicated), skin gliding, skin distraction, and the pinch roll maneuver are often an important part of layer palpation, providing additional information about the extensibility of the subcutaneous tissues.

Structure and Tenderness The superficial soft tissues palpated included fascia, fat, muscles, tendons, joint capsules and ligaments, nerves, and bone. The clinician should palpate for structural deviations as well as tenderness. The region should be assessed for tender points[73] and trigger points.[74] Structural changes such as identification of a gap or loss of tissue continuity might indicate partial or complete tissue rupture. Recall that tenderness to deep palpation is a very unreliable finding. In contrast, superficial structures appear to be much more "honest" tissues: that is, tenderness associated with more superficial structures corresponds more closely with the site of the lesion than does tenderness occurring with more deeply situated pathologic processes. For example, tenderness of the MCL of the knee is a fairly reliable indicator of an MCL sprain.[11]

Gait, Transfers, and Mobility

Although gait, transfers, and mobility were observed during the systems review, a more detailed assessment is performed after the joint-specific examination has been completed. Delaying these higher level tasks ensures the clinician has sufficient information to determine the safety of performing these assessments. It is here that the clinician can piece together all the components of the examination. For example, early heel off and lack of push off may be noted on the cursory gait evaluation. When this information is combined with metatarsal head tenderness and the patient's report of reproduction of plantar midfoot pain at heel off, metatarsalgia should be a key differential diagnosis. It is at this point that the clinician should inspect the patient's footwear, including heel-toe drop and cushioning.

Function

Functional testing, including balance, is a part of the lower quarter screen. Functional assessment plays a very important role in the evaluation of the patient. It is different from the analysis of specific movement patterns of active, passive, and isometric movements. Functional assessment may be as simple as observation of certain patient activities involving the joint or region being examined or attempted performance of a problematic task. Common functional tests carried out at this point for the lower quarter include stair climbing, lifting, balance reach, single-leg squat excursions, and lunge distance. For the upper quarter, functional reaching, overhead lifting, or throwing may be performed. In contrast, far more detailed objective measurement of functional task performance, such as a functional capacity evaluation, may be required. Figure 7-8 provides a summary of the physical examination.

CLINICAL DECISION-MAKING

The clinician must interpret the information gained from the history and physical examination to determine a diagnosis and develop plan of care. Clinical decision-making is not isolated to one point in time but rather has occurred throughout the history and physical examination. During the history, the clinician needed to determine whether the patient's problem appeared to fall within their scope of practice and determine whether it was safe to proceed with the physical examination. The clinician made decisions regarding questions to ask to help formulate a list of differential diagnoses. The clinician needed to determine whether there was an urgent need to rule out significant pathology, such as a fracture. During the physical examination, the clinician had to consider the competing hypotheses and perform tests and measures to assist with proving and disproving each of these.

One of the most critical steps in clinical decision-making is correlation and interpretation of the history and examination findings, requiring that the clinician give meaning and relevance to the data obtained. At times, a pathoanatomic diagnosis is possible. For example, consider a patient who reports hearing and feeling a "pop" after missing a stair. If the patient presents with weak plantarflexion, a positive Thompson test, and a palpable breach in the Achilles region, it is very likely that the patient sustained a ruptured Achilles.[75] A pathoanatomic diagnosis can provide valuable information regarding tissue pathology and can assist with planning interventions. However, this pathoanatomic diagnosis, by itself, is insufficient to guide treatment. In the example of a patient with a torn Achilles tendon, if the injury occurred to a 22-year-old basketball player, surgery would be appropriate. In contrast, for a 72-year-old sedentary individual with diabetes, conservative care would be more appropriate.[76] When there is a new onset of symptoms, generally speaking, clinicians should seek a single source.[2] For example, a patient with a new onset of back pain and foot numbness is more likely to be experiencing lumbar nerve root compression

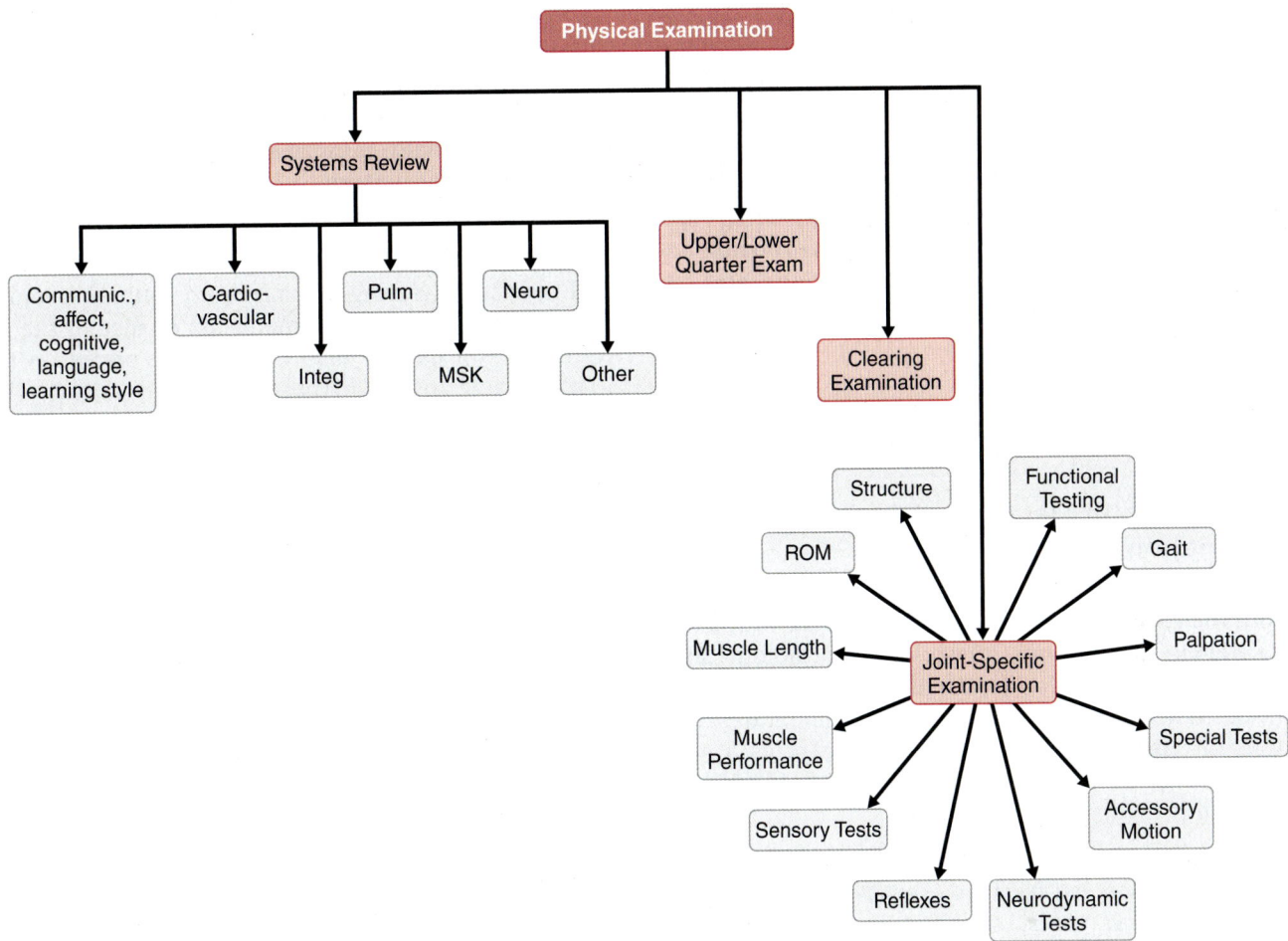

FIGURE 7-8 History and physical examination summary. *ROM*, range of motion; *Communic*, communication; *Integ*, integumentary; *Pulm*, pulmonary; *MSK*, musculoskeletal; *Neuro*, neurological.

than simultaneous occurrences of low back pain and tarsal tunnel syndrome. However, with more chronic conditions, this no longer holds true as patients are likely to adapt compensatory strategies, which, in themselves, can cause symptoms.

Patients often present with a mixture of signs and symptoms that indicates overlapping problems. The novice clinician may recognize the typical feature of an injury, yet fail to exclude other potentially coexisting disorders that may share or predispose the patient to the clinical presentation. When faced with an atypical problem, the decision may be an educated guess; very few problems are textbook perfect. At times, it may not be possible to confirm an anatomic cause for the patient's chief complaint. Indeed, the structural cause of low back pain may not be identifiable.[77] Clinicians should consider a pathokinesiologic approach where the diagnostic classification is related to the movement system impairments.[10,78,79] Subjective and objective reassessment should be built into each patient visit, and these quantifiable data should guide future decisions regarding the intervention strategy and plan of care.

Clinicians must use professional judgment to classify or categorize patients within their legal purview. Such classification should be understood across medical professions and should direct treatment. Therefore, clinicians may choose to use *International Classification of Diseases (ICD-10)* codes that are used for billing purposes but must also include additional key information to direct treatment.[33] Clinicians may also choose to use *International Classification of Functioning, Disability, and Health (ICF)* classification.[80] The *ICF* model involves a multidimensional description of the patient, including the personal factors and comorbidities effecting patient care, body structures involved, and a prioritized problem list, including impairments, activity limitations, and participation restrictions.

Clinicians must also determine the patient's clinical status: is the condition stable, evolving, or unstable?[79] Clinicians must note the patient's stage of healing and irritability,[81,82] as these inform the plan of care. For example, patient with an acute, irritable tendinopathy would benefit from pain modulation and controlled rest, whereas a patient with a nonirritable chronic tendinopathy would benefit from progressive tendon loading.[82,83] The clinician should list any precautions or contraindications. Lastly, the clinician should list any referrals that might be beneficial for the patient. Key components the clinician should document regarding the patient diagnosis include the following:

- Personal factors and comorbidities influencing care
- Prioritized problem list, including impairments, activity limitations, participation restrictions, and environmental and contextual factors
- Clinical status
- Stage of healing
- Irritability
- Precautions or contraindications

Guides to Interpretation of Clinical Information

Clinicians should try to correlate information gained from the history and physical examination with their knowledge of anatomy, physiology, kinesiology, and pathology in order to identify the involved tissue or tissues when possible. The following general descriptions of tissue-level pathologies are meant as a noninclusive guide to assist clinicians with identifying potentially involved tissues.

Bone Radiographs are the first-line diagnostic imaging method for fracture identification.[84] Clinical decision-making tools, such as the Ottawa Ankle Rules, to guide clinicians in determining when imaging studies might be needed to rule out a fracture are discussed in the appropriate chapters. When examining a patient following healing of a fracture, it is important to determine any malunion of bone on inspection of bone structure and alignment, as this may affect eventual functioning of the part. Stress fractures are best identified via magnetic resonance imaging. Dislocations generally occur as a result of trauma but may be the result of progressive joint deterioration in conditions, such as rheumatoid arthritis or diabetic neuropathic osteoarthropathy (e.g., Charcot foot). Dislocations are best detected through radiographs, although they are often obvious on inspection.

Articular Cartilage Degeneration from wearing due to tissue fatigue is the most common lesion affecting articular cartilage. It causes roughening of the normally smooth surface layers of cartilage. Clinically, this is manifested as crepitus on movements in which opposition of joint surfaces is maintained by weight-bearing or other compressive forces. However, considerable degeneration must usually take place before crepitus is detected clinically. A loose body is a fragment of articular cartilage that has broken away and lies free in the joint. This may occur in the late stages of cartilage degeneration or as a result of avascular necrosis of an area of subchondral bone (osteochondrosis). A loose body becomes symptomatic when it alters the mechanical functioning of the joint, usually causing a restriction of movement in a noncapsular pattern.

Intra-articular Fibrocartilage The common disorder affecting intra-articular fibrocartilaginous discs and menisci is tearing, usually from traumatic injury. Forces sufficient to tear a meniscus or disc in the extremities will usually also cause some strain on the joint capsule to which these structures attach. This causes synovial inflammation in the acute stage. Thus, movement is likely to be restricted in a capsular pattern. Minor displacement of a torn fragment of fibrocartilage may simply result in "clicking" of the joint on specific movements. Lower extremity joints, namely, the knee, may "give way" when a piece of a torn meniscus is caught between the articular surfaces, suddenly interfering with the normal mechanics of the joint. A major displacement of a torn fragment may grossly interfere with normal mechanics and block joint movement in a noncapsular pattern. The classic example is a "bucket-handle" tear of a medial meniscus. When the annular ring of an intervertebral disc is torn, secondary neurologic symptoms or signs may result from disc herniation and inflammation against adjacent nerve tissue.

Joint Capsule Fibrosis typically occurs with prolonged immobilization of a joint; in association with a chronic, low-grade inflammatory process such as occurs with DJD; and after resolution of acute synovial inflammation. Joint motion may be limited in a capsular pattern, and there is a capsular end feel at the extremes of movement. Synovial inflammation is commonly caused by rheumatoid arthritis, acute trauma to the joint, and joint infection. There is pain near end ranges and an empty or guarded end feel. Inflammation of the synovium results in an increased production of synovial fluid, causing capsular distention and loss of the capsular laxity necessary for full movement. Joint motion is limited in a capsular pattern. In the more superficial joints, the articular swelling can be observed and palpated. If the effusion persists after resolution of the synovial inflammation, motion will continue to be limited in a capsular manner, with a boggy end feel to movement and pain will be mild or absent. Patients with capsular pathology typically have some combination of fibrosis, synovial inflammation, and effusion. Therefore, end feels are not always distinct.

Occasionally in traumatic injuries, a particular portion of a joint capsule is ruptured, such as the anterior capsule of the shoulder when the humerus dislocates anteriorly. Synovial inflammation and joint effusion usually follow capsular sprains. In the case of a mild sprain, accessory movements (e.g., glides) that stress the involved portion of the capsule will be painful but of normal amplitude. In more severe sprains, the joint may be hypermobile, with a painful muscle-guarding end feel.

Ligaments The history of a sprain invariably includes a traumatic onset. In the case of a mild sprain, motions that stress the ligament (active and passive lengthening) create end-range pain, whereas the accessory movement that stresses the ligament will be painful but of normal amplitude. For more severe sprains (partial ruptures), accessory motions that stress the ligament will be painful and hypermobile. The synovial lining of the adjacent aspect of the joint capsule will often become inflamed, resulting in capsular effusion in the acute stage. For superficial ligaments, there is usually tenderness over the site of the lesion.

With complete ligament ruptures, motions that stress the ligament (active and passive lengthening as well as accessory motions that stretch the ligament) are usually painless and hypermobile because there are no intact fibers from which to elicit pain. Forces sufficient to sprain a ligament usually cause some capsular disruption as well. If adjacent capsular tissue is also sprained, there may be some pain on stress testing during the acute stage. Capsular effusion may not occur with ligament ruptures because synovial fluid leaks through the defect in the capsule. In the chronic stages the patient may give a history of instability.

Bursae The common disorder of bursae is inflammation. Bursitis may be secondary to chronic irritation, infection, gout, or, rarely, acute trauma. Bursae have a rich nerve supply, including free nerve endings.[85] Movement of the nearby joint will cause pain or a noncapsular pattern of restriction of motion or both, due to compression of the inflamed tissue. In some joints, such as the shoulder, there may be a painful arc of movement as well.[86] In acute bursitis, the end feel to movement is often empty due to pain. For superficial bursae, there is local tenderness and edema over the site of the lesion.

Tendons **Tendinopathy** occurs due to exposure to high volume or high loads to a tendon, particularly combined loading of tension, compression, and friction.[87] As such, tendinopathy is often an overuse and degenerative condition. Patients may report a history of repetitive loading, such as running, jumping, or cycling. Clinically, resisted testing of the muscle-tendon unit may be strong but painful. At times, additional stress, such as body weight exercise or repeated contractions, may be required to elicit symptoms. There is seldom a loss of motion, but there may be pain at the extremes of the passive movements that stretch the tendon. There may be palpable tenderness at the site of the lesion or hyperalgesia in the related segment.

Tenosynovitis is an inflammation of the synovial lining of a sheath resulting from friction of a roughened tendon gliding within the sheath. In addition to pain on resisted testing, there is often pain on activity that produces movement of the tendon within the sheath. Thus, active contraction of the musculotendinous structure and passive lengthening may be painful. The classic example occurs with rheumatoid arthritis. There may be palpable and visible swelling of the tendon sheath.

In the case of a partial tendon tear, actual loss of continuity of tendon tissue will result in painful resisted testing and may be strong or weak depending on the percentage of fibers involved. The passive movement that stretches the tendon may be painful. Resisted testing will be weak and painless with a complete tear. With superficial tendons, such as the Achilles, there may be a palpable gap at the site of the rupture.

Muscle Muscle strains are less commonly seen in an outpatient clinic because muscles have an excellent blood supply and tend to heal more rapidly than tendons. When muscle strains do occur, they are generally the result of trauma or delayed-onset muscle soreness. For a minor strain, resisted testing of the involved muscle will be strong and painful. There may be pain on full passive stretch of the muscle and palpable tenderness. In the rare case of a rupture within the muscle belly, the associated resisted test results will be weak and painless and a gap may be palpable, or occasionally visible, at the site of the defect.

Nerves Nerve injuries generally occur at three levels: spinal nerve root, plexus, or peripheral nerve. Nerves can be injured by compression, traction, laceration, and systemic disease processes.[88] Most **radiculopathies** are the caused by nerve root compression. Compression may be the result of disc pathology, ligament hypertrophy, or osteophytes.[89] **Plexopathies**, such as Erb palsy, are the result of a traction injury, whereas thoracic outlet may be the result of compression or traction. Peripheral nerve injuries are commonly caused by compression. These types of nerve injuries are also known as **entrapment neuropathies**,[88] because the nerve undergoes static or dynamic compression as it passes through a narrow path. Carpal tunnel syndrome and tarsal tunnel syndrome are examples of entrapment neuropathies. Nerve lacerations can occur from trauma, such as knife wounds or during surgery. Systemic diseases, such as diabetes, can lead to motor, sensory, and autonomic neuropathy.

The subjective complaints associated with common entrapment disorders can generally be classified as paresthesia (pins and needles), dysesthesia (altered sensation in response to some external stimulus), and pain. Although some patients may describe paresthesia and dysesthesia as painful, pain is usually not a primary complaint when there is pressure on a nerve farther out in the periphery rather than at the nerve root level. With increased or prolonged peripheral nerve compression, muscles innervated distal to the site of compression will be weak. In the case of carpal tunnel syndrome, the patient will experience paresthesias in the median nerve distribution of the hand (radial side of the palmar and the palmar aspect of the first three digits along with the radial half of the 4th digit), thenar eminence atrophy, as well as weakness of the abductor pollicis brevis, opponens pollicis, lumbricals I and II, and the flexor pollicis brevis.

In contrast to peripheral nerve injuries, pain is a common complaint when there is pressure on a nerve root. There is no gold standard for diagnosing radiculopathy.[89] Magnetic resonance imaging may show anatomic areas of nerve compression but should not stand alone as a means of diagnosing radiculopathy.[90] Electromyography and nerve conduction studies may detect nerve abnormalities. However, subtle nerve root involvement is more typical than blatant compression. When a nerve root is compressed, the patient may experience sensory changes in the involved **dermatome**, weakness in the involved myotome, and altered reflex in the involved segment. In isolation, none of these three clinical tests has excellent sensitivity and specificity. However, when considered in combination with the patient history and available imaging and diagnostic studies, the diagnostic accuracy is increased.[91] So, a patient reporting shooting pain into the right upper extremity with right cervical sidebending who also demonstrates decreased sensation of the thumb decreased strength of the biceps, and decreased brachioradialis reflex is likely to be experiencing compression of the C6 nerve root.

PROGNOSIS AND PLAN OF CARE

Following the diagnosis, the clinician determines the prognosis and establishes a plan of care. The patient's prognosis is the highest level of functional improvement that can be expected and the time frame for achieving that level. The prognosis must consider the patient's complexity, acuity, prior level of function, general health status, motivation, and support system. The plan of care includes goals, specific interventions that will be incorporated into treatment, and the frequency and duration of rehabilitation. Any precautions or contraindications should be clearly stated within the plan of care. Determining appropriate treatment goals assists the therapist in planning, prioritizing, and measuring the effectiveness of treatment. The goals are derived from the patient's symptom(s), signs, and diagnosis and from the patient's personal, occupational, and social goals. Rehabilitation goals should be mutually set and agreed upon to maximize patient adherence. Goals may address prevention, impairments, activity limitations, and participation restrictions.[92] Goals must be specific, measurable, attainable, relevant, and time-bound. If a patient is not making consistent and timely progress toward documented goals, the clinician must first consider the implementation of the plan, including intervention choices and patient follow-through. If the plan is being carried out appropriately, then the clinician must reassess the patient to determine whether the diagnosis was correct or if referral is warranted. Daily informal and regular formal reassessment should be performed throughout the plan of care. The plan of care must include discharge plans, such as continuation with an independent home program or transition to a personal trainer.

INTEGRATED APPROACH TO TREATMENT

An integrated approach to rehabilitation optimizes a return to function (Fig. 7-9).

Rehabilitation of acute injuries should focus on progressive stresses to healing tissues. Acute injuries in the inflammatory phase of healing may benefit from a combination of symptom modulation and controlled stress to healing tissues. Symptom modulation may include the use of ice, biophysical agents, and anti-inflammatory medications. Controlled rest, such as modifying painful activities and the use of splinting or assistive devices, can help modify stress to injured tissues. Early motion exercises, including isometric contractions and passive, active-assisted, and AROM exercises, have several positive effects on healing tissues, including:

- Decrease pain by increasing large fiber input
- Decrease edema
- Increase circulation
- Improve joint nutrition
- Promote fiber orientation and organization
- Increase or restore motion
- Prevent contractures and adhesions

Complete immobilization worsens tissue atrophy, amplifies strength loss, and increases the likelihood of DJD. By avoiding immobilization except when medically necessary, the risk of integumentary injury from pressure is decreased and the needless restriction of

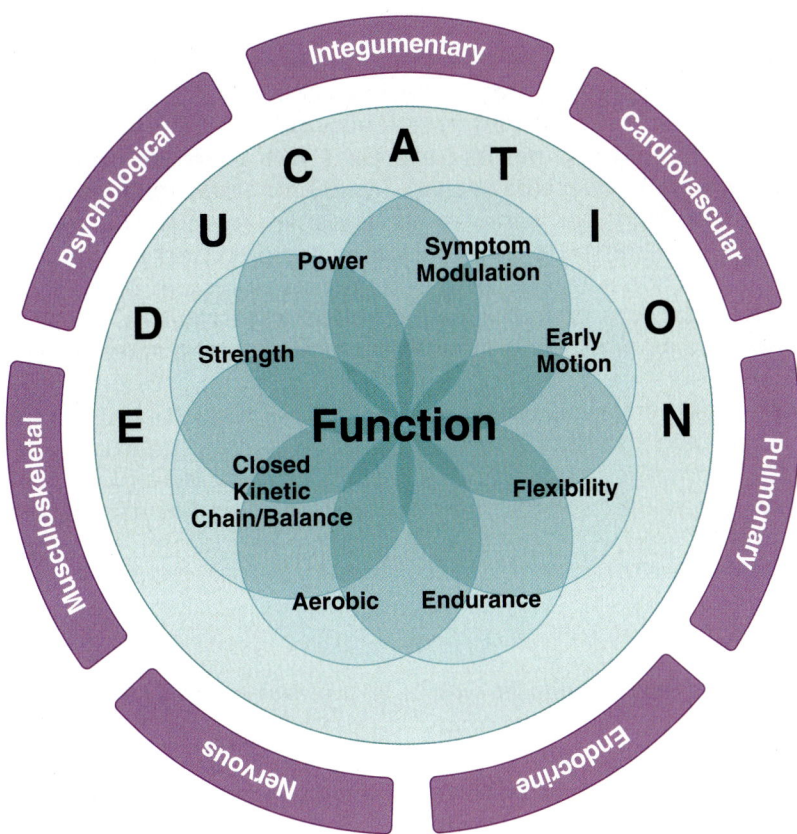

FIGURE 7-9 Integrated approach to rehabilitation.

patient function is also avoided. As healing continues, endurance exercise provides the following:

- Increase recruitment of type 1 muscle fibers
- Improve exchange of oxygen, nutrients, and local waste products
- Increase the number of local capillaries
- Control stress to healing connective tissue
- Improve motor patterns

Aerobic exercise challenges the patient's cardiovascular and pulmonary system while also having positive impacts on the endocrine system. A skilled and intentional progression to strengthening exercises and, when necessary, power and plyometrics further challenges tissues to respond to these controlled increases in demand. Functional activities, or component parts, should be integrated within the rehabilitation plan. Early integration of functional components improves patient adherence and assists with a patient's psychological well-being.

Using an integrated approach to rehabilitation, these steps as not distinct, sequential, or isolated; but rather they are overlapping. See Case Study 7-1 as an example.

CASE STUDY 7-1

Randy: Patient with Lateral Ankle Sprain

Consider the early phases of rehabilitation for Randy, a 17-year-old basketball player, who sustained a left grade 2 lateral ankle sprain yesterday and cannot walk without a limp. Randy's initial home program should include multiple types of protection and exercise simultaneously. Randy may benefit from ice, an ankle brace, and crutches to allow a normal gait pattern partial weight bearing on his left leg. Early motion exercise might consist of active and active-assisted ankle dorsiflexion to assist with edema control and minimize loss of range in this plane that is critical to normal gait. Isometric ankle eversion, inversion, dorsiflexion, and plantarflexion might help with muscle recruitment and pain modulation. Strengthening exercise can be performed on Randy's left hip and knee in the open kinetic chain, whereas his right lower extremity may perform a combination of open- and closed-chain exercise. Randy may perform aerobic exercise on a stationary bike if able or on an upper body ergometer if a bike is painful. Strengthening and aerobic exercises will assist with minimizing deconditioning, while his left ankle is in the acute phase of healing. Randy may participate in basketball "chalk talks," and providing feedback to teammates during drills helps him maintain his identity as an athlete and improve his psychological well-being. He can work on pain-modulated weight shifting and progress to static and then dynamic balance activities. The clinician may perform posterior talar mobilizations[93] and soft-tissue mobilization to the posterior calf.[94] Stretching exercises, particularly of the gastrocnemius, can be incorporated as symptoms allow. Restoration of gastrocnemius muscle length, as well as balance exercises, can decrease the risk of a repeat ankle sprain.[95] Once Randy is able to walk normally on level surfaces, static and walking dribbling drills can be initiated. As he is able to progress to a lunge with little or no pain and good form, then he can participate in passing drills with his team. As Randy improves, a plyometric progression will be started followed by sport-specific rehabilitation. During this phase, Randy may still require continuation of earlier activities, such as balance and stretching, if deficits persist.

The rehabilitation approach for individuals with chronic or degenerative disorders may incorporate additional treatment methods, including activity modification and adaptive equipment. The management of DJD at specific joints is discussed in detail within the appropriate chapters. Rehabilitation of individuals with chronic pain must consider not only pathokinesiologic approach but also a neurophysiologic viewpoint.[96] Progressive exercise can still assist with improving function.[97] However, optimal outcomes are achieved by taking a multidisciplinary approach. Chapter 19, Pain Management, provides additional information on the management of patients with acute and chronic pain.

CHAPTER SUMMARY

The purpose of the physical examination moves beyond just attempting to identify a target tissue. The physical examination also helps identify the presence of red flags, the stage of healing, secondarily involved structures, contributing factors, factors that modulate treatment, and referrals needed. Examination findings also serve as a baseline to compare changes over time. The physical examination begins broadly with the systems review before becoming progressively more focused with the quarter screen, clearing examination, and, finally, the joint-specific examination. Clinicians must integrate information from multiple sources to make clinical decisions regarding diagnosis, prognosis, needed referrals, and the plan of care.

REFERENCES

1. Jones MJ, Rivett DA. *Clinical Reasoning in Musculoskeletal Practice*. Elsevier; 2019.
2. Bikley LS. *Bates' Guide to Physical Examination and History Taking.* 13th ed. Wolters Kluwer; 2021.
3. Hawkins A, Sum J, Kirages D, Sigman E, Sahai-Srivastava S. Pelvic osteomyelitis presenting as groin and medial thigh pain: a resident's case problem. *J Orthop Sports Phys Ther.* 2015;45(4):306–315.
4. Cyriax J, Coldham M. *Textbook of Orthopaedic Medicine: Vol 2. Treatment by Manipulation Massage and Injection.* 11th ed. Bailliere; 1987.
5. Goom TSH, Malliaras P, Reiman MP, Purdam CR. Proximal hamstring tendinopathy: clinical aspects of assessment and management. *J Orthop Sports Phys Ther.* 2016;46(6):483–493.
6. Robinson KA. Tendinopathy and application to hamstring strain injuries. *Orthop Phys Ther Pract.* 2013;25(4):207–214.
7. Willy R, Hoglund L, Barton C, et al. Patellofemoral pain: clinical practice guidelines linked to the international classification of functioning, disability and health from the academy of orthopaedic physical therapy of the American Physical Therapy Association. *J Orthop Sports Phys Ther.* 2019;49(9):CPG1–CPG95.
8. George SZ, Bishop MD. Chronic musculoskeletal pain is a nervous system disorder… Now what? *Phys Ther.* 2018;98(4):209–213.
9. American Physical Therapy Association. *Guide to Physical Therapist Practice 3.0.* 2014. Accessed May 23, 2018. http://guidetoptpractice.apta.org/
10. Davenport T, Kulig K, Sebelski C, Gordon J, Watts H. *Diagnosis for Physical Therapists: A Symptom-Based Approach.* F.A. Davis; 2013.
11. Logerstedt DS, Scalzitti D, Risberg MA, et al. Knee stability and movement coordination impairments: knee ligament sprain revision 2017. *J Orthop Sports Phys Ther.* 2017;47(11):A1–A47.
12. Arundale AJH, Bizzini M, Giordano A, et al. Exercise-based knee and anterior cruciate ligament injury prevention: clinical practice guidelines linked to the International Classification of Functioning, Disability and Health from the Academy of Orthopaedic Physical Therapy and the American Academy of Sports Physical Therapy. *J Orthop Sports Phys Ther.* 2018;48(9):A1–A42.
13. Cyriax J. *Textbook of Orthopedic Medicine: Vol 1. Diagnosis of Soft Tissue Lesions.* 8th ed. W.B. Saunders; 1989.
14. Cyriax JH, Cyriax PJ. *Cyriax's Illustrated Manual of Orthopaedic Medicine.* 2nd ed. Butterworth-Heinemann; 1993.

15. Kaltenborn F. Orthopedic manual therapy for physical therapists Nordic system: OMT Kaltenborn-Evjenth concept. *J Man Manip Ther*. 1993;1(2):47–51.
16. Hengeveld E, Banks K. *Maitland's Vertebral Manipulation*. Vol 1. 8th ed. Churchill Livingstone/Elsevier; 2014.
17. McKenzie R, May S. *The Lumbar Spine: Mechanical Diagnosis and Therapy*. Vol 1. Spinal Publications; 2013.
18. McKenzie R, May S. *The Human Extremities: Mechanical Diagnosis and Therapy*. Spinal Publications; 2017.
19. Sahrmann S. The how and why of the movement system as the identity of physical therapy. *Int J Sports Phys Ther*. 2017;12(6):862–869.
20. Yee J. A case study on differential diagnosis of low back and flank pain in an adult with developmental delay. *Pediatr Phys Ther*. 2004;16(1):67–68.
21. Smyth A, Garovic VD. 25-year-old man with flank pain, hematuria, and proteinuria. *Mayo Clin Proc*. 2009;84(1):72–75.
22. Lovatt P. A case of acute-onset back pain. *Independent Nurse*. 2009:17–17.
23. O'Laughlen MC. Peak technique. Making sense of abdominal assessment. *Nurs Made Incred Easy*. 2009;7(5):15–19.
24. Goodman CC, Heick J, Lazaro R. *Differential Diagnosis for Physical Therapists: Screening for Referral*. 6th ed. Elsevier Science; 2018.
25. Mechelli F, Preboski Z, Boissonault W. Differential diagnosis of a patient referred to physical therapy with low back pain: abdominal aortic aneurysm. *J Orthop Sports Phys Ther*. 2008;38(9):551–557.
26. Blanpied P, Gross A, Elliott J, et al. Neck pain: revision 2017. *J Orthop Sports Phys Ther*. 2017;47(1):A1–A83.
27. Stiell IG, Wells GA, Vandemheen KL, et al. The Canadian C-spine rule for radiography in alert and stable trauma patients. *JAMA*. 2001;286(15):1841–1848.
28. Urch EY, Lee SK. Carpal fractures other than scaphoid. *Clin Sports Med*. 2015;34(1):51–67.
29. Tsyrulnik A. Emergency department evaluation and treatment of wrist injuries. *Emerg Med Clin North Am*. 2015;33(2):283–296.
30. Burrows B, Moreira P, Murphy C, Sadi J, Walton DM. Scaphoid fractures: a higher order analysis of clinical tests and application of clinical reasoning strategies. *Man Ther*. 2014;19(5):372–378.
31. Ochen Y, Peek J, van der Velde D, et al. Operative vs nonoperative treatment of distal radius fractures in adults: a systematic review and meta-analysis. *JAMA Netw Open*. 2020;3(4):e203497–e203497.
32. Cyriax J. *Textbook of Orthopaedic Medicine*. Vol 1. *Diagnosis of Soft Tissue Lesions*. 8th ed. Bailliere Tindall; 1982.
33. Delitto A, George SZ, van Dillen L, et al. Low back pain. *J Orthop Sports Phys Ther*. 2012;42(4):A1–A57.
34. Lam OT, Strenger DM, Chan-Fee M, Pham PT, Preuss RA, Robbins SM. Effectiveness of the McKenzie method of mechanical diagnosis and therapy for treating low back pain: literature review with meta-analysis. *J Orthop Sports Phys Ther*. 2018;48(6):476–490.
35. Hing W, Hall T, Rivett D, Vicenzino B, Mulligan B. *The Mulligan Concept of Manual Therapy: Textbook of Techniques*. Churchill Livingston Elsevier; 2015.
36. Bookhout M. Examination and treatment of muscle imbalance. In: Bourdilon J, Day E, Boohout B, eds. *Spinal Manipulation*. 5th ed. Butterworth-Heinemann; 1992:313–333.
37. Wänman A, Marklund S. Treatment outcome of supervised exercise, home exercise and bite splint therapy, respectively, in patients with symptomatic disc displacement with reduction: a randomised clinical trial. *J Oral Rehabil*. 2020;47(2):143–149.
38. Singh H, McKay M, Baldwin J, et al. Beighton scores and cut-offs across the lifespan: cross-sectional study of an Australian population. *Rheumatology*. 2017;56(11):1857–1864.
39. Hayes KW, Petersen C, Falconer J. An examination of Cyriax's passive motion tests with patients having osteoarthritis of the knee. *Phys Ther*. 1994;74(8):697–708.
40. Cibulka M, Bloom M, Enseki KR, Macdonald C, Woehrle J, McDonough C. Hip pain and mobility deficits—hip osteoarthritis: revision 2017. *J Orthop Sports Phys Ther*. 2017;47(6):A1–A37.
41. Chaya G, Garima A. *An Examination of Cyriax's Passive Motion Tests as a Diagnostic Tool in Patients Having Osteoarthritis of the Knee Joint*. Vol 6. Institute of Medico-legal Publications Pvt Ltd; 2012:32–35.
42. Klässbo M, Harms-Ringdahl K. Examination of passive ROM and capsular patterns in the hip. *Physiother Res Int*. 2003;8(1):1–12.
43. Hayes KW, Petersen CM. Reliability of classifications derived from Cyriax's resisted testing in subjects with painful shoulders and knees. *J Orthop Sports Phys Ther*. 2003;33(5):235–246.
44. Mitsch J, Casey J, McKinnis R, Kegerreis S, Stikeleather J. Investigation of a consistent pattern of motion restriction in patients with adhesive capsulitis. *J Man Manip Ther*. 2004;12(3):153–159.
45. Kelley M, Shaffer M, Kuhn J, et al. Shoulder pain and mobility deficits: adhesive capsulitis. *J Orthop Sports Phys Ther*. 43(5):A1–A31.
46. Wilk KE, Andrews JR, Clancy WG. Nonoperative and postoperative rehabilitation of the collateral ligaments of the knee. *Oper Tech Sports Med*. 1996;4(3):192–201.
47. Bourdilon J, Bookhout M, Day E. *Spinal Manipulation*. 5th ed. Butterworth-Heinemann; 1992.
48. Maitland G. *Vertebral Manipulation*. 5th ed. Butterworth-Heinemann; 1986.
49. Hayes KW, Petersen CM. Reliability of assessing end-feel and pain and resistance sequence in subjects with painful shoulders and knees. *J Orthop Sports Phys Ther*. 2001;31(8):432–445.
50. Kendall FP, McCreary EK, Provance PG, Rogers MM, Romani WA. *Muscles: Testing and Function with Posture and Pain*. 5th ed. Lippincott Williams & Wilkins; 2005.
51. Tawa N, Rhoda A, Diener I. Accuracy of clinical neurological examination in diagnosing lumbo-sacral radiculopathy: a systematic literature review. *BMC Musculoskelet Disord*. 2017;18:1–11.
52. Zasler ND. Validity assessment and the neurological physical examination. *NeuroRehabilitation*. 2015;36(4):401–413.
53. Zimny N, Kirk C. A comparison of methods of manual muscle testing... Kendall method and the Daniels and Worthingham method. *Clin Manag Phys Ther*. 1987;7(2):6–11.
54. Palmer ML. Gross muscle testing: a review. *Clin Manag Phys Ther*. 1985;5(4):18–21.
55. Sahrmann S. *Diagnosis and Treatment of Movement Impairment Syndromes*. Mosby; 2002.
56. Davenport D, Colaco H, Kavarthapu V. Examination of the adult spine. *Br J Hosp Med*. 2015;76(12):C182–C195.
57. Walker H. Deep tendon reflexes. In: Walker H, Hall W, Hurst J, eds. *Clinical Methods: The History, Physical, and Laboratory Examinations*. 3rd ed. Butterworth; 1990.
58. Ertuglu LA, Karacan I, Yilmaz G, Türker KS. Standardization of the Jendrassik maneuver in Achilles tendon tap reflex. *Clin Neurophysiol Pract*. 2017;3:1–5.
59. Zimmerman B, Hubbard J. *Clonus*. StatPearls Publishing; Published 2020. Updated August 13, 2020. Accessed September 16, 2020. https://www.ncbi.nlm.nih.gov/books/NBK534862/

60. Acharya A, Jamil R, Dewey J. *Babinski Reflex*. StatPearls Publishing; Published 2020. Updated January 2020. Accessed September 16, 2020. https://www.ncbi.nlm.nih.gov/books/NBK519009/
61. Grijalva R, Hsu F, Wycliffe N, et al. Hoffman sign: clinical correlation of neurological imaging findings in the cervical spine and brain. *Spine (Phila Pa 1976)*. 2015;40(7):475–479.
62. Staes FF, Banks KJ, De Smet L, Daniels KJ, Carels P. Reliability of accessory motion testing at the carpal joints. *Man Ther*. 2009;14(3):292–298.
63. Alqarni AM, Schneiders AG, Hendrick PA. Clinical tests to diagnose lumbar segmental instability: a systematic review. *J Orthop Sports Phys Ther*. 2011;41(3):130–140.
64. Fritz JM, Piva SR, Childs JD. Accuracy of the clinical examination to predict radiographic instability of the lumbar spine. *Eur Spine J*. 2005;14(8):743–750.
65. Mangus BC, Hoffman LA, Hoffman MA, Altenburger P. Basic principles of extremity joint mobilization using a Kaltenborn approach. *J Sport Rehabil*. 2002;11(4):235–250.
66. Riddle DL. Measurement of accessory motion: critical issues and related concepts. *Phys Ther*. 1992;72(12):865–874.
67. Dawson C, Mudgal CS. Staged description of the Finkelstein test. *J Hand Surg*. 2010;35(9):1513–1515.
68. Sanzarello I, Merlini L, Rosa M, et al. Central sensitization in chronic low back pain: a narrative review. *J Back Musculoskelet Rehabil*. 2016;29:625–633.
69. Plinsinga ML, Brink MS, Vicenzino B, Van Wilgen CP. Evidence of nervous system sensitization in commonly presenting and persistent painful tendinopathies: a systematic review. *J Orthop Sports Phys Ther*. 2015;45(11):864–875.
70. Konarzewska A, Korzon-Burakowska A, Rzepecka-Wejs L, Sudol-Szopinska I, Szurowska E, Studniarek M. Diabetic foot syndrome: Charcot arthropathy or osteomyelitis? Part I: clinical picture and radiography. *J Ultrason*. 2018;18(72):42–49.
71. Berman A, Snyder S. *Skills in Clinical Nursing*. 8th ed. Pearson; 2016.
72. Federman DG, Ladiiznski B, Dardik A, et al. Wound Healing Society 2014 update on guidelines for arterial ulcers. *Wound Repair Regen*. 2016;24(1):127–135.
73. Bourgaize S, Newton G, Kumbhare D, Srbely J. A comparison of the clinical manifestation and pathophysiology of myofascial pain syndrome and fibromyalgia: implications for differential diagnosis and management. *J Can Chiropr Assoc*. 2018;62(1):26–41.
74. Simons DG, Travell JG, Simons LS. *Travell & Simons' Myofascial Pain and Dysfunction: The Trigger Points Manual. Vol 1. Upper Half of Body*, 2nd ed. Williams &Wilkins; 1999.
75. Garras DN, Raikin SM, Bhat SB, Taweel N, Karanjia H. MRI is unnecessary for diagnosing acute Achilles tendon ruptures: clinical diagnostic criteria. *Clin Orthop Relat Res*. 2012;470(8):2268–2273.
76. Deng S, Sun Z, Zhang C, Chen G, Li J. Surgical treatment versus conservative management for acute Achilles tendon rupture: a systematic review and meta-analysis of randomized controlled trials. *J Foot Ankle Surg*. 2017;56(6):1236–1243.
77. Prather H, Cheng A, Steger-May K, Maheshwari V, Van Dillen L. Hip and lumbar spine physical examination findings in people presenting with low back pain, with or without lower extremity pain. *J Orthop Sports Phys Ther*. 2017;47(3):163–172.
78. Ludewig PM, Kamonseki DH, Staker JL, Lawrence RL, Camargo PR, Braman JP. Changing our diagnostic paradigm: movement system diagnostic classification. *Int J Sports Phys Ther*. 2017;12(6):884–893.
79. Alrwaily M, Timko M, Schneiider M, et al. Treatment-based classification system for low back pain: revision and update. *Phys Ther*. 2016;96(7):1057–1066.
80. American Physical Therapy Association. *Physical Therapy Documentation of Patient and Client Management*. Published 2018. Updated January 31, 2018. Accessed September 7, 2020. https://www.apta.org/your-practice/documentation
81. McClure P, Michener L. Staged approach for rehabilitation classification: shoulder disorders (STAR-Shoulder). *Phys Ther*. 2015;95(5):791–800.
82. Martin RL, Chimenti R, Cuddeford T, et al. Achilles pain, stiffness, and muscle power deficits: Midportion Achilles tendinopathy revision 2018: using the evidence to guide physical therapist practice. *J Orthop Sports Phys Ther*. 2018;48(5):425–426.
83. Malliaras P, Cook J, Purdam C, Rio E. Patellar tendinopathy: clinical diagnosis, load management, and advice for challenging case presentations. *J Orthop Sports Phys Ther*. 2015;45(11):887–898.
84. McKinnis L. *Fundamentals of Musculoskeletal Imaging: Contemporary Perspectives in Rehabilitation*. 4th ed. F.A. Davis; 2014.
85. Ide K, Shirai Y, Ito H, Ito H. Sensory nerve supply in the human subacromial bursa. *J Shoulder Elbow Surg*. 1996;5(5):371–382.
86. Kuo Y-C, Hsieh L-F. Validity of Cyriax's functional examination for diagnosing shoulder pain: a diagnostic accuracy study. *J Manipulative Physiol Ther*. 2019;42(6):407–415.
87. Scott A, Backman L, Speed C. Tendinopathy: update on pathophysiology. *J Orthop Sports Phys Ther*. 2015;45(11):833–841.
88. Wahab KW, Sanya EO, Adebayo PB, Babalola MO, Ibraheem HG. Carpal tunnel syndrome and other entrapment neuropathies. *Oman Med J*. 2017;32(6):449–454.
89. Barr K. Electrodiagnosis of lumbar radiculopathy. *Phys Med Rehabil Clin N Am*. 2013;24(1):79–91.
90. Tawa N, Rhoda A, Diener I. Accuracy of magnetic resonance imaging in detecting lumbo-sacral nerve root compromise: a systematic literature review. *BMC Musculoskelet Disord*. 2016;17.
91. Al Nezari NH, Schneiders AG, Hendrick PA. Neurological examination of the peripheral nervous system to diagnose lumbar spinal disc herniation with suspected radiculopathy: a systematic review and meta-analysis. *Spine J*. 2013;13(6):657–674.
92. American Physical Therapy Association. *Documentation: Initial Examination and Evaluation*. Published 2018. Updated January 31, 2018. Accessed September 14, 2020. https://www.apta.org/your-practice/documentation/defensible-documentation/elements-within-the-patientclient-management-model/initial-examination
93. Weerasekara I, Osmotherly P, Snodgrass S, Marquez J, de Zoete R, Rivett DA. Clinical benefits of joint mobilization on ankle sprains: a systematic review and meta-analysis. *Arch Phys Med Rehabil*. 2018;99(7):1395–1412.E5.
94. Truyols-Dominguez S, Salom-Moreno J, Abian-Vicen J, Cleland J, Fernandex-de-las-penas C. Efficacy of thrust and nonthrust manipulation exercise with or without the addition of myofascial therapy for the management of acute inversion ankle sprain: a randomized clinical trial. *J Orthop Sports Phys Ther*. 2013;43(5):300–309.
95. Martin R, Davenport T, Paulseth S, Wukich DK, Godges J. Ankle stability and movement coordination impairments: ankle ligament sprains. *J Orthop Sports Phys Ther*. 2013;43:A1–A73.
96. Courtney CA, Fernández-de-las-Peñas C, Bond S. Mechanisms of chronic pain—key considerations for appropriate physical therapy management. *J Man Manip Ther*. 2017;25(3):118–127.
97. Ambrose KR, Golightly YM. Physical exercise as non-pharmacological treatment of chronic pain: why and when. *Best Pract Res Clin Rheumatol*. 2015;29(1):120–130.

PART III

Lower Quarter

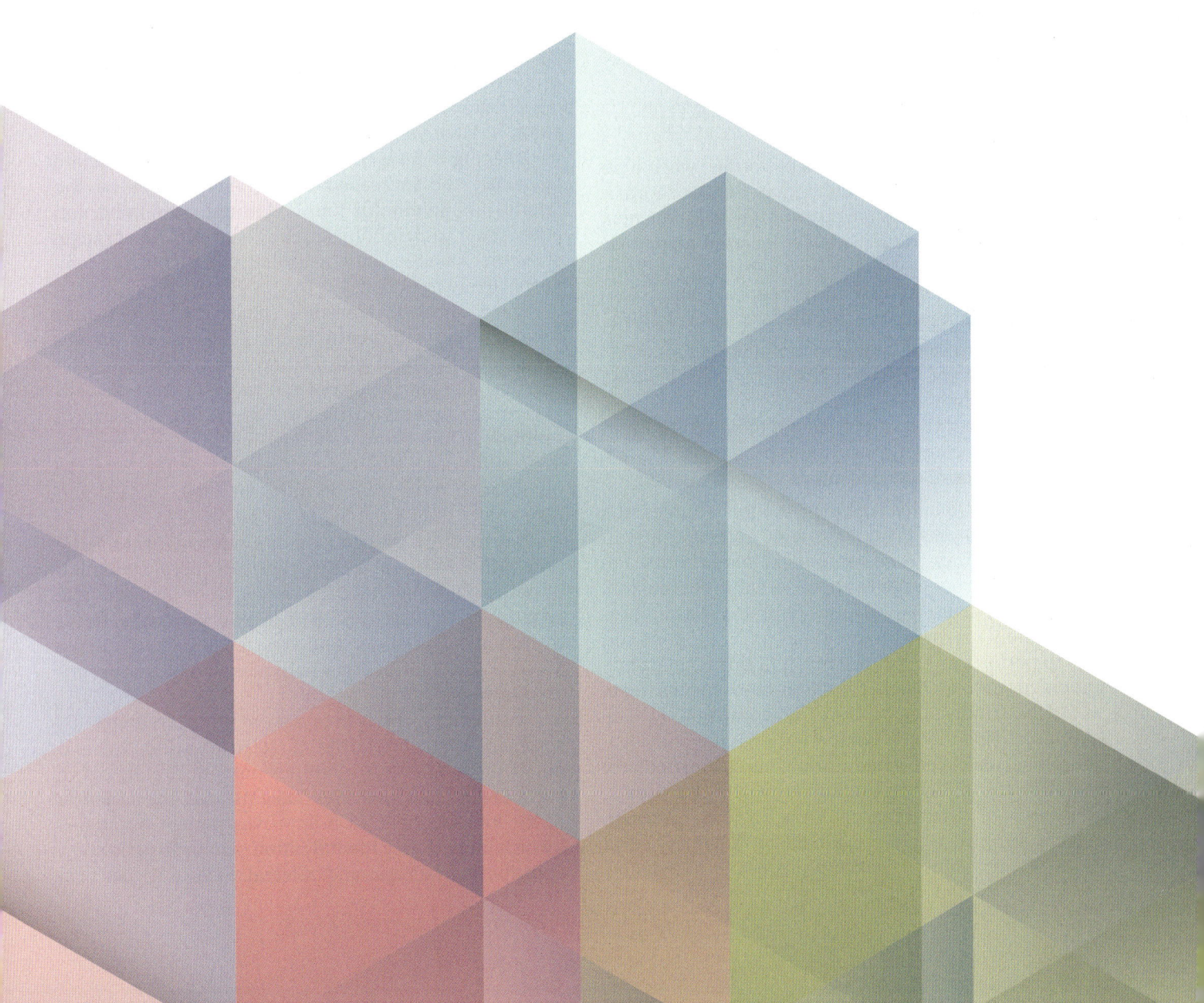

8 | Lower Quarter Screen

Betsy Myers

CHAPTER OBJECTIVES
After reading this chapter, you will be able to:
1. Describe the elements of a lower quarter screen.
2. Describe reasons for performing a lower quarter screen.
3. Identify key anatomic landmarks to screen structural alignment of the lower extremity in weight-bearing and non–weight-bearing positions.
4. Describe the components of a lower quarter neurologic screen.
5. Adapt the lower quarter screen based on patient presentation.

PURPOSE OF THE LOWER QUARTER SCREEN

The lower quarter screen (LQS) is performed when a patient has symptoms in the lower body or lumbar/thoracic region. The LQS includes observation; gross assessment of structure and posture; a lower quarter neurologic screen (LQNS); assessment of lower extremity motion, muscle length, and strength; and functional testing.

The four main purposes for the LQS are as follows:

- Rule out sources of patient symptoms
- Identify relevant deviation and impairments within the kinetic chain
- Identify issues that might alter rehabilitation interventions, precautions, or patient prognosis
- Expedite referral and consultation when needed

First, the LQS helps rule out potential sources of a patient's symptoms. The neurologic screen can help identify pathology related to lumbar nerve roots. Radicular pain[1] from a nerve root, dorsal root ganglion, and dura can cause lateral foot symptoms. If a clinician immediately narrows the examination to the foot and fails to perform an LQNS, the result of this local examination of joint mobility, palpation, and special tests would be fruitless or, at best, noncontributory. The LQS also helps identify competing regional and local neuromuscular pain generators. This is particularly useful in the following situations: vague symptoms, large area of symptoms, multiple regions involved, muscle atrophy, unclear mechanism of injury, or in cases of unexplained weakness or deficits in balance, coordination, and/or gait. Cutaneous pain is quite local; however, pain from somatic structures (e.g., ligaments, joint capsules) tends to be referred to a greater area. When deeper structures are injured, it is harder to localize the pain.

Second, the LQS helps identify relevant deviations and impairments within the kinetic chain. For example, knee pain and effusion may lead to inhibition of not just the quadriceps[2,3] but also the hip.[4] The LQS helps identify these secondarily involved structures. The LQS can identify kinetic chain factors that might be contributing to the patient's chief complaint. This is of particular importance because the lower extremity functions as part of a closed kinetic chain much of the time. For example, a patient with reduced ankle dorsiflexion range of motion may be forced into a position of knee valgus during a jump or cutting maneuver, placing increased strain on the anterior cruciate ligament[5] and increased compressive forces on the lateral patellofemoral joint.[6] Without examining and addressing contributing kinetic chain deficits of range, strength, balance, and neuromuscular control, reinjury is likely to occur.[7,8]

Third, the LQS identifies issues that might alter rehabilitation interventions, precautions, or patient prognosis. A patient with a complaint of knee pain who also has significant loss of hip range consistent with severe hip osteoarthritis may be unable to perform exercise in the prone position. Similarly, the highest level of function that the patient may be predicted to obtain with rehabilitation might be more limited and take longer than if the hip is not involved.

Fourth, the LQS can expedite referral or consultation with additional health care providers. Detection of pathologies, such as the presence of diabetic neuropathy in this same patient, would warrant referral to a medical provider and treatment precautions to avoid any weight-bearing activities without appropriate footwear.

In summary, the LQS is a more global, regional assessment that directs the clinician to a focused and detailed examination, identifies potential spinal nerve pathologies, and provides insights into the function of the kinetic chain. LQS improves patient outcomes by providing timely identification of source pathology, contributing factors, and referral. Failure to perform

LQS can lead to an overreliance on pattern recognition for clinical diagnosis and failure to recognize information that is potentially vital to the plan of care. After the LQS is completed, the examination can be targeted to thoroughly investigate the affected joint and area of involvement, including symptom provocation of the involved joint and a greater exploration and examination of any positive findings within the LQS. For example, if abnormal light touch sensation is noted, more precise investigations, such as monofilament, sharp/dull, temperature, and/or proprioception testing, may need to be pursued.

GENERAL RULES FOR LOWER QUARTER SCREENING

Before performing the LQS, the clinician must have performed a thorough history, including medical history, symptom investigation, and the review of systems. Thus, the clinician is able to make the determination that it is safe to proceed to the physical examination. Next, the clinician must determine the presence of additional red flags that must be investigated. If, for example, based on the history, the clinician suspects the patient might have an ankle fracture, then the next step would be to follow the Ottawa ankle rules (see Chapter 9, Ankle and Foot) in an attempt to determine whether imaging is warranted. If these tests are positive, then further investigation of the patient and kinetic chain are irrelevant, and the patient should be referred for radiographs. Lastly, the clinician must consider contraindications, such as inability to bear weight on the affected side after a particular type of surgery, that would modify the basic components of the LQS. For each LQS component, the patient should be asked to inform the clinician of new symptoms or changes in existing symptoms. The clinician is observing for abnormalities in structure, quantity or quality of motion, end feel, weakness, and discomfort. Although the LQS is a gross screen, it is wise to use traditional test positions for each procedure when possible, allowing for immediate measurement of an abnormality in motion or grade strength without having to repeat the assessment in an official test position.

The LQS is organized by patient position to maximize efficiency. The LQS assessment should proceed from the uninvolved side to the involved side, although some areas, such as great toe extension strength, may be best assessed simultaneously. It is best practice to begin with assessment of joints farther away from the suspected injury/painful area and work toward the affected region. The assessment would, therefore, begin at the hip for a patient with ankle/foot pain and at the ankle for a patient with hip pain. For patients presenting with knee pain, clinicians may choose to begin at the ankle rather than the hip, as the ankle region is smaller and less likely to refer pain to the knee. The LQS progresses from lower levels of tissue stress to higher, assessing active range of motion (AROM) before muscle performance and gait before navigation of stairs.

Not all components of the LQS are needed for every patient. In fact, the experienced clinician will remove portions of the LQS that are not believed to be paramount, given a particular patient's history and area of chief complaint. Consider an ambulatory teenage patient who twisted her ankle 2 days ago playing basketball. If the patient had an unremarkable past medical history and no reports of tingling or numbness, then an LQNS, including trunk range of motion and reflexes, would not be necessary.

COMPONENTS OF THE LOWER QUARTER SCREEN

Figure 8-1 contains the key components of the LQS. The sacroiliac joint is not included as part of this screen because it is significantly less probable as a source of lower extremity symptoms than the ankle, knee, hip, and low back.[9] Should the LQS be negative, the clinician should first examine the spine, followed by the sacroiliac joint, if necessary.

Observation

The LQS begins upon first observation of the patient and continues throughout the patient encounter. How

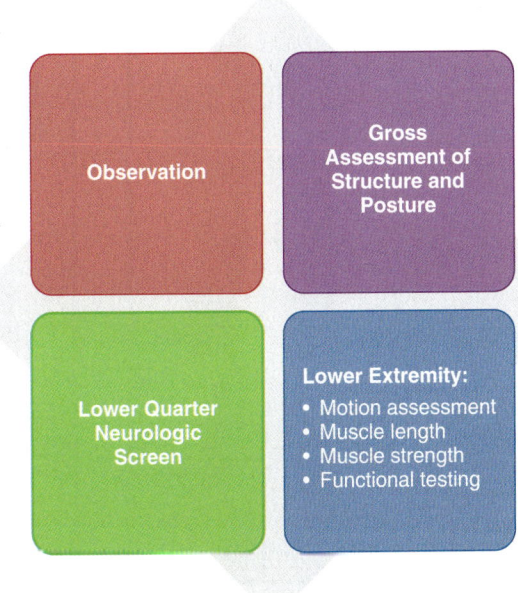

FIGURE 8-1 Components of the lower quarter screen.

is the patient sitting in the waiting room? How does the patient rise from the chair and move into the examination room? What is the patient's positioning during the history? For example, does the patient maintain her painful knee in a loose-packed position of slight flexion indicating possible effusion? Does the patient maintain eye contact during the interview?

Structure and Posture

The clinician should take a cursory view of the patient's overall structure and posture. To maximize exposure of the affected region, the patient should be wearing shorts and be barefoot. It might be useful to have the patient march in place a few steps before stopping in their typical standing posture. With the patient in the standing position (Fig. 8-2), the clinician should make a visual and palpatory examination of bony landmarks, symmetry, atrophy, edema, scars, and skin lesions. Following this big picture approach, the clinician should then proceed from either a top-down or bottom-up approach, observing the patient from posterior, anterior, and lateral views. Table 8-1 provides key standing alignments the clinician should observe along with a description of optimal alignment and possible deviations. From posterior and lateral views, the patient should appear symmetrical from left to right with the line of gravity running through the vertebrae and falling equally between the patient's feet. From a lateral view, an imaginary vertical line should pass through the external auditory meatus, the acromioclavicular joint, and bodies of the lumbar vertebrae, just posterior to the hip joint, slightly anterior to the knee joint and the lateral malleolus.[10] Table 8-2 includes key non–weight-bearing (NWB) structural alignments the clinician should observe.

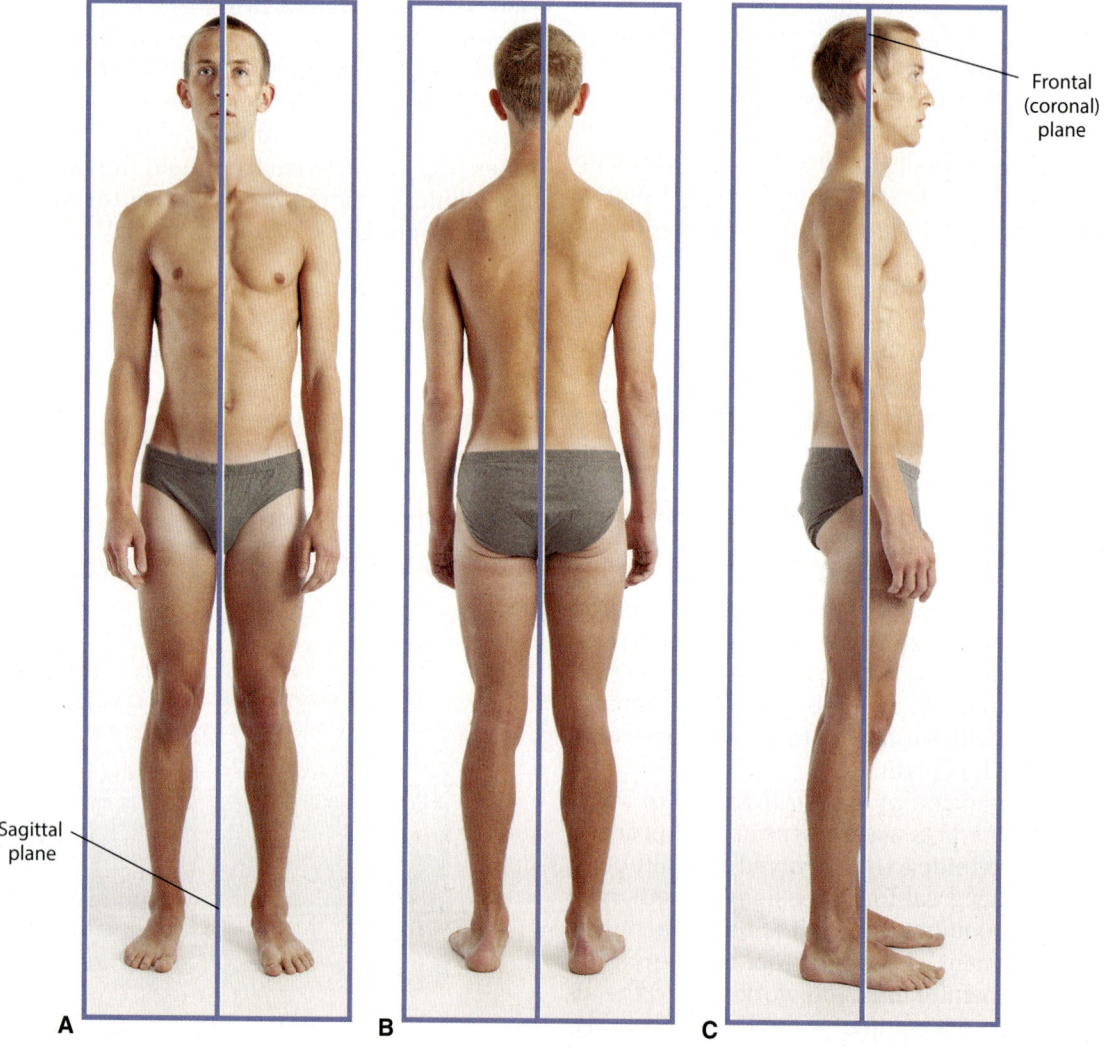

FIGURE 8-2 Assessment of standing alignment. **A.** Anterior view. **B.** Posterior view. **C.** Lateral view. (Allen L, Pounds DM. *Clay and Pounds' Basic Clinical Massage Therapy: Integrating Anatomy and Treatment.* 3rd ed. Wolters Kluwer; 2016: Figures 2.3 and 2.4.)

TABLE 8-1
EXAMINATION OF PATIENT STRUCTURE AND POSTURE IN STANDING

Landmark	Optimal or Typical Alignment
Posterior View	
Foot angle	Normal alignment would be ~5° of toe out. The 5th toe and half of the 4th toe should be visible from the posterior view.
Calcaneal alignment	In the relaxed calcaneal stance position, the calcaneus should be close to vertical.
Talar bulge	The talus should not be visible.
Popliteal crease height	Popliteal crease heights should be even.
Hamstring tendons	Medial and lateral hamstring tendons should be in the frontal plane.
Knee alignment	Knees should be neutral or in slightly varus alignment.
Iliac crest height	Iliac crest heights should be even.
Shoulders	Shoulder heights should be even.
Anterior View	
Toes	Toes should be in neutral position.
Nail beds	Nails should be intact.
Patellae	Patellae should be facing anteriorly.
ASIS height	ASIS height should be symmetrical.
Lateral View	
Medial longitudinal arch height	Observe arch height and compare with NWB arch height later in the screen.
Navicular tubercle	The navicular tubercle should not be clearly visible.
Knee alignment	The knee should be in neutral extension.
Pelvic angle and lumbar lordosis	The ASIS should be slightly lower than the PSIS, and the lumbar spine should have a small lordosis.

ASIS, anterior superior iliac spine; *NWB*, non-weight bearing; *PSIS*, posterior superior iliac spine.

TABLE 8-2
EXAMINATION OF PATIENT STRUCTURE AND POSTURE IN NON–WEIGHT BEARING

Landmark	Optimal or Typical Alignment
Seated	
Medial longitudinal arch height	Observe arch height and compare with weight-bearing posture.
Supine	
Tibial plateau and distal femur	With the patient hooklying supine, observe the patient from a lateral view. The tibial plateaus and distal femurs should appear symmetrical.
Patella position	The inferior pole of the patella should be located approximately at the tibiofemoral joint line.
Prone	
Tibial torsion	With the patient prone and knee flexed 90°, observe the angle between the medial and lateral malleolus and a line perpendicular to the femur (see Fig. 9-20 in Chapter 9, Ankle and Foot). Normal external tibial torsion is 20–30°. Assessment may also be performed in short sitting.
Femoral torsion	With the patient prone, knee flexed 90°, and greater trochanter positioned most laterally, the hip should be internally rotated 8–15° (see Fig. 11-15 in Chapter 11, Hip).

This big picture assessment should be used to begin to understand the patients' overall structure. However, the clinician should be wary of making firm conclusions based on this one-time, static observation. The absence of structural deviations also does not guarantee normal posture or function. Notably, the mere observation of a patient's posture can change patient positioning to his or her perceived ideal posture. A patient who is able to attain optimal alignment during observation may not be able to maintain this alignment for a functional length of time. Static alignment may not predict dynamic alignment.[11–13] For example, a patient may present statically from a posterior view with vertical calcanei and have no talar bulge but ambulate with excessive or prolonged pronation. Patterns of structural deviations, such as excessive out-toeing, lack of a medial longitudinal arch, and a more posterior medial hamstring tendon, indicate a pronated extremity. Deviations such as these may be relevant to the patient's chief complaint and warrant further investigation. However, these structural deviations, although present, may not be contributory to the patient's current (or future) pathology. The structural assessment is just a piece of the information that the clinician must put into context with the patient history and remainder of the physical examination. Further details on structural and postural assessments, as well as the implications of deviations from typical alignment, are covered in the appropriate joint-specific chapters.

Lower Quarter Neurologic Screen

An **LQNS** is required when the patient reports lower extremity neurologic symptoms (e.g., tingling, numbness, burning pain, shooting pain). Because the hip, pelvis, and spine are biomechanically linked, the LQNS is also required if symptoms are present (or pathology is suspected) in the hip, lumbar, or thoracic regions. The LQNS consists of four parts: trunk AROM, myotomes, dermatomes, and reflexes (Fig. 8-3). The LQNS is not an examination of the lumbar spine, but rather a quick screen. If positive, a detailed examination of the spine should follow (see Chapter 12, Lumbar and Sacroiliac Joint).

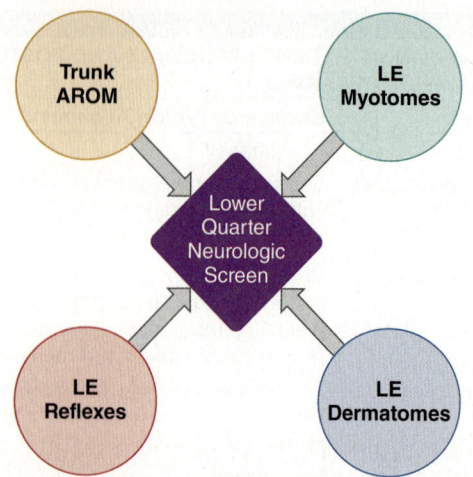

FIGURE 8-3 Components of the lower quarter neurologic screen. *LE*, lower extremity.

Trunk Screen To screen the trunk, the clinician should assess AROM for the following:

- Trunk flexion and extension
- Trunk lateral flexion or side glide
- Quadrant test

Lumbar rotation need not be performed during a screening examination because the frontal plane orientation of lumbar facets allows only 1° to 3° of rotation. To maximally close lateral intervertebral foramen, the patient should perform a quadrant test: a combination of trunk extension with ipsilateral lateral flexion and rotation to each side. The patient's body weight creates sufficient overpressure to these trunk motions, but the clinician can provide manual overpressure at end range if desired.

Myotome Screen The purpose of a myotome screen is to identify neurologic involvement by testing the strength of specific muscles that are *primarily* innervated by one spinal nerve root. Table 8-3 provides a list of lower extremity myotomes. Clinicians need only perform one assessment per myotome. Strength can be assessed using traditional manual muscle testing or functional myotomal testing.[14] When performing myotomal assessment as part of the LQNS, it is wise for clinicians to use specific manual muscle test positions and grading because a detailed measure of strength will still be required to more precisely stress target tissues in the joints at, above, and below the suspected area of complaint. Functional myotomal testing for the lower extremity includes toe walking (S1, S2), heel walking (L4), and performing a squat (L3). Functional myotomal testing requires sufficient balance and ability to weight bear on bilateral lower extremities. As such, this method may prove sufficient only when assessing patients with back pain, when weight bearing is not limited or painful, or when the function of the kinetic chain is deemed unimportant. Refer to Chapter 12, Lumbar and Sacroiliac Joint, for additional details.

Dermatome Screen A **dermatome** screen is used to identify neurologic involvement by testing specific areas of cutaneous sensation that are innervated by one spinal nerve root. To perform a dermatomal assessment, the clinician should assess for the presence of light touch sensation using a wisp of cotton or light contact with a fingertip.[15] Testing should be performed directly on the patient's skin and may be performed simultaneously on both sides. The clinician should ask the patient, "Do these feel the same and normal?" Patient response options include normal, absent, hypoesthesia (reduced light touch sensation), or hyperesthesia (increased sensitivity to light touch). The clinician may touch specific landmarks or sweep across the general dermatomal region (Fig. 8-4).

Reflex Screen The clinician should assess the Achilles reflex (S1, S2) and the patellar tendon reflex (L3) (Table 8-4). Reflexes should be graded using a 0 to 4+ scale or described as normal, hyperreflexive, diminished, or absent. If clonus is noted (4+), the clinician should check the patient's plantar reflex (Babinski reflex). A positive Babinski sign is suggestive of an upper motor neuron lesion.

Lower Extremity Motion, Muscle Length, and Strength

The LQS includes the assessment range of motion and strength of all the major joints of the lower quarter (Table 8-5). These tests are designed to provide stress to the contractile and noncontractile tissues for the purposes of identifying a possible source of the patient's symptoms. These also provide an overall understanding of the patient's lower quarter motion, ability to move, and muscle performance. The patient should perform AROM of each joint for each direction of movement. As with the basic examination of a joint, the clinician should note the quantity and quality of movement as well as any change in symptoms. If the motion is pain free, the clinician

TABLE 8-3
LOWER EXTREMITY MYOTOMAL SCREEN

Spinal Nerve Root	Muscle
S1, S2	Gastrocnemius/soleus Fibularis Hamstrings
L5	Extensor hallucis longus
L4	Tibialis anterior
L3	Quadriceps
L1, L2	Iliopsoas

TABLE 8-4
LOWER EXTREMITY REFLEX SCREEN

Spinal Nerve Root	Tendon Reflex
S1, S2	Achilles
L3	Patellar tendon

CHAPTER 8 | LOWER QUARTER SCREEN   181

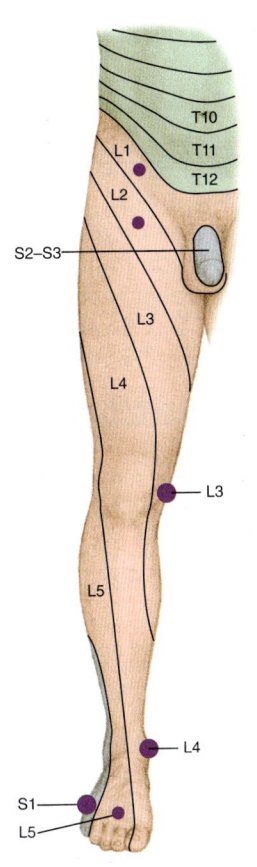
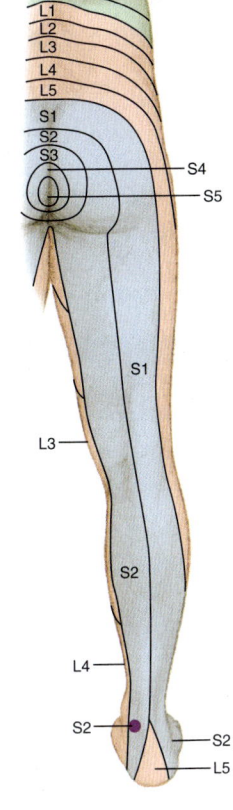

Spinal Nerve Root	Location
S2	Medial calcaneus
S1	Distal lateral fifth ray
L5	Dorsal 3rd metatarsophalangeal joint
L4	Medial malleolus or medial first ray
L3	Medial femoral condyle
L2	Anterior upper thigh
L1	Inguinal region

A. Anterior view   **B. Posterior view**

FIGURE 8-4 Lower extremity dermatomal screen. **A.** Anterior view. **B.** Posterior view. (Modified from Gest TR. *Lippincott Atlas of Anatomy*. 2nd ed. Wolters Kluwer; 2020: Plate 3-70.)

should add gentle overpressure to each motion. The clinician should assess passive range of motion of each joint for each direction, noting quantity, end feel, and any crepitus or changes in movement quality. Manual muscle testing should be performed for each motion. Finally, the clinician should assess muscle length of key multi-joint muscle of the lower extremity (Table 8-5).

TABLE 8-5	
LOWER QUARTER SCREEN FOR MOTION, MUSCLE LENGTH, AND STRENGTH	
Active and Passive Range and Strength	
Joint	Motions
Toes	Flexion, extension
Ankle	Dorsiflexion, plantarflexion Inversion, eversion
Knee	Flexion, extension
Hip	Flexion, extension Abduction, adduction Internal rotation, external rotation
Trunk	Flexor/extensor strength*
Muscle Length	
Gastrocnemius	
Hamstrings	
Hip flexors (iliopsoas, rectus femoris, iliotibial band)	

*Note trunk range of motion was assessed as part of the lower quarter neurologic screen.

Functional Testing

Functional testing during the LQS should begin with a detailed gait assessment with the patient barefoot. To assess the effect of footwear, gait may also need to be assessed with the shoes on. A basic assessment of static balance such as single-leg stance with eyes open, and possibly closed, should be performed. Functional testing in an LQS then may include observing the patient squatting, ascending and descending stairs, and performing a step up and a step down. While this concludes the basic functional testing for an LQS, higher level, more specific functional tasks, such as running, jumping, and hopping, may be required as part of a holistic evaluation on some patients.

Integument

Although technically a part of the systems review, assessment of the integument should be performed as part of the LQS. The integumentary screen includes observing the skin color, integrity, pliability, and for abnormalities such as scars, calluses, and fungal infections.

Vasculature

Although technically a part of the systems review, assessment of the vasculature, including palpation of the dorsalis pedis and posterior tibial arteries, should be performed as part of the LQS.

CASE STUDY 8-1
Hattie and Angelo: Patients With Right Hip and Right Ankle Pain

Hattie is a 64-year-old ambulatory patient who reports right hip pain with hiking and squatting. Angelo is an 18-year-old ambulatory patient who reports right ankle pain after rolling it playing basketball. Neither patient reported tingling or numbness and neither patient had any contraindications for examination based on the patient interview. All tests begin with the uninvolved (left) side first unless otherwise noted. As noted previously, the LQS should be organized by position, provide increasing tissue stress, and start away from and progress toward the area of chief complaint. Table 8-6 provides examples of how an experienced clinician might choose to organize the LQS for two different patients.

TABLE 8-6
SAMPLE LOWER QUARTER SCREENS

Hattie: 64-Year-Old Ambulatory Patient Who Reports Right Hip Pain With Hiking and Squatting		Angelo: 18-Year-Old Ambulatory Patient Who Reports Right Ankle Pain After Rolling It Playing Basketball	
Position	Assessments	Position	Assessments
Observation	Continues from History	Observation	Continues from History
Standing	Structure/posture screen Integument	Standing	Structure/posture screen Integument
Seated	Great toe ext (A, MMT) Ankle DF (A, MMT) Ankle PF (A) Knee ext (A, OP, MMT) Hip flex (A, OP, MMT) Hip ER (A, OP, MMT) Hip IR (A, OP, MMT) Dermatomes L1–S2 Reflexes: patellar, Achilles	Seated	Hip flex (A, MMT) Hip ER (A, MMT) Hip IR (A, OP) Knee ext (A, OP, MMT) Toe ext (A, OP, MMT) Ankle DF (A, OP, P, MMT) Ankle PF (A, OP, P, MMT) Ankle inversion (A, OP, P, MMT) Ankle eversion (A, OP, P, MMT)
Standing	Trunk AROM flex, ext, side glide Trunk quadrant test	Standing	Deferred until completing testing of the proximal kinetic chain
Supine	Muscle length: gastrocnemius, hamstring Hip PROM: rot, flex, abd, add Knee PROM: flex, ext	Supine	Knee PROM MMT: leg lowering abdominal, trunk raise Muscle length: hamstring, gastrocnemius
Right side lying	L hip ext PROM MMT: L hip abd, R hip add	Right side lying	MMT: L hip abd, R hip add
Prone	Trunk ext (prone press up) Hip PROM: ext MMT: hamstring, gluteus maximus, trunk ext Integument	Prone	Trunk ext (prone press up) Hip PROM: ext MMT: trunk ext, gluteus maximus, hamstring Integument
Left side lying	R hip ext PROM MMT: R hip abd, L hip add	Left side lying	MMT: R hip abd, L hip add
Standing	Single leg balance MMT: PF Function: gait, squat, stairs, step up, lateral step down Muscle length: Thomas test Footwear inspection	Standing	Single leg balance MMT: PF Function: gait, squat, stairs, step up, lateral step down Muscle length: Thomas test Footwear inspection
Supine	MMT: leg lowering abdominal, trunk raise Transition to hip-specific examination	Supine	Transition to ankle-specific examination

A, active range of motion; *abd*, abduction; *add*, adduction; *DF*, dorsiflexion; *ER*, external rotation; *ever*, eversion; *ext*, extension; *flex*, flexion; *IR*, internal rotation; *L*, left; *MMT*, manual muscle test; *OP*, overpressure; *PF*, plantarflexion; *R*, right.

The basic framework of the LQS is present for both cases. However, subtle differences in both content and organization make each screen more efficient for the individual patient. For both patients, the clinician began with observation during the history, an overall structural screen, and inspection of all aspects of the integument. For Hattie, the clinician was required to thoroughly investigate the joint proximal to the hip (i.e., the lumbar spine), indicating the need to perform an LQNS. In contrast, an LQNS was not required for Angelo, as the patient did not report any complaints consistent with neurologic involvement and the ankle joint is several joints away from the lumbar spine. Indeed, the clinician did not need to perform passive ankle range at all for Hattie's ankle and foot, assuming the range was full by visual observation of active movement. This is because some tests were performed to assess myotomes (extensor hallucis longus strength) and some to assess the function of the kinetic chain (plantar flexion), rather than to assist with forming a differential diagnosis. Note also how the clinician included all toe and ankle motions in Angelo's screen, but this degree of examination was not required for Hattie. The clinician chose to first assess Hattie's hip extension passive range of motion in sidelying, considering her age and the possibility of very limited hip extension range of motion, that would make assessment of range and strength in prone problematic. However, for Angelo, the clinician assumed more normal hip extension range of motion would be present and only assessed this motion with him in the prone position. The Thomas test was chosen for both patients to assess the length of the iliopsoas, rectus femoris, and iliotibial band. It would have been equally valid for the clinician to have chosen to obtain this same information by using a prone knee flexion test of rectus femoris length, prone hip extension test of iliopsoas length, and Ober's test for iliotibial band assessment.

Core strength testing was performed on both patients for different reasons. For Hattie, these tests were performed to thoroughly investigate the joint proximal to the hip. For Angelo, the tests were performed because poor trunk control places athletes at risk for lower extremity injuries.[8] Neither patient demonstrated reason to assess vasculature or details of specific tibial/femoral length or torsion. If, however, Angelo had a history of diabetes, then circulation testing (along with detailed assessment of protective sensation) would be required. Following the LQS, the clinician will then perform a more focused examination of the hip or ankle for Hattie and Angelo, respectively, including provocative special tests, joint mobility, and local palpation.

There are many acceptable ways to organize the basic lower extremity screen. Clinicians should determine a flow that works best for them and practice this sequence for an inclusive LQS and to maximize efficiency. Once mastering this basic framework, clinicians should consider modifications based on area of chief complaint, as done here. Finally, clinicians must also be ready to adapt this prototypical framework based on individual patient presentation. For example, it might be useful for the new clinician to map how the examination flow might be adapted for a patient with knee pain or a patient who is NWB after ankle surgery.

CHAPTER SUMMARY

The LQS includes observation; gross assessment of structure and posture; an LQNS; assessment of lower extremity motion, muscle length, and strength; and functional testing. The LQS helps rule out areas as sources of a patient's complaint, identify relevant impairments within the kinetic chain, elucidate issues that might alter the plan of care, and expedite referral when needed. Clinicians should adapt the basic LQS based on the patient's history, chief complaint, and presentation. Finally, clinicians should organize the screen to maximize efficiency.

REFERENCES

1. McKenzie R, May S. *The Lumbar Spine. Vol. 1. Mechanical Diagnosis and Therapy.* Spinal Publications; 2013.
2. Delaloye J, Murar J, Vierira T, et al. Knee extension deficit in the early postoperative period predisposes to cyclops syndrome after anterior cruciate ligament reconstruction: a risk factor analysis in 3633 patients from the Santi Study Group database. *Am J Sports Med.* 2020;48(3):565–572.
3. Palmieri-Smith RM, Villwock M, Downie B, Hecht G, Zernicke R. Pain and effusion and quadriceps activation and strength. *J Athl Train.* 2013;48(2):186–191.
4. Wellsandt E, Failla MJ, Snyder-Mackler L. Limb symmetry indexes can overestimate knee function after anterior cruciate ligament injury. *J Orthop Sports Phys Ther.* 2017;47(5):334–338.
5. Kiappour A, Demetropoulos C, Kiapour A, et al. Strain response of the anterior cruciate ligament to uniplanar and multiplanar loads during simulated landings. *Am J Sport Med.* 2016;44(8):2087–2096.
6. Sanchis-Alfonso V, Dye SF. How to deal with anterior knee pain in the active young patient. *Sports Health.* 2017;9(4):346–351.
7. Willy R, Hoglund L, Barton C, et al. Patellofemoral pain: clinical practice guidelines linked to the International

Classification of Functioning, Disability and Health from the Academy of Orthopaedic Physical Therapy of the American Physical Therapy Association. *J Orthop Sports Phys Ther.* 2019;49(9):CPG1–CPG95.

8. Arundale AJH, Bizzini M, Giordano A, et al. Exercise-based knee and anterior cruciate ligament injury prevention: clinical practice guidelines linked to the international classification of functioning, disability, and health from the Orthopaedic and Sports Sections of the American Physical Therapy Association. *J Orthop Sports Phys Ther.* 2018;48(9):A1–A42.

9. Thawrani DP, Agabegi SS, Asghar F. Diagnosing sacroiliac joint pain. *J Am Acad Orthop Surg.* 2019;27(3):85–93.

10. Kendall FP, McCreary EK, Provance PG, Rogers MM, Romani WZ. *Muscles: Testing and Function with Posture and Pain.* 5th ed. Lippincott Williams & Wilkins; 2005.

11. Buldt AK, Levinger P, Murley GS, Menz HB, Nester CJ, Landorf KB. Foot posture is associated with kinematics of the foot during gait: a comparison of normal, planus and cavus feet. *Gait Posture.* 2015;42(1):42–48.

12. Shogo U, Anh-Dung N, Naoko A, Yohei S. Relationship of knee motions with static leg alignments and hip motions in frontal and transverse planes during double-leg landing in healthy athletes. *J Sport Rehabil.* 2017;26(5):396–405.

13. Buldt AK, Murley GS, Butterworth P, Levinger P, Menz HB, Landorf KB. The relationship between foot posture and lower limb kinematics during walking: a systematic review. *Gait Posture.* 2013;38(3):363–372.

14. Davenport D, Colaco H, Kavarthapu V. Examination of the adult spine. *Br J Hosp Med.* 2015;76(12):C182–195.

15. Leighton RD, Sheldon MR. Model for teaching clinical decision making in a physical therapy professional curriculum. *J Phys Ther Educ.* 1997;11(2):23–30.

9 | Ankle and Foot

Betsy Myers, June Hanks, and Jeremiah Tate

CHAPTER OBJECTIVES
After reading this chapter, you will be able to:
1. Describe the basic anatomy and biomechanics of the ankle and foot.
2. Tailor the basic history to a patient with ankle/foot pathology.
3. Describe the components of the physical examination for a patient with ankle/foot pathology.
4. Describe the pathology, history, key examination findings, rehabilitation focus, and expected outcomes of common ankle/foot pathologies.
5. Hypothesize differential diagnoses of ankle/foot symptoms based on location, patient complaint, and onset.
6. Organize the physical examination of a patient with ankle/foot pathology to maximize efficiency.

FUNCTIONAL ANATOMY OF JOINTS

Osteology

The lower leg, ankle, and foot are a complex series of bones and joints (Figs. 9-1 and 9-2). Study of the region is facilitated by groupings into bony regions: leg (tibia and fibula), rearfoot (talus and calcaneus), midfoot (navicular, cuboid, cuneiform), and forefoot (metatarsals, phalanges, and sesamoids). Figure 9-3 demonstrates these groupings of the bones of the foot. Accessory bones and tarsal coalitions must also be considered.

Bones of the Leg

Tibia The tibia is the larger of the two leg bones and transmits most of the body weight to the foot. Next to the femur, the tibia is the longest and heaviest bone in the body.[1] The tibial shaft has three surfaces (anterior, medial, and posterior) separated by anterior, lateral (interosseous), and medial borders. The anterior surface is anterolaterally oriented. The medial surface, between the anterior and medial borders, is broad, smooth, and mostly subcutaneous. The posterior surface is between the medial and lateral borders and is crossed obliquely by the rough soleal line. The anterior border extends from the tibial tuberosity to the anterior portion of the medial malleolus and is easily palpated until its distal portion. The medial border descends from the medial tibial condyle to the posterior portion of the medial malleolus. The lateral border provides attachment for the interosseous membrane, a dense connective tissue joining the tibia to the fibula. Just distal to the soleal line is an obliquely shaped groove that leads to the large nutrient foramen for passage of the main arterial supply to proximal tibia. On cross-section, the more proximal portion of the tibial shaft is triangular whereas the distal portion is more quadrangularly shaped. The tibia is thinnest at the distal third of the bone. Most distally, the tibia projects medially as the medial malleolus. Along the medial side of the distal posterior surface is a groove for the passage of the tibialis posterior tendon. The lateral surface of the medial malleolus articulates with the medial surface of the talus. The distal tibia is saddle-shaped (concave anteroposteriorly and convex mediolaterally) and forms an articular surface for the talus. This distal tibial articular surface, also called the tibial plafond, is slightly wider anteriorly than posteriorly. The posterior lip of the tibial plafond is the posterior malleolus. The distal tibia covers two-thirds of the talus in any position, with one-third remaining uncovered.[2] On the lateral side is the fibular notch, which is concave anteroposteriorly for articulation with the distal end of the fibula.

In adults, the tibia is aligned such that, relative to the proximal end of the tibia, the distal portion is externally rotated in the transverse plane. This transverse twist of the bone is referred to as tibial torsion. The expected amount of tibial torsion changes during development, progressing from slight medial to lateral torsion at birth and progressing to approximately 20 to 30° of external torsion in the adult.[3,4]

Fibula The fibula, the lateral bone of the leg, is more slender than the tibia. The bone consists of a proximal head superior to a small neck; a long, twisted shaft; and a bulbous distal end, the lateral malleolus. The head projects proximally from the posterolateral aspect, forming a blunt apex that is easily palpated. The tibial facet on the head articulates with the fibular

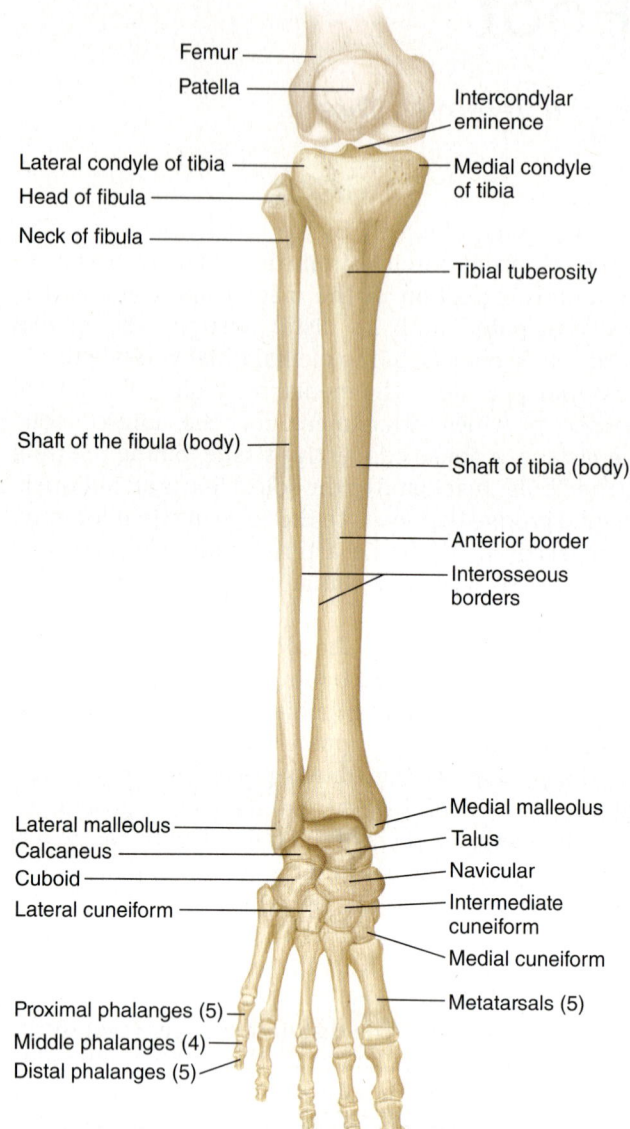

FIGURE 9-1 Leg and foot osteology. Anterior view. (Gest TR. *Lippincott Atlas of Anatomy*. 2nd ed. Wolters Kluwer; 2020: Plate 3-08.)

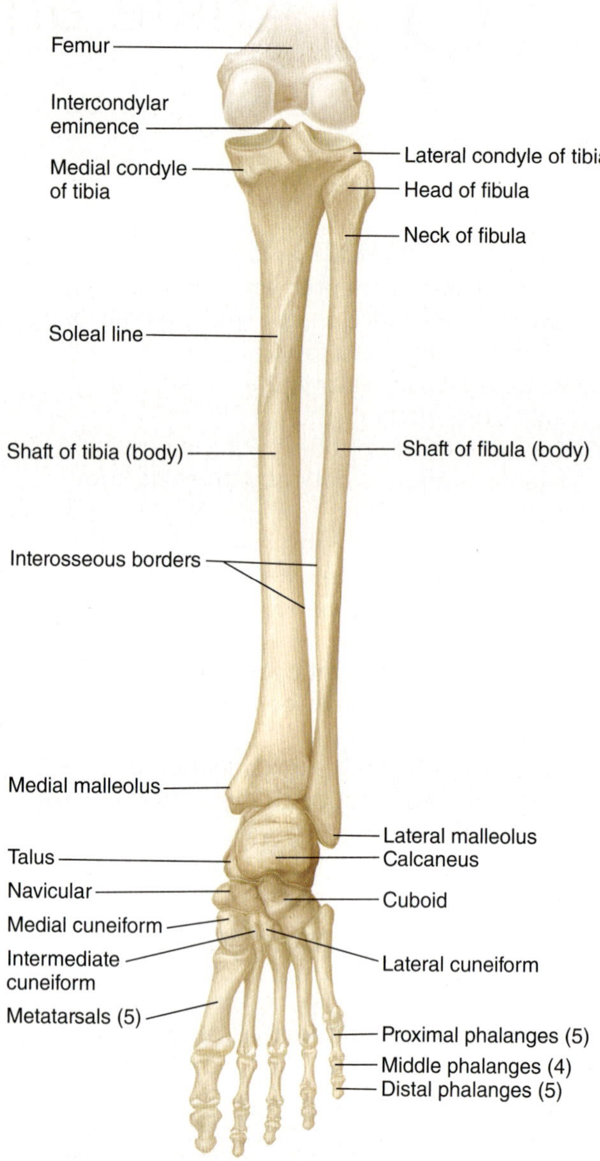

FIGURE 9-2 Leg and foot osteology. Posterior view. (Gest TR. *Lippincott Atlas of Anatomy*. 2nd ed. Wolters Kluwer; 2020: Plate 3-09.)

facet on the inferolateral surface of the lateral tibial condyle, forming the proximal tibiofibular joint.

The common fibular nerve crosses posterolateral to the neck of the fibula and can be pressed against the bone. The lateral malleolus extends farther distally and is situated more posteriorly than the medial malleolus.[2] The medial aspect of the lateral malleolus has a triangularly shaped facet that articulates with the lateral side of the talus. Just superior to this surface, the fibula contacts the tibia in the fibular notch of the tibia. A deep depression in the posteroinferior region of the lateral malleolus is named the malleolar fossa that can be easily palpated. The posterior talofibular (PTF) ligament attaches in this fossa. There is a groove along the posterior aspect of the lateral malleolus through which the fibularis brevis tendon passes.

Bones of the Rearfoot

Talus The talus links the leg and the foot. The talus consists of a large body, anterior to which is the head. The body and head of the talus are connected by a short neck.

The superior surface of the body of the talus is covered with articular cartilage for articulation with the

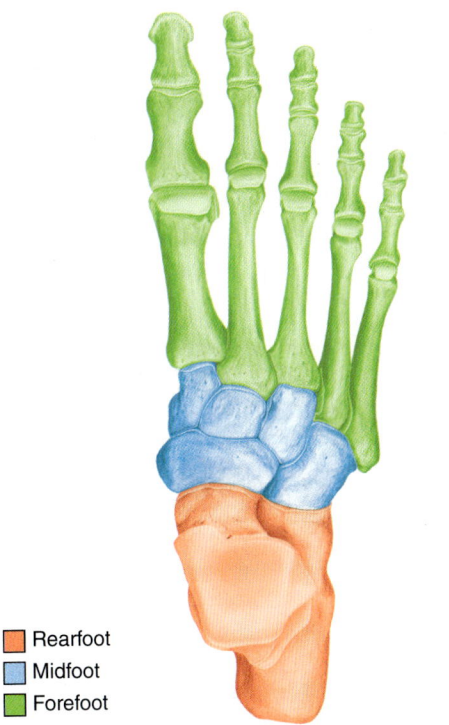

FIGURE 9-3 Bones of the rearfoot, midfoot, and forefoot. (Modified from Gest TR. *Lippincott Atlas of Anatomy*. 2nd ed. Wolters Kluwer; 2020: Plate 3-42.)

inferior surface of the tibia. This articular surface is continuous with the articular surfaces of the medial and lateral aspects of the talus. The superior surface is somewhat wider anteriorly than posteriorly. It is convex anteroposteriorly and slightly concave mediolaterally, corresponding to the opposing saddle-shaped surface of the distal end of the tibia mentioned previously. In this sense, the superior talar articular surface is trochlear, or pulley-like, and is often referred to as the trochlea.

The lateral aspect of the body of the talus is largely covered by articular cartilage for articulation with the distal end of the fibula (Fig. 9-4). This articular surface is triangular, with the apex situated inferiorly. Just below this apex is the lateral process, which is a bony projection to which the lateral talocalcaneal ligament attaches. The articular surface of the medial aspect of the talus (Fig. 9-5) is considerably smaller than that of the lateral side, has a larger radius of curvature than the lateral facet, and faces slightly upward. It contacts the articular surface of the medial malleolus on the tibia. The roughened area below the medial articular surface serves as an attachment for the deltoid ligament. The medial and lateral talar articular surfaces tend to converge posteriorly, leading to the wedge shape of the trochlea. It should be emphasized, however, that the lateral articular surface of the talus is perpendicular to the axis of movement at the ankle joint, whereas the medial surface is not. This asymmetry of the medial and lateral orientation of articular surfaces leads to an obliquity in the ankle joint axis with important biomechanical implications discussed later in this chapter.

Posteriorly, the body of the talus is largely covered by a continuation of the trochlear articular surface as it slopes backward. At the inferior extent of the posterior aspect is the nonarticular posterior process. The posterior process consists of a lateral tubercle and a smaller medial tubercle, with an intervening groove through which passes the tendon of the flexor hallucis longus. The PTF ligament attaches to the lateral tubercle. The medial talocalcaneal ligament and a posterior portion of the deltoid ligament attach to the medial tubercle.

Both the neck and head of the talus are directed slightly inferiorly and medially from the body, contributing to the shape of the medial longitudinal arch. The head is covered with articular cartilage anteriorly for articulation with the navicular and inferiorly for articulation with the spring (plantar calcaneonavicular) ligament.

The inferior (plantar) surface of the talar head has three facets for articulation with the calcaneus. The largest of these is the posterior facet that is concave inferiorly and articulates with the convex posterior facet on the superior middle segment of the calcaneus. The middle and anterior articular facets are convex inferiorly and articulate with the superior aspect of the sustentaculum tali of the calcaneus. A deep groove, the sulcus tali, separates the posterior and middle facets on the inferior aspect of the talus. This groove runs obliquely from posteromedial to anterolateral. Where it is the deepest—posteromedially—it forms the tarsal canal; where it widens and opens out laterally, it is referred to as the sinus tarsi. The interosseous talocalcaneal ligament and the cervical ligament occupy the sinus tarsi.

Calcaneus The calcaneus, the largest of the tarsal bones, is located inferior to the talus, articulating with it superiorly and with the cuboid anteriorly (Figs. 9-4 and 9-5). In standing, the rough plantar surface provides a major contact point with the ground. The calcaneus can be divided into posterior, middle, and anterior segments. The posterior third projects backward, providing considerable leverage for the Achilles tendon that attaches to the posterior aspect. The distal aspect of the posterior segment continues onto the plantar surface as the calcaneal tuberosity, which contacts the ground in standing. The calcaneal tuberosity (tuber calcanei) consists of a lateral and medial tubercle, of which the medial is the larger. Anterior to the tuber

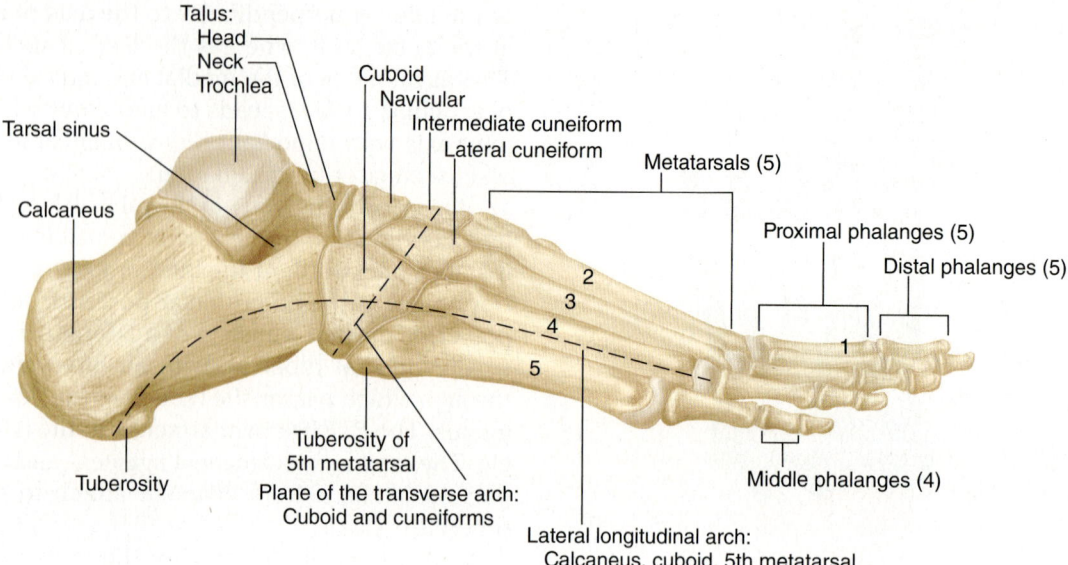

FIGURE 9-4 Foot osteology. Lateral view. (Gest TR. *Lippincott Atlas of Anatomy*. 2nd ed. Wolters Kluwer; 2020: Plate 3-41B.)

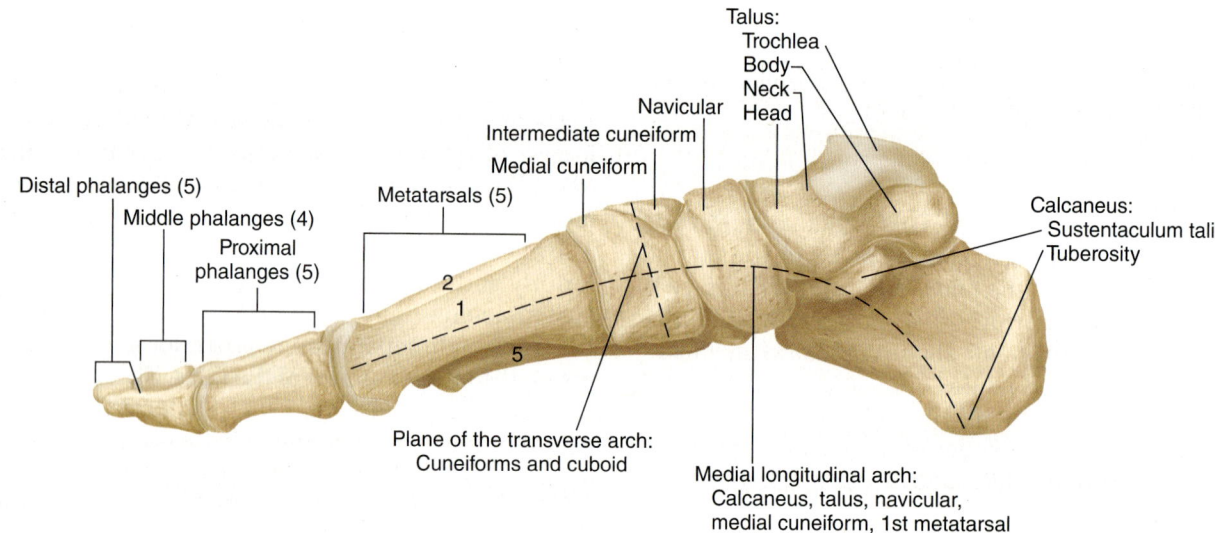

FIGURE 9-5 Foot osteology. Medial view. (Gest TR. *Lippincott Atlas of Anatomy*. 2nd ed. Wolters Kluwer; 2020: Plate 3-41A.)

calcanei is a roughened surface for the attachment of the long and short plantar ligaments. At the anterior extent of the inferior surface of the calcaneus is the anterior tubercle, which also serves as a point of attachment for the long plantar ligament.

The middle segment of the calcaneus has on its superior surface a large posterior facet that articulates with the posterior facet of the talus. The superior surface of the anterior segment bears a middle and anterior facet that articulates with the middle and anterior talar facets. These facets are separated from the posterior facet by the sulcus calcanei, which forms the inferior (bottom) of the sinus tarsi and tarsal canal.

The anterior surface of the anterior segment is nearly entirely articular, forming a saddle-shaped surface for the cuboid.

The lateral aspect of the calcaneus is nearly flat with a small prominence, the fibular trochlea, located just distal to the lateral malleolus. The fibularis brevis tendon travels inferior and anterior, just superior to this trochlea, whereas the fibularis longus tendon passes inferior to it. The calcaneofibular ligament (CFL) attaches just posterior and slightly superior to the fibular trochlea.

From the anterosuperior extent of the medial aspect of the calcaneus, the sustentaculum tali projects in a medial direction. On the inferior aspect of the sustentaculum tali is a groove by which the flexor hallucis longus tendon passes. On the narrowed anterior aspect of the calcaneus is the cartilage-covered, saddle-shaped articular surface that contacts the cuboid bone.

Bones of the Midfoot Distally, the three cuneiform bones are interposed between the navicular proximally, the first three metatarsals distally and the cuboid laterally (Fig. 9-3).

Navicular The crescent-shaped navicular bone has a biconcave posterior surface that articulates with the convex-shaped head of the talus proximally and is an integral part of the talotarsal joint.

The convex anterior articular surface articulates with the cuneiforms distally. The navicular has little to no articular contact with the cuboid and is firmly bound to the calcaneus by ligaments. The medial surface projects the navicular tuberosity that provides attachment for the tibialis posterior tendon.

Cuboid The cuboid is a wedge-shaped bone interposed between the calcaneus and the base of the 4th and 5th metatarsals. Medially, the cuboid has a fossa for the navicular and lateral cuneiform bones. A groove for the fibularis longus tendon is located on the lateral and plantar surface. Proximally, the articular surface with the calcaneus is saddle-shaped.

Cuneiforms The cuneiforms are primarily wedge-shaped.[2] Each cuneiform articulates with the navicular proximally. The cuneiforms articulate distally with metatarsal bones. The lateral cuneiform also articulates with the cuboid. Distally, the intermediate cuneiform is shorter than the others, providing a recess (mortise) for the base of the 2nd metatarsal, increasing the stability of the joint. The cuneiforms have facets on proximal, distal, medial, and lateral surfaces for articulation with adjacent bones.

Bones of the Forefoot
Metatarsals The five metatarsals articulate proximally with the three cuneiforms and the cuboid and form the tarsometatarsal joints. Each metatarsal has a proximal base, shaft, and distal head (Fig. 9-6A). The 1st metatarsal is shorter than the 2nd and 3rd and is the thickest of all the metatarsals. A tubercle at the junction of the medial and plantar surface provides attachment for the tibialis anterior tendon. The tuberosity at the junction of the plantar and lateral surface provides attachment for the fibularis longus tendon. The 2nd metatarsal is thinner and longer than the others and is securely wedged in place by the cuneiforms and the adjacent metatarsals. The 5th metatarsal projects farther proximally and provides attachment for the fibularis brevis tendon. Shafts of the metatarsals are curved longitudinally so as to be slightly convex superiorly and concave inferiorly. The heads of the metatarsals are convex, presenting as oblong from superior to inferior and extending farther posteriorly in the inferior portion. The sides of the heads are flattened but with a small tubercle for ligamentous attachment. The plantar surfaces are grooved anteroposteriorly for passage of the flexor tendons.

The functional unit of the forefoot is described as a "ray." Each of the three medial rays consist of the metatarsal, associated proximal cuneiform, and distal phalangeal bones. For example, the 1st ray is composed of the medial cuneiform, 1st metatarsal, and associated phalanges of the great toe. The 4th and 5th rays consist of the respective metatarsal and phalanges.[5,6] It should be noted that some consider a ray to consist of the metatarsal and associated phalanges without including the proximal articulating cuneiform.[7]

Phalanges There are three phalanges in each of the lateral four toes and two in the great toe. Each phalanx has a proximal base and distal head. The bases of the proximal phalanges are an oval, biconcave shape to fit the trochlear-shaped metatarsal heads. Similarly, the bases of the middle and distal phalanges have a central ridge to accommodate the trochlear-shaped proximal and middle phalanges.

Sesamoids The sesamoids are small, round bones embedded, partially or totally, in the substance of a corresponding tendon juxtaposed to articulations and are anatomically a part of a gliding or pressure-absorbing mechanism (Fig. 9-6B). Structurally, some sesamoids always ossify, whereas others remain cartilaginous or fibrocartilaginous. The medial and lateral sesamoids of the flexor hallucis brevis are commonly present plantar to the 1st metatarsal head.[8] Other locations where sesamoids may be found are in the plantar plates of the metatarsophalangeal (MTP) and interphalangeal joints, the intrinsic tendons of the lesser toes, or the tendons of the tibialis anterior, tibialis posterior, or fibularis longus.

Accessory Bones and Tarsal Coalitions Accessory (extra) bones and tarsal coalitions (abnormal unions among tarsal bones) are common developmental variations in the foot and ankle.[9,10] Accessory bones, such as naviculare secundarium, os peroneum, os trigonum, and os intermetatarseum, may become a source of irritation, fracture, dislocation, degenerative change, avascular necrosis, or impingement of adjacent tissues and require immobilization or excision.[11] The os trigonum, associated with the posterior lateral tubercle of the talus, connected to it by a fibrous band,[12]

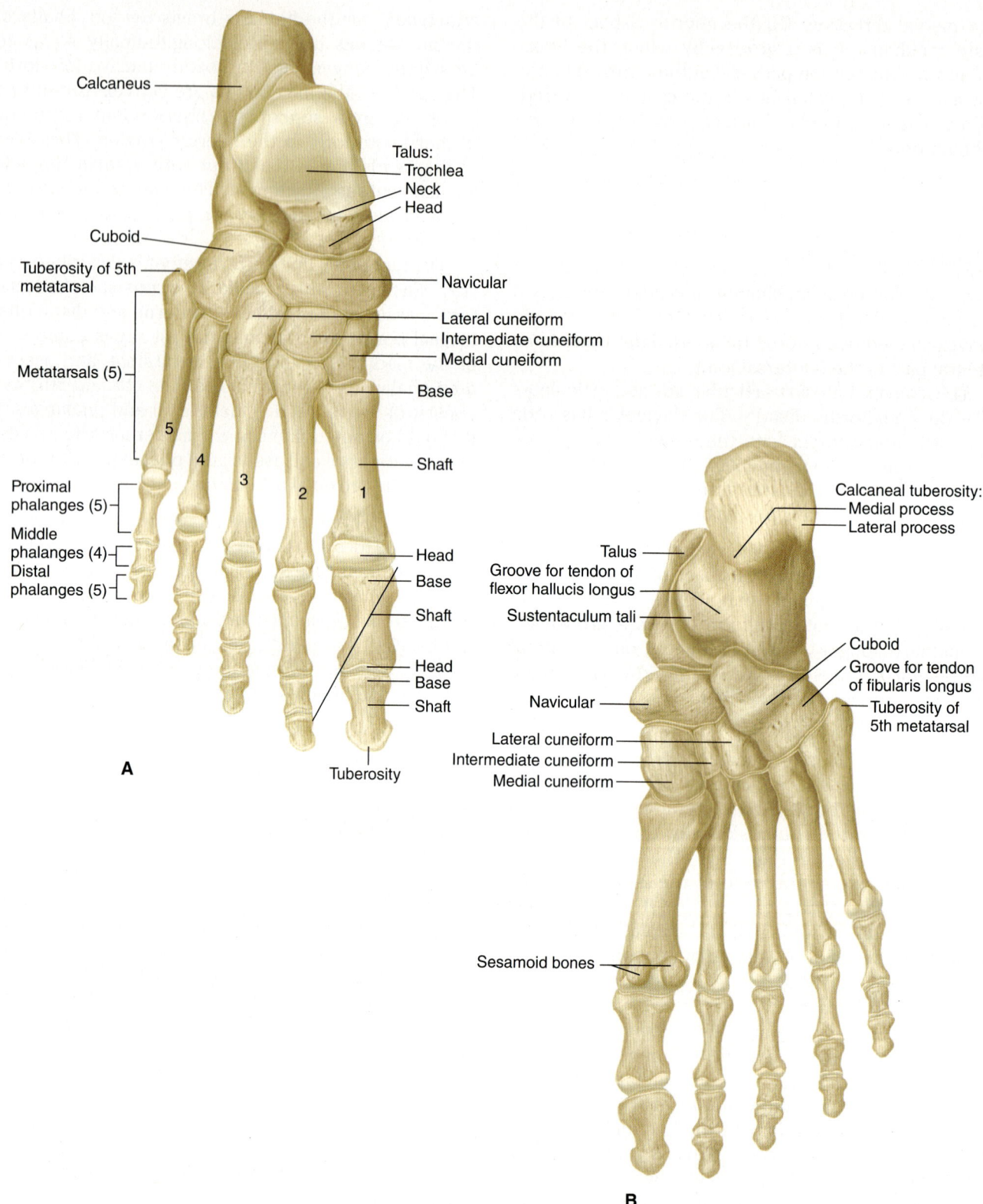

FIGURE 9-6 Foot osteology. **A.** Dorsal view. **B.** Plantar view. (Gest TR. *Lippincott Atlas of Anatomy*. 2nd ed. Wolters Kluwer; 2020: Plate 3-40.)

may become irritated with excessive plantar flexion activities, such as ballet. Tarsal coalitions are complete or partial osseous, fibrous, or cartilaginous connections among tarsal bones that restrict movement between adjacent bones. Calcaneonavicular and talocalcaneal coalitions are the most common.[13,14] Tarsal coalitions may go undetected and be asymptomatic or lead to pain, stiffness, or deformity.[9]

Joints, Ligaments, and Capsules

The articulations, associated connective tissues, and muscles/tendons of the leg, ankle, and foot afford the mobility and stability necessary for human ambulation. The talus articulates with the distalmost portion of the tibia and fibula, forming the talocrural joint. The bones of the rearfoot form the subtalar joint. The articulations of the bones of the midfoot form the midtarsal and distal intertarsal joints. The forefoot is composed of the tarsometatarsal, intermetatarsal, MTP, and interphalangeal joints. This section presents key considerations of articulations of the lower leg and foot that will be further developed throughout the remainder of the chapter.

Proximal Tibiofibular Joint The proximal tibiofibular joint is a gliding synovial joint formed by the articulation of the head of the fibula with the posterolateral aspect of the tibia. The joint is supported by the thicker anterior and thinner posterior proximal tibiofibular ligaments.[15] The interosseous membrane binds the tibia and fibula and provides support to the proximal and distal tibiofibular joints. Inferiorly, the interosseous membrane is continuous with the interosseous ligament of the distal tibiofibular syndesmotic joint and also thickens and divides, forming the anteroinferior and posteroinferior tibiofibular ligaments surrounding the joint.

The anterior, lateral, and posterior compartments of the leg are formed by the tibia, fibula, interconnecting interosseous membrane, and deep connective tissue of the leg. The muscles in each compartment serve common functions and share common blood supply and innervation. The inelastic properties of the deep connective tissue create the relatively close space of the compartments that permit little expansion with muscle contraction, thus aiding venous return. Swelling within the compartments because of trauma or overuse may increase intracompartmental pressure impairing blood flow and compressing neural structures[16,17] and may require a fasciotomy.

Distal Tibiofibular Joint The distal tibiofibular joint is a syndesmosis and lacks articular cartilage and synovium, except for a small area at the base.[18,19] The distal fibula is situated in the fibular notch of the lateral aspect of the distal tibia and is bound to it by several ligaments. The interosseous ligament, a continuation of the interosseous membrane, extends between the adjacent surfaces of the bones at the syndesmosis. The anterior and posterior tibiofibular ligaments pass in front of and behind the syndesmosis. The inferior transverse ligament passes from the posterior margin of the inferior tibial articular surface downward and laterally to the malleolar fossa of the fibula. The tibia and fibula are separated at the syndesmosis by a fat pad.

The asymmetrical shape of the talar dome leads to motion, albeit minimal, of the fibula in relation to the tibia during ankle dorsiflexion and plantar flexion. Displacement of the lateral malleolus is medial and anterior during plantar flexion and lateral and posterior during dorsiflexion. The orientation of the surrounding ligaments serves to restrict movement of the fibula with these movements and with forceable rotation on the tarsus.[20,21] Instability of the distal tibiofibular joint may lead to chronic ankle dysfunction.[22,23]

Talocrural (Ankle) Joint The talocrural joint is formed by the superior portion of the body of the talus fitting within a cavity formed by the combined distal ends of the tibia and fibula. The articulation is often referred to as a mortise because of its resemblance to the mortise used by a carpenter. All articular surfaces within the mortise are continuous (the medial, superior, and lateral articular surfaces of the talus and the combined surfaces of the medial malleolus, distal end of the tibia, and the lateral malleolus). The wide anterior surface of the talar trochlea contributes to the tight articular fit, especially with dorsiflexion. The fibrous capsule attaches at the margins of the articular surfaces of the talus below and to the tibia and fibula above, except anteriorly, where a portion of the dorsal aspect of the neck of the talus is enclosed within the joint cavity. The capsule extends somewhat superiorly between the distal ends of the tibia and fibula, to just below the syndesmosis. A synovial membrane lines the fibrous capsule throughout its entirety. The capsule is well supported by ligaments, especially medially and laterally.

The medial ankle ligamentous complex, consisting of blended superficial and deep layers, is collectively referred to as the deltoid ligament (Fig. 9-7A). The shape is somewhat triangular, with the apex at its proximal attachment to the medial malleolus and distal attachments to the navicular, talus, and calcaneus. The anterior portion of the deltoid ligament consists of the tibionavicular ligament, superficially, and the deeper anterior tibiotalar fibers. The tibionavicular ligament blends with the spring ligament inferiorly. The middle fibers of the deltoid ligament constitute the tibiocalcaneal ligament, with some tibiotalar fibers deep into it. The posterior tibiotalar ligament forms

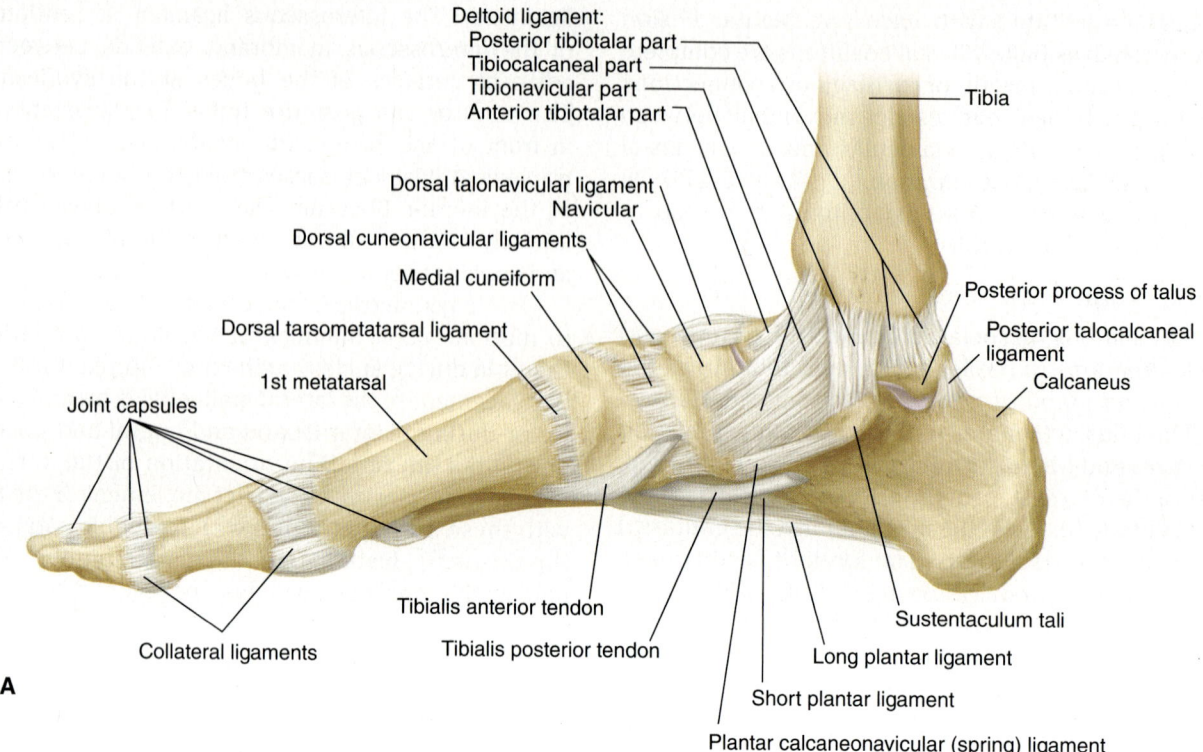
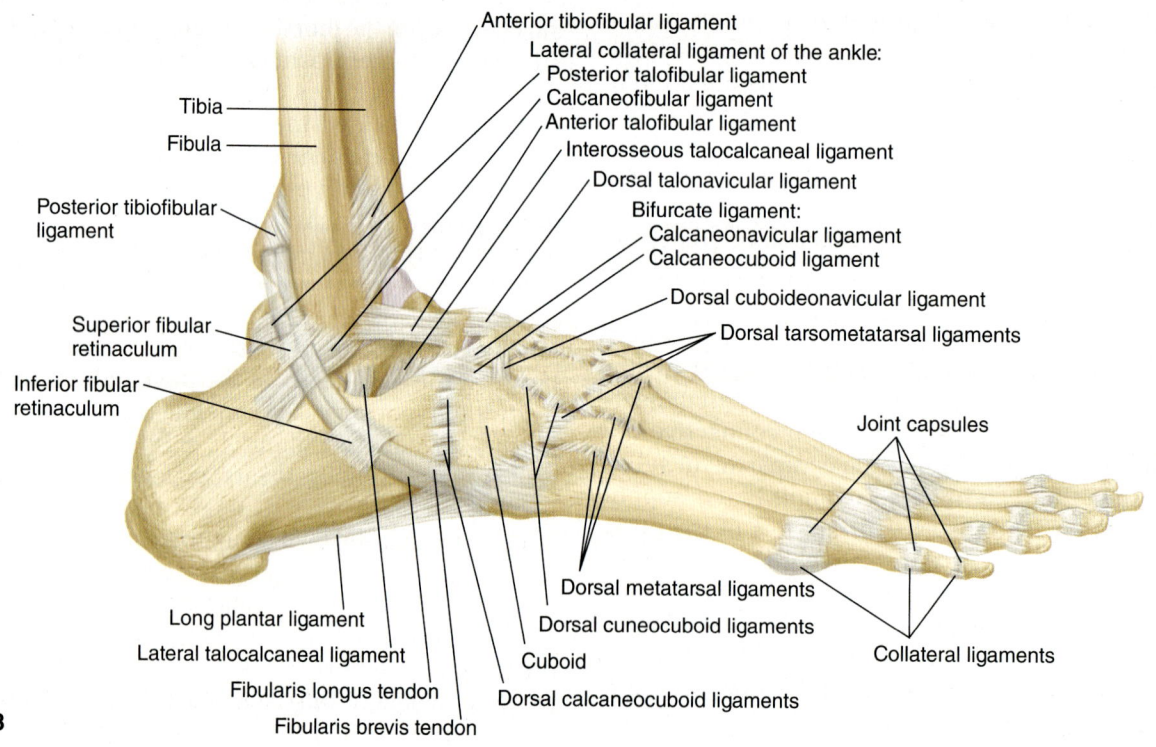

FIGURE 9-7 Ligaments of the ankle and foot. **A.** Medial view. **B.** Lateral view. (Gest TR. *Lippincott Atlas of Anatomy*. 2nd ed. Wolters Kluwer; 2020: Plate 3-60.)

the posterior portion of the deltoid ligament. The deltoid ligament primarily helps support the medial ankle and subtalar joint against valgus stresses.

The lateral ligamentous complex (Fig. 9-7B), unlike those of the medial side, are separate bands of fibers diverging from their proximal attachment at the distal end of the fibula. The anterior talofibular (ATF) ligament passes medial, anterior, and inferior from the anterior aspect of the fibula to the lateral aspect of the neck of the talus. The CFL runs from the tip of the lateral malleolus inferior and posterior to the fibular tuberosity, a small prominence on the upper lateral surface of the calcaneus. It is longer and narrower than the anterior and PTF ligaments. The PTF ligament passes from the malleolar fossa medially and slightly inferior and posterior to the lateral tubercle of the talus.

The ligaments about the talocrural joint primarily function to restrict tilting and rotation of the talus within the mortise and to restrict anterior or posterior displacement of the leg on the tarsus. The main exception to this is the tibiocalcaneal portion of the deltoid ligament, which is so oriented as to help check eversion at the subtalar joint as well as an "eversion tilt" of the talus in the mortise.

In the neutral position during weight bearing, the ATF ligament can check posterior movement of the leg on the tarsus and external rotation of the leg on the tarsus because it is directed forward and medially. With the foot in plantar flexion, the ATF ligament becomes more vertically oriented and is in a position to check inversion of the talus in the mortise. This ligament is the most commonly injured of the ligaments of the ankle, the mechanism of injury usually being a combined plantar flexion–inversion motion.

The CFL is directed downward and posterior when the foot is in the neutral position. When the foot is dorsiflexed, the ligament assumes a more vertical orientation and is better positioned to check inversion of the tarsus with respect to the leg. The PTF ligament is oriented so as to check internal rotation and anterior displacement of the leg on the tarsus.

Subtalar Joint Functionally, the subtalar joint includes the articulation between the facets of the talus and the opposing articular surfaces of the calcaneus. These articulations move in conjunction with one another. Anatomically, the anterior and medial articulation of the talus and calcaneus are enclosed within a joint capsule separate from that of the posterior talocalcaneal articulation. Separating these two subtalar joint capsules is the interosseous talocalcaneal ligament that runs from the underside of the talus, at the sulcus tali, posterior and lateral to the dorsum of the calcaneus, at the sulcus calcanei.

Because the interosseous talocalcaneal ligament is situated medial to the axis of motion of inversion–eversion at the subtalar joint, it checks eversion.

More laterally, in the sinus tarsi is the cervical talocalcaneal ligament that passes from the inferolateral aspect of the talar neck inferiorly and laterally to the dorsum of the calcaneus. It occupies the anterior aspect of the sinus tarsi. Because the cervical ligament lies lateral to the subtalar joint axis, it restricts inversion of the calcaneus on the talus.

Also, within the lateral aspect of the sinus tarsi, bands from the inferior aspect of the extensor retinaculum pass inferiorly and medially to the calcaneus. These bands are considered part of the talocalcaneal ligament complex and help check inversion at the subtalar joint.

Midtarsal Joint The midtarsal joint, also referred to as the transverse tarsal joint or Chopart joint, is a combined articulation of the medial talonavicular joint and the lateral calcaneocuboid joint. The midtarsal joint represents the functional articulation between the rearfoot (talus and calcaneus) and the midfoot (navicular and cuboid).[24]

Talonavicular Joint The talonavicular joint includes the articulation between the convex-shaped head of the talus and the reciprocal concave-shaped navicular bone. The head of the talus and its large navicular socket are enclosed by the same joint capsule as the anterior and middle facets of the subtalar joint. This joint capsule is reinforced medially by the tibionavicular portion of the deltoid ligament, dorsally by the medial band (i.e., calcaneonavicular) of the bifurcate ligament and inferiorly by the spring ligament (Fig. 9-8). The superomedial portion of the spring ligament contains a concave fibrocartilaginous facet that corresponds to the plantar surface of the talar head, allowing the ligament to act as a sling for the talar head[25,26] and helping to maintain the normal arched configuration of the foot.[26] The anatomic and functional relationships of the talus to the talonavicular and subtalar joint lead some to refer to the articulations as the talocalcaneonavicular joint.

Calcaneocuboid Joint The calcaneocuboid joint, comprising the lateral portion of the midtarsal joint, is a saddle-shaped joint in that the calcaneal joint surface is concave superoinferiorly and convex mediolaterally; the adjoining cuboid surface is reciprocally shaped. This joint is enclosed in a joint capsule distinct from that of the talonavicular joint. The joint capsule is reinforced dorsally by the lateral band (i.e., calcaneocuboid) of the bifurcate ligament and inferiorly by the short and long plantar ligaments. The short plantar ligament runs from the anterior tubercle of the plantar aspect of

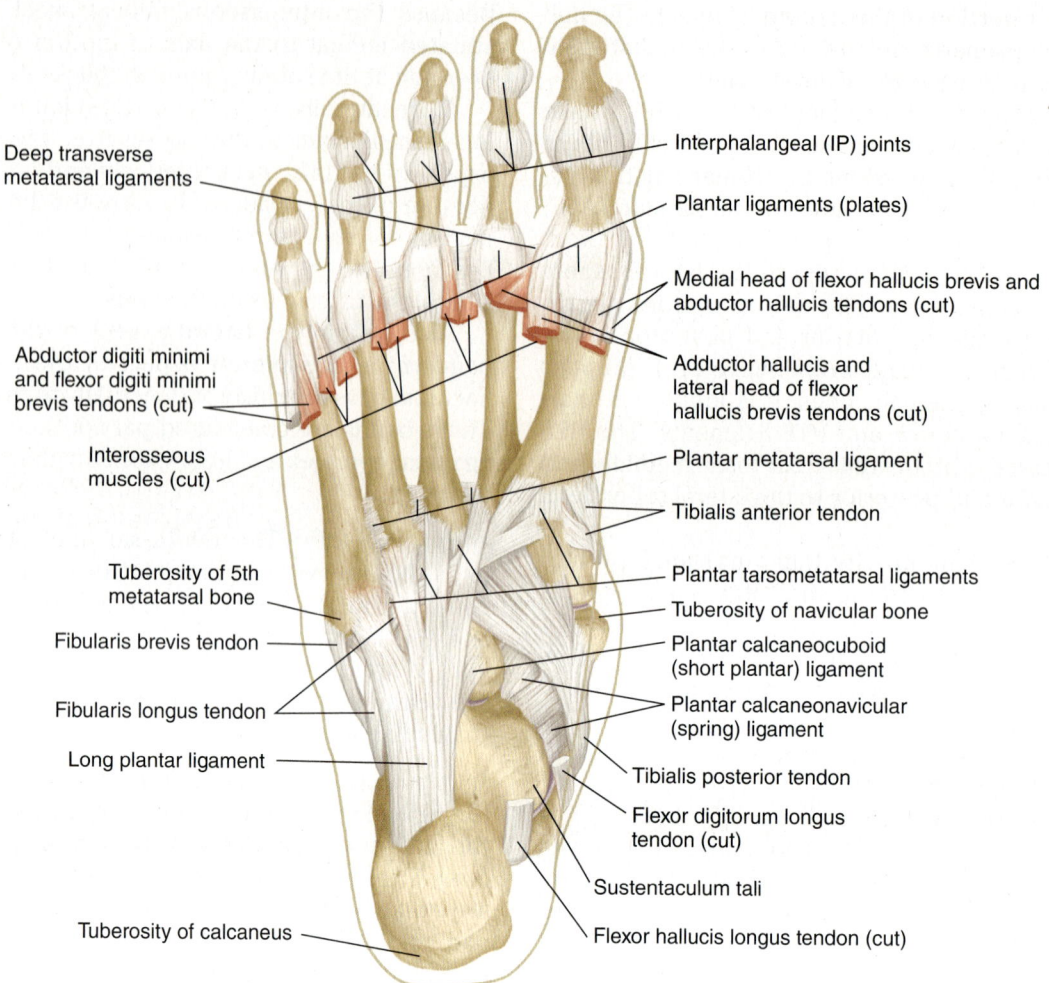

FIGURE 9-8 Deep ligaments of foot. (Gest TR. *Lippincott Atlas of Anatomy*. 2nd ed. Wolters Kluwer; 2020: Plate 3-61A.)

the calcaneus to the underside of the cuboid. The long plantar ligament runs from the posterior tubercles of the calcaneus anterior to the bases of the 5th, 4th, 3rd, and sometimes 2nd metatarsals. Both the short and long plantar ligaments support the normal arched configuration of the foot.

Intertarsal Joints The medial cuneiform and 1st metatarsal articulation has a separate cavity, as does the cuboid articulation with the 4th and 5th metatarsals. A common joint cavity encapsulates the cuboid, navicular, three cuneiforms, and 2nd and 3rd metatarsals. Interosseous, dorsal, and plantar ligaments strengthen all of these small joints.

The cubonavicular joint is usually a fibrous joint, but not infrequently the syndesmosis is replaced by a synovial joint of an almost plane variety, with the capsule and cavity continuous with the cuneonavicular joint. Ligaments include the plantar cubonavicular ligament, interosseus ligament, and dorsal cubonavicular ligament, which strongly unite the cuboid and the navicular.

The cuneonavicular, cuneocuboid, and intercuneiform joints have a common joint capsule. The navicular articulates with the three cuneiform bones and may be considered convex distally, being divided by low ridges into three facets that articulate with the medial, intermediate, and lateral cuneiforms to form the cuneonavicular joint. The cuboid articulates with the lateral cuneiform and the cuneiforms articulate with each other. The articulations between adjacent tarsal bones are sometimes referred to as intertarsal joints.

Tarsometatarsal Joints The tarsometatarsal joints lie in somewhat of a straight line, except for the shallow mortises created by the middle cuneiform and cuboid. The ligaments connecting the cuboid and the cuneiforms to the metatarsal bases are the dorsal, plantar, and interosseous ligaments.

The 1st tarsometatarsal joint (the articulation between the 1st metatarsal and medial cuneiform) has its own articular capsule. The 2nd tarsometatarsal joint is stronger, and its motion is more restricted than the other tarsometatarsal joints. The 3rd tarsometatarsal joint shares its capsule with the 2nd tarsometatarsal joint, whereas the 4th and 5th tarsometatarsal joints share a capsule with their articulation with the cuboid. A Lisfranc injury occurs when there is displacement between the tarsal and metatarsal bones.

The relatively flat articulations between the bases of the metatarsals permit slight gliding and rotation motions of one metatarsal on the next. Although there is little movement between the individual tarsals and metatarsals, their collective movement can enhance either the foot's stability or flexibility. Dorsal and plantar ligaments join the bones. The plantar ligaments of the cuneocuboid and intercuneiform joints are strengthened by slips from the tendons of the tibialis posterior.

Metatarsophalangeal Joints The metatarsal heads that are condylar in shape articulate with the accommodating concave phalangeal bases and are reinforced by collateral ligaments (medial and lateral) and MTP ligaments. The dorsal capsule is reinforced by the extensor hood expansion. The fibrocartilaginous plantar plates are attached to the metatarsal heads and the bases of the phalanges. The plates are pulled distally with hyperextension of the toes to protect the distal aspect of the articular surface. A plantar MTP ligament is continuous with the plantar aponeurosis, so that toe dorsiflexion (extension) tenses the plantar aponeurosis and stabilizes the foot's longitudinal arches.

Proximal Phalangeal Joint of Great Toe The two sesamoids, embedded in the thick fibrous plantar plate and united to the proximal phalanx of the great toe, form an anatomic and functional unit called the sesamophalangeal apparatus. The sesamoids are foci of insertion: the flexor hallucis brevis inserts on the proximal segment of each sesamoid, the abductor hallucis inserts on the medial sesamoid, and the lateral sesamoid gives insertion to the oblique and transverse components of the adductor hallucis muscle. The deep transverse metatarsal ligament attaches longitudinally along the lateral sesamoid. The sesamophalangeal apparatus moves backward or forward relative to the fixed metatarsal head; in hallux valgus (HV) the sesamoids follow the proximal phalanx and are displaced with the phalanx, not with the metatarsal head.

Interphalangeal Joints In the lateral four toes, the interphalangeal joints accommodate heads and bases of associated phalanges as do the MTP joints. The joints are supported by a joint capsule that is reinforced dorsally by the extensor tendons, medially and laterally by collateral ligaments, and inferiorly by the plantar plate covering the plantar surface of the joints. Sesamoid bones, when present, are an integral part of the plantar plate.

Plantar Aponeurosis

Dense fibrous connective tissue on the sole of the foot consists of plantar fascia with the thickest central portion, the plantar aponeurosis, originating at the medial and lateral tuberosities of the calcaneus and passing anteriorly to split into five fibrous bands that attach to the digits in the following manner: each splits at the level of the corresponding MTP joint, to allow passage of the short and long plantar flexor tendons, and attaches at both sides of these joints and their ligaments. From the margins of the plantar aponeurosis, vertical septa extend deeply to form the three compartments (medial, central, and lateral) of the sole of the foot. Inferior to the metatarsal heads, fascial fibers running transversely form the superficial transverse metatarsal ligament, which blends with the aponeurosis. The relationship between the MTP joints and the plantar aponeurosis is described as resembling a "windlass mechanism." A windlass is a cylinder that rotates by a crank to pull on a chain or rope that wraps around the cylinder, such as to lift a heavy anchor or raise a bucket from a well. The distal connection of the plantar aponeurosis to the MTP joints is such that when the MTP joints extend, the plantar aponeurosis becomes taut, pulling the MTP bones and tarsal bones together and causing a rise in the longitudinal arches (Fig. 9-9). This plantar aponeurotic support is reinforced by the contraction of intrinsic and extrinsic muscles. This windlass mechanism can be seen with passive extension of the 1st MTP joint.

Relationships and Palpation by Region

Medial Aspect The medial malleolus is easily palpated and observed as a large prominence medially. Just inferior to the medial malleolus, the sustentaculum tali can be felt, especially if the rearfoot is held in an everted position. Superficial portions of the deltoid ligament can be palpated in this region as it passes from the malleolus to the navicular, talus, and calcaneus. The tendons of the tibialis posterior, flexor digitorum longus, and flexor hallucis longus muscles pass behind the medial malleolus just deep to the flexor retinaculum. The tibialis posterior is the most anterior of these and can be visualized and palpated when plantar flexion and inversion are performed against slight resistance. Posterior to the tibialis posterior tendon is the flexor digitorum longus tendon, which is less prominent. Palpation of the flexor digitorum is facilitated by providing some resistance to toe flexion. The flexor hallucis longus tendon is deeper and runs farther posteriorly; it is not usually palpable. Between

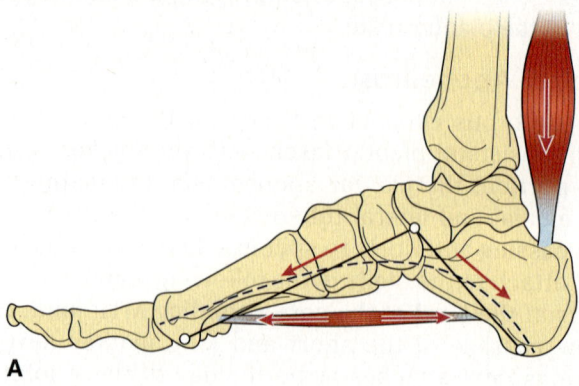

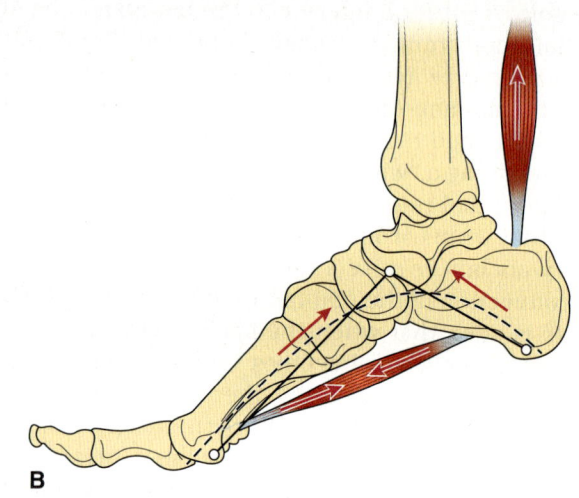

FIGURE 9-9 Windlass mechanism. **A.** Great toe neutral. **B.** Great toe extended. (Adapted from Gest TR. *Lippincott Atlas of Anatomy*. 2nd ed. Wolters Kluwer; 2020: Plate 3-41A.)

the flexor digitorum and flexor hallucis longus tendons runs the posterior tibial artery. Its pulse is palpable behind the malleolus. The tibial nerve, which usually cannot be palpated, runs deep and posterior to the artery.

The navicular tubercle, a prominent bone on the medial aspect of the medial longitudinal arch of the foot, can be palpated by moving anterior and inferior to the medial malleolus. The medial aspect of the talar head can be palpated as a less prominent bony landmark by everting the rearfoot. The spring ligament can be palpated as it fills the gap between the sustentaculum tali and the inferior margin of the posterior articular surface of the navicular.

Palpating farther distally along the medial side of the foot, the 1st tarsometatarsal joint can be felt, in particular the outflaring of the base of the 1st metatarsal bone. From the joint, one should probe distally along the medial shaft of the 1st metatarsal bone to the articulation with the proximal phalanx of the great toe. The 1st MTP joint is the site of the common pathologic condition, HV (also called a bunion), characterized by lateral deviation of the great toe.

Dorsal Aspect At the level of the malleoli, the anterior aspects of the distal ends of the tibia and fibula can be felt. The junction of the two bones, at the syndesmosis, can usually be distinguished, although it is considerably obscured by the distal tibiofibular ligament that overlies it. With the foot relaxed in some degree of plantar flexion, the dorsal aspect of the talar neck can be felt just distal to the end of the tibia. With the foot held inverted and plantar-flexed, the anterolateral aspect of the articular surface of the talus can be easily felt just distal and somewhat lateral to the syndesmosis. The dorsal aspect of the navicular bone can be palpated between the dorsal aspect of the talar neck and the medial cuneiform, which is the most prominent aspect of the dorsum of the foot farther distally.

The intermediate and lateral cuneiform may be felt distal to the dorsal surface of the navicular. The cuboid can be palpated by moving laterally from the lateral cuneiform or proximally from the styloid process at the base of the 5th metatarsal. By moving distally on the dorsum of the foot, the metatarsals and the phalangeal joints of each toe may be palpated.

Running along the medial side of the dorsum of the ankle is the tendon of the tibialis anterior, which is the most prominent tendon crossing the dorsal aspect of the foot and made especially prominent by resisting inversion and dorsiflexion of the foot. It attaches to the medial aspect of the base of the 1st metatarsal. Just lateral to the tibialis anterior tendon, the extensor hallucis longus tendon can easily be seen and palpated as the subject extends the big toe. Lateral to the extensor hallucis longus tendon, passing distally from where it emerges at the ankle, is the dorsalis pedis artery; the pulse can best be palpated over the dorsum of the foot, at about the level of the navicular and medial cuneiform bones. Farther laterally, the common tendon of the extensor digitorum longus is seen and felt when the subject extends the toes; the four branches can be distinguished where they develop, just distal to the ankle, and each palpated as they pass toward their distal attachments. If the subject everts and dorsiflexes the foot, the tendon of the fibularis tertius is usually observable just proximal to its insertion at the dorsum of the base of the 5th metatarsal. On the lateral side of the foot dorsum, the thin muscle bellies of the extensor hallucis and extensor digitorum brevii can be palpated when the toes are extended. Returning to the area between the medial and lateral malleoli, one may follow the crest of the tibia superiorly while palpating the muscles of the lateral compartment (fibularii and posterior tibialis) and anterior compartment (tibialis anterior and long extensors).

Lateral Aspect The lateral malleolus lies subcutaneously and is easily palpated. Just distal to the tip of the lateral malleolus the fairly flat lateral aspect of the calcaneus can be felt throughout its extent. A small prominence, the fibular tubercle, can be palpated. The CFL attaches to the tubercle, whereas the fibularis brevis tendon passes superiorly and the fibularis longus passes inferiorly.[27] Some resistance should be applied to plantar flexion and eversion of the foot when palpating the fibularii tendons. The distal fibular retinaculum, which holds the fibular tendons in place, may be palpated in this area.

Just distal, and slightly anterior, to the lateral malleolus, a rather marked depression can be felt if the foot is relaxed; this is the lateral opening of the sinus tarsi. Traversing the lateral aspect of the sinus tarsi are the inferior bands of the extensor retinaculum and the cervical talocalcaneal ligament. If the palpating finger is moved dorsally and slightly superiorly from the sinus tarsi, the lateral aspect of the neck of the talus can be felt, where the ATF ligament attaches. The other lateral ligaments (anterior tibiofibular, CFL, PTF, and posterior tibiofibular) and the bifurcate ligament may be palpated at and in the segments between their attachments.

From the sinus tarsi, approximately one finger's width distally, one may palpate the lateral aspect of the cuboid to the styloid process at the base of the 5th metatarsal bone. Proximal to the flare of the styloid one can appreciate the depression of the cuboid and the groove for the fibularis longus tendon as it runs to the medial plantar surface of the foot. As one probes distally along the lateral shaft of the 5th metatarsal to the head, the lateral aspect of the 5th head may demonstrate a prominence if a bunionette deformity, called tailor toe or tailor's bunion, is present.

Posterior Aspect At the posterior aspect of the heel is a prominent crest running horizontally between the upper and lower posterior calcaneal surfaces. The Achilles tendon is quite prominent and is easily seen and felt proximal to its insertion on the posterosuperior surface of the crest. Just proximal and anterior to the insertion of the Achilles tendon is a triangular fat pad named Kager triangle.[28] Palpation of the posterior aspect of the talus is obscured by the Achilles tendon, which overlies it before inserting on the calcaneus.

Though not palpable unless inflamed, the retrocalcaneal bursa is located between the calcaneus and Achilles tendon and serves to lubricate and cushion the tendon during propulsion.[29,30]

Plantar Aspect Palpation of the inferior aspect of the calcaneus is made difficult by the thick skin and fat pad that cover it to provide a distribution of load during weight bearing.[31] The medial tubercle may be distinguished posteriorly in some individuals. The long and short plantar ligaments and the spring ligament are difficult to differentiate in palpation of the plantar aspect of the foot. The long plantar ligament passes from the plantar surface of the calcaneus to the cuboid, with some of its fibers continuing to the bases of the metatarsals forming a tunnel for the fibularis longus tendon. The short plantar ligament extends from the anterior aspect of the inferior calcaneus to the cuboid and is located between the long plantar and spring ligaments. The intrinsic foot muscles and plantar aponeurosis should be palpated for tenderness and nodules.[32,33] Maintaining extension of the toes will facilitate palpation. Superficial nodules in the central or medial bands of the plantar aponeurosis may be a manifestation of plantar fibromatosis, a benign fibroblastic disorder.[34,35] Nodules on the ball of the foot, particularly in non–weight-bearing areas, may be plantar warts.[36]

Medially, on the plantar aspect of the 1st metatarsal, one may identify and palpate the two sesamoid bones just proximal to the head of the 1st metatarsal. This may be facilitated by extending the big toe. In a similar fashion, the heads of the remaining four toes are palpated, and while doing so, it should be determined whether any are disproportionately prominent. If one is more prominent, it may bear an unaccustomed amount of weight, characterized by excessive calluses as a result of increased pressure. The various causes of plantar keratoses are numerous, and a significant differential diagnosis exists that needs to be taken into account when evaluating the patient.[37]

BIOMECHANICS OF ANKLE-FOOT COMPLEX

Structural Relationships

The structural relationships and movement at the ankle and rearfoot are complex. The joints of the foot and ankle constitute the first movable pivots in the weight-bearing extremity once the foot becomes fixed to the ground. Considered together, these joints must permit mobility in all planes to allow for minimal displacement of a person's center of gravity with respect to the base of support when walking over flat or uneven surfaces. In this sense, maintenance of balance and economy of energy consumption are, in part, dependent on proper functioning of the ankle–foot complex. Adequate mobility and proper structural alignment of these joints are also necessary for normal attenuation of forces transmitted from the ground to the weight-bearing extremity. Deviations in alignment and changes in mobility are likely to cause abnormal stresses to the joints of the foot and ankle and to the other weight-bearing joints. It follows that detection of biomechanical alterations in the ankle–foot region is often necessary for adequate interpretation of painful conditions affecting the foot and ankle, as well as conditions affecting the knee, hip, or lower spine.

In the normal standing position, the patella faces straight forward, the knee joint axis lies in the frontal plane, and the tibial tubercle is in line with the midline or lateral half of the patella. In this position, a line passing between the tips of the malleoli should make an angle of about 20 to 25° with the frontal plane,[2] representing the normal amount of external tibial torsion. Because the lateral malleolus is positioned inferiorly with respect to the medial malleolus such that the intermalleolar line makes an angle of about 10° with the transverse plane,[38] the joint axis of the ankle mortise corresponds approximately to the intermalleolar line. With the patellae facing straight forward, the feet should be pointed outward about 5 to 10°.

If, when the feet are in normal standing alignment, the patellae face inward (described as "squinting"), increased femoral anteversion, increased lateral tibial torsion, or both may be present. Clinically, the fault can be differentiated by assessing rotational range of motion of the hips and estimating the degree of tibial torsion by assessing the thigh–foot angle.[4] In the presence of increased hip anteversion, the total range of hip transverse plane motion will be normal but skewed such that internal rotation is excessive and external rotation is restricted proportionally. Similar considerations hold for a situation in which the patellae face outward (described as "frog eye") when the feet are normally aligned; femoral retroversion, medial tibial torsion, or both are likely to exist.

With respect to the frontal plane, normal knee alignment may vary from slight genu valgum to some degree of genu varum. Because in most persons the medial femoral condyle extends farther distally than the lateral condyle, slight genu valgum tends to be more prevalent. The rearfoot should be positioned vertically relative to the leg. A valgus or varus heel can usually be observed as a bowing of the Achilles tendon. A valgus positioning of the rearfoot is associated with pronation at the subtalar joint, whereas a varus rearfoot involves supination.

Terminology of Ankle–Foot Motions

Terminology-related motions at the ankle–foot complex of the body differ from standard descriptions. Throughout this chapter the following definitions will be used:

- Inversion/eversion: Movement about an anterior/posterior axis lying in the sagittal plane. Functionally, pure inversion and eversion rarely occur at any of the joints of the ankle or foot. More often they occur as a component of supination or pronation.
- Abduction/adduction: Movement of the forefoot about a vertical axis.
- Internal/external rotation: Movement between the leg and foot occurring about a vertical axis. Pure rotations do not occur functionally but rather occur as components of pronation and supination.
- Plantar flexion/dorsiflexion: Movement about a medial/lateral axis lying in the plane corresponding to the intermalleolar line. Functionally, these movements usually occur in conjunction with other movements.
- Pronation/supination: Functional movements occurring around the obliquely situated subtalar or midtarsal joint axis. At both of these joints, pronation involves abduction, eversion, and some dorsiflexion; supination involves adduction, inversion, and plantar flexion of the distal segment on the proximal segment. This is because these joint axes are declined posteriorly, inferiorly, and laterally.
- Pronated foot/supinated foot: Traditionally, a pronated foot (in the standing position) is one in which the medial longitudinal arch is reduced; the rearfoot is pronated and the forefoot is relatively supinated. In a supinated foot (in the standing position) the arch is high, the rearfoot is supinated, and the forefoot is relatively pronated.
- Valgus/varus: Terms used for frontal plane alignment of segments. Valgus denotes inclination away from the midline of a segment with respect to its proximal neighbor, whereas varus is inclination toward the midline.

Ankle Complex

The talocrural, subtalar, and midtarsal joints that compose the ankle complex represent articulations of varying shapes and orientations that allow the movements of dorsiflexion/plantar flexion in the sagittal plane, abduction/adduction in the transverse plane, and eversion/inversion in the frontal plane, resulting in triplanar motions described as pronation and supination, respectively. Although all components of pronation/supination occur at these joints, some components predominate at particular joints. The predominant motion of the talocrural joint is dorsiflexion/plantar flexion, whereas the subtalar joint permits primarily inversion/eversion and abduction/adduction. All component motions are equally represented in movement at the midtarsal joint. The path of motion of the entire foot is impacted by the functional relationship among the joints and surrounding structures of the ankle complex.[39]

Ankle (Talocrural) Joint The primary motion of the ankle joint is 20° of dorsiflexion and 50° of plantar flexion,[40] though large variations exist.[41] The axis of rotation at the talocrural joint is obliquely oriented, passing inferiorly and posteriorly from medial to lateral in the frontal plane. Although changing somewhat throughout the talocrural joint's range of motion,[42,43] the axis runs close to a central point in the trochlea of the talus.[43] The joint axis is inclined approximately 10° in the frontal plane and 6° to the transverse plane (Fig. 9-10).[6,44]

Although the predominate motions are dorsiflexion/plantar flexion, movement at the joint is multiplanar.[45] The shape of the trochlea and the obliquity of the joint axis indicate the joint does not function simply as a hinge. With dorsiflexion, there is a slight abduction and eversion (components of pronation) about the joint axis. Similarly, slight adduction and inversion (components of supination) are demonstrated with plantar flexion. Additionally, internal and external rotation of the tibia and fibula occur simultaneously with the sagittal plane movements of dorsiflexion and plantar flexion, respectively.[46] From a superior view, the trochlea of the talus is shaped like a cone lying on its side, with either end cut off at slightly different angles. The talus is widest anteriorly, such that the tightest fit of the talus in the mortise occurs with weight-bearing dorsiflexion as the tibia rotates over the talus. As the

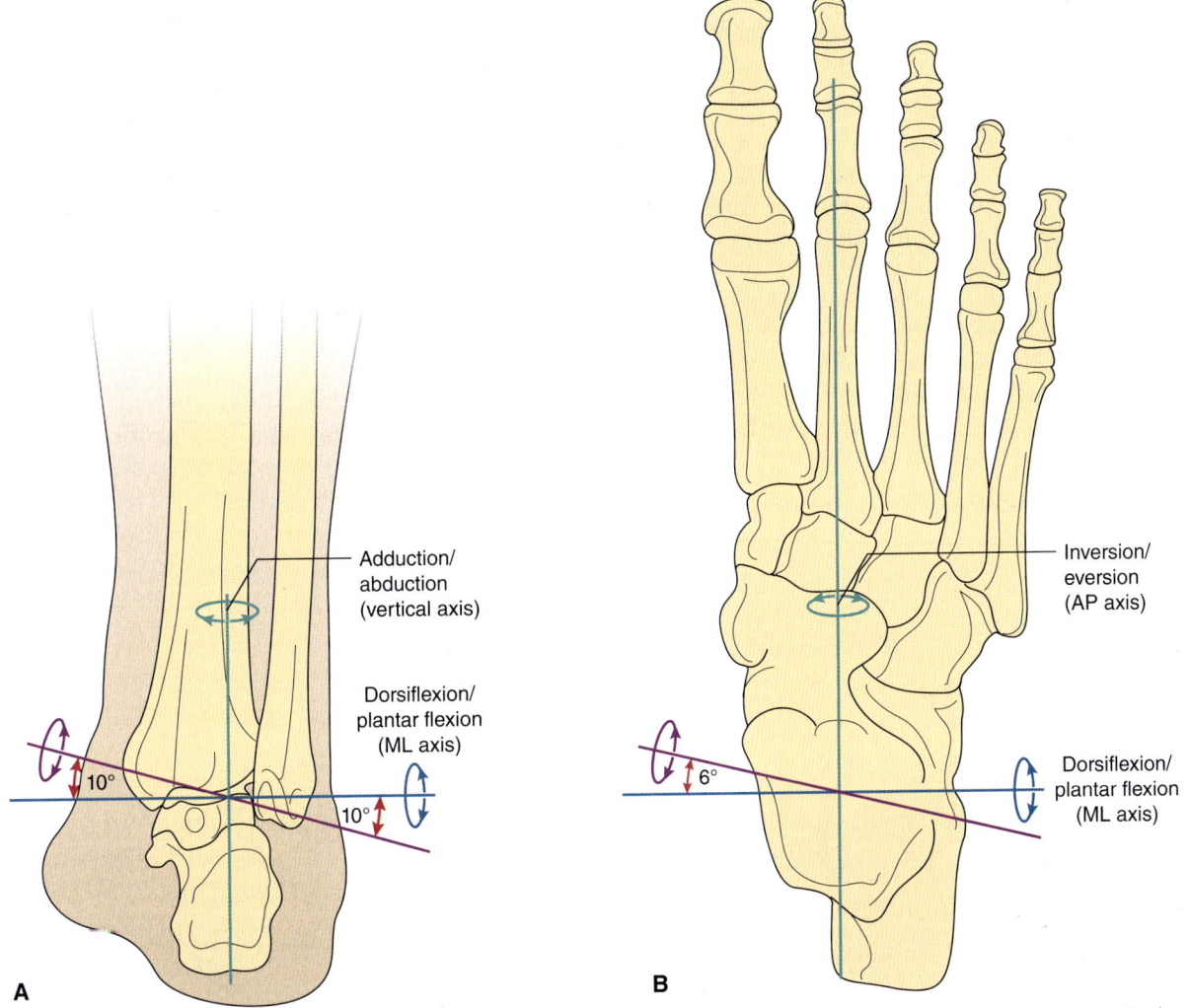

FIGURE 9-10 Talocrural joint axis. **A.** Viewed posteriorly. (Adapted from Gest TR. *Lippincott Atlas of Anatomy*. 2nd ed. Wolters Kluwer; 2020: Plate 3-33.) **B.** Viewed superiorly. (Adapted from Gest TR. *Lippincott Atlas of Anatomy*. 2nd ed. Wolters Kluwer; 2020: Plate 3-40A.) *AP*, anteroposterior; *ML*, mediolateral.

tibia and fibula move together during weight-bearing dorsiflexion, the lateral malleolus undergoes greater displacement on the larger, more obliquely oriented lateral talar facet than does the tibial malleolus on the medial talar facet,[47–49] influencing lower leg rotation during movement.

At the beginning of the gait cycle at initial contact, the talocrural joint plantar flexes to lower the rest of the foot to the ground. When the foot is flat, the leg begins to rotate forward (dorsiflex) over the planted foot until the heel rises. During this dorsiflexion phase, the talocrural joint is stabilized by the collateral ligaments, tension in the ankle plantar flexors, and bony articulation as the talar head is wedged within the ankle mortise. As push-off is initiated, the dorsiflexed talocrural joint is in its stable, close-packed position.

In the open kinetic chain, such as would be used in many joint mobilization techniques, the talus rolls and slides within the talocrural mortise following the convex–concave pattern of movement. With dorsiflexion, the talus rolls anteriorly and slides posteriorly (Fig. 9-11A). With plantar flexion, the talus rolls posteriorly and slides anteriorly (Fig. 9-11B).

Subtalar Joint The subtalar joint axis is obliquely oriented passing from the posterolateral calcaneus in an anterosuperior and medial direction, passing through the talar neck.[2] Substantial variability in reported outcomes exists in the literature regarding the precise axis of the subtalar joint.[6,50] Some studies describe motion around one axis,[51,52] whereas others describe motion as occurring around multiple axes.[53–55]

Despite the differing methodologies, the general location and direction of the axis are similarly reported at about 40 to 45° from the horizontal plane and 16 to 25° medial to the long axis of the foot (Fig. 9-12).[2,5,6,50,51,53,56,57]

The motions of pronation and supination occur in an arc perpendicular to the axis of rotation. Because of the degree of obliquity of the subtalar joint axis, the inversion/eversion and adduction/abduction components of pronation and supination are most evident.[43,51,53] That is, at the subtalar joint, eversion and abduction are the primary components of pronation, whereas inversion and adduction are the main components of supination.[7]

In weight-bearing pronation and supination, such as during the stance phase of gait, pronation and supination occur as the talus and leg move over the relatively fixed calcaneus. With the calcaneus fixed under the load of body weight, a significant portion of pronation and supination involves rotation of the talus in the horizontal plane (abduction/adduction). Because the body of the talus can rotate only minimally within the tight-fitting mortise, rotation of the talus can occur only if the superimposed mortise moves with the talus.[44] That is, rotation of the lower leg accompanies movement of the talus in weight-bearing supination/pronation.[7]

Midtarsal Joint The midtarsal joint represents the functional articulation between the rearfoot (talus and calcaneus) and the midfoot (navicular and cuboid). The medial (talonavicular) articulation of the midtarsal joint resembles a ball-and-socket articulation and allows significant movement, contributing to the mobility of the medial longitudinal arch. The lateral (calcaneocuboid) articulation is saddle-shaped, forming interlocking joint surfaces that resist sliding and contributes to the stability of the lateral longitudinal arch. The naviculocuboid articulation is relatively fixed because of the bony and ligamentous arrangement. The medial and lateral components of the midtarsal

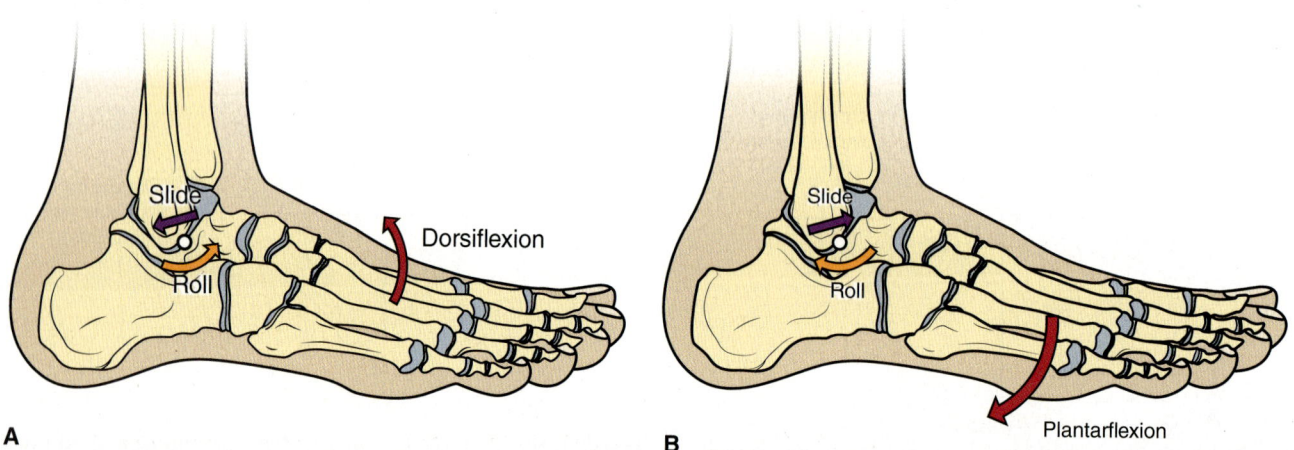

FIGURE 9-11 Talocrural joint accessory motions: roll and glide. **A.** Dorsiflexion. **B.** Plantarflexion. (Adapted from Gest TR. *Lippincott Atlas of Anatomy*. 2nd ed. Wolters Kluwer; 2020: Plate 3-60A.)

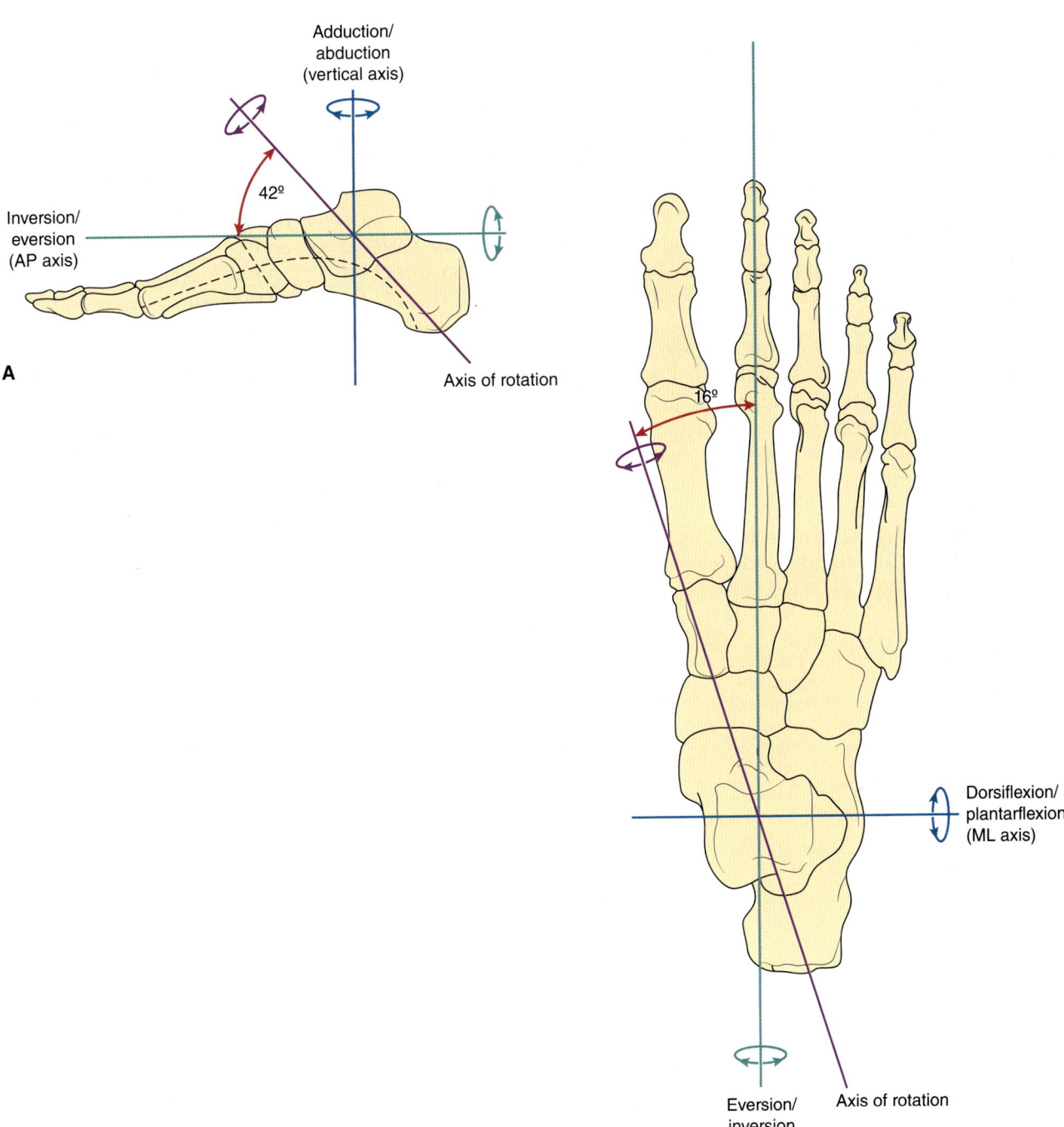

FIGURE 9-12 Subtalar joint axis. **A.** Viewed medially. (Adapted from Gest TR. *Lippincott Atlas of Anatomy*. 2nd ed. Wolters Kluwer; 2020: Plate 3-41A.) **B.** Viewed superiorly. (Adapted from Gest TR. *Lippincott Atlas of Anatomy*. 2nd ed. Wolters Kluwer; 2020: Plate 3-40A.) *AP*, anteroposterior; *ML*, mediolateral.

joint move together, such that movement at one is accompanied by movement at the other. Movement at the midtarsal joint is synchronous with movement of the subtalar joint. The interrelated movements are complex and remain the subject of intense research.

In classic studies of the midtarsal joint, two axes of rotation are described: the longitudinal and oblique.[6,50,58] The longitudinal axis is inclined superiorly approximately 15° from the transverse plane and angled 9° medially from the sagittal plane, thus closely approximating a true anterior–posterior axis. Though all component motions of pronation/supination are present, the predominant motion is inversion/eversion about the longitudinal axis. The oblique axis is inclined 52° superiorly from the transverse plane and 57° medially from the sagittal plane (Fig. 9-13). About the oblique axis, the coupled motions of abduction/dorsiflexion and adduction/plantar flexion predominate over inversion/eversion. Though described separately here, the functional movements are blended across both axes, demonstrating all components of pronation and supination.[59] Although the range of motion at the midtarsal joint is difficult to quantify and isolate from the adjacent joints, the total range of pronation/supination at the midtarsal joint is about twice that of the subtalar joint.[6,44]

The linkage between the subtalar and midtarsal joints is such that when the subtalar joint moves into supination, the midtarsal joint moves in the same direction—into supination. Likewise, pronation of the subtalar joint results in pronation of the midtarsal joint. The summation of the component movements across the subtalar and midtarsal joints allows the foot to accommodate greater variability in changes with the terrain during standing and walking.

A study of arthrokinematics of the midtarsal joint requires an initial separate investigation of its two components: the talonavicular and calcaneocuboid joints. Movement at the talonavicular joint involves the distal concave navicular moving on the more proximal convex talus. Following the convex/concave pattern of movement, as the navicular rolls on the talus, it slides in the same direction. The calcaneocuboid articular surfaces are saddle-shaped. In a flexion/extension direction, the cuboid is concave, much like the navicular, and the articulating convex surface of the calcaneus is much like the convex surface of the talus. As such, the roll and slide for the talonavicular and calcaneocuboid joints are the same for dorsiflexion and plantar flexion motions. Clinicians mobilizing the midtarsal joint have the option of mobilizing the midtarsal joints together as one or individually to achieve the same outcomes. For motion in abduction/adduction, the cuboid is convex and the calcaneus is concave; therefore, roll and slide are in opposite directions. The close-packed position for the midtarsal joint

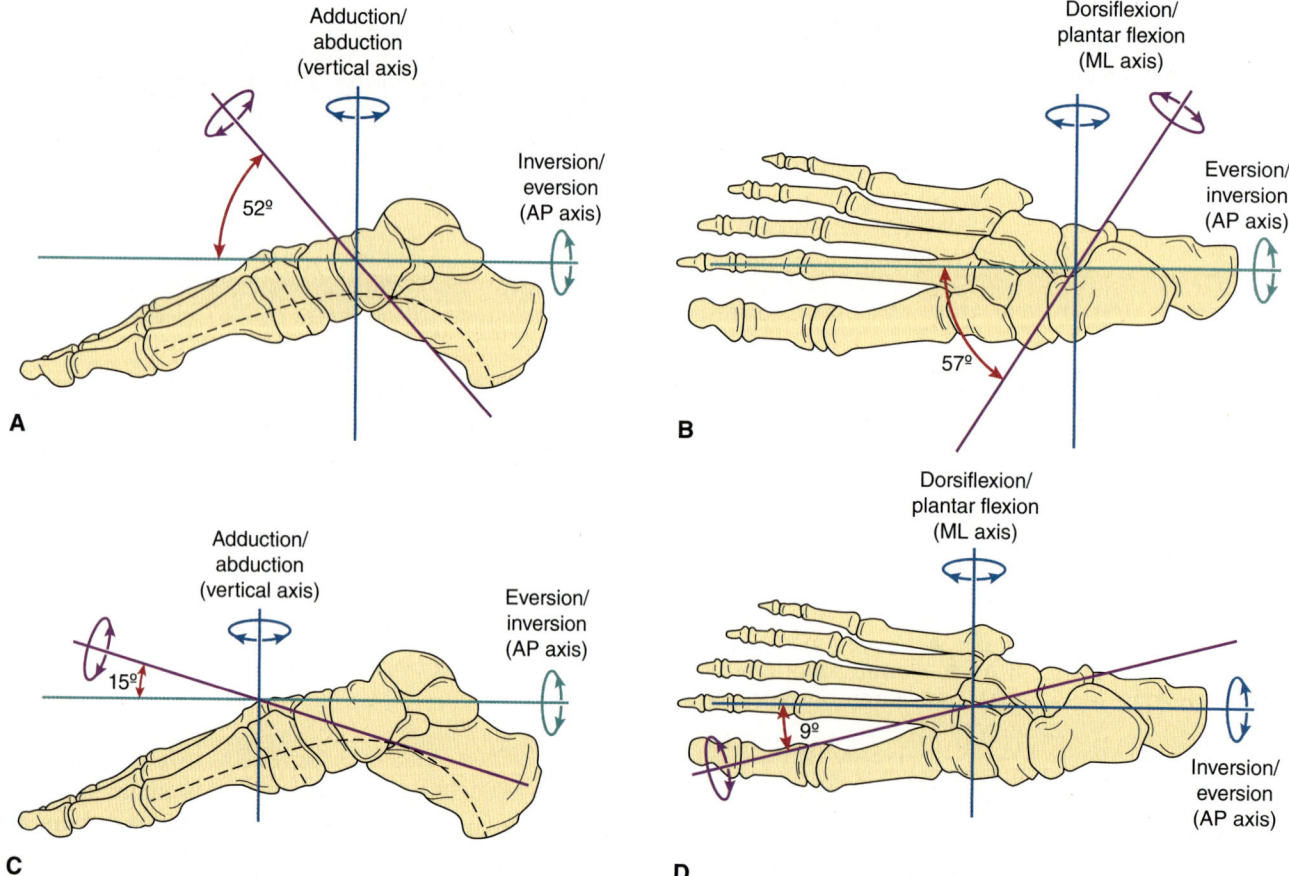

FIGURE 9-13 Midtarsal joint axes: oblique axis (*purple*), longitudinal axis (*green*), vertical axis (**A,C**) and medial-lateral axis (**B,D**) (*blue*). **A.** Viewed medially. **B.** Viewed superiorly. **C.** Viewed medially. **D.** Viewed superiorly. (**A and C:** Adapted from Gest TR. *Lippincott Atlas of Anatomy*. 2nd ed. Wolters Kluwer; 2020: Plate 3-41A. **B and D:** Adapted from Gest TR. *Lippincott Atlas of Anatomy*. 2nd ed. Wolters Kluwer; 2020: Plate 3-40A.) *AP*, anteroposterior; *ML*, mediolateral.

is full supination. In pronation, the individual articulations are more freely movable.

Distal Intertarsal, Tarsometatarsal, Metatarsophalangeal, and Phalangeal Joints

Distal Intertarsal Joints The distal intertarsal joints (cuneonavicular, cuboideonavicular, intercuneiform, and cuneocuboid joints) occupy a part of the midfoot and, as a group, assist the midtarsal joint in pronation and supination of the midfoot. The movement at these joints is small. The transverse arch formed by the distal intertarsal joints contributes to the stability of the midfoot. Though movement is minimal, the intertarsal joints can be moved in dorsal and plantar sliding movements when one bone is stabilized and the adjacent bone is moved.

Tarsometatarsal Joints The tarsometatarsal joints are formed by articulations of the three cuneiforms and the cuboid with the metatarsals. These relatively flat synovial joints allow flexion and extension of the metatarsal bones and a certain degree of supination and pronation (longitudinal axial rotations) of the medial and lateral sides for the forefoot. The 2nd tarsometatarsal joint is the most stable; thus, the 2nd ray, of which the 2nd metatarsal is a part, is used as the reference point for motions of the forefoot. Overall mobility is greatest in the 1st, 4th, and 5th tarsometatarsal joints. Motion of the 1st tarsometatarsal joint includes dorsiflexion (extension) and plantar flexion (flexion), with little inversion/eversion and even less abduction/adduction. The movement of dorsiflexion is combined with slight inversion, and plantar flexion is combined with slight eversion.[60]

Intermetatarsal Joints Similar to the intertarsal joints, dorsal and plantar sliding movements occur when one metatarsal base is stabilized and the adjacent metatarsal base is moved on it. The 1st and 2nd metatarsal bases are interconnected by ligaments, but rarely form a true joint, which increases the relative movement of the 1st ray. The deep transverse metatarsal ligaments interconnecting the heads of the metatarsal bones help limit movement at the intermetatarsal joints.

Metatarsophalangeal and Interphalangeal Joints The five MTP joints allow flexion/extension and abduction/adduction, whereas the interphalangeal joint allows flexion and extension. A large range of extension is required at the MTP joint during the late phase of stance after heel rise. In the weight-bearing foot, toe extension permits the body to pass over the foot while the toes dynamically balance the superimposed body weight as they press into the supporting surface through activity of the toe flexors.

The MTP joints serve primarily to allow the foot to hinge at the toes so that the heel may rise off the ground. This function is enhanced by the effect of MTP extension on the plantar aponeurosis, contributing to the windlass mechanism. The toes participate in weight bearing in giving hold against the ground and in stabilizing the longitudinal arch by tensing the plantar aponeurosis during the push-off phase of the walking cycle.

Weight-bearing forces to the toes are attenuated by the tension in the toe flexor tendons and the tendon sheaths. The interosseous and lumbrical muscles dynamically stabilize the toes on the floor. Failure of these muscles to function accounts for toe deformities such as claw toe. The long flexors of the toes act as plantar flexors of the talocrural joint and invertors of the talocalcaneonavicular joint, whereas the long extensors of the toes act as dorsiflexors of the talocrural joint and evertors of the talocalcaneonavicular joint.

ARCHES OF THE FOOT

The bones of the foot and associated ligaments form three arches: two longitudinal (medial and lateral) arches and the transverse arch. The arches serve several purposes to include absorption of shock during impact with the ground, protection of neurovascular structures and muscles during weight bearing, and improving the efficiency of locomotion. The arches are formed by the tarsal and metatarsal bones and are supported passively by the plantar aponeurosis, long and short plantar ligaments and spring ligament, and dynamically by muscles whose tendons attach in the foot. The longitudinal arches are primarily concave along the length of the foot, with the medial being longer and higher than the lateral. The transverse arch is concave medial to lateral, with the arch disappearing in the normal foot at the heads of the metatarsal bones in standing.

Most of the arching on the medial side of the foot is dependent on static maintenance by the short and long plantar ligaments and dynamic contribution of the anterior and posterior tibialis muscles. In contrast, the lateral longitudinal and transverse arches are more reliant on their bony configurations for support: the lateral longitudinal arch from the wedging of the cuboid between the calcaneus and metatarsals and the transverse arch from the wedge-shaped contours and relationships of the tarsals and metatarsals. This bony support is greatest for the transverse arch, with the keystone being the middle cuneiform.

The arches have been compared to a curved beam supported by a tie-rod, forming a truss to prevent the separation of the ends of the curved beam. The concave plantar surface of the metatarsals resembles a curved beam and the plantar aponeurosis resembles the tie-rod forming the truss. As the metatarsals are loaded during weight-bearing activities, tension builds on the plantar concave surfaces. The plantar aponeurosis becomes taut, allowing acceptance of large forces and supporting the arches of the foot. As stated previously, the plantar aponeurosis is reinforced by intrinsic and extrinsic foot muscles, which provide dynamic support to the arches.

The structure of the foot as a whole has been compared to a twisted plate with the calcaneus, at one end, positioned vertically when contacting the ground and the metatarsal heads positioned horizontally when making contact with a flat surface.[61,62] Thus, in the normal standing position on a flat, level surface, the metatarsal heads are twisted 90° with respect to the calcaneus. To demonstrate this, a model can be constructed by taking a thin rectangular piece of cardboard and twisting it so that one end lies flat on a table and the opposite end is perpendicular to the tabletop. Note the arching of the cardboard. This is analogous to the arching of the human foot. Notice that when the cardboard is allowed to untwist—by changing the inclination of the vertical end in one direction and keeping the other end flat on the table—the arch either flattens (becomes less) or heightens as the twist/untwist will decrease or increase the arch.

In the foot, inclination of the calcaneus will result in similar untwisting or twisting; this results in a respective decrease or increase in the arching of the foot, if the metatarsal heads remain in contact with the ground. The person who stands with the rearfoot in a valgus position will have a relatively flat or untwisted foot, whereas a person who stands with the rearfoot in a varus position will appear to have a high arch because of increased twisting between rearfoot and forefoot. The former situation is often termed a pronated foot or pes planus (flatfoot), and the latter is termed a supinated foot or pes cavus (arched foot). In the situation of the rearfoot remaining in a vertical position but the metatarsal heads inclined, as on an uneven surface, the effect will also be to twist or untwist the foot, thereby raising or lowering the arch, allowing the foot to accommodate to the uneven terrain.

INTRODUCTION TO THE EXAMINATION OF THE ANKLE AND FOOT

The foot has four basic functions.[63] First, the foot serves as a base of support for gait and other activities. Second, it must be able to adapt to changes in the support surface. For example, when walking on the left side of a typical road, a person's right limb requires increased pronation range, whereas the left requires less. Third, the foot must serve as a torque converter, altering motion of the primarily sagittal plane motion of the hip, knee, and ankle into the frontal and transverse planes of the subtalar and midtarsal joints. Last, the foot must be able to function as a rigid lever for effective push-off during gait.

The common lesions affecting the ankle are of generally acute, traumatic onset, whereas those affecting the foot are more likely to be chronic disorders resulting from stress overload. The biomechanical interdependency of the weight-bearing joints (discussed in Chapter 8, Lower Quarter Screen) necessitates attention to the structure and function of more proximally situated joints, particularly when examining patients with chronic or subtle foot disorders. Similarly, examination of the ankle and foot may well be in order for patients with disorders affecting more proximal regions.

Dysfunction in proximal segments, such as the L4, L5, S1, and S2 region, commonly refers to the ankle and foot, perhaps the most common being paresthesias arising from the lumbar spine. Pain arising from tissues of the foot or ankle may be referred to a short distance proximally but almost never to the knee or above.

PATIENT HISTORY: ANKLE AND FOOT JOINT

A patient interview designed to elicit specific information related to the patient's health history and demographics, symptoms, and review of systems should be conducted (refer to Chapter 6, Patient History). Given that the foot functions in a closed kinetic chain a large portion of the time, clinicians must specifically ask the patient to discuss any prior foot, ankle, knee, or hip injuries or surgeries on either extremity. The clinician must understand the patient's symptoms and determine the acuity, severity, irritability, stability, and functional implications of the patient's condition. The following are general concepts that apply to information that may be elicited when interviewing patients with common foot or ankle disorders. Limb dominance may be applicable for athletes, particularly in certain sports, such as soccer or golf.

If the condition is of an acute, traumatic onset, an attempt should be made to determine the exact mechanism of injury. Plantar flexion–inversion stresses are more likely to result in capsuloligamentous injury, whereas forces moving the foot into dorsiflexion and external rotation (abduction) are more likely to produce a fracture. A traumatic injury may involve injury to multiple structures, such as ligament, muscle, articular cartilage, and bone. If the disorder is of a more chronic nature and of insidious onset, the clinician should attempt to determine whether a change in activity level may be associated with the onset of the problem. Chronic stress overload (fatigue) disorders may be caused by an abnormal stress on normal tissue where the rate of tissue breakdown exceeds the rate of

TABLE 9-3
FOOT STRUCTURE

Landmark	Pronated Foot	Supinated Foot
Calcaneus	Inverted	Everted
Talar bulge	Present	Absent
Navicular tuberosity	Closer to the support surface	Elevated
Medial longitudinal arch	Flattened	Prominent arch

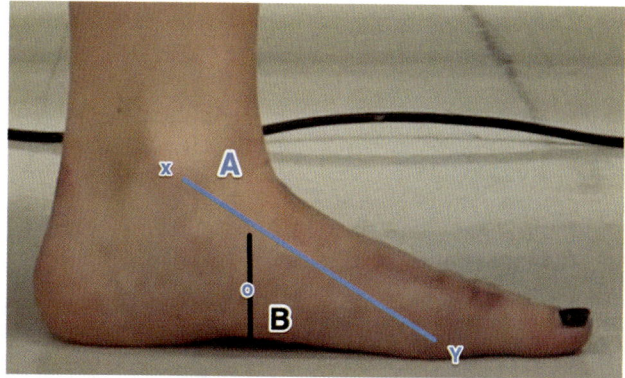

FIGURE 9-15 Feiss line (A), medial malleolus (X), plantar aspect of the first metatarsophalangeal joint (Y), line perpendicular to the floor through the navicular head (B).

position of plantar flexion, inversion, and adduction. A supple or mobile flatfoot will have signs of excessive pronation in standing but will take on a more normal configuration in sitting with the force of weight bearing relieved. In contrast, a fixed or structural flatfoot will maintain its planus (untwisted or flat) state in both weight bearing and non–weight bearing.

Feiss line (Fig. 9-15) may also be used to assess for a pronated foot.[72] A line is drawn connecting the medial malleolus with the plantar aspect of the first metatarsophalangeal joint with the patient in a relaxed calcaneal stance position. In a neutral foot, the navicular head should fall on or near this line. A line is drawn through the navicular head and perpendicular to the floor. If the navicular head is more than one third of the distance to the floor, the patient has a pronated or flat foot. Therefore, because the navicular head lies roughly half way between the Feiss line and the floor, the patient in Figure 9-15 has a pronated foot.

Hyperpronation, regardless of the cause, leads to hypermobility of the midtarsal joint and the 1st ray, increased 2nd ray weight bearing, increased shearing forces on the foot, and greater demand on the plantar ligaments of the foot and the foot intrinsic muscles to create a rigid lever for push-off. The effects of hyperpronation are not limited to the foot. In the closed kinetic chain, excessive pronation leads to increased tibial internal rotation, knee flexion and adduction, as well as increased hip internal rotation. Limited pronation, or excessive supination, leads to a more rigid foot, preventing normal shock absorption and increasing the risk of bone stress injuries. Patients who supinate excessively may develop callusing on the plantar posterolateral heel. Following this up the kinetic chain, supination leads to tibial external rotation, knee extension, and hip external rotation.

The clinician should note deformities such as claw toes, hammertoes, and varus–valgus deviations (Fig. 9-16). Claw toes are usually associated with a pes cavus deformity (high-arched foot) and may accompany certain neurologic disorders. The MTP joints are positioned in extension and the interphalangeal joints in flexion. Contracture of the long toe extensors causes extension of the toes, which increases the passive tension on the long toe flexors. The intrinsic muscles are

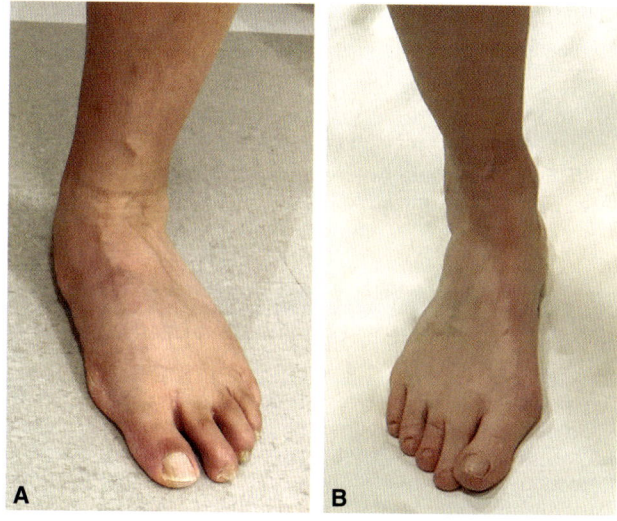

FIGURE 9-16 Toe deformities. **A.** Claw toe (3rd digit) and mallet toe (2nd digit). **B.** Hallux valgus with overlapped 2nd toe.

overbalanced, both actively and passively, by these muscle groups. Hammertoes are a result of capsular contracture of the proximal interphalangeal joints placing the involved joint in some degree of flexion. Typically, there is hyperextension of the MTP joint and distal interphalangeal joints and flexion of the proximal interphalangeal joint. Hammertoes are most often seen in the 2nd toe, although occasionally the 3rd toe is involved. The hyperextension of the MTP joints of claw toes and hammertoes results in increased pressure under the metatarsal heads. Both these deformities are frequently seen in RA.[65] Mallet toe is a flexion deformity of the distal interphalangeal joint. The MTP joint and proximal interphalangeal joints usually are normal. There is usually a callus formation under the tip of the toe or a deformity of the nail.

Tailor bunions (bunionette deformity) are caused by irritation and pressure of the 5th metatarsal head. There may be an overlapping 5th toe or digiti quinti

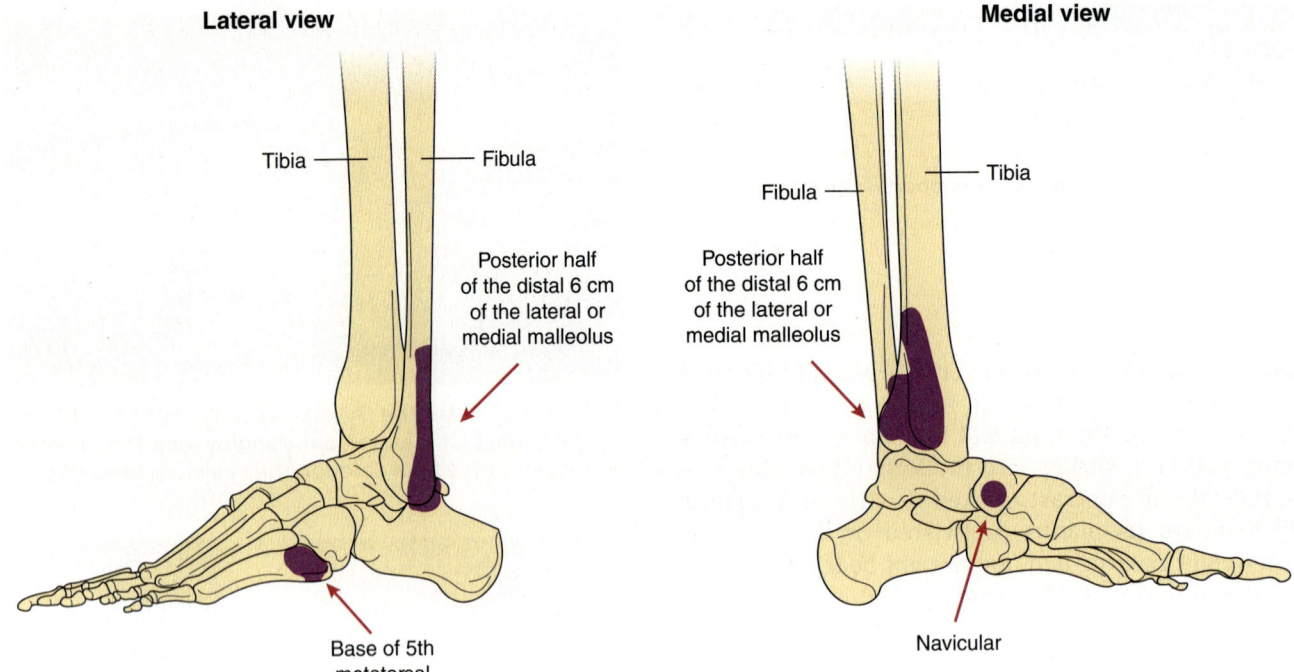

FIGURE 9-14 Ottawa Ankle Rules. (Adapted from Gest TR. *Lippincott Atlas of Anatomy*. 2nd ed. Wolters Kluwer; 2020: Plates 3-41A, B and 3-60A, B.)

TABLE 9-2	
CLINICAL ASSESSMENT GUIDELINE FOR DEEP VEIN THROMBOSIS (DVT)	
	Points
One point is awarded for each of the following clinical parameters: • Cancer currently or treated for cancer in the past 6 months • Paralysis, paresis, or recent lower extremity immobilization • Recently bed-bound for more than 3 days or major surgery within 1 month • Localized tenderness along the distribution of the deep vein system • Swelling of the entire leg • Calf swelling >3 inches when measured 10 cm below the tibial tuberosity • Pitting edema (greater in the symptomatic leg) • Collateral superficial veins	
Two points are deducted from this score if an alternative diagnosis is as likely or more likely than a DVT.	
Total score	
If total score is 3 or higher, consult physician	

potentially contributing factors have been identified. All components of the joint-specific examination need not be performed on every patient. Like the LQS, the experienced clinician will titrate the joint-specific examination based on the patient's history, presentation, and goals. In practice, the joint-specific examination is organized by position and should proceed from uninvolved (or less involved) to involved side but is presented here by category for aiding conceptualization.

Structure

Observe the patient's general appearance and body structure. Examine the lower extremities for edema or atrophy.

Bony Structure and Alignment Perform a lower quarter structural examination as discussed in Chapter 8, Lower Quarter Screen (see Tables 8-1 and 8-2). Any structural deviations or asymmetries should be noted, and the possible effects on the biomechanics of the ankle and foot considered. When assessing patients with ankle/foot pathology, a more detailed assessment of the foot can be beneficial, particularly with patients with chronic conditions or overuse injuries.

The clinician should examine general configuration of the foot in both non–weight bearing and weight bearing (unless contraindicated). Assess for signs of excessive pronation or supination in weight bearing (Table 9-3). When sitting, the foot should relax into a

- Bony tenderness
  - Posterior half of the distal 6 cm of either malleolus (ankle radiograph)
  - Navicular or base of the 5th metatarsal (foot radiograph)

The Ottawa Ankle Rules has a sensitivity of 99%,[70] so, if negative, a fracture can reasonably be ruled out. This avoids unnecessary exposure to radiation, cost, and delay of proper treatment.

If based on the history or systems review a DVT is suspected, the clinician should utilize a clinical assessment guideline (Table 9-2).[71] Patients scoring 3 or more should be considered to have a high probability of DVT and referred for additional medical assessment.

Once the patient has been cleared of any red flags and the history and systems review have been performed, the clinician should perform a lower quarter screen (LQS) and a clearing examination (in this case active and passive knee flexion and extension) to ensure that the area of pathology has been narrowed down to the ankle/foot region and any proximal

TABLE 9-1

COMMON OUTCOME TOOLS FOR PATIENTS WITH ANKLE/FOOT PATHOLOGIES

Tool	Tool Basics
Lower Extremity Function Scale (LEFS)	• Covers global lower extremity function • Scoring: 0-80 • 20 items rated 0-4 with higher scores indicating greater function • MDC* 9 points • May have a ceiling effect for higher functioning individuals • Common diagnoses: total knee/hip replacement, anterior cruciate ligament reconstruction, lower extremity fracture
Foot and Ankle Ability Measure (FAAM)	• Scoring: 0-100% function • 2 subscales: ADL (21 items) and Sports (8 items) • Scored 0-4 with higher scores indicating greater function • Total score for each section generally reported as a percentage of function • 9 items specifically relating to walking abilities • MDC* 5.7 points for ADL, 12.3 for Sports • Common diagnoses: various foot and ankle musculoskeletal disorders
Foot and Ankle Disability Index (FADI) and FADI Sport	• Scoring: 0-104 • 26 items rated 0-4 with higher scores indicating worse function • Generally reported as a percentage with higher scores indicating greater dysfunction • Items are similar to LEFS but also include 4 items regarding pain levels • FADI Sport contains 8 items • MDC* 4.5 points, FADI Sport MDC 6.4 points • Common diagnoses: ankle sprains
Foot Function Index (FFI)	• Scoring: 0-100% • 23 items in 3 subscales (pain, disability, activity limitations) rated 0-10 with higher scores indicating worse function • MDC* 2.4 points • Common diagnoses: plantar fasciopathy, ankle sprain, metatarsalgia, rheumatoid arthritis, ankle/foot fracture
Victorian Institute of Sports Assessment-Achilles (VISA-A)	• Scoring: 0-100, commonly reported as a percentage • 8 items in 3 domains: pain, ADL, sports rated 0-10 with higher scores indicating greater function • MDC* 18.5 points • Common diagnoses: Achilles tendinopathy
Cumberland Ankle Instability Tool (CAIT)	• Scoring: 0-30 • 9 items rated variously from −3 to +5 with higher scores indicating greater function • Cutoff of ankle instability for ankle instability is <27.5 • MDC* 7.6% • Common diagnoses: ankle sprain

ADL, activities of daily living; MDC, minimal detectable change.
*MDC may differ for various subpopulations and is provided for a global frame of reference.
Adapted from Shirley Ryan Ability Lab. Rehabilitations Measures Database. Accessed December 15, 2020. Vuurberg G, Kluit L, van Dijk CN. The Cumberland Ankle Instability Tool (CAIT) in the Dutch population with and without complaints of ankle instability. *Knee Surg Sports Traumatol Arthrosc.* 2018;26(3):882–891. Hiller CE, Refshauge KM, Bundy AC, Herbert RD, Kilbreath SL. The Cumberland Ankle Instability Tool: a report of validity and reliability testing. *Arch Phys Med Rehabil.* 2006;87(9):1235–1241.

repair and the tissue gradually fatigues. For example, a sedentary individual who initiates a running program by running 5 miles daily for the first month is likely underprepared for this dramatic increase in stress to the tissues with no time for recovery. Tissues may also be overloaded with normal activity levels if there is a structural or biomechanical abnormality. For example, without proper footwear, a patient with suboptimal bony alignment, such as forefoot varus or ligamentous laxity, will require increased foot intrinsic strength and endurance. With prolonged walking, this can cause intrinsic muscle fatigue, added tension to the plantar ligaments, and ultimately may lead to pain. Small amounts of stress over a period of time may induce tissue hypertrophy. The body may respond by laying down an excessive amount of tissue in an attempt to strengthen itself against these abnormal stresses. Tissue hypertrophy, such as corns and calluses, may, in itself, lead to pain by allowing localized areas of stress concentration.

The effect of footwear on the patient's condition must be ascertained (refer to Chapter 5, Gait and Footwear). For example, a clinician should determine the effect of variations in heel height and whether the problem is affected, for better or for worse, by going barefoot. Footwear may provide support for the twisted or arched configuration of the foot to varying degrees. Footwear with a high heel causes the toes to extend when standing with the feet in contact with the ground. This raises the arch by tightening the plantar aponeurosis that extends proximally to the MTP joints. Wearing footwear with a higher heel also decreases the passive tension on the Achilles tendon complex. Shoes with a contoured base of support for the foot may help optimize foot contact area and distribute weight-bearing stresses. Proper footwear contouring also minimizes the amount of tension that needs to be developed by the passive and active support systems of the foot.

The clinician should investigate non-musculoskeletal systems that can create ankle/foot symptoms. Complaints of cramping in the presence of muscular fatigue are usually associated with some biomechanical disturbance. However, cramping may also accompany intermittent claudication from arterial insufficiency. Claudication should always be suspected when the patient relates a history of pain or cramping of the lower leg, or sometimes the feet, after walking some distance, but the pain is relieved shortly after stopping this activity. Complaints of calf fatigue may also be the result of chronic venous insufficiency. In such a case, the patient may have leg swelling or skin changes, such as hemosiderin deposition. Case reports in the literature have noted that even a condition as seemingly straightforward as a calf strain requires careful clinician assessment for the possibility of a deep vein thrombosis (DVT).[64]

The clinician should consider the potential for systemic disease processes to cause or exacerbate ankle and foot conditions. Peripheral neuropathy, as a consequence of diabetes or idiopathic, can cause sensory, motor, or autonomic dysfunctions affecting the foot. For these individuals, symptoms may occur as paresthesias or a painless, progressive decrease in function. Likewise, there is an extremely high lifetime risk of foot problems in individuals with rheumatoid arthritis (RA).[65] Other systemic conditions, such as gout, frequently involve the hallux, with hallux pain being the first presenting sign in many cases. Therefore, gout should be considered for patients presenting with a red, painful, and swollen 1st MTP joint even if the patient has no history of the condition.[66] Sickle cell disease and osteomyelitis may also result in ankle and foot pain. Complex regional pain syndrome may occur after a rather inconsequential ankle sprain.[67-69] Without proper medical management, patients with systemic conditions are unlikely to attain optimal results. Therefore, interprofessional communication and collaboration are crucial.

Chapter 6, Patient History, introduced the use of common outcome tools. Although the Patient-Specific Functional Scale and the Global Rating of Change might be applicable to any patient population, clinicians should choose outcome tools specific to the lower extremity (e.g., the Lower Extremity Function Scale or LEFS) or tools that are specific to the ankle and foot. Table 9-1 provides an introduction to commonly used outcome tools for individuals with ankle and foot pathologies.

PHYSICAL EXAMINATION OF THE ANKLE AND FOOT

As noted earlier in the text, the physical examination is composed of the systems review, the quarter screen, the clearing examination, and the joint-specific examination. However, the clinician must first be alert to any potential red flags, such as a fracture or DVT. Foot and ankle fractures can result from minor trauma, such as stepping in a hole, athletic participation, such as landing awkwardly from a jump or contact with another player, or from massive trauma, such as motor vehicle accidents or falls from a height. If the patient history raises suspicion for fracture, the clinician should proceed directly to using the Ottawa Ankle Rules to determine if radiographs are warranted. According to the Ottawa Ankle Rules (Fig. 9-14), ankle or foot radiographs are warranted if there is a history of trauma and:

- Inability to take at least four steps both immediately after injury and at the place of examination
  or

varus deformity. Digiti quinti varus is often congenital. HV is the most common deformity of the 1st MTP joint. HV is a lateral deviation of the proximal phalanx and medial deviation of the 1st metatarsal. It may be associated with a pronated foot and is found most frequently in older women. Note the presence of any bursa over the medial aspect of the 1st MTP joint and whether active inflammatory changes are present. The great toe may be rotated with the toenail pointed inward.

Subtalar Joint Neutral The subtalar joint neutral theory, also known as the foot morphology theory, was first conceptualized by Root et al.[73] in 1971 and has been used as a reference point for normal foot structure and as a basis for orthotic fabrication for decades. The **subtalar joint neutral** theory is a concept that there is a theoretical neutral position of the subtalar joint where the joint is neither pronated nor supinated. Although the measurement of subtalar joint neutral has been shown to be unreliable and there are validity concerns with the use of static foot alignment to predict dynamic foot function, there are no alternate methods currently available.[74] Given the limitations of the subtalar joint neutral theory, clinicians should consider the result of this assessment with some skepticism.

The subtalar joint neutral position can be found in a non–weight-bearing position using the palpation method.

- Have patient prone in a figure 4 position (Fig. 9-17A).
- The clinician's lateral hand should grasp the patient's 4th and 5th ray.
- The clinician should use the thumb and index finger of the medial hand to palpate the medial and lateral talar head, respectively.
- The clinician's lateral hand should invert and evert the foot until the talus is felt equally by the index finger and thumb.
- The clinician should then use the lateral hand to dorsiflex the foot to neutral or until resistance is felt to lock the midfoot.
- The clinician should visually examine the relationship of the calcaneus to the lower leg as well as the calcaneus to the forefoot (Fig. 9-17B).

Alternatively, non–weight-bearing subtalar joint neutral can be found by moving the calcaneus through the arc of inversion and eversion. Subtalar joint neutral is described as the position that is two-thirds of the way to the fully inverted position of the calcaneus.

Subtalar joint neutral can also be found in the weight-bearing position. This method is used for the navicular drop test discussed in the Special Tests section.

- Have patient stand barefoot.
- The clinician's thumb and index finger should be in the region of the talar head.
- The clinician should guide the patient's leg into internal and external rotation until the talus is felt equally by the index finger and thumb.

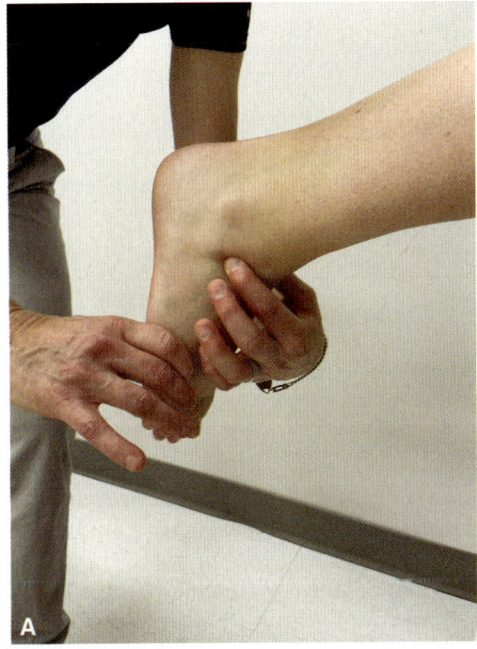
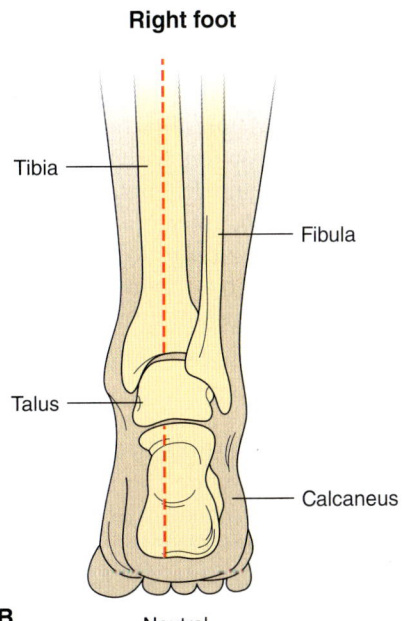

FIGURE 9-17 Assessment of subtalar joint neutral. **A.** Patient positioning for assessment of subtalar joint neutral. **B.** As viewed by the clinician, right foot neutral foot alignment: the calcaneus is vertical and the forefoot is perpendicular to it. (Adapted from Hamill J, Knutzen KM, Derrick TR. *Biomechanical Basis of Human Movement.* 5th ed. Wolters Kluwer; 2022: Figure 6-34B.)

- The clinician should visually examine the relationship of the calcaneus to the lower leg as noted previously.

Rearfoot varus is when the calcaneus is inverted when the subtalar joint is in the neutral position (Fig. 9-18A). As a result, at heel strike, the calcaneus lands more inverted than normal, contacting only the lateral condyle. To attain full contact with the support surface, the calcaneus needs to evert, or pronate, earlier and more than would occur with a more neutral foot posture (Fig. 9-18B).[4] Rearfoot valgus is when the calcaneus is in a more everted position (Fig. 9-18C). This may lead to a more supinated foot posture.[4]

Resting (or relaxed) calcaneal stance position is the position the foot naturally adopts during static standing. It appears that resting calcaneal stance position may be a better indicator of dynamic foot function than subtalar joint neutral.[75]

Forefoot Varus and Valgus Once subtalar joint neutral is found in non-weightbearing, the clinician can compare the relationship between the calcaneus and the forefoot. In a neutral foot, the forefoot should be perpendicular to the rearfoot in both the weight-bearing and non–weight-bearing positions. If the forefoot is in a varus position (Fig. 9-19A), in order for the medial side of the foot to contact the support surface, the rearfoot will need to pronate excessively. The effects of forefoot varus can include an overall increase in pronation. In contrast, if the forefoot is in a valgus position (Fig. 9-19B), the lateral border of the foot will contact the support surface sooner in the gait cycle than normal, limiting rearfoot pronation.

First Ray Position and Mobility

With patient prone and the foot in subtalar joint neutral, assess the position and mobility of the 1st ray. The 1st metatarsal should be in line with the 5th metatarsal, whereas the 2nd, 3rd, and 4th metatarsal heads form a dome-like shape. The 1st metatarsal should glide equally dorsally and plantarly. A plantar-flexed ray may develop in response to a forefoot varus in an attempt to bring the medial forefoot into contact with the ground.[4]

Distal Tibial Alignment

As noted previously, the distal tibia is externally rotated relative to the proximal end. The tibial torsion test (Fig. 9-20) is generally performed in prone but may also be performed with the patient in the seated position.[4] The clinician should examine the alignment of the distal 3rd of the tibia relative to the vertical.[4] Tibial varum is a frontal plane deformity in which there is a medial inclination of the distal tibia. Tibial varum is normal until the age of 2, giving toddlers a bow-legged appearance. If tibial varum continues through

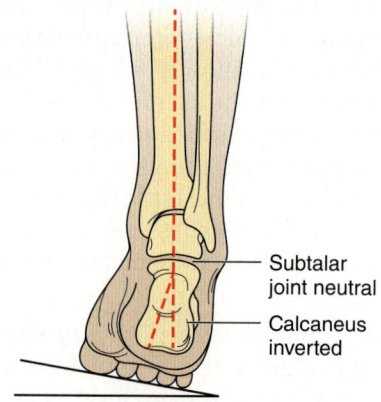

A Non–weight bearing

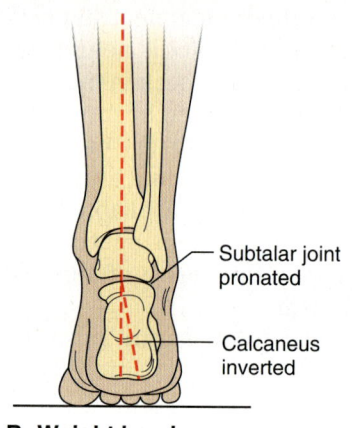

B Weight bearing

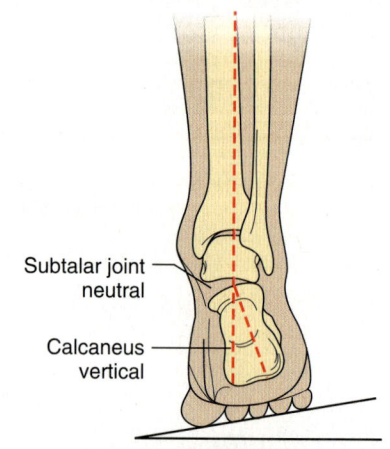

C Non–weight bearing

FIGURE 9-18 Rearfoot varus and valgus alignment. Posterior view of right foot. **A.** Rearfoot varus. **B.** Compensatory pronation in weight bearing because of rearfoot varus. **C.** Rearfoot valgus. (Adapted from Hamill J, Knutzen KM, Derrick TR. *Biomechanical Basis of Human Movement*. 5th ed. Wolters Kluwer; 2022: Figures 6-34 and 6-35.)

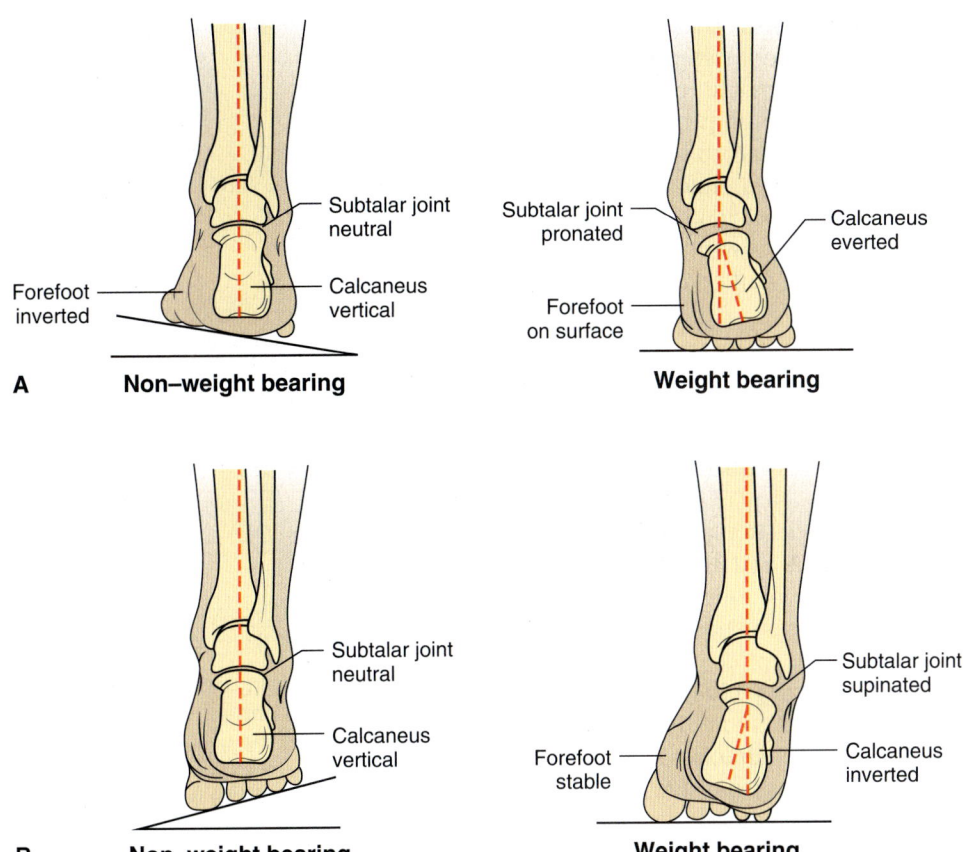

FIGURE 9-19 Forefoot varus and valgus alignment. Posterior view of right foot. Forefoot varus **(A)** and forefoot valgus **(B)** in non–weight-bearing and weight-bearing positions. (Adapted from Hamill J, Knutzen KM, Derrick TR. *Biomechanical Basis of Human Movement*. 5th ed. Wolters Kluwer; 2021: Figure 6-35.)

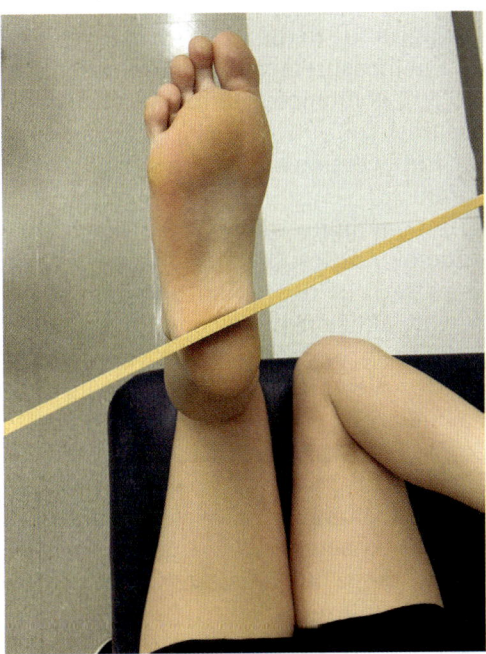

FIGURE 9-20 Tibial torsion test. With the patient prone with the knee 90° flexed, compare the line formed by the edge of the table (representing the proximal tibia) with a line drawn through the malleoli (stick). The resulting angle should be approximately 20 to 30° of external tibial torsion.

adulthood, this deformity leaves the medial border of the foot elevated without compensatory foot pronation.[76] In contrast, tibial valgum is a lateral inclination of the distal tibia, which elevates the lateral border of the foot unless compensatory supination occurs.

Skin and Nails

Diffuse ecchymosis may be associated with common ankle sprains as well as more serious trauma such as fracture. Excessive dryness or moisture may suggest abnormal vascularity or abnormal sympathetic activity to the area or both. If areas of abnormal callosities, redness, or actual skin breakdown are noted, suggesting excessive shear or compression forces, document the size of the involved area to serve as a baseline measurement. Note the site and size of hypertrophic skin changes, such as corns and calluses, which suggest shearing or compression. In many instances, callus formation can provide insights into how the foot functions. Patients with HV tend to develop calluses along the plantar medial 1st MTP joint and the plantar medial 1st interphalangeal joint.[77] Patients with excessive pronation are more likely to develop a callus under the 2nd metatarsal head, whereas those who lack pronation are more likely to develop a callus under the 5th metatarsal head.[78] However, callus patterns in populations have not been consistently linked to foot type.[77] Keep in mind that a painful callus is one in which the underlying tissue is in the process of breaking down. Nail deformities can lead to gait deviations and may provide insights on systemic disease processes such as diabetes. The clinician should inspect the toenails for splitting, overgrowth, inappropriate trimming, and thickening of the nail beds.

Range of Motion

Active physiologic ankle and toe motions with passive overpressure should be assessed and compared with the motions with the American Academy of Orthopaedic Surgeons (AAOS) normative values (Table 9-4).[79-81] However, clinicians should be wary of the potential for poor neuromuscular control, particularly of the lesser toes. With the patient seated and the legs hanging freely, visually compare range of motion of one foot/ankle to the other. Passive motion should be assessed noting any abnormal end-feels.

The clinician should note any changes in patient symptoms or crepitus with each motion. Although not objectively measured, the clinician should hold the rearfoot inverted and assess passive transverse tarsal joint pronation and supination. Measuring weight-bearing dorsiflexion may be a better indicator of functional dorsiflexion range.[82] This can be measured with the patient barefoot using a goniometer,

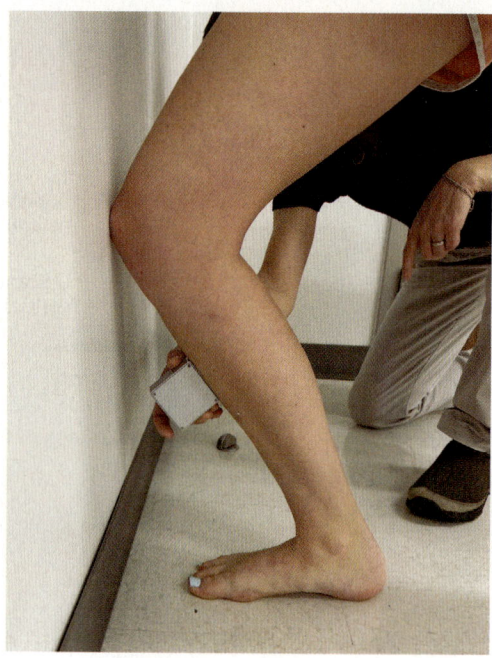

FIGURE 9-21 Weight-bearing dorsiflexion test using an inclinometer. The patient maintains the foot facing forward and heel on the ground, while lunging forward into dorsiflexion toward to touch the knee to the wall. The foot is moved away from the wall to the furthest point that the knee can contact the wall while maintaining heel contact with the ground.

inclinometer (Fig. 9-21), or measuring the distance from the longest toe to the wall. Normative values vary based on the measurement technique used: inclinometer 35 to 50°, goniometer 40 to 45°, or distance from wall to nearest toe (9 to 10 cm).[83,84] Passive rearfoot inversion and eversion should be performed with the patient prone.

Joint hypomobility may be the result of edema, sprain, immobilization, or degenerative changes. A capsular pattern of restriction is commonly seen in patients with effusion or degenerative joint disease (DJD). Refer to Table 7-2 in Chapter 7, The Physical Examination, for the capsular patterns of ankle and foot joints. Pain near the end of passive range may indicate minor damage of the tissue being elongated. Joint hypermobility may represent systemic hypermobility or a structural deviation such as ligamentous rupture. A patient with an acute ATF ligament sprain will have pain with end-range inversion. However, a patient with a chronic ATF rupture is likely to have excessive inversion range of motion.

Patients with ankle pathology frequently present with a lack of dorsiflexion. Loss of dorsiflexion range can be both the result of ankle trauma, such as edema,

TABLE 9-4
PASSIVE RANGE OF MOTION NORMATIVE VALUES

Joint	Motion	Normative Value (Degrees)
Ankle	Dorsiflexion	0–20
	Plantar flexion	0–50
	Inversion	0–35
	Eversion	0–15
Rearfoot/subtalar	Inversion	5
	Eversion	5
Great toe MTP	Extension	0–70
	Flexion	0–45
Lesser toe MTP	Extension	0–40
	Flexion	0–40
Great toe IP	Extension	0
	Flexion	0–90
Lesser toe PIP	Extension	0
	Flexion	35
Lesser toe DIP	Extension	0
	Flexion	60

DIP, distal interphalangeal; *IP*, interphalangeal; *MTP*, metatarsophalangeal; *PIP*, proximal interphalangeal.

and the cause of ankle pathologies, such as ankle sprains. Likewise, great toe extension can be limited due to DJD, HV, or hallux rigidus (HR). A loss of dorsiflexion or great toe extension range can significantly impact gait and function.

Muscle Length

Because restrictions in flexor hallucis longus length can affect terminal stance, flexor hallucis longus length should be measured by passively extending the 1st MTP with the ankle in neutral dorsiflexion (Fig. 9-22). Normal flexor hallucis longus length is 70° of 1st MTP extension with the IP joint extended. Gastrocnemius length should be measured with the knee in 0° of extension (Fig. 9-23). Normal gastrocnemius length is 10° of dorsiflexion. Additional lower extremity flexibility testing, including hamstring and hip flexor length, may be performed as part of the LQS.

Muscle Performance

Muscle performance of the ankle and foot may be assessed using manual muscle testing[85] or handheld dynamometry. Clinicians should recall that painless weakness of the tibialis anterior (L4), extensor hallucis longus (L5), fibularis (S1, S2), semimembranosus and semitendinosus (S1), or gastrocnemius (S1, S2) may indicate myotomal involvement. Pain with active motion that increases with resistive testing is consistent with a muscle strain or tendinopathy. Note that in the case of a gastrocnemius/soleus complex strain, manual resistance may not be enough stress to elicit pain and weight-bearing testing may be required. The inability to perform weight-bearing heel raises, particularly unilaterally, has been linked to functional limitations in gait, stair climbing, and higher level activities in patients with Achilles tendinopathy (AT), ankle sprain, tibialis posterior insufficiency, and the elderly. Given the significant strength and endurance required for functional activities, it is recommended that clinicians utilize 25 repetitions of heel raises as a normative value for weight-bearing testing.[86] The use of handheld dynamometry has been found to be reliable[87] and accurate[87] and may provide a more precise gauge for changes over time. Additionally, this measure has been found to be correlated with both static and dynamic balance.[88]

Given that a primary function of the toe flexors is to assist with stabilizing the foot and assist with push-off while the foot is in contact with the ground rather than in the open kinetic chain, functional strength of the great toe flexors may best be assessed using the paper grip test (Fig. 9-24).[89]

- With the patient seated and foot flat on the ground, the clinician places an index card under the patient's great toe.

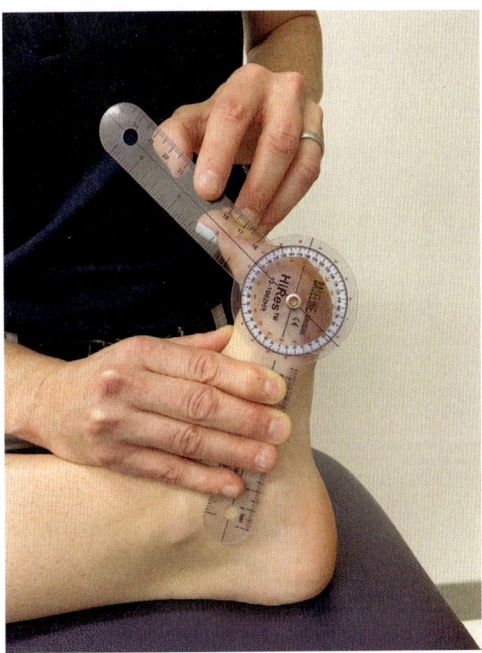

FIGURE 9-22 Assessment of flexor hallucis longus length.

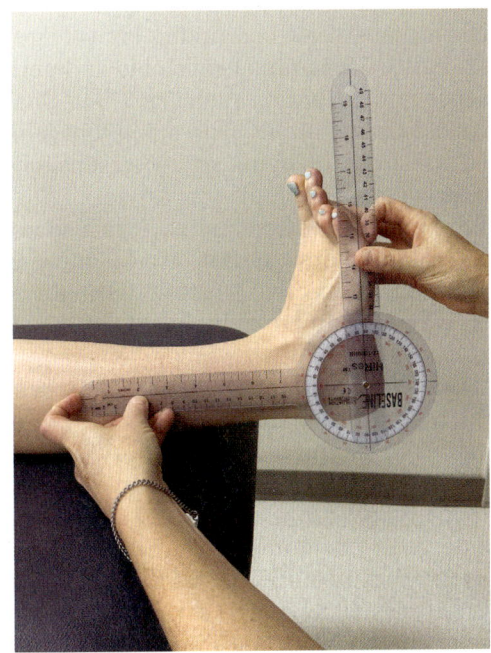

FIGURE 9-23 Assessment of gastrocnemius length performed with the knee extended.

- The patient is instructed to try to grip the card by pressing the great toe into the support surface.
- The clinician gradually tries to pull out the paper with a gradual increase in force.
- The patient passes if the clinician is unable to pull the paper from underneath the patient's toe.

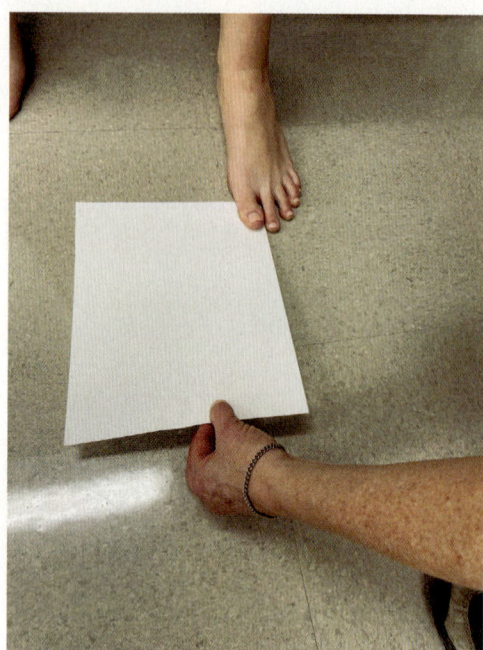

FIGURE 9-24 Paper grip test.

Sensory Tests

The clinician must have a working knowledge of the lower extremity dermatomal segments and peripheral nerve sensory distribution (see Fig. 7-5 in Chapter 7, The Physical Examination). The ankle/foot should be assessed for areas of hypo- or hypersensitivity. Decreased sensation on the plantar aspect of the foot is common in patients with diabetes. It is also common to have areas of altered sensation near incisions. Patients who lack protective sensation should be educated on proper footcare guidelines and encouraged to wear appropriate footwear. Hypersensitivity can be one of the signs of complex regional pain syndrome but may occur after HV surgery.

Paresthesias in the lower extremity, and particularly the foot, can stem from systemic sources, for example, patients with diabetes and individuals who have undergone chemotherapy treatment. Paresthesias may be due to lumbosacral nerve root pathology or compression along the sciatic nerve. Although less common, the clinician should assess for local sources of foot paresthesias when other areas have been ruled out. The tibial nerve can be compressed at the tarsal tunnel and interdigital nerves of the foot can be compressed near the metatarsal heads, creating numbness, tingling, burning, and pain within their respective areas of innervation within the foot.

Reflexes

If a patient reports paresthesias, the clinician should assess Achilles and patellar reflexes to assess possible upper or lower motor neuron involvement.

Neurodynamic Testing

Neurodynamic testing should be performed on patients reporting paresthesias to help with ruling out the lumbar spine as a source.

Accessory Motion

Joints should be assessed for hyper- or hypomobility, and the presence or absence of pain. Patients with increased pronation typically have increased mobility of the joints of the foot and decreased talocrural joint mobility. Foot hypomobility is common in the supinated foot and following fracture, immobilization, and edema. The method used to assess joint mobility may also be used for treatment following the guidelines reviewed in Chapter 3, Arthrology. When used for assessment purposes, the mobilization is generally performed in the open-packed position and the full range of joint mobility is noted. When used for assessment or pain modulation, grade I and II mobilizations are generally performed in the open-packed position. When used for improving motion, grade III and IV mobilizations may begin in the open-packed position but are progressed to being performed near the end of the range that is being facilitated.

Proximal Tibiofibular Joint

Purpose: To increase joint play at the proximal tibiofemoral joint. Anterior glide facilitates plantar flexion. Posterior glide facilitates dorsiflexion.

Patient: Supine, with knee flexed about 90°, the foot flat on the plinth.

Clinician: Grasps the head and neck of the proximal fibula with the mobilizing hand, the thumb contacting anteriorly, the index and long finger pads contacting posteriorly taking care to avoid direct pressure to the common fibular nerve. Alternatively, the clinician can use the heel of the hand to perform the mobilization.

Mobilization: The mobilizing hand moves the proximal fibula posteriorly or anteriorly (Fig. 9-25).

Distal Tibiofibular Joint Mobilization

Purpose: Anterior glide facilitates plantar flexion. Posterior glide facilitates dorsiflexion.

Patient: Supine with the calcaneus hanging over the end of the plinth and the ankle in 10° of plantar flexion.

Clinician: Cradles the ankle in the stabilizing hand, fixing the patient's leg to the plinth and wrapping the fingers around the heel posteriorly. For the posterior glide, the mobilizing hand contacts the lateral malleolus anteriorly with the heel of the hand. For the anterior glide, the clinician hooks the index finger posteriorly around the lateral malleolus (Fig. 9-26). Alternately, the anterior glide can be

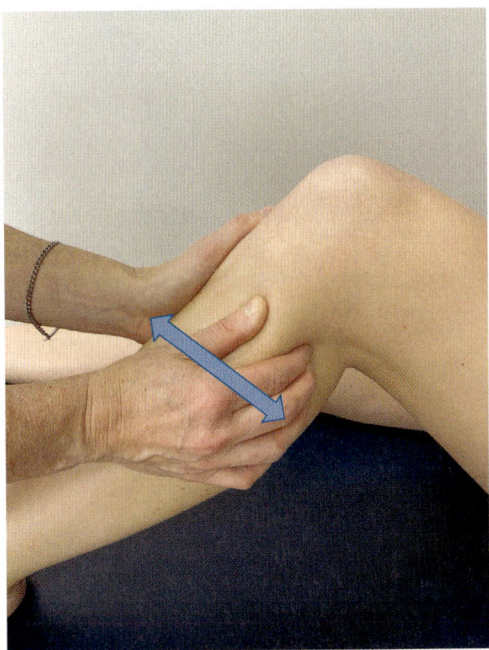

FIGURE 9-25 Assessment of proximal tibiofibular joint.

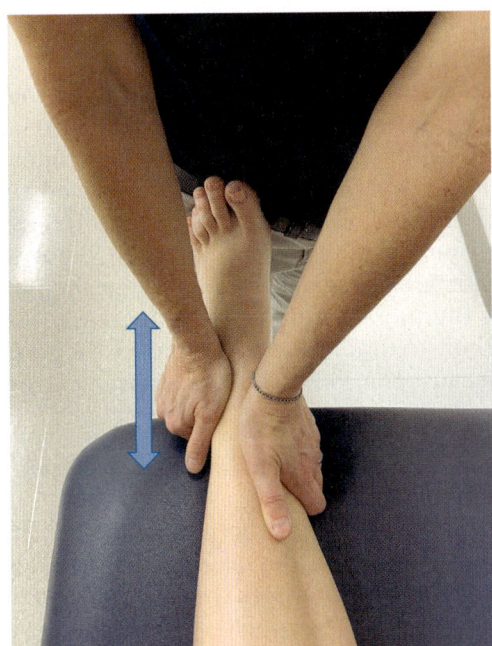

FIGURE 9-26 Assessment of distal tibiofibular joint.

performed in prone using the heel of the hand for the mobilization.

Mobilization: The mobilizing hand moves the proximal fibula posteriorly or anteriorly.

Talocrural Joint Mobilization: Posterior Glide

Purpose: Anterior glide facilitates plantar flexion. Posterior glide facilitates dorsiflexion.

Patient: Supine with the calcaneus hanging over the end of the plinth and the ankle in 10° of plantar flexion.

Clinician: Stabilizes the distal tibia against the plinth by grasping it with the hand, wrapping the fingers around posteriorly. The stabilizing forearm rests over the dorsum of the patient's lower leg to prevent it from rising up from the plinth during the movement. The clinician contacts the neck of the talus dorsally with the web of the mobilizing hand, bringing the thumb and the index finger around the sides of the foot. The remaining three fingers of the mobilizing hand wrap around the sole of the foot for support and control of the degree of plantar flexion. Alternatively, the clinician may stand facing the patient at the foot of the plinth, supporting the patient's foot in about 10° of plantar flexion with her thigh to deliver the posterior glide.

Mobilization: The mobilizing hand glides the talus posteriorly on the tibia (Fig. 9-27).

Talocrural Joint Mobilization: Anterior Glide

Purpose: Anterior glide facilitates plantar flexion. Posterior glide facilitates dorsiflexion.

Patient: Supine with the calcaneus hanging over the end of the plinth and the ankle in 10° of plantar flexion.

Clinician: Stabilizes the distal tibia against the plinth by grasping it with the hand, wrapping the fingers around posteriorly. The stabilizing forearm rests over the dorsum of the patient's lower leg to prevent it from rising up from the plinth during the movement. The clinician contacts the posterior talus with the index finger and web space of the mobilizing hand. The clinician's leg (or remaining fingers) controls the degree of plantar flexion.

Mobilization: The mobilizing hand glides the talus anteriorly on the tibia (Fig. 9-28).

Talocrural Joint Mobilization: Distraction

Purpose: To assess or improve global talocrural joint mobility.

Patient: Supine with the calcaneus hanging over the end of the plinth and the ankle in 10° of plantar flexion.

Clinician: The patient's bodyweight stabilizes the tibia. The clinician contacts the anterior and posterior talus with the web space of both hands. The hands control the degree of plantar flexion.

Mobilization: Both hands impart a distraction force (Fig. 9-29).

Subtalar Joint Mobilizations

Purpose: A lateral glide of the calcaneus facilitates inversion and global joint mobility.

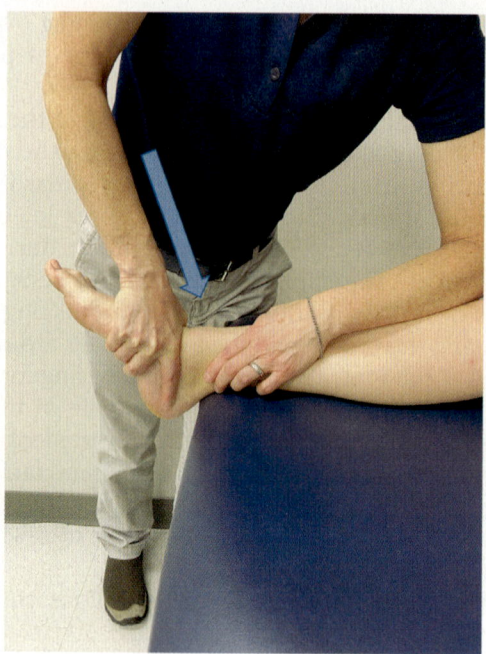

FIGURE 9-27 Posterior talocrural joint mobilization.

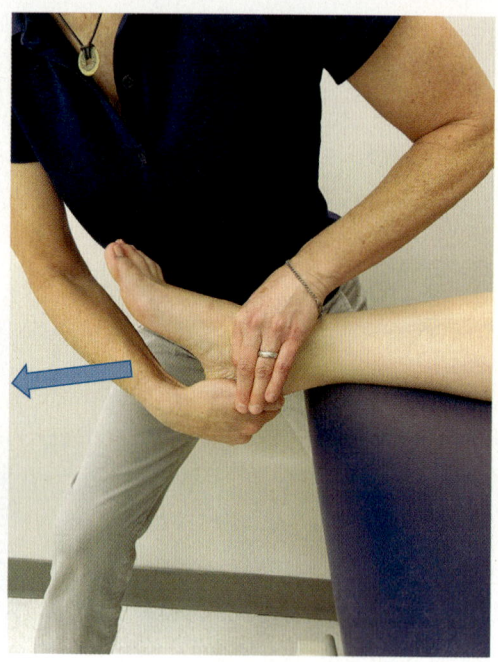

FIGURE 9-29 Distraction of the talocrural joint.

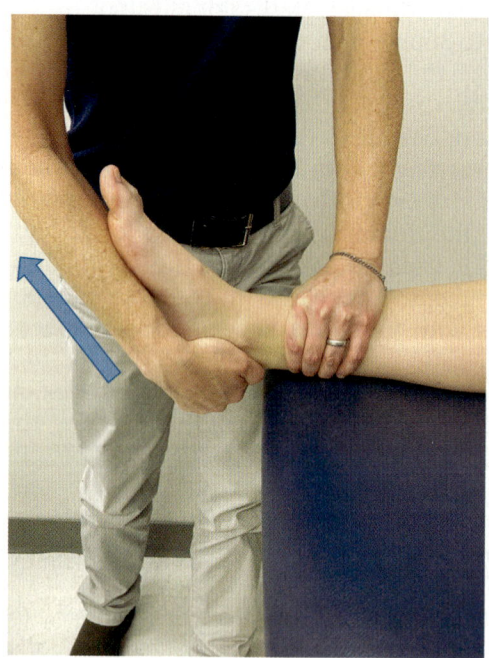

FIGURE 9-28 Anterior talocrural joint mobilization.

Patient: Ipsilateral side-lying with calcaneus off the edge of the plinth and the ankle dorsiflexed.

Clinician: Stabilizes the ankle with the superior hand and wraps the fingers around the lateral talus to stabilize it. The clinician contacts the medial calcaneus with the mobilizing hand and loosely wraps the fingers around the heel.

Mobilization: The mobilizing hand glides the calcaneus laterally (toward the floor) (Fig. 9-30).

A medial glide of the calcaneus to facilitate eversion and general joint mobility is performed similarly but with the patient lying on the contralateral side.

The mobilizations are frequently performed in supine for assessment. However, when the patient is supine, the mobilization requires increased clinician effort both to stabilize and to impart the mobilizing force because the glide is no longer assisted by gravity.

Intertarsal Joint Mobility

Purpose: Dorsal and plantar glides facilitate global joint mobility.
Patient: Supine with the foot in a neutral position.
Clinician: Facing the dorsal aspect of the foot, the stabilizing hand encircles the midfoot. The mobilizing hand grasps the cuboid.
Mobilization: The mobilizing hand glides the cuboid dorsally or plantarly.

Mobilizations between each tarsal are carried out in a similar manner: stabilizing one segment, while mobilizing the adjacent bone. Figure 9-31 demonstrates a cuboid–metatarsal mobilization.

Intermetatarsal Joint Mobility

Purpose: Dorsal and plantar glides facilitate global joint mobility.
Patient: Supine with the foot in a neutral position.

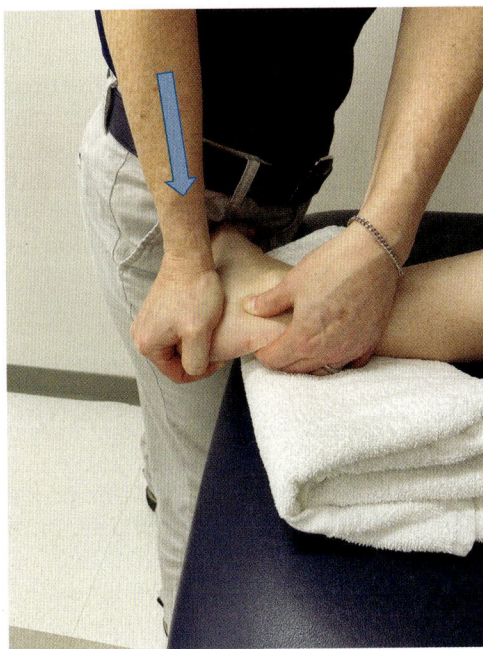

FIGURE 9-30 Lateral glide of calcaneus.

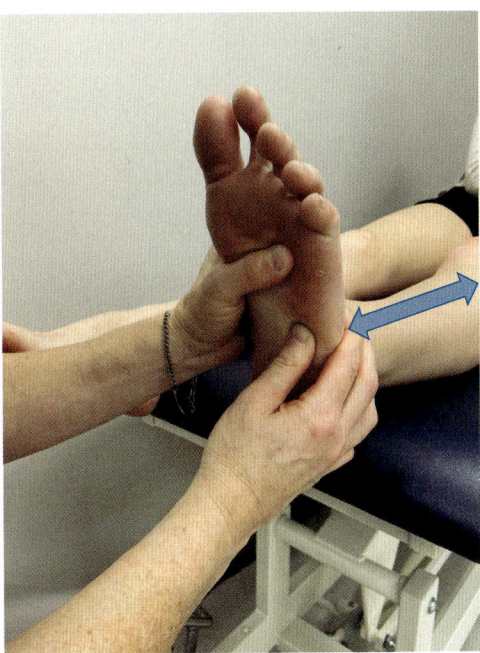

FIGURE 9-31 Cuboid–metatarsal mobilization.

Clinician: Facing the plantar aspect of the foot, the stabilizing hand holds midshaft of one metatarsal with the thumb on the plantar and fingers on the dorsal aspect. The mobilizing hand grasps the midshaft of the adjacent metatarsal in the same manner as the stabilizing hand.

Mobilization: The mobilizing hand glides the metatarsal dorsally or plantarly (Fig. 9-32). Movements can be performed between the 2nd and 1st, the 2nd and 3rd, the 3rd and 4th, and the 4th and 5th metatarsal bones. The mobilizations can also be performed in reverse, with the clinician facing the dorsal aspect of the patient's foot.

Metatarsophalangeal Joint Mobility

Purpose: Dorsal glide facilitates extension. Plantar glide facilitates flexion. Distraction facilitates global joint mobility. Movements will simultaneously take place in the tarsometatarsal joints and between the MTPs.

Patient: Position of comfort.

Clinician: The stabilizing hand holds the metatarsal. The mobilizing hand grasps the proximal phalanx.

Mobilization: The mobilizing hand glides the distal segment dorsally, plantarly, or creates a distraction force (Fig. 9-33).

Interphalangeal Joint Mobilizations

Interphalangeal joint mobilizations are performed similarly to MTP joint mobilizations, with the clinician stabilizing the proximal or middle phalanx and mobilizing the distal segment. A glove or athletic prewrap can be

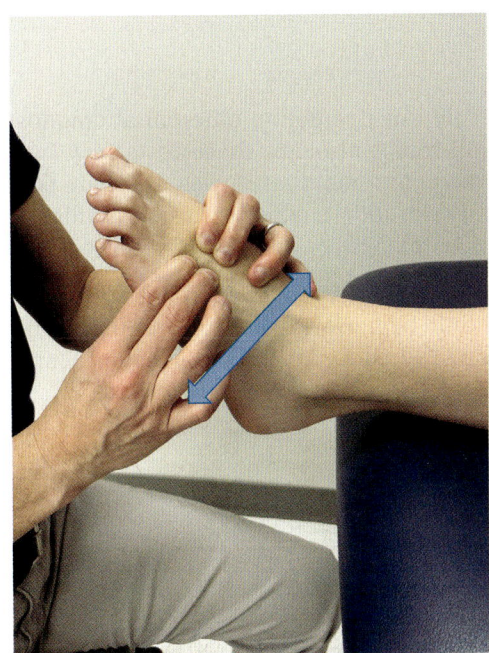

FIGURE 9-32 Intermetatarsal mobilization.

used to assist the clinician in obtaining a firmer grasp by reducing slippage.

Special Tests/Provocative Testing

Clinicians should choose which special/provocative tests to perform based on the patient history and physical examination to this point in order to help rule

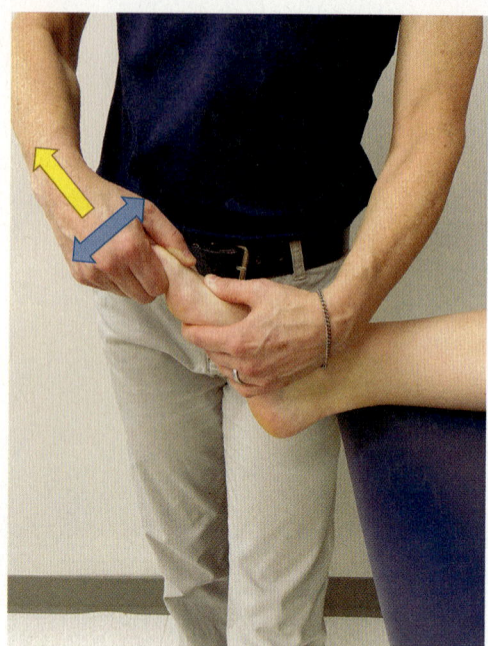

FIGURE 9-33 First metatarsophalangeal mobilization demonstrating dorsal glide/plantar glide (*blue arrow*) and distraction (*yellow arrow*).

index finger squeeze test, Mulder sign, and the dorsal and plantar Tinel test. All Tinel tests are performed in the same manner as noted for interdigital neuroma—the examiner simply taps over the superficial nerve in an attempt to provoke the patient's symptoms. The following special tests should be performed to rule in/out tarsal tunnel syndrome (TTS): Tinel test at the tarsal tunnel and the dorsiflexion–eversion stress test.

Metatarsal Compression Test

Purpose: Assess for the presence of an interdigital neuroma.
Method: The clinician encircles the metatarsal heads and compresses them together.[90]
Interpretation: A positive test is if this produces or exacerbates the patient's report of pain, burning, or tingling in the region or the adjacent two toes. This test is reported to have a positive predictive value of 95% (Fig. 9-35).[91]

Thumb Index Finger Squeeze Test

Purpose: Assess for the presence of an interdigital neuroma.[91]
Method: The clinician compresses the intermetatarsal space from the plantar and dorsal aspects with the thumb and index finger.
Interpretation: A positive test is if this compression produces or exacerbates the patient's report of pain, burning, or tingling in the region or the adjacent two toes (Fig. 9-36).

Mulder Sign

Purpose: Assess for the presence of an interdigital neuroma.

in and rule out competing differential diagnoses. For ankle and foot pathology, these tests may be grossly grouped into four main categories. Tests are performed to identify the source of paresthesias, sprains/instability, Achilles pathology, and hypermobility (Fig. 9-34).

Special Tests for Paresthesias The following special tests should be performed to rule in/out an interdigital neuroma: the metatarsal compression test, thumb

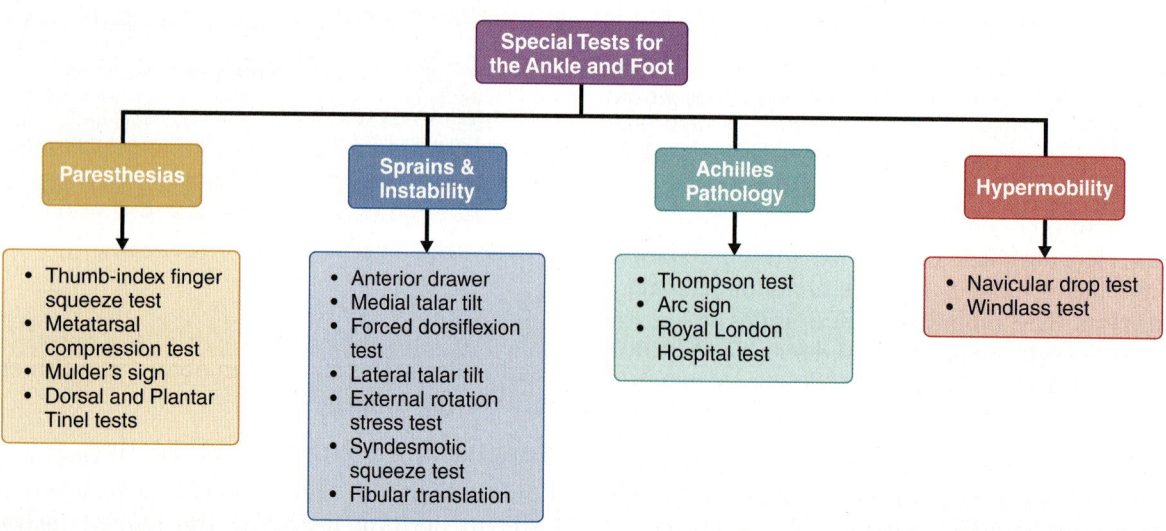

FIGURE 9-34 Special tests for ankle/foot pathology.

CHAPTER 9 | ANKLE AND FOOT

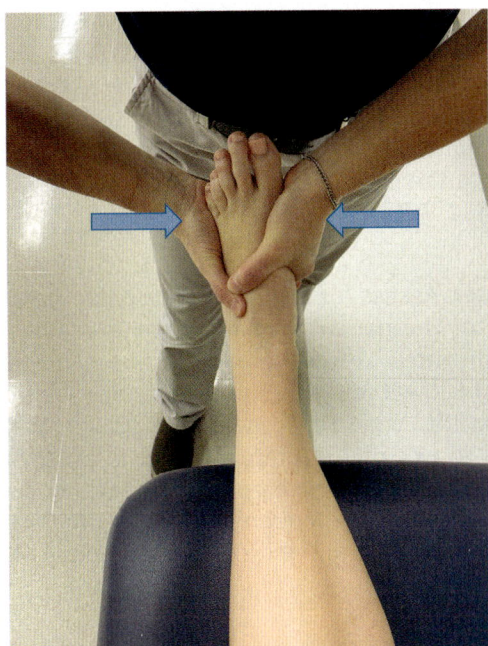

FIGURE 9-35 Metatarsal compression test.

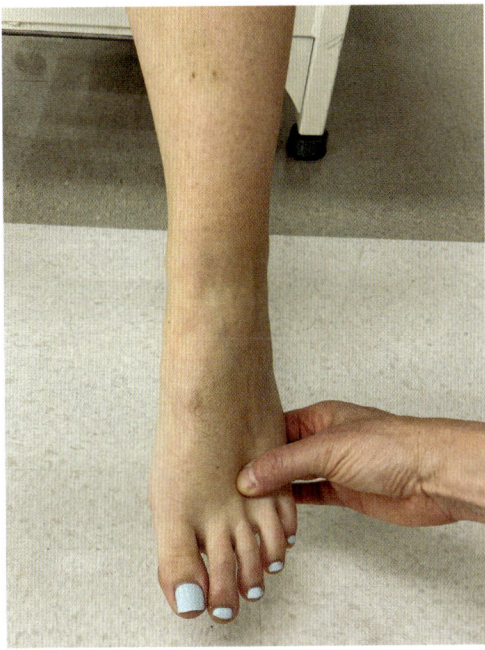

FIGURE 9-36 Thumb index finger squeeze test.

Method: The clinician uses the thumb of one hand to provide dorsal pressure in the area of the suspected interdigital neuroma. The other hand then compresses the metatarsal heads.

Interpretation: A positive test is if this produces or exacerbates the patient's report of pain, burning, or tingling in the region or the adjacent two toes. The clinician may notice a palpable click.[91]

Dorsal and Plantar Tinel Test

Purpose: Assess for the presence of an interdigital neuroma.

Method: The clinician taps on the dorsal and plantar aspect of the foot in the region of the intermetatarsal nerve.

Interpretation: A positive test is if this produces or exacerbates the patient's report of pain, burning, or tingling in the region or the adjacent two toes. Because this test has high specificity but is not very sensitive,[91] a positive test helps rule in the diagnosis.

Special Tests for Sprains and Instability The following special tests should be performed to rule in/out a lateral ankle sprain: anterior drawer test and, medial talar tilt test. Because anterolateral impingement may be a sequela of lateral ankle sprain, the forced dorsiflexion test is included here. The lateral talar tilt test helps rule in/out a medial ankle sprain. The following special tests should be performed to rule in/out a syndesmotic sprain: external rotation stress test, the syndesmotic squeeze test, and the fibular translation test.

Anterior Drawer Test

Purpose: Assess the integrity of the ATF ligament.[92]

Method: With the patient's ankle in 10° of plantar flexion, the clinician stabilizes the distal lower leg with one hand, whereas the contralateral hand grasps the calcaneus. The clinician then tries to draw calcaneus and talus anteriorly.

Interpretation: A positive test is if there is more than approximately 3 to 4 mm of movement.[92,93] The clinician should also note if the test is painful and if the end-feel is firm or soft. Laxity with the anterior drawer test has a sensitivity of 80 to 95% and a specificity of 74 to 84%[92] (Fig. 9-37).

Medial Talar Tilt Test

Purpose: Assess the integrity of the CFL.[92]

Method: Position the patient in side-lying and neutral dorsiflexion. While stabilizing the lower leg, the clinician grasps the calcaneus and talus and thrusts them medially (toward the floor).

Interpretation: A positive test for CFL involvement is if there is hypermobility or excessive motion compared to the contralateral side. The clinician should also note if the test is painful (Fig. 9-38).

Forced Dorsiflexion Test

Purpose: Assess for anterolateral ankle impingement.[92]

Method: Starting with the ankle in plantar flexion, the clinician places a thumb in the lateral gutter in the region of the ATF ligament, then forcefully dorsiflexes and everts the patient's ankle.

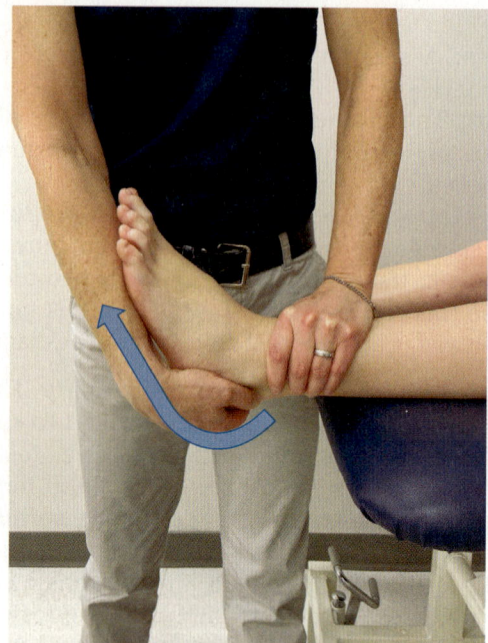

FIGURE 9-37 Anterior drawer test.

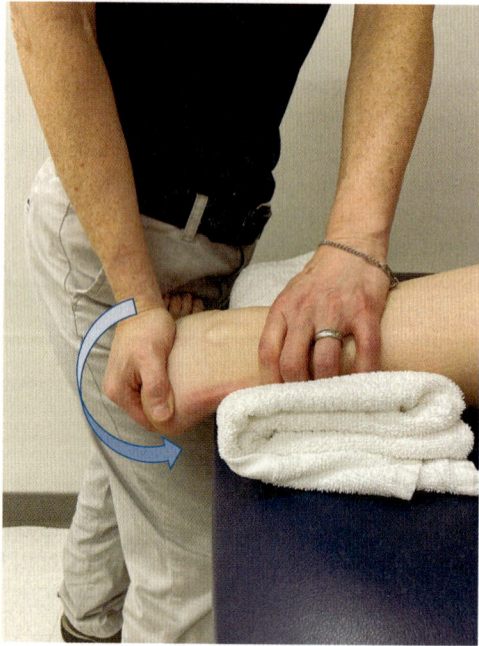

FIGURE 9-38 Medial talar tilt test.

Interpretation: A positive test is reproduction of pain in the anterolateral ankle with the maneuver (Fig. 9-39).

Lateral Talar Tilt Test (aka Eversion Stress Test)
Purpose: Assess the integrity of the deltoid ligament.[92]
Method: With the patient side-lying on the side to be tested, place the ankle in neutral dorsiflexion. The clinician stabilizes the lower leg and then everts the ankle. To bias the test toward various parts of the deltoid ligament, the clinician can vary the degree of ankle dorsiflexion and plantar flexion.
Interpretation: A positive test is if there is excessive motion compared to the contralateral side. The clinician should also note if there is any pain created in the region of the deltoid ligament with testing (Fig. 9-40).

External Rotation Stress Test (aka the Kleiger Test)
Purpose: Assess for a syndesmotic ankle sprain.[92]
Method: The patient's ankle is positioned in neutral dorsiflexion. The clinician uses one hand to stabilize the lower leg without compressing the tibia and fibula together. The other hand grasps the calcaneus to externally rotate the foot in an attempt to use the talus to wedge open the syndesmosis.
Interpretation: A positive test is reproduction of pain in the area of the syndesmosis (Fig. 9-41).

Syndesmotic Squeeze Test (aka the Distal Tibiofibular Compression Test)
Purpose: Assess for a syndesmotic ankle sprain.[92]
Method: The clinician compresses the tibia and fibula together. The clinician should begin several centimeters proximal to the malleolus. If the test is not painful, then the clinician should move the force distally.
Interpretation: A positive test is reproduction of pain in the area of the syndesmosis (Fig. 9-42).

Fibular Translation Test
Purpose: Assess for a syndesmotic ankle sprain.[92]
Method: The patient's ankle is positioned in loose-packed position of about 10° of plantar flexion.

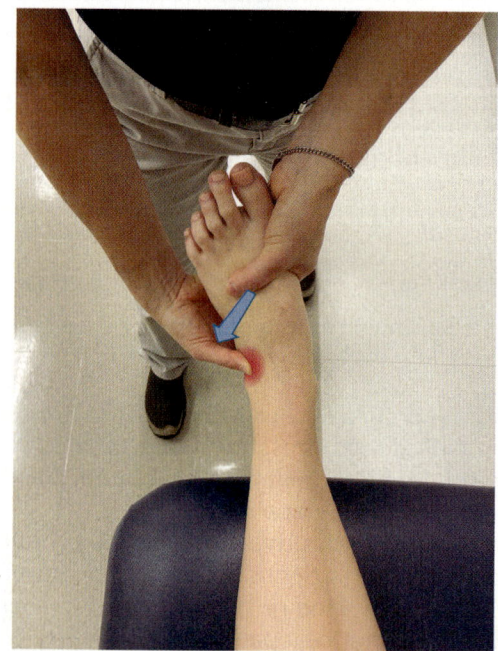

FIGURE 9-39 Forced dorsiflexion test.

CHAPTER 9 | ANKLE AND FOOT

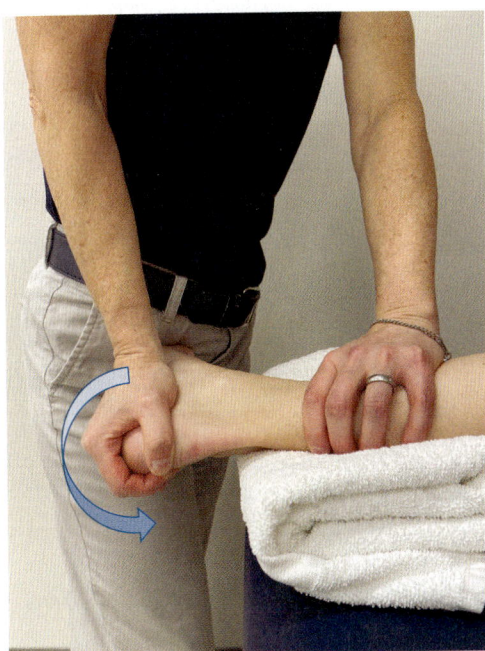

FIGURE 9-40 Lateral talar tilt test.

Special Tests for Achilles Pathology The following special tests should be performed to rule in/out Achilles pathology: Thompson test, Arc sign, and the Royal London Hospital test.

Thompson Test
Purpose: Assess the integrity of the Achilles tendon.[94]
Method: With the patient prone and ankle off the edge of the table, the clinician squeezes the muscle belly of the gastrocnemius.
Interpretation: A positive test is if the ankle fails to plantarflex when the muscle belly is squeezed.

Arc Sign
Purpose: Assess for AT.[94]
Method: With the patient prone and ankle off the edge of the table, the clinician should examine the Achilles for an area of swelling. The patient then dorsiflexes the ankle.
Interpretation: A positive test is if the swollen portion of the tendon moves when the patient performs dorsiflexion.

Royal London Hospital Test
Purpose: Assess for AT.[94]
Method: With the patient prone and ankle off the edge of the table, the clinician should palpate the Achilles approximately 3 cm proximal to the distal attachment to the calcaneus. The patient then dorsiflexes the ankle, and the clinician palpates in the same location.
Interpretation: A positive test is if the Achilles tendon is less tender when the same location is palpated after the patient moves into dorsiflexion.

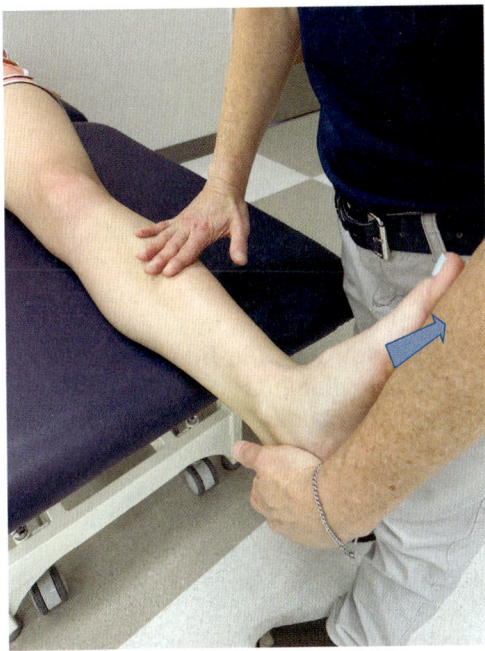

FIGURE 9-41 External rotation stress test.

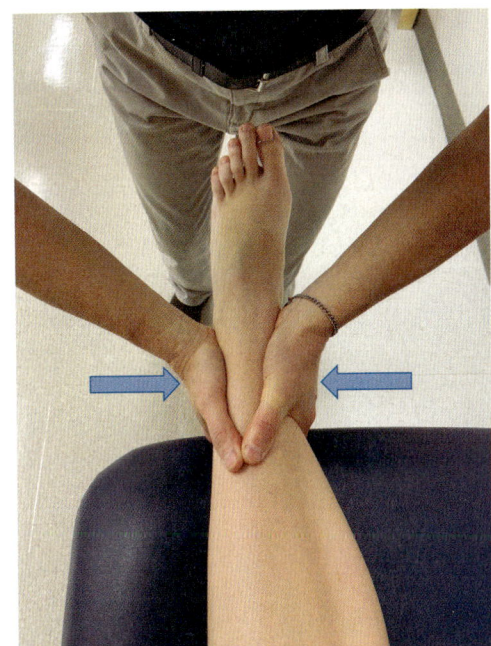

FIGURE 9-42 Syndesmotic squeeze test.

The clinician stabilizes the tibia with one hand and performs a posterior fibular mobilization with the other hand. Note that the test is also a distal tibiofibular joint mobilization (see Fig. 9-26).
Interpretation: A positive test is reproduction of pain in the area of the syndesmosis.

Special Tests for Hypermobility Both the navicular drop test and the windlass test assess foot mobility. The windlass test is also used to assess for plantar fasciitis.

Navicular Drop Test

Purpose: Assess foot mobility.[95,96]

Method: With the patient seated, place the foot in subtalar neutral position and measure the height of the navicular tuberosity. Repeat the measurement with the patient standing in relaxed calcaneal stance position. The navicular drop is the difference between these two measurements.

Interpretation: A normal navicular drop is about 5 mm. A hypomobile foot is if the navicular drop is less than 3 to 5 mm. A hypermobile foot is if the drop is greater than 10 mm (Fig. 9-43).

Windlass Test

Purpose: Assess foot hypermobility or for plantar fasciitis.[97]

Method: With patient standing, the clinician passively extends the MTP joint to wind the plantar fascia around the MTP joint.

Interpretation: A positive test for hypermobility is if the medial longitudinal arch fails to rise with great toe extension, a positive test for plantar fasciitis is if arch pain is created with great toe extension (Fig. 9-44).

Palpation

The region should be palpated for swelling, hydration, temperature, pulses, and tenderness. Global unilateral lower extremity edema may indicate chronic venous insufficiency, whereas bilateral edema may indicate congestive heart failure. Generalized foot edema may follow trauma or immobilization or a period of non–weight bearing because of the dependent nature of the lower leg and lack of ankle pump. Localized extra-articular swelling generally accompanies ankle sprains, usually involving the lateral aspect of the ankle below the malleolus. Local edema in the area of a known bursa is consistent with bursitis. The skin should be palpated for moisture or dryness. Dry cracked skin is common with aging and also accompanies the autonomic neuropathy of diabetes. Skin temperature and texture should be noted. Local warmth may indicate an inflammatory process or sign of infection. Vascular changes and complex regional pain syndrome may result in an increase or decrease in skin temperature of one side compared with another. Arterial insufficiency and aging may lead to thinning of the skin, whereas venous insufficiency may lead to thickening or a rash. If present, scar thickness and mobility should be assessed. The pulse of the dorsalis pedis artery may be palpated just lateral to the tendon of the extensor hallucis longus over the dorsum of the foot. The pulse of the posterior tibial artery is palpated behind the tendons of the flexor digitorum longus and flexor hallucis longus posterosuperior to the medial malleolus. Patients should be asked to try to point to the area of symptoms. This can serve as an initial guide for palpating potentially involved ligaments, joints, tendon, and muscles.

Clinicians should palpate structures for tenderness as described previously. Bony tenderness with

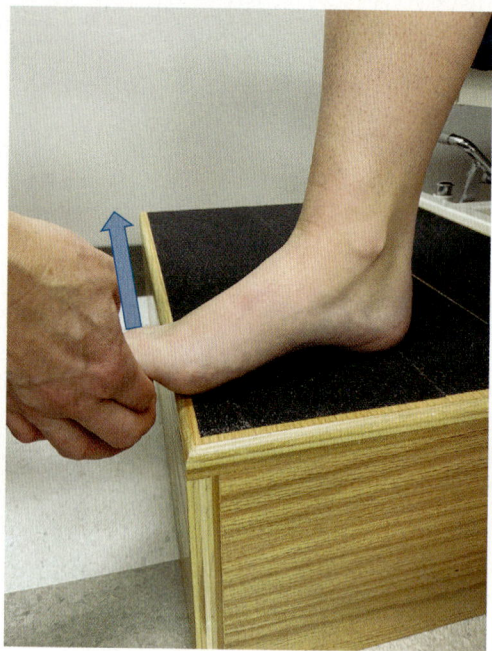
FIGURE 9-44 Windlass test.

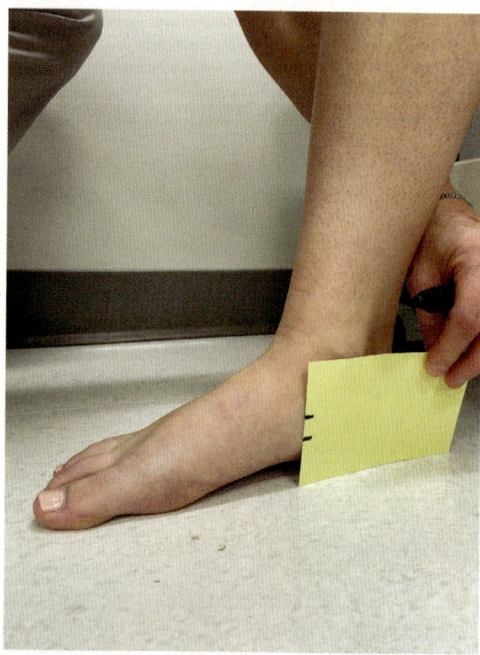
FIGURE 9-43 Navicular drop test.

a history of trauma may indicate fracture.[70] After an acute sprain or strain, tenderness of the involved structure can be expected. In cases of rupture, such as the Achilles,[98] the clinician may feel a palpable breach of gap in the involved tissue.

Footwear and Gait

The patient's footwear should be inspected. Shoes should be inspected for type, fit, signs of excessive wear, and wear patterns that may offer clues as to the presence of persistent biomechanical disturbances and localized areas of pressure. The inside of the patient's footwear should also be inspected. Is the patient using over-the-counter or custom orthotics? Are there any nails protruding through the insole or prominent seams that can be contributing to the patient's complaint? Clinicians may need to enquire about typical footwear the patient uses on a daily basis as well as any specialized footwear, running shoes, cleats, work or dress shoes, etc. The clinician should determine if these alternate shoes should be brought in and inspected at a future visit.

The patient should be observed walking with and without shoes, noting any deviations or symptoms. The amount and timing of pronation and supination should be noted. Caution should be used when interpreting the effects of excessive pronation or supination as abnormal motion may not be related to pathology. An antalgic gait associated with foot or ankle pathology may affect heel strike or push-off. For example, a patient with plantar fasciopathy (PFasc) may avoid heel strike and instead make initial contact with the foot flat. In contrast, after an ankle fracture, a patient may exhibit an early heel rise, indicating a lack of dorsiflexion range or gastrocnemius length. Patients with HR or HV may report pain during terminal stance. Asking patients to adopt different gait patterns may help identify impairments (Table 9-5).

If appropriate, running mechanics can be evaluated. The use of video analysis and a treadmill can be particularly helpful in recognizing more subtle deviations. For patients whose symptoms are not highly irritable or do not occur until a prolonged plyometric activity such as running 3 miles, endurance testing (as described in Chapter 7, The Physical Examination) might be appropriate. Refer to Chapter 5, Gait and Footwear, for additional information.

Functional Testing

General transverse plane motion can be assessed with the patient standing barefoot with feet hip distance apart and asking the patient to rotate to the left keeping the feet fixed. Left rotation should cause left foot supination, rising of the left arch, and left lower extremity external rotation. Left rotation should cause the opposite to occur in the right foot: pronation, lowering of the right arch, and right lower extremity pronation. The test should be repeated with the patient rotating to the right. Compare motion of one foot to the other and total amount of pronation and supination available. General frontal plane motion can be assessed with the patient standing with the knees extended and inverting the feet by standing on the lateral borders of the feet. Repeat with everting the feet and standing on the medial borders of the feet.

Functional balance testing can be performed by assessing a patient's reach, a part of the Y-balance test, or the Star Excursion Balance Test (Fig. 9-45).[99] Having more than a 4 cm difference in anterior reach between sides has been linked to an increased risk of lower extremity injury.[100]

There are several plyometric functional tests that can be used for patients with ankle pathology (Fig. 9-46). The single hop for distance[101] or single vertical hop[102] can be used to compare the uninvolved side to the involved side or to normative values. The lateral hop for distance and the timed side hop test are commonly used for patients with ankle instability because they require a greater amount of balance and control of frontal plane motion.[103,104]

TABLE 9-5	
ALTERNATE GAIT PATTERNS TO ASSESS	
Pattern	Clinical Insights to Be Gained
Long strides	May expose deficits in dorsiflexion or great toe extension
Slow walking	May help identify balance deficits
Backward walking	May help identify deficits in balance, gastrocnemius length, or ankle dorsiflexion
Toe walking	May expose plantar flexor weakness/strain, Achilles or hallux pathology, or balance deficits
Heel walking	May expose tibialis anterior weakness, loss of gastrocnemius length or dorsiflexion range, or balance deficits
Walking on the lateral borders of the foot	May expose invertor weakness. May be painful or difficult with lateral ankle or midfoot ligament injury or instability
Walking on the medial borders of the foot	May expose evertor weakness, deltoid ligament injury

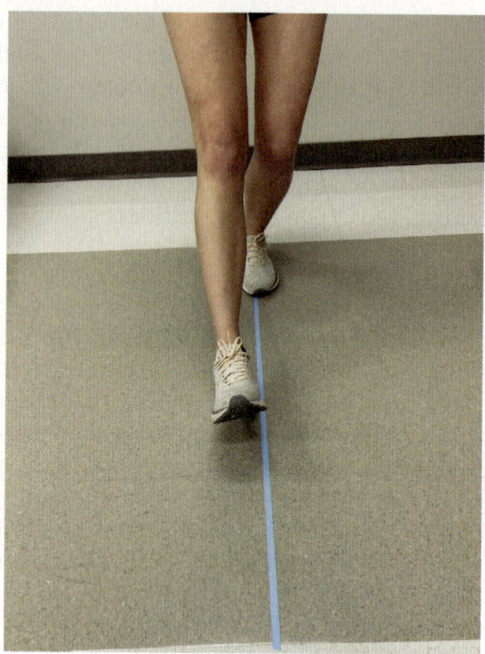

FIGURE 9-45 Anterior reach assessment.

COMMON FOOT PATHOLOGIES

This section contains details on the most common or most problematic foot pathologies a clinician may see in an outpatient setting: HV, HR, metatarsalgia, interdigital neuroma, PFasc, and bone stress injuries.

Hallux Valgus

Pathology HV deformity (Fig. 9-47) is the result of angulations of the 1st metatarsal and the proximal phalanx of the great toe. This condition is significantly more common in women than men.[105] For females HV is more likely to be the result of footwear choices including shoes with a narrow toe box or high heels. For males, the condition is more likely to be hereditary.[106] HV can be congenital.

Once the angle of the 1st MTP joint reaches 45°, the lines of pull of the flexor hallucis brevis, flexor hallucis longus, and adductor hallucis all exacerbate this valgus deformity (Fig. 9-48).[107] Likewise, the abductor hallucis is unable to create sufficient counterforce to prevent deformity progression. Over time, the medial collateral ligament of the 1st MTP becomes lengthened and the lateral collateral ligament becomes shortened. The widening of the forefoot leads to increased soft tissue compression of the medial 1st metatarsal from footwear, resulting in calluses and soft tissue thickening in this region.

As a result of the HV deformity, rather than plantar flexing firmly into the support surface during terminal stance, the 1st metatarsal becomes insufficient,[108] and it is no longer able to function as a rigid lever for push-off. This leads to a more mobile foot and increased 2nd metatarsal pressures during gait.

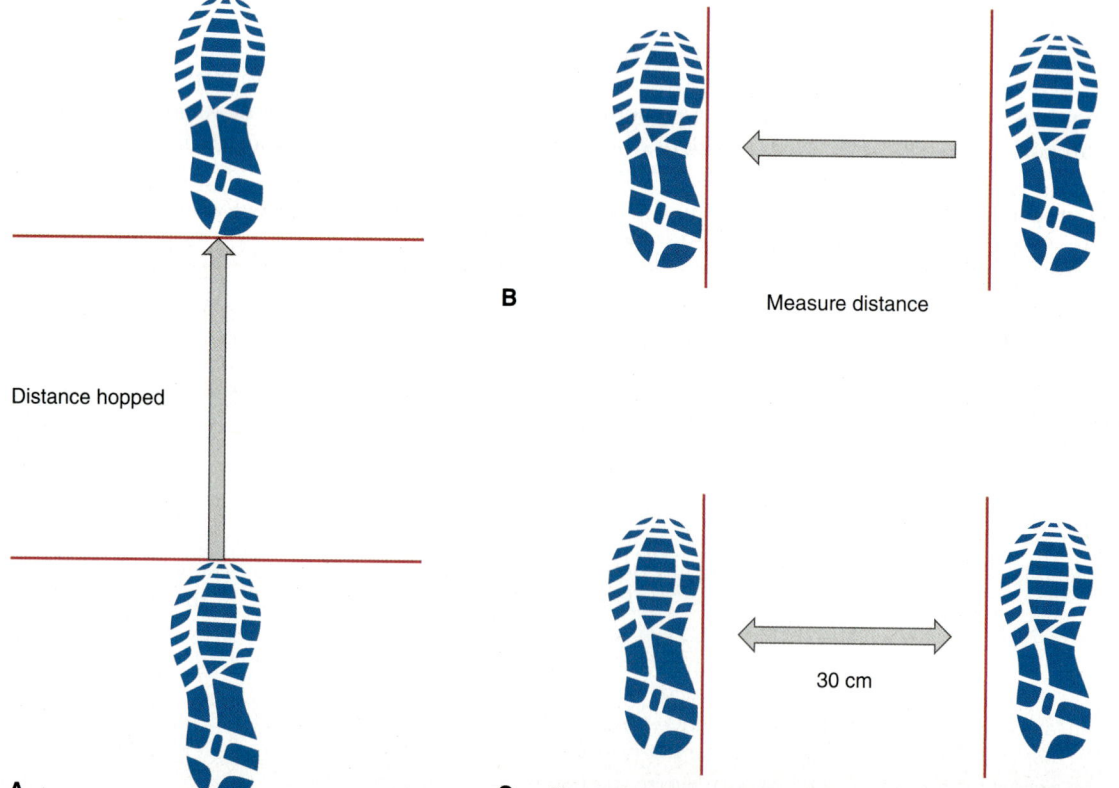

FIGURE 9-46 Hop testing for patients with ankle/foot injuries. **A.** Single hop for distance. **B.** Lateral hop for distance. **C.** Timed side hop test.

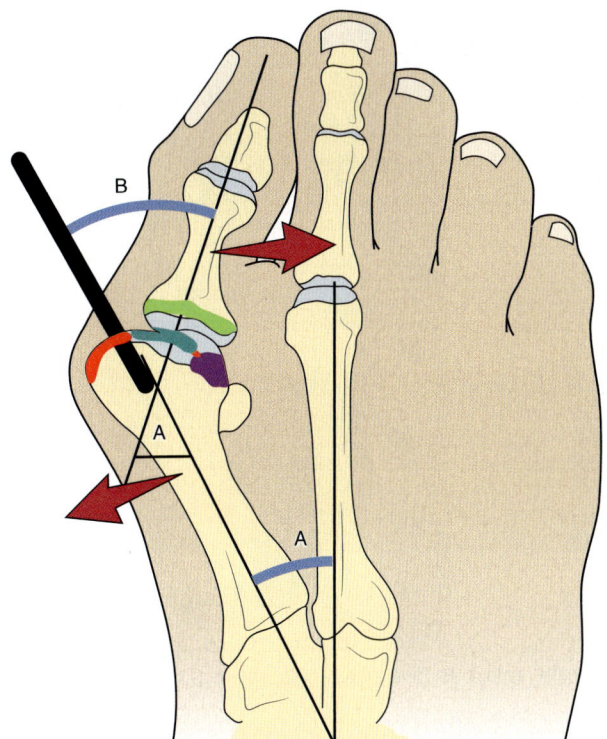

FIGURE 9-47 A hallux valgus deformity is a combination of medial angulation of the first metatarsal (angle A >15°) and lateral angulation of the proximal phalanx of the great toe (angle B >40°). As a result, the distal metatarsal now has exposed articular cartilage (*red*) and an area of non-articular cartilage (*purple*) that is now in contact with the joint surface of the proximal phalanx.

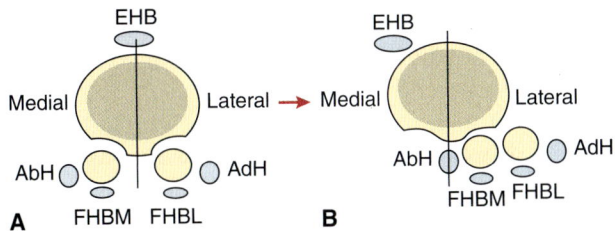

FIGURE 9-48 Changes in tendon line of pull as a result of right hallux valgus. Cross-section of right great toe looking distally. **A.** Normal tendon alignment. **B.** Changes in tendon location and therefore line of pull as a result of the bony changes of hallux valgus. The AdH, FHB, and FHL have a greater mechanical advantage to adduct the great toe, while the ability of the AbH to abduct the great toe is lost. *AbH*, abductor hallucis; *AdH*, adductor hallucis; *EHB*, extensor hallucis longus; *FHB*, flexor hallucis brevis; *FHBL*, flexor hallucis brevis and longus. (Adapted from Nordin M, Frankel VH. *Basic Biomechanics of the Musculoskeletal System*. 5th ed. Wolters Kluwer; 2022: Figure 9-26.)

History Patients with HV report 1st MTP pain, likely because of the changes in articular contact surface as a result of the HV deformity. Pain is exacerbated during terminal stance when there is greater weight-bearing forces through the great toe and the need for end-range great toe extension. Patients may also complain of pain at the plantar 2nd metatarsal head secondary to the increased weight-bearing forces in this region resulting from 1st metatarsal insufficiency.[109] Patients frequently complain of difficulty finding comfortable footwear because of the widening of the forefoot and increased pressure on the medial 1st MTP. Patients with HV report lower function on outcome tools, such as the Foot and Ankle Abilities Measure.[110,111]

Key Examination Findings First and foremost, patients with HV must have an HV deformity. Patients with HV are more likely to have excessive pronation. Females with HV are more likely to have increased lower extremity range and flexibility including having excessive hip internal rotation range, genu valgus, and greater amounts of rearfoot eversion.[108] The altered articular surface contact between the great toe and the 1st metatarsal leads to a loss of great toe extension range. Gait may be altered to avoid great toe extension during terminal stance by shifting weight more laterally during weight bearing on the affected side.[111] The patient may exhibit a greater toe-out and increased double limb support time along with reduced push-off on the affected side.[107] Patients with HV typically have decreased cadence and decreased gait speed.[112] As a result of the increased foot mobility and excessive pronation,[107] patients with HV may have limited dorsiflexion range and gastrocnemius muscle length. These patients also tend to have worse balance.

Differential Diagnoses Differential diagnoses to consider include HR, sesamoid pathology, metatarsalgia, and neuropathy.

Rehabilitation Focus and Key Points Rehabilitation for HV, like so many lower extremity pathologies, should include a local and a regional approach. Locally, night splints can be used to hold the patient's toe in a more neutral position (Fig. 9-49A).[113] This can provide pain relief and may prevent soft tissue changes from progressing. Likewise, a toe spacer or taping can assist with toe alignment during the day (Fig. 9-49B, C).[107] Pain relief can be attained by over-the-counter inserts to reduce foot pronation and/or choosing more rigid footwear to reduce 1st MTP extension. Choosing footwear with a lower heel will decrease the need for great toe extension and reduce MTP weight-bearing forces. Shoes with a wider toe box and more flexible material can decrease medial MTP soft tissue soreness. Rehabilitation should focus on restoring ankle dorsiflexion and gastrocnemius length if limited. Strengthening of the foot intrinsics, the fibularii, and the tibialis posterior can all provide needed dynamic support for the foot as well as increased stabilization of the 1st metatarsal.[114] However, caution should be used when strengthening toe flexors. Exercises such as open kinetic chain toe flexion, towel scrunches, and picking up marbles with the toes may exacerbate the

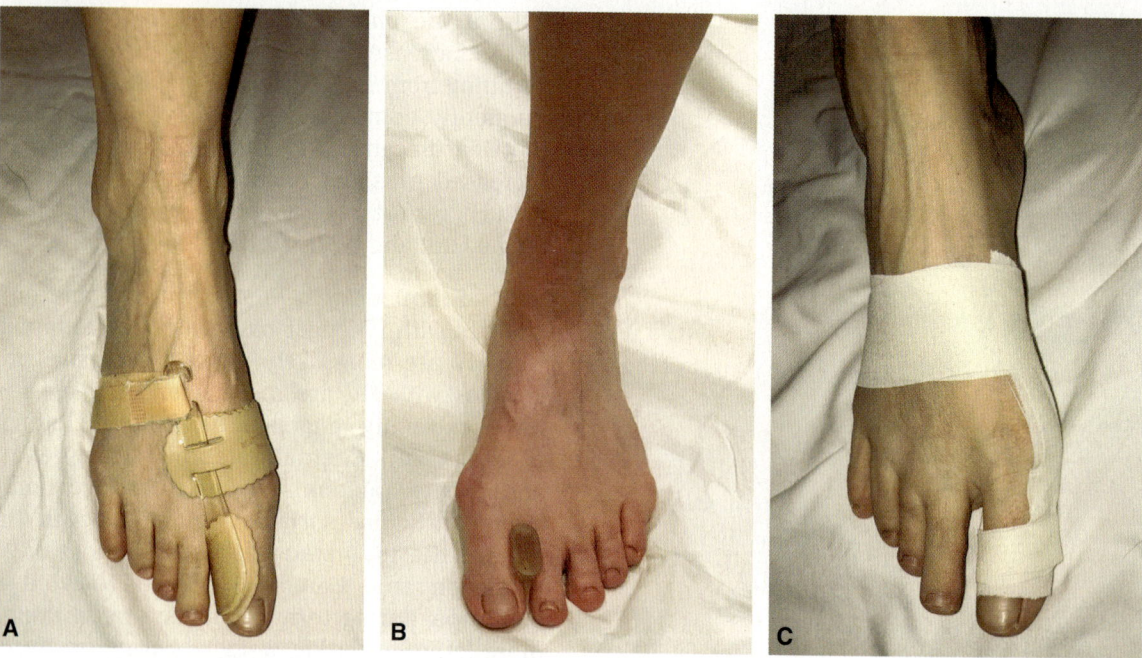

FIGURE 9-49 Methods of improving hallux valgus positioning. **A.** Night splint. **B.** Toe spacer. **C.** Taping. Note the patient also has a digiti quinti varus deformity.

HV deformity if the 1st MTP angle is greater than 45°. A simple toe gripping exercise, where the patient has the feet in contact with the ground and tries to flex the toes down into the support surface, may provide a safer alternative. Clinicians may consider strengthening additional muscle groups that control pronation, including the gluteus maximus and hip external rotators. This may be particularly important for women with HV.[105] Hip extensor weakness may occur as a result of years of gait changes, such as decreased push-off and decreased gait speed. Balance training should be used to improve any deficits noted and reduce the risk for falls. Last, patients may require gait retraining to improve 1st MTP weight bearing during push-off.

Expected Outcomes Physical therapy outcomes are equivalent to surgical outcomes.[114] Sadly, however, many patients with HV are not seen by physical therapy until after surgery.

Rehabilitation after Hallux Valgus Surgery There are multiple surgical approaches to address HV. As such, there is no one "best" HV surgical procedure for all patients. Common procedures include Chevron, Mitchell, Austin, Wilson, and Scarf procedures.[115–118] The method chosen depends on the degree of HV deformity, age of the patient, foot functional demands, and surgeon expertise. HV surgery generally includes an osteotomy, where a wedge is cut out of the shaft of the 1st metatarsal. The bone may be stabilized with locking plates or by impaction (grinding the removed bone and using this to facilitate healing of the cut bone). Soft tissue balancing procedures, such as a lateral MTP capsular release and release of the lateral metatarsosesamoid suspensory ligament, may need to be performed because of adaptive tissue changes from prolonged malpositioning. Many times, HV surgery is performed simultaneously bilaterally and additional procedures are performed to correct any lesser toe deformities present.

Postoperative precautions generally include about 6 weeks of weight bearing as tolerated using a rigid postoperative shoe to prevent weight bearing the 1st MTP extension and allow the tissues to heal. During this early healing time, patients should be encouraged to ice and elevate the foot to minimize pain and edema. Ankle pumping and active toe wiggling should also be encouraged. Physical therapy generally begins 6 weeks after surgery when weight-bearing precautions are lifted. Rehabilitation after surgery is then very similar to rehabilitation without surgery: restoring motion in the sagittal plane, including great toe extension, ankle dorsiflexion, and gastrocnemius length. The clinician should also assess and address flexor hallucis longus length, as the tendon may have adaptively shortened preoperatively and now postoperatively is in a more anatomic position. First MTP, talocrural joint, and midfoot/rearfoot joint mobility should be assessed and addressed via joint mobilizations if needed. Scar mobilization and desensitization may be required. Strengthening should focus on foot intrinsics, flexor hallucis longus, and 1st metatarsal stabilizers. As with nonoperative treatment, clinicians may need to address weakness within the entire kinetic chain. Balance exercises and gait retraining should focus on improved weight transfer to the 1st metatarsal and active push-off using the intrinsics and long toe flexors.[112,119,120]

HV surgery has a 10% complication rate.[121] Overall, the surgery leads to decreased pain, improved self-reports of function, improved pressure distribution,[112,113] and improved push-off, but therapeutic rehabilitation appears to be required to attain maximal benefits.[110] Interestingly, there is no correlation between angular improvement and clinical improvement.[122] Although the greatest improvements occurred in the first 6 months of surgery, patients may continue to have improved function up to 2 years after surgery.[110] Clinicians should be aware that rehabilitation alone demonstrated equivalent outcomes to surgery plus rehabilitation for reducing pain and improving function.[114,119,120]

Hallux Rigidus

HR is a condition characterized by progressive loss of 1st MTP extension because of the presence of a dorsal osteophyte. HR may result from osteoarthritis or prior trauma.[123] Initially there is a functional loss of great toe extension, but over time the joint motion becomes more and more restricted by both bony and soft tissue changes (Fig. 9-50), including a loss of 1st MTP capsular mobility and great toe flexor length. Differential diagnoses include gout, HV, and sesamoid pathology.

Physical therapy may have short-term benefits via joint mobilization and stretching. Footwear modifications, such as reducing heel heights and use of shoes with a rigid sole,[124] will predictably reduce pain with gait by reducing or eliminating the need for 1st MTP extension.[125] Nonsteroidal anti-inflammatories may also be beneficial.[124]

In later stages of the condition, minimally invasive surgical procedures such as a dorsal cheilectomy (removal of the bony block to 1st MTP extension), with or without debridement of the articular surface, has a 90% success rate.[126] Surgery results in improvements in pain, increased 1st MTP extension range, tolerance of more "fashionable" footwear, improved gait mechanics, and patient reports of improved function.[123,127] However, patients with severe osteoarthritis may require a partial or total joint arthroplasty.[128] Rehabilitation after HR surgery is quite similar to that of HV.

Metatarsalgia

Pathology Metatarsalgia, as the name implies, is pain on the plantar aspect of the metatarsal heads, most commonly the 2nd, 3rd, or 4th metatarsals. Metatarsalgia may be the result of structural abnormalities (such as HV), systemic conditions, or training errors. Structurally, a long 2nd metatarsal can lead to metatarsalgia of the 2nd metatarsal.[129] Metatarsalgia may result from a supinatory foot type[129] because the rigid foot architecture is unable to absorb shock. However, individuals with a pronatory foot type[129] may develop metatarsalgia because of the increased stress placed on the 2nd and 3rd metatarsal heads when the foot fails to become a rigid lever for push-off. Individuals with RA[130] may experience metatarsalgia because of fat pad atrophy and distal fat pad migration, which uncovers the metatarsal heads. Gout is also associated with metatarsalgia.[130] A hammertoe deformity may lead to pain in the associated metatarsal because hyperextension of the MTP increases pressure on the metatarsal head.[131]

History Patients with metatarsalgia report pain on the plantar aspect of the foot, specifically at the plantar metatarsal head. The pain is typically described as if stepping on stones and is typically increased from heel-off to push-off phase of gait as well as when walking barefoot. The onset may be slow or the result of an acute overload, such as a sudden increase in running or new military recruits marching in boots with loaded packs.

Key Examination Findings The key examination finding for patients with metatarsalgia is pain upon palpation of one or more plantar metatarsal heads. The skin should be examined for calluses indicative of non-neutral foot mechanics. Further inspection may reveal prominent metatarsal heads, particularly in patients with RA. A hammertoe deformity may be present. Gait assessment may result in deviations such as reduced push-off, decreased dorsiflexion range, or simply the patient reporting pain during the later phases of gait.

Differential Diagnoses Differential diagnoses include sesamoiditis, osteochondrosis, stress fracture, plantar plate rupture, Morton neuroma, and PFasc.[131] Clinicians

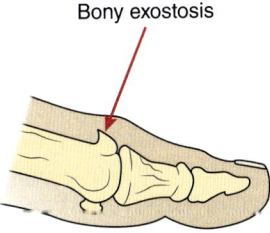

FIGURE 9-50 Hallux rigidus. Note the bony exostosis on the dorsal aspect of the distal 1st metatarsal that is characteristic of hallux rigidus. (Adapted from Nordin M, Frankel VH. *Basic Biomechanics of the Musculoskeletal System*. 5th ed. Wolters Kluwer; 2022: Figure 9-17A.)

should consider if there is a need for management of any systemic disease, such as gout or RA.[132]

Rehabilitation Focus and Key Points Interventions for metatarsalgia should focus on reducing the cause of increased plantar metatarsal pressure. Training modifications are needed if symptom onset coincided with an increase in activity, such as marathon training or military basic training. Footwear modifications,[133] such as a metatarsal pad, can distribute forces over a larger surface area, thus reducing pain (Fig. 9-51A). Likewise, pressure-reducing insoles[134] or shoes with improved shock absorption or a rocker bottom shoe may provide relief.[132] For hammertoes, taping[129] or over-the-counter orthotic devices can be used to reduce MTP hyperextension, thus reducing plantar metatarsal head pressure (Fig. 9-51B).

If plantar pressures are the result of limited dorsiflexion or limited MTP flexion, talocrural or MTP joint mobilizations and stretching should be considered. Likewise, stretching should address any loss of gastrocnemius or toe extensor length. Shaving down prominent calluses can provide relief[129] and may need to be repeated if the cause of callus cannot be rectified. Anti-inflammatory agents may provide short-term relief but should not be used for long-term management.[131]

Expected Outcomes Conservative interventions generally lead to full recovery. If conservative treatment fails, surgical interventions to address a structural root cause of metatarsalgia, such as gastrocnemius lengthening[135] or an osteotomy of a disproportionately long 2nd metatarsal, have proven effective in reducing pain and improving function.[132,136]

Interdigital or Morton Neuroma

Pathology Interdigital neuroma, also known as Morton or intermetatarsal neuroma, is an irritation and fibrous enlargement of a terminal branch of the medial and lateral plantar nerves (Fig. 9-52). About two-thirds of cases occur in the 3rd webspace and one-third in the 2nd webspace.[137] The 3rd webspace may be more commonly affected because the 3rd interdigital nerve contains a communicating branch from the lateral plantar nerve that increases the size of this nerve.[138] The nerve may become entrapped as it runs deep to the transverse metatarsal ligament.[139] The nerve may become irritated by repetitive trauma from dance or running,[140] particularly in a hyperpronated foot. This is because a hyperpronated foot is more mobile and can create increased shearing forces between the metatarsals, which irritate the interdigital nerve.[138,139] Compression from wearing a shoe with a narrow toe box can also irritate the nerve.[140] It is likely that a symptomatic patient may present with a combination of these factors.

History Patients report sharp or dull pain, tingling, or a burning sensation in the intermetatarsal region that radiates into two adjacent toes. Patients may report it feels like they have a pebble in their shoes. Symptoms are worse with gait or when wearing tight-fitting shoes with a narrow toe box. Women are 10 times more likely to have an interdigital neuroma than men.[137,139] The condition is also more common in middle-aged individuals.[138]

Key Examination Findings Key examination findings to rule in an interdigital neuroma include the following positive special tests: thumb index finger squeeze test, metatarsal compression test, dorsal and plantar Tinel test, and Mulder sign. Additionally, intermetatarsal glides[138] may recreate the patient's chief complaint by compressing and shearing the affected nerve. Patients with an intermetatarsal neuroma may have

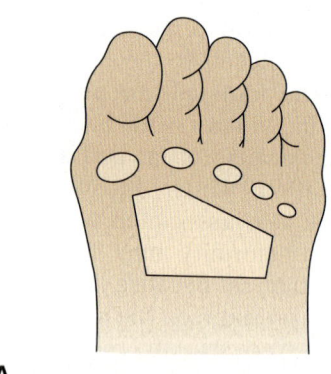

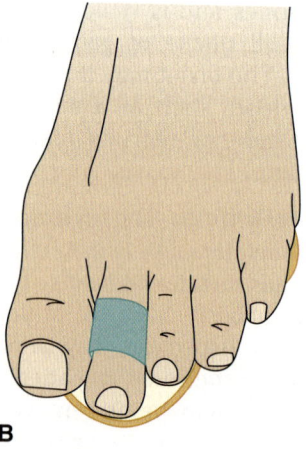

FIGURE 9-51 Footwear modification for metatarsalgia. **A.** Metatarsal pad. **B.** Over-the-counter orthotic device to improve hammertoe alignment. The band decreases proximal interphalangeal flexion. This decreases metatarsophalangeal hyperextension, thereby reducing pressure under the metatarsal head.

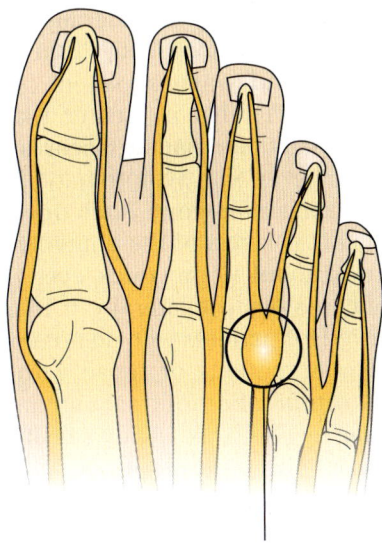

FIGURE 9-52 Interdigital neuroma. Note the enlarged interdigital nerve between the 3rd and 4th metatarsals. (Adapted from Gest TR. *Lippincott Atlas of Anatomy*. 2nd ed. Wolters Kluwer; 2020: Plate 3-68A.)

reduced dorsiflexion range of motion that leads to compensatory increase in pronation.

Differential Diagnoses Differential diagnoses include TTS, PFasc, lumbar radiculopathy, and diabetic neuropathy.

Rehabilitation Focus and Key Points Rehabilitation for patients with an interdigital neuroma should focus on footwear modification and restoring dorsiflexion range.

Expected Outcomes Conservative treatment has about a 40% success rate and is more likely to be successful in acute cases. Patients with chronic complaints are more likely to require a staged approach[141] beginning with local injections of alcohol, steroids, or anesthetics. Injections have up to an 82% success rate, although patients may require more than one injection and many may still require surgical intervention at some point in the future.[90,142] Radiofrequency ablation appears to result in about a 50% reduction in pain within the first week and symptoms remain stable for at least 1 year postprocedure.[143] Should these interventions fail, surgical excision of the affected nerve results in an 83% success rate.[139] Rehabilitation is seldom required after surgery.

Plantar Fasciopathy

Pathology PFasc constitutes 10 to 15% of all foot problems.[144] The peak onset is between 40 and 70 years of age. However, 5 to 10% of runners will also have PFasc,[144] and it is the most common foot injury in athletic populations.[97] The cost of PFasc (in 2007 dollars) has been estimated to be $200 to $375 million.[145] PFasc, also known as plantar fasciitis, was thought to only be an inflammatory condition of the plantar fascia. However, tissue biopsies of patients with chronic PFasc have shown an absence of inflammatory cells. Therefore, PFasc is best categorized as being acute, chronic, or plantar fascia rupture.

Acute PFasc does have areas of tissue inflammation and is most commonly because of a sudden increase in activity, such as a transition from a sedentary job to one requiring significant walking or when an athlete has a substantial increase in training. More commonly, PFasc is seen within the clinical setting when it has become a chronic degenerative condition marked by tissue fibrosis and immature vascularization.[146] Chronic PFasc is characterized by a thickening of the plantar fascia in response to prolonged overload. Patients with PFasc may have a horizontal calcaneal spur that is thought to develop from the body's attempt to manage the repeated tensile forces on the plantar fascia. Whereas 89% of patients with PFasc had a calcaneal spur, 32% of asymptomatic patients also had a calcaneal spur,[147] bringing into question whether the spur was the cause, the result, or only associated with PFasc pain. The symptoms of PFasc may resolve, while the spur remains unchanged. For these reasons, radiographs are not a recommended imaging modality for this pathology.

Patients with PFasc have atrophy of the plantar heel fat pad.[147] Heel forces during gait are dissipated by the plantar fascia, the fat pad, the intrinsics, and footwear. The fat pad is thought to play a protective role in absorbing impact loads and protecting deeper structures. With PFasc, changes in the fat pad, including an increase in collagen linking and lower proteoglycan content, make it less able to dissipate heel forces.[148] The cause of these fat pad changes is unclear, but it appears that these changes occur after plantar fascia fibrosis.[148]

Individuals with high-arched feet are at increased risk for PFasc, likely because the structure of the foot prevents the necessary pronation to absorb forces, placing increased strain on the plantar fascia. Excessive pronation, loss of dorsiflexion range, loss of great toe extension range, intrinsic muscle weakness, and high body mass index (BMI) all increase the load on the plantar fascia and, therefore, are risk factors for PFasc. Individuals with tight hamstrings are almost nine times more likely to have PFasc than those with normal hamstring flexibility.[149] Likewise, occupations that require prolonged standing, such as teachers or bank tellers, or a recent job change that requires increased standing and walking increase the risk of PFasc. In the athletic population, PFasc is commonly due to a sudden increase in training, particularly an increase in speed work as plantar fascia stress is greater with greater amounts of MTP extension. Patients with a history of corticosteroid injection in the plantar fascia have a significantly increased risk for plantar fascia rupture, with one study noting that 88% of patients with plantar fascia rupture had received a prior injection.[150]

Although much less frequent, rupture of the plantar fascia does occur and is generally the result of either a one-time sudden high force (such as landing from a high jump) or quick loading to a damaged plantar fascia, such as when an athlete with PFasc was treated with a steroid injection[97,146] and then goes to strongly push off the affected foot. Plantar fascia rupture should be considered for patients who report hearing a pop or feeling a tearing sensation after trauma, particularly a patient with a history of steroid injection to the plantar fascia. If seen acutely, the patient will present with ecchymosis, swelling, and may have a palpable breach in the plantar fascia.[146] Ruptures are generally treated with immobilization and 4 to 6 weeks of non–weight bearing.

History Patients with PFasc report plantar heel pain with gait, particularly the first few steps in the morning or after prolonged sitting, or if walking in bare feet.[151] Patients report the pain causes them to alter their gait, sometimes walking only on the forefoot to avoid pain. After the initial steps, the pain typically subsides but may return with prolonged weight bearing. Patients with more severe PFasc may have constant pain with weight-bearing activities. Patients may report a recent change in activity level as noted earlier. Paresthesias are uncommon.

Key Examination Findings Key examination findings include reproduction of the patient's pain complaint with deep palpation of the plantar medial calcaneal tubercle, the proximal attachment site of the plantar fascia. Palpation along the plantar fascia reveals fibrotic tissue. In milder cases, tenderness may only be noted after passive extension of digits, which tightens the plantar fascia. The patient may have a positive windlass test. To rule out TTS, the patient should have a negative Tinel test at the tarsal tunnel and sustained dorsiflexion and eversion should not reproduce symptoms.

Clinicians should assess dorsiflexion and great toe extension range, gastrocnemius and hamstring length, as well as weight-bearing versus non-weight-bearing foot posture. Trigger points may be present along the plantar aspect of the foot, in the soleus or gastrocnemius. Gait assessment may reveal pain at heel contact, increased time spent at midfoot and forefoot contact,[151] hyperpronation or limited pronation.

The diagnosis of PFasc is generally made based on clinical examination alone. The PFasc can be confirmed via ultrasound when a patient has a symptomatic plantar fascia that is greater than or equal to 4 mm.[145] Normally, the plantar fascia is only about 3.3 mm thick; however, with symptomatic PFasc the involved plantar fascia averages 6.7 mm thickness. Interestingly, the plantar fascia of the uninvolved foot has been found to be about 4.2 mm thick, even though only about 30% of cases occur bilaterally.[152] Diagnostic imaging is reserved for patients who do not improve with conservative interventions or those with suspected plantar fascia rupture. Both ultrasound and magnetic resonance imaging (MRI) are highly sensitive for diagnosing PFasc, but MRI is more specific.[153]

Differential Diagnoses Differential diagnoses include calcaneal insufficiency fracture, Achilles pathology, tibialis posterior pathology, metatarsalgia, neuropathy, S1 radiculopathy, and TTS.[144,147] Additionally, clinicians should consider the possibility of systemic inflammatory conditions such as RA.[144]

Rehabilitation Focus and Key Points Rehabilitation for patients with PFasc should emphasize reducing plantar fascia load and stretching. Activity modification, particularly for athletes, can provide a necessary load reduction to the plantar fascia. Changing to a more supportive or shock-absorbing shoe can provide substantial relief. Taping to support the plantar fascia (Fig. 9-53A) may be beneficial for short-term relief.[154,155] Off-the-shelf orthotic devices that provide cushioning and/or support to the medial longitudinal arch may also be beneficial in the short term.[154] A heel cup (Fig. 9-53B) provides shock absorption and may assist patients with pain because of fat pad atrophy. Short-term use of night splints (Fig. 9-53C) may be useful for patients who have been symptomatic for more than 6 months[156] by preventing the plantar fascia and posterior calf from becoming shortened overnight.

Strengthening of the foot intrinsics and tibialis posterior can unload the plantar fascia. Individuals with PFasc have been shown to have decreased intrinsic strength and muscle volume, further limiting their ability to unload the plantar fascia.[157] Foot intrinsic strengthening, sometimes referred to as foot core training or toe yoga, can also be used preventatively, reducing the risk of running-related injury by more than twofold.[158] Figure. 9-54A to D provides examples of toe yoga. Figure 9-54D and E is sometimes called a short foot exercise. The patient attempts to actively elevate the arch while maintaining 1st MTP contact with the floor. This supinatory action essentially shortens the foot. Patients with hyperpronation may

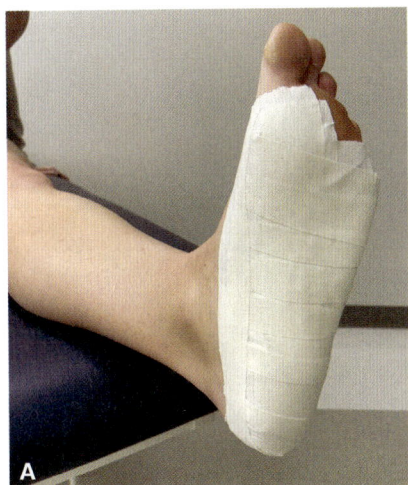 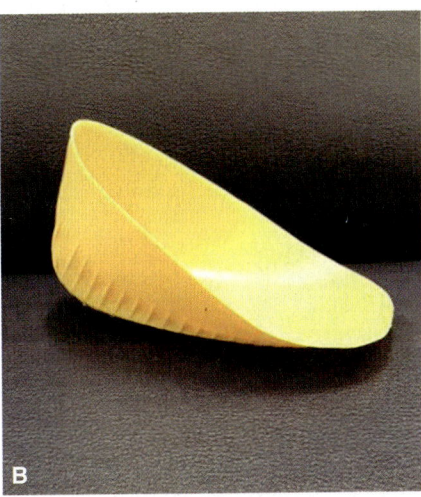 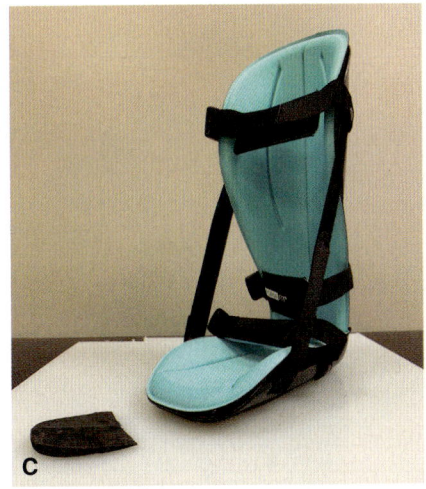

FIGURE 9-53 Possible adjunctive interventions for plantar fasciopathy. **A.** Plantar fascia taping. **B.** Heel cup. **C.** Night splint with removable wedge for metatarsophalangeal extension. (Photo courtesy of Jim Rogers, CPO, FAAOP.)

benefit from strengthening of more proximal muscles that control pronation, such as the gluteus maximus and hip external rotators. The combination of strength training and stretching appears to be superior to either approach in isolation.[159] Weight loss can help with long-term management of PFasc.

Five key structures, if restricted, should be addressed with stretching and soft tissue mobilization[154,160]: the plantar fascia, flexor hallucis longus, soleus, gastrocnemius, and hamstrings. Manual and instrumented soft tissue mobilization to the plantar fascia (Fig. 9-55) can assist with tissue remodeling, hastening recovery.[161] Patients or significant others can be taught self-mobilization of the plantar fascia as part of a home program.

Modalities may be beneficial adjuncts in the treatment of PFasc. Patients with acute plantar fasciitis may benefit from ice's anti-inflammatory effects, whereas those with more chronic condition may benefit from its analgesic effects. Two to four weeks of iontophoresis may help with acute plantar fasciitis.[144] Extracorporeal shockwave therapy may be beneficial for recalcitrant cases by destroying unmyelinated sensory nerve fibers and the microtrauma caused may promote tissue healing.[154,162]

Expected Outcomes PFasc does not appear to be a progressive condition. Overall, 80% of cases resolve within 1 year and 90% have a full recovery within 6 to 12 months.[156]

Surgical Interventions Endoscopic release of the medial 3rd of the central band of the plantar fascia, with a gastrocnemius release if a contracture is present,[163] should be considered for patients who fail to improve with conservative care. This surgery has a 60 to 90% success rate,[164] with smaller gains seen in patients whose symptoms have been present for a longer period of time. Patients are weight bearing as tolerated in a controlled ankle motion (CAM) boot until the stitches are removed, about 2 weeks after surgery.[165] Then the patients transition into a regular shoe. A night splint is recommended for the first month. Generally speaking, patients return to normal activity, including sports, within 3 to 6 months of surgery.[144]

Bone Stress Injuries

Bone stress injuries (also known as stress fractures) can be divided into two categories: fatigue fractures and insufficiency fractures. Fatigue fractures occur because of repeated stress to normal bone, whereas insufficiency fractures occur because of normal stress on weakened bone, such as osteoporosis. Training errors, such as a significant increase in running that can be seen in new runners or military recruits,[166,167] increase the risk for bone stress injuries.[168] Additional bone stress injury risk factors include low bone mineral density, relative energy deficiency in sport (RED-S), and vitamin D deficiency.[168]

Bone stress injuries occur in less than 1% of the athletic population but may be as high as 15% in runners.[169] Stress fractures are more common in female than male athletes, with the highest rates in National Collegiate Athletic Association athletes occurring in cross country, track, and gymnastics.[170] The metatarsals are the most common site for stress fractures (38%) followed by the tibia (22%) and spine/pelvis (12%).[170] Up to one-fifth of bone stress injuries are recurrent and season-ending.[170]

A bone stress injury should be considered in patients with local bony tenderness, swelling, and

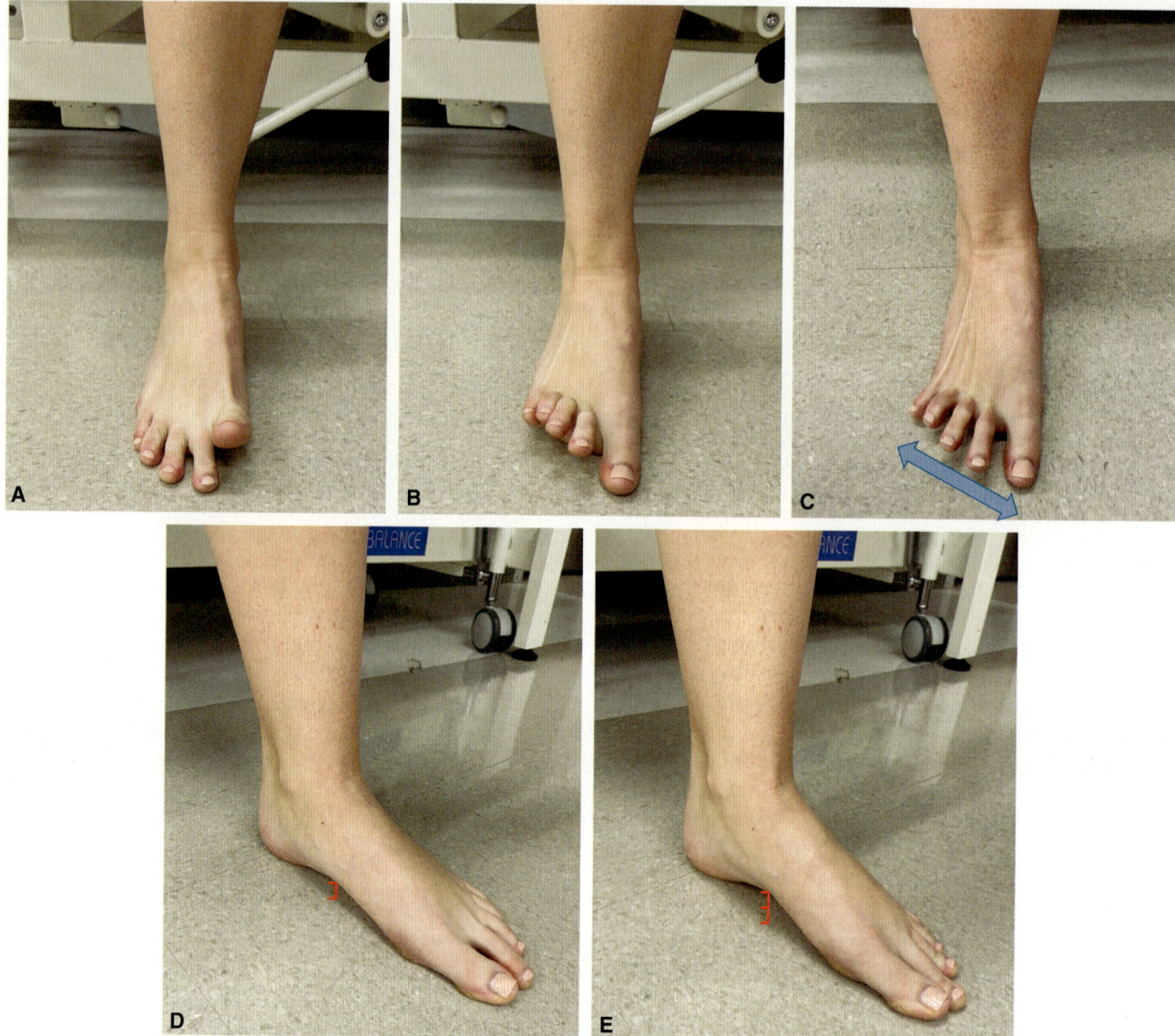

FIGURE 9-54 Foot intrinsic strengthening. **A.** Great toe extension with lesser toe flexion. **B.** Great toe flexion with lesser toe extension. **C.** Toe abduction and adduction. **D.** Short foot exercise (also known as doming) where the patient moves the foot from a relaxed position **(D)** to a high-arched position **(E)**.

exertional pain.[166] A higher index of suspicion should be given to females, athletes, and military recruits with poor preparticipation conditioning[167] and those with a prior history of bone stress injuries.

Delayed identification of bone stress injuries can lead to poor results and prolonged disability. If a bone stress injury is suspected, the patient should be sent for radiographs. If the radiograph is negative for a bone stress injury and there is still a concern for a high-risk fracture (see below), then an MRI should be ordered. If the radiograph is negative for a bone stress injury and symptoms persist for 2 to 3 weeks, an MRI is warranted.

The majority of bone stress injuries are low-risk and treated with activity modification and symptom-modulated rehabilitation followed by a gradual progression of bone loading. However, high-risk bone stress injuries include those involving the navicular, the 5th metatarsal, the hallux sesamoids, the medial malleolus, and the anterior distal tibia.[168] Injuries to these areas are at risk for delayed healing or nonunion and, therefore, are treated more aggressively, including periods of restricted weight bearing. Open reduction and internal fixation may be required for bone stress injuries that do not respond to conservative management. The reader should refer

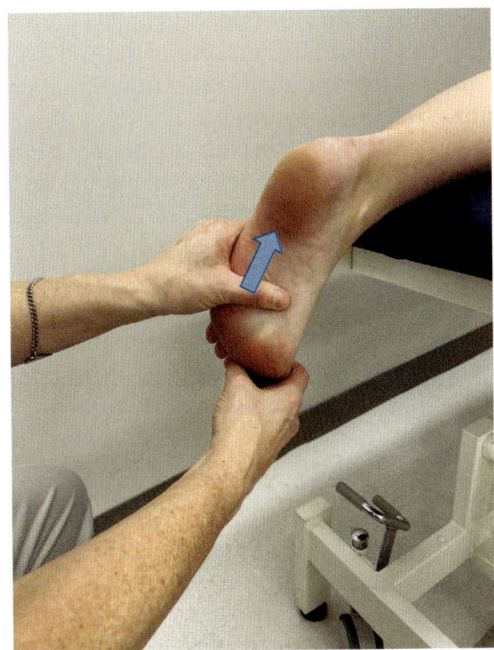

FIGURE 9-55 Soft tissue mobilization of plantar fascia.

to additional resources for more detailed examination and treatment of specific bone stress injuries.[166,167]

COMMON ANKLE PATHOLOGIES

This section contains details on the most common or most problematic foot pathologies a clinician is likely to see in an outpatient setting: fractures, sprains, Achilles tendon pathology, retrocalcaneal bursitis, tibialis posterior insufficiency, TTS, medial tibial stress syndrome (MTSS), and chronic exertional compartment syndrome.

Ankle and Foot Fractures

Pathology Ankle and foot fractures may result from falls; athletic activities; direct trauma, such as stubbing one's toe or an object landing on the foot; and high-velocity events, such as motor vehicle accidents. Typical healing times are 3 to 4 weeks for phalanx fractures, 4 to 6 weeks for metatarsal fractures, and 6 to 8 weeks for distal fibula and tibia fractures. Fractures of the remaining tarsals are much less common. Additionally, healing times and fracture management for these are quite varied. A unimalleolar fracture is typically a fracture of the distal fibula but may also be used for a fracture of the distal tibia. A bimalleolar fracture involves both the distal fibula and tibia. A trimalleolar fracture involves the fibula, tibia, and the posterior malleolus of the tibia. Trimalleolar fractures and ankle dislocations are twice as likely to have associated chondral lesions than bimalleolar fractures.[171] Chondral lesions may be a direct result of the original trauma or may result indirectly over time from fracture malalignment.

Fracture management is dependent upon fracture type and location. Short-term immobilization in a rigid-soled shoe (distal foot/toe fractures) or below-knee cast or CAM walker (ankle fractures) is the norm for simple, nondisplaced fractures. Open reduction and internal fixation is generally indicated for displaced fractures, open fractures, complex fractures, and nonunion fractures. Weight bearing initially may be restricted until bone healing has occurred. However, most fractures, such as simple fibular fractures or surgically managed fractures, are stable and not prone to migration with weight bearing.[172] For surgically managed fractures, early (within 2 weeks) weight bearing in a CAM walker and early range-of-motion exercises appear to be more convenient for the patient, improve motion, and improve function without any increase in complications.[173] For surgically managed ankle fractures, early active-controlled motion has led to superior results, even when partial weight bearing is required because of concomitant ligamentous injury.[174] Ankle immobilization consistently results in 20 to 33% reduction in gastrocnemius/soleus cross-sectional areas, 50% loss of gastrocnemius strength on the involved side, and a 28% reduction in strength on the uninvolved calf.[175] Additionally, immobilization after ankle fracture increases the risk of DJD.[176] When compared with cast immobilization, the use of a removable CAM walker resulted in fewer DVTs, less atrophy, less edema, less pain, better range of motion, better strength and endurance, less functional limitations, and a faster return to work.[177-179] Although early protected weight bearing and early motion are the emerging standard for simple and surgically managed ankle fractures, clinicians should be sure to discuss postoperative restrictions with the managing medical professional to ensure individual patients are managed properly and safely.

History When taking a history after a fracture, clinicians should strive to understand the mechanism of injury, involved structures, management, and timeline of events. Clinicians should ascertain prefracture mobility, including perceived sense of balance and stability. Access to imaging and operative reports provides vital management information, such as involved structures and fracture alignment, influence treatment, recovery time, and outcomes.

Key Examination Findings After ankle and foot fractures, patients typically present with edema, stiffness, and weakness. Minimizing ankle and foot edema early on via positioning, compression, and ice can assist with pain control and enhance recovery of motion. In the early stages of healing, ankle and foot edema and pain may be minimized utilizing positioning, compression, and ice, enhancing recovery of motion. Gait and balance deficits are common, even if no deficits were present prior to fracture.

Differential Diagnoses Clinicians should assess for associated soft tissue damage, such as ligament rupture, as this damage may not be evident on the initial radiograph identifying the fracture. Clinicians must also consider that diagnosed or undiagnosed chondral lesions may be present.

Rehabilitation Focus and Key Points Early rehabilitation interventions should focus on resolving effusion and restoring ankle dorsiflexion range. Foot joint mobilizations may be needed after ankle or foot fractures considering the tendency for development of stiffness. Talocrural joint mobilization and posterior calf soft tissue mobilization are typically required to minimize joint stiffness and musculotendinous length deficits.[180,181] Balance and gait training will help with improving function and reducing fall risk. When weaning off of the CAM walker, short-term use of adjustable, layered heel lifts may improve gait by compensating for the lack of weight-bearing dorsiflexion. Unloaded gait training in a pool or with an antigravity treadmill, such as the AlterG (Freemont, CA), may improve weight-bearing tolerance and gait form (Fig. 9-56). Four-direction ankle strengthening is important, but particular emphasis should be placed on the plantar flexors given their functional role and their known decline after fracture.[173,182]

Long-term patients who are unable to attain functional dorsiflexion may benefit from a rocker bottom shoe or bilateral heel lifts (Fig. 9-57). If using a heel lift, it is wise to have the patient perform prophylactic gastrocnemius stretches on the contralateral side to prevent contracture formation. Weight-bearing dorsiflexion, single-leg balance, and functional capacity for unilateral heel raises are all correlated with function. Weight loss strategies may be beneficial for overweight/obese patients with chondral damage or suboptimal fracture alignment by reducing ankle joint loads.

Expected Outcomes Approximately 2 months after an ankle fracture, most patients are able to walk normally on level surfaces. By 3 months, such patients will likely return to normal activities of daily living.[183,184] At 6 months, most patients will report up to 80% of normal function and by 1 year postfracture 90% of patients have restored 90% of function.[185] Although patients will make quick gains the first 3 months postfracture, they should expect to continue to improve up to 2 years after surgery. Patients who are younger, nondiabetic, and without less than 10% of articular surface involvement have better outcomes.[186] Chondral lesions may result in long-term posttraumatic DJD and persistent ankle pain.[171]

Ankle Sprain

Pathology Acute ankle sprains account for about 5% of all emergency room visits and 20% of injuries in sports.[187] Multiple structures can be injured in an ankle sprain (Fig. 9-58). Because the ATF ligament has the smallest load to failure, nearly 70% of lateral ankle sprains involve only the ATF. Roughly half of ATF injuries are an avulsion from the fibula, whereas the other half are mid-substance tears.[188] About 20% of lateral ankle sprains involve both the ATF ligament and the CFL, whereas 5% also involve the PTF.[92] Because the CFL crosses both the talocrural and subtalar joints, damage to this ligament may lead to more functional deficits. The PTF primarily provides rotatory stability. The PTF is the strongest of the three lateral ankle ligaments and, therefore, is less likely to be injured. Because the deltoid ligament is significantly more robust than the lateral ankle ligament complex, the vast majority of ankle sprains affect the lateral structures.

Lateral ankle sprains typically involve the plantar-flexed ankle moving into inversion. In response to this motion, the fibularii forcefully contract to attempt to limit ankle inversion. This can result in a

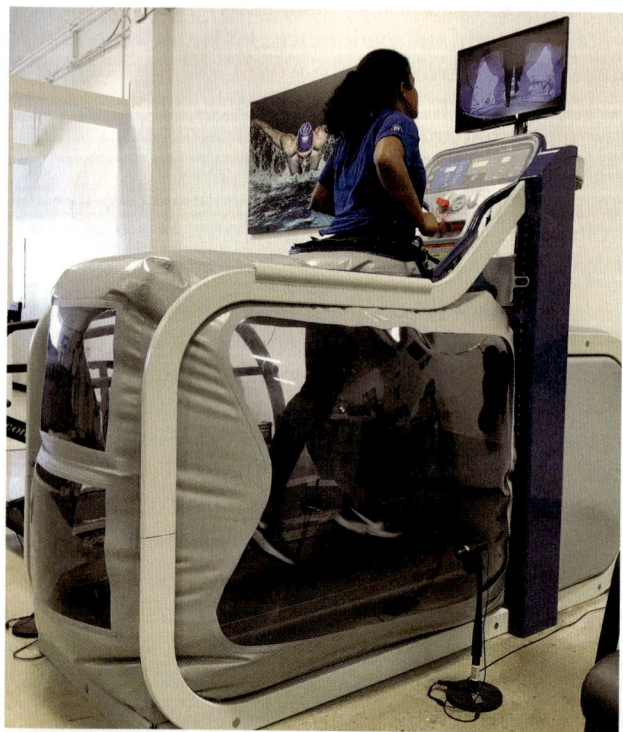

FIGURE 9-56 Patient running with reduced body weight on an unloaded treadmill.

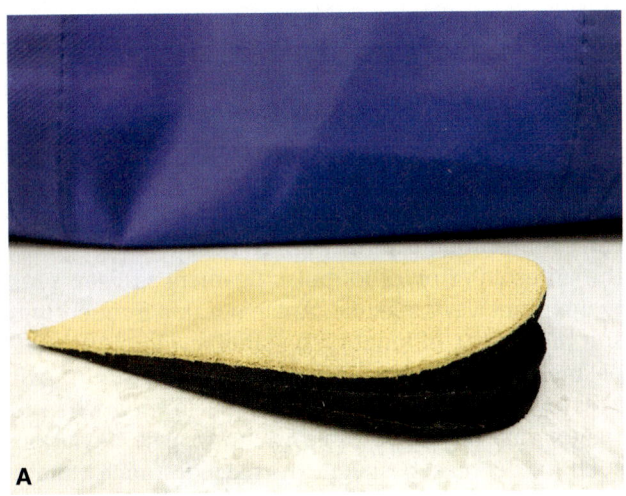
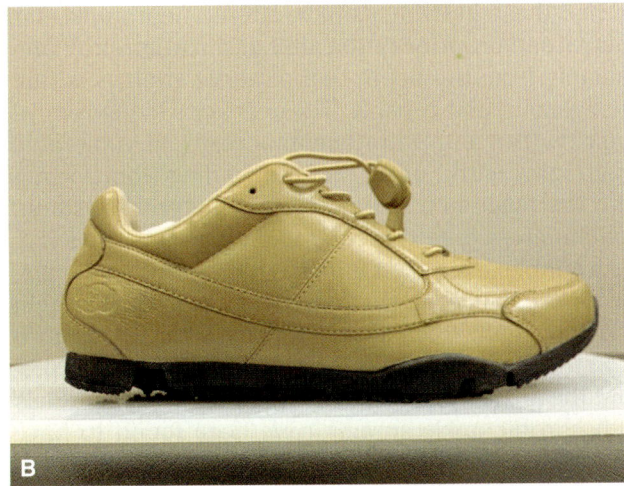

FIGURE 9-57 Footwear modifications for loss of dorsiflexion. **A.** Multilayered heel lift. **B.** Rocker bottom shoe. (Image B: Photo courtesy of Jim Rogers, CPO, FAAOP.)

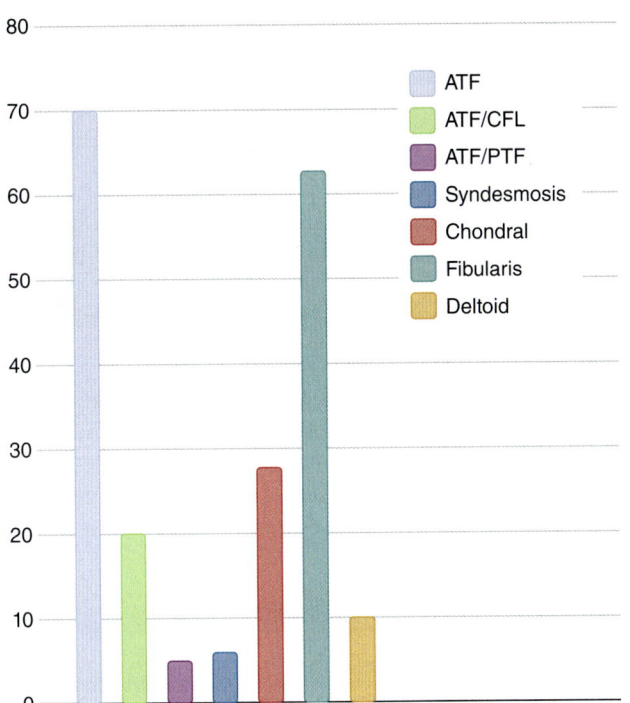

FIGURE 9-58 Structures involved in ankle sprains. *ATF*, anterior talofibular ligament; *CFL*, calcaneofibular ligament; *PTF*, posterior talofibular ligament.

combination sprain/strain injury. Occasionally, an individual will overcorrect for ankle inversion, moving suddenly into full eversion. In such a case, the patient may also sustain a deltoid ligament sprain. Osteochondral lesions can occur with ankle sprains, particularly on the talus.[189] Ankle sprains may also occur from extreme external rotation of leg on a fixed foot. Deltoid ligament sprains occur with ankle eversion with or without external rotation. Syndesmotic ankle sprains, sometimes referred to as "high ankle sprains," involve the inferior tibiofibular joint. The weaker anteroinferior tibiofibular ligament is injured first, followed by the stronger posteroinferior tibiofibular ligament, the interosseous and transverse tibiofibular ligament. Syndesmotic ankle sprains typically occur as a result of forceful external rotation of the dorsiflexed foot and, as such, the deltoid ligament may also be injured.[92]

The biggest risk factor for ankle sprains is a history of prior sprain. Other risk factors include decreased balance and proprioception as well as limited ankle dorsiflexion range that puts the ankle in a vulnerable position (closer to open-packed position). There is moderate evidence that lack of a brace in high-risk sports such as football and basketball increases the risk of an ankle sprain.

For recurrent ankle sprains, a distinction must be made between mechanical instability and functional instability. Mechanical instability is described in terms of anatomic laxity. Cadaver studies have shown that cutting of the ATF yields a 50% increase in anterior talocrural laxity. Hence, the anterior drawer test is a good assessment of ATF integrity. Sectioning of the ATF and CFL led to a 100% increase in anterior talocrural laxity. Laxity was greatest in a plantar-flexed position, followed by the neutral position. The least amount of laxity was noted in dorsiflexion (close-packed position). In contrast to mechanical instability, functional instability is the patient's perception of the ankle giving way.

Functional ankle instability (also called chronic ankle instability) occurs in up to 40% of individuals post-sprain.[100,190] However, sprain severity does not predict who will go on to have chronic ankle sprains or instability. The majority of individuals with chronic ankle instability do not, in fact, have mechanical instability.

Rather, these individuals have altered neuromuscular control and proprioception after an ankle sprain,[92] presumably from the disruption of nerve endings within the ligament and capsule. These deficits in neuromuscular control and proprioception result in vulnerable positioning with a load, such as landing from a jump with the ankle in a more inverted, high-risk position. Deficits are worse closer to end-range positions. So, for example, even if an individual has good static single limb balance on the floor, when put closer to an at-risk position, such as stepping on the side of a curb or in a divot in a field, the individual is unable to prevent the ankle from inverting. Additionally, individuals with chronic ankle sprains have been found to have weakness, decreased muscle endurance, and a loss of dorsiflexion range.

History Nearly half of all ankle sprains occur during athletic activity,[191] such as an athlete landing on another player's foot. Patients with chronic ankle sprains are likely to report a feeling of "giving way" or instability and frequently "rolling" their ankles with seemingly inconsequential stresses, such as stepping on a crack in the sidewalk.

Key Examination Findings The clinician should examine ankle active and passive motion. Table 9-6 presents the most common grading scale, involved structures, and characteristics for lateral ankle sprains.[191] Stress testing for the lateral ankle ligaments should be performed. Although the term "sprain" is specific to a ligament or joint capsule injury, recall that more than one structure is commonly injured with ankle sprains. Therefore, clinicians should also assess fibularii muscle strength to assess for a strain and stress testing for the deltoid ligament to ensure that the patient has not sustained both an inversion and eversion sprain. Patients with a syndesmotic sprain are likely to have pain with the following special tests: fibular translation test, external rotation stress test, and syndesmosis squeeze test.[189]

When assessing an acute injury, the clinician should check for local edema and ecchymosis (Fig. 9-59) and palpate the ankle ligaments for tenderness. For syndesmotic injuries, tenderness in the region of the anteroinferior tibiofibular ligament is very sensitive but not very specific. Ankle sprains frequently result in the loss of functional stability; therefore, static balance assessments such as single-leg stance with eyes open and closed should be performed when full weight bearing is possible. Acutely, gait deviations, such as decreased speed, decreased stance time on the affected side, and pain near end-range dorsiflexion, are common. Less acute patients may only have difficulty with higher level tasks such as descending stairs, squatting, running, or cutting.

Patients with recurrent or with less acute ankle sprains may present with little to no ecchymosis. Edema may be minimal or may be chronically present. These patients are likely to have positive ligament stress testing, a loss of dorsiflexion range, as well as balance and muscle performance deficits.

Differential Diagnoses Differential diagnoses include differentiating sprain location (lateral, medial, syndesmotic, or midfoot), fibularii strain, lateral ankle impingement, cuboid syndrome, osteochondral lesions, and fracture.

Rehabilitation Focus and Key Points The focus of early rehabilitation for an acute ankle sprain should focus on edema management (ice, elevation, compression wrapping, manual lymph drainage, etc.) and early weight bearing with support of an assistive

TABLE 9-6
GRADES OF LATERAL ANKLE SPRAINS

Grade	Involved Structures	Characteristics	General Timeline to Recovery
I	ATF	• ATF is tender • A/P inversion if painful • Anterior drawer may be painful but there is no laxity • Little swelling, little ecchymosis • Small loss of motion and swelling	• 7 days
II	ATF • Possible concomitant fibularii involvement	• Positive anterior drawer test indicating torn or significant stretching of the ATF • More ecchymosis and swelling • Greater loss of motion and functional deficits	• 15 days
III	ATF and CFL Concomitant fibularii involvement likely	• Positive anterior drawer test indicating torn ATF • Positive talar tilt test indicating CFL involvement • More ecchymosis and swelling • Significant loss of motion and functional deficits	• 31-55 days

A, active; *ATF*, anterior talofibular ligament; *CFL*, calcaneofibular ligament; *P*, passive.

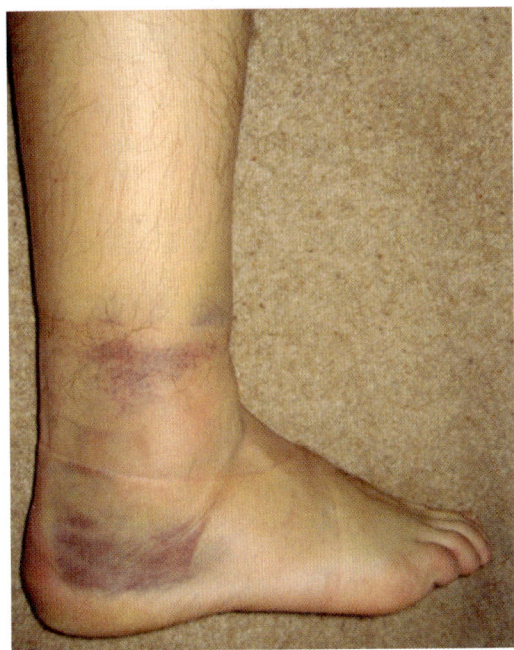

FIGURE 9-59 Acute lateral ankle sprain.

device if needed. Grade III ankle sprains may benefit from short-term use of a CAM walker.[189] An ankle brace may help decrease pain and provide ankle support until evertor muscles and balance have improved. Bracing helps prevent ankle inversion but not the combined motions of inversion, plantar flexion, and internal rotation.[192] Early controlled motion, particularly moving from end-range dorsiflexion to 30° of plantar flexion, and four-direction isometric ankle exercises have been found to be superior to immobilization without increasing strain on the injured ankle ligaments.[193] Short-term use of a heel lift may be beneficial to compensate for a loss of dorsiflexion range early on. Manual therapy, including posterior talar glides, talocrural distraction, and posterior calf soft tissue mobilization, can help improve weight-bearing dorsiflexion range of motion.[92,181,194,195]

Local strengthening should focus on ankle evertors, plantar flexors, and invertors in the open and closed kinetic chain.[187] Because individuals post–ankle sprain frequently have decreased gluteal activation and decreased core strength,[196,197] these areas should be assessed and addressed as well. Balance training should be incorporated throughout rehabilitation,[190,198] progressing from single to multiple planes, eyes open to eyes closed or head turns, flat/stable to irregular/unstable surfaces, and expected to reactive activities. Dual-task training is paramount to successful recovery of balance and proprioceptive deficits and may include cognitive tasks (counting backward by 7's) or physical tasks (reacting to a ball).[199,200] Figure 9-60 provides an example of dual-task balance training for a soccer player.

For athletes, rehabilitation should progress to include plyometric training including multidirectional jumps and hops.[187,201] An ankle brace (Fig. 9-61A) is typically recommended during high-risk activities, such as sports that require cutting or jumping, for 6 to 12 months after an ankle sprain, to help prevent recurrence.[199] Alternatively, athletes may use ankle taping (Fig. 9-61B). Taping with white coaches tape appears to be superior to other types of tape,[202] especially when incorporating heel locks.

Expected Outcomes Because the presence of laxity with ligamentous stress testing does not predict functional outcomes,[92] conservative interventions are largely successful, with 90% of individuals with complete ATF ruptures regaining functional stability with rehabilitation alone.[191] Restoration of dorsiflexion range and balance is critical to recovery.[100] Table 9-6 provides a general timeline for recovery from lateral ankle sprains.[92,189,203] Individuals with syndesmotic injuries are more likely to have residual deficits and take longer to return to sporting activities.

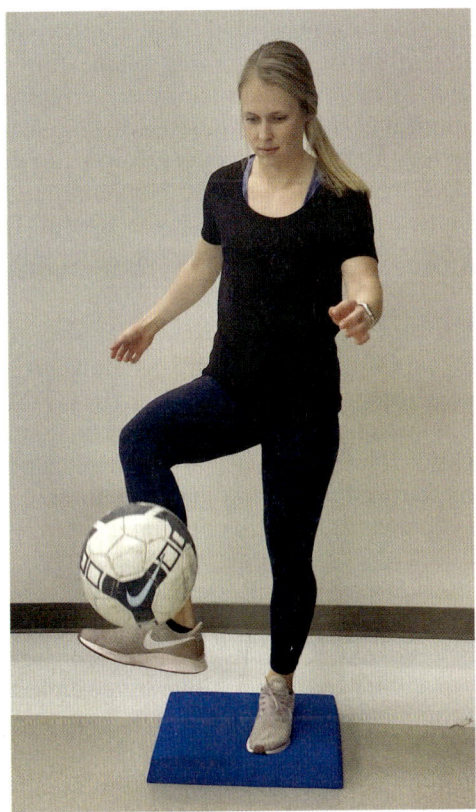

FIGURE 9-60 Static balance exercise with secondary task.

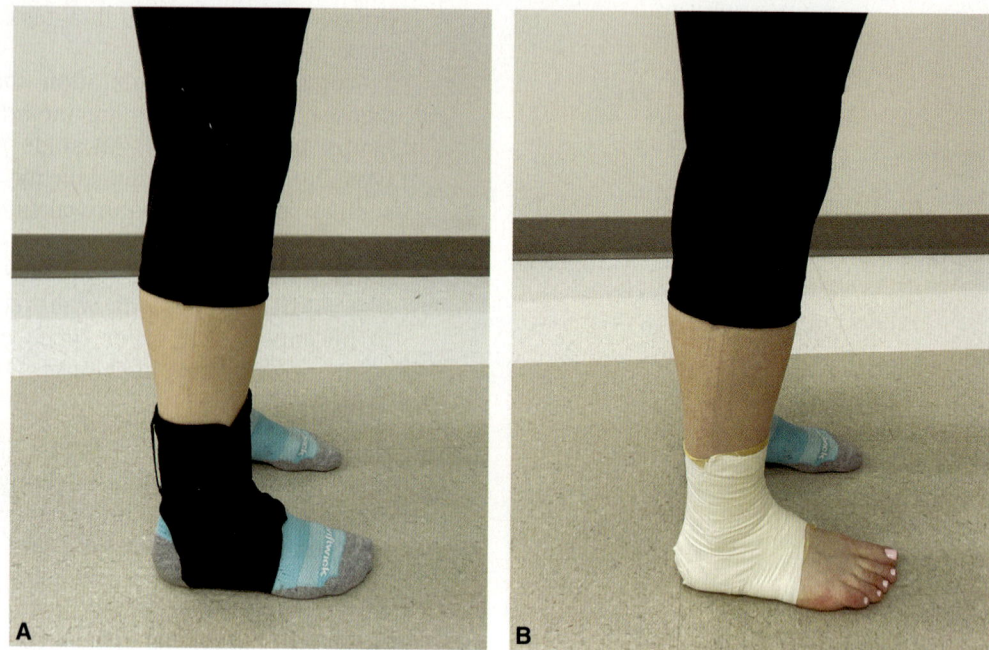

FIGURE 9-61 Ankle brace (A) or ankle taping (B) for managing ankle sprains.

Surgical Interventions At this time, surgery cannot be recommended over conservative interventions for the management of ankle sprains.[199] Individuals who fail conservative treatment may receive anatomic reconstructive surgery such as the Brostrom or the modified Brostrom method where the capsule is opened to allow inspection and treatment of osteochondral lesions.[204] These procedures tend to provide good functional recovery, lower incidence of DJD, and greater return to sport.[92] Nonanatomic repairs or augmented repairs,[204] such as the Watson-Jones or Evans procedures, may be better for larger athletes or those who have failed reconstructions.

Rehabilitation after Lateral Ankle Surgery After lateral ankle surgery, individuals are generally progressed from partial weight bearing for 2 weeks in a CAM walker followed by weight bearing as tolerated in a brace for 4 to 8 weeks.[205] Rarely, non–weight bearing in a posterior splint for the first week may be used to help accommodate effusion. Ankle active motion generally begins within 2 to 4 weeks of surgery.[205] Ankle inversion and plantar flexion beyond 30° should be limited for the first 6 weeks to prevent overstressing the repair.[205] Other than these precautions, rehabilitation after ankle surgery is similar to conservative interventions. Generally, individuals can be expected to start light plyometrics at 8 to 12 weeks, straight plane running at 12 weeks,[205] and cutting around 16 weeks after surgery.

Surgical Outcomes After surgery, reinjury is higher in those returning to high-level activities,[206] which suggests the need for high-quality, progressive rehabilitation. Re-rupture a year after surgery is rare, and ankle function can be expected to improve for up to 2 years after surgery.[207] About 94% of athletes are able to return to high-level sports after ankle surgery. In contrast to lateral ligament surgery, surgery for syndesmotic injuries has a 75% success rate.[208]

Ankle Impingement

Anterior ankle impingement is a relatively uncommon condition that occurs roughly 3% of the time after an ankle sprain.[209] Anterior impingement can occur from scarring of a previously injured ATF, osteophyte formation in the anterior distal tibia or anterior talus, or ankle synovitis (Fig. 9-62).[210,211] Patients with anterior impingement typically report anterior or anteromedial ankle pain with activities requiring increased dorsiflexion range, such as squatting or descending stairs. They may have a loss of dorsiflexion range and a positive forced dorsiflexion test. Posterior ankle impingement can occur in individuals who undergo repeated or forceful plantar flexion, such as ballet dancers and soccer players. Posterior impingement may occur from scarring of the flexor hallucis longus, posterior ankle ligament complex, an os trigonum, and/or posterior osteophytes.[212] Individuals with posterior impingement report posteromedial ankle pain with end-range plantar flexion motions.

Soft tissue impingement may resolve with conservative interventions such as manual therapy to restore motion and cross-friction to break down scar tissue.[212]

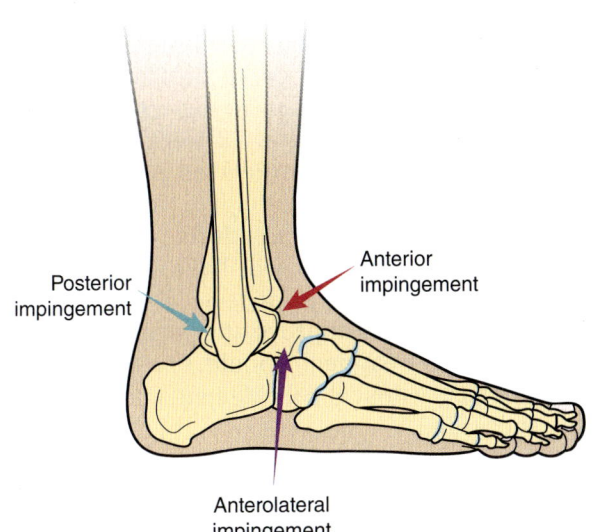

FIGURE 9-62 Common ankle impingement sites. (Adapted from Gest TR. *Lippincott Atlas of Anatomy*. 2nd ed. Wolters Kluwer; 2020: Plate 3-36.)

Bony impingement limiting function can be treated successfully with arthroscopic debridement.[213,214]

Degenerative Joint Disease

Ankle DJD is relatively rare and is usually secondary to prior trauma such as an ankle fracture that resulted in chondral damage.[215,216] The talocrural joint is most often involved, but damage may progress to the talonavicular and subtalar joints as well. Patients with ankle DJD present with a loss of motion, decreased dorsiflexion, and resulting gait deviations, which lead to a loss of plantar flexion strength. They will also have decreased balance. Interventions for DJD are impairment-related, including working on improving range and strength,[217] and may also include footwear modifications and/or an assistive device.[218,219] Pharmacologic interventions such as nonsteroidal anti-inflammatories, steroid injections, and hyaluronic acid may be useful.[220] Surgical interventions, for those failing conservative treatment, include ankle replacement or arthrodesis.[216]

Achilles Tendinopathy

Pathology Achilles tendon pathology should be described by location, chronicity, and irritability. AT primarily affects the midportion of the tendon. The Achilles tendon may be at increased risk for tendinopathy because of the high tensile loads it must accept, a potentially poor blood supply, and the shear forces that result from the 90° twist the tendon undergoes from proximal to distal attachment. Insertional tendinopathy is less common and may occur because of the addition of compression of the anterior portion of the tendon against the posterosuperior aspect of the calcaneus as the individual moves into dorsiflexion.[221,222] Interestingly, in the case of AT, abnormal tendon structure has been identified in the contralateral, asymptomatic Achilles tendon as well as the symptomatic one.[223] AT should be classified as either acute (<3 months) or chronic (>3 months).[94]

Risk factors for AT include excessive pronation, as shear forces are increased with greater pronation.[224,225] Loss of gastrocnemius length requires compensatory pronation and is also a risk factor. Weak plantar flexion and comorbidities such as diabetes, hypertension, hypercholesterolemia, obesity, and systemic inflammatory diseases are also risk factors.[94,224–227] The use of statin drugs increases the risk for AT.[228] Training errors including a significant increase in running mileage, footwear changes, or quickly changing from a rearfoot to a forefoot strike pattern increase the risk for AT. Lastly, there seems to be a genetic component to AT as individuals with a family history of AT are five times more likely to have AT.

History Patients with AT report a gradual increase in Achilles pain and stiffness. For midportion AT, the patient is tender 2 to 6 cm proximal to the insertion, and for insertional tendinopathy tenderness is at the calcaneus. Patients with highly irritable conditions may report difficulty with walking and stairs, whereas those who are less irritable may only report difficulty with higher level tasks such as running, hopping, and sports.

Key Examination Findings Hallmarks of AT are tendon thickening (>6 mm) and tenderness to palpation (Fig. 9-63). Patients may have a positive Arc sign and positive Royal London Hospital test. Heel raising may be weak, painful, or lack endurance.[226,229] The patient may have a loss of dorsiflexion range or gastrocnemius length.[94] Gait assessment or running analysis may reveal increased or prolonged pronation. Patients with AT have been found to have about a 30% decreased hip strength on the involved side[230,231] and decreased balance.[232] Higher functioning patients may have an increase in ground contact time and up to a 20% decrease in hop height.[233]

Differential Diagnoses Differential diagnoses include partial or complete Achilles rupture, bursitis, plantaris pathology, and posterior ankle impingement.

Rehabilitation Focus and Key Points The first rehabilitation decision is to determine if the patient's condition is reactive and acute or chronic. Reactive tendons are red, warm, and inflamed and require

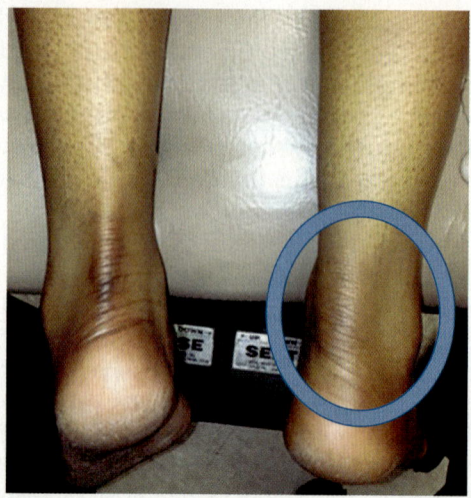

FIGURE 9-63 Patient with right midportion Achilles tendinopathy.

activity modification, ice, and, if severe, may benefit from the short-term use of a CAM walker or partial weight bearing. In contrast, chronic conditions present with tendon thickening and require progressive tendon loading. A classic tendon loading strategy progression is listed in Table 9-7.[234]

Stretching and joint mobilizations should be included to improve deficits in dorsiflexion range and gastrocnemius length.[235–237] Soft tissue mobilization, including instrument-assisted soft tissue mobilization, appears to be effective in combination with tendon loading exercises.[222] Controlling excessive pronation can be accomplished via taping, intrinsic strengthening, and neuromuscular training.[94,225] Strengthening of the tibialis posterior and hip is recommended. Custom orthotics do not appear to have an added benefit for most individuals with AT.[222] Dry needling and night splints do not appear to provide additional benefits.[94,238]

Expected Outcomes Progressive tendon loading can lead to improved collagen alignment, decreased tendon thickness, nerve and vessel regression, and a more normal stress/strain curve profile.[239] Clinically relevant decreases in pain can be expected in 4 weeks with maximal improvement at 12 weeks.[239] However, for some, recovery may be delayed as athletes will frequently continue to participate in their sport, particularly if the injury occurs during season. Ninety percent of the individuals will have minimal or no pain and return to their prior level of function.[239–241] Individuals who fail to improve after at least 6 months of conservative treatment should consider surgical interventions.[240] Surgical debridement and/or repair is highly successful.

Achilles Tendon Rupture

More than 80% of Achilles tendon ruptures occur during athletic activities.[242] Ruptures are typically the result of a one-time rapid dorsiflexion, such as landing from a jump. Males, typically 30 to 49 years of age, are more likely to rupture their Achilles. The individual will report feeling and/or hearing a pop at the time of rupture. Less than 4% of patients with chronic AT go on to rupture. Those that do rupture are generally older individuals and may be diabetic or obese. Certain medications, such as statins, fluoroquinolones, and steroid injections into the tendon, increase the risk for Achilles rupture.

Clinically, an Achilles rupture is identified by a visible deformity, palpable gap in the tendon, weak plantar flexion, and a positive Thompson test.

TABLE 9-7	
ACHILLES TENDON LOAD PROGRESSION	
Stage	**Characteristics**
Isometrics	Pain-modulating exercise 45–60″ holds for 5 repetitions, one to three times per day Increase load to supra-bodyweight before progressing to next phase
Weight-bearing PF	Progress bilateral to unilateral to external weight If insertional tendinopathy, perform on floor rather than edge of step to prevent DF 3 or more sets of 15 (~65% of 1 RM) Can progress to next phase once able to complete 4 sets with pain <5/10
Heavy slow resistance	Progress load of weight-bearing exercise from 3 to 4 sets of 15 repetitions to 4 sets of 6–8 repetitions at 6 seconds per repetition (increase from 65 to 85% intensity) Consider progressing to next phase once able to perform 25 unilateral heel raises without pain
Energy storage	Fast weight-bearing PF Progress to plyometrics: stairs, skipping, jumping, hopping Perform every third day, continue isometric exercise on off days Consider progressing to the next phase once tolerating 2 weeks of plyometric activities
Sport-specific training	Increase tendon loads toward sport-specific volume, intensities, and angles

1 RM, one-repetition maximum; *DF*, dorsiflexion; *PF*, plantar flexion.

Currently, conservative management of Achilles rupture may be best suited for older, less active individuals without tendon retraction. Those managed conservatively tend to have worse active heel raise, take longer to reach maximal function, and are two to four times more likely to rerupture.[243,244] Conservative interventions include prolonged immobilization in a CAM boot followed by gradual calf strengthening and balance and gait training.

Postoperative Rehabilitation Postoperatively, surgeons vary on the amount and timing of stress to the repaired Achilles. It appears that active dorsiflexion as early as the day after surgery results in better collagen fiber orientation and strength.[245] Immediate weight bearing as tolerated in a CAM walker appears to be superior to non–weight bearing.[246] At 3 to 6 weeks postsurgery, individuals can progress gradually from the CAM boot to a shoe with a heel lift. Once walking normally with the heel lift, slowly remove layers of the heel lift to provide a gradual increase in stress to the repaired Achilles.[247] Gentle stretching of the Achilles should be performed only if there is motion loss and should not begin until 6 weeks postsurgery.[248] Overstretching the Achilles can lengthen the repair. A lengthened Achilles alters the plantar flexor length–tension relationship, leaving the patient without power for an active push-off in gait and an inability to run or hop.

Strengthening of the remaining kinetic chain, hips, quads, etc. can occur immediately after surgery. However, plantar flexor strengthening with light resistance bands should not begin until about 4 weeks postoperatively.[248] Once the patient is 6 to 8 weeks after surgery and able to walk painfree on level surfaces without a heel lift, weight-bearing plantar flexion progression can begin bilaterally before shifting to unilateral strengthening. Athletes may begin a basic running progression as early as 10 weeks postsurgery;[249] however, this time frame depends heavily on the athlete having been allowed to progress as noted earlier.

Surgical Outcomes Persistent Achilles pain is an early sign of delayed outcomes, whereas calf muscle endurance is key for functional recovery.[250] Overall, about 90% of athletes are able to return to sport after an Achilles tendon repair, with most returning by 4 to 6 months.[251,252] However, many will be competing at a lower level than prior to their injury.[251]

Retrocalcaneal Bursitis

Retrocalcaneal bursitis can result from compression from poorly fitting footwear or the presence of a Haglund deformity, an enlarged posterosuperior border of the calcaneus.[253] Bursitis is readily identifiable by local swelling that is painful to palpation. Individuals with retrocalcaneal bursitis can generally find relief from ice and avoiding shoes with tight or rigid heel counters.[254] In rare cases, steroid injection or surgical removal of the inflamed bursa and the deformity resolves the issue.[253]

Tibialis Posterior Insufficiency

Pathology The tibialis posterior has several key functions.[255] It is a powerful muscle that works eccentrically to control pronation. Through its broad distal attachment to eight bones in the foot, the tibialis posterior is the primary stabilizer of the medial longitudinal arch. It is a dynamic stabilizer during gait, locking the midtarsal joint and everting the hindfoot so the Achilles acts as a rigid lever for push-off. The total excursion of the tibialis posterior is only 2 cm, so if it becomes elongated, or insufficient, the muscle–tendon unit will no longer perform these functions effectively.

Tibialis posterior dysfunction (TPD) is a progressive condition with a 3% prevalence rate and is the leading cause of acquired adult flat foot.[256] There are many intrinsic and extrinsic risk factors for TPD (Table 9-8). TPD is likely the result of osseous, soft issue, and vascular failures.[256] Bony structural abnormalities, such as excessive pronation, a shallow malleolar grove, an accessory navicular and preexisting flat feet, appear to increase the risk of TPD. Soft tissue abnormalities, such as age-related collagen degeneration or a tight flexor retinaculum, also place the tendon at risk for injury. The tendon's multiple insertion points create intratendinous shear forces, generating combined loading of tensile and shear forces during gait, which can adversely affect the tendon. Last, the tendon is prone to micro- and macrovascular abnormalities from diabetes, hypertension, steroid use, obesity, and trauma. There also appears to be a hypovascular region near the medial malleolus, approximately 4 cm proximal to the distal attachment of the tibialis posterior.[255,257] Tissue biopsies from patients with TPD demonstrate tissue degeneration, neovascularization, increased number of fibroblasts, and tendon thickening. Risk factors for TPD include being over 50 years

TABLE 9-8
RISK FACTORS FOR TIBIALIS POSTERIOR DYSFUNCTION

Intrinsic	• Bony structural abnormalities • Soft tissue abnormalities • Age • Female gender • Vascular abnormalities
Extrinsic	• Sedentary lifestyle • Occupation requiring prolonged standing • Inappropriate footwear

of age, female gender,[258] having bony abnormalities or ligamentous laxity, having micro- or macrovascular conditions, obesity,[258] and having an inflammatory condition, such as RA.[256] Extrinsic risk factors include being sedentary, occupations that require prolonged standing, and use of inappropriate footwear.

Because tibialis posterior insufficiency is progressive and has a significant impact on gait, it is important to identify the condition early. TPD is described in terms of stages (Table 9-9).[255,257,259] Initially, tendon overload appears similar to a strain (stage I). Manual muscle testing of the tibialis posterior will be painful as will attempts to perform a single-leg heel raise (because of the tibialis posterior's need to invert the hind foot).[260] With continued degeneration, the tendon becomes elongated and, therefore, incompetent, as even maximal shortening of the lengthened tendon will not create the force necessary to supinate the foot. This leads to rearfoot valgus and flattening of the medial longitudinal arch[260] during weight bearing because of the attenuation of the spring ligament (stage IIa) but the ability to passively reposition the foot in non–weight bearing (Fig. 9-64).[256] As the condition progresses, fibularii forces will be left unopposed, leading to forefoot abduction and a "too many toes" sign is noted (more than the 5th toe is visible when viewed from behind). Without intervention, over time these flexible deformities will become fixed and even passive attempts at correcting non–weight-bearing rearfoot valgus will be unsuccessful (stage III). Ultimately, foot pronation will drive the talus into a valgus tilt within the ankle mortise, the deltoid ligament will be attenuated, and the ankle will show signs of early degenerative changes (stage IV). Once the hindfoot moves into further valgus, the Achilles now becomes a powerful hindfoot evertor, further perpetuating foot deformity.[255]

History Patients with TPD generally complain of pain at the distal tibialis posterior tendon attachment and/or medial calf. During later stages, the patient may also complain of pain in the region of the ATF/CFL/anteroinferior tibiofibular joint because of lateral impingement,[261] the deltoid ligament, or the ankle. Although a sudden onset of flat foot is possible, most patients will note a progressive flattening of the arch. Patients will report pain with gait and possibly a slowing of gait. Patients with diabetic neuropathy may be painfree and are more likely to present later in the disease process.[257]

Key Examination Findings Clinicians should examine weight-bearing and non–weight-bearing foot posture to determine if there is a deformity and, if present, if it is possible to manually reposition the foot into rearfoot inversion. Careful palpation should be performed along

TABLE 9-9

STAGES OF TIBIALIS POSTERIOR DYSFUNCTION

Stage	Characteristics
I	Pain, tenderness to palpation, and edema in the tendon region
II	Tendon incompetence resulting in a flexible deformity IIa: rearfoot valgus IIb: rearfoot valgus and forefoot abduction
III	Fixed deformity
IV	Early ankle degenerative changes

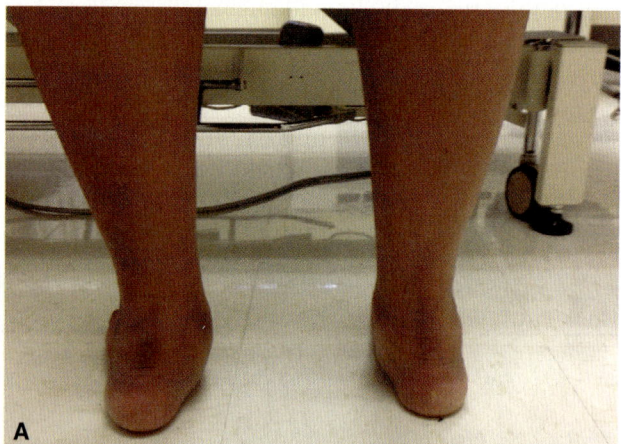
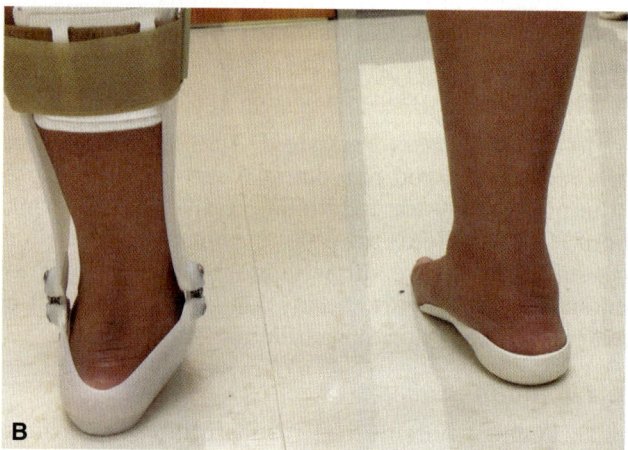

FIGURE 9-64 Patient with stage IIa tibialis posterior insufficiency. **A.** When standing barefoot, note the patient's bilateral calcaneal valgus (left more than right), left talar bulge, flattening of the medial longitudinal arch, and the left forefoot is beginning to abduct. **B.** An articulated ankle–foot orthotic is needed to control the left foot positioning. In contrast, the right foot can be managed with a simple in-shoe orthosis to control rearfoot valgus and support the medial longitudinal arch.

the length of the tibialis posterior tendon assessing for tenderness, edema, and thickening. Specific manual muscle testing of the tibialis posterior should be performed in long sitting with the hip externally rotated, placing the ankle into inversion with plantar flexion.[85] The clinician should have the patient attempt to perform bilateral and then unilateral heel raises.[261] Although technically an assessment of gastrocnemius/soleus function, observing for the inability of the tibialis posterior to invert the rearfoot and lock the midfoot to allow a rigid lever to fully rise onto the toes, and pain with testing are all signs of TPD.

Single limb balance should be assessed in patients with TPD, as they have been shown to be significantly less likely to perform single-leg stance for 10 seconds and, if successful, have much greater postural sway.[262] Clinicians should assess dorsiflexion range and gastrocnemius length as both may become limited in patients with TPD and further exacerbate the condition. Gait should be assessed noting both pain and deviations present. Patients with TPD have increased and prolonged pronation and may lack resupination. It has been shown that although typically individuals use about 60% of their available pronation, patients with TPD use nearly 92% of their available pronation range.[263] Because patients with TPD have been found to have weakness and decreased endurance in the foot intrinsics, gastrocnemius/soleus, and hip extensors, clinicians should assess muscle performance of these structures.

Differential Diagnoses TPD is a clinical diagnosis with no single definitive test. However, ultrasound and MRI can be used to identify changes within the tibialis posterior tendon.[257] Differential diagnoses to consider include structural malalignment (such as rearfoot/forefoot varus), concomitant PFasc, deltoid sprain, fracture, neuropathic osteoarthropathy (also known as Charcot foot), concomitant lateral ankle impingement, and ankle DJD.[257,259,264]

Rehabilitation Focus and Key Points Rehabilitation for patients with TPD should focus on footwear, stretching, strengthening, and balance training.[261,265] Arch taping may be beneficial for stage I.[262,266] For stage I and IIa, off-the-shelf orthotics provide pain relief and may stop deformity progression.[257] Acute, severe TPD may benefit from a CAM walker with an orthotic insert for 2 to 6 weeks to allow inflammation to subside. Individuals with stage IIb or higher severity should be referred to an orthotist.[256] Stretching to improve or restore ankle dorsiflexion and gastrocnemius length[267] will help prevent compensatory pronation for individuals in the early stages of TPD and will allow optimal positioning in orthotics for those in the later stages. Strengthening should focus on foot intrinsics and hip external rotators to provide dynamic foot stability, whereas hip extensors and plantar flexor strengthening can help improve gait.[267] Tibialis posterior strengthening (Fig. 9-65), with and without neuromuscular electrical stimulation, can be beneficial pending the degree of tendon elongation.[262,265] Balance training may assist with gait as well as reducing the risk for falls. Activity modification and weight loss programs for individuals who are overweight or obese will decrease tibialis posterior load. Nonsteroidal anti-inflammatory medications appear to reduce pain, likely because of an analgesic action.[257]

Expected Outcomes Nearly 90% of patients with stage I or II TPD can be managed successfully via conservative measures, achieving improvements in pain, strength, and gait within 4 months.[268] Patients with more advanced TPD may require surgical interventions, such as a flexor hallucis longus transfer, calcaneal osteotomy, or arthrodesis.[256,257]

Tarsal Tunnel Syndrome

TTS is entrapment of the tibial nerve as it passes through the fibro-osseous space of the tarsal tunnel, a region that is posterior to the medial malleolus, medial to the talus and calcaneus, and covered by the flexor retinaculum.[269] The contents of the tarsal tunnel (from posterior to anterior) include the tibialis posterior, the flexor digitorum longus, the posterior tibial artery and vein, the tibial nerve, and the flexor hallucis

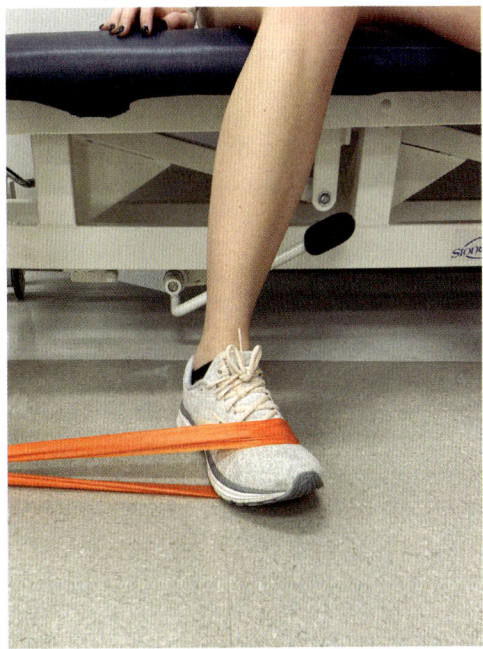

FIGURE 9-65 Elastic resistance exercise targeting the tibialis posterior muscle. Performing the exercise with footwear on provides additional support to the patient's foot.

longus. Within the tunnel, the tibial nerve divides into three main branches: the medial plantar, lateral plantar, and medial calcaneal nerves. Tibial nerve entrapment within the tarsal tunnel can be caused by repetitive hyperpronation or compression caused by edema, soft tissue restrictions, or osteophytes.[140,270] Patients with TTS report paresthesias and dysesthesias in the distribution of the posterior tibial nerve and in the medial ankle and plantar aspect of the foot. Symptoms typically increase with gait and decrease with rest. Patients with TTS may have a positive Tinel sign and a positive dorsiflexion–eversion stress test.[270] Differential diagnoses for TTS include more proximal nerve compression, such as lumbar radiculopathy, diabetes, PFasc, and interdigital neuroma. It is common for individuals with diabetes to also have TTS.

Conservative management of TTS includes manual therapy to address soft tissue restrictions, exercise, and footwear modifications to control hyperpronation.[271,272] Medical management can include oral, topical, and injected nonsteroidal and steroidal anti-inflammatories as well as tricyclic antidepressants.[270,271] Patients not responding to conservative interventions should be referred for surgical management, which results in about a 90% success rate.[270]

Medial Tibial Stress Syndrome

Pathology MTSS, sometimes known as shin splints, is the third most common running-related injury[273] and is common among military recruits. This condition is multifactorial and poorly understood, as such clinical understanding of the condition continues to evolve. Three main theories exist. Originally, MTSS was thought to be part of a continuum of shin splints to overt stress fracture.[274] The traction injury theory postulates that repeated contraction of the plantar flexor muscle group leads to periosteal edema, periostitis, and myositis.[275,276] However, although symptomatic runners were nearly twice as likely to have periosteal and tendinous abnormalities, 37% of asymptomatic control runners also had these structural changes.[275] The third theory is that MTSS may be a response to repeated tibial bending and bowing.[277]

Risk factors for MTSS include the following[95,276,278–280]:

- Female gender
- History of MTSS or running-related injury
- Higher BMI
- Greater navicular drop
- Prolonged rearfoot eversion
- Great hip external rotation
- Greater stiffness of the flexor digitorum longus or tibialis posterior
- Muscle imbalances: hip abductor weakness or evertor dominance
- Running less than 5 years
- Altered running mechanics such as excessive pelvis motion and less knee flexion

There may be some connection with MTSS and hypermobility given the condition is more prevalent in females and that individuals with MTSS appear to have prolonged pronation and increased hip external range.[278,281]

History Individuals with MTSS report diffuse posteromedial tibial border pain that is related to activity. More than half of the patients note a recent increase in training (runners) or activity (military recruits).[282] Frequently, patients will report a prior history of MTSS.

Key Examination Findings The posteromedial tibia should be palpated for tenderness. Manual muscle testing may reveal pain or weakness of the tibialis posterior, soleus, or flexor digitorum longus. Given the association between MTSS and hip abductor weakness, hip strength testing should be performed. Commonly, patients will have a positive navicular drop test and excessive or prolonged pronation with gait or running. Patients may have a loss of dorsiflexion range. A running analysis, including assessment of footwear, should be performed on runners with MTSS, particularly if no training errors have been noted.

Differential Diagnoses Differential diagnosis includes stress fracture, tibialis posterior strain, and compartment syndrome.

Rehabilitation Focus and Key Points Mild cases of MTSS respond well to activity modification and 7 to 10 days of rest.[283] Severe, recurrent, or recalcitrant cases may require 3 to 8 weeks of partial weight bearing. Stretching to improve dorsiflexion range and decrease stiffness of the flexor digitorum longus and tibialis posterior may be beneficial. Strengthening of the invertors, tibialis anterior, plantar flexors, and hip should be considered.[282] Footwear modifications may be used to help control pronation. A weight loss program may be beneficial for overweight or obese individuals.[284] Most importantly, rehabilitation must include a progressive return to activities, such as running.

Expected Outcomes Overall, conservative interventions lead to 30% of individuals recovering in a month and 92% in 4 months.[283] Patience and consistency should be emphasized as runners may require about 3 to 4 months to complete a return to running program.[283]

Surgical Interventions Individuals who fail to improve after 6 months of conservative care may benefit from extracorporeal shock wave therapy or fasciotomy.[285]

Chronic Exertional Compartment Syndrome

Compartment syndrome is caused by an increase in pressure within one or more of the four leg compartments (anterior, lateral, posterior, deep posterior). Normal compartment pressure is at least 30 mm Hg lower than diastolic pressure. A sudden increase in pressure can result from a large burn, bleeding disorders, or creatine supplementation. Athletes, particularly runners, field athletes, and military recruits, may have a gradual increase in compartment pressure during activity, called chronic exertional compartment syndrome.[286] Compartment syndrome is recognized by the "5Ps": pain, paresthesias, paresis, pallor, and pulselessness, affecting structures within the affected compartment(s). Risk factors for chronic exertional compartment syndrome include a sudden increase in training, chronic overuse,[287] abnormal gait mechanics, decreased strength, and decreased gastrocnemius flexibility. Manual therapy, stretching, and strengthening may be beneficial. The addition of gait retraining in combination with these interventions has led to positive results.[286] Most athletes, however, will require a fasciotomy of the involved compartment(s) to obtain a full recovery.[288]

DIFFERENTIAL DIAGNOSIS

The novice clinician may be a bit overwhelmed by the number and type of pathologies within the ankle and foot region. Because it is not feasible nor efficient to perform every diagnostic test, clinicians may choose to start narrowing down differential diagnoses by symptom location (Fig. 9-66), patient symptoms (Table 9-10), and onset (Fig. 9-67).

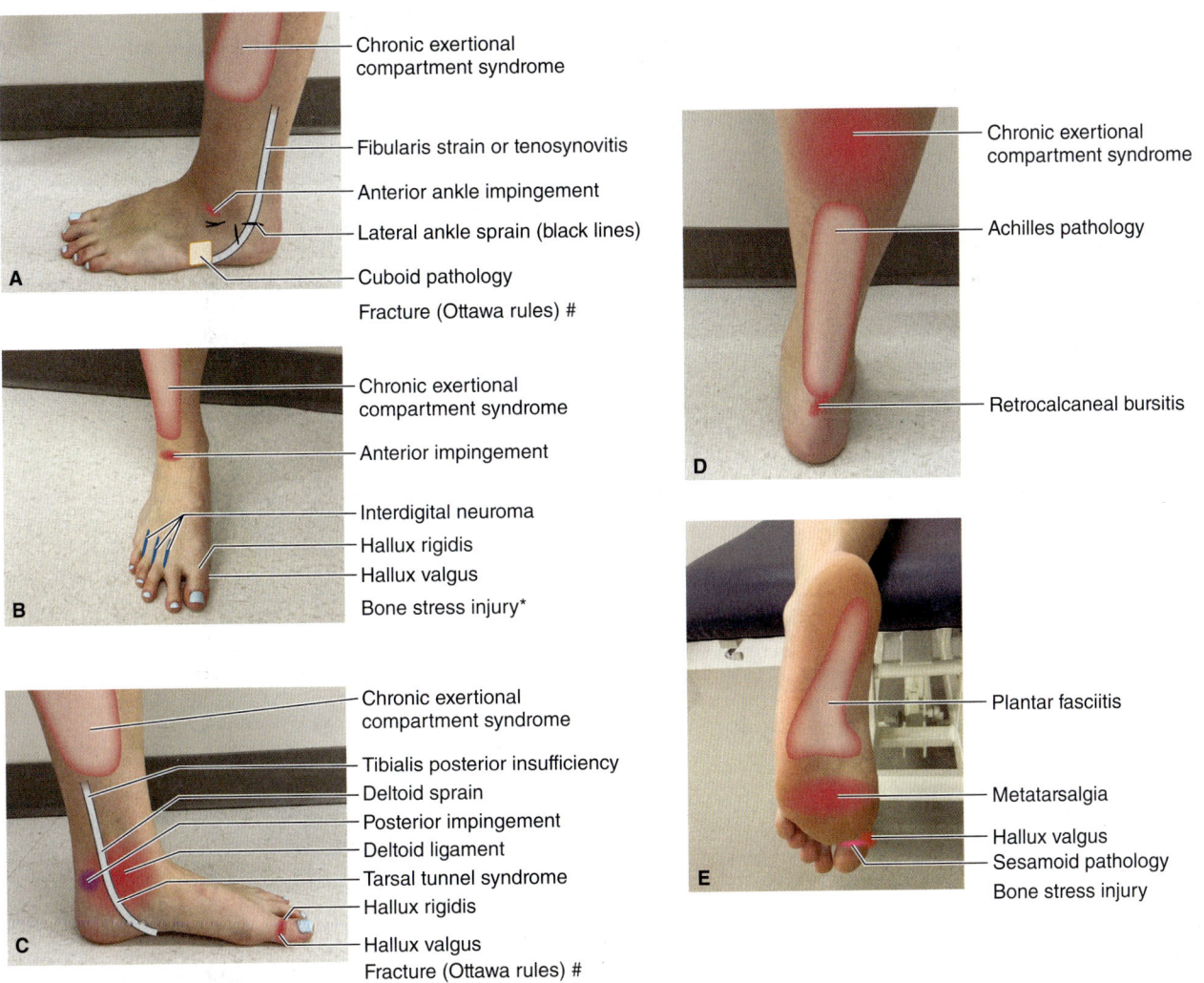

FIGURE 9-66 The location of ankle/foot symptoms can be used to begin to hypothesize possible differential diagnoses. **A.** Lateral ankle/foot. **B.** Dorsal ankle/foot. **C.** Medial ankle/foot. **D.** Posterior ankle/foot. **E.** Plantar foot. *Bone stress injury may be indicated by tenderness to bony palpation. # See Ottawa ankle rules.

TABLE 9-10
DIFFERENTIAL DIAGNOSIS OF ANKLE/FOOT PATHOLOGY BY COMPLAINT

Complaint	Differential Diagnoses
Paresthesias: numbness, tingling, burning	Proximal structure (e.g., lumbar spine, sciatic nerve) Systemic pathology (e.g., diabetes) Chronic exertional compartment syndrome Tarsal tunnel syndrome Interdigital neuroma
Instability	Ankle sprain
Plantar pain on first few steps	Plantar fasciopathy
Clicking, catching	Degenerative joint disease Osteochondral lesion

ADDITIONAL JOINT MOBILIZATION TREATMENT TECHNIQUES

When used for assessment or pain modulation, pain-modulating mobilizations are generally performed in the open-packed position or other positions of comfort. When used for improving motion, grade III and IV mobilizations are used and may begin in the open-packed position but are progressed to being performed near the end of the range that is being facilitated. The patient or family member can easily be taught self-mobilizations for the toes.

Mobilizations with Movement

Mobilizations with movement, initially described by Mulligan, are a combination of clinician-facilitated arthrokinematic motion performed with dynamic osteokinematic motion.[289]

Posterior Talocrural Joint Mobilization with Movement in Supine

Purpose: Increase ankle dorsiflexion.
Patient: Supine with the calcaneus hanging over the end of the plinth and the ankle in 10° of plantar flexion.
Clinician: The clinician contacts the patient's dorsal talus with the web space of the superior hand. The clinician's inferior hand grasps the calcaneus with the forearm against the plantar aspect of the patient's foot.
Mobilization: The clinician glides the talus posteriorly with the superior hand while the inferior hand pulls the calcaneus distally. While sustaining those forces, the clinician uses the forearm of the inferior hand to move the patient's ankle into dorsiflexion (Fig. 9-68). The motion is rhythmic with release of range, then glide, then repeated. A sustained hold may also be used.

Posterior Talocrural Joint Mobilization with Movement in Step Standing

Purpose: Increase ankle dorsiflexion. This technique is more aggressive than the supine technique.

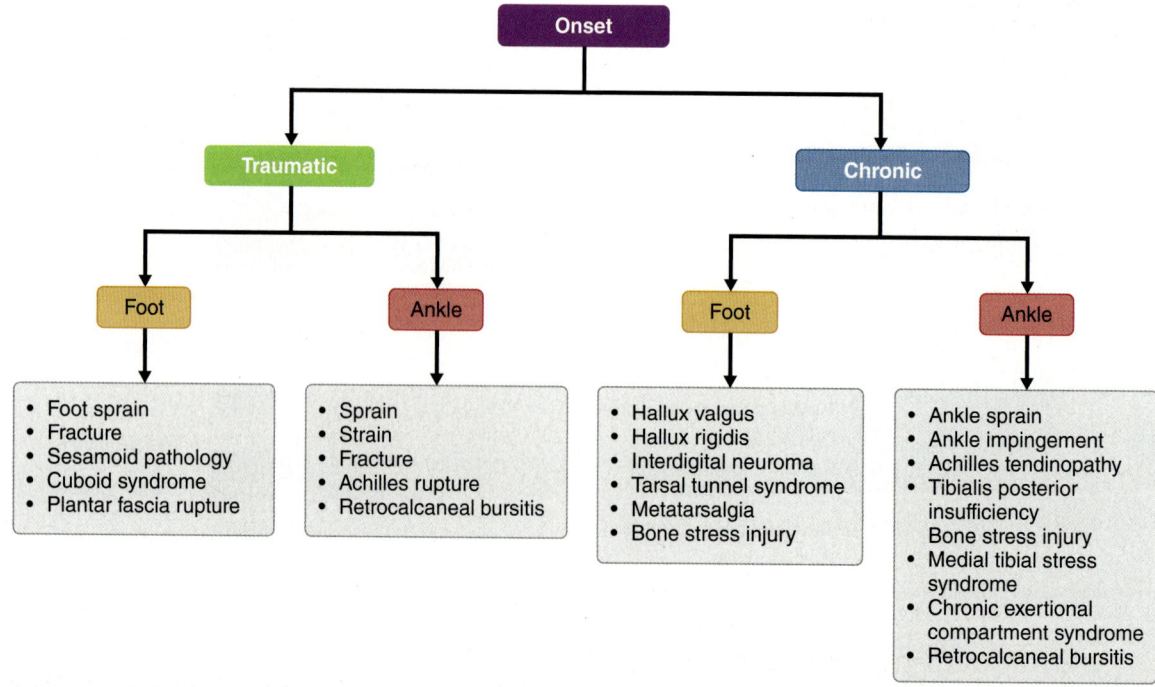

FIGURE 9-67 Ankle and foot pathology based on typical onset.

CHAPTER 9 | ANKLE AND FOOT

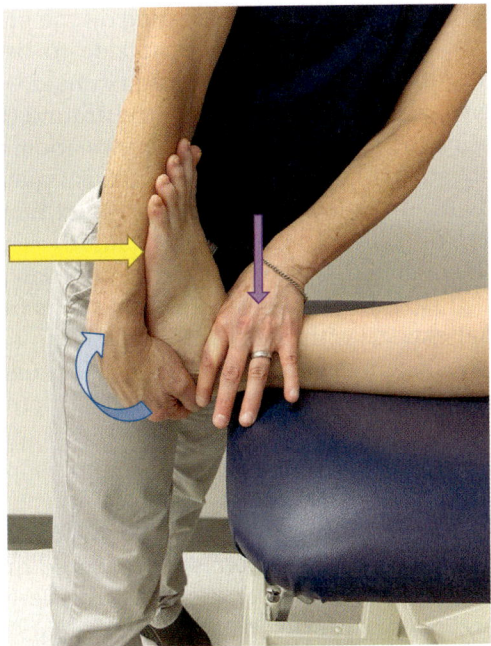

FIGURE 9-68 Posterior talocrural joint mobilization with movement in supine.

Patient: Step standing with the ankle to be mobilized on a tall step in slight plantar flexion.
Clinician: The clinician is half-kneeling lateral to the extremity to be mobilized. The clinician contacts the patient's anterior talus with the web space of one or both hands.

Mobilization: The clinician holds the talus posteriorly with one or both hands while the patient weight shifts to increase the amount of dorsiflexion (Fig. 9-69A). As with the non–weight-bearing mobilization with movement, this can be repeated rhythmically on/off or sustained.

A progression of forces can be created using a mobilization belt around the patient's distal tibia to create an anterior tibial glide during the mobilization (Fig. 9-69B).

Subtalar Joint Mobilization: Distraction

Purpose: Improve global subtalar joint mobility.
Patient: Prone with a towel roll under the patient's talus.
Clinician: Stabilizes the tibia, while the towel roll stabilizes the talus. The heel of the mobilizing hand contacts the posterior calcaneus.
Mobilization: The clinician glides the calcaneus distally, parallel to the sole of the foot (Fig. 9-70).

Cuboid Whip Manipulation

Purpose: The cuboid may be dislocated or subluxed plantarly in an inversion sprain. This technique is an attempt to reposition the cuboid more dorsally.
Patient: Prone with the knee flexed at least 45°. A pillow can be placed under the lower leg if there is any discomfort with knee extension range.
Clinician: Standing at the foot end of the table, the clinician encircles the foot with both hands and

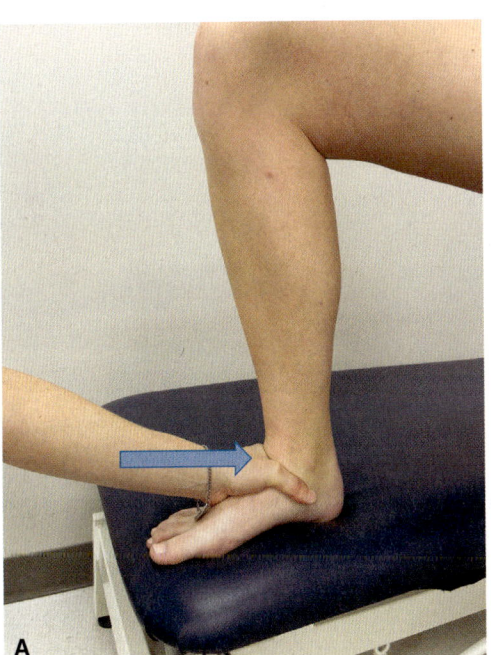
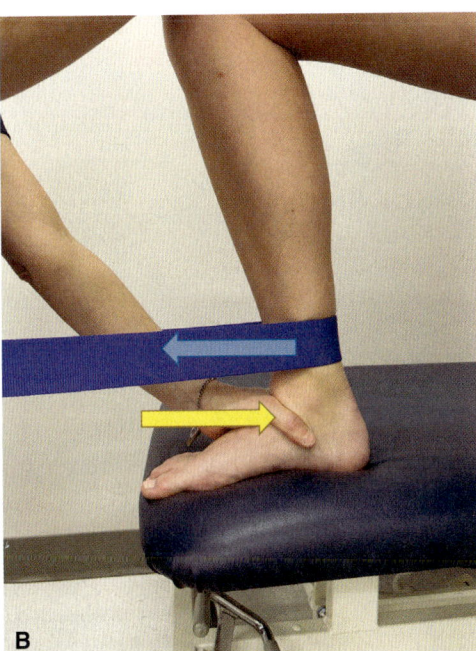

FIGURE 9-69 Posterior talocrural joint mobilization with movement in step standing **(A)** and using a mobilization belt **(B)**.

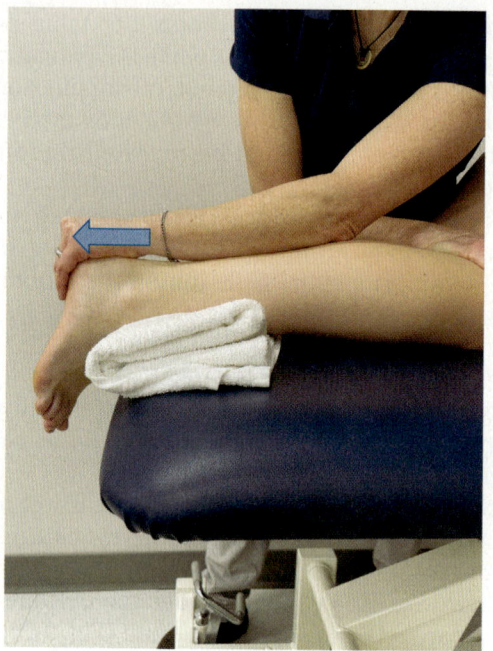

FIGURE 9-70 Distraction of the subtalar joint.

places thumb over thumb on the plantar aspect of the cuboid.

Mobilization: The clinician maximally dorsiflexes the foot, then rapidly moves the patient into knee extension, plantar flexion, and supination while performing a dorsal and lateral glide on the cuboid (Fig. 9-71).

Rotation of Tarsometatarsal Joint
Purpose: Improve pronation and supination.

Patient: Supine with the heel resting on the plinth.
Clinician: Positioned lateral to the side to be mobilized, stabilizes the cuneiforms and cuboid with the superior hand, the thumb wrapping around the foot dorsally, the fingers plantarly. For pronation, the clinician's distal hand grasps the proximal metatarsal shafts from the lateral aspect, with the thumb contacting dorsally and the fingers plantarly. The forearm is supinated. For supination, the clinician's distal hand grasps the proximal metatarsal shafts from the medial aspect, with the thumb contacting dorsally and the fingers plantarly. The forearm is pronated.
Mobilization: The mobilizing hand rotates the metatarsals, as a unit, into pronation or supination (Fig. 9-72).

ADDITIONAL THERAPEUTIC EXERCISES

Many of the therapeutic exercises presented throughout this chapter may be beneficial for a variety of patients and diagnoses. Flexibility exercises, particularly those helping to regain dorsiflexion range of motion (Fig. 9-73) and gastrocnemius muscle length (Fig. 9-74), are important for many patients with ankle/foot injuries. A Biomechanical Ankle Platform System, or BAPS board, is useful for gaining or control of multiplanar motion in the ankle (Fig. 9-75). The BAPS board can also be used for balance in a standing position. Calf weakness is common after ankle/foot injuries. Strengthening should progress to bilateral then unilateral weight bearing as able. Supramaximal weight can be achieved by having the patient hold a dumbbell or wear weighted backpack.

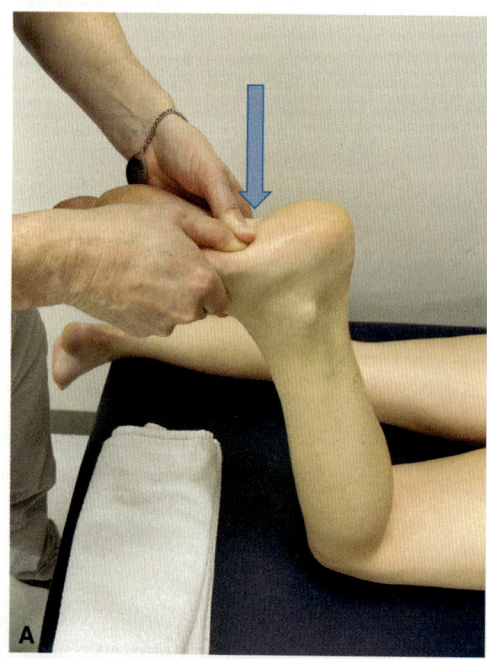
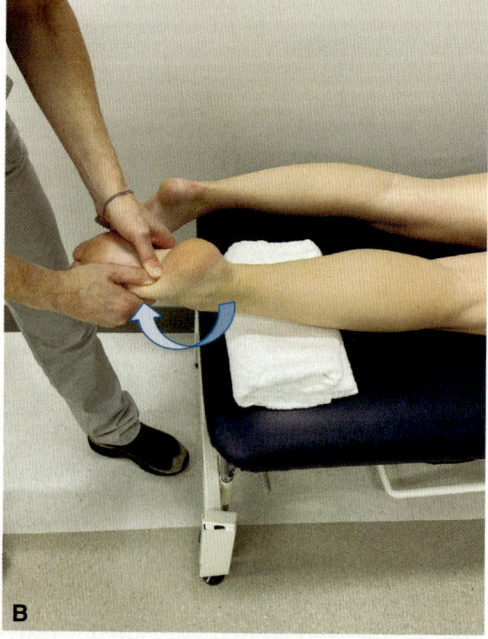

FIGURE 9-71 Cuboid whip. **A.** Starting position. **B.** Ending position.

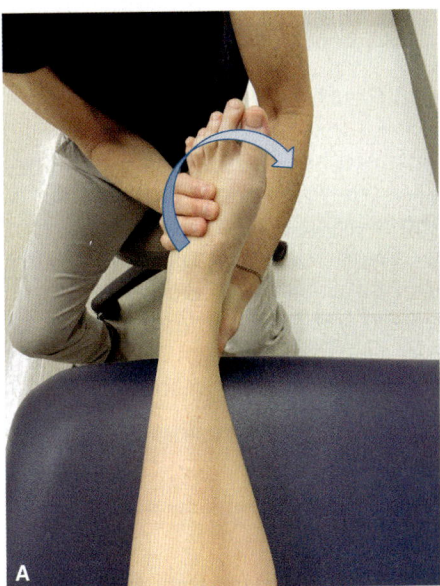 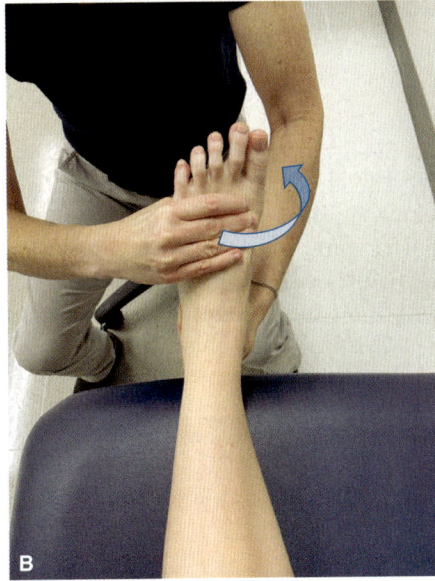

FIGURE 9-72 Rotation of tarsometatarsal joint into pronation **(A)** and supination **(B)**.

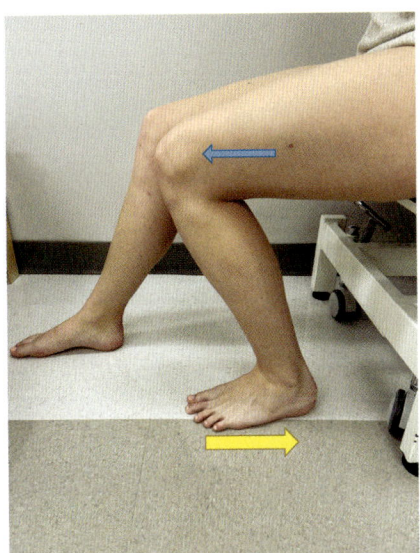

FIGURE 9-73 Seated left ankle dorsiflexion stretch.

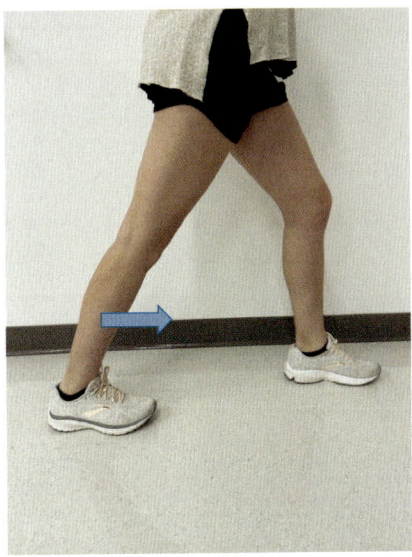

FIGURE 9-74 Standing right gastrocnemius stretch.

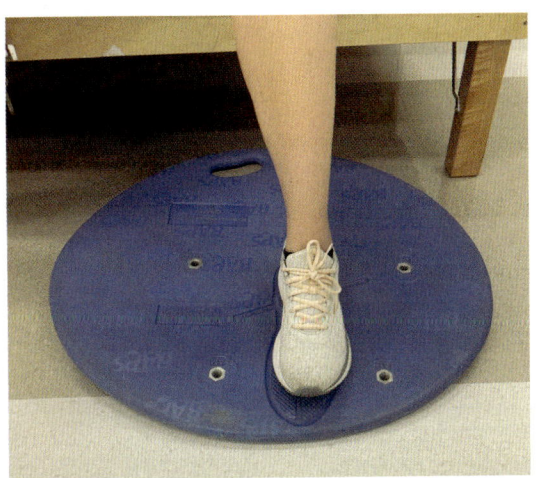

FIGURE 9-75 Seated Biomechanical Ankle Platform System board.

CASE STUDY 9-1
Shavonne: Patient with Fractured Right Ankle

Shavonne is a 59-year-old social worker who fractured her right ankle when she accidently missed a step on a friend's back porch. She is being seen for the first time 4 weeks after a right ankle open reduction and internal fixation. She has been weight bearing as tolerated (WBAT) in a CAM walker for 2 weeks and performing ankle pumps and icing her ankle/foot multiple times a day. All tests begin with the uninvolved (left) side unless otherwise noted. As noted previously, the examination should be organized by position, begin away and progress toward the involved area, and provide increasing stress to injured or potentially involved structures. Table 9-11 provides an example of how an experienced clinician might organize the physical examination after performing the history and systems review.

TABLE 9-11
SAMPLE ANKLE/FOOT EXAMINATION
Shavonne: 59-year-old social worker 4 weeks s/p R ankle open reduction and internal fixation

Position	Assessments
Observation	Continues from history
Seated	Hip ER (A*) Hip IR (A*) Knee ext (A, OP, MMT) Toe ext (A, OP, MMT) Ankle DF (A, OP, P, MMT) Ankle PF (A, OP, P, MMT) Ankle inversion (A, OP, P, MMT) Ankle eversion (A, OP, P, MMT)
Supine	Knee flex (P) Knee ext (P) Muscle length: gastrocnemius, hamstring
Right side-lying	MMT: L hip abd
Prone	Muscle length: rectus femoris Hip PROM: ext MMT: hamstring, gluteus maximus Integument
Left side-lying	MMT: R hip abd
Supine	Sensory assessment Palpation Accessory motion (talocrural, foot) Integument including incision mobility and nails Footwear inspection
Standing	Structure/posture screen barefoot Weight shifting to assess WBing tolerance Single-leg balance L Single-leg balance R if able to full WB on RLE with minimal pain MMT: PF L, consider B pending earlier examination findings Function: gait#

A, active range of motion; *DF*, dorsiflexion; *ER*, external rotation; *ext*, extension; *flex*, flexion; *IR*, internal rotation; *L*, left; *MMT*, manual muscle test; *OP*, overpressure; *P*, passive range of motion; *PF*, plantar flexion; *R*, right; *WB*, weight bearing, #, in parallel bars or with assistive device barefoot.
*If more than slightly limited additional assessment, such as passive motion and strength, would be indicated.

Shavonne's physical examination begins in the seated position, as she has been seated during the history. Because she has not borne weight on her right ankle outside of her CAM walker, the non–weight-bearing portion of the examination is completed prior to moving on to this more challenging activity. Hip assessment is limited to screening to ensure no gross deficits are present in rotation and assessing the functionally relevant strength of the hip extensors and abductors. The joints adjacent to the ankle, the knee and toes, are fully assessed (cleared) via active/passive motion and muscle performance testing. Sensory assessment and scar inspection and mobility are performed because she had surgery and the incision should be healed by this time. Weight-bearing assessment is progressed gradually from simple weight shifting up to a trial of gait using an assistive device or parallel bars to ensure safety. Balance and bilateral weight-bearing plantar flexion strength may or may not be assessed pending her abilities on lower level activities.

In this scenario, the patient had a known injury that was thoroughly investigated and treated operatively. Further investigation for possible ligamentous disruption (deltoid, lateral, or inferior tibiofibular ligaments) is unlikely to be needed at this time. First, any instability may be masked by edema and 4 weeks of immobilization. However, this may be required later in the rehabilitation process. For Shavonne, a highly skilled clinician may be even more efficient by initiating treatment of some impairments as they are noted. For example, during the seated examination, if noting a loss of dorsiflexion range, the clinician might provide a seated dorsiflexion stretch (see Fig. 9-73). If ankle weakness is found, the patient would be instructed in self-resisted ankle isometrics, active or resisted ankle exercises. If gastrocnemius length, balance, or weight bearing was problematic, then appropriate activities would be integrated into a home program as these were assessed as well. Note that deficits found at the knee and hip may, or may not, be addressed during this first visit. If knee/hip deficits are minor, the priority for now should be placed on the ankle/foot. However, if knee/hip deficits prevent normal gait and transfers, these might become a higher priority.

In a different scenario, the clinician is likely to need to gather all necessary information prior to initiating treatment. Consider the case of an individual being assessed for ankle pain after twisting it in a fall. If the clinician is the first practitioner to evaluate this patient and begins to prescribe range and strengthening exercises prior to clearing the patient of possible fracture via the Ottawa Ankle Rules, increased tissue damage and patient mistrust may ensue.

CHAPTER SUMMARY

The examination and treatment of patients with ankle or foot symptoms begin with a thorough history to determine if the symptoms stem from local tissues. An LQS further elucidates the source of the patient's complaint and helps identify relevant issues within the kinetic chain. The clinician must clear the joints proximal and distal to the presumed pathology and thoroughly investigate the ankle and foot. Assessment of accessory motion within the pathologic area can help identify joint hypo- and hypermobility if present. The judicious selection of special and provocative tests based on the patient history and basic examination findings may help clinicians fine-tune competing differential diagnoses. Acute, traumatic onset of symptoms is common for ankle injuries, whereas foot symptoms are more likely to be chronic injuries. Global rehabilitation strategies provided for ankle and foot pathologies should be individualized for each patient to maximize patient outcomes.

REFERENCES

1. Williams PL. *Gray's Anatomy: The Anatomical Basis of Medicine and Surgery*. 38th ed. Churchill Livingstone; 1995.
2. Kelikian AS. *Sarrafian's Anatomy of the Foot and Ankle*. 3rd ed. Lippincott Williams & Wilkins; 2011.
3. Thomas AC, Simon JE, Evans R, Turner MJ, Vela LI, Gribble PA. Knee surgery is associated with greater odds of knee osteoarthritis diagnosis. *J Sport Rehabil*. 2019;28(7):716–723.
4. Gross MT. Lower quarter screening for skeletal malalignment—suggestions for orthotics and shoewear. *J Orthop Sports Phys Ther*. 1995;21(6):389–405.
5. Houglum PA, Bertoti DB. *Brunnstrom's Clinical Kinesiology*. 6th ed. F.A. Davis; 2012.
6. Hicks J. The mechanics of the foot. I. The joints. *J Anat*. 1953;87(4):345–357.
7. Neumann DA. *Kinesiology of the Musculoskeletal System: Foundations for Rehabilitation*. 3rd ed. Elsevier; 2017.
8. Sun T, Zhao H, Wang L, Wu W, Hu W. Distribution patterns and coincidence of sesamoid bones at metatarsophalangeal joints. *Surg Radiol Anat*. 2017;39(4):427–432.
9. Zaw H, Calder J. Tarsal coalitions. *Foot Ankle Clin*. 2010;15(2):349–364.
10. Lee J, Kyung M, Cho Y, Go T, Lee D. Prevalence of accessory bones and tarsal coalitions based on radiographic findings in a healthy, asymptomatic population. *Clin Orthop Surg*. 2020;12(2):245–251.
11. Keles-Celik N, Kose O, Sekerci R, Aytac G, Turan A, Güler F. Accessory ossicles of the foot and ankle: disorders and a review of the literature. *Cureus*. 2017;9(11):e1881.
12. Nault M, Kocher M, Micheli L. Os trigonum syndrome. *J Am Acad Orthop Surg*. 2014;22(9):545–553.
13. Solomon L, Ruhli F, Taylor J, Ferris L, Pope R, Henneberg M. A dissection and computer tomograph study of tarsal coalitions in 100 cadaver feet. *J Orthop Res*. 2003;21(2):352–358.
14. Ruhli F, Solomon L, Henneberg M. High prevalence of tarsal coalitions and tarsal joints variants in a recent cadaver sample and its possible significance. *Clin Anat*. 2003;16(5):411–415.
15. Anavian J, Daniel C, Moatshe G, et al. The forgotten joint: quantifying the anatomy of the proximal tibiofibular joint. *Knee Surg Sports Traumatol Arthrosc*. 2018;26(4):1096–1103.

16. Knight J, Daniels M, Robertson W. Endoscopic compartment release for chronic exertional compartment syndrome. *Arthrosc Tech.* 2013;2(2):e187–e190.
17. Merle G, Harvey E. Pathophysiology of compartment syndrome. In: Mauffrey C, Hak D, Martin M III, eds. *Compartment Syndrome.* Springer; 2019.
18. Hermans J, Beumer A, de Jong T, Kleinrensink G. Anatomy of the distal tibiofibular syndesmosis in adults: a pictorial essay with a multimodality approach. *J Anat.* 2010;217(6):633–645.
19. Bartoníček J. Anatomy of the tibiofibular syndesmosis and its clinical relevance. *Surg Radiol Anat.* 2003;25(5–6):379–386.
20. Rammelt S, Manke E. Syndesmotic injuries. *Trauma Surg.* 2018;121:693–703.
21. Rammelt S, Obruba P. An update on the evaluation and treatment of syndesmotic injuries. *Eur J Trauma Emerg Surg.* 2015;41(6):601–614.
22. Ataoğlu M, Tokgöz M, Köktürk A, Ergişi Y, Hatipoğlu M, Kanatlı U. Radiologic evaluation of the effect of distal tibiofibular joint anatomy on arthroscopically proven ankle instability. *Foot Ankle Int.* 2020;41(2):223–228.
23. Chun K, Choi Y, Lee S, et al. Deltoid ligament and tibiofibular syndesmosis injury in chronic lateral ankle instability: magnetic resonance imaging evaluation at 3T and comparison with arthroscopy. *Korean J Radiol.* 2015;16(5):1096–1103.
24. Tweed J, Campbell J, Thompson R, Curran M. The function of the midtarsal joint: a review of the literature. *Foot.* 2008;18(2):106–112.
25. Davis W, Sobel M, DiCarlo E, et al. Gross, histological, and microvascular anatomy and biomechanical testing of the spring ligament complex. *Foot Ankle Int.* 1996;17(2):95–102.
26. Patil V, Ebraheim N, Frogameni A, Liu J. Morphometric dimensions of the calcaneonavicular (spring) ligament. *Foot Ankle Int.* 2007;28(8):927–932.
27. Kafka R, Aveytua I, Choi P, et al. Anatomico-radiological study of the bifurcate ligament of the foot with clinical significance. *Cureus.* 2019;8(11):e3847.
28. Longo U, Ronga M, Maffulli N. Achilles tendinopathy. *Sports Med Arthrosc Rev.* 2018;26(1):16–30.
29. Pękala P, Henry B, Pękala J, Piska K, Tomaszewski K. The Achilles tendon and the retrocalcaneal bursa: an anatomical and radiological study. *Bone Joint Res.* 2017;6(7):446–451.
30. Doral M, Alam M, Bozkurt M, et al. Functional anatomy of the Achilles tendon. *Knee Surg Sports Traumatol Arthrosc.* 2010;18(5):638–643.
31. Ledoux W, Blevins J. The compressive material properties of the plantar soft tissue. *J Biomech.* 2007;40(13):2975–2981.
32. Okano J, Arakawa A, Ogino S, Suzuki Y. Bilateral plantar fibromatosis complicated by Dupuytren's contracture. *J Surg Case Rep.* 2020;2:rjz402.
33. Akdag O, Yildiran G, Karamese M, Tosun Z. Dupuytren-like contracture of the foot: Ledderhose disease. *Surg J.* 2016;2(3):e102–e104.
34. Carroll P, Henshaw R, Garwood C, Raspovic K, Kumar DA. Plantar fibromatosis: pathophysiology, surgical and nonsurgical therapies: an evidence-based review. *Foot Ankle Spec.* 2018;11(2):168–176.
35. Fuiano M, Mosca M, Caravelli S, et al. Current concepts about treatment options of plantar fibromatosis: a systematic review of the literature. *Foot Ankle Surg.* 2019;25(5):559–564.
36. Witchey D, Witchey N, Roth-Kauffman M, Kauffman M. Plantar warts: epidemiology, pathophysiology, and clinical management. *J Am Osteopath Assoc.* 2018;118(2):92–105.
37. Plascencia G, Vega M, Torres TM, Rodríguez C. Skin disorders in overweight and obese patients and their relationship with insulin. *Actas Dermosifiliogr.* 2014;105(2):178–185.
38. Nordin M, Frankel V. *Basic Biomechanics of the Musculoskeletal System.* 4th ed. Wolters Kluwer; 2012.
39. Kleipool R, Balankevoort L. The relation between geometry and function of the ankle joint complex: a biomechanical review. *Knee Surg Sports Traumatol Arthrosc.* 2010;18(5):618–627.
40. American Academy of Orthopaedic Surgeons. *Joint Motion: Method of Measuring and Recording.* AAOS; 1965.
41. Martin RL, McPoil TG. Reliability of ankle goniometric measurements: a literature review. *J Am Podiatr Med Assoc.* 2005;95(6):564–572.
42. Zhao D, Huang D, Zhang G, et al. Talar dome investigation and talocrural joint axis analysis based on three-dimensional (3D) models: implications for prosthetic design. *Biomed Res Int.* 2019;2019:8634159.
43. Lundberg A, Svensson O, Nemeth G, Selvik G. The axis of rotation of the ankle joint. *J Bone Joint Surg Br.* 1989;71(1):94–99.
44. Levangie PK, Norkin CC. *Joint Structure and Function: A Comprehensive Analysis.* 5th ed. F.A. Davis; 2011.
45. Sheehan F, Seisler A, Siegel K. In vivo talocrural and subtalar kinematics: a non-invasive 3D dynamic MRI study. *Foot Ankle Int.* 2007;28(3):323–335.
46. Sarrafian S. Biomechanics of the subtalar joint complex. *Clin Orthop Relat Res.* 1993;290:17–26.
47. Siegler S, Toy J, Seale D, Pedowitz D. The Clinical Biomechanics Award 2013—presented by the International Society of Biomechanics: new observations on the morphology of the talar dome and its relationship to ankle kinematics. *Clin Biomech (Bristol, Avon).* 2014;29(1):1–6.
48. Belvedere C, Siegler S, Ensini A, et al. Experimental evaluation of a new morphological approximation of the articular surfaces of the ankle joint. *J Biomech.* 2017;53:97–104.
49. Huang J, Liu H, Wang D, Griffith J, Shi L. Talar dome detection and its geometric approximation in CT: sphere, cylinder or bi-truncated cone? *Comput Med Imaging Graph.* 2017;57:62–66.
50. Manter J. Movements of the subtalar and transverse tarsal joints. *Anat Rec.* 1941;80(4):397–410.
51. Goto A, Morimoto H, Itohara T, Watanabe T, Sugamoto K. Three dimensional in vivo kinematics of the subtalar joint during dorsi-plantarflexion and inversion-eversion. *Foot Ankle Int.* 2009;30(5):432–438.
52. Taylor K, Bojescul J, Howard R, Mizel M, McHale K. Measurement of isolated subtalar range of motion: a cadaver study. *Foot Ankle Int.* 2001;22(5):426–432.
53. Leardini A, Stagni R, O'Connor J. Mobility of the subtalar joint in the intact ankle complex. *J Biomech.* 2001;34(6):805–809.
54. Siegler S, Chen J, Schneck C. The three-dimensional kinematics and flexibility characteristics of the human ankle and subtalar joints—part I: kinematics. *J Biomech Eng.* 1988;110(4):364–373.
55. Wong Y, Kim W, Ying N. Passive motion characteristics of the talocrural and the subtalar joint by dual Euler angles. *J Biomech.* 2005;38(12):2480–2485.
56. Jastifer J, Gustafson P. The subtalar joint: biomechanics and functional representations in the literature. *Foot.* 2014;24(4):203–209.
57. Inman VT. *The Joints of the Ankle.* Williams & Wilkins; 1976.
58. Elftman H. The transverse tarsal joint and its control. *Clin Orthop.* 1960;16:41–46.
59. Lundgren P, Nester C, Liu A, et al. Invasive in vivo measurement of rear-, mid- and forefoot motion during walking. *Gait Posture.* 2008;28(1):93–100.
60. Glasoe W, Yack H, Saltzman C. Anatomy and biomechanics of the first ray. *Phys Ther.* 1999;79(9):854–859.

61. Richie D. *Pathomechanics of Common Foot Disorders.* Springer; 2021.
62. Sarrafian S. Functional characteristics of the foot and plantar aponeurosis under tibiotalar loading. *Foot Ankle.* 1987;8(1):4–18.
63. McPoil TG, Knecht H. Boimechanics of the foot in walking: a function approach. *J Orthop Sports Phys Ther.* 1985;7(2):69–72.
64. Theiss J, Fink M, Gerber J. Deep vein thrombosis in a young marathon athlete. *J Orthop Sports Phys Ther.* 2011;41(12):942–947.
65. Walker R, Wong F, Singh S, Ajuied A. The foot in systemic disease: management of the patient with rheumatoid arthritis or diabetes mellitus. *Orthop Trauma.* 2019;33(4):249–262.
66. Poratt D, Rome K. Surgical management of gout in the foot and ankle. A systemic review. *J Am Podiatr Med Assoc.* 2016;106(3):182–188.
67. Mohamed M, Wong CK. More than meets the eye: clinical reflection and evidence-based practice in an unusual case of adolescent chronic ankle sprain. *Phys Ther.* 2011;91(9):1395–1402.
68. Harris J, Fallat L, Schwartz S. Characteristic trends of lower-extremity complex regional pain syndrome. *J Foot Ankle Surg.* 2004;43(5):296–301.
69. Walia KS, Muser DE, Raza SS, Griech T, Khan YN. A management of early CRPS I caused by ankle sprain: a case report. *Pain Pract.* 2004;4(4):303–306.
70. Bachmann LM, Kolb E, Koller MT, Steurer J, Riet GT. Accuracy of Ottawa ankle rules to exclude fractures of the ankle and mid-foot: systematic review. *Br Med J.* 2003;326(7386):417.
71. Anand SS, Wells PS, Hunt D, Brill-Edwards P, Cook D, Ginsberg JS. Does this patient have a deep vein thrombosis? *JAMA.* 1998;279(14):1094–1099.
72. Nilsson M, Friss K, Nichaelsen M, Jakobsen P, Nielsen R. Classification of the height and flexibility of the medial longitudinal arch of the foot. *J Foot Ankle Res.* 2012;5(3):1–9.
73. Root M, Orien W, Weed J. *Normal and Abnormal Function of the Foot.* Vol 1. Clinical Biomechanics Corporation; 1971.
74. Harradine P, Gates L, Bowen C. If it doesn't work, why do we still do it? The continuing use of subtalar joint neutral theory in the face of overpowering critical research. *J Orthop Sports Phys Ther.* 2018;48(3):130–132.
75. McPoil TG, Cornwall M. Relationship between neutral subtalar joint positoin and the pattern of rearfoot motion during walking. *Foot Ankle Int.* 1994;15(4):141–145.
76. Tomaro J. Measurment of tibiofibular varum in subjects with unilateral overuse symptoms. *J Orhtop Sports Phys Ther.* 1995;21(2):86–89.
77. Spink MJ, Menz HB, Lord SR. Distribution and correlates of plantar hyperkeratotic lesions in older people. *J Foot Ankle Res.* 2009;2(1):8.
78. Tiberio D. Pathomechanics of sturctural foot deformities. *Phys Ther.* 1988;68(12):1840–1849.
79. American Academy of Orthopaedic Surgeons. *Joint Motion: Method of Measuring and Recording.* Churchill Livingstone; 1965.
80. Clarkson HM. *Musculoskeletal Assessment: Joint Range of Motion, Muscle Testing, and Function.* 4th ed. Wolters Kluwer; 2021.
81. Astrom M, Arvidson T. Alignment and joint motion in the normal foot. *J Orhtop Sports Phys Ther.* 1995;22(5):216–222.
82. Smith M, Lee D, Russell T, Matthews M, Macdonald DA, Vicenzino B. How much does the talocrural joint contribute to ankle dorsiflexion range of motion during the weightbearing lunge test? A cross-sectional radiographic validity study. *J Orthop Sports Phys Ther.* 2019;49(12):934–941.
83. Rabin A, Kozol Z, Spitzer E, Finestone AS. Weight-bearing ankle dorsiflexion range of motion-can side-to-side symmetry be assumed? *J Athl Train.* 2015;50(1):30–35.
84. Konor MM, Morton S, Eckerson JM, Grindstaff TL. Reliability of three measures of ankle dorsiflexion range of motion. *Int J Sports Phys Ther.* 2012;7(3):279–287.
85. Kendall FP, McCreary EK, Provance PG, Rogers MM, Romani WA. *Muscles: Testing and Function with Posture and Pain.* 5th ed. Lippincott Williams & Wilkins; 2005.
86. Lunsford B, Perry J. The standing heel-rise test for ankle plantar flexion: criterion for normal. *Phys Ther.* 1995;75(8):964–698.
87. Moraux A, Canal A, Ollivier G, et al. Ankle dorsi-and plantar-flexion torques measured by dynamometry in healthy subjects from 5 to 80 years. *BMC Musculoskelet Disord.* 2013;14(1):104.
88. Oskouei ST, Malliaras P, Jansons P, et al. Is ankle plantar flexor strength associated with balance and walking speed in healthy people? A systematic review and meta-analysis. *Phys Ther.* 2021;101(1):pzab018.
89. Menz HB, Zammit GV, Munteanu SE, Scott G. Plantarflexion strength of the toes: age and gender differences and evaluation of a clinical screening test. *Foot Ankle Int.* 2006;27(12):1103–1108.
90. Ata AM, Onat ŞŞ, Özçakar L. Ultrasound-guided diagnosis and treatment of Morton's neuroma. *Pain Physician.* 2016;19(2):E355–E358.
91. Mahadevan D, Venkatesan M, Bhatt R, Bhatia M. Diagnostic accuracy of clinical tests for Morton's neuroma compared with ultrasonography. *J Foot Ankle Surg.* 2015;54(4):549–553.
92. Chen ET, McInnis KC, Borg-Stein J. Ankle sprains: evaluation, rehabilitation, and prevention. *Curr Sports Med Rep.* 2019;18(6):217–223.
93. Vaseenon T, Gao Y, Phisitkul P. Comparison of two manual tests for ankle laxity due to rupture of the lateral ankle ligaments. *Iowa Orthop J.* 2012;32:9–16.
94. Martin R, Chimenti R, Cuddeford T, et al. Achilles pain, stiffness, and muscle power deficits: midportion Achilles tendinopathy revision 2018: using the evidence to guide physical therapist practice. *J Orthop Sports Phys Ther.* 2018;48(5):425–426.
95. Reinking MF, Austin TM, Richter RR, Krieger MM. Medial tibial stress syndrome in active individuals: a systematic review and meta-analysis of risk factors. *Sports Health.* 2017;9(3):252–261.
96. Buldt AK, Levinger P, Murley GS, Menz HB, Nester CJ, Landorf KB. Foot posture is associated with kinematics of the foot during gait: a comparison of normal, planus and cavus feet. *Gait Posture.* 2015;42(1):42–48.
97. Martin R, Davenport T, Reischl SF, et al. Heel pain-plantar fasciitis: revision 2014. *J Orthop Sports Phys Ther.* 2014;44(11):A1–A33.
98. Maffulli N. The clinical diagnosis of subcutaneous tear of the Achilles tendon. *Am J Sports Med.* 1998;26(2):266–270.
99. Gribble PA, Hertel J, Plisky P. Using the Star Excursion Balance Test to assess dynamic postural-control deficits and outcomes in lower extremity injury: a literature and systematic review. *J Athl Train.* 2012;47(3):339–357.
100. Doherty C, Bleakley V, Hertel J, Caulfield B, Ryan J, Delahunt E. Recovery from a first-time lateral ankle sprain and the predictors of chronic ankle instability: a prospective cohort analysis. *Am J Sports Med.* 2016;44(4):995–1003.
101. Myers BA, Jenkins WL, Killian C, Rundquist P. Normative data for hop tests in high school and collegiate basketball and soccer players. *Int J Sports Phys Ther.* 2014;9(5):596–603.

102. Hu H, Whitney S, Irrgang J, Janosky J. Test-retest reliability of the one-legged vertical jump test and the one-legged standing hop test. *J Orthop Sports Phys Ther.* 1992;15:51.
103. Madsen LP, Booth RL, Volz JD, Docherty CL. Using normative data and unilateral hopping tests to reduce ambiguity in return-to-play decisions. *J Athl Train.* 2020;55(7):699–706.
104. Madsen LP, Hall EA, Docherty CL. Assessing outcomes in people with chronic ankle instability: the ability of functional performance tests to measure deficits in physical function and perceived instability. *J Orthop Sports Phys Ther.* 2018;48(5):372–380.
105. Steinberg N, Finestone A, Noff M, Zeev A, Dar G. Relationship between lower extremity alignment and hallux valgus in women. *Foot Ankle Int.* 2013;34(6):824–831.
106. Nery C, Coughlin MJ, Baumfeld D, Ballerini FJ, Kobata S. Hallux valgus in males—part I: demographics, etiology, and comparative radiology. *Foot Ankle Int.* 2013;34(5):629–635.
107. Glasoe W, Nuckley D, Ludewig P. Hallux valgus and the first metatarsal arch segment: a theoretical biomechanical perspective. *Phys Ther.* 2010;90(1):110–120.
108. Greisberg J, Sperber L, Prince DE. Mobility of the first ray in various foot disorders. *Foot Ankle Int.* 2012;33(1):44–49.
109. Slullitel G, López V, Pablo Calvi J, Seletti M, Bartolucci C, Pinton G. Effect of first ray insufficiency and metatarsal index on metatarsalgia in hallux valgus. *Foot Ankle Int.* 2016;37(3):300–306.
110. Nilsdotter A, Coster M, Bremander A, Coster M. Patient-reported outcome after hallux valgus surgery—a two year follow up. *Foot Ankle Surg.* 2019;25(4):478–481.
111. Eshraghi S, East R, Mohagheghi A. Characterization of gait using plantar force transfer trajectory in individuals with hallux valgus deformity. *Gait Posture.* 2018;62:186–190.
112. Canseco K, Long J, Smedberg T, Tarima S, Marks RM, Harris GF. Multisegmental foot and ankle motion analysis after hallux valgus surgery. *Foot Ankle Int.* 2012;33(2):141–147.
113. Guo J, Wang L, Mao R, Chang C, Wen J, Fan Y. Biomechanical evaluation of the first ray in pre-/post-operative hallux valgus: a comparative study. *Clin Biomech (Bristol, Avon).* 2018;60:1–8.
114. Mortka K, Lisiński P. Hallux valgus—a case for a physiotherapist or only for a surgeon? Literature review. *J Phys Ther Sci.* 2015;27(10):3303–3307.
115. Park CH, Jang JH, Lee SH, Lee WC. A comparison of proximal and distal chevron osteotomy for the correction of moderate hallux valgus deformity. *Bone Joint J.* 2013;95-B(5):649–656.
116. Nery C, Coughlin MJ, Baumfeld D, Ballerini FJ, Kobata S. Hallux valgus in males—part 2: radiographic assessment of surgical treatment. *Foot Ankle Int.* 2013;34(5):636–644.
117. Kalender AM, Uslu M, Bakan B, et al. Mitchell's osteotomy with mini-plate and screw fixation for hallux valgus. *Foot Ankle Int.* 2013;34(2):238–243.
118. Smith SE, Landorf KB, Butterworth PA, Menz HB. Scarf versus chevron osteotomy for the correction of 1-2 intermetatarsal angle in hallux valgus: a systematic review and meta-analysis. *J Foot Ankle Surg.* 2012;51(4):437–444.
119. Schuh R, Adams JS, Hofstaetter SG, Krismer M, Trnka H-J. Plantar loading after chevron osteotomy combined with postoperative physical therapy. *Foot Ankle Int.* 2010;31(11):980–986.
120. Schuh R, Hofstaetter S, Adams SJ, Pichler F, Kristen K, Trnka H. Rehabilitation after hallux valgus surgery: importance of physical therapy to restore weight bearing of the first ray during the stance phase. *Phys Ther.* 2009;89(9):934–945.
121. Moon J-Y, Lee K-B, Seon JK, Moon E-S, Jung S-T. Outcomes of proximal chevron osteotomy for moderate versus severe hallux valgus deformities. *Foot Ankle Int.* 2012;33(8):637–643.
122. Ajmi Q, Maguire P, Barlas K, Giannakou A, Dunkow P. Comparison of radiological improvement in hallux valgus toe deformity after different corrective surgeries and its correlation with patient satisfaction score. *Int Musculoskelet Med.* 2008;30(1):23–28.
123. Nawoczenski DA. Nonoperative and operative intervention for hallux rigidus. *J Orthop Sports Phys Ther.* 1999;29(12):727–735.
124. Miner S, Foote G, Cheskis D, McGuire J. Conservative care recommendations for the stages of hallux limitus/rigidus. *Podiatry Today.* 2017;30(12):48–52.
125. Kon Kam King C, Loh SYJ, Zheng Q, Mehta KV. Comprehensive review of non-operative management of hallux rigidus. *Cureus.* 2017;9(1):e987.
126. Teoh KH, Tan WT, Atiyah Z, Ahmad A, Tanaka H, Hariharan K. Clinical outcomes following minimally invasive dorsal cheilectomy for hallux rigidus. *Foot Ankle Int.* 2019;40(2):195–201.
127. Hickey BA, Siew D, Nambiar M, Bedi HS. Intermediate-term results of isolated minimally invasive arthroscopic cheilectomy in the treatment of hallux rigidus. *Eur J Orthop Surg Traumatol.* 2020;30(7):1277–1283.
128. Stibolt RD, Patel HA, Lehtonen EJ, et al. Hemiarthroplasty versus total joint arthroplasty for hallux rigidus: a systematic review and meta-analysis. *Foot Ankle Spec.* 2019;12(2):181–193.
129. DiPreta JA. Metatarsalgia, lesser toe deformities, and associated disorders of the forefoot. *Med Clin North Am.* 2014;98(2):233–251.
130. Chahal GS, Davies MB, Blundell CM. Treating metatarsalgia: current concepts. *Orthop Trauma.* 2020;34(1):30–36.
131. Harvey M. Metatarsalgia. *Podiatry Rev.* 2016;73(1):9–11.
132. Charen DA, Markowitz JS, Cheung ZB, Matijakovich DJ, Chan JJ, Vulcano E. Overview of metatarsalgia. *Orthopedics.* 2019;42(1):e138–e143.
133. Anwar F. Morton's neuroma—outcome of surgical excision. *J Orthop.* 2010;7(3):e8.
134. Chang B-C, Liu D-H, Chang JL, Lee S-H, Wang J-Y. Plantar pressure analysis of accommodative insole in older people with metatarsalgia. *Gait Posture.* 2014;39(1):449–454.
135. Morales-Muñoz P, De Los Santos Real R, Barrio Sanz P, Pérez JL, Varas Navas J, Escalera Alonso J. Proximal gastrocnemius release in the treatment of mechanical metatarsalgia. *Foot Ankle Int.* 2016;37(7):782–789.
136. Haque S, Kakwani R, Chadwick C, Davies MB, Blundell CM. Outcome of minimally invasive distal metatarsal metaphyseal osteotomy (DMMO) for lesser toe metatarsalgia. *Foot Ankle Int.* 2016;37(1):58–63.
137. Ettehadi H, Saragas NP, Ferrao P, Khademi MA, Khorshidi A. First webspace Morton's neuroma case report with literature review. *Foot.* 2020;45.
138. Pérez-Domínguez B, Casaña-Granell J. The effects of a combined physical therapy approach on Morton's Neuroma. An N-of-1 Case Report. *Foot.* 2020;44.
139. Jain S, Mannan K. The diagnosis and management of Morton's neuroma: a literature review. *Foot Ankle Spec.* 2013;6(4):307–317.
140. Ferkel E, Hodges Davis W, Ellington JK. Entrapment neuropathies of the foot and ankle. *Clin Sports Med.* 2015;34(4):791–801.
141. Santos D, Morrison G, Coda A. Sclerosing alcohol injections for the management of intermetatarsal neuromas: a systematic review. *Foot.* 2018;35:36–47.
142. Pabinger C, Malaj I, Lothaller H, Samaila E, Magnan B. Improved injection technique of ethanol for Morton's neuroma. *Foot Ankle Int.* 2020;41(5):590–595.

143. Masala S, Cuzzolino A, Morini M, Raguso M, Fiori R. Ultrasound-guided percutaneous radiofrequency for the treatment of Morton's neuroma. *Cardiovasc Intervent Radiol.* 2018;41(1):137–144.
144. Petralgia F, Ramazzina I, Costantino C. Plantar fasciitis in athletes: diagnostic and treatment strategies. A systematic review. *Muscles Ligaments Tendons J.* 2017;7(1):107–118.
145. Radwan A, Wyland M, Applequist L, Bolowsky E, Klingensmith H, Virag I. Ultrasonography, an effective tool in diagnosing plantar fasciitis: a systematic review of diagnostic trials. *Int J Sports Phys Ther.* 2016;11(5):663–671.
146. Peerbooms JC, van Laar W, Faber F, Schuller HM, van der Hoeven H, Gosens T. Use of platelet rich plasma to treat plantar fasciitis: design of a multi centre randomized controlled trial. *BMC Musculoskelet Disord.* 2010;11:69.
147. Boayke L, Chambers M, Carney D, Yan A, Hogan M, Ewalefo S. Management of symptomatic plantar fasciitis. *Oper Tech Orthop.* 2018;28:73–78.
148. Wearing S, Smeathers J, Urry S, Sullican P, Yates B, Dubois P. Plantar enthesopathy: thickening of the enthesis is correlated with energy dissipation of the plantar fat pad during walking. *Am J Sports Med.* 2010;38(12):2522–2527.
149. Labovitz JM, Yu J, Kim C. The role of hamstring tightness in plantar fasciitis. *Foot Ankle Spec.* 2011;4(3):141–144.
150. Acevedo J, Beskin J. Comlications of plantar fascia rupture associated with corticosteroid injections. *Foot Ankle Int.* 1998;19(2):91–97.
151. Phillips A. Gait deviations associated with plantar heel pain: a systematic review. *Clin Biomech (Bristol, Avon).* 2017;42:55–64.
152. Tahririan MA, Motififard M, Tahmasebi MN, Siavashi B. Plantar fasciitis. *J Res Med Sci.* 2012;17(8):799–804.
153. Xu Z, Duan X, Yu X, Wang H, Dong X, Xiang Z. The accuracy of ultrasonography and magnetic resonance imaging for the diagnosis of Morton's neuroma: a systematic review. *Clin Radiol.* 2015;70(4):351–358.
154. Salvioli S, Guidi M, Marcotulli G. The effectiveness of conservative, non-pharmacological treatment, ofplantar heel pain: a systematic review with meta-analysis. *Foot.* 2017;33:57–67.
155. Verbruggen L, Thompson M, Durall C. The effectiveness of low-dye taping in reducing pain associated with plantar fasciitis. *J Sport Rehabil.* 2018;27(1):94–98.
156. Luffy L, Grosei J, Thonas R. Plantar fasciitis: a review of treatments. *J Am Acad Phys Assist.* 2018;31(1):20–24.
157. Osborne J, Menz H, Whittaker G, Landorf K. Muscle function and muscle size differences in people with and withou plantar heel pain: a systematic review. *J Orthop Sports Phys Ther.* 2019;49(12):925–933.
158. Taddei UT, Matias AB, Duarte M, Sacco ICN. Foot core training to prevent running-related injuries: a survival analysis of a single-blind, randomized controlled trial. *Am J Sports Med.* 2020;48(15):3610–3619.
159. Huffer D, Hing W, Newton R, Clair M. Strength training for plantar fasciitis and the intrinsic foot musculature: a systematic review. *Phys Ther Sport.* 2017;24:44–52.
160. Mischke J, Jayaseelan D, Sault J, Kavchak E. The symptomatic and functional effects of manual physical therapy on plantar heel pain: a systematic review. *J Man Manip Ther.* 2017;25(1):3–10.
161. Sillevis R, Shamus E, Mouttet B. The management of plantar fasciitis with a musculoskeletal ultrasound imaging guided approach for instrument assisted soft tissue mobilization in a runner: a case report. *Int J Sports Phys Ther.* 2020;15(2):274–286.
162. Wang Y-C, Chen S-J, Huang P-J, Huang H-T, Cheng Y-M, Shih C-L. Efficacy of different energy levels used in focused and radial extracorporeal shockwave therapy in the treatment of plantar fasciitis: a meta-analysis of randomized placebo-controlled trials. *J Clin Med.* 2019;8(9):1497.
163. Abbassian A, Kohls-Gatzoulis J, Solan MC. Proximal medial gastrocnemius release in the treatment of recalcitrant plantar fasciitis. *Foot Ankle Int.* 2012;33(1):14–19.
164. Healey K, Chen K. Plantar fasciitis: current diagnostic modalities and treatments. *Clin Podiatr Med Surg.* 2010;27(3):369–380.
165. Morton TN, Zimmerman JP, Lee M, Schaber JD. A review of 105 consecutive uniport endoscopic plantar fascial release procedures for the treatment of chronic plantar fasciitis. *J Foot Ankle Surg.* 2013;52(1):48–52.
166. Mandell J, Khurana B, Smith S, Mandell JC, Smith SE. Stress fractures of the foot and ankle, part 2: site-specific etiology, imaging, and treatment, and differential diagnosis. *Skeletal Radiol.* 2017;46(9):1165–1186.
167. Welck MJ, Hayes T, Pastides P, Khan W, Rudge B. Stress fractures of the foot and ankle. *Injury.* 2017;48(8):1722–1726.
168. Mandell J, Khurana B, Smith S, Mandell JC, Smith SE. Stress fractures of the foot and ankle, part 1: biomechanics of bone and principles of imaging and treatment. *Skeletal Radiol.* 2017;46(8):1021–1029.
169. Greaser MC. Foot and ankle stress fractures in athletes. *Orthop Clin North Am.* 2016;47(4):809–822.
170. Rizzone KH, Ackerman KE, Roos KG, Dompier TP, Kerr ZY. The epidemiology of stress fractures in collegiate student-athletes, 2004–2005 through 2013–2014 academic years. *J Athl Train.* 2017;52(10):966–975.
171. Regier M, Petersen JP, Hamurcu A, et al. High incidence of osteochondral lesions after open reduction and internal fixation of displaced ankle fractures: medium-term follow-up of 100 cases. *Injury.* 2016;47(3):757–761.
172. Tan EW, Sirisreetreerux N, Paez AG, Parks BG, Schon LC, Hasenboehler EA. Early weightbearing after operatively treated ankle fractures. *Foot Ankle Int.* 2016;37(6):652–658.
173. Dehghan N, McKee MD, Jenkinson RJ, et al. Early weight-bearing and range of motion versus non-weightbearing and immobilization after open reduction and internal fixation of unstable ankle fractures: a randomized controlled trial. *J Orthop Trauma.* 2016;30(7):345–352.
174. Jansen H, Jordan M, Frey S, Hölscher-Doht S, Meffert R, Heintel T. Active controlled motion in early rehabilitation improves outcome after ankle fractures: a randomized controlled trial. *Clin Rehabil.* 2018;32(3):312–318.
175. Shaffer MA, Okereke E, Esterhai JL, et al. Effects of immobilization on plantar-flexion torque, fatigue resistance, and functional ability following an ankle fracture. *Phys Ther.* 2000;80(8):769–780.
176. Farsetti P, Caterini R, Potenza V, De Luna V, De Maio F, Ippolito E. Immediate continuous passive motion after internal fixation of an ankle fracture. *J Orthop Trauma.* 2009;10(2):63–69.
177. Lehtonen H, Jarvinen T, Honkonen S, Nyman M, Vihtonen K, Jarvinen M. Use of a cast compared with a functional ankle brace after operative treatment of an ankle fracture: a prospective, randomized study. *J Bone Joint Surg Am.* 2003;85(2):205–211.
178. Lin Chung-Wei C, Moseley AM, Refshauge KM. Rehabilitation for ankle fractures in adults. *Cochrane Database Syst Rev.* 2008; (3).
179. Thomas G, Whalley H, Modi C. Early mobilization of operatively fixed ankle fractures: a systematic review. *Foot Ankle Int.* 2009;30(7):666–674.
180. Albin S, Koppenhaver S, Marcus R, Dibble L, Conrwall M, Fritz J. Short-term effects of manual therapy in patietns after surgical fixation of ankle and/or hindfoot fracture:

181. Painter EE, Deyle GD, Allen C, Petersen EJ, Croy T, Rivera KP. Manual physical therapy following immobilization for stable ankle fracture: a case series. *J Orthop Sports Phys Ther.* 2015;45(9):665–674.

180. a randomized clinical trial. *J Orthop Sports Phys Ther.* 2019;49(5):310–319.

182. Suciu O, Onofrei RR, Totorean AD, Suciu SC, Amaricai EC. Gait analysis and functional outcomes after twelve-week rehabilitation in patients with surgically treated ankle fractures. *Gait Posture.* 2016;49:184–189.

183. Simanski CJP, Maegele MG, Lefering R, et al. Functional treatment and early weightbearing after an ankle fracture: a prospective study. *J Orthop Trauma.* 2006;20(2):108–114.

184. Papachristou G, Efstathopoulos N, Levidiotis C, Chronopoulos E. Early weight bearing after posterior malleolar fractures: an experimental and prospective clinical study. *J Foot Ankle Surg.* 2003;42(2):99–104.

185. Egol KA, Tejwani NC, Walsh MG, Capla EL, Koval KJ. Predictors of short-term functional outcome following ankle fracture surgery. *J Bone Joint Surg Am.* 2006;88(5):974–979.

186. Meijer DT, Gevers Deynoot BDJ, Stufkens SA, et al. What factors are associated with outcomes scores after surgical treatment of ankle fractures with a posterior malleolar fragment? *Clin Orthop Relat Res.* 2019;477(4):863–869.

187. Bleakley CM, Taylor JB, Dischiavi SL, Doherty C, Delahunt E. Rehabilitation exercises reduce reinjury post ankle sprain, but the content and parameters of an optimal exercise program have yet to be established: a systematic review and meta-analysis. *Arch Phys Med Rehabil.* 2019;100(7):1367–1375.

188. van den Bekerom MP, Jan Oostra R, Alvareez P, van Dijk C. The anatomy in relation to injury of the lateral collateral ligaments of the ankle: a current concepts review. *Clin Anat.* 2008;21(7):619–626.

189. Kaminski T, Hertel J, Amendola N, et al. National Athletic Trainers' Association position statement: conservative management and prevention of ankle sprains in athletes. *J Athl Train.* 2013;48(4):528–545.

190. Burcal CJ, Sandrey MA, Hubbard-Turner T, McKeon PO, Wikstrom EA. Predicting dynamic balance improvements following 4-weeks of balance training in chronic ankle instability patients. *J Sci Med Sport.* 2019;22(5):538–543.

191. Martin R, Davenport T, Paulseth S, et al. Ankle stability and movement coordination impairments: ankle ligament sprains. *J Orthop Sports Phys Ther.* 2013;43(9):A1–A40.

192. Burger M, Dreyer D, Fisher RL, et al. The effectiveness of proprioceptive and neuromuscular training compared to bracing in reducing the recurrence rate of ankle sprains in athletes: a systematic review and meta-analysis. *J Back Musculoskelet Rehabil.* 2018;31(2):221–229.

193. Kerkhoffs GM, van den Bekerom MP, Elders LAM, van Beek P, Hullefie WAM, Bloemers G. Diagnosis, treatment, and prevention of ankle sprains: an evidence-based clinical guideline. *Br J Sports Med.* 2012;46(12):854–860.

194. Willems T, Witvrouw E, Verstuyft J, Vaes P, De Clercq D. Proprioception and muscle strength in subjects with a history of ankle sprains and chronic instability. *J Athl Train.* 2002;37(4):487–493.

195. Truyols-Dominguez S, Salom-Moreno J, Abian-Vicen J, Cleland J, Fernandex-de-las-penas C. Efficacy of thrust and nonthrust manipulation exercise with or without the addition of myofascial therapy for the management of acute inversion ankle sprain: a randomized clinical trial. *J Orthop Sports Phys Ther.* 2013;43(5):300–309.

196. Webster KA, Gribble PA. A comparison of electromyography of gluteus medius and maximus in subjects with and without chronic ankle instability during two functional exercises. *Phys Ther Sport.* 2013;14(1):17–22.

197. Dejong A, Koldenhoven R, Hertel J. Proximal adaptations in chronic ankle instability: systematic review and meta-analysis. *Med Sci Sports Exerc.* 2020;52(7):1563–1575.

198. Galleher C, Carson M, Ford S, Harne A, Norris T. Applying the clinical practice guidelines and the literature on ankle instability: a case series. *Orthop Pract.* 2020;32(4):230–236.

199. McKeon PO, Donovan L. A perceptual framework for conservative treatment and rehabilitation of ankle sprains: an evidence-based paradigm shift. *J Athl Train.* 2019;54(6):628–638.

200. Webster KA, Gribble PA. Functional rehabilitation interventions for chronic ankle instability: a systematic review. *J Sport Rehabil.* 2010;19(1):98–114.

201. Ismail MM, Ibrahim MM, Youssef EF, El Shorbagy KM. Plyometric training versus resistive exercises after acute lateral ankle sprain. *Foot Ankle Int.* 2010;31(6):523–530.

202. Briem K, Sdottir H, Magnusdottir R, Palmarsson R, Runardottir T, Sveinsson T. Effects of Knesio Tape with nonelastic sports tape and the untaped ankle during a sudden inversion perturbation in male athletes. *J Orthop Sports Phys Ther.* 2011;41(5):328–335.

203. Malliaropoulos N, Papalexandris S, Papacostas E, Maffulli N. Acute lateral ankle sprains: healing process and acceleration of rehabilitation. *Arch Int J Med.* 2008;1(1):39–43.

204. Ferkel E, Nguyen S, Kwong C. Chronic lateral ankle instability: surgical management. *Clin Sports Med.* 2020;39(4):829–843.

205. Hermanns C, Coda R, Cheema S, et al. Review of variability in rehabilitation protocols after lateral ankle ligament surgery. *Kans J Med.* 2020;13:152–159.

206. Haraguchi N, Tokumo A, Okamura R, et al. Influence of activity level on the outcome of treatment of lateral ankle ligament rupture. *J Orthop Sci.* 2009;14(4):391–396.

207. Li X, Killie H, Guerrero P, Busconi BD. Anatomical reconstruction for chronic lateral ankle instability in the high-demand athlete: functional outcomes after the modified Brostrom repair using suture anchors. *Am J Sports Med.* 2009;37(3):488–494.

208. Valkering KP, Vergroesen DA, Nolte PA. Isolated syndesmosis ankle injury. *Orthopedics.* 2012;35(12):e1705–e1710.

209. Waldén M, Hägglund M, Ekstrand J. Time-trends and circumstances surrounding ankle injuries in men's professional football: an 11-year follow-up of the UEFA Champions League injury study. *Br J Sports Med.* 2013;47(12):748–753.

210. Cannon LB, Hackney RG. Anterior tibiotalar impingement associated with chronic ankle instability. *J Foot Ankle Surg.* 2000;39(6):383–386.

211. Lee JW, Suh J, Huh Y, Moon E, Kim SJ. Soft tissue impingement syndrome of the ankle: diagnostic efficacy of MRI and clinical results after arthroscopic treatment. *Foot Ankle Int.* 2004;25(12):896–902.

212. Sharpe B, Stegisnky B, Suhling M, Vora A. Posterior ankle impingement and flexor hallucis longus pathology. *Clin Sports Med.* 2020;39(4):911–930.

213. El-Sayed AMM. Arthroscopic treatment of anterolateral impingement of the ankle. *J Foot Ankle Surg.* 2010;49(3):219–223.

214. Calder JD, Sexton SA, Pearce CJ. Return to training and playing after posterior ankle arthroscopy for posterior impingement in elite professional soccer. *Am J Sports Med.* 2010;38(1):120–124.

215. Horisberger M, Valderrabano V, Hintermann B. Posttraumatic ankle osteoarthritis after ankle-related fractures. *J Orthop Trauma*. 2009;23(1):60–67.
216. Nwankwo EC Jr, Labaran LA, Athas V, Olson S, Adams SB. Pathogenesis of posttraumatic osteoarthritis of the ankle. *Orthop Clin North Am*. 2019;50(4):529–537.
217. Al-Mahrouqi MM, Macdonald DA, Vicenzino B, Smith MD. Physical impairments in adults with ankle osteoarthritis: a systematic review and meta-analysis. *J Orthop Sports Phys Ther*. 2018;48(6):449–459.
218. Huang Y-C, Harbst K, Kotajarvi B, et al. Effects of ankle-foot orthoses on ankle and foot kinematics in patient with ankle osteoarthritis. *Arch Phys Med Rehabil*. 2006;87(5):710–716.
219. Martin R, Stewart G, Conti S. Postraumatic ankle arthritis: an update on conservative and surgical management. *J Orthop Sports Phys Ther*. 2007;37(5):253–259.
220. Paterson KL, Gates L. Clinical assessment and management of foot and ankle osteoarthritis: a review of current evidence and focus on pharmacological treatment. *Drug Aging*. 2019;36(3):203–211.
221. Chimenti RL, Cychosz CC, Hall MM, Phisitkul P. Current concepts review update: insertional Achilles tendinopathy. *Foot Ankle Int*. 2017;38(10):1160–1169.
222. Cook JL, Stasinopoulos D, Brismée J-M. Insertional and mid-substance Achilles tendinopathies: eccentric training is not for everyone—updated evidence of non-surgical management. *J Man Manip Ther*. 2018;26(3):119–122.
223. Docking SI, Rosengarten SD, Daffy J, Cook J. Structural integrity is decreased in both Achilles tendons in people with unilateral Achilles tendinopathy. *J Sci Med Sport*. 2015;18(4):383–387.
224. Edama M, Kubo M, Onishi H, Takabayashi T, Inai T, Yokoyama E. The twisted structure of the human Achilles tendon. *Scand J Med Sci Sports*. 2015;25(5):e497–e503.
225. Wezenbeek E, Willems TM, Mahieu N, Van Caekenberghe I, Witvrouw E, De Clercq D. Is Achilles tendon blood flow related to foot pronation? *Scan J Med Sci Sports*. 2017;27(12):1970–1977.
226. O'Neill S, Barry S, Watson P. Plantarflexor strength and endurance deficits associated with mid-portion Achilles tendinopathy: the role of soleus. *Phys Ther Sport*. 2019;37:69–76.
227. Noback PC, Freibott CE, Tantigate D, et al. Prevalence of asymptomatic Achilles tendinosis. *Foot Ankle Int*. 2018;39(10):1205–1209.
228. Tilley BJ, Cook JL, Docking SI, Gaida JE. Is higher serum cholesterol associated with altered tendon structure or tendon pain? A systematic review. *Br J Sports Med*. 2015;49(23):1504–1509.
229. McAuliffe SÁ, Tabuena A, McCreesh K, et al. Altered strength profile in Achilles tendinopathy: a systematic review and meta-analysis. *J Athl Train*. 2019;54(8):889–900.
230. Habets B, van den Broek AG, Huisstede BMA, Backx FJG, van Cingel REH. Return to sport in athletes with mid-portion Achilles tendinopathy: a qualitative systematic review regarding definitions and criteria. *Sports Med*. 2018;48(3):705–723.
231. Creaby MW, Honeywill C, Franettovich Smith MM, Schache AG, Crossley KM. Hip biomechanics are altered in male runners with achilles tendinopathy. *Med Sci Sports Exerc*. 2017;49(3):549–554.
232. Scholes M, Stadler S, Connell D, et al. Men with unilateral Achilles tendinopathy have impaired balance on the symptomatic side. *J Sci Med Sport*. 2018;21(5):479–482.
233. Silbernagel KG, Gustavsson A, Thomee R, Karlsson J. Evaluation of lower leg function in patients with Achilles tendinopathy. *Knee Surg Sports Traumatol Arthrosc*. 2006;14(11):1207–1217.
234. Malliaras P, Cook J, Purdam C, Rio E. Patellar tendinopathy: clinical diagnosis, load management, and advice for challenging case presentations. *J Orthop Sports Phys Ther*. 2015;45(11):887–898.
235. Syvertson P, Dietz E, Matocha M, et al. A treatment-based classification algorithm to treat Achilles tendinopathy: an exploratory case series. *J Sport Rehabil*. 2017;26(3):260–268.
236. Jayaseelan DJ, Kecman M, Alcorn D, Sault JD. Manual therapy and eccentric exercise in the management of Achilles tendinopathy. *J Man Manip Ther*. 2017;25(2):106–114.
237. Youdas J, Krause D, Egan K, Therneau T, Laskowski E. The effect of static stretching of the cal mucle-tendon unit on active ankle dorsiflexion range of motion. *J Orthop Sports Phys Ther*. 2003;33(7):408–417.
238. Chaudhry FA. Effectiveness of dry needling and high-volume image-guided injection in the management of chronic mid-portion Achilles tendinopathy in adult population: a literature review. *Eur J Orthop Surg Traumatol*. 2017;27(4):441–448.
239. Murphy M, Rio E, Debenham J, Docking S, Travers M, Gibson W. Evaluating the progress of mid-portion Achilles tendinopathy during rehabilitation: a review of outcome measures for self-reported pain and function. *Int J Sports Phys Ther*. 2018;13(2):283–292.
240. Aicale R, Tarantino D, Maffulli N. Surgery in tendinopathies. *Sports Med Arthrosc Rev*. 2018;26(4):200–202.
241. Kearney RS, Achten J, Lamb SE, Plant C, Costa ML. A systematic review of patient-reported outcome measures used to assess Achilles tendon rupture management: what's being used and should we be using it? *Br J Sports Med*. 2012;46(16):1102–1109.
242. Khan RJ, Carey Smith RL. Surgical interventions for treating acute Achilles tendon ruptures. *Cochrane Database of Syst Rev*. 2010; (9).
243. Deng S, Sun Z, Zhang C, Chen G, Li J. Surgical treatment versus conservative management for acute Achilles tendon rupture: a systematic review and meta-analysis of randomized controlled trials. *J Foot Ankle Surg*. 2017;56(6):1236–1243.
244. Lantto I, Heikkinen J, Flinkiilia T, Ohtonen P, Siira P, Laine V. A prospective randomized trial comparing surgical and nonsurgical treatments of acute Achilles tendon ruptures. *Am J Sports Med*. 2016;44(9):2406–2414.
245. Maffulli N, Testa V, Capasso G, et al. Surgery for chronic Achilles tendinopathy produces worse results in women. *Disabil Rehabil*. 2008;30(20–22):1714–1720.
246. Majewski M, Schaeren S, Kohlhaas U, Ochsner PE. Postoperative rehabilitation after percutaneous Achilles tendon repair: early functional therapy versus cast immobilization. *Disabil Rehabil*. 2008;30(2–22):1726–1732.
247. Wulf M, Wearing S, Hooper S, Bartold S, Reed L, Brauner T. The effect of an in-shoe orthotic heel lift on loading of the achilles tendon during shod walking. *J Orthop Sports Phys Ther*. 2016;46(2):79–86.
248. Hrnack SA, Crates JM, Barber FA. Primary achilles tendon repair with mini-dorsolateral incision technique and accelerated rehabilitation. *Foot Ankle Int*. 2012;33(10):848–851.
249. Silbernagel KG, Willy R, Davis I. Preinjury and postinjury running analysis along with measurements of strength and tendon length in a patient with a surgically repaired

Achilles tendon rupture. *J Orthop Sports Phys Ther.* 2012;42(6):521–529.
250. Bostick GP, Jomha NM, Suchak AA, Beaupre LA. Factors associated with calf muscle endurance recovery 1 year after Achilles tendon rupture repair. *J Orthop Sports Phys Ther.* 2010;40(6):345–351.
251. Olsson N, Nilsson-Helander K, Karlsson J, et al. Major functional deficits persist 2 years after acute Achilles tendon rupture. *Knee Surg Sports Traumatol Arthrosc.* 2011;19(8):1385–1393.
252. Chiodo CP, Glazebrook M, Bluman EM, et al. Diagnosis and treatment of acute Achilles tendon rupture. *J Am Acad Orthop Surg.* 2010;18(8):503–510.
253. Ortmann FW, McBryde AM. Endoscopic bony and soft-tissue decompression of the retrocalcaneal space for the treatment of haglund deformity and retrocalcaneal bursitis. *Foot Ankle Int.* 2007;28(2):149–153.
254. Money W. Haglund's deformity—a review. *Br J Podiatr.* 2002;5(1):19–24.
255. Yao K, Yang TX, Yew WP. Posterior tibialis tendon dysfunction: overview of evaluation and management. *Orthopedics.* 2015;38(6):385–391.
256. Smyth N, Aiyer A, Kaplan J, Carmody C, Kadakia A. Adult-acquired flatfoot deformity. *Eur J Orthop Surg Traumatol.* 2017;27(4):433–439.
257. Soliman SB, Spicer PJ, van Holsbeeck MT. Sonographic and radiographic findings of posterior tibial tendon dysfunction: a practical step forward. *Skeletal Radiol.* 2019;48(1):11–27.
258. Reb CW, Schick FA, Karanjia HN, Daniel JN. High prevalence of obesity and female gender among patients with concomitant tibialis posterior tendonitis and plantar fasciitis. *Foot Ankle Spec.* 2015;8(5):364–368.
259. Ikoma K, Ohashi S, Maki M, Kido M, Hara Y, Kubo T. Diagnostic characteristics of standard radiographs and magnetic resonance imaging of ruptures of the tibialis posterior tendon. *J Foot Ankle Surg.* 2016;55(3):542–546.
260. Kamiya T, Uchiyama E, Watanabe K, Suzuki D, Fujimiya M, Yamashita T. Dynamic effect of the tibialis posterior muscle on the arch of the foot during cyclic axial loading. *Clin Biomech (Bristol, Avon).* 2012;27(9):962–966.
261. Albano D, Martinelli N, Bianchi A, et al. Posterior tibial tendon dysfunction: clinical and magnetic resonance imaging findings having histology as reference standard. *Eur J Radiol.* 2018;99:55–61.
262. Kulig K, Lee S-P, Reischl SF, Noceti-DeWit L. Effect of posterior tibial tendon dysfunction on unipedal standing balance test. *Foot Ankle Int.* 2015;36(1):83–89.
263. Rabbito M, Pohl MB, Humble N, Ferber R. Biomechanical and clinical factors related to stage I posterior tibial tendon dysfunction. *J Orthop Sports Phys Ther.* 2011;41(10):776–784.
264. Hope R, Prescott D. Practice based evidence versus evidence based practice: reviewing the clinical tests currently used to diagnose posterior tibial tendon dysfunction. The 4th European Congress of the European Region of the World Confederation of Physical Therapy (ER-WCPT) Abstracts, Liverpool, UK, 11–12 November 2016. *Physiotherapy.* 2016;102:e216–e217.
265. Bek N, Simsek IE, Erel S, Yakut Y, Uygur F. Home-based general versus center-based selective rehabilitation in patients with posterior tibial tendon dysfunction. *Acta Orthop Traumatol Turc.* 2012;46(4):286–292.
266. Franettovich MM, Murley GS, David BS, et al. A comparison of augmented low-Dye taping and ankle bracing on lower limb muscle activity during walking in adults with flat-arched foot posture. *J Sci Med Sport.* 2012;15(1):8–13.
267. Houck J, Neville C, Tome J, Flemister A. Randomized controlled trial comparing orthosis augmented by either stretching or stretching and strengthening for stage ii tibialis posterior tendon dysfunction. *Foot Ankle Int.* 2015;36(9):1006–1016.
268. Espinosa N, Maurer MA. Stage I and II posterior tibial tendon dysfunction. *Clin Sports Med.* 2015;34(4):761–768.
269. Pomeroy G, Wilton J, Anthony S. Entrapment neuropathy about the foot and ankle: an update. *J Am Acad Orthop Surg.* 2015;23(1):58–66.
270. McSweeney SC, Cichero M. Tarsal tunnel syndrome—a narrative literature review. *Foot.* 2015;25(4):244–250.
271. Gallas J, Gearhart M. Conservative management of tarsal tunnel syndrome in a competitive distance runner. *Orthop Phys Ther Pract.* 2015;27(2):84–91.
272. Kavlak Y, Uygur F. Effects of nerve mobilization exercise as an adjunct to the conservative treatment for patients with tarsal tunnel syndrome. *J Manipulative Physiol Ther.* 2011;34(7):441–448.
273. De la Fuente C, Henriquez H, Andrade DC, Yañez A. Running footwear with custom insoles for pressure distribution are appropriate to diminish impacts after shin splints. *Asian J Sports Med.* 2019;10(3):1–7.
274. Mattock J, Steele J, Mickle K. Does tibial bone mineral status quality differ between medial tibial stress syndrome symptomatic and asymptomatic long-distance runners? *J Sci Med Sport.* 2019;22:S20–S20.
275. Winters M, Bon P, Bijvoet S, Bakker EWP, Moen MH. Are ultrasonographic findings like periosteal and tendinous edema associated with medial tibial stress syndrome? A case-control study. *J Sci Med Sport.* 2017;20(2):128–133.
276. Kinoshita K, Okada K, Saito I, et al. Alignment of the rearfoot and foot pressure patterns of individuals with medial tibial stress syndrome: a cross-sectional study. *Phys Ther Sport.* 2019;38:132–138.
277. Edama M, Onishi H, Kubo M, et al. Gender differences of muscle and crural fascia origins in relation to the occurrence of medial tibial stress syndrome. *Scand J Med Sci Sports.* 2017;27(2):203–208.
278. Becker J, James S, Wayner R, Osternig L, Chou L-S. Biomechanical factors associated with achilles tendinopathy and medial tibial stress syndrome in runners. *Am J Sports Med.* 2017;45(11):2614–2621.
279. Saeki J, Nakamura M, Nakao S, Fujita K, Yanase K, Ichihashi N. Muscle stiffness of posterior lower leg in runners with a history of medial tibial stress syndrome. *Scand J Med Sci Sports.* 2018;28(1):246–251.
280. Becker J, Nakajima M, Wu W. Factors contributing to medial tibial stresssyndrome in runners: a prospective study. *Med Sci Sports Exerc.* 2018;50(10):2092–2100.
281. Garnock C, Witchalls J, Newman P. Predicting individual risk for medial tibial stress syndrome in navy recruits. *J Sci Med Sport.* 2018;21(6):586–590.
282. Yüksel O, Özgürbüz C, Ergün M, et al. Inversion/eversion strength dysbalance in patients with medial tibial stress syndrome. *J Sports Sci Med.* 2011;10(4):737–742.
283. Moen MH, Holtslag L, Bakker EW, Marten C, Weir A, Tol JL. The treatment of medial tibial stress syndrome in athletes: a randomized clinical trial. *Sports Med Arthrosc Rehabil Ther Technol.* 2012;4(12):1–8.
284. Moen MH, Bongers T, Bakker EW, et al. Risk factors and prognostic indicators for medial tibial stress syndrome. *Scand J Med Sci Sports.* 2012;22(1):34–39.

285. Gomez Garcia S, Ramon Rona S, Gomez Tinoco MC, et al. Shockwave treatment for medial tibial stress syndrome in military cadets: a single-blind randomized controlled trial. *Int J Surg.* 2017;46:102–109.
286. Rynkiewicz KM, Fry LA, DiStefano LJ. Demographic characteristics among patients with chronic exertional compartment syndrome of the lower leg. *J Sport Rehabil.* 2020;29(8):1214–1217.
287. Roberts A, Franklyn-Miller A. The validity of the diagnostic criteria used in chronic exertional compartment syndrome: a systematic review. *Scand J Med Sci Sports.* 2012;22(5):585–595.
288. Murray MC, Heckman MM. Chronic exertional compartment syndrome: diagnostic techniques and management. *Tech Orthop.* 2012;27(1):75–78.
289. Hing W, Hall T, Rivett D, Vicenzino B, Mulligan B. *The Mulligan Concept of Manual Therapy: Textbook of Techniques.* Churchill Livingston/Elsevier; 2015.

10 | Knee

Betsy Myers and June Hanks

CHAPTER OBJECTIVES

After reading this chapter, you will be able to:
1. Describe the anatomy of the knee and patellofemoral joints.
2. Describe the biomechanics of the knee and patellofemoral joints, including joint stabilization.
3. Tailor the basic history to a patient with knee pathology.
4. Describe the components of the physical examination for a patient with knee pathology.
5. Describe the pathology, history, key examination findings, rehabilitation focus, and expected outcomes of common knee pathologies.
6. Hypothesize differential diagnoses of knee symptoms based on location, patient complaint, and onset.
7. Organize the physical examination of a patient with knee pathology to maximize efficiency.

FUNCTIONAL ANATOMY

The knee joint is the largest joint in the body and one of the most commonly injured. The knee joint complex includes articulation between two long bones, the femur and tibia (forming the knee [tibiofemoral] joint), and between the patella and distal femur (forming the patellofemoral joint). Although these joints are contained within a single joint capsule, the condylar-shaped knee joint and sellar-shaped patellofemoral joints can be considered separately. Knee joint stability is provided by the bony configuration, ligaments, muscular forces, and meniscocapsular aponeuroses.[1]

Osteology

Femur The femur, the more proximal long bone forming the knee joint, is the longest and strongest bone in the body.[2] In standing, the shaft of the femur is varied in its oblique orientation, being generally greater in women owing to the wider pelvis and shorter femoral length. The distal end of the femur forms medial and lateral condyles separated inferiorly and posteriorly by the intercondylar fossa. Anteriorly, the condyles merge and form a shallow depression, the patellar fossa, for articulation with the patella. In the anatomic position, the condyles are in the same horizontal plane. The femoral condyles articulate with the medial and lateral tibial condyles and associated menisci (Fig. 10-1). Projecting from the femur as a rounded eminence at the lateral portion of the lateral condyle is the lateral epicondyle. The medial surface of the medial condyle bears an even larger medial epicondyle. Superior to the medial epicondyle is the adductor tubercle that serves as an attachment for the adductor magnus muscle. The medial and lateral epicondyles serve as proximal attachments for the medial (tibial) and lateral (fibular) collateral ligaments.

Tibia The tibia is the second longest bone in the body. The medial and lateral condyles of the proximal tibia form the weight-bearing surface for the femur. The condyles of this superior tibial articular surface, called the *tibial plateau*, are separated by intercondylar eminences (Fig. 10-2). The medial tibial condyle is large with a concave oval-shaped articular surface. The lateral tibial condyle articular surface has an anteroposterior convexity and is nearly circular in shape. The anterior surfaces of the condyles merge centrally toward a triangularly shaped area that extends distally to the tibial tuberosity. The smooth proximal portion of the tibial tuberosity serves as an attachment for the patellar ligament (Fig. 10-3). The rough distal portion is easily palpable, with the infrapatellar bursa separating it from the skin. The anterior intercondylar area is broadest in the most anterior aspect. A depression on the anterior portion of the anterior intercondylar area serves as an attachment for the anterior horn (cornu) of the medial meniscus. Just posterior is the attachment of the anterior cruciate ligament (ACL). Lateral to the ACL and anterior to the intercondylar eminence, the anterior horn of the lateral meniscus attaches to the tibia. More posteriorly, the posterior horns of the menisci attach. Most posterior is the attachment for the posterior cruciate ligament (PCL). Attached to the posterolateral (PL) portion of the proximal tibia are the capsular and posterior portions of the medial collateral ligament (MCL) (Fig. 10-3). The posteromedial (PM) proximal portion of the medial tibial condyle serves as

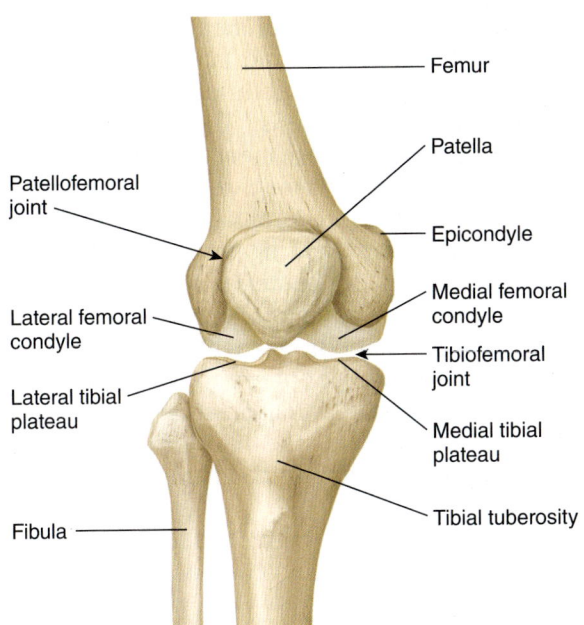

FIGURE 10-1 Anterior view. Medial and lateral femoral condyles, menisci, and proximal tibial condyles. (Gest TR. *Lippincott Atlas of Anatomy*. 2nd ed. Wolters Kluwer; 2020: Plates 3-6 and 3-8.)

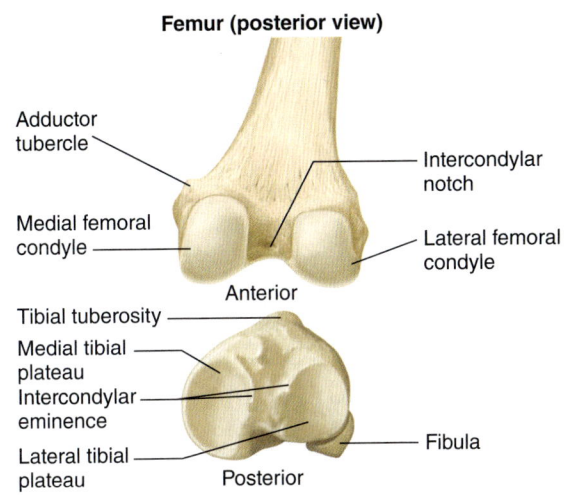

FIGURE 10-2 Distal end of femur demonstrating asymmetrical condyles and intercondylar notch. Superior view of tibia showing asymmetrical condyles with intercondylar eminence. (Gest TR. *Lippincott Atlas of Anatomy*. 2nd ed. Wolters Kluwer; 2020: Plate 3-7 and Flynn JM, Sankar WN. *Operative Techniques in Pediatric Orthopaedic Surgery*. 3rd ed. Wolters Kluwer; 2022.)

attachment for the semimembranosus. The facet for articulation of the tibia with the fibula is located on the lateral tibial condyle. The popliteus muscle attaches to the posterior proximal tibia between and just

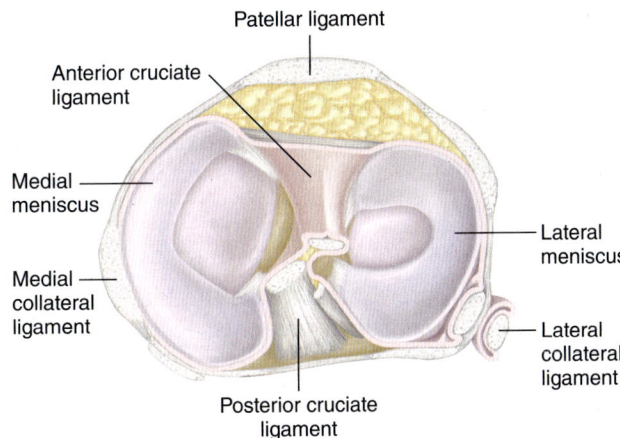

FIGURE 10-3 Superior view of proximal tibia with cruciate and collateral ligaments, menisci, and tibial tuberosity. (Gest TR. *Lippincott Atlas of Anatomy*. 2nd ed. Wolters Kluwer; 2020: Plate 3-58C.)

distal to the fibular facet and the semimembranosus attachment.

Patella The flat and somewhat triangularly shaped patella is the largest sesamoid bone in the body. The patella articulates with the distal femur in a sulcus formed by the medial and lateral femoral condyles.[1] The superior border is curved and embedded within the quadriceps tendon. The anterior surface is covered by the connective tissue expansion of the quadriceps tendon, which blends distally with the patellar ligament, commonly referred to as the *patellar tendon* that attaches to the tibial tubercle. The posterior surface of the patella has proximal oval-shaped smooth articular area, with a vertical ridge creating a larger lateral facet and a smaller medial odd facet (Fig. 10-4). The most medial portion of the medial facet articulates with the femur during extreme flexion. The infrapatellar fat pad covers the posterior surface just distal to the articular portion. The patellar ligament attaches to the most distal portion of the apex.

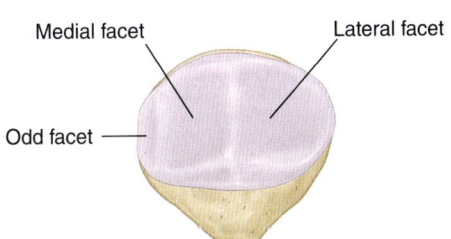

FIGURE 10-4 Facets of patella (posterior view). (Modified from Gest TR. *Lippincott Atlas of Anatomy*. 2nd ed. Wolters Kluwer; 2020: Plate 3-58C.)

Fibula

The long, slender fibula articulates with the tibia at the fibular facet, forming the proximal tibiofibular joint. The lateral collateral ligament (LCL) and the biceps femoris muscle attach to the proximal fibula. The proximal tibiofibular joint is discussed in Chapter 9, Ankle and Foot.

Menisci and Associated Ligaments

The medial and lateral menisci of the knee joint are composed of fibrocartilage attached to the proximal tibia. The function of the meniscus is to stabilize, distribute loads, and promote nutrition to the knee joint. The menisci help protect the tibial plateau articular cartilage by limiting fluid loss during joint loading, minimizing stress by increasing the contact area of the articulation.[3]

The wedge shape of the menisci deepen the articular tibial surface, providing some stability for the femoral condyles and load distribution for the joint (Fig. 10-5).[4] The medial meniscus is larger than the lateral meniscus, consistent with the larger size of the medial tibial condyle. The lateral meniscus covers a greater percentage of the smaller lateral tibial condyle. Thicker on the periphery, the menisci taper toward the center and are unattached at the interior edges on their respective tibial condyles. The firm attachment of the menisci to the tibia is critical for attenuation of joint loads.[5,6] Multiple collagen fibril interfaces called *entheses* anchor the meniscal body to the subchondral bone[7,8] and are located at the medial anterior, lateral anterior, medial posterior, and lateral posterior portions of the menisci. The anterior horn attaches to the tibia by a typical enthesis.[9] The anterior and posterior ends (horns) of the menisci firmly attach to the intercondylar portion of the tibia.[6] The anterior and posterior meniscofemoral ligaments (named the ligament of Humphrey and ligament of Wrisberg, respectively) connect the posterior horn of the lateral meniscus to the medial femoral condyle near the PCL insertion, adding stability to meniscus.[10,11] Each meniscus attaches at the periphery to the tibial condyle by coronary (meniscotibial) ligaments. The transverse ligament of the knee joins the anterior portions of the menisci, helping to stabilize the menisci during knee movements (Fig. 10-6).

The medial meniscus is attached to the medial portion of the joint capsule and the deep portion of the MCL. The lateral meniscus covers a greater portion of the tibial plateau and demonstrates more variation in size, shape, and mobility than the medial meniscus.[4,12] The medial meniscus is more commonly torn than the lateral. However, lateral meniscus tears result in greater degeneration and activity impairment.[13,14]

The menisci can be divided into zones based on vascularity and innervation. The outermost region

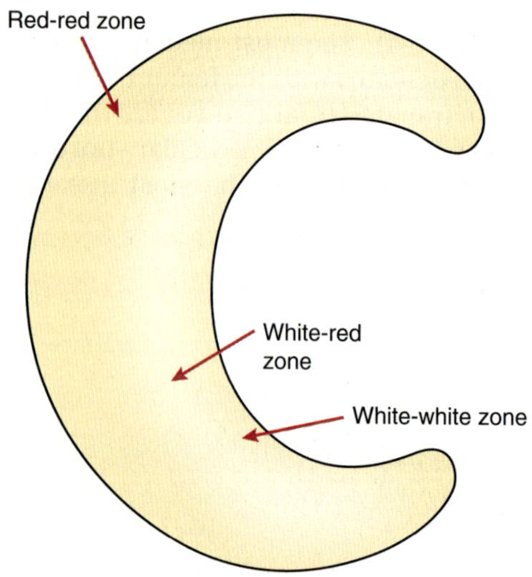

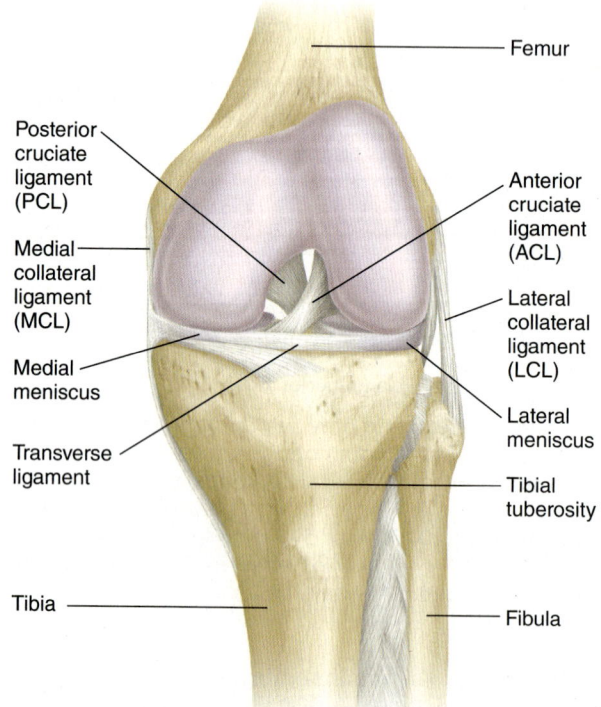

FIGURE 10-5 Menisci shape and regional vascularization. (Adapted from Makris EA, Hadidi P, Athanasiou KA. The knee meniscus: structure-function, pathophysiology, current repair techniques, and prospects for regeneration. *Biomaterials*. 2011;32(30):7411-7431: Figure 3.)

FIGURE 10-6 Menisci positioning between femur and tibia with ligaments. (Gest TR. *Lippincott Atlas of Anatomy*. 2nd ed. Wolters Kluwer; 2020: Plate 3-59A.)

(red-red zone) has the most vascularity and innervation, whereas the innermost portion (white-white zone) is completely avascular and aneural. The intervening region (red-white zone) has some vascular/neural supply. The healing potential of each zone is based on vascularity, leaving the innermost region most susceptible to permanent damage, if injured.[12,15] Tears to the menisci are categorized by the zone torn (e.g., red-red), thickness (e.g., partial or full thickness), or tear pattern (e.g., vertical/longitudinal, including bucket handle; flat/oblique, and horizontal/complex).[4,16]

Owing to decreased vascularity with aging, tears to the meniscus, as well as recovery following surgical intervention, are less favorable among older adults than younger individuals.[17] Lateral meniscus tears result in greater degeneration and activity impairment.[13,14] The injured menisci can be surgically repaired, partially or completely removed, or replaced with an allograft. However, these interventions do not halt the progression of meniscus-derived osteoarthritis (OA).[18,19]

Collateral Ligaments

The collateral ligaments of the knee are located on the medial and lateral sides of the knee, resisting valgus and varus stresses, respectively. The MCL demonstrates nearly twice the ultimate tensile strength of the LCL, but no significant difference in stiffness.[20] The components of both collateral ligaments blend with other knee ligaments, adding to their contribution to knee stability (Fig. 10-6).

Medial (Tibial) Collateral Ligament
The MCL is composed of superficial and deep components with no firm connection between them. The superficial MCL (sMCL) attaches superiorly to the medial femoral epicondyle and the anterior portion of the semimembranosus tendon.[21] The broad distal attachment of the sMCL includes a bony insertion just anterior to the posteromedial tibial crest along with insertion to the pes anserine bursae and distal semimembranosus tendon attachment.[21] The deep layer of the MCL (dMCL) is a thickening of the anteromedial (AM) joint capsule, with the deepest portions contributing to the meniscofemoral (ligament of Humphrey) and meniscotibial (coronary) ligaments.[21,22] The dMCL posterior border blends with the central portion of the popliteal oblique ligament,[21] which attaches to the semimembranosus muscle, joint capsule, and medial meniscus.[18,23] Together, the sMCL and dMCL contribute to valgus and rotational stability,[18] though the fibers of the dMCL are shorter, weaker, and exhibit less ultimate strength when subjected to valgus forces. However, the sMCL contributes the majority of valgus stability. Thus, a rupture of the dMCL may go undetected, whereas an injury leading to rupture of the sMCL will likely also tear the dMCL with resulting marked knee laxity. The anterior border of the fanlike MCL is palpable at the medial joint line when the knee is flexed.

Lateral (Fibular) Collateral Ligament
The LCL attaches proximally to the femoral epicondyle, deep to the iliotibial tract, and distally to the lateral side of the fibular head.[24] The LCL provides ligamentous restraint against varus, particularly with knee flexion around 30°[25,26] and, along with the popliteus muscle tendon and the popliteofibular ligament, provides PL stability to the knee.[27] Although the LCL is most taut with the knee in extension and becomes progressively less taut as the knee flexes, the relative contribution of the LCL to varus stability is greatest at approximately 30° of flexion. The cordlike LCL can be palpated laterally when a varus force is applied to the slightly flexed knee.

Cruciate Ligaments

The ACL and PCL are critical for knee stability and mobility. Located within the knee joint capsule between the synovial and fibrous layers, the ligaments are intracapsular, but extrasynovial. The cruciate ligaments are composed of multiple fiber bundles, with each bundle providing slightly different contributions to the ligament as a whole.

Anterior Cruciate Ligament
The ACL attaches proximally to the PM surface of the lateral femoral condyle and distally to the tibia just anterior and lateral to the intercondylar eminence (Fig. 10-7).[28] The ACL is composed of two primary bundles, the AM and PL bundles, named for their relative tibial attachments.[28] The ACL primarily limits anterior translation of the tibia on the femur, and the two

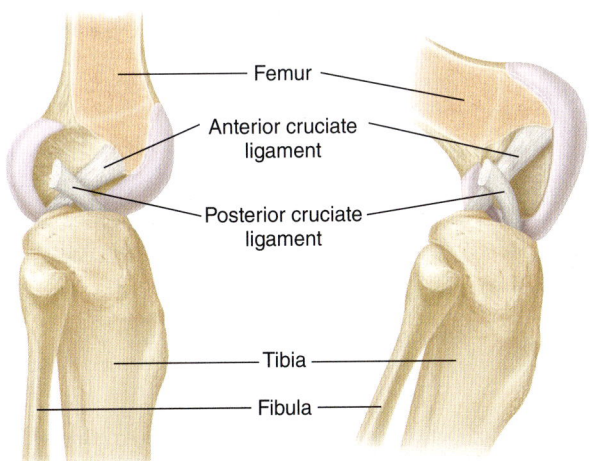

FIGURE 10-7 Attachments of anterior and posterior cruciate ligaments to femur and tibia. (Gest TR. *Lippincott Atlas of Anatomy*. 2nd ed. Wolters Kluwer; 2020: Plate 3-59C, D.)

bundles serve to reinforce knee stability at different angles of knee flexion. The AM bundle is most taut during flexion, whereas the PL bundle is most taut during extension.[1,28,29] In addition, the ACL limits medial and lateral rotation.[30,31]

Posterior Cruciate Ligament The PCL attaches superiorly to the lateral surface of the medial femoral condyle within the intercondylar notch (Fig. 10-7)[1] and distally on the posterior intercondylar fossa of the tibia.[32] The PCL is larger and stronger than the ACL.[33] The PCL is the primary ligamentous structure limiting posterior translation of the tibia on the femur at all angles of flexion,[1] but, in an extended position, limits all translational movements along with adduction/abduction at the knee.[1] Like the ACL, the PCL is composed of multiple bundles, including the PM bundle and the anterolateral (AL) bundle.[1,32,33] The AL and PM bundles of the PCL both contribute throughout the flexion arc to limit posterior translation of the tibia.[33,34]

Other Knee Ligaments

While the primary ligaments of the knee are the collateral and cruciate ligaments (Table 10-1), other ligaments blend with these ligaments or exist separately and provide additional stability.

Of particular note are the popliteofibular, fabellofibular, and AL ligaments that, together with the PCL and LCL, provide support to the posterior and lateral aspect of the knee, called the "posterolateral corner."

The posterolateral corner (Fig. 10-8) has been described as a three-layered (superficial, middle, and deep) complex of soft-tissue structures. Fibers from the iliotibial band (ITB), vastus lateralis, and biceps femoris form the superficial layer.[35] The middle layer is composed of fibers from the ITB and vastus lateralis, along with ligaments formed by thickenings of the joint capsule, namely, the lateral patellofemoral ligament and patellomeniscal ligaments.[36] The more superficial portion of the deep layer is composed of the LCL, fabellofibular, and arcuate ligaments (defined later). The fabella is a sesamoid bone not present in all individuals. However, when present, it is located in the lateral head of the gastrocnemius muscle and is accompanied by the fabellofibular ligament that runs alongside the LCL attaching distally to the fibula.[1,37,38] The deepest component of the deep layer is composed

TABLE 10-1

PRIMARY LIGAMENTOUS RESTRAINTS TO KNEE MOTION, DESCRIBED AS THE MOVEMENT OF THE TIBIA ON THE FEMUR

Ligament	Attachments	Functions
ACL	• Medial surface lateral femoral condyle • Anterior intercondylar area of tibia	Anterior translation* Valgus and varus rotation†; medial (and lateral) rotation; hyperextension
PCL	• Medial surface lateral femoral condyle • Anterior tibial intercondylar area	Posterior translation* Valgus and varus rotation†; lateral (and medial) rotation
MCL	• Medial femoral epicondyle • Medial tibial condyle and medial meniscus	Valgus* Medial and lateral rotation†; anterior and posterior translation
LCL	• Lateral femoral epicondyle • Fibular head	Varus* Lateral rotation†; anterior and posterior translation

ACL, anterior cruciate ligament; *LCL*, lateral collateral ligament; *MCL*, medial collateral ligament; *PCL*, posterior cruciate ligament.
*, primary; †, secondary.

Modified from Dutton M. *Dutton's Orthopedic Examination: Evaluation and Intervention.* 5th ed. McGraw Hill; 2020; Hamill J, Knutzen KM, Derrick TR. *Biomechanical Basis of Human Movement.* 5th ed. Wolters Kluwer; 2022; Neumann DA. *Kinesiology of the Musculoskeletal System: Foundations for Rehabilitation.* 3rd ed. Elsevier; 2017.

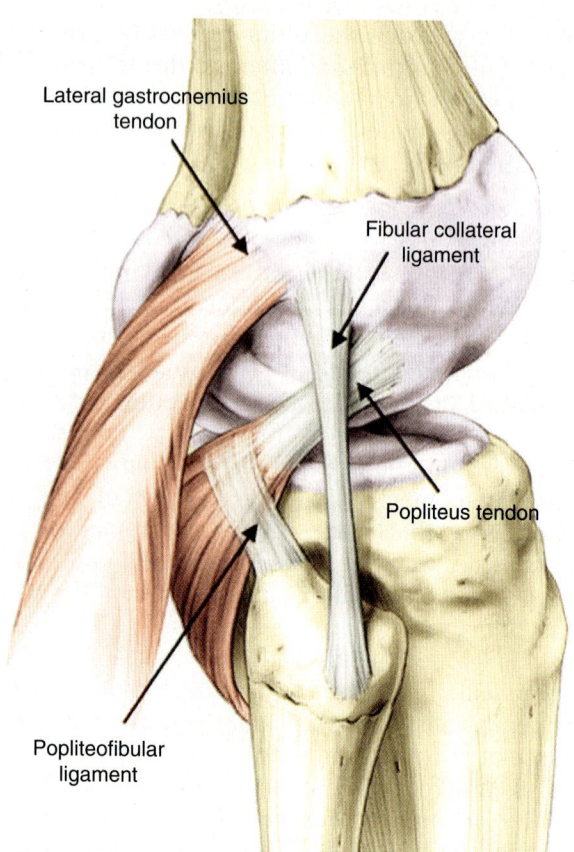

FIGURE 10-8 Structures of posterolateral corner of knee. (Adapted from James EW, LaPrade BA, LaPrade RF. Anatomy and biomechanics of the lateral side of the knee and surgical implications. *Sports Med Arthrosc Rev.* 2015;23(1):2–9, Figure 1.)

of the popliteus musculotendinous unit and the popliteofibular ligament passing from the popliteus tendon to the fibula.[1,37–39]

Additional support to the posterior joint capsule is provided by the arcuate-popliteal complex, formed by two ligaments.[40] The oblique popliteal ligament lies in the floor of the popliteal fossa and attaches to the semimembranosus tendon, portions of the posterior joint capsule and lateral femoral condyle. The Y-shaped arcuate ligament arches over the popliteal surface of the joint capsule with attachments to the fibular head, lateral femoral epicondyle, and posterior tibia.[2] The arcuate-popliteal complex limits anterior tibial displacement, hyperextension, hyperflexion, and varus and external rotation.[40]

The shared attachments of ligaments, retinacula, and dynamic structures in the posterolateral corner contribute to the stability,[38,41] particularly in limiting varus and external rotation.[38]

Joint Capsule and Synovium

The thin outer fibrous layer of the knee joint capsule attaches to the femur superiorly and anteriorly just proximal to the articular portion of the condyles. Posteriorly, the capsule encloses the condyles and the intercondylar fossa with a gap near the lateral tibial condyle for passage of the popliteus tendon. Inferiorly, the capsule attaches to the tibial plateau, except in the region of the popliteus tendon. Anteriorly, the capsule is continuous with the quadriceps tendon, patellar ligament, and the medial and lateral portions of these structures. An internal synovial membrane lines the inner surface of the fibrous layer, except in the central portion where the two separate. The synovial membrane attaches to the nonarticular portion of the knee joint, attaching to the periphery of the articular cartilage of the femoral and tibial condyles, as well as the posterior patella and edge of the menisci. The synovial membrane covers the two cruciate ligaments and infrapatellar fat pad, creating a vertically oriented infrapatellar synovial fold that extends anteriorly to the posterior aspect of the patella, occupying the majority of the intercondylar space and creating two femorotibial articular cavities.

Plicae are inward folds in the synovial lining of the knee, forming a pouch or band between the synovium of the patella and knee joint. The thin tissue forming the plicae may be partially or fully resorbed in embryologic development and is, therefore, inconsistently present in the adult.[42,43] The suprapatellar, medial patellar, and infrapatellar plicae often blend to form one pouch.[44,45] Trauma to plicae may cause inflammation and thickening, resulting in a painful disorder named plica syndrome. Treatment includes rest, activity modification, muscle strengthening and stretching, and surgical excision.[46]

Bursae

There are many bursae around the knee joint (Fig. 10-9), with some communicating with the knee joint capsule and others remaining contained.[47] Table 10-2 describes several of the larger bursae. The suprapatellar bursa is formed as the knee joint cavity extends superiorly, deep to the vastus intermedius muscle, thus making the suprapatellar bursa and knee joint cavity continuous. The synovial membrane lines both cavities. Infection of the bursa may spread to the knee joint cavity. The subcutaneous prepatellar and infrapatellar bursae are located anterior to the patella and facilitate skin mobility during knee movements. Irritation of the pes anserine bursa, formed where the tendons of the semitendinosus, gracilis, and sartorius muscles insert at the medial proximal tibia, commonly presents clinically as pain along the medial joint line that may mimic a tear in the medial meniscus.[48] The gastrocnemius and semimembranosus bursae may combine to form a gastrocnemio-semimembranosus bursa that communicates with the knee joint and often has unidirectional flow of fluid contributing to the formation of popliteal cysts (Baker cysts).[49]

The infrapatellar fat pad consists of adipose tissue with small blood vessels from the inferior genicular arteries coursing through its substance. When injured, the fat pad may fibrose, leading to impairment in patellar movement and patellar tendon function.[1]

BIOMECHANICS

Mobility and stability of the knee joint complex results from the interaction between static and dynamic influences. During functional activity, movements of the

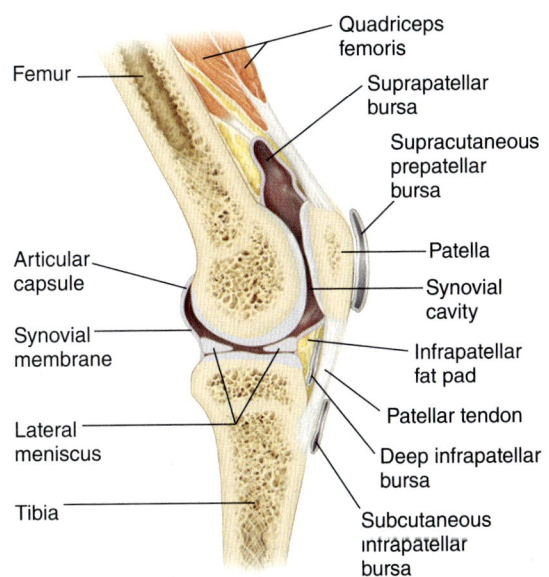

FIGURE 10-9 Bursae of knee joint. Medial view of knee. (Modified from Wingerd BD. *The Human Body: Concepts of Anatomy and Physiology*. 3rd ed. Lippincott Williams & Wilkins; 2014: Figure 4.19.)

TABLE 10-2
BURSAE AROUND THE KNEE JOINT

Bursae	Location	Description
Suprapatellar	Between distal femur and quadriceps femoris tendon	Communicates with knee joint cavity
Subcutaneous prepatellar	Between skin and anterior patellar surface	Allows free skin movement over patella during knee movement
Subcutaneous infrapatellar	Between skin and tibial tuberosity	Assists to withstand pressure when kneeling
Deep infrapatellar	Between patellar ligament and anterior proximal tibia	Separated from knee joint by infrapatellar fat pad
Popliteal	Between popliteus tendon and lateral tibial condyle	Communicates with knee joint cavity
Pes anserine	Between tendons of sartorius, gracilis, and semitendinosus and tibia near insertion	Limits friction of tendons against tibia
Gastrocnemius	Deep to attachment of medial head of gastrocnemius to distal femur	Communicates with knee joint cavity; considered an extension of synovial cavity into knee joint
Semimembranosus	Between gastrocnemius medial head and semimembranosus tendon	Often combines with gastrocnemius bursa; communicates with knee joint cavity

Adapted from Moore KL, Dalley AF, Agur AMR. *Moore's Clinically Oriented Anatomy*. 8th ed. Wolters Kluwer, 2018:Table 7.17.

knee and patellofemoral joints occur in conjunction with movements of the hip and ankle. The muscles crossing the knee include two joint muscles that also cross the hip or the ankle. Although many muscles influence movement, the quadriceps accounts for the majority of muscle force acting on knee joint complex. The patella provides a mechanical advantage to the quadriceps by increasing the moment arm of the patellar tendons and thereby improving torque production (Fig. 10-10). The quadriceps works concentrically to produce knee extension and eccentrically to decelerate the knee as it moves into flexion. Working concentrically, the hamstrings flex the knee and eccentrically decelerate knee extension. The quadriceps reduces posterior translation of the tibia on the femur, and the hamstrings reduce anterior translation. Stability is promoted through the interconnection among tendinous, ligamentous, and capsular connective tissue elements.[1]

Knee Joint

Knee Joint Alignment
Movement of the knee occurs in three planes concurrently, with movement in the sagittal plane predominating. The knee joint load consists of the superimposed weight of all structures above it (head, arms, trunk or HAT) and the opposite lower extremity. Stress to the knee joint results from malalignment of other joints as well as from muscle imbalances and other tissue abnormalities.[34,50]

Knee joint alignment in the frontal plane is described by the degree of varus and valgus. The normal anatomic knee joint alignment, using the long axes of the femur and tibia, is 5° to 8° of valgus. Genu

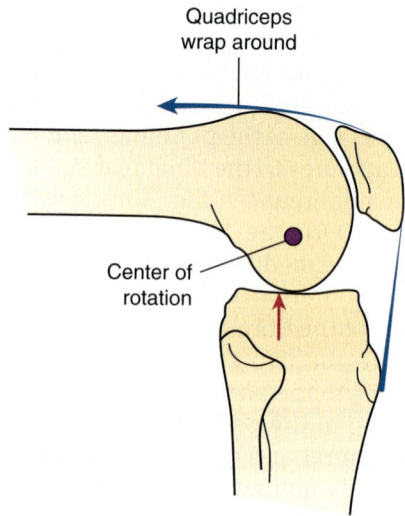

FIGURE 10-10 Lateral view of knee joint at 90° flexion. Patella provides mechanical advantage increasing force capacity of quadriceps muscle. (Adapted from Nordin M, Frankel VH. *Basic Biomechanics of the Musculoskeletal System*. 5th ed. Wolters Kluwer; 2022: Figure 7-21.)

valgus (or valgum—knock knee) and genu varus (or varum—bow legs) are used to describe frontal plane malalignment of valgus or varus that is greater than normal (Fig. 10-11). In erect standing, the knee is at 0° of flexion/extension in the sagittal plane. Movement toward hyperextension is called *genu recurvatum*. Genu valgus and genu recurvatum occur more commonly in women, whereas genu varus is more common in men.[51] Both genu valgus and genu varus increase loading of the knee joint[52] and may lead to the

gait, the knee moves from near-complete extension at midstance to 65 to 75° in mid-swing. Activities such as climbing/descending stairs[61,62] and siting/rising from a chair require approximately 110° of flexion. Flexion greater than 110° is required for squatting and getting in/out of the bathtub.[60,62] The available knee movement is the same whether the tibia is moving on the femur (as occurs during the swing phase of gait) or whether the femur is moving on a fixed tibia (as occurs in the lead leg when going up steps in a step-over-step movement pattern).

The flexion-extension rotation of the knee moves along a curved path, called the "evolute." The evolute exists because the femoral condyles are not spherical, but rather ovoid in shape (Fig. 10-12). Thus, the knee demonstrates a migrating axis of rotation in sagittal plane movements, explaining in part why muscle forces acting across the knee vary across a ROM. The contact surface area changes with flexion and loading (non–weight bearing [NBW] versus weight bearing). Devices such as a goniometer or a hinged knee brace move about a fixed axis. Therefore, it is important when assessing knee flexion-extension ROM that goniometer axis and knee brace hinge align closely to lateral epicondyle of the knee, the location of the "average" axis of rotation.

Data supporting the amount of rotational motion and abduction/adduction at the knee are varied,

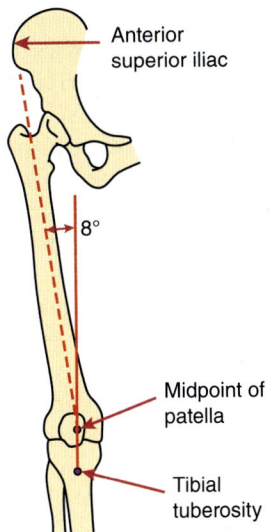
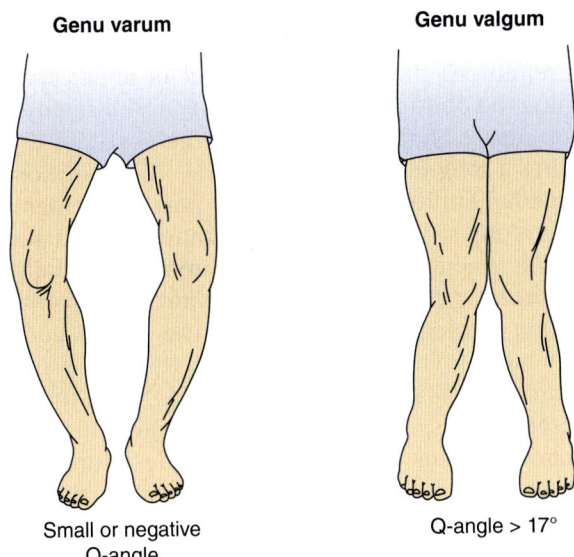

FIGURE 10-11 Genu varus and valgus. Q angle is demonstrated. (Adapted from Hamill J, Knutzen KM, Derrick TR. *Biomechanical Basis of Human Movement*. 5th ed. Wolters Kluwer; 2022: Figure 6-22.)

development of OA.[53] In normal alignment in the transverse plane, described as 0° of rotation (or version), the axis of the tibial plateau and femoral condyles are parallel,[54] though varying degrees are demonstrated between races and sexes.[55,56]

Knee Joint Osteokinematics Normal knee movement is predominately in the sagittal plane about a mediolateral axis and ranges from 5 to 10° of hyperextension to approximately 150° of flexion,[57,58] or to soft-tissue approximation of the posterior thigh and leg musculature.[59] The knee range of motion (ROM) necessary for function depends on the task.[60] During

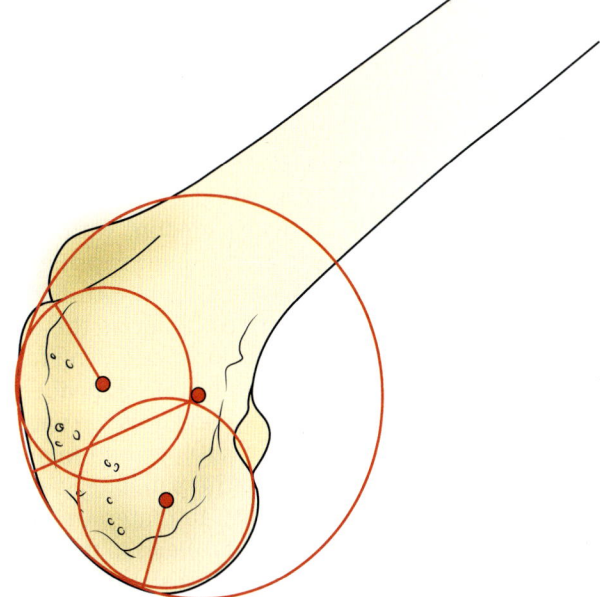

FIGURE 10-12 Sagittal view of knee demonstrating varied position of center of rotation about the knee. (Adapted from Oatis CA. *Kinesiology: The Mechanics and Pathomechanics of Human Movement*. 3rd ed. Wolters Kluwer; 2017: Figure 41.4.)

perhaps because these movements are small, technically difficult to measure, and studied using varied methodologies. The reported mean excursion in medial/lateral rotation ranges from 12 to 80°,[63–65] with an average expected rotation of approximately 40 to 45° with the knee flexed. The amount of external rotation exceeds internal rotation.[66,67] There is little to no internal/external rotation excursion with the knee completely extended.[63,66–68] During walking, little axial rotation occurs, with ranges from 8 to 15°. Medial rotation occurs in stance and lateral rotation in swing.[69,70]

Most commonly, the medial/lateral rotation (also called *axial rotation*) is assessed based on movement of the tibial tuberosity relative to the distal femur, with no distinction as to whether the end position is based on the tibia moving on the femur (tibial-on-femur) or the femur moving on the tibia (femur-on-tibia). When communicating axial rotation movement, it is important to distinguish knee joint rotation and bony (tibial or femoral) rotation, the first communicating an osteokinematic motion and the second communicating an arthrokinematic motion.

MUSCLES ABOUT THE KNEE AND PATELLOFEMORAL JOINT

The extensor mechanism of the knee is considered the quadriceps muscle, patella, and patellar tendon. All components of the quadriceps muscle group narrow distally toward the knee, with fibers forming portions of the quadriceps tendon and attaching to the patella. The rectus femoris attaches the central portion of the base of the patella. The distal portion of the vastus lateralis forms a flattened tendon, attaching to the base and lateral portion of the patella with fibers extending to the lateral joint capsule, lateral tibial condyle, and ITB (Fig. 10-13). The vastus medialis forms an aponeurosis distally that attaches to the medial patellar border and quadriceps tendon, with an expansion that reinforces the medial joint capsule. The distal fibers are nearly horizontal (Fig. 10-14). The distal portion of the vastus intermedius forms the deepest portion of the quadriceps tendon, attaching to the lateral patella and lateral tibial condyle. Many fibers of the quadriceps tendon continue distally as the patellar ligament, attaching to the patellar apex and margins, with superficial fibers covering the patella and fibers extending distally on the medial and lateral sides of the patellar ligament (Fig. 10-15).[2,71] Deep to the vastus intermedius is the articularis genu, a small muscle attaching to the distal anterior femur and anterior joint capsule. The articularis genu acts to pull the knee joint capsule superiorly during knee extension. The vasti muscles contribute 80% and the rectus muscle 20% to the extension torque of the knee.

The medial and lateral heads of the gastrocnemius muscle serve as weak flexors of the knee. All other muscles crossing the posterior aspect of the knee joint (i.e., hamstrings, sartorius, gracilis, and popliteus) may flex and axially rotate the knee and are referred to as *flexor rotators*. The hamstrings muscle group (i.e., semimembranosus, semitendinosus, and biceps femoris long head) are located posteriorly (Fig. 10-16) and attach proximally to the ischial tuberosity. The biceps femoris short head attaches proximally to the lateral lip of the linea aspera of the femur and, along with the long head, passes distally to insert on the fibular head, the LCL, and associated ligaments and, along with the iliotibial tract, to the lateral side of the tibia. When the knee is flexed, the biceps femoris and tensor facia latae (via the iliotibial tract) contribute to lateral rotation of the tibia at the knee joint.[71,72] The semimembranosus attaches directly to the posterior aspect of the medial tibial condyle, with additional attachment to the popliteal fascia and a reflected portion that blends with and reinforces the posterior aspect of joint capsule, forming the oblique popliteal ligament. The semitendinosus passes on the medial side of the posterior thigh, forming a long cordlike tendon near the insertion to the medial surface of the tibia as part of the pes anserine along with the distal attachment of the sartorius and gracilis.[73] The popliteus attaches distally to the posterior surface of the tibia and proximally via a strong intracapsular tendon to the lateral surface of the lateral femoral condyle, with fibers passing to the lateral meniscus and fibular head.[74] Together, the semitendinosus, semimembranosus, sartorius, gracilis, and popliteus contribute to medial rotation of the tibia when the knee is flexed. Active tension in the pes anserine muscle group in concert with the MCL and PM joint capsule resists external rotation and valgus stresses to the knee,[75] with some regarding the pes anserine muscle group as "dynamic MCL."[76]

The flexor-rotator muscles control tibia-on-femur osteokinematics when the foot is free, as in the swing phase of walking or running. In this example, the flexor-rotator muscles act to accelerate or decelerate the lower leg. More complex and greater demands are placed on the flexor-rotator muscle group during femur-on-tibia motions when the foot is in contact with the ground. For example, when running to catch a ball over the left shoulder, a player plants the right foot on the ground whereas the right femur and pelvis are rotated to the left. The biceps femoris short head moves the femur toward internal rotation, whereas the pes anserinus muscle group eccentrically contracts to limit external rotation of the tibia and decelerate femoral internal rotation. In addition, the popliteus stabilizes the lateral side of the knee by providing resistance to the imposed varus load.

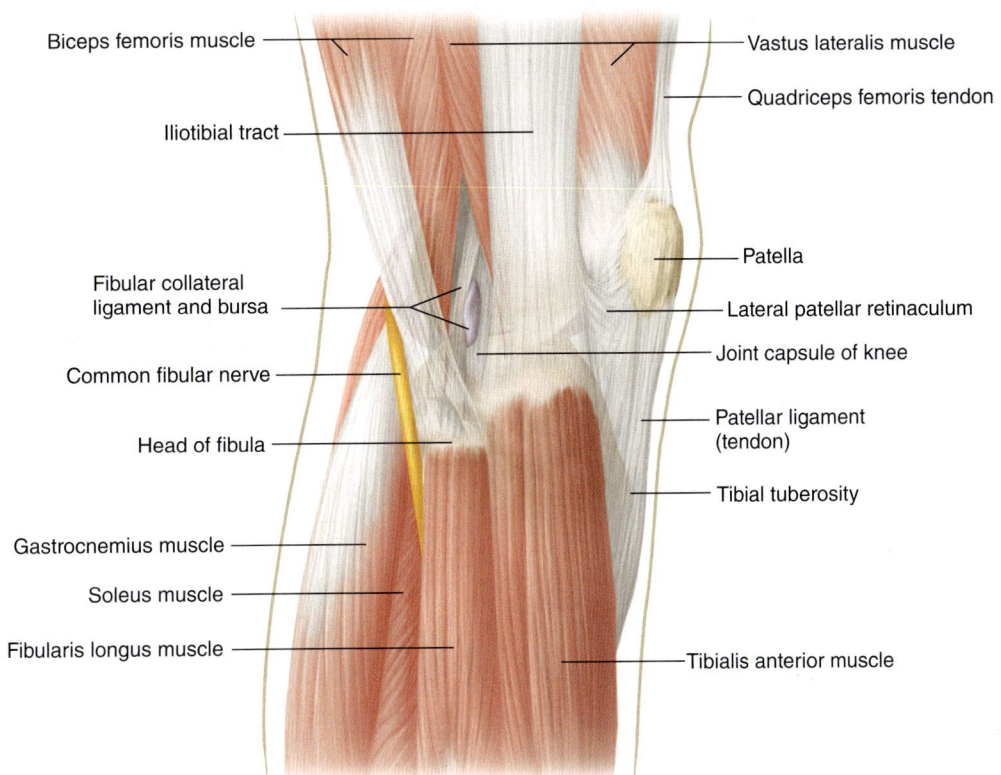

FIGURE 10-13 Muscles and bony structures about the lateral knee. Lateral view. (Gest TR. *Lippincott Atlas of Anatomy*. 2nd ed. Wolters Kluwer; 2020: Plate 3-57B.)

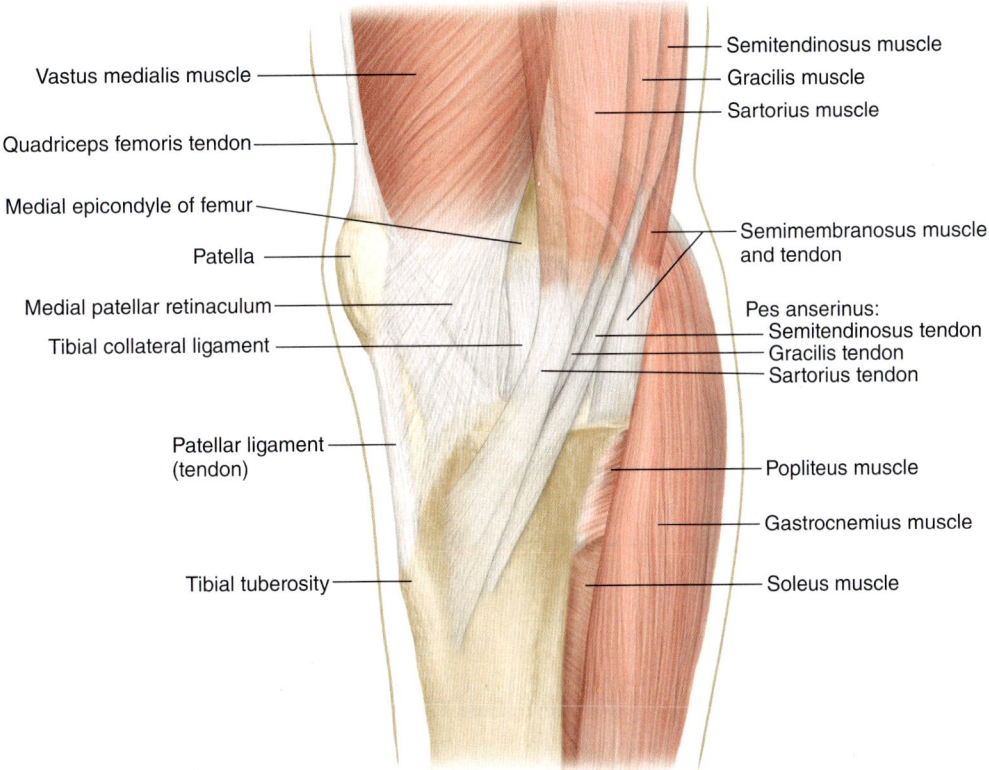

FIGURE 10-14 Muscles and bony structures about the medial knee. Medial view. (Gest TR. *Lippincott Atlas of Anatomy*. 2nd ed. Wolters Kluwer; 2020: Plate 3-57A.)

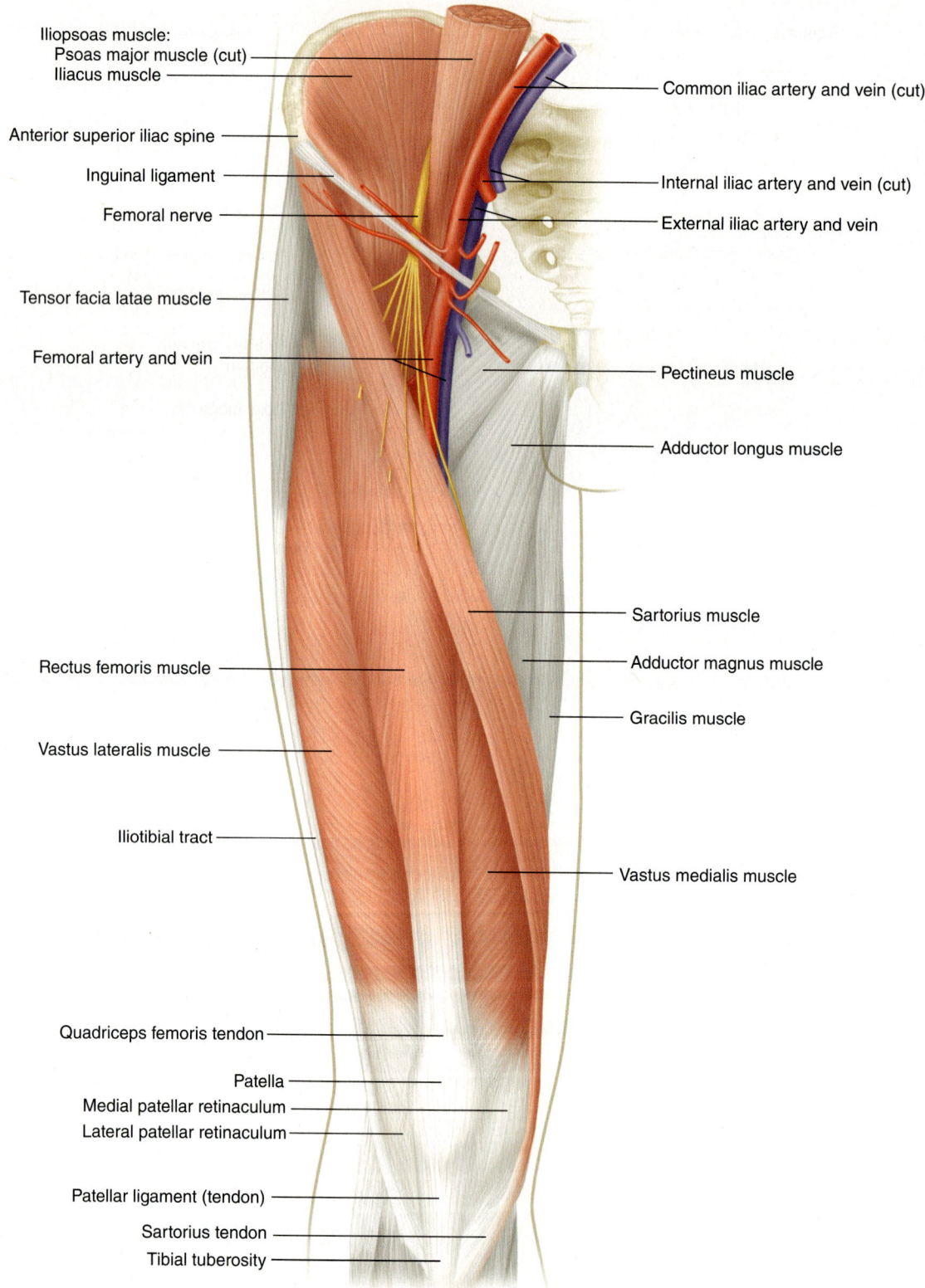

FIGURE 10-15 Muscles of the anterior thigh. Anterior view. (Gest TR. *Lippincott Atlas of Anatomy*. 2nd ed. Wolters Kluwer; 2020: Plate 3-16.)

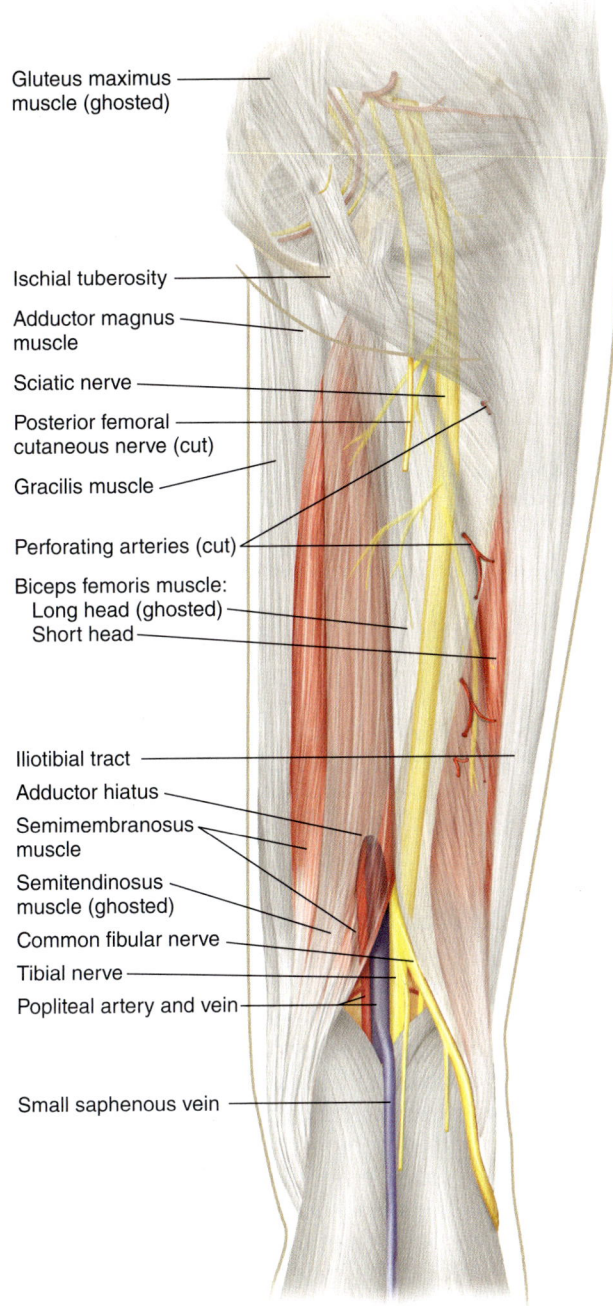

FIGURE 10-16 Muscles of the posterior thigh. Posterior view. (Gest TR. *Lippincott Atlas of Anatomy*. 2nd ed. Wolters Kluwer; 2020: Plate 3-29B.)

PALPATION

Many of the bony and connective tissue structures about the knee are easily palpated. Relevant palpable structures include:

- Lateral femoral condyle and epicondyle
- Medial femoral condyle and epicondyle
- Adductor tubercle of the femur
- Tibial plateaus
- Tibial tuberosity
- Patella base, apex, and borders
- Head of the fibula
- Joint line
- Margins of menisci
- LCL and MCL
- Tendons: quadriceps, sartorius, gracilis, semitendinosus, semimembranosus, biceps femoris

The structures about the knee are easiest to palpate when the knee is somewhat flexed. The patient should sit on the edge of the examination table with the legs hanging freely at approximately a 90°. The clinician should sit in front of the patient or a little to the side. The clinician may start palpation by placing the thumbs in the depression on either side of the patellar ligament and allowing the fingers to wrap lightly around the patient's leg with fingertips in/toward the popliteal fossa. Moving the thumbs inferiorly and centrally, the patellar tendon can be palpated as it passes toward its insertion on the tibial tuberosity. Just medial and distal to the tibial tubercle below the tibial plateau is the pes anserine region, the insertional area for the sartorius, gracilis, and semitendinosus. Returning to the depression on the medial side of the patellar tendon, the clinician can apply firm pressure into the soft tissue and palpate medially to identify the bony boundaries of the medial joint space: the medial tibial plateau and the inferior margin of the medial femoral condyle. Within the joint space, the anterior border of the medial meniscus can be palpated. Moving the fingers slightly inferiorly, the sharp edge of the medial tibial plateau can be palpated. Moving the fingers superiorly adjacent to the medial patella, the medial femoral condyle can be felt. Continuing palpation medially along the medial femoral condyle, the large protruding medial femoral epicondyle is evident. The adductor tubercle can be palpated just posterior to the medial femoral epicondyle. The relatively flat MCL passes from the medial femoral epicondyle and the proximal medial tibia and can be palpated as it passes superficial to the joint line.

Just lateral to the depression on the lateral side of the patellar tendon, the clinician can palpate the lateral joint line. Pushing slightly inferiorly, the lateral tibial plateau can be felt. The lateral tibial tubercle is felt just distal to the plateau. Returning to the depression of the joint line and pressing superiorly, the lateral femoral condyle can be felt. With firm pressure in the joint space just lateral to the patellar tendon, the iliotibial tract can be palpated, especially when the patient contracts the tensor facia latae and vastus lateralis. On the lateral side of the femoral condyle, the prominence of the lateral femoral epicondyle can be felt. Moving the fingers directly inferiorly across the joint line and distally, the head of the fibula can be felt. The LCL runs from the lateral femoral epicondyle to the head of the fibula and can be most easily palpated if the patient's leg is crossed over the opposite one with the ankle resting on the knee and the hip flexed, abducted, and laterally rotated. In this position, a varus tension is placed on the LCL, making the ligament more prominent and easier to palpate.

To palpate the tendons of the major muscles about the knee, the clinician should sit in front of the patient who is sitting on a table with the leg draped over the side and the knee flexed to 90°. The clinician should locate the apex of the patella and palpate on either side and distally to identify the patellar tendon as it passes to attach to the tibial tuberosity. With the clinician's thumbs on either side of the patellar tendon and the fingers wrapped around the knee on either side, the posterior aspect of the knee can be felt. On the PM side of the knee, the tendons of the pes anserinus muscle group (sartorius, gracilis, and semitendinosus) can be palpated as a group. To differentiate among these muscles, palpation should be accompanied by resisted knee flexion along with additional selective resisted actions at the hip joint: hip flexion, adduction, and extension for differential palpation of the sartorius, gracilis, and semitendinosus, respectively. The semitendinosus tendon is the most prominent and easily palpated as the palpating fingers are moved from the middle of the popliteal fossa and medially. The semimembranosus tendon is deep to the pes anserine muscle group on the posterior tibia. The biceps tendon creates the lateral superior border of the popliteal fossa and can be easily palpated as it courses distally to attach to the fibular head.

Knee Joint Arthrokinematics

During active tibia-on-femur knee extension with the foot free, the relatively concave articular surface of the tibia rolls and slides anteriorly on the femoral condyles, with the quadriceps muscle pulling the menisci anteriorly. With femur-on-tibia extension, such as when moving from sitting to a standing position, the relatively convex femoral condyles simultaneously roll anteriorly and slide posteriorly on the fixed tibia. As the knee moves toward full extension, external rotation of the tibia relative to the femur occurs simultaneously, placing the knee joint surfaces in a position of greatest contact at full extension (Fig. 10-17). This combined movement of extension and external rotation, often referred to as the "screw-home mechanism," is an example of conjunct rotation (see Chapter 3, Arthrology). In conjunct rotation at the knee, the axial rotation cannot be performed, independent of the flexion/extension; that is, the movements are coupled.[77] The screw-home rotation is influenced by the tension

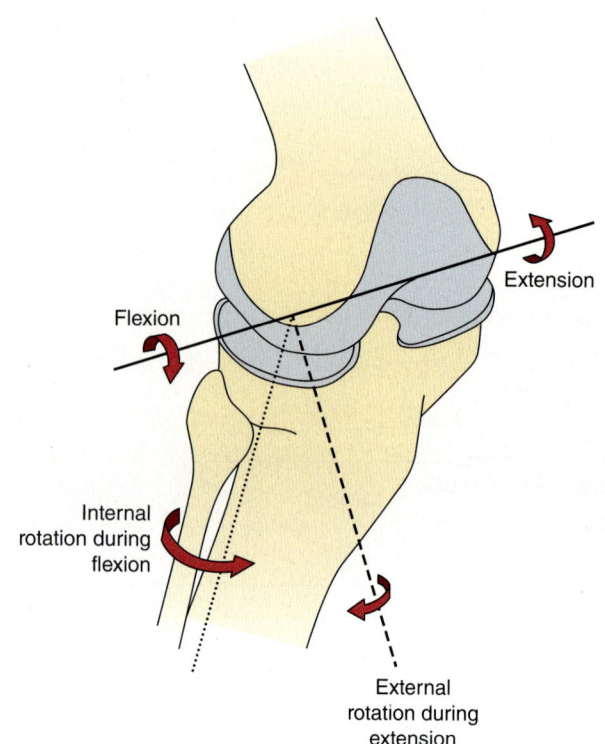

FIGURE 10-17 Screw-home mechanism of knee. (Adapted from Helfet AJ. Anatomy and mechanics of movement of the knee joint. In: Helfet A, ed. *Disorders of the Knee*. JB Lippincott Co; 1974:1-17, Fig. 7.9.)

in the ACL, the slightly lateral angled pull of the quadriceps muscle,[76,78] and the shape of the medial femoral condyle.[1] The medial femoral condyle extends farther anteriorly than the lateral femoral condyle and also curves laterally from posterior to anterior as the trochlear groove is approached. In tibia-on-femur extension, the tibia follows this lateral path, with an obvious tibial external rotation demonstrated. In femur-on-tibia extension, the medial femoral condyle is guided on a medial path on the tibia, such that at full knee extension, the relative position of the tibia is one of external rotation. To "unlock" the knee from the fully extended position, the popliteus muscle rotates the tibia slightly medially when the foot is free or the femur laterally when the foot is fixed. Independent medial and lateral rotation at the knee joint can occur when the knee is in a flexed position, and most commonly does so as a spin between the menisci and the tibia and femur articular surfaces.[76]

Patellofemoral Joint

The patella contributes to knee extension by serving as a connector and force transmitter between the quadriceps muscles to the tibia. Proper motion of the patella within the femoral trochlear groove is critical to the function of the patellofemoral joint itself as well as the knee joint. Pathology of the patellofemoral and knee joints can occur either in isolation or in conjunction with each other. The patellar surface can be located centrally or offset to the medial or lateral direction (see Fig. 10-1). The patella connects the knee extensor muscles (vastus medialis, vastus intermedius, vastus lateralis, and rectus femoris) to the tibia and contributes to knee extension by transferring the quadriceps force to the tibia via the patellar tendon.

Patellofemoral Joint Alignment

The mediolateral position of the patella with respect to the femur is one of slight lateral deviation as the patella moves (tracks) within the groove formed by the femoral trochlea.[79] The shape of the trochlea plays a significant role in patella stability.[80,81] The lateral trochlea projects farther anteriorly, helping to maintain the position of the patella within the groove as the knee moves into flexion from an extended position (Fig. 10-18). Beyond 30° of knee flexion, the patella is less confined by the bony configuration and its stability is gained from soft-tissue structures connecting to it, such as tendons, fascia, and retinacula. The contact surface of the patella with the femoral trochlea varies with knee flexion, with the greater contact occurring as maximum flexion is approached.[82] The articular cartilage on the posterior aspect of the patella varies in thickness and conformity. The cartilage covering the medial and lateral facets is among the thickest in the body, serving to minimize friction between the patella and joint surfaces.[83] Excessive tracking of the patella in the medial, or more commonly lateral direction, may result in pain, subluxation, or dislocation.[84] An markedly lateral insertion of the patellar tendon to the tibial tuberosity tends to pull the patella laterally, increase the patellar contact pressure, and contribute to instability.[85,86]

The proximal-distal alignment is defined by the position of the patella relative to the trochlear groove. Patella alta (high-riding patella) is associated with reduced patellofemoral stability during knee movement and is a risk factor for patellofemoral OA.[87,88] Both patella alta and patella baja (low-riding patella) are associated with patellofemoral pain.

Angular alignment considerations include patellar tilt and sulcus angle. Patellar tilt is described as a rotation about a superoinferior axis. The sulcus angle is formed by lines drawn from the deepest aspect of the trochlear groove (sulcus) to the highest point of the medial and lateral femoral condyles. Clinical measurement of these angular alignments is unreliable and demonstrates wide variations.[34,89–91]

Patellofemoral Kinematics

With the knee extended, the patella is positioned above the trochlear groove, with the minimal contact with the femur. In initial flexion, the patella moves slightly medially, influenced by lateral trochlear groove, the medial retinacula, and medial patellofemoral ligament (MPFL).[92–94] The patella translates laterally as knee flexion proceeds toward than 20 to 30° and greater,[92,95] while also laterally tilting and medially rotating.[94] During knee flexion, the patella moves distally on the femur, with bony contact increasing as flexion progresses.[94] There is normal variation in contact between patellar surfaces and the interplay between static and dynamic structures that influence patellar position during knee movement. This suggests that abnormalities in structural alignment, bony configuration, muscular strength, and forces to which the complex is subjected play a role in pathology at the joint.

The portion of the patella in contact with the femur varies throughout knee ROM, with similar outcomes reported from in vivo[96–98] and in vitro studies.[52,99,100] In near-full flexion, the patella rests below the trochlear groove with the lateral edge of the lateral facet and the odd facet in contact with the femur. Between 60 and 90° of flexion, the contact area of the patella shifts from the superior pole toward the inferior pole and the patella becomes well seated in the trochlear groove, demonstrating the greatest amount of contact and the highest compressive forces when in this position. As the knee moves farther toward extension, the inferior pole of the patella rests against the femur, but with

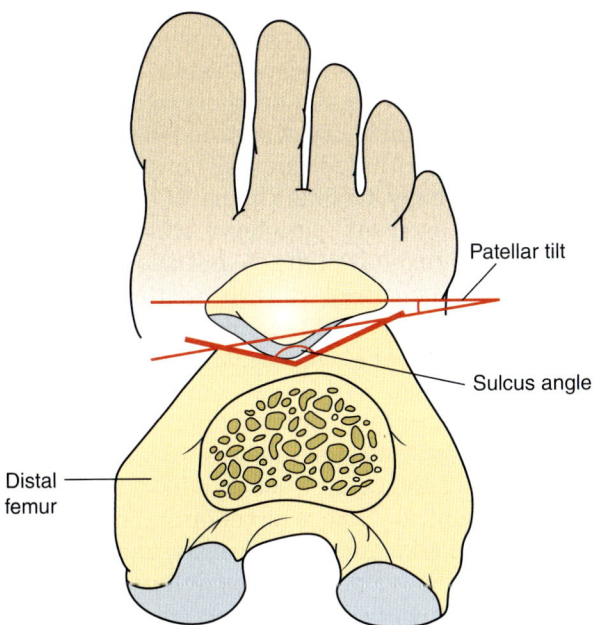

FIGURE 10-18 Patellar tilt and sulcus angle for patella. (Adapted from Oatis CA. *Kinesiology: The Mechanics and Pathomechanics of Human Movement.* 3rd ed. Wolters Kluwer; 2017: Figure 41.35.)

less contact than at 60°. At full extension, the patella is entirely proximal to the trochlear groove, where it rests on a suprapatellar fat pad against the femur. In full extension, the patella is very mobile if the quadriceps is relaxed. Most chronic subluxations or dislocations of the patella occur with the knee in the extended position.[101]

The amount and direction of force from the overlying quadriceps muscle plays a major role in patellofemoral joint mechanics. As the knee moves from a flexed to extended position, the quadriceps muscles pull the patella superiorly, slightly laterally, and posteriorly. The angle of the femur relative to the tibia, known as the *quadriceps* or *Q angle*, is sometimes used as a clinical measure of the line of pull of the quadriceps on the patella, even though research indicates poor association between the degree of Q angle and pathology of the patellofemoral joint.[102,103] Differences in methodology and populations studied may explain the apparent controversy in the association between the Q angle and anterior knee pain.[104,105] The Q angle is commonly assessed as the angle formed by the intersection of lines at the center of the patella, with one line along the long axis of the femur and another from the tibial tuberosity to the patella (see Fig. 10-11). The measured Q angle is impacted by torsional deformities of the long bones or malalignment of the tibial tuberosity relative to the shaft of the tibia and may not affect the valgus alignment of the knee.

The fiber direction of the vastus medialis, particularly the oblique portion, suggests that the muscle may play a major role in dynamic stabilization of the patella against the lateral pull of the other quadriceps muscles or lateral structures. However, the results of in vivo studies are controversial.[106,107] The muscles of the quadriceps group work in concert to produce knee extension; thus, it is difficult to study the impact of isolated vastus medialis weakness.[34] Rather, weakness of the entire quadriceps group is correlated with anterior knee pain.[106,108]

INTRODUCTION TO THE EXAMINATION OF THE KNEE

Many common lesions affect the knee joint. Athletes as well as more sedentary persons may sustain traumatic injuries. Symptomatic degenerative disorders involving the knee are not uncommon in middle-aged or older persons, and overuse syndromes may affect virtually any age group. The approach to the evaluation of knee disorders must be flexible enough to accommodate such a broad spectrum of disorders. An assessment scheme that includes most of the evaluative procedures needed to perform a thorough clinical examination common knee disorders is presented in the subsequent section.

HISTORY: KNEE JOINT

The key to an efficient yet comprehensive evaluation of a patient with knee pain is the history. A patient interview should elicit specific information related to the patient's health history and demographics, symptoms, and review of systems (refer to Chapter 6, Patient History). The clinician must understand the patient's symptoms and determine the acuity, severity, irritability, stability, and functional implications of the patient's condition. The following are general concepts that apply to information that may be elicited when interviewing patients with common knee disorders. Additional questions may be required based on the nature of the specific disorder. Limb dominance may be applicable for athletes.

Prior Ankle, Knee, or Hip Pathology

Patients should be asked if they have had prior ankle, knee, or hip injuries or surgeries on either lower extremity. As noted in Chapter 8, Lower Quarter Screen, the lower extremity functions in the closed kinetic chain, and therefore, pathology at one joint can impact other joints. Likewise, the left and right lower extremities are linked, with impairments on one limb having a potential impact on the other. For example, decreased right lower extremity strength results in increased stress to the left lower extremity when landing from a jump. Patients who have had knee surgery are more likely to have OA in the surgical knee than those who have had knee injuries that were treated conservatively.[109]

Onset

Injuries caused by trauma are common, particularly in sports activities involving contact or a change of direction. An attempt should be made to determine the exact mechanism of injury. A sudden twisting injury, in which the tibia is rotated externally on the femur, may tear either the capsular fibers of the MCL (grade I tear), the coronary ligament (peripheral attachment of the meniscus), or the body of the medial meniscus. If some external force is involved with this twisting injury, such as in contact sports, and the knee is also forced into valgus position, the PM capsule, MCL, or ACL may also be damaged. Valgus injuries are common and may be due to contact by another player from the unprotected lateral side. However, the majority of valgus injuries are noncontact and occur when an athlete lands from a jump or attempts to change direction and moves into a position of hip adduction, genu valgus, and tibial internal rotation. This "valgus collapse" injury may damage the ACL, MCL, and/or either meniscus. A hyperextension injury may damage the posterior capsule. If severe, the ACL may rupture, followed by the PCL. Posterior forces on the tibia, which might occur when the tibia hits the dashboard, stress the PCL.

For symptoms that are nontraumatic and gradual in onset, clinicians should attempt to rule out symptomatic degenerative joint disease (DJD) if the patient is middle aged or older. Pain from DJD is typically initially noticed near the end of the day or after long periods of walking. Later, pain and stiffness are felt on rising in the morning, easing somewhat after getting up and about. Possible precipitating factors, such as recent immobilization, alteration in activities, past injuries, and previous surgeries, should be considered. In contrast, if the patient is younger, patellofemoral pain syndrome (PFPS) should be considered. Pain from PFPS is typically worse with prolonged sitting or activities requiring increased quadriceps activation, such as going down stairs. For patients with recurrent knee pain (reporting a history of similar symptoms), patellar tendinopathy, meniscal pathology, and DJD should be considered.

Swelling

Patients should be asked about the amount and timing of knee swelling. A large effusion minutes to hours after an acute injury, such as an injury occurring from making a sharp turn on a planted foot, is indicative of a **hemarthrosis** and may represent an ACL rupture or intra-articular fracture. In contrast, a smaller effusion that develops over 6 to 24 hours is indicative of synovial effusion and commonly occurs with meniscal lesions.[110] Intermittent mild knee joint swelling is not uncommon in patients with knee DJD, occurring with increased levels of activity and resolving after joint stress is reduced. Isolated areas of local swelling can be a sign of bursal irritation, particularly for the anterior knee (patellar bursitis) or medial knee (pes anserine bursitis).

Knee-Specific Symptoms

Patients with suspect knee pathology should be asked about symptoms such as grating, grinding, or clicking, as these should make the clinician suspect possible meniscal involvement or DJD. Knee stiffness may represent DJD or a low-level inflammatory condition. Patients reporting the knee feels unstable, or "gives way," may have sustained an ACL or meniscal injury. Reports of knee locking or catching might be the result of pathology of the meniscus, plica, or patellofemoral joint. Pain with prolonged sitting or going up and down stairs may indicate patellofemoral pathology. The patient should be asked about functional activities, such as rising, walking, squatting, stairs, turning, running, and cutting.

Location of Symptoms

The knee joint receives innervation from the L3 through S2 segments of the spinal column. In the patient with nontraumatic onset of pain about the knee, lesions located elsewhere in the L3 through S2 segments must be ruled out. The two common sources of referred pain to the knee are the lumbosacral region and the hip region. The L3 segment innervates both the anterior hip and the anterior and medial knee. Therefore, a patient with a hip joint problem may complain of "knee pain." This is most commonly seen in children with a slipped capital femoral epiphysis (SCFE) (see Chapter 11, Hip). The medial knee is primarily innervated by L3. Therefore, pain derived from medial knee structures does not extend much below the knee. In contrast, pain from posterior knee structures may be felt in the posterior knee and may extend some distance distally because they are innervated by the S1 and S2 segments.

Bilateral symptoms may be related to OA, rheumatoid arthritis (RA), or systemic diseases, such as Lyme disease or systemic lupus erythematosus. Both sides are affected, though one side may exhibit more severe symptoms at a given time.

Outcome Measures

The Patient-Specific Outcome Tool and Lower Extremity Function Scale (LEFS) introduced in Chapter 6, Patient History, and Chapter 9, Ankle and Foot, respectively, might be applicable to any patient with a lower extremity disorder. However, the clinician should also consider the use of outcome tools that are specific to the knee (Table 10-3) or that assess higher level activities.

PHYSICAL EXAMINATION OF THE KNEE

As noted earlier in the text, the physical examination is composed of the systems review, the quarter screen, the clearing examination, and the joint-specific examination. However, the clinician must first be alert to any potential red flags. If the patient history raises suspicion for fracture, the clinician should proceed directly to using the Ottawa Knee Rules or the Pittsburg Knee Rules (Table 10-4) to determine whether radiographs are warranted. Both tests are highly sensitive; however, the Pittsburgh Knee Rules are much more specific.[111] Despite this, the Ottawa Knee Rules tend to be utilized more often. Therefore, it is wise for clinicians to be comfortable using both systems.

Once the patient has been cleared of any red flags and the history and systems review have been performed, the clinician should perform a lower quarter screen (LQS) and a clearing examination (in this case, active and passive hip and ankle ROM) to ensure that the area of pathology has been narrowed down to the knee region and any proximal potentially contributing factors have been identified. Practically speaking, the clinician will rarely use all the tests and procedures outlined here for any one patient. However, the

TABLE 10-3
COMMON OUTCOME TOOLS FOR PATIENTS WITH KNEE PATHOLOGIES

Tool	Tool Basics
Lower Extremity Function Scale (LEFS)	• Addresses global lower extremity function • Scoring: 0-80 • 20 items rated 0-4, with higher scores indicating greater function • MDC* 9 points • May have a ceiling effect for higher functioning individuals • Common diagnoses: total knee/hip arthroplasty, anterior cruciate ligament reconstruction, lower extremity fracture
WOMAC	• Addresses lower level global lower extremity function • Scoring: 0-100 • 24 items are rated 0-4, with higher scores indicated worse pain/function • Points from 3 scales: pain (5 question), stiffness (2 questions), and function (17 questions) • Points are summed and converted to a percentage • MDC* 3.94 points for knee degenerative joint disease and 10.9 points for total knee arthroplasty at 6 months • Common diagnoses: hip/knee degenerative joint disease, total knee/hip arthroplasty, rheumatoid arthritis
International Knee Documentation Committee 2000 Subjective Knee Evaluation Form (IKDC)	• Addresses global lower extremity function • Scoring: 0-100 • Points from 3 scales: symptoms (37 points), sports (0-40 points), and function (20 points), with higher scores indicating greater function • Points are summed and converted to a percentage • MDC* 11.5 • Common diagnoses: wide variety of knee disorders including ligament, meniscus, cartilage, and general knee pain
Knee injury and Osteoarthritis Score (KOOS)	• Addresses a wide range of common knee complaints and activities • Scoring: 0-100 • 42 items ranked 0-4 in 5 domains (pain, symptoms, activities of daily living, sports/recreation, and quality of life), with higher scores indicating greater function • MDC* 5-8 varies based on domain and population • Common diagnoses: knee ligament, meniscus, degenerative joint disease, total knee arthroplasty
Lysholm Knee Score	• Scoring: 0-100 • 8 weighted items with scores ranging from 0 to 25, with higher scores indicating greater function. The patient also marks the amount of pain in one or both knees on a line ranging from no pain to worst possible pain. • MDC* 15 points • Half of all points are determined by patient report of knee pain and giving way • May not be able to detect changes over time • Common diagnoses: knee ligament, meniscus, patellofemoral pain syndrome, degenerative joint disease
Victorian Institute of Sport Assessment-Patella (VISA-P)	• Addresses higher level activities, with 40% of points derived from sport-like activities • Scoring: 0-100 • 8 weighted items with scores ranging from 0 to 30, with lower scores indicating worse pain and function • MDC† 11 points • Common diagnoses: patellar tendinopathy
SANE (Single Assessment Numerical Evaluation)	• Scoring: 0-100 • Patient rates knee function on a scale of 0-100 • MCID‡ 7 points • Does not provide details as to what the patient is having difficulties with • Common diagnoses: knee ligament, meniscus, ankle, shoulder

MCID, minimal clinically important difference; MDC, minimally detectable change.
Adapted from Shirley Ryan Ability Lab. *Rehabilitations Measures Database.* Accessed December 15, 2020. sralab.org

*Collins NJ, Misra D, Felson DT, Crossley KM, Roos EM. Measures of knee function: International Knee Documentation Committee (IKDC) Subjective Knee Evaluation Form, Knee Injury and Osteoarthritis Outcome Score (KOOS), Knee Injury and Osteoarthritis Outcome Score Physical Function Short Form (KOOS-PS), Knee Outcome Survey Activities of Daily Living Scale (KOS-ADL), Lysholm Knee Scoring Scale, Oxford Knee Score (OKS), Western Ontario and McMaster Universities Osteoarthritis Index (WOMAC), Activity Rating Scale (ARS), and Tegner Activity Score (TAS). *Arthritis Care Res.* 2011;63 suppl 11:S208-S228.

†Hernandez-Sanchez S, Hidalgo M, Gomez A. Responsiveness of the VISA-P scale for patellar tendinopathy in athletes. *Br J Sports Med.* 2014;48:453-457.

‡Winterstein AP, McGuine TA, Carr KE, Hetzel SJ. Comparison of IKDC and SANE Outcome measures following knee injury in active female patients. *Sports Health.* 2013;5(6):523-529.

TABLE 10-4	
SCREENING FOR KNEE FRACTURES	
Ottawa Knee Rules	*Pittsburgh Knee Rules*
Knee radiographs are warranted if there is a history of trauma and ...	
• The patient is >54 years of age OR • Isolated bony tenderness of the patella or fibular head OR • Unable to flex knee at least 90° OR • Unable to take at least 4 steps both immediately after injury and at the place of examination	• The patient is >50 or <12 years of age OR • Unable to take at least 4 steps both immediately after injury and at the place of examination

clinician should become proficient in all the tests and must know the rationale for each. Likewise, for the LQS, the experienced clinician will titrate the joint-specific examination based on the patient history, presentation, and goals. Clinically, the joint-specific examination is organized by position and should proceed from uninvolved (or less involved) to involved side but is presented here by category to aide conceptualization.

Structure

Observe the patient's general appearance and body structure. Examine the lower extremities for edema, ecchymosis, or atrophy. Perform a lower quarter structural examination as discussed in Chapter 8, Lower Quarter Screen (see Tables 8-1 and 8-2). In standing, the knee should be in full extension, and there should be a slight amount of genu valgum. Note abnormal or asymmetrical genu recurvatum, valgum, or varum. Excessive genu valgum can be documented by measuring the distance between the malleoli with the knees in contact with each other. The reverse is true for excessive genu varum, which can be documented by measuring the distance between the knees with the malleoli in contact with each other. Alternatively, the angulation can be measured with a goniometer with the patient in supine.

With the patient in short sitting, observe the tibial tuberosity. An excessively prominent tibial tuberosity suggests current or prior apophysitis (current or previous stress injury to the proximal tibia growth plate). The tibial tuberosity should line up with the middle or lateral half of the patella. If one tuberosity is more lateral, this may represent laxity of the PM capsule. With the patient supine, the clinician should assess the position of the patella relative to the tibiofemoral joint:

- Normal: Inferior patellar pole is approximately at the level of the tibiofemoral joint line.
- Patella alta: Inferior patellar pole is greater than 20 mm above the tibiofemoral joint line.
- Patella baja: Inferior patellar pole is below the tibiofemoral joint line.

Patella alta (a high-riding patella) or laterally facing patella may be significant in terms of patellofemoral joint problems.[112,113]

Skin and Soft Tissue

Observe for obvious signs of knee effusion or swelling. A localized area of swelling within the popliteal fossa, known as a *popliteal cyst* (Baker cyst), is suggestive of a meniscal tear or OA. Ecchymosis within the thigh is most commonly associated with either a strain or contusion but may also be seen in recent patellar dislocations.

Range of Motion

Active physiologic knee motions with passive overpressure should be assessed and compared the motions with the American Academy of Orthopaedic Surgeons (AAOS) normative values (Table 10-5).[114,115] Although the primary motion at the knee is flexion and extension, it may be useful to assess tibial rotation with the patient short sitting as the greatest amount of motion occurs in this position. The clinician should note the endfeel and any changes in patient symptoms. If crepitus is noted during movement, the clinician should try to determine whether this arises from the tibiofemoral joint or the patellofemoral joint via palpation and patient questioning. If pain is noted, the clinician should note the point in the range this is felt.

TABLE 10-5	
PASSIVE RANGE OF MOTION NORMATIVE VALUES	
Motion	Normative Value (degrees)
Knee flexion	0-135
Knee extension	0-10*
Tibial internal rotation	30
Tibial external rotation	40

*Symmetrical knee hyperextension of up to 15° may be considered normal, particularly in females. De Carlo MS, Sell KE. Normative data for range of motion and single-leg hop in high school athletes. *J Sport Rehabil.* 1997;6(3):246-255.

A capsular pattern of restriction for the tibiofemoral joint is a gross limitation of flexion and slight limitation of extension. This is commonly seen in patients with effusion or tibiofemoral DJD. Loss of extension in the presence of full knee flexion is most often caused by an internal derangement, such as a bucket-handle meniscus tear.

Loss of even a small amount of knee extension can have significant impacts on function. During midstance and terminal stance, the knee is near-full extension.[116] Pain with end range knee extension or inability to fully extend will lead to the patient walking on a flexed knee. This, in essence, shortens the extremity and requires significantly more quadriceps activation, which may lead to early fatigue.

Although there is roughly 40° of tibiofemoral rotation, this is not typically measured.[115] Assess for normal tibial external rotation on the femur by observing the position of the tibial tuberosity. In 90° of knee flexion, the tibial tuberosity should be near the midline of the patella. During knee extension, the tibia externally rotates, and at end range, the tibial tuberosity should line up with the lateral border of the patella. This is sometimes called the modified Helfet test.[117] Loss of tibial external rotation may reflect tightness of the medial capsuloligamentous structures, which can occur following immobilization, whereas rupture of these same structures can lead to excessive tibial external rotation. Lack of tibial external rotation may also be indicative of meniscal or cruciate ligament injury.[117] Pain with active (or resisted) tibial internal rotation or with passive tibial external rotation may be indicative of a popliteal strain or tendinopathy.[118,119]

Muscle Length

There are several multi-joint muscles that cross the knee joint. Table 10-6 provides normative values for key multi-joint muscles that should be assessed.[115] The clinician must, therefore, consider how the position of the neighboring hip and ankle joints can affect knee motion in the case of a lack of normal muscle length. For example, a patient may appear to have a loss of knee joint ROM if knee extension is assessed in the seated position because the hamstring is not capable of fully lengthening simultaneously across both the hip and the knee joints. Failure to distinguish between this loss of muscle length and loss of joint motion would lead the clinician to inappropriately perform joint mobilizations and joint stretching procedures, such as prone knee extension hangs, rather than hamstring stretching. The Thomas test (Fig. 10-19) can be used to assess the length of the three main hip flexors: the iliopsoas, rectus femoris, and tensor facia latae/ITB. The modified Ober test (Fig. 10-20) can be used to assess the length of the tensor facia latae/ITB.

Muscle Performance

After performing the LQS, knee-specific muscle performance testing should be performed. Knee extensor and flexor strength may be assessed using manual muscle testing (MMT).[120] Any symptoms with testing should be further investigated and correlated with the patient history. Table 10-7 lists symptoms and potential diagnostic hypotheses based on symptoms with quadriceps MMT. For example, a patient with anterior thigh pain with quadriceps MMT who also has a history of being hit in the thigh with a lacrosse ball

TABLE 10-6	
MUSCLE LENGTH NORMATIVE VALUES	
Motion	Normative Value (degrees)
Hamstring: straight leg raise*	≥68° hip flexion with knee in full extension
Hamstring: popliteal angle test*	≤20° of knee flexion with hip flexed 90°
Rectus femoris: prone knee flexion*	125°
Thomas test†	• With clinician overpressure, patient's thigh is parallel with support surface in neutral ABD/ADD and knee flexed 80°. • If abnormal, record hip flexion/extension angle with the knee flexed (rectus femoris length) and extended (iliopsoas length). • If the hip moves into further extension when allowed to abduct, denotes ITB/TFL tightness (there is generally no numerical measurement associated with this portion of the test).
Modified Ober test#†	With clinician overpressure, the patient's thigh is at least 10° adducted.
Gastrocnemius#†	10° of ankle DF

ABD, abduction; ADD, adduction; ITB, iliotibial band; TFL, tensor facia latae.
*Clarkson HM. Musculoskeletal Assessment: Joint Range of Motion, Muscle Testing, and Function. 4th ed. Wolters Kluwer; 2021.
†Kendall FP, McCreary EK, Provance PG, Rogers MM, Romani WA. Muscles: Testing and Function with Posture and Pain. 5th ed. Lippincott Williams & Wilkins; 2005.

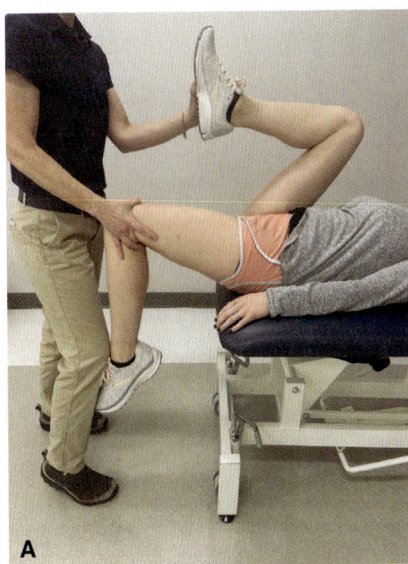
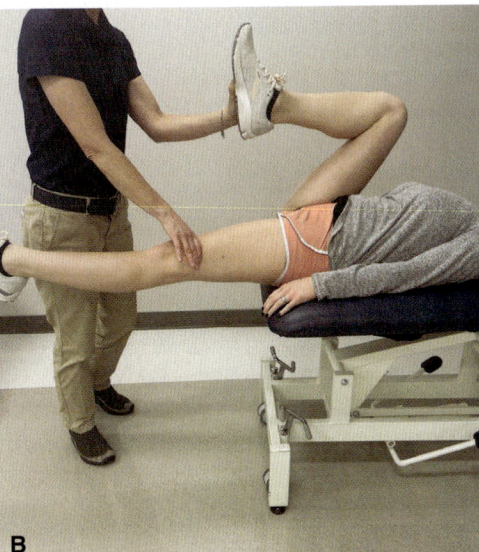
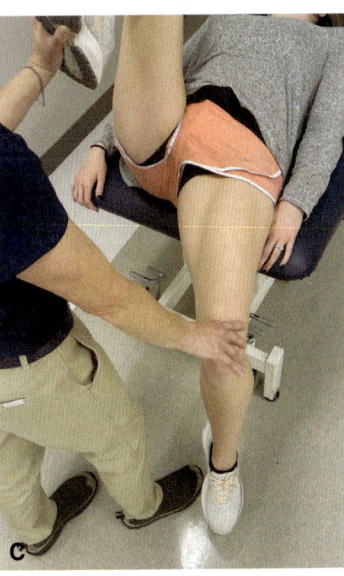

FIGURE 10-19 Thomas test. **A**. Assessment of rectus femoris. **B**. Assessment of iliopsoas length. **C**. Assessment of tensor facia latae/iliotibial band length.

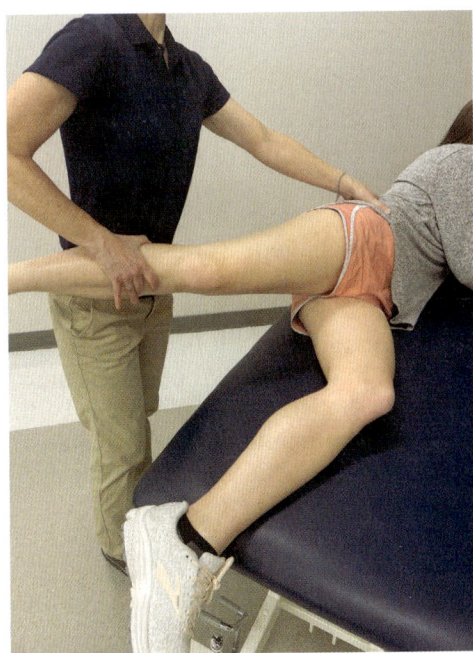

FIGURE 10-20 Modified Ober test.

2 days prior is likely to have a contusion and may also have ecchymosis in the region. In contrast, a patient whose symptoms began after attending his first high-intensity interval training program with a significant number of weighted squats is likely experiencing a quadriceps strain from acute overuse. It may be possible to differentiate between the various heads of the quadriceps via symptoms location and palpation. For a rectus femoris strain, the clinician must consider that the rectus femoris is a two-joint muscle. Therefore, resisted hip flexion is likely to be painful. Similar methods can be utilized to differentiate between the semitendinosus, semimembranosus, and biceps femoris and gastrocnemius.

For lower functioning patients, such as those who have had recent knee surgery, clinicians may describe the patient's ability to perform a quadriceps set. Is the patient able to make a strong contraction and lock the knee (Fig. 10-21)? If so, can the patient maintain full knee extension while performing a straight leg raise? One can also compare the amount of passive knee extension to active extension maintained against gravity and document any extensor lag if present.

The gluteus maximus is the strongest hip external rotator. The hip external rotators can assist with controlling excessive lower extremity internal rotation and dynamic valgus. For athletes, clinicians may choose to supplement the standard MMT assessment of hip external rotator performance in short sitting with assessment in the prone position (Fig. 10-22).

In order to detect and quantify subtle losses in muscle strength, a handheld dynamometer can be employed for specific muscle groups. This can be performed with the clinician holding the handheld dynamometer (Fig. 10-23A). For stronger patients, the handheld dynamometer can be placed underneath a strap anchored to the table and looped around the

TABLE 10-7
SYMPTOMS AND DIAGNOSTIC HYPOTHESES IF QUADRICEPS MANUAL MUSCLE TEST IF PAINFUL

Symptom	Potential Diagnostic Hypotheses
Anterior thigh pain	Quadriceps strain Quadriceps contusion
Pain "in" the knee joint	Tibiofemoral degenerative joint disease Patellofemoral degenerative joint disease
Pain "behind" or "under" the patella	Patellofemoral pain syndrome Osteochondral defect of the patellar or femoral trochlea
Patellar tendon pain	Patellar tendinopathy
Pain near the tibial tubercle	Apophysitis
Painless weakness	L3 nerve pathology Femoral nerve pathology Quadriceps rupture

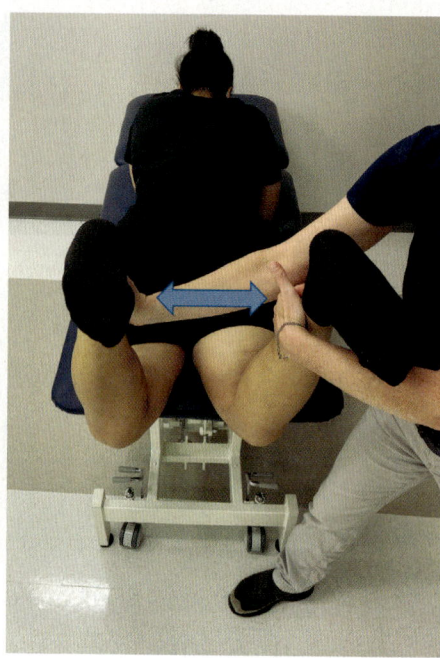

FIGURE 10-22 Muscle performance assessment of the hip external rotators in prone. Clinician resists patient's attempt to externally rotate bilateral lower extremities.

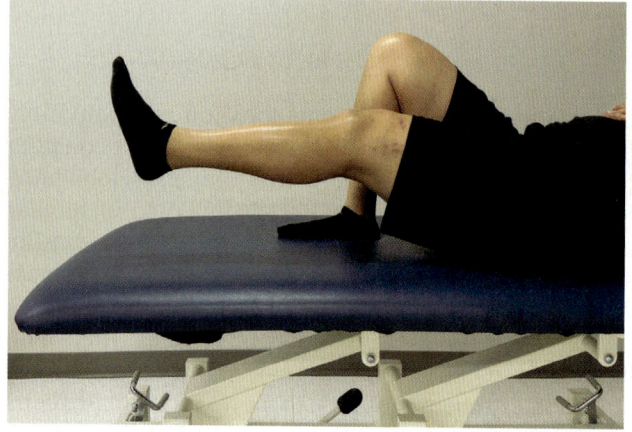

FIGURE 10-21 Straight leg raise with lag indicating poor quadriceps muscle performance.

patient's distal tibia. In addition, various pieces of exercise equipment can be used. For example, a leg extension machine (Fig. 10-23B) can be used to compare the strength of the involved and uninvolved quadriceps muscles or a leg press machine can be used for a comparison of multi-joint strength either between limbs or with normative data. Some facilities will have access to isokinetic machines (Fig. 10-23C), such as those made by Biodex and Cybex. As noted in Chapter 6, Patient History, such devices provide insights into the patient's ability to generate force at various speeds. Muscle endurance can be assessed using fatigue testing, such as comparing the number of repetitions of leg extension or leg curls each limb can perform with a given load until failure or with a 30-second or 1-minute isokinetic test at a medium or high speed.

Sensory Tests

The clinician must have a working knowledge of the lower extremity dermatomal segments and peripheral nerve sensory distribution (see Fig. 7-5 in Chapter 7, The Physical Examination). It is not uncommon after knee surgery to have a loss of cutaneous sensation in the region of the incision due to damage to the small branches of the saphenous nerve. The size of the insensate area is likely to decrease over time and usually completely resolves.

Reflexes

If a patient reports paresthesias, the clinician should assess patellar and Achilles reflexes to assess possible upper or lower motor neuron involvement.

Neurodynamic Testing

Neurodynamic testing, particularly the straight leg raise,[121] should be performed on patients reporting paresthesias in the posterior or lateral thigh and leg to help with ruling out the lower lumbar spine as a source. The anterior thigh equivalent of the straight leg raise is the femoral nerve stretch test (alternately referred to as Ely test, femoral nerve tension test, or

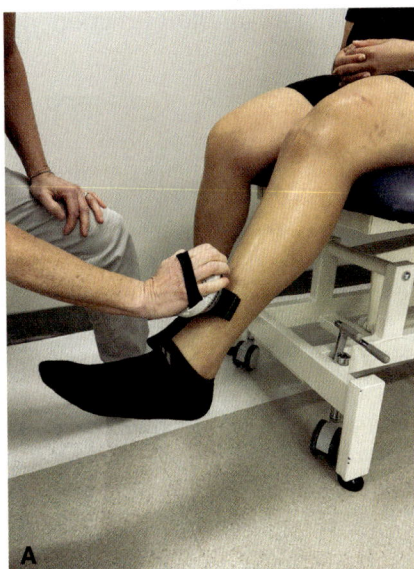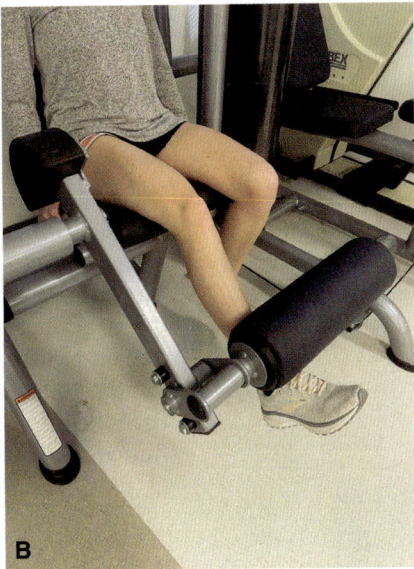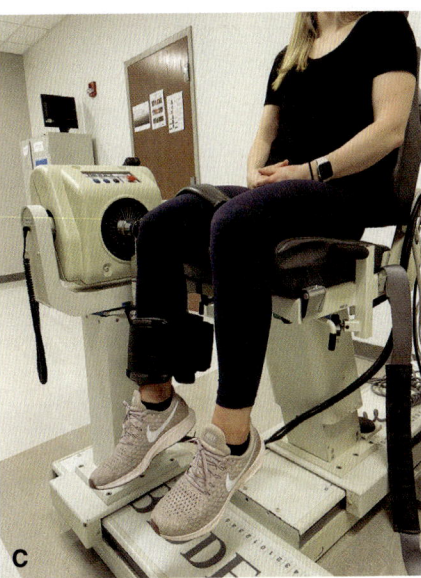

FIGURE 10-23 Objective methods of assessing quadriceps muscle performance. **A.** Leg extension machine. **B.** Handheld dynamometer. **C.** Isokinetic quadriceps strength testing.

prone knee flexion test). Although less often involved than the lower lumbar segments, the femoral nerve stretch test should be used to assess tension in the L1-3 nerve roots and the femoral nerve.[121] The reader is referred to Chapter 12, Lumbar Spine and Sacroiliac Joint, for further details.

Accessory Motion

Joints should be assessed for hypermobility or hypomobility and the presence or absence of pain. Tibiofemoral joint anterior (Fig. 10-24) and posterior (Fig. 10-25) glides should be assessed along with distraction (Fig. 10-68) and rotation (Figs. 10-63 and 10-66). These mobilizations can be used for both assessment and treatment purposes. For a quick assessment, all of these mobilizations can be performed in supine or the seated positions with the knee in the open-packed position of about 25° of knee flexion. When used for treatment, positioning is usually changed to optimize clinician's body mechanics. The tibiofemoral joint frequently becomes hypomobile with DJD, after immobilization, and after surgery. Tibiofemoral joint hypermobility may represent systemic hypermobility or significant capsular or ligamentous damage. Patellofemoral joint mobility should be considered because hypomobility can lead to increased patellofemoral joint compressive forces as well as restrict end range motion. Patellofemoral joint hypermobility can be seen after patellar dislocation, MPFL rupture, systemic hypermobility, and in certain anatomic anomalies (such as a patellar dysplasia or a low or flat lateral femoral epicondyle).[122]

Tibiofemoral Joint Mobilization: Anterior Glide

Purpose: To assess joint-play movement necessary for knee extension.
Patient: Supine with the knee in loose pack position.
Clinician: The cranial hand stabilizes the distal femur. The caudal mobilizing hand contacts the posterior tibia just distal to the tibiofemoral joint.
Mobilization: Keeping the arm straight, the mobilizing hand glides the tibia anteriorly (Fig. 10-24).

Tibiofemoral Joint Mobilization: Posterior Glide

Purpose: To increase joint-play movement necessary for flexion.
Patient: Seated with knee slightly flexed.
Clinician: The clinician uses one hand to support the lower leg and places the mobilizing hand on the anterior tibia just distal to the tibiofemoral joint.
Mobilization: The mobilizing hand moves the tibia posteriorly (Fig. 10-25). Note this patient position is generally also used for assessing anterior glide of the tibia. The clinician would simply change to contacting the posterior tibia and drawing the tibia anteriorly.

Patellofemoral Joint Mobilization: Superior and Inferior

Purpose: Superior glide is used to increase mobility for knee extension. Inferior glide is used to increase mobility for knee flexion.
Patient: Supine with the knee extended.

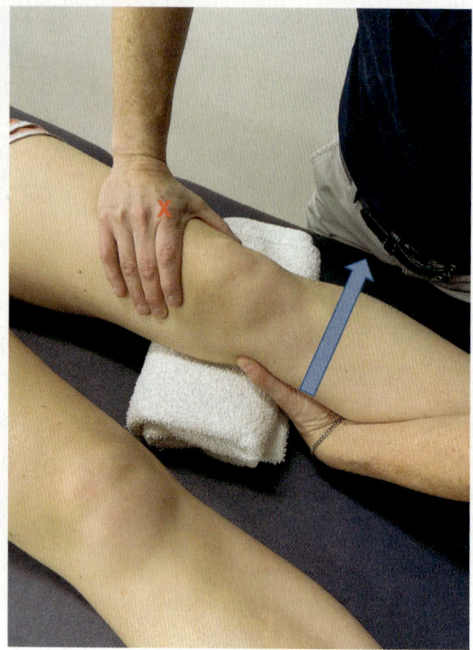

FIGURE 10-24 Assessment of tibiofemoral joint mobility: anterior glide.

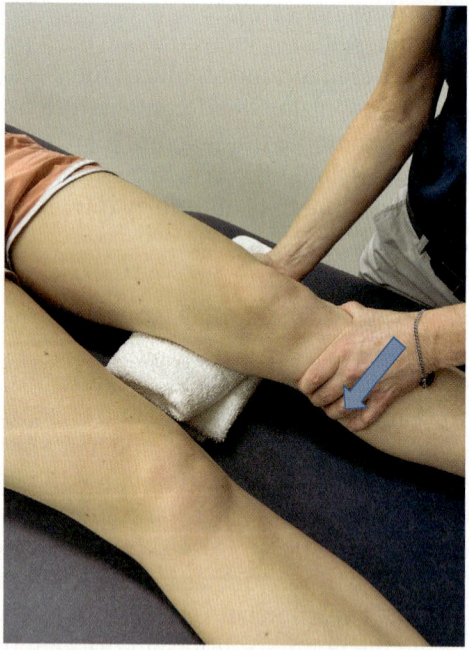

FIGURE 10-25 Assessment of tibiofemoral joint mobility: posterior glide.

hand glides the patella in an inferior direction, parallel to the femur (Fig. 10-26).

Patellofemoral Joint Mobilization: Medial and Lateral

Purpose: To decrease pain and increase patellofemoral joint mobility.

Patient: Supine with the knee extended.

Clinician: Contacts the lateral patellar border with the thumb pads with the index fingers contacting the medial patella. The remaining fingers rest over the anterior aspect of the patient's leg. Alternately, the heel of the hand can be used.

Mobilization: A medial glide of the patella is produced with both thumbs. A lateral glide is produced by using the pads of the index fingers (Fig. 10-27).

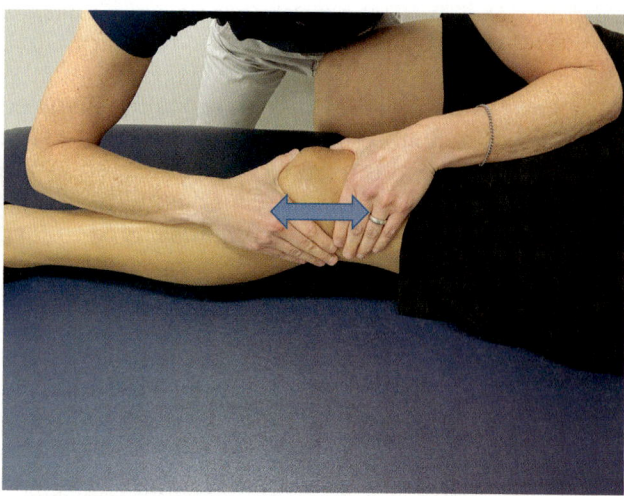

FIGURE 10-26 Assessment of patellofemoral joint superior/inferior mobility.

Clinician: The web space or heel of the caudal hand contacts the inferior pole of the patella. The web space of the cranial hand contacts the superior pole of the patella.

Mobilization: The caudal hand glides the patella in a superior direction, parallel to the femur. The cranial

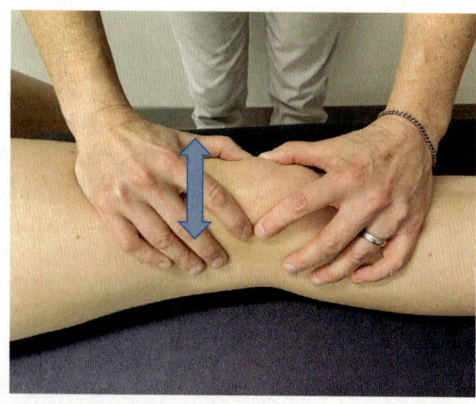

FIGURE 10-27 Assessment of patellofemoral joint medial/lateral mobility.

Special Tests/Provocative Testing

Clinicians should choose which special/provocative tests to perform based on the patient history and physical examination to this point in order to help rule in and rule out competing differential diagnoses. For knee pathology, these tests may be grossly grouped into five main categories (Fig. 10-28): tests to identify effusion, meniscal pathology, ligament pathology, patellofemoral pathology, and ITB pathology. Recall, special tests are best chosen based on patient history and clinical presentation.

Special Tests for Effusion

Either the modified stroke test and the ballottement test should be performed to assess for the presence of effusion.[110,123] Effusion may be documented as being present of absent. To objectify the assessment, the clinician can compare circumferential measurements of the involved and uninvolved legs at the knee joint line and 8 cm proximal to identify effusion within the joint capsule. Identification of knee effusion is important for several reasons. First, effusion can limit knee joint ROM. Second, effusion may inhibit the quadriceps muscle, which may limit function.[124–126] Third, the onset, or return of, knee join effusion during rehabilitation indicates that the tissues are not able to tolerate the current workload or exercise intensity.[127]

Modified Stroke Test (aka the Bulge Sign or the Sweep Test)

Purpose: To identify knee joint effusion.
Method: With the patient lying supine, the clinician should perform several sweeps superiorly and laterally from the inferomedial knee joint line toward the suprapatellar pouch in an attempt try to milk any effusion present into the suprapatellar pouch. The examiner then strokes downward and medially from the superolateral knee toward the medial knee joint line (Fig. 10-29).
Interpretation: A positive test is if a bulge of fluid is seen in the medial knee, a wave of fluid is seen returning medially with the downward strokes, or if there is so much fluid, it is not possible to milk the fluid superiorly in the initial portion of the test.
Grading: Rather than grading the test as positive or negative, the modified stroke test has also been graded reliably using a 5-point scale as follows[128]:
- 0: No fluid wave
- Trace: Small fluid wave seen on downstroke
- 1+: Large medial fluid bulge noted on downstroke
- 2+: Fluid returns spontaneously without downstroke
- 3+: Fluid cannot be removed from the medial knee with upstroke

Ballottement Test (aka the Patella Tap Test)

Purpose: To identify knee joint effusion.
Method: With the patient lying supine, the clinician should apply several downward strokes from about 10 cm proximal to the knee joint line to the patella to try to milk any fluid within the suprapatellar pouch inferiorly into the main compartment of the knee. On the last repetition, while maintaining contact with the patient's proximal thigh, the clinician uses the contralateral hand to provide a gentle posterior (downward) pressure on the patella (Fig. 10-30).
Interpretation: A positive test is when the clinician can feel a tap when the patellar pressure is applied because the effusion has raised the patella up away from the femur.

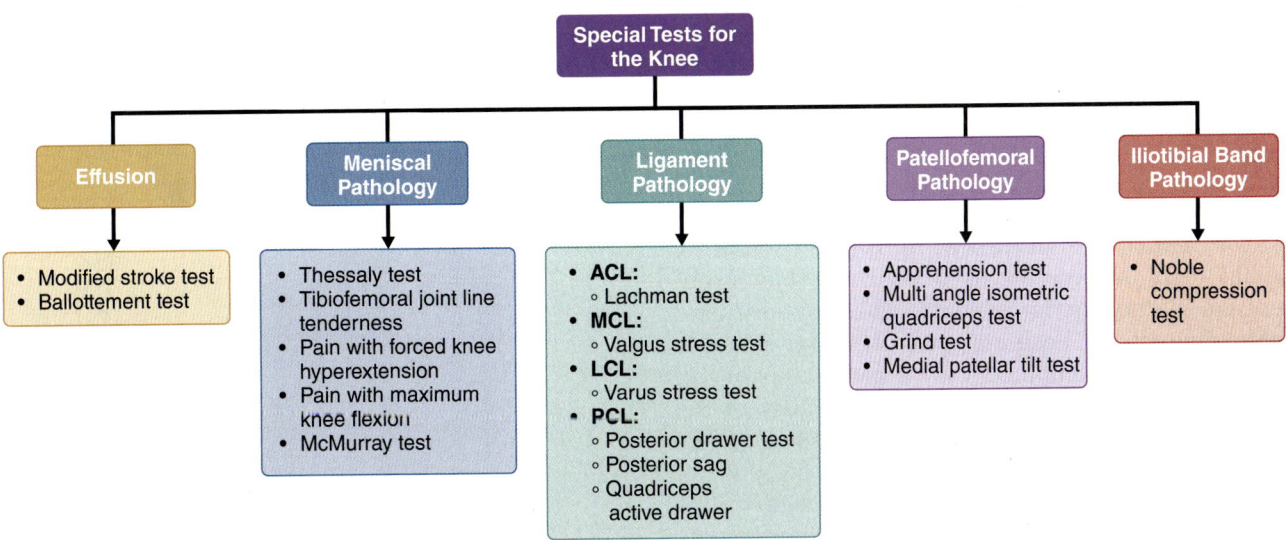

FIGURE 10-28 Knee special tests. *ACL*, anterior cruciate ligament.

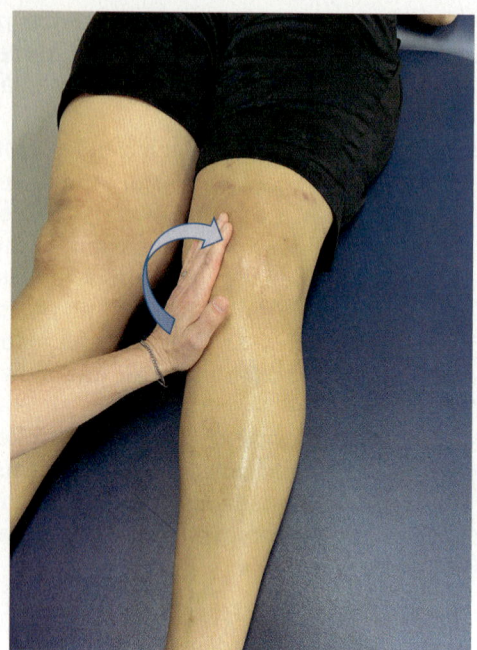

FIGURE 10-29 Modified stroke test.

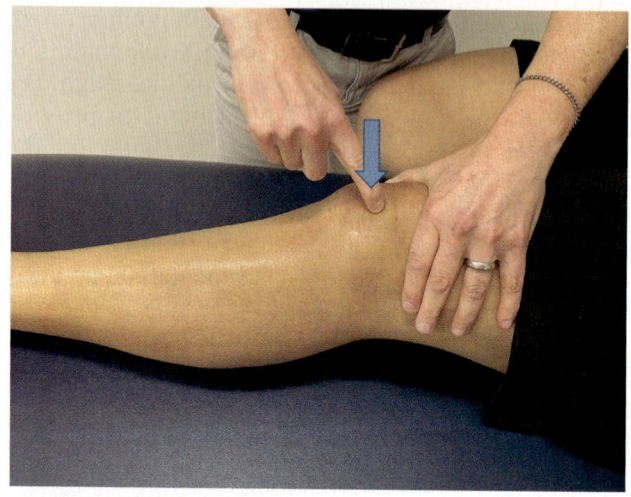

FIGURE 10-30 Ballottement test.

Special Tests for Meniscal Pathology The following special tests should be used to help rule in/out meniscal pathology in patients: Thessaly test and McMurray test.[129] These are most useful for ruling in pathology when combined with a patient history of knee catching or locking or a twisting injury of the knee.[110] A cluster of tests should be performed to rule in meniscal pathology: Thessaly test, the presence of tibiofemoral joint line tenderness, pain with forced knee hyperextension, pain with maximum knee flexion, and McMurray test.

Thessaly Test
Purpose: To identify a meniscal lesion.
Method: With the patient single limb standing on the limb to be tested with the knee unlocked in about 5° of flexion, the clinician rotates the patient's pelvis as far as possible to the left and right three times, creating a twisting motion in the knee. If no symptoms are created, the test is repeated in about 20° of knee flexion.
Interpretation: A positive test is reproduction of the patient's complaint of clicking, catching, or locking (Fig. 10-31).

McMurray Test (aka McMurray Maneuver)
Purpose: To identify a meniscal lesion.
Method: With the patient supine, maximally flex the patient's knee, maximally externally rotate the tibia, then extend the patient's knee. Repeat the test with the tibia internally rotated. Variations of this test include providing a varus or valgus stress while extending the knee, but this does not seem to improve the test's diagnostic value.[130]
Interpretation: A positive test is pain or an audible click with testing (Fig. 10-32).

Special Tests for Ligament Pathology Several special tests exist to identify knee ligament pathology. Clinicians should use the Lachman test to identify ACL pathology.[127] Although many alternative tests exist (such as the pivot shift test), the Lachman test is the most accurate when assessing acute and chronic ACL tears in a conscious patient.[131-133] The historic

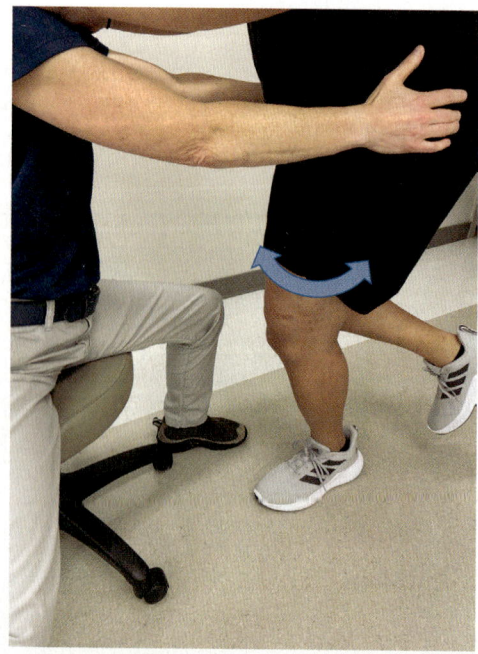

FIGURE 10-31 Thessaly test.

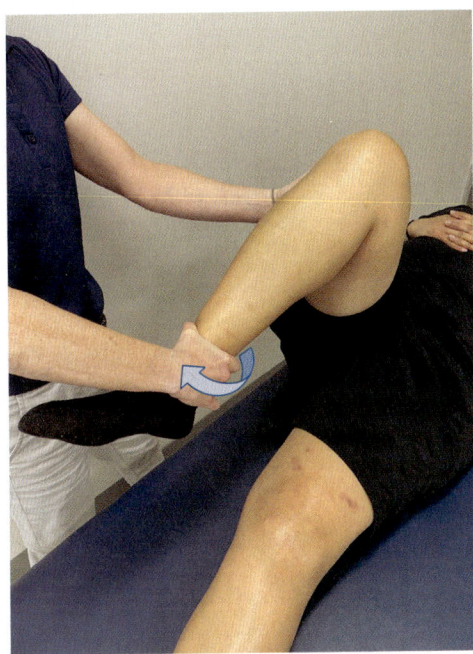

FIGURE 10-32 McMurray test.

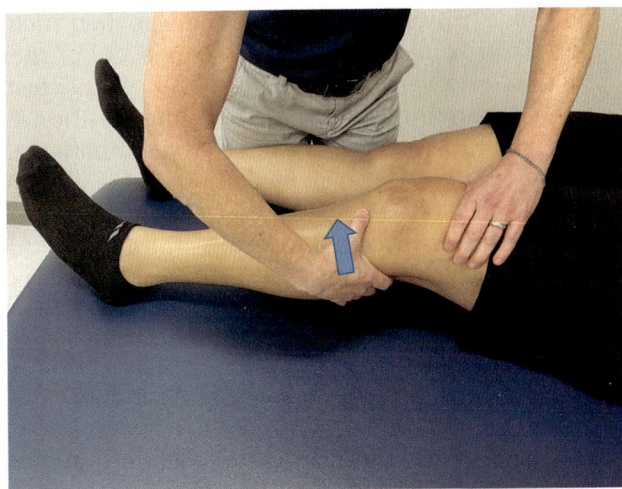

FIGURE 10-33 Lachman test.

use of the anterior drawer test and its variations for identifying ACL injuries should be discontinued.[131,134] To identify PCL pathology, clinicians may choose to use one or more of the following special tests: the posterior drawer, the posterior sag, or the quadriceps active drawer test.[127] To identify MCL or LCL pathology, the valgus or varus stress tests.[127] Acutely, MCL and LCL lesions will also have local tenderness to palpation.

Lachman Test
Purpose: To identify an ACL lesion.
Method: With the patient supine, flex the knee 30°, stabilize the distal femur with the superior hand, and use the inferior hand to glide the tibia anteriorly. This test can also be performed reliably as an instrumented assessment using a device such as the KT-2000 arthrometer.[135]
Interpretation: A positive test is if the clinician appreciates an increase in anterior tibial glide and/or a soft endfeel.
Grading: Rather than grading the test as positive or negative, the Lachman test has also been graded using a 1 to 3 scale[132] (Fig. 10-33) as follows:
- Grade 1: 1 to 5 mm anterior translation compared to the uninjured knee
- Grade 2: 6 to 10 mm anterior translation compared to the uninjured knee
- Grade 3: greater than 10 mm anterior translation compared to the uninjured knee

Posterior Sag Test (aka Godfrey Test)
Purpose: To identify a PCL lesion.
Method: Position the patient supine, then prop the heels on a support surface such as a chair to create 90° of hip and knee flexion. Using a lateral view, the clinician then observes the relative positions of the tibial tuberosities.
Interpretation: A positive test is if the tibial tuberosity of the involved side appears at least 2 mm inferior (sagged posteriorly) because of a lack of PCL restraint (Fig. 10-34).

Posterior Drawer Test
Purpose: To identify a PCL lesion.
Method: With the patient hook-lying supine with the knee flexed 90°, the clinician stabilizes the patient's

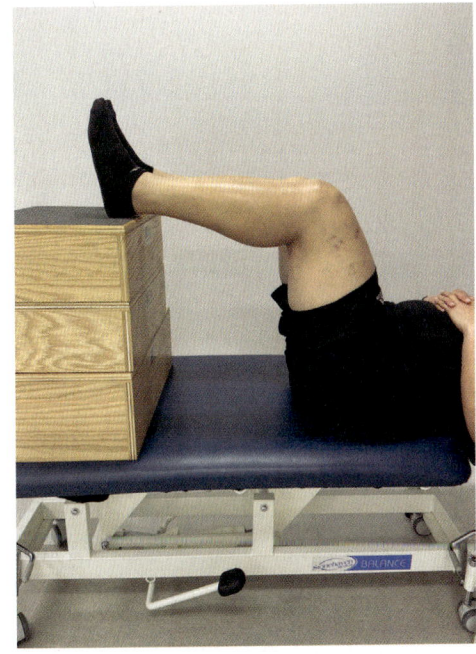

FIGURE 10-34 Posterior sag test.

foot, usually by sitting on it. The clinician then encircles the proximal tibia with both hands and pushes the tibia backward. To prevent a false-negative test, the clinician should first observe the position of the tibial tuberosity of the affected and unaffected knees, as a PCL tear may result in the tibia already being sagged posteriorly.

Interpretation: A positive test is if the tibia glides posteriorly or if there is a soft endfeel (Fig. 10-35).

Quadriceps Active Drawer Test

Purpose: To identify a PCL lesion.
Method: Position the patient hooklying supine in 90° of knee flexion. Stabilize the patient's distal tibia. Ask the patient to attempt to straighten the knee. The clinician then observes the position of the tibial tuberosity.
Interpretation: A positive test is if the clinician observes the tibial tuberosity moving anteriorly when the patient attempts to straighten the knee. This is because the superior tibia sagged posteriorly due to of the lack of PCL restraint (Fig. 10-36).

Valgus Stress Tests

Purpose: To identify an MCL lesion.
Method: With the patient supine, the clinician places the superior hand at the patient's lateral knee joint line to create a medial force. The clinician's inferior hand or arm cradles the patient's lower leg to create a lateral force. The clinician then creates a valgus stress on the knee first with the knee in full extension, then with the knee in about 20° of flexion.

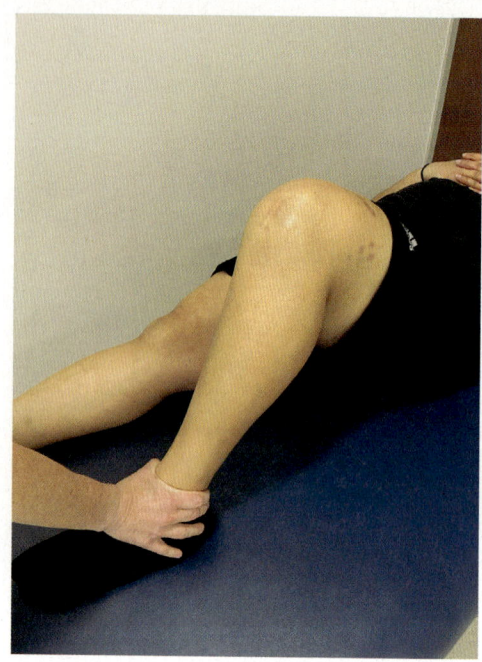

FIGURE 10-36 Quadriceps active drawer test.

Interpretation: A positive test is if there is an increase in motion (gapping of the medial joint line) and/or a soft endfeel. If laxity is noted with the knee in extension, the MCL, medial capsule, and at least one cruciate ligament are likely involved.[132] If there is gapping only in the flexed position, the MCL is likely to be involved. Pain in the region of the MCL without laxity represents a mild MCL sprain.

Grading: Although several grading scales exist for the valgus stress test, this amount of detail is less useful and less reliable than simply noting hypermobility and endfeel.[132,136,137] In addition, the amount of perceived gapping with testing has not been shown to correlate with stress radiographs[138] (Fig. 10-37).

Varus Stress Test

Purpose: To identify an LCL lesion.
Method: With the patient supine, the clinician places the superior hand at the patient's medial knee joint line to create a lateral force. The clinician's inferior hand or arm cradles the patient's lower leg to create a medial force. The clinician then creates a varus stress on the knee first with the knee in full extension, then with the knee in about 20° of flexion.
Interpretation: A positive test is if there is an increase in motion (gapping of the lateral joint line) and/or a soft endfeel. If laxity is noted with the knee in extension, the LCL, posterolateral corner and at least

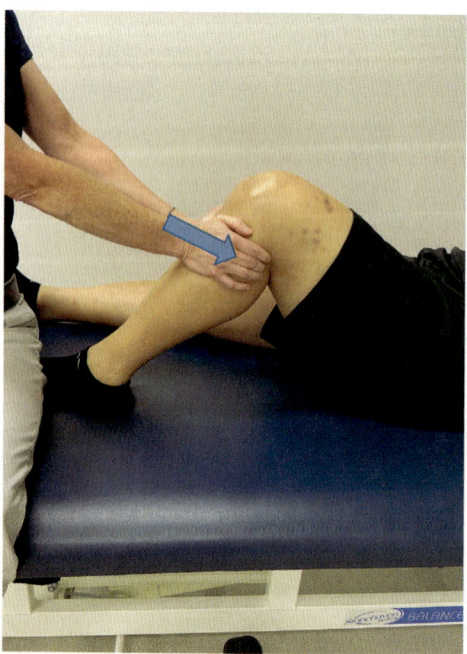

FIGURE 10-35 Posterior drawer test.

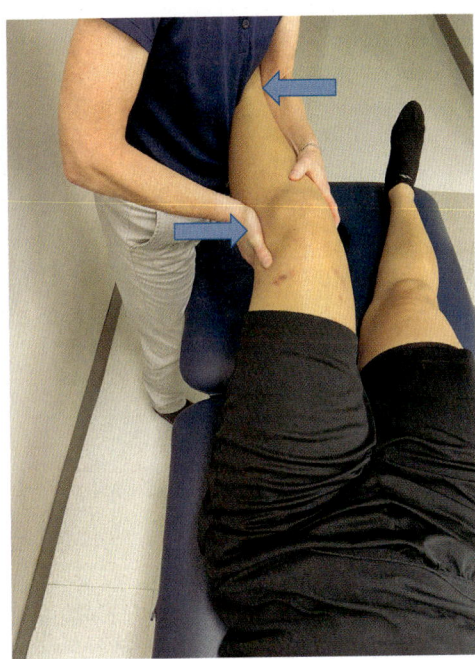

FIGURE 10-37 Valgus stress test.

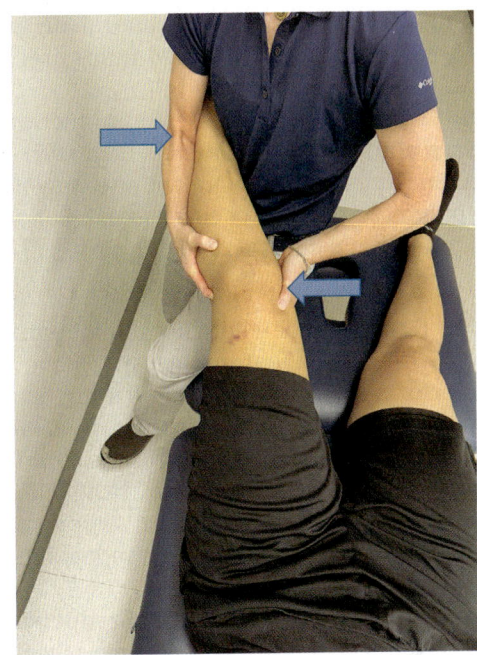

FIGURE 10-38 Varus stress test.

one cruciate are likely involved. If there is gapping only in the flexed position, the LCL is likely to be involved. Pain in the region of the LCL without laxity represents a mild LCL sprain.

Grading: Although several grading scales exist, this amount of detail is less useful and less reliable than simply noting hypermobility and endfeel[136] (Fig. 10-38).

Special Tests for Patellofemoral Pathology The following special tests should be performed to identify patellofemoral pathology: apprehension test, multiangle isometric quadriceps test, grind test, and patellar tilt tests.[139–143] While a positive grind and patellar tilt test can help rule in PFPS,[129] this condition is primarily diagnosed via patient history and exclusion of other diagnostic hypotheses.[144]

Apprehension Test

Purpose: To identify lateral patellar instability after a lateral patellar dislocation.

Method: With the patient supine and the quadriceps relaxed, the clinician performs a lateral patellar glide. Note some authors have recommended performing this test in 20 to 30° of knee flexion. In this flexed position, a lack of bony stability from a low medial femoral epicondyle or a flat patella will allow increased lateral glide. The position also more closely simulates the position of most patellar dislocations.

Interpretation: A positive test is if the patient verbalizes apprehension or involuntarily contracts the quadriceps in an attempt to stabilize the patella (Fig. 10-39).

Multiangle Isometric Quadriceps Test

Purpose: To identify patellofemoral joint pathology.

Method: With the patient seated, the clinician manually resists knee extension at various angles (90°, 75°, 60°, etc.). The change in knee flexion angle changes the contact surfaces between the patella and the femur. With the knee in 90° of flexion, there is a large amount of surface area to dissipate joint reaction forces, whereas there is much less surface area in around 15° of knee flexion. In addition,

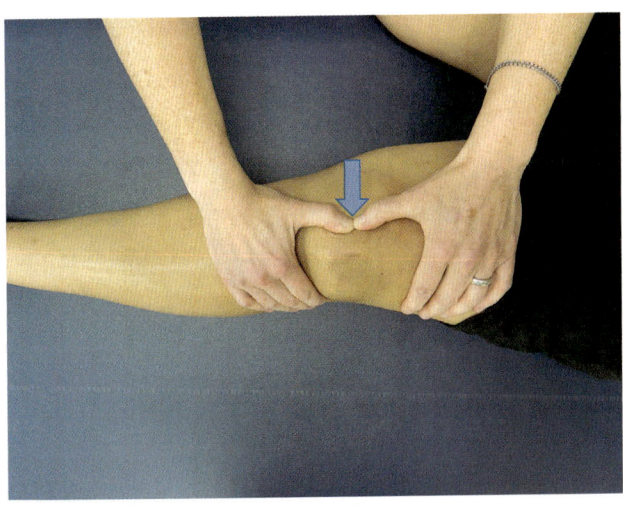

FIGURE 10-39 Apprehension test.

there may be a local osteochondral or articular cartilage defect that is stressed more precisely at a certain angle.

Interpretation: A positive test is reproduction of the patient's anterior or subpatellar pain with testing. The clinician should document the angle(s) that were painful as this represents the patellar and femoral joint surface contact area.

Grind Test (aka Clarke Sign)

Purpose: To identify patellofemoral joint pathology.
Method: With the patient supine, first have the patient perform a quadriceps set and note the amount of pain while performing if present. Next, with the patient relaxed, the clinician performs a partial inferior glide to the patella inferiorly, being careful not to reach end range of the glide or compress the patella posteriorly. The patient then repeats the quadriceps set.
Interpretation: A positive test is reproduction of the patient's anterior or subpatellar pain when testing with the inferior patellar glide. Any crepitus with testing should be noted. Note that this test is often painful in asymptomatic patients, making comparison between sides critical (Fig. 10-40).

Medial Patellar Tilt Test

Purpose: To identify tightness in the lateral retinaculum, which may increase the risk for patellofemoral joint pathology.
Method: With the patient supine and the knee 20° flexed, the clinician attempts to tilt the patella medially by elevating the lateral border of the patella. Normally, the patella should be able to be tilted above the horizontal.
Interpretation: A positive test is the inability to tilt the patella to at least horizontal (Fig. 10-41).

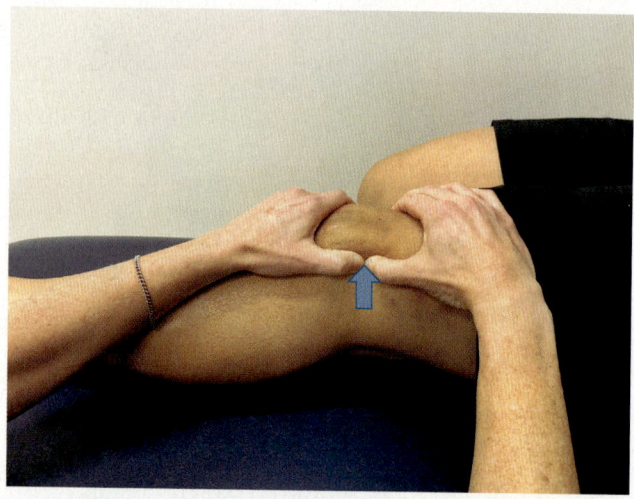

FIGURE 10-41 Medial patellar tilt test.

Special Test for Iliotibial Band Pathology The Noble Compression Test[145] is an assessment for ITB syndrome.

Noble Compression Test

Purpose: To identify ITB syndrome.
Method: With patient supine and knee 90° flexed, the clinician applies pressure on the lateral femoral epicondyle, compressing the distal ITB. The clinician then extends the knee while maintaining compression.
Interpretation: A positive test is reproduction of the patient's lateral knee pain around 30° of knee flexion (Fig. 10-42).

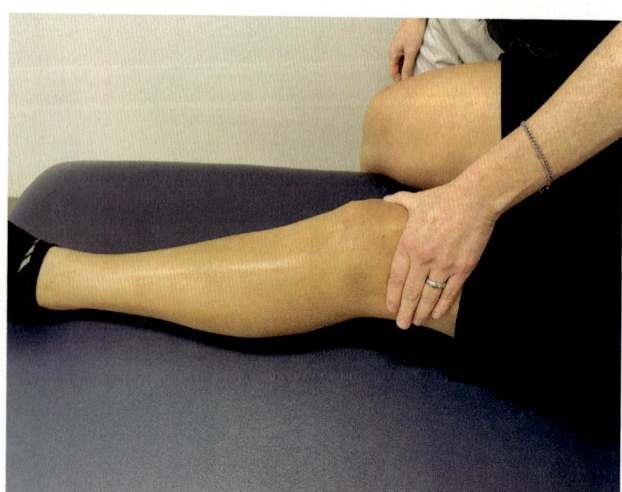

FIGURE 10-40 Grind test.

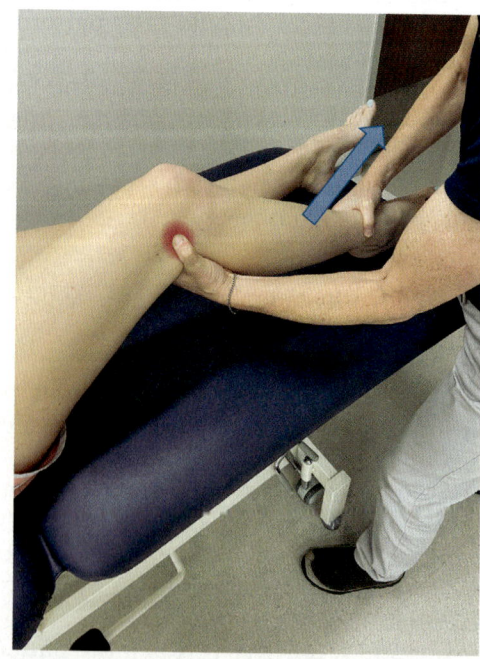

FIGURE 10-42 Noble compression test.

Palpation

The region should be palpated for tenderness, temperature, and swelling. The mobility of any scars should be assessed. Clinicians should palpate structures for tenderness, as noted in the "Palpation" section. Bony tenderness with a history of trauma may indicate fracture.[146] After an acute sprain or strain, tenderness of the involved structure can be expected. In cases of significant superficial sprains or strains, there may be a loss of fiber continuity that can be felt or identified as a palpable breach of gap in the involved tissue. Palpation should also be used to assess local tissue temperature and swelling.

Gait

The patient's gait should be assessed with and without footwear, noting any deviations or symptoms. Common gait abnormalities and their causes are discussed in Chapter 5, Gait and Footwear. Commonly, patients with knee effusion are unable to achieve full knee extension and, therefore, walk on a flexed knee throughout stance phase. In contrast, patient with quadriceps weakness may ambulate with the knee held somewhat rigid in extension during stance phase in an attempt to allow the bony structures to compensate for the lack of dynamic stability. Having the patient attempt alternate gait patterns may provide insights into patient pathology. For example, to increase patellofemoral joint compressive forces in an attempt to provoke symptoms, patients may be asked to lunge walk or walk in a semi-squat position. Footwear should be assessed for appropriateness and wear patterns. If appropriate, running mechanics can be evaluated. The use of video analysis and a treadmill can be particularly helpful in recognizing more subtle deviations.

Functional Testing

Myriad functional tests can be performed for patients with knee pathology. Single leg balance should be assessed. Progressions to testing with eyes closed or on a soft surface may be appropriate. Additional key tests include the squat, single leg squat, forward step-down test, and the four hop tests described in Chapter 9, Lower Leg, Ankle, and Foot.[147] To assess patient's squatting abilities, the patient is asked to stand with their feet hip distance apart and squat, noting any change in symptoms and at what point in the movement they occur. The clinician should note any deviations present, such as a valgus collapse (Fig. 10-43) or increase in pronation. If present, the clinician should ask if the patient can correct these deviations and if any changes in symptoms ensued. The use of specific descriptors of proper form and a dichotomous rating system (e.g., good/poor, normal/deviation) helps improve inter-rater reliability and the ability to detect change over time.[147] A progression to the squat is a single leg squat. Quadriceps weakness can be identified by a lack of symmetry in single leg squat depth.[148]

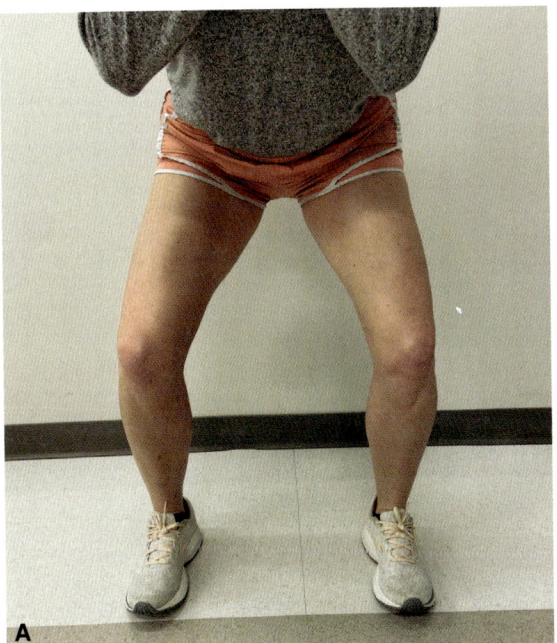
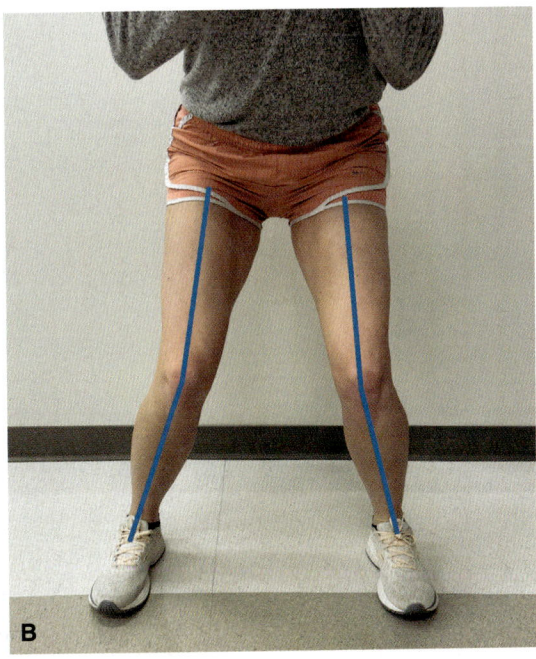

FIGURE 10-43 Squat. **A.** Squat with good form with knees over the second toe. **B.** Squat with right greater than left knee valgus.

For the forward step-down test (Fig. 10-44A), the patient stands on the limb to be assessed on top of an 8-inch step. The patient then slowly lowers down until the contralateral heel lightly taps the floor and then returns to the start position. As with the squat, the clinician should note changes in symptoms and if deviations, such as a contralateral pelvic drop, are present (Fig. 10-44B), and how far the patient can descend before deviation or symptoms. The clinician should note if the patient can correct any deviations with cueing along with any changes in symptoms. The clinician should document form, depth (if not 8-inch), symptoms, and when they occur. This test requires a modicum of balance to perform. To take away the balance component in a patient with known balance deficits, the patient can perform with fingertip support, with this testing method documented.

Quadriceps endurance strength and patellofemoral joint compressive forces can be challenged by having the patient try to maintain a wall sit. Advanced plyometric testing, including the four hop tests (Fig. 10-45), may be indicated for higher level patients.

COMMON KNEE PATHOLOGIES

This section contains details on the most common or most problematic musculoskeletal knee pathologies, including meniscal and chondral injuries; ligamentous pathology; patellar disorders such as patellar tendinopathy, patellar instability, and PFPS; OA and total joint arthroplasty; ITB syndrome; apophysitis; plica syndrome; quadriceps contusion; and bursitis.

Meniscal Injuries

Pathology Meniscal injuries account for 25% of all knee injuries. For younger individuals, isolated meniscal damage commonly arises from a twisting or rotational-type injury. These injuries are typically noncontact and result from cutting or landing from a jump. Soccer and wrestling are considered the highest risk sports for sustaining a meniscal injury.[149] For wrestling, the damage appears to be due to rotational forces on a hyperflexed knee. The meniscus may also be injured in combination with other structures. For example, the medial or lateral meniscus is torn in about half of all ACL ruptures.[150] For patients with chronic (unrepaired) ACL ruptures, these numbers are even higher because without the stability of the ACL, the knee undergoes higher levels of shear forces, which are attenuated by the meniscus.[151] Older individuals are likely to have a degenerative meniscal tear. As examples, a 40-year-old is four times as likely to have a meniscal tear as a 20-year-old, and about 60% of 60-year-olds have a meniscal tear. It is important to note that degenerative meniscal tears may be asymptomatic. Patients who are obese or in kneeling occupations are also more likely to have meniscal pathology due to the increased loading of the knee joint.[110,149,152,153] Medial meniscal tears are more common than lateral meniscal tears,[149] in part due to its reduced mobility: as the knee moves into full flexion, the medial meniscus moves about half as much as the lateral meniscus.[152] Meniscal tears can be categorized by zone, pattern, and location (Table 10-8).

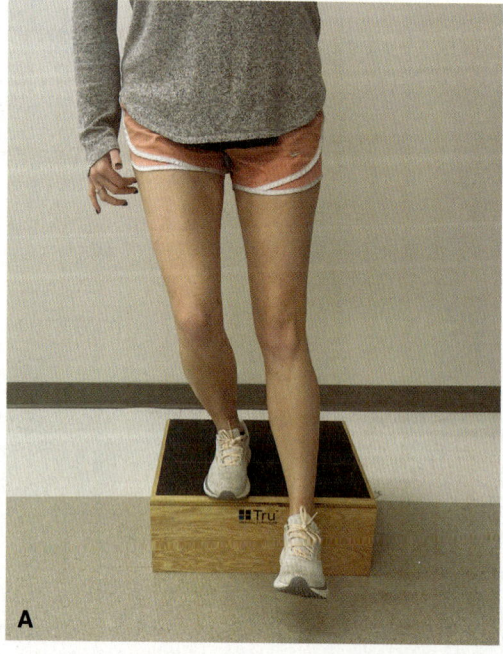 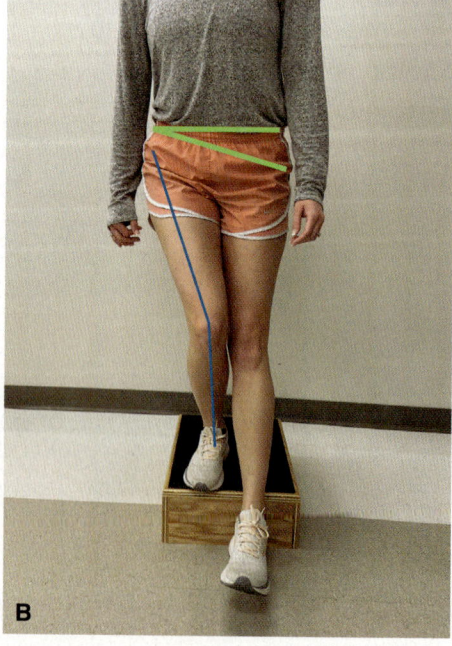

FIGURE 10-44 Forward step-down test. **A.** Proper form with knee in line with second toe, pelvis level, and trunk upright. **B.** Poor form with valgus collapse and contralateral pelvic drop.

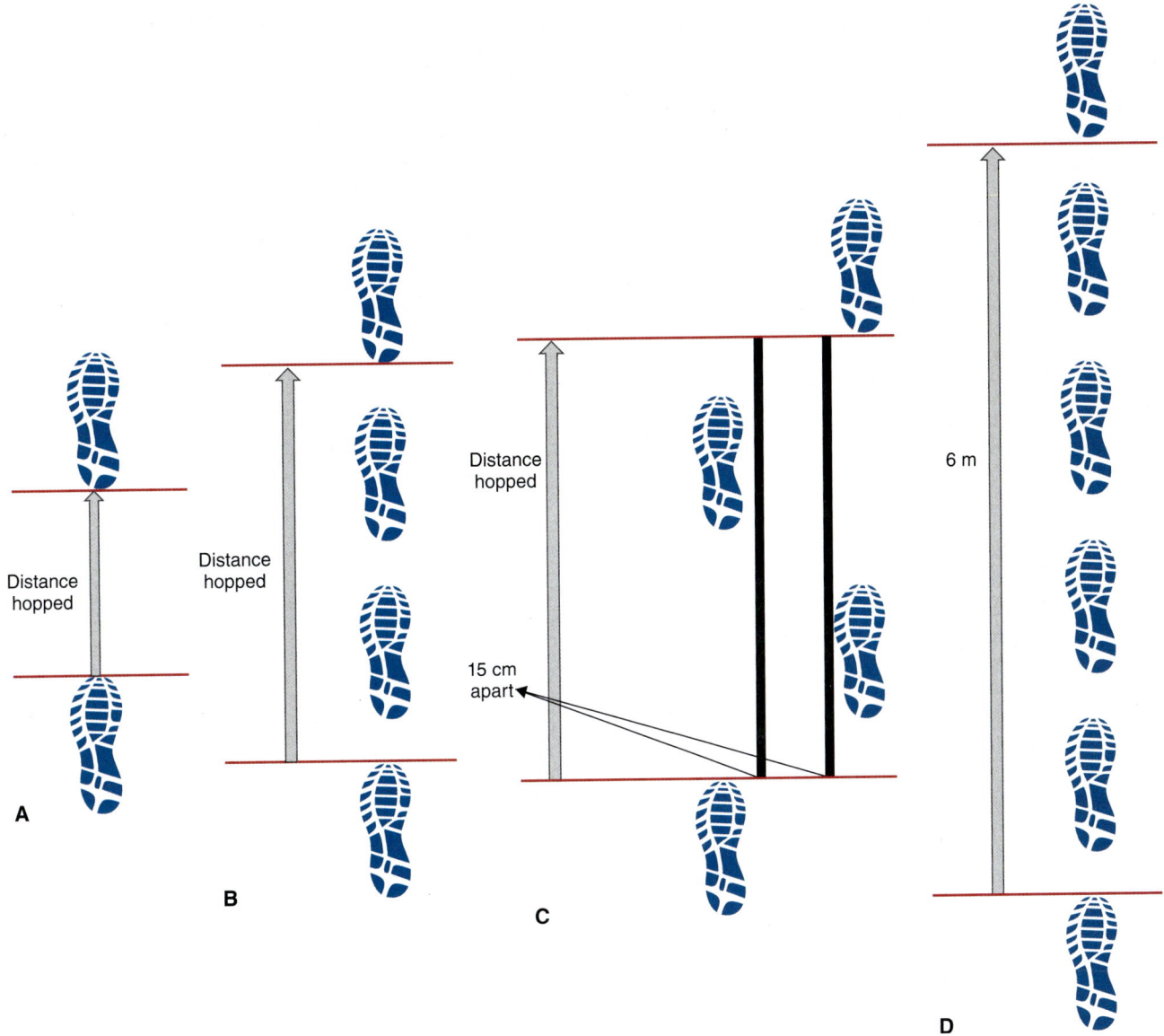

FIGURE 10-45 Hop testing. **A.** Single hop for distance. **B.** Triple hop for distance. **C.** Crossover hop for distance. **D.** 6-m timed hop.

History Patients with acute meniscus injuries report a history of a twisting or hyperflexion injury and may have felt a tearing sensation at the time of injury. They will report knee effusion beginning 6 to 24 hours after injury. Some will report the inability to fully bend or straighten their knee. This is likely due to the meniscus tear blocking the motion. Patients with chronic meniscal tears are likely to report mild intermittent knee swelling. Patients will knee catching, locking, or popping.

Key Examination Findings Meniscal injuries are best identified using a cluster of positive findings:

- History as noted above
- Mild, delayed knee effusion
- Pain with passive end range flexion
- Pain with passive end range extension
- Knee joint line tenderness
- Positive Thessaly test
- Positive McMurray test

The more positive findings, the more likely the patient has a meniscal tear.[110,129,154] Because meniscal tears commonly occur in combination with ligament rupture, the clinician should also perform ligamentous stress testing in individuals with acute meniscal lesions.

An arthroscopic examination is the gold standard for diagnosing meniscal lesions. For isolated meniscal lesions, the history and physical examination has been shown to be as accurate as a magnetic resonance imaging (MRI) in identifying symptomatic meniscal tears.[155]

TABLE 10.8 TYPES OF MENISCAL TEARS

Tear Type	Examples	Implication
Zone	Red-red Red-white White-white	Red zone tears occur in the highly vascular outer portions of the meniscus, as such they have the potential to heal. White zone tears are thought to be nonhealing because there is no direct blood supply. Red-white zone tears occur in the transition area.
Pattern	Radial Horizontal Vertical Flap or bucket handle Complex	Acute tears more likely to be radial or vertical and may be more amenable to repair Chronic tears more likely horizontal or complex Bucket-handle tears frequently limit knee motion. Complex tears associated with osteoarthritis
Location	Horn Body Root Ramp	Location can affect symptoms as well as potential for repair.

Because nearly one-third of athletes[156] and over half of patients over 50 years of age[157] have been shown to have asymptomatic meniscal tears, clinicians should not rely solely on imaging results for determining an appropriate treatment plan.

Differential Diagnoses Differential diagnosis should include OA, chondral lesions, and ligament injuries.

Rehabilitation Focus and Key Points The role of surgical treatment for the management of isolated meniscal tears is controversial.[154,158,159] Current research is also unable to identify a subgroup of patients with meniscal tears who are more likely to benefit from surgery.[160,161] Therefore, conservative intervention should be the first line of treatment for all patients with meniscal tears.[162] Early rehabilitation should focus initially on reducing effusion, regaining knee range, and improving quadriceps activation. Neuromuscular electrical stimulation (NMES) can help improve quadriceps function.[110] An assistive device should be used if the patient is unable to ambulate without a gait deviation or pain.[159] Low-intensity cycling can assist with joint nutrition, effusion, and cardiovascular fitness. Isolated hamstring resistive exercises should be avoided for the first 4 to 6 weeks, given its relationship to the meniscus. Rehabilitation should include progressive strengthening of the hip, core, and plantarflexors as well as balance/proprioceptive exercises.[163] Weight-bearing stresses should be progressed as tolerated[163] with careful monitoring for production of, or increase in, effusion. Once gait is possible without deviation or pain, aerobic exercise can be progressed to an elliptical device. Aquatic therapy or an unloaded treadmill may be beneficial. Athletes should participate in a supervised, progressive return to sport-specific activity.[110]

Expected Outcomes Patients can be expected to return to prior level of function in 3 to 6 weeks.[164] Patients with continued symptoms, including a loss of motion, should be referred for possible surgical intervention.

Rehabilitation after Meniscal Surgery Surgical interventions for meniscal tears that continue to be symptomatic despite conservative rehabilitation include partial meniscectomies, meniscal repair, and meniscal transplants. Partial meniscectomies should preserve as much meniscus as possible to try to limit increased joint contact stress.[165] Rehabilitation after partial meniscectomy should follow the same steps as conservative interventions. However, after surgery, patients will require more substantial efforts to reduce knee effusion caused by surgery and to regain knee ROM. Knee extension range should be prioritized. The patient should have at least 90° of flexion within the first week, followed by a gradual increase to full flexion within a month. In addition, quadriceps strength deficits typically profound, likely requiring an assistive device for up to 2 weeks due to quadriceps inhibition. In fact, these deficits have been shown to continue up to 1 year after surgery.[154] Therefore, clinicians should strongly consider quadriceps neuromuscular stimulation. Anecdotally, after knee surgery, patients appear to have a substantial decrease in plantarflexor and hip strength. For example, it is not uncommon for patients to be unable to perform a unilateral heel raise after knee surgery even if weight bearing is not painful. It is possible that this is due to inhibition of the plantarflexors. Open kinetic chain hamstring strengthening should continue to be avoided for the first 4 to 6 weeks after surgery. As with conservative care, clinicians should provide a graded progression to sport-specific training while monitoring for signs of excessive joint stress, such as production or worsening of knee effusion. Most patients can be expected to ambulate without deviation or assistive device in 1 to 2 weeks, and athletes can return to sports in 5 to 7 weeks.[166] Patients with medial meniscectomies appear to return to function faster than those with lateral meniscectomies.[165] After a partial medial or lateral meniscectomy, patients are at increased risk of developing knee OA.[153,159]

Meniscal repairs were developed in an attempt to preserve meniscal function and reduce the chances of developing knee OA. The failure rate of isolated meniscal repairs is as high as 40%.[167] This low success rate may be partially due to lack of knowledge of which type and location of meniscal tear is most likely to be repairable, variability in repair methods (all inside, inside-out, outside-in), and a steep learning curve in perfecting surgical technique.[167,168] Further complicating factors include the distinct lack of prospective studies describing the rehabilitation process after meniscal repair. Most literature supports that weight bearing in knee extension provides a compressive force on vertical and bucket-handle tears, and therefore, gait with an assistive device and a knee brace locked in extension should be allowed immediately postoperatively for repairs of these tears for the first 6 weeks.[153] After this point, the brace can be discontinued once the patient demonstrates satisfactory knee control for gait. In addition, most rehabilitation guidelines support knee ranging from 0 to 90° for the first 3 to 6 weeks[153,165–167] to assist with effusion, joint nutrition, and prevent contracture while not overstressing the repair. After this, a gradual progression of knee flexion range is allowed. Isolated hamstring strengthening is generally not begun until 6 to 12 weeks postrepair.[165] In addition to the high failure rate, a return to sporting activities is not expected until roughly 4.5 to 10 months after surgery.[166,169]

Articular Cartilage Injuries

Most articular cartilage injuries can occur as a result of either acute trauma or repetitive minor trauma.[110] These injuries usually occur in combination with meniscus or ACL injuries. Patients with articular cartilage injuries typically report intermittent knee pain and swelling and that the knee catches or locks.[110] The examination may reveal joint line tenderness.[110] Conservative interventions are similar to that for meniscal injuries but more drawn out with progression to full weight bearing over 6 to 8 weeks.[110] There are a variety of surgical interventions for chondral lesions. Microfracture was historically the norm for small lesions. However, this procedure relies on the formation of scar tissue rather than a more anatomic repair that can be achieved with biologic interventions such as osteochondral autograft transplantation (OAT) or matrix-induced autologous chondrocyte implantation (MACI). There is limited research to guide rehabilitation after these procedures.

Anterior Cruciate Ligament Injuries

Pathology There are over a quarter of a million ACL injuries in the United States annually.[170] For professional athletes, around 90% are able to return to sport in around 9 to 14 months albeit with decreased performance, decreased playing time, and a shortened career.[171] Unfortunately, for lower level athletes, the numbers are much worse, with as little as half returning to competitive sports at their preinjury level.[172,173]

The vast majority of ACL injures are noncontact. The key mechanisms of injury are as follows[110,174]:
- Dynamic knee valgus
- Poor landing form
- Deceleration
- Knee hyperextension

Dynamic valgus (sometimes referred to as *valgus collapse*) includes combinations of hip adduction, hip internal rotation, tibial abduction, tibial rotation, and foot pronation.[175] When occurring unilaterally, this may also include ipsilateral trunk flexion and contralateral pelvic drop.[176] Poor landing form might include dynamic valgus but may also involve asymmetrical landing, placing greater stresses on one extremity. Deceleration, as occurs with a sudden stop or change of direction, requires significant quadriceps force, which can result in increased anterior shear if not counterbalanced by hamstring co-contraction. Knee hyperextension directly increases ACL strain.

ACL injuries rarely occur in isolation (Fig. 10-46).[150,177–179] The ACL is highly loaded with combined forces that occur with dynamic valgus, especially in combination with tibial rotation. Because the ACL has a lower

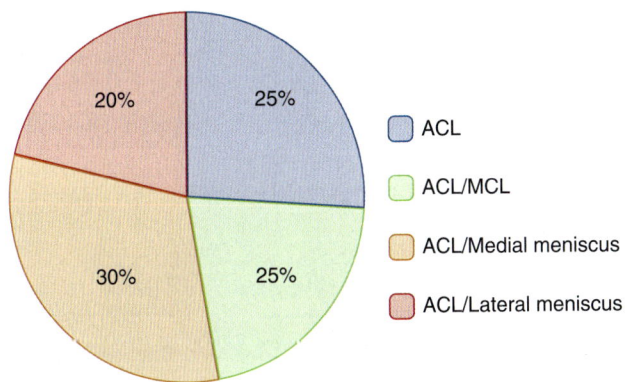

FIGURE 10-46 Structures involved in anterior cruciate ligament ruptures. *ACL*, anterior cruciate ligament; *MCL*, medial collateral ligament.

load to failure, the ACL is typically torn first. If the force is large enough, the MCL is also torn, and this occurs in roughly a quarter of all cases. One or both menisci are torn roughly half of the time.

Risk factors for ACL injuries include[110,174,180,181]:

- Prior ACL injury
- Participating in a pivoting or cutting sport
- Female gender
- Core or lower extremity strength deficits
- Poor single limb balance
- Fatigue

History

Patients with ACL ruptures report an acute onset of pain, usually after a cutting motion or landing from a jump. They may report feeling or hearing a snap or pop. Most individuals will be unable to walk without assistance or a significant limp. Although rare, some athletes may be able to continue to finish their athletic event. Patients usually report the knee swelled significantly within hours of the injury. A hemarthrosis occurs within hours of the injury.

Post–Anterior Cruciate Ligament Rupture Evaluation and Differential Diagnosis

The clinician should perform a Lachman test to rule in an ACL rupture. Instrumented testing, such as the KT-2000, can objectively quantify knee laxity both preoperatively and postoperatively.[182,183] However, this is rarely required. Because ACL injuries infrequently occur in isolation, the clinician should also assess the menisci, MCL, and LCL. If seen more than a few hours after injury, patients are likely to have a hemarthrosis (bleeding within the knee joint) along with a positive stroke test or ballottement test. After rupture, patients have decreased weight-bearing tolerance, quadriceps inhibition, and difficulty fully straightening the knee. MRI can assist with identifying tissue injury.

Conservative Management versus Prehabilitation

There was a push for several years to try conservative management for patients with ACL ruptures to see if they could "cope" with the resulting loss of stability. However, these individuals have gluteus biased movement patterns (Fig. 10-47)[184,185] and worse ratings of knee function, and well over half of these individuals will go on to surgery.[186,187] In addition, delaying ACL reconstruction more than 6 months results in a significant increased risk of new or worsening meniscal tears.[151] Therefore, with the exception of less active or older individuals, ACL reconstruction is the path most often chosen by individuals with ACL ruptures.[187]

Rehabilitation after ACL rupture is similar for both a nonoperative (rehabilitation) and an operative (prehabilitation) plan. Prehabilitation is the phrase used for rehabilitation between ACL rupture and

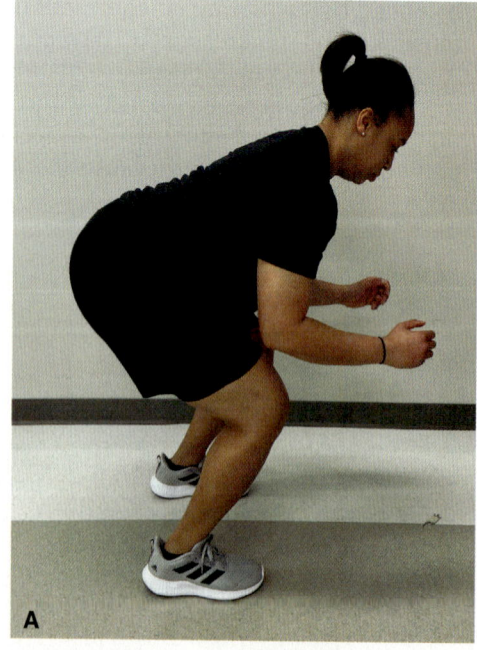 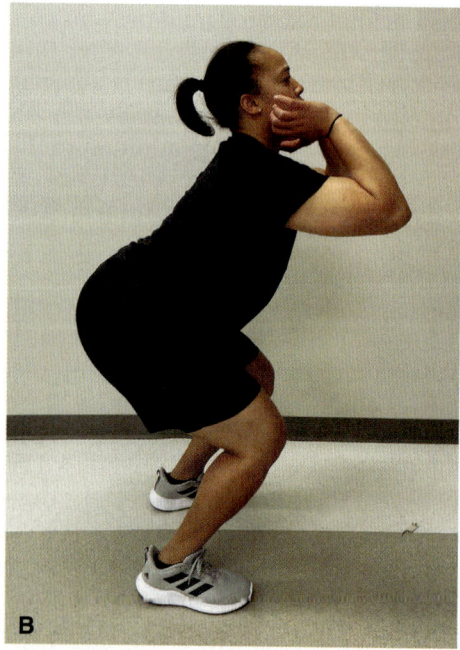

FIGURE 10-47 Gluteal- and quadriceps-dominant movement patterns. **A.** A gluteal-dominant (also known as quadriceps avoidance) squat is characterized by increased hip flexion moving the center of mass closer to the knee joint axis reducing the need for quadriceps activation. **B.** A quadriceps-dominant squat is characterized by a more upright trunk requiring greater quadriceps strength.

reconstruction. There are six main goals of rehabilitation after ACL rupture[188]:
- Resolve knee effusion.
- Regain knee ROM.
- Activate the quadriceps muscle.
- Normalize gait.
- Slow decline of unaffected tissues.
- Educate the patient.

Table 10-9 includes a basic outline of prehabilitation. Prehabilitation has several advantages. It allows surgery to be performed on a quiet, uninflamed knee and allows the patient to prepare mentally and physically for the rehabilitation process. Those individuals who participated in a prehabilitation program were more likely to return to sport.[189] By the end of this phase, the patient should have little or no knee effusion, full knee extension, and as much flexion as is possible. The patient should be able to perform a straight leg raise without a lag (Fig. 10-48), ambulate normally without an assistive device, and understand the postoperative plan of care. This process generally takes 3 to 4 weeks.

Anterior Cruciate Ligament Reconstruction Surgery A graft is used to reconstruct the torn ACL. An autograft comes from the patient's own tissues, generally the ipsilateral quadriceps or hamstring, whereas an allograft is cadaver tissue. Table 10-10 lists the advantage and disadvantages of each. The graft, irrespective of type, must be protected from excessive strain. The ACL, and hence the graft, is relatively unstressed with most activities, including weight

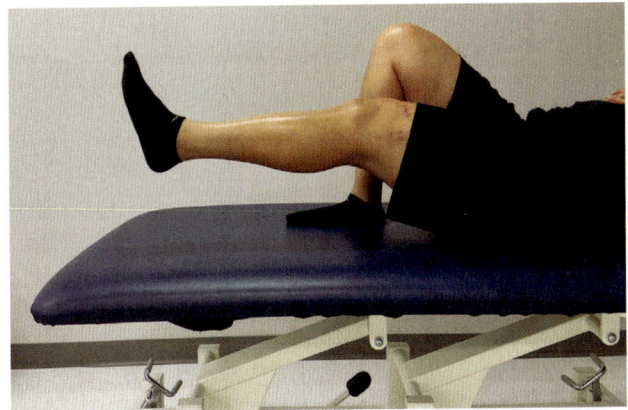

FIGURE 10-48 Straight leg raise with a lag. A lag during a straight leg raise is indicative of poor quadriceps strength.

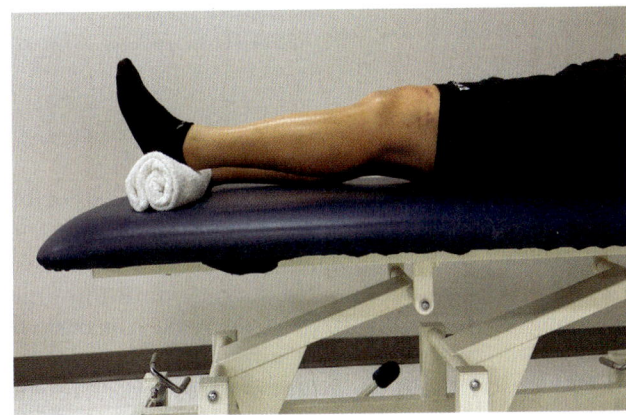

FIGURE 10-49 Heel prop.

TABLE 10-9	
PREHABILITATION AFTER ANTERIOR CRUCIATE LIGAMENT RUPTURE	
	Examples
Resolve knee effusion	• Ice • Elevation • Knee ROM exercises
Regain knee ROM	• Heel prop (Fig. 10-49) • Prone hang (Fig. 10-50) • Patellar mobilizations (superior/inferior) • Active/active assisted knee flexion range
Activate the quadriceps	• Quad sets • SLR • "Low" arc quads (active knee extension from 90 to 45°) • Squats • Leg press bilateral to unilateral
Normalize gait	• Gait with an assistive device to promote a more normal pattern • Balance exercises bilateral to unilateral
Slow decline of unaffected tissues	• Strengthening: involved limb, involved limb, and core • Cardiovascular fitness as able (Bike, elliptical, pool upper body ergometer)
Educate the patient	• Rehabilitation process and rationale

ROM, range of motion; *SLR*, straight leg raise.

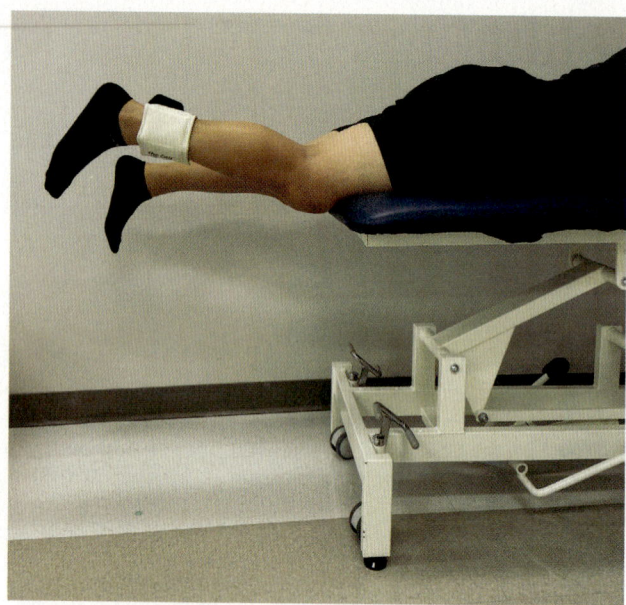

FIGURE 10-50 Prone hang.

bearing and ROM. However, resisted knee extension between 45 and 0° causes anterior tibial shear and stresses the graft. Therefore, this is contraindicated for the first few months after surgery until the graft is strong enough. However, to decrease the risk of anterior knee pain after ACL surgery, clinicians may choose to continue to avoid resisted open kinetic chain knee extension and, instead, work in the 90 to 45° arc to reduce patellofemoral joint stress.

All grafts are stronger than the native ACL.[190] Patellar tendon grafts were the first grafts used for ACL reconstruction. However, postoperatively, many patients had anterior knee pain and quadriceps weakness. Hamstring grafts and allografts were used to try to mitigate this. However, it is now clear that these symptoms were less related to the donor site than to the injury and surgery[191] as quadriceps weakness is the norm after ACL reconstruction, regardless of graft choice.[192] Additional quadriceps dysfunction frequently results from the use of a femoral nerve block for perioperative pain management.[193] The technically more difficult adductor block results in similar pain control while preserving quadriceps function.[193] Unfortunately, graft choice does not reduce the risk of future knee OA,[194] which may be as high as 50%.[172]

It is pivotal that physical therapists read the operative report to learn what graft was chosen, what additional injuries were found (e.g., meniscal tear, chondral lesions, ligament damage), and how they were managed. For example, if a meniscal debridement was performed, open chain resisted hamstring exercises should not begin before 6 weeks postsurgery. If a meniscal repair was performed, additional details are needed from the surgeon regarding the type of tear and type of repair. Given the high failure rate of meniscal repairs, physical therapists should communicate with the surgeon for individual patient precautions. Likewise, chondral lesions may be managed with various techniques including microfracture, which may require additional precautions on motion and weight bearing.[195] European surgeons are far more likely to choose the patellar tendon graft over other options and to debride, rather than repair, the meniscus.[189] In the United States, the choices are much more varied and may be based on surgeon preference.

Postoperative Rehabilitation Focus and Key Points The following section discusses ACL reconstruction rehabilitation with or without a meniscal debridement. Clinicians must observe any and all postoperative precautions based on the injuries sustained and the procedures performed (Table 10-10). While immediate postoperative and functional knee braces were once the norm, it is now known that these devices do not influence outcomes. Some patients after ACL reconstruction may lack confidence in their knee and demonstrate kinesiophobia.[196] It is possible that this subpopulation may feel more confident with the use of postoperative and/or functional bracing. Though typical in the early phase of rehabilitation, fear of movement and reinjury well into the rehabilitation process reduces chances for maximal return to function.[197] To assess kinesiophobia, clinicians should utilize tools such as the Tampa Kinesiophobia Scale (TSK) or the Knee Self-Efficacy Scale.[127]

Rehabilitation should be based on specific criteria rather than time postsurgery.[189] The key criteria for progression are decreasing or lack of effusion and demonstrating the range, strength, and neuromuscular control required for the task. In addition, the Knee Soreness Rules help guide progression (Table 10-11). The Knee Soreness Rules are not specific to ACL rehabilitation and can be used for other knee pathologies.

The focus of the first 2 weeks after surgery is the same as that for prehabilitation. Effusion should resolve within 1 to 3 months, although this may be longer with allografts. Superior and inferior patellar mobilizations can assist with pain modulation and restoring knee extension. These mobilizations are particularly important for patients with patellar tendon grafts to prevent patellar baja.[198] Patients can be taught how to self-mobilize the patella as part of a home program. Knee extension range should be prioritized because failure to gain knee extension by 3 weeks post-op may indicate scarring within the joint (a cyclops lesion) and need for surgical intervention to regain extension range.[199] There is strong evidence to support the

TABLE 10-10
ANTERIOR CRUCIATE LIGAMENT RECONSTRUCTION GRAFTS AND PRECAUTIONS

	Patellar Tendon	*Hamstring*	*Allograft*
Method	• Central third of the patellar tendon with 2 bone plugs	• Quadrupled semitendinosus and possibly gracilis tendons	• Cadaver patellar tendon, hamstring, Achilles tendon, or tibialis posterior
Advantages	• Bone plugs provide faster/greater stability • Better functional outcome[336] • Reduced risk of second ACL injury[224] • Better for females	• Evidence that donor site may regenerate	• Avoids donor site morbidity
Disadvantages	• Short term may have pain with kneeling • 1% chance of patellar fracture	• Takes longer to incorporate into tunnel than bone plug graft • Potential for knee flexion contracture without knee extension brace early on • Tends to stretch out over time • Graft failure rate higher than patellar tendon[224,337] • HS weakness possible	• Highest failure rate[188,338] • Prolonged inflammatory response • Takes longer to mature
Postoperative precautions based on graft	• No aggressive rectus femoris stretching for ~6 weeks	• No isolated open kinetic chain resisted hamstring strengthening for 6-8 weeks[189] • No aggressive hamstring stretching for 6 weeks	• Slow rehabilitation given disadvantages noted[188]
ACL precautions	• No resisted open kinetic chain knee extension 45–0°[188] for 12+ weeks*		

ACL, anterior cruciate ligament; HS, hamstring.
*To decrease the risk of anterior knee pain after ACL surgery, clinicians may choose to continue to avoid resisted open kinetic chain knee extension and, instead, work in the 90 to 45° arc to reduce patellofemoral joint stress.

TABLE 10-11
KNEE SORENESS RULES

Knee Soreness Status	Action
During warm-up that continues or redevelops during session	2 days off from knee exercises*, decrease 1 level
During warm-up that goes away	No change
Day after exercise	1 day off from knee exercises*
None	May advance if consistent with goals

*Gentle range of motion exercises can continue and may assist with resolving soreness.
Adapted from Fees M, Decker T, Snyder-Mackler L, Axe M. Upper extremity weight-training modifications for the injured athlete. A clinical perspective. *Am J Sports Med.* 1998;26(5):732-742.

use of quadriceps NMES during the first 2 months or rehabilitation to facilitate quadriceps function.[127,200] Table 10-12 provides a roadmap of typical milestones after an ACL reconstruction. Time frames, when given, should be considered approximate times the average patient might reach the criteria.

The intermediate phase of rehabilitation can shift toward maintaining knee extension and gaining the final degrees of knee flexion. Strengthening progressions for both lower extremities must include not just quadriceps but also the gluteals, hip external rotators, hamstrings, and ankle plantarflexors.[195,201–203] Exercises should include both open and closed kinetic chain activities. As with hip strengthening, core exercises including plank variations and supine or quadruped progressions should also be included to decrease the potential for high-risk positioning, such as dynamic valgus. Balance exercises should progress from static to dynamic and single to multiplanar and dual task. Cardiovascular fitness should be incorporated

TABLE 10-12
TYPICAL MILESTONES AFTER ACL RECONSTRUCTION

Time Frame*	Milestone
Week 1	0–90° SLR without lag Single limb balance on level surfaces
Week 2	Full hyperextension, 110° Full revolutions on bike at appropriate seat position
Week 2–4	Full knee range Gait without deviation without assistive device Bike for cardiovascular fitness
Week 4–6	Stairs without deviation Elliptical for cardiovascular fitness
Week 6–12	Walk 1 mile at pace without deviation or increase in effusion Begin a running progression, if consistent with patient goals, starting with straight line running

ACL, anterior cruciate ligament; SLR, straight leg raise.
*Time frames represent when the average patient might reach the criteria.

as part of the overall program with activities chosen based on patient goals and overall progression. Functional activities, including sport-specific drills, should be added based on the patient's ability. For example, a basketball player can walk through a dribbling maze once ambulating without deviation or practice passing drills once able to perform a lunge with good form.

Plyometrics can begin with reduced loading using a total gym, unloading treadmill (Fig. 10-51), or in a pool.[204] Plyometrics can be performed two to three times per week and begin bilaterally with a low number of foot contacts progressing, as able, in number of contacts and to include unilateral exercises.

Common impairment and functional tests rely on limb symmetry index (LSI), where the involved limb is required to achieve a certain percentage of the uninvolved limb. The clinician should consider the following criteria, developed from several sources,[189,195,205,206] to determine if a patient is ready to begin a return to running program:

- Pain less than 2/10
- No/trace knee effusion
- Full knee extension range
- At least 95% flexion range
- Normal gain on levels and stairs
- Walk 1 mile in 18 minutes
- Quadriceps MMT at 45° of 5/5
- 30 single leg heel raises with fingertips for balance
- 30 single leg squats to 45° with good balance
- At least 70% LSI for quadriceps at 45° using handheld dynamometry, leg extension machine, or isokinetics
- At least 70% LSI for unilateral leg press
- 1-minute bilateral jump rope
- Able to single leg jump rope
- Symmetrical jump for height and distance at 25% effort

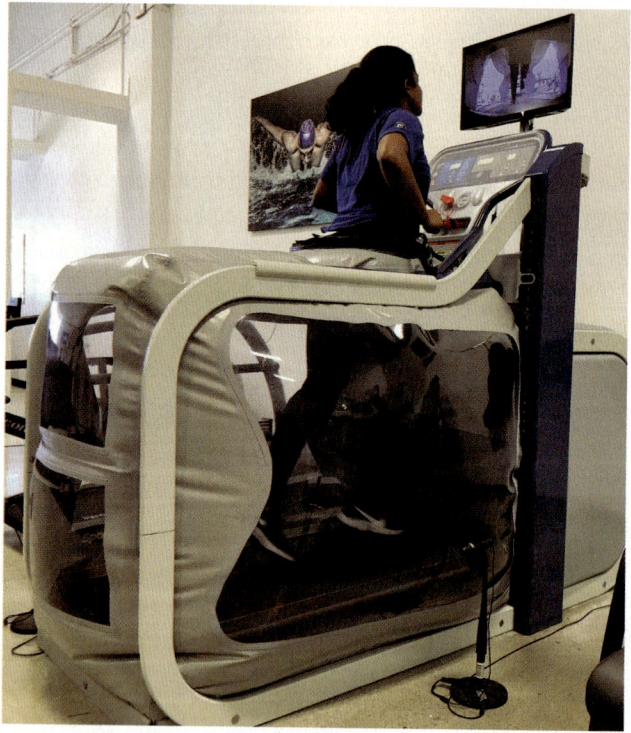

FIGURE 10-51 Unloaded treadmill.

These criteria are meant to ensure the patient has the requisite range, strength, neuromuscular control, and endurance for running. A sample running progression might begin with five repetitions of 0.1 miles jogging and 0.1 miles walking. Distance jogged is gradually progressed until the athlete is able to run 2 miles without pain, effusion, or deviation at which point traditional conditioning rules should be followed. Running should be performed initially every other or every third day to ensure adequate recovery between sessions. Running on an unloaded treadmill at less than body weight may reasonably begin sooner and may improve athlete confidence and self-efficacy.

For athletes, advanced rehabilitation and transition to return-to-play activities should be considered once a running program has begun. Resistance training and plyometrics should continue to be progressed and include both bilateral and unilateral exercises.[207] Acceleration drills should begin with short distances (e.g., 20 m) and progress in distance and intensity to replicate the athlete's sport. Deceleration and change of direction drills should begin at a slow pace and gentle angles before progressing to full speed cutting, making 90° turns and eventually all 180° turns. During cutting drills, clinicians should carefully observe for proper form, including not more than 5° of knee valgus and optimal trunk alignment.[208] Preplanned activities should be progressed to reactive drills. Activities should then provide the athlete with a progressive cognitive load—such as adding a ball or decision an athlete must make as to when and where to cut using visual or auditory cues.[209]

At this time, the optimal test battery for safe return to sport is unknown.[210,211] Four key points for return to sport progressions are patient self-reports, impairment and functional performance testing, the development of a chronic training load, and increasing sport specificity. Sample return-to-play criteria include[188,207,212–216]:

- Patient self-report questionnaire indicating psychological readiness to return to play
- 90 to 110% LSI for quadriceps at 45° using handheld dynamometry, leg extension machine, or isokinetics
- 90 to 110% LSI for unilateral leg press
- 90 to 100% LSI for single, triple, crossover, 6-m timed hop tests (Chapter 9, Ankle and Foot)
- Safe form with sport-specific tasks in a simulated environment
- Form does not degrade with sport-specific training load
- Comparison with known normative data when possible

One should be cautious about solely relying on LSI for making judgments for two reasons. First, LSI does not predict safe form. Second, the uninvolved limb of patients with ACL reconstructions has been shown to undergo significant decline during the rehabilitation process and LSI has not been found to correlate with optimal form.[217–219] Therefore, when possible, clinicians should compare patient scores with preoperative values[220] or known normative data available for hop tests,[221] isokinetic performance, and sport-specific drills, such as jump height and change of direction tests.

For team sports, athletes should advance from sprint drills, unopposed skills, one-on-one, small field/court, full team partial practice and then to full practice participation.[212,213] It should be noted that return to competition before 10 to 12 months is associated with a significant increase in risk of ipsilateral and contralateral ACL injury,[212,222] regardless of the individual's impairment and functional testing results, and, therefore, should be discussed in concert with the patient's entire medical team.

Expected Outcomes Outcomes after ACL reconstruction continue to be suboptimal with low return to sport, reduced sports performance, and significant ipsilateral or contralateral ACL ruptures.[171,173,223,224] This can be partly explained by clinicians failing to provide progressive, holistic rehabilitation programs with objective criteria for return to sport beyond time postsurgery. In addition, a large proportion of these individuals will go on to have OA within 5 to 10 years of injury.[172] Athletes who return to sport earlier than 9 months post-ACL reconstruction have seven times the rate of new injuries than those who return later.[225] The recommended activity progression at this time is for gradual incorporation of sport-specific skills and return to sport no sooner than 10 months, with the understanding the sports performance will likely be lessened for up to 2 years postsurgery (Fig. 10-52).

Anterior Cruciate Ligament Injury Prevention Because of the frequency of ACL injuries in sport and the devastating consequence they can have in terms of loss of playing time, future injury risk, and limited ability to return to competitive activity, much attention has been drawn to ACL injury prevention programs.

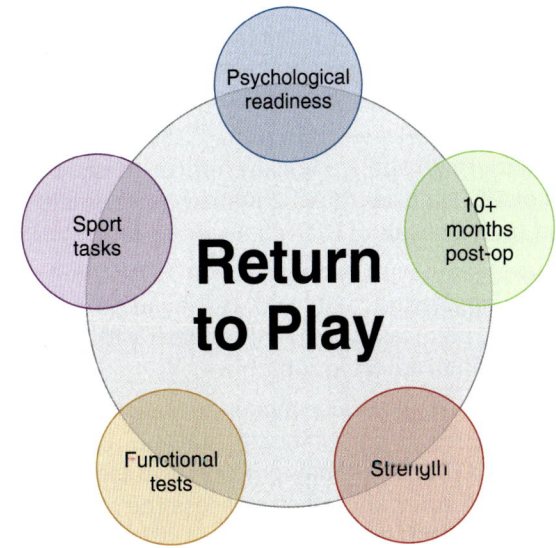

FIGURE 10-52 Anterior cruciate ligament reconstruction postoperative interventions.

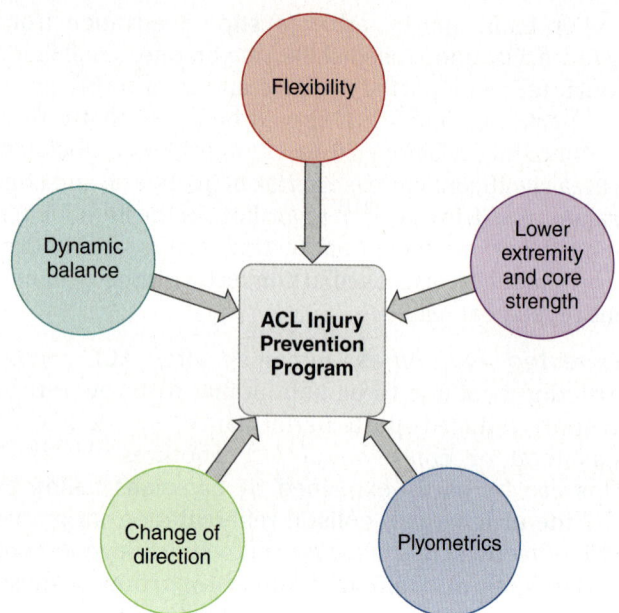

FIGURE 10-53 Anterior cruciate ligament (ACL) injury prevention program.

Figure 10-53 includes the key components of an ACL injury prevention program. However, the ideal injury prevention program is unknown and likely should contain sport-specific activities as are seen in FIFA 11+ and the PEP (Prevent injury to Enhance Performance) Program designed for American soccer (football).[226] Prevention programs, when fully implemented, do appear to reduce high-risk positioning,[227–229] reduce ACL injuries,[230–232] as well as other lower extremity injuries.[233,234]

Medial Collateral Ligament Injuries

In contrast to ACL injuries, most MCL injuries are the result of direct contact causing a valgus stress at the knee.[235] Less frequently, MCL injuries are the result of noncontact dynamic valgus, particularly when combined with excessive pronation.[236] Skiing, American soccer, football, and ice hockey appear to have higher rates of MCL injuries.[235] MCL injuries are graded 1 to 3 based on the result of the valgus stress test.[127,235]

- Grade 1: pain with testing at 20 to 30° without laxity
- Grade 2: pain and laxity with testing at 20°
- Grade 3: pain, laxity, and soft endfeel with testing at 20°, lax tibial external rotation

The MCL is generally tender to palpation. With a grade 3 injury, a palpable gap may be appreciated. Because MCL injuries may not occur in isolation, the physical therapist should also assess the status of the ACL and menisci.

Grade 1 and 2 MCL injuries are treated nonoperatively with excellent results. Most patients have no residual deficits and are able to return to sports in 1 to 4 weeks.[127] In addition, there does not appear to be any increased risk of long-term OA.[235] Rehabilitation of grade 1 to 2 injuries includes controlling effusion, immediate knee ROM, and weight bearing as tolerated. Valgus stresses should be avoided for at least 2 weeks to allow tissue healing. For example, side-lying hip adduction would be contraindicated early in the program. These forces can be gradually increased as pain resolves. While quadriceps strength deficits are not as severe with MCL injuries as with ACL injuries, quadriceps neuromuscular stimulation may still be beneficial.

Management of grade 3 injury is somewhat controversial. It appears that nonoperative and surgical management leads to similar results, albeit a much faster return to sport with conservative treatment (5–7 weeks vs. 6–9 months). For grade 3 injuries, patients should use a hinged brace to prevent valgus stress that allows knee motion from 0 to 90°. This range has been found to be safe without overstretching the repair. In fact, strict immobilization is now believed to result in weaker scar formation.[138] If MCL reconstruction is performed, the patient is generally NWB for a period of 4 to 6 weeks using the same range precautions noted earlier.

Posterior Cruciate Ligament Injuries

PCL injuries are less common than ACL or MCL injuries, possibly due to the larger size of the ligament. Nearly all PCL injuries are the result of trauma,[237] such as a motor vehicle accident in which the passenger hits the tibia on the dashboard or a fall in which the individual lands on the flexed knee with the ankle in plantarflexion driving the tibia posteriorly (Fig. 10-54). Patients with PCL injuries will commonly have positive posterior drawer, the posterior sag, and quadriceps active drawer tests.[127]

In contrast to ACL injuries, after a PCL injury, patients do not normally have an effusion.[237] Isolated PCL injuries rarely lead to functional instability.[238] This can lead to patients not seeking treatment or being undiagnosed. It is not uncommon to see a patient with a chronic, undiagnosed PCL injury. Individuals with chronic PCL deficiency may have an increased risk of future medial knee OA due to persistent knee joint laxity.[239] The standard of care of PCL injuries is conservative management. Rehabilitation should strive to limit posterior shear forces, such as open kinetic chain hamstring exercises. A knee brace may be beneficial for PCL injuries, and particularly for combined injuries.[127]

The PCL can also be injured in combination with the ACL from knee hyperextension. In these situations, the ACL is typically reconstructed, but the PCL may or may not be. The PCL and multiple other structures are

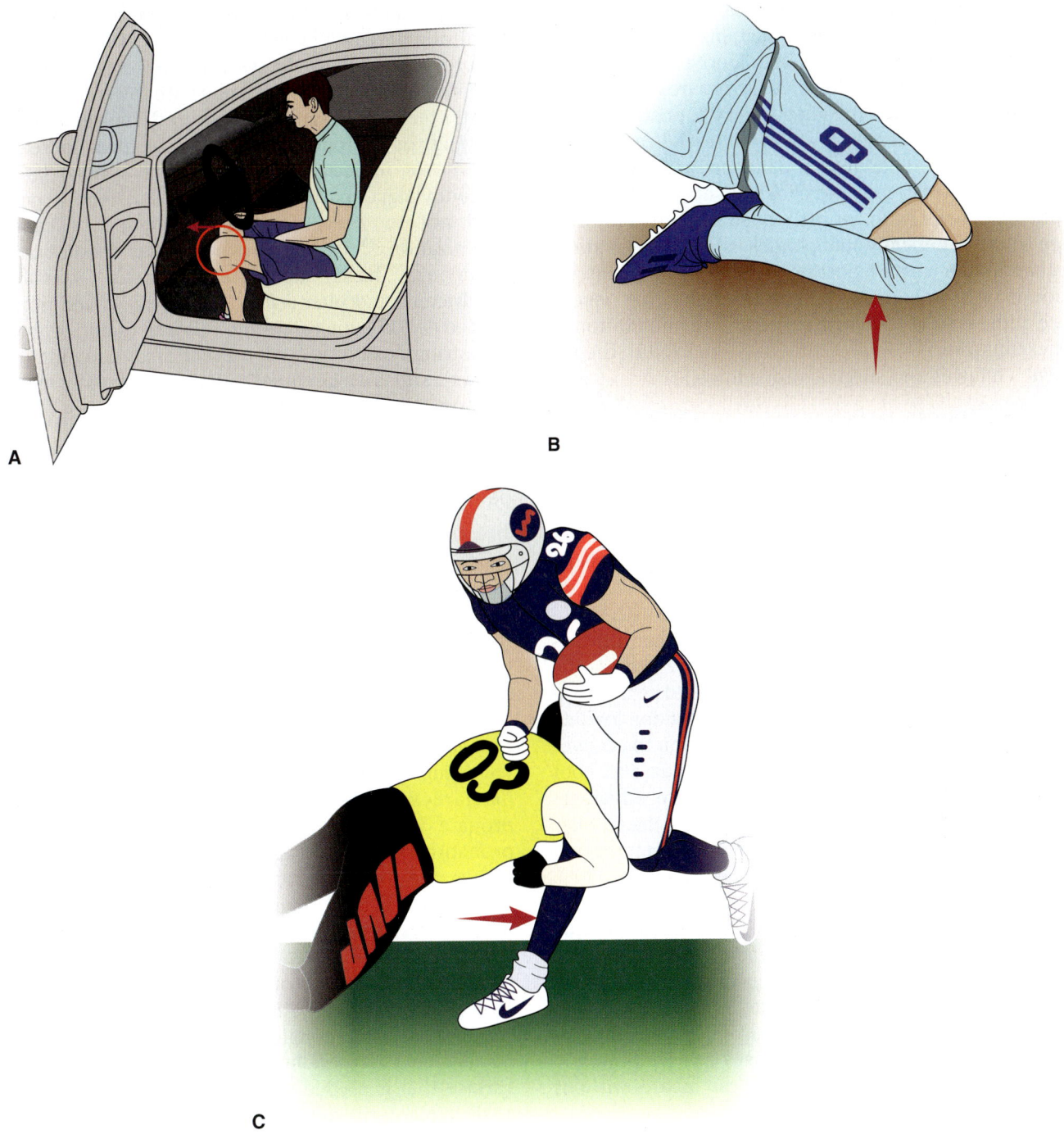

FIGURE 10-54 Common mechanisms of posterior cruciate ligament injuries. **A.** Dashboard injury. **B.** Landing on the lower leg with the ankle plantarflexed. **C.** Direct posterior blow to the lower leg.

typically injured with a knee dislocation. Management of these injuries is typically surgical with individualized rehabilitation based on the involved structures.

Lateral Collateral Ligament Injuries

LCL injuries result from a sudden varus stress. These injuries are identified by local tenderness to palpation along the LCL and varus stress testing.[240]

- Grade 1: pain with testing at 20 to 30° without laxity
- Grade 2: pain and laxity with testing at 20°
- Grade 3: pain, laxity, and soft endfeel with testing at 20°

Grade 1 LCL injuries may benefit from knee bracing to prevent varus stresses along with management of effusion, gentle progressive ROM, quadriceps strengthening, and short-term use of an assistive device.

LCL injuries are rare, particularly in isolation.[127] More commonly, the patient sustains a catastrophic knee injury, such as a collision in football or in a wrestling match, involving the many structures in the posterolateral corner of the knee: the LCL, posterolateral capsule, biceps femoris, and/or lateral head of the gastrocnemius. Therefore, if pain and laxity are noted with varus stress test, the clinician should request an MRI or consult with an orthopaedist. These injuries are treated surgically, many times using a staged surgical approach where a portion of the repair/reconstruction is performed early on and the remaining tissues are addressed at a second surgery.[241] Rehabilitation of these injuries is complex and individualized to the patient's injuries and surgical procedures.

Patellar Tendinopathy

Pathology Patellar tendinopathy is sometimes referred to as *jumper's knee* as the condition is common in basketball players, volleyball players, and other jumping and pivoting sports where the tendon must act like a spring repeatedly storing and releasing energy. Patellar tendinopathy appears to be more common in single sport athletes compared with those who participate in multiple sports.[242] Younger athletes (15–30-year-olds) and males are also more likely to be affected. Tissue injury appears to be due to an increase in the frequency or intensity of patellar tendon loading or insufficient rest time to allow the tendon to recover and remodel. Recall from Chapter 9, Ankle and Foot (Achilles tendinopathy), that tendons are adversely affected by combined loading. In the case of the patellar tendinopathy, the tendon is vulnerable to compression against the femoral condyle with knee flexion[243] (>90°). This may explain why runners are less affected than those who routinely jump and pivot in a more athletic or defensive position. Histologically, affected tendons have an increase in fibroblasts and neovascularization.[242] While MRI and ultrasound imaging can identify tissue structural changes, these abnormalities can also be found in a high percentage of knees in asymptomatic athletes. In addition, symptoms can abate without accompanying changes on imaging.[244]

History Patients with patellar tendinopathy report pain with activities that load the patellar tendon: jumping, hopping, running, and deep squatting. When severe or irritable, descending stairs will be painful owing to the increased load on the patellar tendon compared to ascending stairs. Initially, the patient may report that the pain may subside after sufficient warm-up.

Key Examination Findings Two key features of patellar tendinopathy are tenderness and pain with loading. The majority of patients have tenderness of the patellar tendon attachment at inferior pole of the patella,[245] but tenderness may also be located at the tibial attachment.[242] Tests such as quadriceps MMT or a forward step-down are likely to recreate patient symptoms. However, in patients with lower irritability, greater tendon loads may be required, such as running, jumping, or hopping. In either case, pain increases will mirror increases in tendon load. Unlike lateral epicondylalgia, patients with patellar tendinopathy tend not to have significant evidence of central sensitization.[246] Patients with patellar tendinopathy commonly have decreased gluteus maximus, quadriceps, and plantarflexor strength, in addition to limited dorsiflexion range and reduced quadriceps and hamstring flexibility.[247] Movement analysis commonly shows a stiff knee landing.[245] All of these factors lead to an increase in patellar tendon load.

Differential Diagnoses Differential diagnosis includes PFPS, fat pad irritation,[242] and bursa or plica pathology.

Rehabilitation Focus and Key Points Passive treatments to the patellar tendon, such as manual therapy, ultrasound, phonophoresis,[242] and injections, should be used sparingly.[245] Cryotherapy may be beneficial. Tendon load can be reduced by altering training if possible.[242] However, this can be difficult to do for in-season athletes. For these individuals, the pain-modulating effects of isometric patellar tendon loading[248–250] may be particularly useful. Tendon unloading can also be achieved by hip extensor and plantarflexor strengthening.[251] Patients who hyperpronate may benefit from an orthotic to control pronation[242] because this may reduce shear forces within the tendon. Lastly, training the patient to increase hip flexion during landing has been shown to result in an immediate decrease in pain[252] owing to a reduction in patellar tendon load.

Ultimately, satisfactory outcomes require progressive tendon loading. Historically, the decline squat (Fig. 10-55) was considered central to successful management for patellar tendinopathy. Standing on a surface that is sloped downward places the patient's ankle in plantarflexion. This allows the patient to move into greater amounts of knee flexion before being limited by the available motion at the ankle. Standing on a 15° declined surface allows the knee to flex to 60° while maintaining an upright trunk, thus increasing the patellar tendon force by 40%.[253] This allows high tendon tensile forces without the compressive forces found at higher knee flexion angles. Although this exercise can be beneficial, in isolation, it is insufficient to restore the spring-like qualities the tendon requires for jumping sport. Table 10-13 provides a sample patellar tendon loading strategy progression[245] that might lead to improved success and a more rapid return to sport.

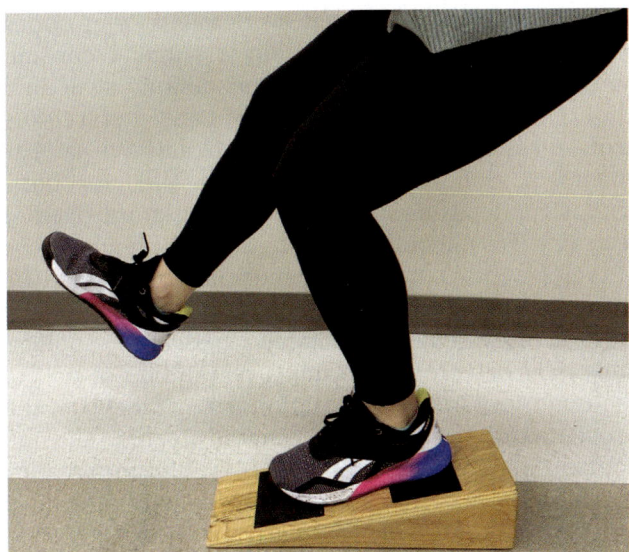

FIGURE 10-55 Single leg decline squat.

Expected Outcomes Maximal recovery time for patients with patellar tendinopathy is highly variable and may depend on whether the athlete is in or out of season. Progressive loading programs can be expected to take 8[251] to 12 weeks for maximal benefit.

Patellar Fracture

Patellar fractures constitute about 1% of all fractures and are commonly the result of a direct blow, such as a fall in which the patient lands on the patella[254] or a motor vehicle accident. Nonoperative treatment is reserved for closed, nondisplaced fractures. These patients are immobilized in knee extension and allowed to weight bear as tolerated in a locked brace. Effusion can be significant and should be treated with ice and compression. Quadriceps setting and straight leg raising can be performed immediately as soreness allows.[255] Gentle knee ROM is started once fracture callus is evident. Quadriceps strength deficits are to be expected. Resisted quadriceps exercises should not be started for at least 6 weeks. To decrease the risk of falls, balance training should be emphasized once range restrictions are discontinued. Patellar mobilizations may be beneficial in gaining range; however, patients are unlikely to regain much more than 100° of knee flexion ROM.[256] Patients have an increased risk of patellofemoral joint arthritis long term.

Operative management may entail various fixation devices, including wires, tension bands, and/or plates, based on the fracture pattern, the degree of displacement, and surgeon preference. Rehabilitation generally follows the same progression as conservative interventions noted earlier with the addition of scar mobilization as needed. The vast majority of elderly patients return to their prior level of function with open reduction internal fixation (ORIF) and rehabilitation.[257] However, frequently, the hardware must be removed 6 to 12 months postfracture due to superficial irritation.

Patellar Instability

Pathology Patellar instability can be the result of dislocation or structural anomalies. Acute lateral patellar dislocation can result from a direct blow to the patella or from a noncontact cut or rapid twist of

TABLE 10-13
PATELLAR TENDON LOAD PROGRESSION

Stage	Characteristics
Isometrics	Pain-modulating exercise Possible exercises: wall sit, leg press, decline squat, or leg extension machine in 60–30° of knee extension 45-60 second holds for 5 repetitions, 1–3 times per day Consider progressing to next phase when can tolerate isotonic exercise
Heavy slow resistance	Leg press (performed from 0 to 60° of knee extension) or leg extension (performed from 60 to 30° of knee extension) Progress load of weight-bearing exercise from 3 to 4 sets of 15 repetitions to 4 sets of 6–8 repetitions at 6 seconds per repetition (increase from 65 to 85% intensity) Consider progressing to next phase when strength approximates other side, minimal pain with exercise/activities that lasts <24 hours
Energy storage	Progress to plyometrics (jumping to hopping and split jumps) as well as deceleration drills Perform every third day, continue isometric exercise on off days Consider progressing to the next phase once tolerating 2 weeks of plyometric activities
Sport-specific training	Increase tendon loads toward sport-specific volume, intensities, and angles
Reduce intensity or return to the last successful phase if pain is increased > 24 hours after exercise.	

the leg.[258] The patella may remain dislocated requiring emergent medical intervention or may relocate spontaneously. First-time dislocators are most often adolescents participating in sports or recreation.

Lateral patellar dislocation stretches or ruptures the medial patellar retinaculum and the MPFL. The MPFL is a fanlike structure attaching to the medial femoral epicondyle to the medial border of the patella that provides the main restraining force to lateral patellar translation in the first 30° of knee flexion.[113] Rupture or attenuation of the MPFL results in lateralization of the patella and delayed capture within the trochlear groove. While it is theorized that this may lead to an increased risk of recurrent lateral patellar dislocation,[258] this has not been consistently found within the literature.[112] It is possible that these patients may feel "unstable" and have a sense that the patella is sliding, shifting, or catching, particularly in the early part of knee flexion. Individuals with trochlear dysplasia and patella alta[112] are also at risk for patellar dislocation, recurrent dislocations, and patellar instability because the patella is less constrained during the initial 30° of knee flexion.

Key Examination Findings Patients with patellar instability may have mild, intermittent knee effusion.[113] They will have excessive lateral patellar glide with the patella gliding more than three-fourths of its width laterally. The patient may have a positive apprehension test as this test simulates the position of dislocation. The patient may have a positive grind test due to chondral trauma from instability or dislocation. If acute, the MPFL may be tender to palpation.

Differential Diagnoses Differential diagnoses include PFPS and fracture.

Rehabilitation Focus and Key Points Conservative treatment is the recommended first line of treatment for both first-time dislocation and patellar instability. During the acute phase, treatment should focus on effusion control and quadriceps activation. An assistive device may be needed short term to normalize gait. A brace with a patellar cutout and lateral buttress may be beneficial early on and provide the patient with a sense of security. Isometric and resisted quadriceps exercises are generally better tolerated between 90 and 45° of flexion to maximize patellofemoral contact. As inflammation subsides and quadriceps function improves, rehabilitation can focus on maximizing motor control with squats, lunges, and sport-related activities.

Expected Outcomes It is estimated that about one-third of first-time dislocators will have a recurrence,[112] mostly those who are younger with open physes. Patients who have repeated dislocations or episodes of instability may benefit from a surgical consult, particularly if they have concomitant structural abnormalities. Multiple bony and soft-tissue procedures can be performed to try to improve patellar alignment. Soft-tissue repair of the MPFL or bony reconstruction can assist with restoring lateral patellar restraint. Trochleoplasties (surgery to accentuate the lateral trochlea) may be beneficial for individuals with trochlear dysplasia. The tibial tuberosity can be elevated and rotated medially (modified Fulkerson osteotomy) to improve the line of pull of the quadriceps.[259] Rehabilitation is dependent on the procedure(s) performed but generally include effusion control, a period of protected ROM, superoinferior patella mobilizations, and progressive strengthening. Most patients are able to return to regular activities including sports within 4 to 6 months.[113]

Patellofemoral Pain Syndrome

Pathology PFPS (also known as *anterior knee pain*) is a complex condition, ultimately due to increased stress on the patellofemoral joint. Willy et al.[139] developed a classification system (Fig. 10-56) for PFPS. Quite often, patients fit into more than one category. For example, a patient may have a loss of ankle dorsiflexion range and gastrocnemius length, forcing the patient into excessive pronation. This excessive tibial rotation results in increase patellofemoral compressive forces.[260] Likewise, the patient may also have gluteal weakness or poor neuromuscular control, leading to dynamic valgus and increased patellofemoral compressive forces.[260] This classification system provides the clinician with a partial checklist of interview questions to ask and examination procedures to investigate.

History PFPS is largely a diagnosis of exclusion for patients with anterior knee, retropatellar, or peripatellar pain.[144] However, there are a few key inclusion criteria for PFPS[139,144,261,262]:
- Insidious onset of anterior knee pain
- Participation in activities that repetitively load the patellofemoral joint, such as running, cycling, and jumping
- Pain during or after activity that loads the patellofemoral joint
- Pain with prolonged sitting (commonly referred to as a *positive "movie-goer's sign"*)
- Pain with ascending and/or descending stairs
- Pain with squatting
- Pain with palpation of the patellar facets

The greater number of factors present in the patient's history, the more likely the diagnosis of PFPS is correct.[261] Patients may report a sense of "giving way" during activities that load the patellofemoral joint.

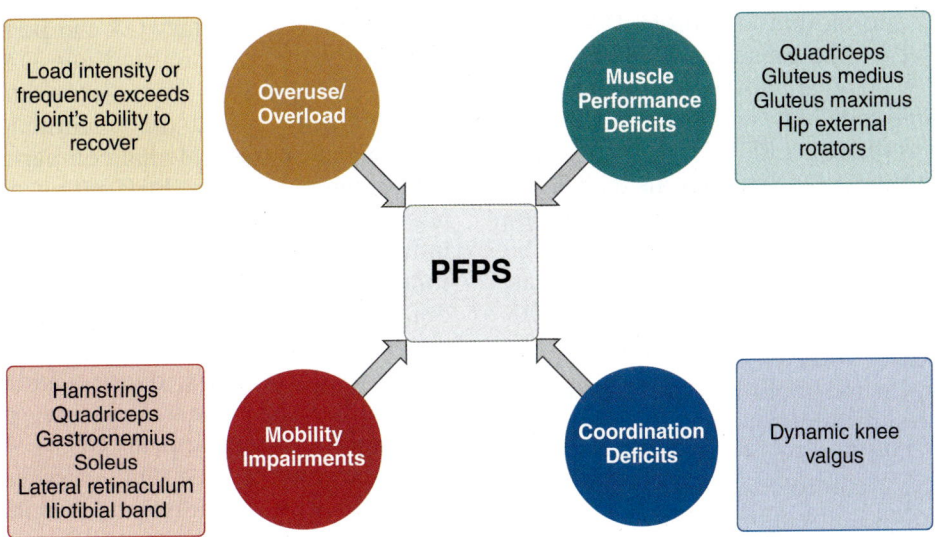

FIGURE 10-56 Patellofemoral pain syndrome (PFPS).

The physical therapist should ask about any recent changes in activity. Athletes should be asked about changes in training and footwear. Patients with PFPS are typically younger, less than 40 years of age, and female.[263] Most patients with PFPS continue to function at high levels and participate at high physical activity levels despite reporting long-standing knee pain.[264]

Key Examination Findings The multifactorial nature of PFPS indicates care should be taken to examine the entire kinetic chain, including dorsiflexion range; lower extremity flexibility; and strength of the quadriceps, hips, trunk, and antipronation musculature such as the tibialis posterior and foot intrinsics. A positive navicular drop test indicates excessive pronation and possibly the patient's inability to control the amount of pronation present. The clinician should observe the patient's motor control with functional tasks such as squatting, single leg squat, jumping, and running as appropriate. Patients with PFPS have been found to have impaired balance and proprioception.[265] The clinician should palpate the posterior aspect of the patella (Fig. 10-57) for tenderness. Special tests for the patellofemoral joint including multiangle isometric quadriceps test, the grind test, and patellar tilt tests are likely to be positive in patients with PFPS. Effusion is unusual and, if present, will be mild. Patients with chronic PFPS may have allodynia and hyperalgesia as well as psychological factors such as catastrophizing.[262]

Adolescents with PFPS are more likely to have anatomic abnormalities, such as trochlear or patellar dysplasia. However, there does not appear to be a correlation between morphology and pain.[266] Historically, a patient's static Q-angle measurement was thought to be related to PFPS, but this is now known to be incorrect.[267]

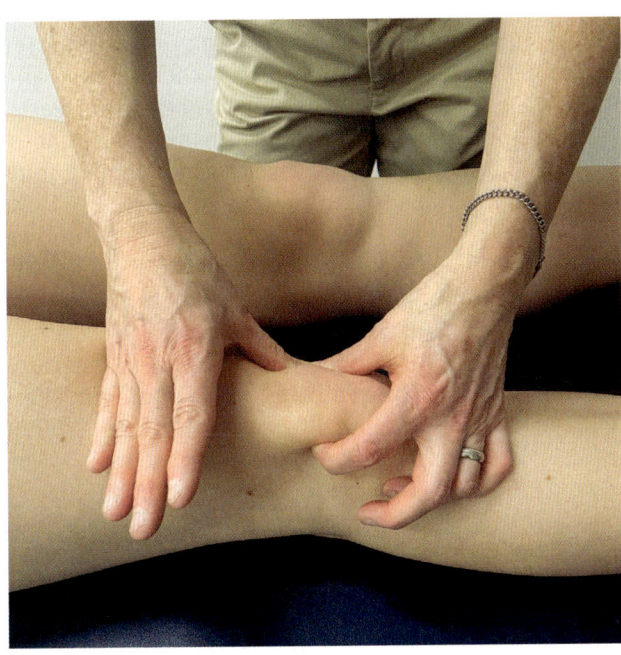

FIGURE 10-57 Retropatellar palpation. Palpation of posterior portions of the patella is best performed by first gliding the patella laterally and then palpating the exposed posterolateral patellar surface. This is then repeated with a medial glide.

Differential Diagnoses

A history of trauma and bony tenderness would suggest possible fracture. Tenderness of alternate structures such as the patellar tendon, tibial tuberosity, the inferior pole of the patella, or a cordlike structure should make the clinician consider tendinopathy, or tibial or femoral apophysitis or plica syndrome. Knee or thigh pain with hip motion in a 10- to 14-year-old child is concerning for the presence of an SCFE (see Chapter 11, Hip). A positive apprehension test or excessive lateral patellar glide is suggestive of the presence of instability rather than PFPS.[142]

While some authors place patellar instability as a subclassification of PFPS, most consider this as a separate entity. Patellar instability is discussed later in this section. Older individuals with anterior knee pain are more likely to have patellofemoral or tibiofemoral OA.

Rehabilitation Focus and Key Points

The rehabilitation focus should be based on the patient history and examination findings, and in particular the diagnostic classification of the patient's PFPS as described by Willy[139]: controlling patellofemoral joint loads, motion/flexibility, strength, and neuromuscular control.[263,268] On first glance, one might think it beneficial to avoid quadriceps strengthening in patients with PFPS fearing excessive patellofemoral joint loading. However, research supports the use of both open kinetic chain quadriceps exercise (e.g., resisted knee extension) between 90 and 45° of knee flexion and closed kinetic chain (e.g., leg press, squatting variations) between 0 and 45°.[139,261,269] These exercises actually limit patellofemoral joint stress by affecting joint surface or internal and external moment arms.[270] Both quadriceps and hip strengthening have been shown to reduce pain and improve function.[271] Core strengthening should be incorporated for higher functioning patients.[261] Balance and motor control exercises should be incorporated as needed. Manual therapy, with an emphasis on restoring lower extremity flexibility or medial patellar tilt, may be needed.[263] Foot orthotics may help control excessive pronation, when present.[139] There is no evidence to support the use of knee braces[272]; however, given the potential role psychological factors may play in PFPS, the use of braces, such as those with a patellar cutout, should be considered on an individual basis. Interestingly, the use of aspirin and nonsteroidal anti-inflammatory medications is no better than placebo, indicating that modulating inflammation is not of primary importance for patients with PFPS.[273]

Expected Outcomes
When using a multimodal, individualized approach to manage load and address the impairments of the patient's diagnostic classification(s), a high percentage of patients have good to excellent results within 4 to 6 weeks.[139,261]

Knee Osteoarthritis

Pathology
Knee OA is a chronic degenerative condition characterized by joint pain, motion loss, and decreased function. OA most frequently effect the knee, hip, and hand/finger.[274] Primary OA has no known cause; secondary OA can be traced to altered mechanics or prior injury. Knee OA may affect the medial tibiofemoral joint (also known as *medial compartment*), lateral tibiofemoral joint, and/or the patellofemoral joint. Medial compartment OA may be more common in individuals with genu varus, whereas lateral compartment OA may be more common in individuals with genu valgus. Traditionally, it was thought the knee OA began in the tibiofemoral joint, but it is now believed that the patellofemoral arthritis develops first.[275] Risk factors for knee OA include age, prior joint injury, obesity, and lower extremity malalignment.[274] General sports participation or running[276] do not appear to be linked with the development of knee OA. However, participation in competitive long-distance running, elite soccer, and wrestling may be associated with knee OA later in life.[277] Individuals with a history of prior knee surgery, including ACL reconstruction,[172] meniscal surgery,[153,159] or patellar fracture, are at increased risk for future knee OA.[109]

History
Patients with knee OA are likely to report diffuse knee pain with squatting, stairs, transfers, and weight bearing.[159] Patients with patellofemoral OA are likely to report anterior knee pain with stairs.[278] Patients may report pain at night and/or at rest. Knee stiffness, particularly in the morning,[279] and intermittent swelling,[159] especially after activities that increase knee loads, are common. They may report catching, grating, or grinding with knee motion.

Key Examination Findings
The primary diagnostic criteria for knee OA are knee pain, age over 50, radiographic evidence of joint space narrowing, and/or osteophytes.[274,275] Radiographic changes are associated with decreased knee ROM, but do not appear to be related to pain or function.[280]

Key physical examination findings include bony enlargement of the knee,[129] intermittent effusion, and warmth.[279] There is typically a loss of knee ROM[275] that may be in a capsular pattern with flexion more limited than extension. For example, the patient's passive knee motion may be 20 to 100°. Crepitus may be noticed in the tibiofemoral joint, the patellofemoral joint, or both during motion,[129,278,279,281] particularly with squatting.[275] A capsular endfeel and end range pain are common. Joint accessory motions are typically hypomobile. Patients with knee OA have been shown to have weakness in both the knee and the hip musculature.[282] These patients also tend to have reduced balance.[282] While OA may affect only one joint, it is common for patients with knee arthritis to have bilateral symptoms and concomitant hip arthritis. Therefore, a thorough LQS, including single limb balance and the Berg Balance test, should be performed.

Common gait changes include increased affected knee flexion during midstance, decreased stance time on the affected side, Trendelenburg sign, and decreased gait speed.

Patients may have knee joint line tenderness.[129,275] Patients with patellofemoral OA are likely to have pain with the grind test.[275] Patients may have asymmetrical knee wear, which can lead to knee instability. For example, lateral compartment OA can lead to significant knee valgus, resulting in MCL insufficiency and laxity with valgus stress testing.[283] The reverse would be true for patients with significant medial compartment involvement. Therefore, varus and valgus stress testing should be performed.[279]

Differential Diagnoses Differential diagnosis includes meniscal or chondral pathology, RA, inflammatory arthritis, gout, and joint infection. Some distinguishing factors between OA and RA are listed in Table 10-14.[284]

Rehabilitation Focus and Key Points Education is critical for patients with knee OA (Table 10-15).[285] Without a clear understanding of what is causing their pain, patients with OA do not know what is safe or harmful and, as a result, may avoid activity. There is strong evidence for the use of self-efficacy and self-management programs for patients with knee OA,[286] including diet and exercise are effective in promoting weight loss, decreasing pain, and improving function in patients who are overweight or obese.[286,287]

The use of an assistive device[286] can help reduce pain and improve mobility. Shock-absorbing footwear may decrease knee pain with ambulation, but the use of medial or lateral wedged insoles in an attempt to redistribute knee loads has not been shown to be effective.[286,288] There is conflicting evidence on the effectiveness of knee braces, including those designed to unload the medial or lateral compartment of the knee.[286,288,289] Both ice and heat appear to assist with pain modulation.[286]

There is strong evidence to support the use of exercise for the management of knee OA.[285,286] Exercise may improve self-efficacy, reduce depression, decrease pain, and improve function.[290] Exercise should include strength training and balance exercises.[286,291] Aquatic exercise appears to reduce pain and improve the quality of life[291,292] and should be part of the initial

TABLE 10-14

FACTORS ASSOCIATED WITH OSTEOARTHRITIS AND RHEUMATOID ARTHRITIS

Osteoarthritis	Rheumatoid Arthritis
• Degenerative condition with progressive loss of joint cartilage space • Slowly progressive • Onset: insidious, may be genetically linked, repetitive injury, obesity, prior joint injury/surgery • Age over 50 • Morning stiffness < 30 minutes • Motion loss common • May have small effusion • Bony enlargements • May be tender • May affect individual joints to varying degrees • Commonly affects knees, hips, fingers/hand, and spine	• Autoimmune disease with chronic inflammation of synovial membranes and secondary erosion of cartilage • Progressive, often chronic with exacerbations and remissions • More common in women • Morning stiffness > 30 minutes • Motion loss common • Synovial swelling • Tenderness • May have associated symptoms such as fatigue or weight loss • Tends to be symmetrical pattern • Commonly initially affects hand (PIP, MCP), wrist, MTP, knees, elbows, ankles • Concomitant medical management recommended

MCP, metacarpophalangeal; *MTP*, metatarsophalangeal; *PIP*, proximal interphalangeal.

TABLE 10-15

EDUCATION FOR INDIVIDUALS WITH OSTEOARTHRITIS

Education Concept	Example
Activity modification	Consider biking or swimming rather than jogging and walking.
Pacing	Spreading activities out over the day to allow time for rest to prevent flare-ups
Prioritizing	Do tasks that need to be accomplished first, then move on to less urgent tasks. If needed, put tasks off for another day.
Protecting joint	Using proper mechanics for functional activities, using equipment (e.g., a wheelbarrow rather than carrying loads of soil for gardening), and getting help when needed
Unloading	Attaining and maintaining a proper weight, using an assistive device when needed, strengthening muscles
Joint nutrition	Move affected joint(s) repeatedly through pain-modulated range of motion.

phase of treatment for individuals with high pain ratings.[279] Active ROM exercises can help joint nutrition and maintain range. Progressive hip, knee, and plantarflexor strengthening are most important for patients with knee OA; however, a full body program should be included. Manual therapy, including joint mobilizations, when combined with exercise, can assist with maximizing joint motion and is recommended for the management of knee OA.[293] Exercise programs should be at least two times per week to be effective, and both land-based and aquatic exercise may require 8 to 12 weeks to create substantial changes in pain, function, and quality of life.[292,294] Both low- and high-intensity exercise programs appear to be effective, however, lower intensity exercises are less likely to have adverse effects,[295] such as postexercise joint or muscle soreness or effusion. This should be viewed with caution as clinicians traditionally underdose exercise, particularly in older adults. Long-term participation in yoga or tai chi may be beneficial.[286] It appears that the benefits of land-based exercises may continue for up to 6 months after cessation of an exercise program.[296] Therefore, patients should be educated on the benefits of developing an exercise habit to maintain improvements and possibly continue to improve over time. Aerobic exercise, such as cycling, an elliptical machine, or swimming, should be encouraged. There is evidence that booster sessions spaced across several months may be beneficial and cost-effective.[297] This may be an additional tool to increase patient adherence to needed lifestyle changes.

Table 10-16 highlights some of the American College of Rheumatology's recommendations for exercise therapy for patients with knee and hip OA.[279] Exercises should include areas to address individual patient deficits and be progressed gradually. For example, many patients may need to begin with 10-minute aerobic exercise sessions or may require rest breaks. Exercise intensity for the next session should be reduced if joint pain increases after a workout or lasts longer than 2 hours after exercise completion.

Medical management of patients with knee OA may include oral or topical nonsteroidal anti-inflammatory medication, acetaminophen, COX-2 inhibitors, and steroid injections.[286,291]

Expected Outcomes Improvements in pain, ROM, strength, gait, and function can be expected. Improvements in strength are associated with improvements in function.[298] However, knee OA is a progressive condition. In addition, rehabilitation can do little to directly affect damaged joint surfaces. There are limits to how much range can be regained or function can be restored in cases of severe joint disease. Patients who fail conservative management should be referred to an orthopaedist for additional interventions.

Total Knee Arthroplasty

Total knee arthroplasty (TKA) is the mainstay treatment for end-stage knee OA and RA and may also be indicated in certain cases of severe trauma or cancer. It is one of the most commonly performed orthopaedic procedures.[299] TKA is the resection of the distal femur, proximal tibia, and posterior patella joint surfaces and replacement with metal and polyethylene prosthetic components. Components are most frequently cemented in place using polymethyl methacrylate to immediately fixate them,[299] allowing immediate weight bearing. However, for younger patients, a porous, coated prosthesis may be used that is press fit (uncemented) into the residual bone. This fixation method relies on bony ingrowth. This takes time and good bone stock to occur and, therefore, requires a period of partial weight bearing. Most cemented TKAs fail because of the bone cement wearing down over time, creating micromotion between the residual bone and the prosthesis. The benefits of uncemented components are that they are a more durable bone-prosthetic interface and ease of revision. Surgical techniques and components continue to evolve, including smaller incisions creating less tissue trauma with the use of mini-open procedures and in components, including joint resurfacing. The TKA procedure may take place in a hospital or surgery center. While the majority of patients at this time are hospitalized for about 2 to 3 days, 24-hour stays and outpatient surgery are becoming more

TABLE 10-16

EXERCISE RECOMMENDATIONS FOR PATIENTS WITH KNEE AND HIP OSTEOARTHRITIS

Strength Training	Aerobic Exercises	Additional Inclusions
2+ times/week Starting intensity: 50-60% 1RM or 12-13 RPE Target intensity: 60-80% 1RM or 14-17 RPE Large muscle groups especially: knee flexors/extensors, hip extensors/abductors	5+ times per week for 30+ minutes Starting intensity: 40-60% 1RM or 12-13 RPE Target intensity: >60% max heart rate or 14-17 RPE Consider exercises/activities with low joint loads (cycling, walking, aquatics)	Warm-up and cool-down activities Balance exercises Stretching/active range of motion to improve or maintain motion Functional components (stairs/steps)

common for individuals with few/no comorbidities, good mobility, and a sound support system.

Preoperative rehabilitation is cost-effective[300] and should include education and exercise. The patient should be educated regarding the procedure, patient expectations for the procedure, likely outcomes, perioperative rehabilitation, mobility training, postoperative positioning, and discharge planning. Caregiver or significant other involvement is recommended. A preoperative exercise program should be individualized based on the timing of surgery and include strengthening and ROM exercises as well as immediate postoperative exercises, including preventive exercises of deep breathing, ankle pumps, and quad sets. Given that preoperative strength, range, function, and social support are positively correlated with outcomes,[301] clinicians should strive to maximize these through exercise and preoperative planning. Depression is common in individuals with chronic conditions and negatively correlated with outcomes[301] after TKA. Therefore, patients should be screened for depression and appropriate referrals made. While higher body mass index is related to worse postoperative outcomes,[301] clinicians must consider that patients are best served not going into a major surgery in a caloric deficit. Preoperative physical therapy, even in patients with end-stage disease, results in improvements in knee range, strength, balance, functional activity, and quality of life in addition to lower pain ratings with no reported adverse effects.[301]

Postoperative physical therapy can begin as soon as the day of surgery, but should be no later than 24 hours after surgery,[301] and may take place in a variety of settings, including acute care, home health, and outpatient clinic, pending the patient's abilities and personal factors. Rehabilitation should include[301,302]:

- Cryotherapy[303]
- Early aggressive passive, active assisted, active knee ROM[303]
- Quadriceps NMES
- Progressive, high-intensity lower extremity resistance exercises
- Balance exercises
- Mobility training

NMES is most beneficial when initiated within the first month of surgery.[304] Manual therapy, including joint mobilizations, in the early phase of rehabilitation may assist with improving knee ROM and scar mobility.

Arthrofibrosis (excessive scar tissue formation limiting motion) is a well-known potential complication of TKA requiring surgical release and manipulation.[305,306] Manipulation under anesthesia is one of the most common reasons for readmission after a TKA.[306] Even a 5° loss of knee extension leads to a significant increase in quadriceps force for gait. Therefore, clinicians should strive for early, full knee extension, or at least as much as was obtained in surgery. Generally, speaking, knee range should be 0 to 90° in the first week, with an ultimate goal of 0 to 110° or more. This will allow more normal gait and comfortable, symmetrical transfers from a variety of surfaces. Should the patient not be on target for range goals, the clinician should reassess the plan of care and its implementation to identify and remove barriers. Pharmacologic interventions may be useful adjuncts along with more intensive patient education. Patients who lack 10° or more of extension or who have less than 90° of flexion may be the candidates for surgery.[305] While optimal timing for surgery is unknown, it appears that 6 weeks after TKA is the most common recommended time frame.[305]

Continuous passive motion (CPM) machines were once considered the norm after a TKA. While there may be individual patients or subgroups that benefit from CPM use, at this time, the literature clearly states that CPMs should not be used for patients with uncomplicated TKA[302] because their use increases bed rest and cost without improving outcomes.[301]

Clinicians should utilize functional performance tests, such as the Berg Balance test, Timed Up and Go, and 30-Second Sit-to-Stand test, as well as patient-reported outcome measures such as the WOMAC, Knee Injury and Osteoarthritis Outcome Score (KOOS), or Short-Form 36 to plan interventions and track changes over time. Lastly, as rehabilitation progresses to self-management, physical therapists should have patients strive to reach the Academy of Sports Medicine's (ACSM) guidelines for physical activity.[301] This may represent a lifestyle change for patients with knee OA, as their prior condition may have contributed to lack of adherence. Unfortunately, surgically addressing the arthritic joint has not been consistently linked with an increase in physical activity long term.[307]

After TKA, patients can expect a reduction in pain, improvements in knee range, improved function, and an enhanced sense of well-being.[308,309] The current life expectancy of a TKA is around 25 years.[310]

Iliotibial Band Syndrome

ITB syndrome is a common overuse injury of runners and cyclists characterized by poorly localized lateral knee pain. Symptoms are due to friction between the lateral femoral epicondyle and the ITB. Specifically, there appears to be a zone of impingement when the knee is about 30° flexed, which occurs during the early stance phase of running as well as during cycling.[311,312] Pain occurs as the patient's knee flexes and extends through this zone and can be exacerbated by the clinician by compressing over the lateral femoral epicondyle (the Noble compression test).[145] Patients may have minimal local swelling and tenderness near the lateral femoral epicondyle. Thickening of the distal ITB and crepitus or snapping may be noted as the knee moves through the impingement zone.[145]

The current literature seems to support that runners with ITB syndrome have greater rearfoot eversion at heel strike and greater hip adduction during the stance phase of running, which may contribute to symptoms.[313] In addition, having a more prominent lateral femoral epicondyle[314] and dynamic knee varus[315] may also be contributory. The condition is more common in males than females. Hip abductor weakness[316,317] or fatigue[318] may be contributory, particularly for female runners,[311] but this has not been consistently found in studies with more diverse populations.[319,320]

Interventions for ITB syndrome include short-term restriction of exacerbating activities along with ice and nonsteroidal anti-inflammatory medications to decrease inflammation. Hip abductor strengthening, hip abductor endurance training,[311] and ITB stretching appear to help improve symptoms and prevent recurrence.[313] Running form assessment and retraining may be beneficial for runners. Cyclists may benefit from careful assessment of saddle setback as well as modifying pedaling technique to decrease hip adduction and knee rotation.[312]

Apophysitis

Apophysitis is irritation and inflammation of a secondary ossification center (apophysis) in skeletally immature individuals. The condition generally occurs in active individuals during periods of rapid growth where the bone grows faster than the muscle-tendon unit, causing traction on the apophysis.[321] As such, the condition occurs in girls between the ages of 8 and 13 and boys between the ages of 12 and 15 years.[322] Apophysitis typically occurs at the tibial tuberosity (sometimes referred to as Osgood-Schlatter), the inferior pole of the patella (Sinding-Larsen-Johansson), and the calcaneus (Sever), but can also occur in areas around the hip and pelvis.

Individuals with apophysitis about the tibial tuberosity or inferior pole of the patella present with a bony enlargement of the apophysis with local tenderness. The patient may report pain with stairs, jumping, running, and, possibly, with resisted quadriceps activities. Patients with apophysitis should have negative tests for instability and effusion. Individuals with Osgood-Schlatter continue to participate in high levels of activities despite reports of knee pain.[264] The condition is benign and self-limiting and resolves completely once the growth plate closes.[323] However, symptoms can be modulated sooner by the use of ice, nonsteroidal anti-inflammatories, activity modification, and quadriceps and hamstring stretching.[322,323] Preventive measures include a warm-up followed by regular stretching.[321]

Plica Syndrome

As noted previously, synovial plica is shelflike membranes between the synovium and the synovial folds. Their presence and location are variable, but the suprapatellar, medial, and inferior are most common. Plicae can be identified via palpation as a cordlike structure. Plica syndrome is a symptomatic inflammation and thickening of a plica, most commonly the medial plica, between the patella and the medial femoral condyle.[324] Plica syndrome is thought to be caused by repeated knee flexion and extension, such as in cycling, running, and swimming. The condition is more common in females and teenagers.

Patients with plica syndrome will report local pain, clicking, or snapping. The patient may report a catching or pseudolocking of the patella.[325] A mild effusion may be present. Quadriceps weakness or atrophy is common. The key diagnostic finding is a tender, palpable cordlike structure.[324] Treatment is aimed at reducing information via cryotherapy or potentially pharmacologic interventions, including nonsteroidal anti-inflammatory medication or steroid injections, along with short-term reduction of repetitive knee motion. Short term (up to 3 days) of bracing in extension has shown to have positive effects. Once inflammation is controlled, progressive quadriceps strengthening and quadriceps stretching should be prescribed. Conservative management is nearly always successful,[324] but if not, surgical resection yields highly positive results.[326,327]

Quadriceps Contusion

Contusions are common in sports due to contact from another player, stick, or ball. Although quadriceps contusions (Fig. 10-58) occur frequently, they should not be taken lightly because improper management of a quadriceps contusion with a large hematoma can lead to prolonged time loss and potential surgical intervention. Early treatment of a quadriceps contusion should include ice, compression, and knee ROM as tolerated.[328] Manual lymph drainage may be useful in reducing swelling. An assistive device should be used if gait is painful or if deviations are present. Recovery time after a quadriceps contusion is related to the amount of knee flexion present. Those with at least 90° of knee flexion typically return to play within 2 weeks, whereas those with less motion generally require an additional week.[329]

Somewhere between 9[329] and 20%[330] of quadriceps contusions with large hematomas progress to myositisossificans, a condition in which there is a proliferation of bone at the site of trauma. Delaying treatment

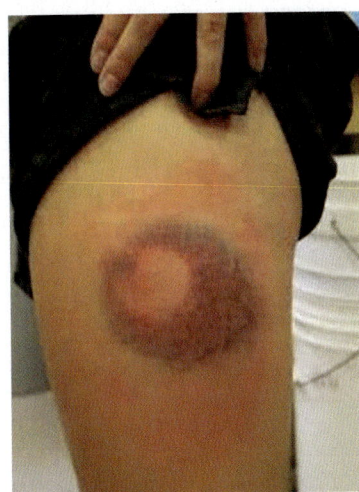

FIGURE 10-58 Quadriceps contusion after being hit in the thigh with a field hockey ball. Note the area of ecchymosis. The pink discoloration is from an ice pack that was recently removed.

of the initial contusion for more than 3 days and a history of prior contusion in the same location are associated with an increased risk of myositis ossificans.[329] Preventive measures include the use of padding as is seen in the typical American football player's equipment. The most common sites for myositis ossificans are the quadriceps, brachialis, and adductors.[331] In the quadriceps, the condition is diagnosed clinically when there is a loss of knee ROM, pain with active knee extension, a palpable firm mass in the previously injured area, and quite often pain with gait.[332] Imaging studies to confirm the presence of myositis ossificans include diagnostic ultrasound, MRI, and computed tomography (CT) scan.[331] Radiographs may initially be negative. Myositis ossificans is typically treated with gentle ROM exercises, an assistive device as needed, extracorporeal shock wave therapy, and progressive strengthening. Patients who fail to improve may have the lesion surgically excised. A return to light activity can be expected in about 3 months, but a full return to prior level of function is not expected for a year.[331]

Bursitis

As noted earlier, there are numerous bursae in the knee region. The prepatellar bursa may become inflamed as a result of an acute direct trauma, such as a fall. However, more commonly, the prepatellar bursa is irritated by repeated occupation-related activities,[333] such as prolonged kneeling and crawling required for bricklaying. The pes anserine bursa can become inflamed as a result of swimming, particularly breast stroke, or in runners who have repeated valgus collapse. Bursitis can be recognized by local swelling in the area of a bursa, and activities that put pressure or tension on the bursa increase symptoms. For example, kneeling exacerbates prepatellar bursitis.

Ice, compression, and short-term avoidance of the irritating activity typically allow the inflammation to subside.[47] Nonsteroidal anti-inflammatory medications may be beneficial.[47] For prepatellar bursitis, the use of knee pads may be beneficial to cushion the region, and these are often used prophylactically in workers who must crawl frequently and in volleyball players. For swimmers, correction of stroke form and improvement in flexibility are indicated. Steroid injections may be beneficial for recalcitrant cases.[334]

Most cases of bursitis are acute, occupational, or recreation related. However, bursae may also be inflamed in patients with gout and RA. In addition, patients may have septic bursitis from bacteria entering breaks in the skin,[335] such as kneeling on a contaminated sharp object. Patients with nonseptic and septic bursitis will both have localized bursal inflammation, bogginess to palpation, and local tenderness. However, patients with septic bursitis generally feel unwell and have a fever and may have skin lesions, such as eczema.[335] Differential diagnosis is made by a physician aspirating the bursa, and appropriate antibiotic interventions are initiated.[47,335]

DIFFERENTIAL DIAGNOSIS

Because it is neither feasible nor necessary to perform every diagnostic test, clinicians should begin narrowing down differential diagnoses by symptom location (Fig. 10-59), patient symptoms (Table 10-17), and onset (Fig. 10-60).

ADDITIONAL JOINT MOBILIZATION TECHNIQUES

The accessory motion procedures described earlier can be used to treat knee hypomobility, particularly when using grade III and IV mobilizations and/or performing closer to end range. However, at times, additional techniques can be valuable.

Mobilizations to Improve Knee Extension Range of Motion

Knee extension can be most directly improved by performing an anterior tibial glide or by providing a posterior glide of the femur. External tibial rotation mobilization may assist with end range extension by facilitating normal conjunct rotation that takes place with the screw-home mechanism of the knee.

Tibiofemoral Joint Mobilization: Anterior Glide

Purpose: To increase joint-play movement necessary for knee extension.

Patient: Prone with the knee in loose pack position (for assessment) or near end range extension for increasing motion.

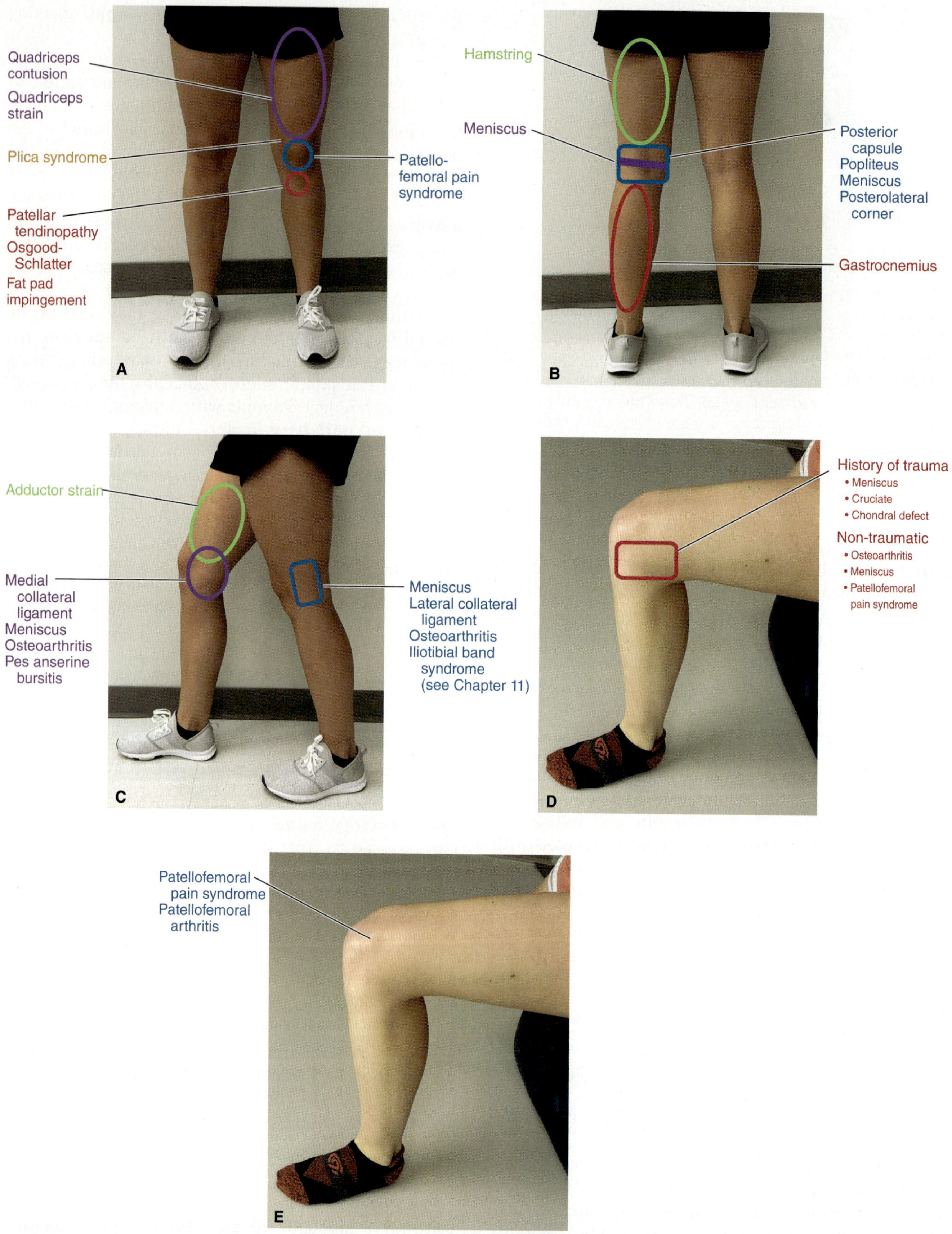

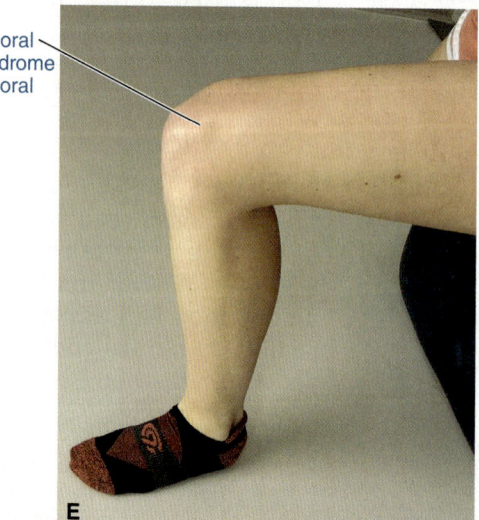

FIGURE 10-59 Knee pathology by symptom location. **A.** Anterior knee pain. **B.** Posterior knee pain. **C.** Medial/lateral knee pain. **D.** Retropatellar pain or pain in the knee. **E.** Pain "In the knee".

TABLE 10-17
DIFFERENTIAL DIAGNOSIS OF KNEE PATHOLOGY BY COMPLAINT

Complaint/Symptom	Differential Diagnoses
Instability	Patellar instability
	Anterior cruciate ligament
	Articular cartilage injury
Clicking, catching	Meniscus pathology
	Knee osteoarthritis
Difficulty with stairs	Patellofemoral pain syndrome
	Knee osteoarthritis
	Patellar tendinopathy
Pain with prolonged sitting	Patellofemoral pain syndrome
Effusion	Fracture
	Anterior cruciate ligament
	Articular cartilage injury
Minor or local swelling	Patellar instability
	Knee osteoarthritis
	Meniscus pathology
	Plica syndrome
	Bursitis

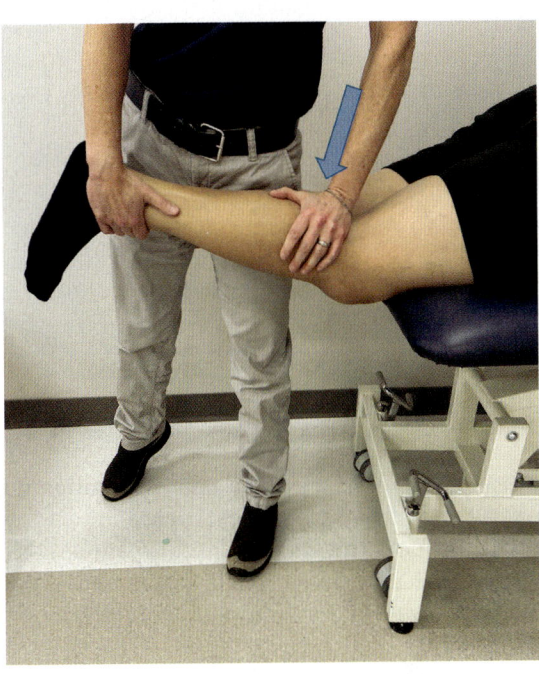

FIGURE 10-61 Tibiofemoral joint mobilization: anterior glide.

Clinician: The caudal hand supports the leg at the distal tibia. The cranial mobilizing hand contacts the posterior tibia just distal to the tibiofemoral joint.

Mobilization: Keeping the arm straight, the mobilizing hand glides the tibia anteriorly (Fig. 10-61).

Posterior Glide of Femur

Purpose: To increase joint-play movement necessary for knee extension.

Patient: Supine with the knee near end range extension with a towel roll placed under the proximal tibia.

Clinician: The caudal hand stabilizes the proximal tibia. The cranial mobilizing hand contacts the anterior femur just proximal to the tibiofemoral joint.

Mobilization: Keeping the arm straight, the mobilizing hand glides the femur posteriorly (Fig. 10-62).

Tibiofemoral Joint Mobilization: External Rotation

Purpose: To facilitate conjunct tibial external rotation.

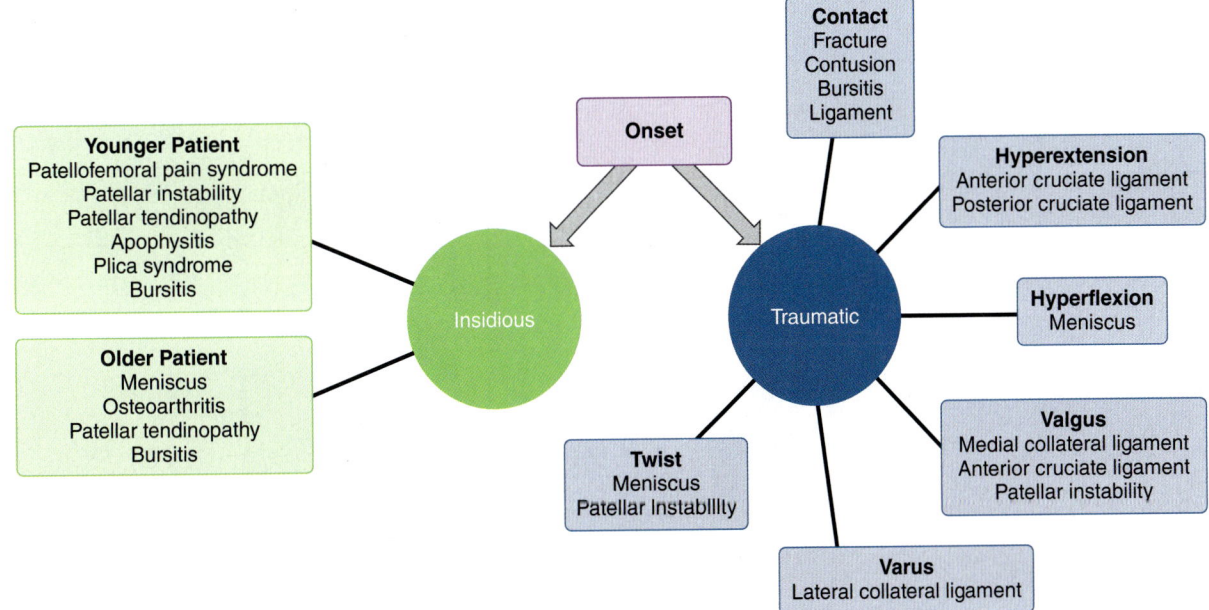

FIGURE 10-60 Knee pathology based on typical onset.

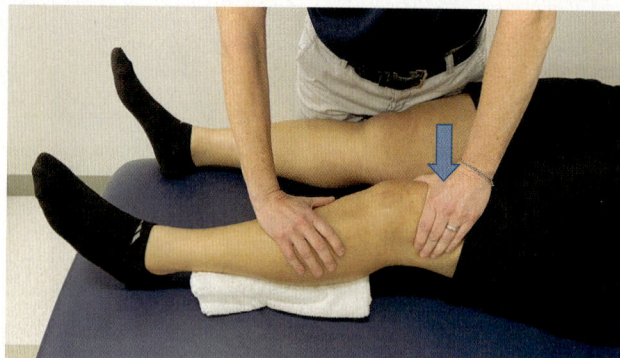

FIGURE 10-62 Posterior glide of femur.

Patient: Supine with the knee near end range extension. A towel roll can be placed behind the patient's knee to support the knee near end range.
Clinician: The clinician's hands grasp the proximal tibia with the fingers wrapped around posteriorly (Fig. 10-63).
Mobilization: Both hands rotate the proximal tibia laterally gaining purchase on the tibial spine and the posterior leg.

Mobilizations to Improve Knee Flexion Range of Motion

Knee flexion can be most directly improved by performing a posterior tibial glide near end range flexion with the patient seated or prone. Internal tibial rotation mobilization may assist with end range flexion. Patients can be taught how to perform a posterior tibial glide or self-distraction.

Tibiofemoral Joint Mobilization: Posterior Glide in Sitting

Purpose: To increase joint-play movement necessary for flexion.
Patient: Seated with knee slightly flexed.
Clinician: The clinician uses one hand to support the lower leg and places the mobilizing hand on the anterior tibia just distal to the tibiofemoral joint.
Mobilization: The mobilizing hand moves the tibia posteriorly (Fig. 10-64). Note this patient position is generally also used for assessing anterior glide of the tibia. The clinician would simply change to contacting the posterior tibia and drawing the tibia anteriorly.

Tibiofemoral Joint Mobilization: Posterior Glide in Prone

Purpose: To increase joint-play movement necessary for flexion.
Patient: Prone with the knee near end range flexion.
Clinician: The clinician supports the lower leg with the shoulder. The thenar eminences are placed on the anterior tibia just distal to the joint line, while the fingers wrap around the patient's posterior calf.
Mobilization: The mobilizing hands move the tibia posteriorly (Fig. 10-65).

Tibiofemoral Joint Mobilization: Internal Rotation

Purpose: To facilitate conjunct tibial internal rotation.

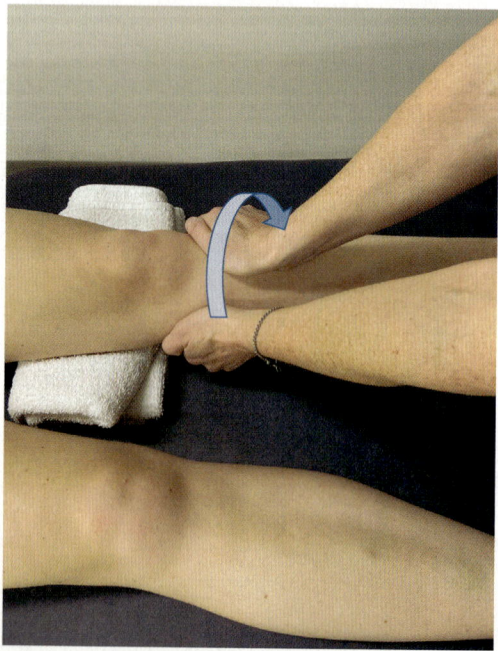

FIGURE 10-63 Tibiofemoral joint mobilization: external rotation.

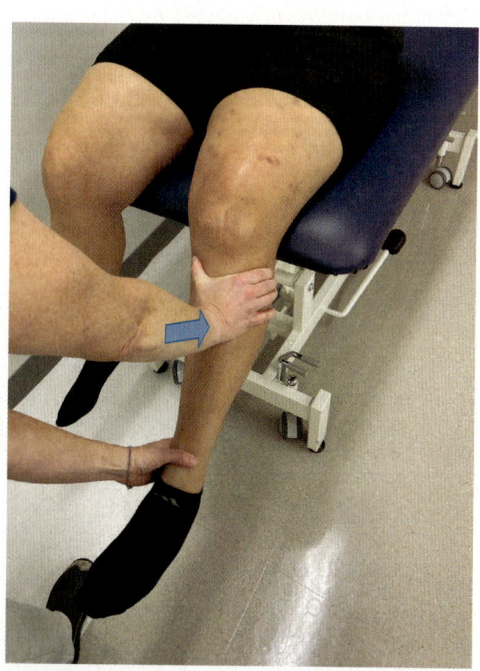

FIGURE 10-64 Tibiofemoral joint mobilization: posterior glide in sitting.

CHAPTER 10 | KNEE

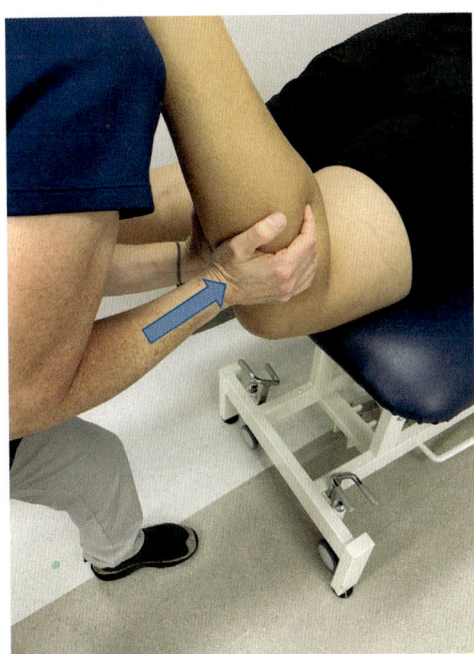

FIGURE 10-65 Tibiofemoral joint mobilization: posterior glide in prone.

Patient: Seated with the knee flexed to near end range.
Clinician: The clinician's hands grasp the proximal tibia with the fingers wrapped around posteriorly.
Mobilization: Both hands rotate the proximal tibia medially gaining purchase on the tibial spine and the posterior leg (Fig. 10-66). The mobilization can also be performed in prone.

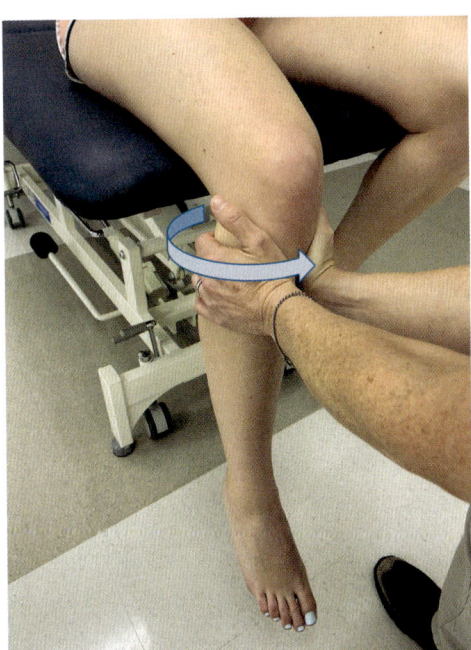

FIGURE 10-66 Tibiofemoral joint mobilization: internal rotation.

Self-Mobilization of Knee into Flexion
Patient: Seated with the knee near end range knee flexion.
Mobilization: The patient interlocks the fingers around the proximal tibia and then provides a posterior force (Fig. 10-67).

Distraction Mobilizations to Improve Global Knee Range of Motion

Tibiofemoral distraction can be performed by the clinician in sitting or in prone to provide a global joint capsular stretch. Although generally performed in the open-packed position, any angle can be used. The patient can perform self-distraction with the use of a towel roll to help gap the joint surfaces.

Tibiofemoral Joint Distraction in Sitting
Purpose: To improve global tibiofemoral joint mobility.
Patient: Seated with the knee comfortably flexed.
Clinician: Gently grasps the proximal leg with both hands. The clinician may use the knees to control the angle of knee flexion.
Mobilization: Distraction is applied on the long axis of the tibia by pulling down with the hands. The clinician's knees can provide additional distraction force (Fig. 10-68).

Tibiofemoral Joint Distraction in Prone
Purpose: To improve global tibiofemoral joint mobility.
Patient: Prone with the knee comfortably flexed. A mobilization belt is wrapped around the table to stabilize the patient's thigh.

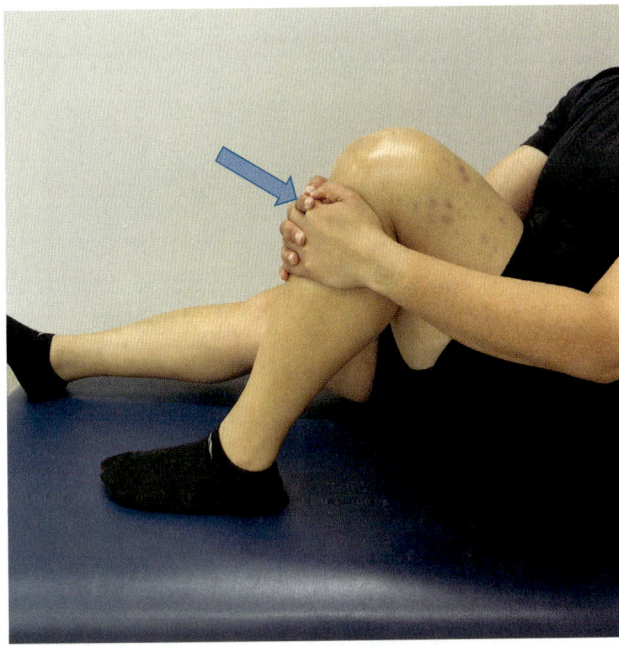

FIGURE 10-67 Self-mobilization into knee flexion.

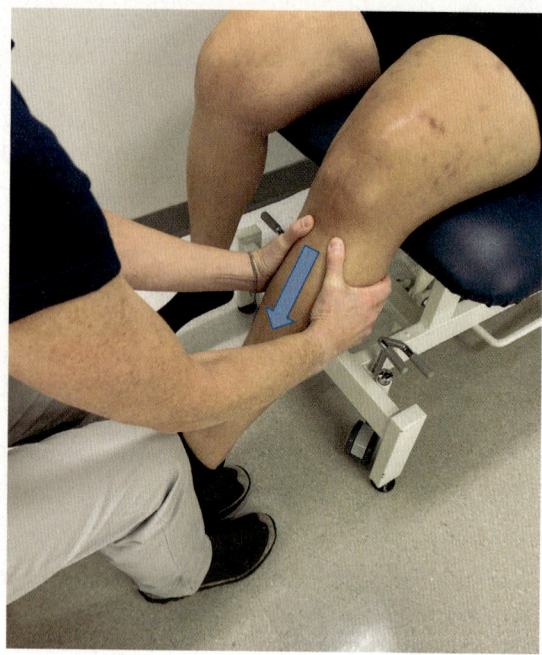

FIGURE 10-68 Tibiofemoral joint distraction in sitting.

Clinician: Gently grasps proximal to the malleoli with both hands.

Mobilization: Distraction is applied on the long axis of the tibia by shifting weight from the cranial foot to the caudal foot (Fig. 10-69).

Self-Distraction of the Knee

Patient: Seated with the knee near end range knee flexion.

Mobilization: The patient interlocks the fingers around the proximal tibia and then provides a posterior force (Fig. 10-70).

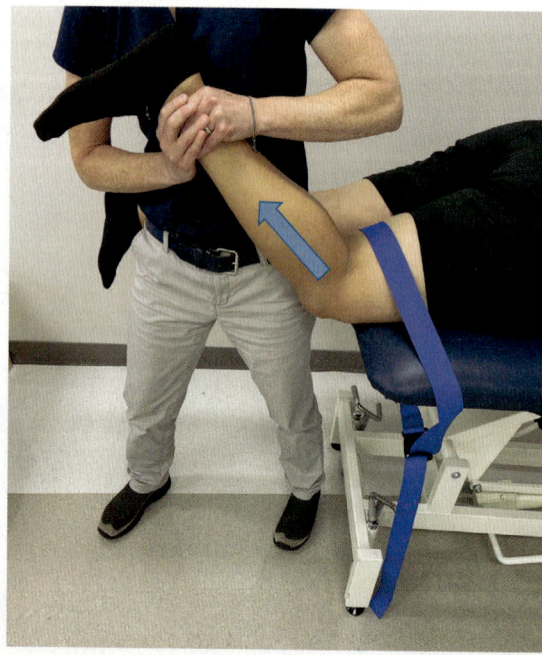

FIGURE 10-69 Tibiofemoral joint distraction in prone.

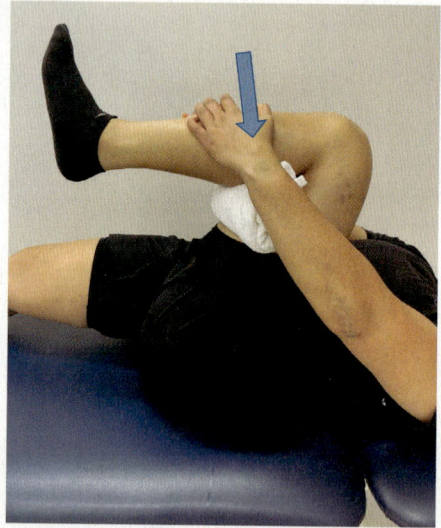

FIGURE 10-70 Self-distraction of the knee.

ADDITIONAL THERAPEUTIC EXERCISES

Many of the exercises that have been presented throughout this chapter may be beneficial for a variety of patients and diagnoses. While knee extension ROM has been emphasized due to its critical role in gait, knee flexion ROM is required for stairs, car transfers, and dressing. Knee flexion range can be facilitated in several ways. Early postoperative patients may benefit from simply allowing their leg to relax into flexion while short sitting (this is also known as the "drop-and-dangle" exercise). The patient can rock forward and backward on a stationary bicycle, adjusting the seat closer once able to perform a full repetition without compensation. Self-assisted flexion can be performed with a belt in lying or the patient can prop the heel up on a wall and allow gravity or the contralateral leg to assist with bending the knee (Fig. 10-71).

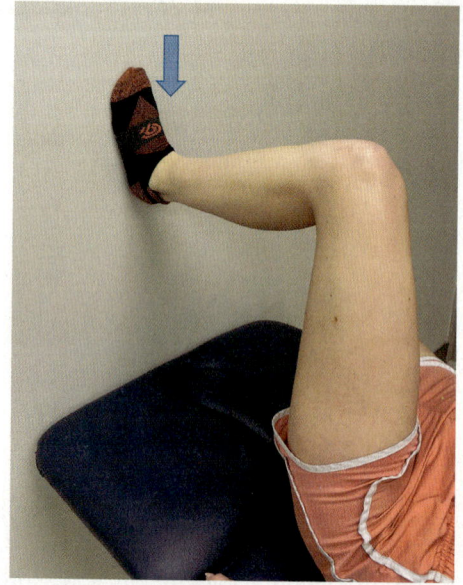

FIGURE 10-71 Wall slide for knee flexion range.

Balance assessments can also be used as interventions to improve balance. In addition to changing base of support and vision, the support surface can be altered, and a secondary task can be added (Fig. 10-72).

Resistance bands can provide additional challenges in both NWB and weight-bearing positions (Fig. 10-73).

Lastly, in the later phases of rehabilitation, power and plyometric exercises can be incorporated, including movements in the frontal and sagittal planes (Fig. 10-74).

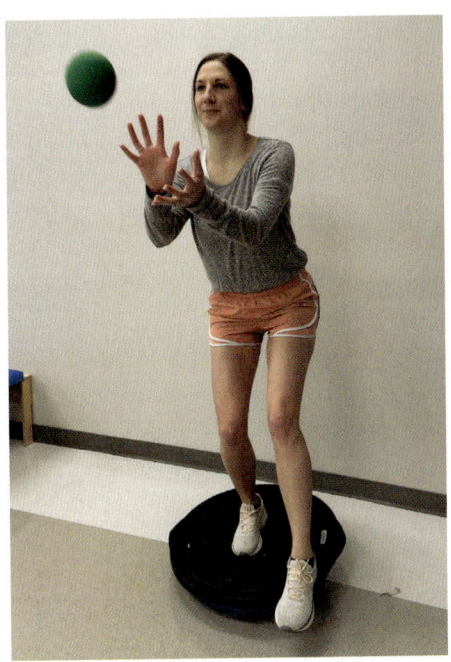

FIGURE 10-72 Single leg balance on an unstable surface with a secondary task.

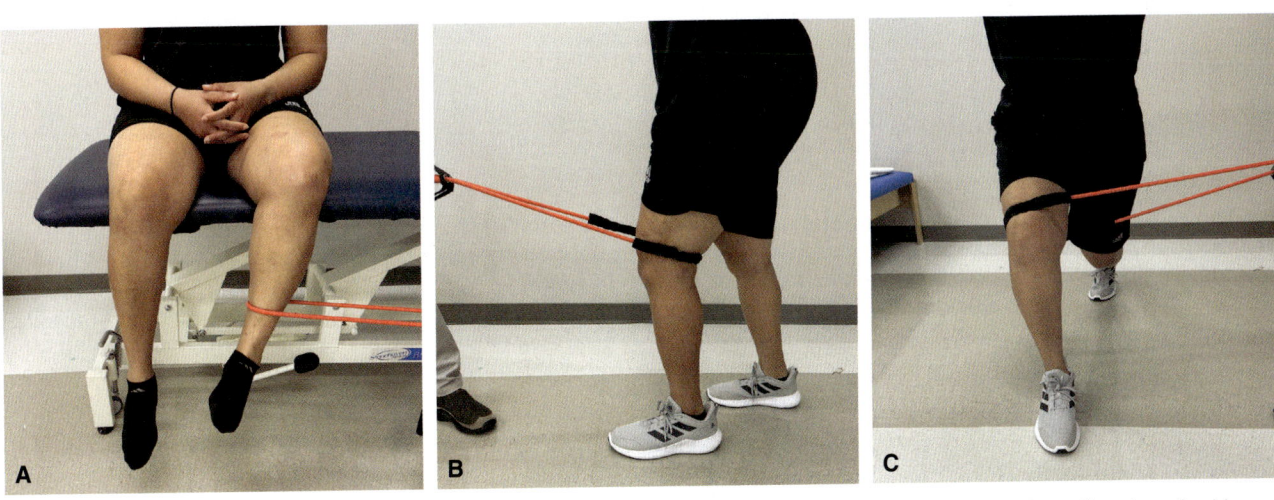

FIGURE 10-73 Band resisted exercises. **A.** Seated hip external rotation with resistance band. **B.** Standing terminal knee extension with resistance band to facilitate use of end range knee extension. **C.** Split squat with a medial vector to facilitate hip abductors and external rotators.

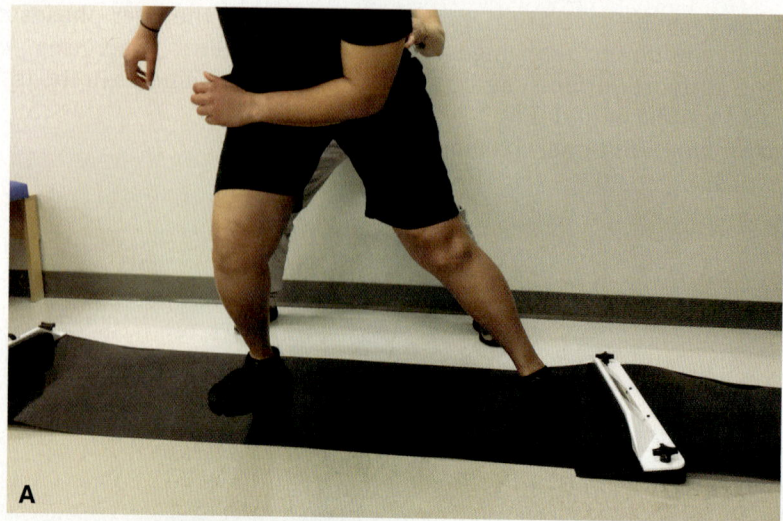

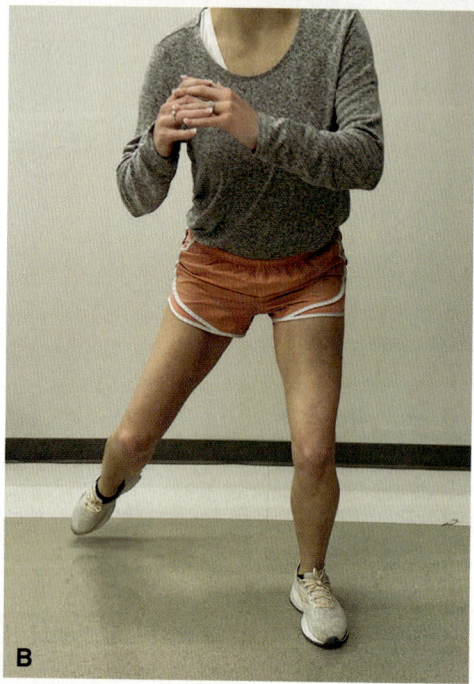
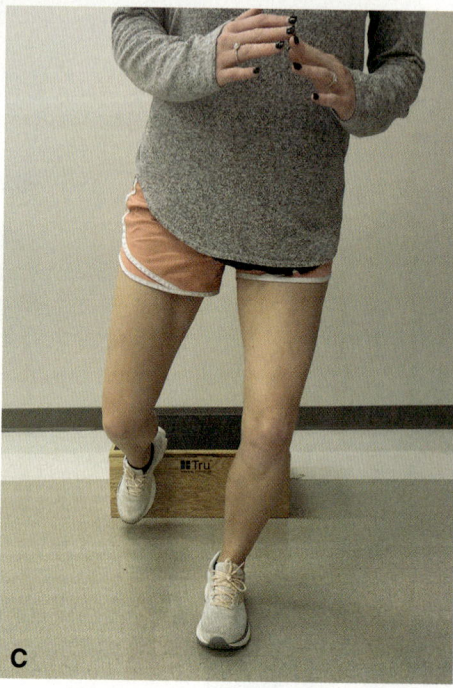

FIGURE 10-74 Late-phase frontal and sagittal plane exercises. **A.** Lateral slide exercise is performed by the patient by repeatedly pushing into hip abduction to slide side to side for repetitions or for time. **B.** Lateral skater exercise where the patient leaps side to side controlling lower extremity and trunk positioning. **C.** Forward single limb drop jump in which the patient first drops from a height landing with control on a single limb before progressing to performing a single leg depth jump (performing a vertical hop immediately upon landing). The exercise can be made easier by performing on both limbs.

CASE STUDY 10-1
Padma: Patient with Right Anterior Knee Pain

Padma is a 16-year-old field hockey player who reports a 4-month history of right anterior knee pain. She does not recall a particular injury or event that caused her symptoms to begin. She reports initially only noticing her symptoms during practice, particularly running and weight training. However, now she has symptoms while sitting in class as well. All tests begin with the uninvolved (left) side unless otherwise noted. As noted previously, the examination should be organized by position, begin away and progress toward the involved area, and provide increasing stress to injured or potentially involved structures. Table 10-18 provides an example of how an experienced clinician might organize the physical examination after performing the history and systems review.

TABLE 10-18
SAMPLE KNEE EXAMINATION
Padma: 16-year-old field hockey player with reports of right anterior knee pain

Position	Assessments
Observation	Continues from history
Seated	Ankle dorsiflexion (A, OP, MMT) Ankle plantarflexion (A, OP, MMT) Ankle inversion (A, OP, MMT) Ankle eversion (A, OP, MMT) Hip flexion (A, OP, MMT) Hip external rotation (A, OP, MMT) Hip internal rotation (A, OP, MMT) Knee extension (A, OP, MMT) Special tests: multiangle isometric quadriceps
Supine	Hip flexion, abduction (P) Knee flexion (P) Knee extension (P) Muscle length: gastrocnemius, hamstring, Thomas test (iliopsoas, rectus femoris, and iliotibial band) Integument
Right-side lying	MMT: L hip abduction, R hip adduction
Prone	Hip PROM: hip extension MMT: hamstring, gluteus maximus Muscle performance: resisted hip external rotation Integument
Left-side lying	MMT: R hip abduction, L hip adduction
Supine	MMT: trunk raise, leg-lowering abdominal test Accessory motion: patellofemoral joint, tibiofemoral joint Special tests: modified stroke test, apprehension test, medial patellar tilt test, McMurray Palpation including patellar tendon, peripatellar and retropatellar with attention also to the presence of plicae that are tender
Standing	Structure/posture screen barefoot Single leg balance: eyes open, eyes closed MMT: plantarflexion Special test: Thessaly Function: gait, squat, forward step-down, possible running analysis or hopping Footwear inspection

A, active; *L*, left; *MMT*, manual muscle test; *OP*, overpressure; *P*, passive range of motion; *R*, right.

Based on the history, there are no red flags that require immediate assessment. The patient's history of no known trauma or mechanism of injury in a young female athlete participating makes the clinician have an initial hypothesis of PFPS, patellar tendinopathy, or plica syndrome as potential reasons for her anterior knee pain. Padma's physical examination begins in the seated position with testing of the ankle and hip, as a thorough investigation of both knee-adjacent joints is required. The seated examination ends with the assessment of quadriceps strength. Because the clinician has an initial hypothesis based on the history that the patient may have PFPS, the clinician performs resisted quadriceps testing at multiple angles to see if this changes her symptoms to try to help differentiate between PFPS and patellar tendinopathy. Should quadriceps testing create or increase Padma's knee pain, then this would reinforce the need to assess at different angles as well. The examination progresses to lying positions and includes core strength assessment and prone hip external rotation testing because the patient is an athlete and deficits in these regions may contribute to the patient's symptoms. Dorsiflexion range and muscle length of the gastrocnemius, hamstring, and key hip flexors are assessed, given the known association of limitations in muscle length to PFPS.

The clinician chose to perform special tests for effusion, PFPS, and meniscal pathology. Given the patient participates in a cutting sport, meniscal testing was included to rule out meniscal pathology despite her not reporting any episodes of catching or giving way. Higher level functional testing, such as running or hopping, is possible given the patient's current high level of physical activity. However, these may eventually need to be performed on the basis of the results of the tests outlined above. ACL, PCL, and collateral ligament testing were ruled out on the basis of the patient's history and location of symptoms. A lower extremity neurologic screen is not necessary given the patient has no neurologic complaints and the patient does not report symptoms in the hip region.

CHAPTER SUMMARY

The examination and treatment of patients with knee symptoms begins with a thorough history. Patients should be asked about the effect of activities that load the knee and about the presence of effusion. Symptom description and location can assist differential diagnosis to help target the examination to identify injured tissues. A LQS is required because, many times, the ultimate cause of knee pathology may stem from impairments of proximal or distal joints. Therefore, rehabilitation strategies must include management of knee symptoms and knee loading, and resolution of these associated factors.

REFERENCES

1. Flandry F, Hommel G. Normal anatomy and biomechanics of the knee. *Sports Med Arthrosc Rev.* 2011;19(2):82–92.
2. Williams P, Warwick R, Myson M, Bannister L, eds. *Gray's Anatomy.* 37th ed. Churchill Livingstone; 1989.
3. Haemer J, Carter D, Giori N. The low permeability of healthy meniscus and labrum limit articular cartilage consolidation and maintain fluid load support in the knee and hip. *J Biomech.* 2012;45(8):1450–1456.
4. Makris E, Hadidi P, Athanasiou K. The knee meniscus: structure-function, pathophysiology, current repair techniques, and prospects for regeneration. *Biomaterials.* 2011;32(30):7411–7431.
5. Andrews S, Shrive N, Ronsky J. The shocking truth about meniscus. *J Biomech.* 2011;44(16):2737–2740.
6. Hauch K, Oyen M, Odegard G, Haut Donahue T. Nanoindentation of the insertional zones of human meniscal attachments into underlying bone. *J Mech Behav Biomed Mater.* 2009;2(4):339–347.
7. Benjamin M, Toumi H, Ralphs J, Bydder G, Best T, Milz S. Where tendons and ligaments meet bone: attachment sites ("entheses") in relation to exercise and/or mechanical load. *J Anat.* 2006;208(4):471–490.
8. Abraham A, Haut Donahue T. From meniscus to bone: a quantitative evaluation of structure and function of the human meniscal attachments. *Acta Biomater.* 2013;9(5):6322–6329.
9. Wang Y, Yu J, Luo H, et al. An anatomical and histological study of human meniscal horn bony insertions and peri-meniscal attachments as a basis for meniscal transplantation. *Chin Med J (Engl).* 2009;122(5):536–540.
10. Kim Y-M, Joo Y-B, Yeon K-W, Lee K-Y. Anterolateral meniscofemoral ligament of the lateral meniscus. *Knee Surg Relat Res.* 2016;28(3):245–248.
11. Soejima T, Murakami H, Tanaka N, Nagata K. Anteromedial meniscofemoral ligament. *Arthroscopy.* 2003;19(1):90–95.
12. Clark C, Ogden J. Development of the menisci of the human knee joint. Morphological changes and their potential role in childhood meniscal injury. *J Bone Joint Surg Am.* 1983;65(4):538–547.
13. Beaufils P, Pujol N. Management of traumatic meniscal tear and degenerative meniscal lesions. Save the meniscus. *Orthop Traumatol Surg Res.* 2017;103(8S):S237–S244.
14. Chatain F, Adeleine P, Chambat P, Neyret P. A comparative study of medial versus lateral arthroscopic partial meniscectomy on stable knees: 10-year minimum follow-up. *Arthroscopy.* 2003;19(8):842–849.
15. Arnoczky S, Warren R. Microvasculature of the human meniscus. *Am J Sports Med.* 1982;10(2):90–95.
16. Posadzy M, Joseph G, McCulloch C, et al. Natural history of new horizontal meniscal tears in individuals at risk for and with mild to moderate osteoarthritis: data from osteoarthritis initiative. *Eur Radiol.* 2020;30(11):5971–5980.
17. Barrett G, Field M, Treacy S, Ruff C. Clinical results of meniscus repair in patients 40 years and older. *Arthroscopy.* 1998;14:824–829.
18. Lind M, Jakobsen B, Lund B, Hansen M, Abdallah O, Christiansen S. Anatomical reconstruction of the medial collateral ligament and posteromedial corner of the knee in patients with chronic medial collateral ligament instability. *Am J Sports Med.* 2009;37(6):1116–1122.
19. Magnussen R, Mansour A, Carey J, Spindler K. Meniscus status at anterior cruciate ligament reconstruction associated with radiographic signs of osteoarthritis at 5- to 10-year follow-up: a systematic review. *J Knee Surg.* 2009;22(4):347–357.
20. Wilson W, Deakin A, Payne A, Picard F, Wearing S. Comparative analysis of the structural properties of the collateral ligaments of the human knee. *J Orthop Sports Phys Ther.* 2012;42(4):345–351.

21. LaPrade R, Engebretsen A, Ly T, Johansen S, Wentorf F, Engebretsen L. The anatomy of the medial part of the knee. *J Bone Joint Surg Am.* 2007;89(9):2000–2010.
22. Andrews K, Lu A, McKean L, Ebraheim N. Review: medial collateral ligament injuries. *J Orthop.* 2017;14(4):550–554.
23. Griffith C, LaPrade R, Johansen S, Armitage B, Wijdicks C, Engebretsen L. Medial knee injury: part 1, static function of the individual components of the main medial knee structures. *Am J Sports Med.* 2009;37(9):1762–1770.
24. James E, LaPrade C, LaPrade R. Anatomy and biomechanics of the lateral side of the knee and surgical implications. *Sports Med Arthrosc Rev.* 2015;23(1):2–9.
25. Coobs B, LaPrade R, Griffith C, Nelson B. Biomechanical analysis of an isolated fibular (lateral) collateral ligament reconstruction using an autogenous semitendinosus graft. *Am J Sports Med.* 2007;35(9):1521–1527.
26. Veltri D, Deng X, Torzilli P, Warren R, Maynard M. The role of the cruciate and posterolateral ligaments in stability of the knee. A biomechanical study. *Am J Sports Med.* 1995;23(4):436–443.
27. Lim H, Bae J, Bae T, Moon B, Shyam A, Wang J. Relative role changing of lateral collateral ligament on the posterolateral rotatory instability according to the knee flexion angles: a biomechanical comparative study of role of lateral collateral ligament and popliteofibular ligament. *Arch Orthop Trauma Surg.* 2012;132(11):1631–1636.
28. Siegel L, Vandenakker-Albanese C, Siegel D. Anterior cruciate ligament injuries: anatomy, physiology, biomechanics, and management. *Clin J Sport Med.* 2012;22(4):349–355.
29. Marieswaran M, Jain I, Garg B, Sharma V, Kalyanasundaram D. A review on biomechanics of anterior cruciate ligament and materials for reconstruction. *Appl Bionics Biomech.* 2018;2018:4657824.
30. Shin C, Chaudhari A, Andriacchi T. Valgus plus internal rotation moments increase anterior cruciate ligament strain more than either alone. *Med Sci Sports Exerc.* 2011;43(8):1484–1491.
31. Monaco E, Ferretti A, Labianca L, et al. Navigated knee kinematics after cutting of the ACL and its secondary restraint. *Knee Surg Sports Traumatol Arthrosc.* 2012;20(5):870–877.
32. Bowman KJ, Sekiya J. Anatomy and biomechanics of the posterior cruciate ligament, medial and lateral sides of the knee. *Sports Med Arthrosc Rev.* 2010;18(4):222–229.
33. Pache S, Aman Z, Kennedy M, et al. Posterior cruciate ligament: current concepts review. *Arch Bone Jt Surg.* 2018;6(1):8–18.
34. Oatis C. *Kinesiology: The Mechanics and Pathomechanics of Human Movement.* 3rd ed. Wolters Kluwer; 2016.
35. Terry G, Hughston J, Norwood L. The anatomy of the iliopatellar band and iliotibial tract. *Am J Sports Med.* 1986;14(1):39–45.
36. Merican A, Amis A. Anatomy of the lateral retinaculum of the knee. *J Bone Joint Surg Br.* 2008;90(4):527–534.
37. Seebacher J, Inglis A, Marshall J, Warren R. The structure of the posterolateral aspect of the knee. *J Bone Joint Surg Am.* 1982;64(4):536–541.
38. Nannaparaju M, Mortada S, Wiik A, Khan W, Alam M. Posterolateral corner injuries: epidemiology, anatomy, biomechanics and diagnosis. *Injury.* 2018;49(6):1024–1031.
39. Covey D. Injuries of the posterolateral corner of the knee. *J Bone Joint Surg Am.* 2001;83(1):106–118.
40. Anderson J, Williams AE, Nester CJ. A narrative review of musculoskeletal problems of the lower extremity and back associated with the interface between occupational tasks, feet, footwear and flooring. *Musculoskelet Care.* 2017;15(4):304–315.
41. Shon O, Park J, Kim B. Current concepts of posterolateral corner injuries of the knee. *Knee Surg Relat Res.* 2017;29(4):256–268.
42. Nakayama A, Sugita T, Aizawa T, Takahashi A, Honma T. Incidence of medial plica in 3,889 knee joints in the Japanese population. *Arthroscopy.* 2011;27(11):1523–1527.
43. Dandy D. Anatomy of the medial suprapatellar plica and medial synovial shelf. *Arthroscopy.* 1990;6:79–85.
44. Patel D. Arthroscopy of the plicae—synovial folds and their significance. *Am J Sports Med.* 1978;6(5):217–225.
45. Hughston J, Whatley G, Dodelin R, Stone M. The role of the suprapatellar plica in internal derangement of the knee. *Am J Orthop.* 1963;5:25–27.
46. Schindler O. "The Sneaky Plica" revisited: morphology, pathophysiology and treatment of synovial plicae of the knee. *Knee Surg Sports Traumatol Arthrosc.* 2014;22(2):247–262.
47. Aaron DL, Patel A, Kayiaros S, et al. Four common types of bursitis: diagnosis and management. *J Am Acad Orthop Surg.* 2011;19(6):359–367.
48. Rennie W, Saifuddin A. Pes anserine bursitis: incidence in symptomatic knees and clinical presentation. *Skeletal Radiol.* 2005;34(7):395–398.
49. Herman A, Marzo J. Popliteal cysts: a current review. *Orthopedics (Online).* 2014;37(8):e678–e684.
50. Lucha-López M, Tricás-Moreno J, Gaspar-Calvo E, et al. Relationship between knee alignment in asymptomatic subjects and flexibility of the main muscles that are functionally related to the knee. *J Int Med Res.* 2018;46(8):3065–3077.
51. Fahlman L, Sangeorzan E, Chheda N, Lambright D. Older adults without radiographic knee osteoarthritis: Knee alignment and knee range of motion. *Clin Med Insights Arthritis Musculoskelet Disord.* 2014;7:1–11.
52. Sharma P, Maffulli N. Tendon injury and tendinopathy: healing and repair. *J Bone Joint Surg Ser A.* 2005;87(1):187–202.
53. Tetsworth K, Paley D. Malalignment and degenerative arthropathy. *Orthop Clin North Am.* 1994;25(3):367–377.
54. Eckhoff D. Effect of limb malrotation on malalignment and osteoarthritis. *Orthop Clin North Am.* 1994;25(3):405–414.
55. Weinberg D, Park P, Morris W, Liu R. Femoral version and tibial torsion are not associated with hip or knee arthritis in a large osteological collection. *J Pediatr Orthop.* 2017;37(2):e120–e128.
56. Hovinga K, Lerner A. Anatomic variations between Japanese and Caucasian populations in the healthy young adult knee joint. *J Orthop Res.* 2009;27(9):1191–1196.
57. Roach K, Miles T. Normal hip and knee active range of motion: the relationship to age. *Phys Ther.* 1991;71(9):656–665.
58. American Academy of Orthopaedic Surgeons. Instruments AAoOSO. Normative Values from the General Population, Norms Base Scoring and Original Standard Raw Scores; 2000.
59. Dutton M. *Dutton's Orthopedic Examination: Evaluation and Intervention.* 5th ed. McGraw Hill; 2020.
60. Hyodo K, Masuda T, Aizawa J, Jinno T, Morita S. Hip, knee, and ankle kinematics during activities of daily living: a cross-sectional study. *Braz J Phys Ther.* 2017;21(3):159–166.
61. Nadeau S, McFadyen B, Malouin F. Frontal and sagittal plane analyses of the stair climbing task in healthy adults aged over 40 years: what are the challenges compared to level walking? *Clin Biomech (Bristol, Avon).* 2003;18(10):950–959.
62. Rowe P, Myles C, Walker C, Nutton R. Knee joint kinematics in gait and other functional activities measured using flexible electrogoniometry: how much knee motion is sufficient for normal daily life? *Gait Posture.* 2000;12(2):143–155.
63. Andersen H, Dyhre-Poulsen P. The anterior cruciate ligament does play a role in controlling axial rotation in the knee. *Knee Surg Sports Traumatol Arthrosc.* 1997;5(3):145–149.

64. Brage M, Draganich L, Pottenger L, Curran J. Knee laxity in symptomatic osteoarthritis. *Clin Orthop Relat Res.* 1994(304):184–189.
65. Lundberg M, Thuomas K, Messner K. Evaluation of knee-joint cartilage and menisci ten years after isolated and combined ruptures of the medial collateral ligament. Investigation by weight-bearing radiography, MR imaging and analysis of proteoglycan fragments in the joint fluid. *Acta Radiol.* 1997;38(1):151–157.
66. Mossberg K, Smith L. Axial rotation of the knee in women. *J Orthop Sports Phys Ther.* 1983;4(4):236–240.
67. Osternig L, Bates B, James S. Patterns of tibial rotary torque in knees of healthy subjects. *Med Sci Sports Exerc.* 1980;12(3):195–199.
68. Mills O, Hull M. Rotational flexibility of the human knee due to varus/valgus and axial moments in vivo. *J Biomech.* 1991;24(8):673–690.
69. Kettelkamp D, Johnson R, Smidt G, Chao E, Walker M. An electrogoniometric study of knee motion in normal gait. *J Bone Joint Surg Am.* 1970;52(4):775–790.
70. Lafortune M, Cavanagh P, Sommer Hr, Kalenak A. Three-dimensional kinematics of the human knee during walking. *J Biomech.* 1992;25(4):347–357.
71. Drake R, Vogl A, Mitchell A. *Gray's Anatomy for Students.* 3rd ed. Churchill Livingstone/Elsevier; 2015.
72. Moore KL, Dalley AF, Agur AMR. *Clinically Oriented Anatomy.* 8th ed. Wolters Kluwer; 2018.
73. Olewnik L, Gonera B, Podgórski M, Polguj M, Jezierski H, Topol M. A proposal for a new classification of pes anserinus morphology. *Knee Surg Sports Traumatol Arthrosc.* 2019;27(9):2984–2993.
74. Jadhav S, More S, Riascos R, Lemos D, Swischuk L. Comprehensive review of the anatomy, function, and imaging of the popliteus and associated pathologic conditions. *Radiographics.* 2014;34(2):496–513.
75. Mochizuki T, Akita K, Muneta T, Sato T. Pes anserinus: layered supportive structure on the medial side of the knee. *Clin Anat.* 2004;17(1):50–54.
76. Neumann D. *Kinesiology of the Musculoskeletal System: Foundations for Rehabilitation.* 3rd ed. Elsevier; 2017.
77. Patel V, Hall K, Ries M, et al. A three-dimensional MRI analysis of knee kinematics. *J Orthop Res.* 2004;22(2):283–292.
78. Jeon JW, Hong J. Comparison of screw-home mechanism in the unloaded living knee subjected to active and passive movements. *J Back Musculoskelet Rehabil.* 2021;34(4):589–595.
79. Ota S, Nakashima T, Morisaka A, Ida K, Kawamura M. Comparison of patellar mobility in female adults with and without patellofemoral pain. *J Orthop Sports Phys Ther.* 2008;38(7):396–402.
80. Amis A, Oguz C, Bull A, Senavongse W, Dejour D. The effect of trochleoplasty on patellar stability and kinematics: a biomechanical study in vitro. *J Bone Joint Surg Br.* 2008;90(7):864–869.
81. Senavongse W, Amis A. The effects of articular, retinacular, or muscular deficiencies on patellofemoral joint stability: a biomechanical study in vitro. *J Bone Joint Surg Br.* 2005;87(4):577–582.
82. Boström A. Fracture of the patella. A study of 422 patellar fractures. *Acta Orthop Scand Suppl.* 1972;143:1–80.
83. Luo T, Marino D, Pilson H. Patella fractures. In: *StatPearls.* StatPearls Publishing; 2021.
84. Esfandiarpour F, Lebrun CM, Dhillon S, Boulanger P. In-vivo patellar tracking in individuals with patellofemoral pain and healthy individuals. *J Orthop Res.* 2018;36(8):2193–2201.
85. Askenberger M, Janarv P, Finnbogason T, Arendt E. Morphology and anatomic patellar instability risk factors in first-time traumatic lateral patellar dislocations: a prospective magnetic resonance imaging study in skeletally immature children. *Am J Sports Med.* 2017;45(1):50–58.
86. Stephen J, Lumpaopong P, Dodds A, Williams A, Amis A. The effect of tibial tuberosity medialization and lateralization on patellofemoral joint kinematics, contact mechanics, and stability. *Am J Sports Med.* 2015;43(1):186–194.
87. Haj-Mirzaian A, Guermazi A, Pishgar F, et al. Association of patella alta with worsening of patellofemoral osteoarthritis-related structural damage: data from the Osteoarthritis Initiative. *Osteoarthritis Cartilage.* 2019;27(2):278–285.
88. Tanaka M, D'Amore T, Elias J, Thawait G, Demehri S, Cosgarea A. Anteroposterior distance between the tibial tuberosity and trochlear groove in patients with patellar instability. *Knee.* 2019;26(6):1278–1285.
89. Watson CJ, Propps M, Galt W, Redding A, Dobbs D. Reliability of McConnell's classification of patellar orientation in symptomatic and asymptomatic subjects. *J Orthop Sports Phys Ther.* 1999;29(7):378–393.
90. Tecklenburg K, Dejour D, Hoser C, Fink C. Bony and cartilaginous anatomy of the patellofemoral joint. *Knee Surg Sports Traumatol Arthrosc.* 2006;14(3):235–240.
91. Tomsich D, Nitz A, Threlkeld A, Shapiro R. Patellofemoral alignment: reliability. *J Orthop Sports Phys Ther.* 1996;23(3):200–208.
92. Amis A, Firer P, Mountney J, Senavongse W, Thomas N. Anatomy and biomechanics of the medial patellofemoral ligament. *Knee.* 2003;10(3):215–220.
93. Lin F, Makhsous M, Chang A, Hendrix R, Zhang L. In vivo and noninvasive six degrees of freedom patellar tracking during voluntary knee movement. *Clin Biomech (Bristol, Avon).* 2003;18(5):401–409.
94. Wheatley M, Rainbow M, Clouthier A. Patellofemoral mechanics: a review of pathomechanics and research approaches. *Curr Rev Musculoskelet Med.* 2020;13(3):326–337.
95. Philippot R, Boyer B, Testa R, Farizon F, Moyen B. The role of the medial ligamentous structures on patellar tracking during knee flexion. *Knee Surg Sports Traumatol Arthrosc.* 2012;20(2):331–336.
96. Borotikar B, Sheehan F. In vivo patellofemoral contact mechanics during active extension using a novel dynamic MRI-based methodology. *Osteoarthritis Cartilage.* 2013;21(12):1886–1894.
97. Kobayashi K, Hosseini A, Sakamoto M, Qi W, Rubash H, Li G. In vivo kinematics of the extensor mechanism of the knee during deep flexion. *J Biomech Eng.* 2013;135(8):81002.
98. LaPrade RF, Bollom TS, Wentorf FA, Wills NJ, Meister K. Mechanical properties of the posterolateral structures of the knee. *Am J Sports Med.* 2005;33(9):1386–1391.
99. Goodfellow J, Hungerford D, Zindel M. Patello-femoral joint mechanics and pathology. 1. Functional anatomy of the patello-femoral joint. *J Bone Joint Surg Br.* 1976;58(3):287–290.
100. Amis A, Senavongse W, Bull A. Patellofemoral kinematics during knee flexion-extension: an in vitro study. *J Orthop Res.* 2006;24(12):2201–2211.
101. Amis A. Current concepts on anatomy and biomechanics of patellar stability. *Sports Med Arthrosc Rev.* 2007;15(2):48–56.
102. Lankhorst N, Bierma-Zeinstra S, van Middelkoop M. Risk factors for patellofemoral pain syndrome: a systematic review. *J Orthop Sports Phys Ther.* 2012;42(2):81–94.
103. Caylor D, Fites R, Worrell TW. The relationship between quadriceps angle and anterior knee pain syndrome. *J Orthop Sports Phys Ther.* 1993;17(1):11–16.

104. Smith TO, Davies L. When should open reduction and internal fixation ankle fractures begin weight bearing? A systematic review. *Euro J Trauma Emerg Surg.* 2008;34(1):69–76.
105. Lankhorst N, Bierma-Zeinstra S, van Middelkoop M. Factors associated with patellofemoral pain syndrome: a systematic review. *Br J Sports Med.* 2013;47(4):193–206.
106. Powers CM, Landel R, Perry J. Timing and intensity of vastus muscle activity during functional activities in subjects with and without patellofemoral pain. *Phys Ther.* 1996;76(9):946–967.
107. Chen S, Chang W, Wu J, Fong Y. Electromyographic analysis of hip and knee muscles during specific exercise movements in females with patellofemoral pain syndrome: an observational study. *Medicine (Baltimore).* 2018;97(28):e11424.
108. Mohr KJ, Kvitne RS, Pink MM, Fideler B, Perry J. Electromyography of the quadriceps in patellofemoral pain with patellar subluxation. *Clin Orthop Relat Res.* 2003;415:261–271.
109. Thomas AC, Simon JE, Evans R, Turner MJ, Vela LI, Gribble PA. Knee surgery is associated with greater odds of knee osteoarthritis diagnosis. *J Sport Rehabil.* 2019;28(7):716–723.
110. Logerstedt DS, Scalzitti DA, Bennell KL, et al. Knee pain and mobility impairments: meniscal and articular cartilage lesions revision 2018. *J Orthop Sports Phys Ther.* 2018;48(2):A1–A50.
111. Cheung TC, Tank Y, Breederveld RS, Tuinebreijer WE, de Lange-de Klerk ES, Derksen RJ. Diagnostic accuracy and reproducibility of the Ottawa Knee Rule vs the Pittsburgh Decision Rule. *Am J Emerg Med.* 2013;31(4):641–645.
112. Huntington LS, Webster KE, Devitt BM, Scanlon JP, Feller JA. Factors associated with an increased risk of recurrence after a first-time patellar dislocation: a systematic review and meta-analysis. *Am J Sports Med.* 2020;48(10):2552–2562.
113. Manske R, Prohaska D. Rehabilitation following medial patellofemoral ligament reconstruction for patellar instability. *Int J Sports Phys Ther.* 2017;12(3):494–511.
114. Surgeons AAOO. *Joint Motion: Method of Measuring and Recording.* Churchill Livingstone; 1965.
115. Clarkson HM. *Musculoskeletal Assessment: Joint Range of Motion, Muscle Testing, and Function.* 4th ed. Wolters Kluwer; 2021.
116. Houglum P, Bertoti D. *Brunnstrom's Clinical Kinesiology.* 6th ed. F.A. Davis; 2012.
117. Bhagia S, Weinik M, Xin S. What is the role of the modified Helfet test in the physical exam of meniscal injury. *WebMD LLE.* Medscape Web site. Published 2020. Updated April 24, 2020. Accessed December 30, 2020. https://www.medscape.com/answers/308054-158718/what-is-the-role-of-the-modified-helfet-test-in-the-physical-exam-of-meniscal-injury
118. Nyland J, Lachman N, Kocabey Y, Brosky J, Altun R, Caborn D. Anatomy, function, and rehabilitation of the popliteus musculotendinous complex. *J Orthop Sports Phys Ther.* 2005;35(3):165–179.
119. Petsche TS, Selesnick FH. Popliteus tendinitis: tips for diagnosis and management. *Phys Sportsmed.* 2002;30(8):27–31.
120. Kendall FP, McCreary EK, Provance PG, Rogers MM, Romani WA. *Muscles: Testing and Function with Posture and Pain.* 5th ed. Lippincott Williams & Wilkins; 2005.
121. Tawa N, Rhoda A, Diener I. Accuracy of clinical neurological examination in diagnosing lumbo-sacral radiculopathy: a systematic literature review. *BMC Musculoskelet Disord.* 2017;18:1–11.
122. Manske RC, Davies GJ. Examination of the patellofemoral joint. *Int J Sports Phys Ther.* 2016;11(6):831–853.
123. Cibere J, Guermazi A, Nicolaou S, et al. Association of knee effusion detected by physical examination with bone marrow lesions: cross-sectional and longitudinal analyses of a population-based cohort. *Arthritis Care Res.* 2019;71(1):39–45.
124. Palmieri-Smith RM, Villwock M, Downie B, Hecht G, Zernicke R. Pain and effusion and quadriceps activation and strength. *J Athl Train.* 2013;48(2):186–191.
125. Bolgla LA, Keskula DR. A review of the relationship among knee effusion, quadriceps inhibition, and knee function. *J Sports Rehabil.* 2000;9(2):160–168.
126. Konin J, Lebscak D, Snyder Valier A. *Special Tests for Orthopaedic Examination.* SLACK Incorporated; 2016.
127. Logerstedt DS, Scalzitti D, Risberg MA, et al. Knee stability and movement coordination impairments: knee ligament sprain revision 2017. *J Orthop Sports Phys Ther.* 2017;47(11):A1–A47.
128. Sturgill LP, Snyder-Mackler L, Manal TJ, Axe MJ. Interrater reliability of a clinical scale to assess knee joint effusion. *J Orthop Sports Phys Ther.* 2009;39(12):845–849.
129. Décary S, Ouellet P, Vendittoli P-A, Desmeules F. Reliability of physical examination tests for the diagnosis of knee disorders: evidence from a systematic review. *Man Ther.* 2016;26:172–182.
130. Bronstein RD, Schaffer JC. Physical examination of the knee: meniscus, cartilage, and patellofemoral conditions. *J Am Acad Orthop Surg.* 2017;25(5):365–374.
131. Squillantini R, Ringle B, Cavallario J. Comparing the diagnostic accuracy of two selective tissue tests for anterior cruciate ligament injuries: a critically appraised topic. *Int J Athl Ther Train.* 2019;24(4):145–150.
132. Bronstein RD, Schaffer JC. Physical examination of knee ligament injuries. *J Am Acad Orthop Surg.* 2017;25(4):280–287.
133. Leblanc M-C, Kowalczuk M, Andruszkiewicz N, et al. Diagnostic accuracy of physical examination for anterior knee instability: a systematic review. *Knee Surg Sports Traumatol Arthrosc.* 2015;23(10):2805–2813.
134. Huang W, Zhang Y, Yao Z, Ma L. Clinical examination of anterior cruciate ligament rupture: a systematic review and meta-analysis. *Acta Orthop Traumatol Turc.* 2016;50(1):22–31.
135. Ruzbarsky JJ, Konin G, Mehta N, Marx RG. MRI arthroscopy correlations: ligaments of the knee. *Sports Med Arthrosc Rev.* 2017;25(4):210–218.
136. Yoo J, Ahn J, Sung K-S, et al. Measurement and comparison of the difference in normal medial and lateral knee joint opening. *Knee Surg Sports Traumatol Arthrosc.* 2006;14(12):1238–1244.
137. Aronson PA, Gieck JH, Hertel J, Rijke AM, Ingersoll CD. Tibiofemoral joint positioning for the valgus stress test. *J Athl Train.* 2010;45(4):357–363.
138. Logan C, O'Brien L, LaPrade R. Post-operative rehabilitation of grade III medial collateral ligament injuries: evidence based rehabilitation and return to play. *Int J Sports Phys Ther.* 2016;11(7):1177–1190.
139. Willy R, Hoglund L, Barton C, et al. Patellofemoral pain. *J Orthop Sports Phys Ther.* 2019;49(9):CPG1–CPG95.
140. Manal T, Sturgill L. The knee: physical therapy patient management utilizing current evidence. In: *Independent Study Course 16.2: Current Concepts of Orthopedic Physical Therapy.* American Physical Therapy Association; 2008.
141. Buchanan G, Torres L, Czarkowski B, Giangarra CE. Current concepts in the treatment of gross patellofemoral instability. *Int J Sports Phys Ther.* 2016;11(6):867–876.
142. Nijs J, Van Geel C, Van der Auwera C, Van de Velde B. Diagnostic value of five clinical tests in patellofemoral pain syndrome. *Man Ther.* 2006;11(1):69–77.

143. Décary S, Frémont P, Pelletier B, et al. Validity of combining history elements and physical examination tests to diagnose patellofemoral pain. *Arch Phys Med Rehabil.* 2018;99(4):607–614.e601.
144. Leibbrandt DC, Louw Q. The development of an evidence-based clinical checklist for the diagnosis of anterior knee pain. *S Afr J Physiother.* 2017;73(1):1–10.
145. Noble CA. Iliotibial band friction syndrome in runners. *Am J Sports Med.* 1980;8(4):232–234.
146. Bachmann LM, Kolb E, Koller MT, Steurer J, Riet Gt. Accuracy of Ottawa ankle rules to exclude fractures of the ankle and mid-foot: systematic review. *Br Med J.* 2003;326(7386):417.
147. Whatman C, Hume P, Hing W. The reliability and validity of visual rating of dynamic alignment during lower extremity functional screening tests: a review of the literature. *Phys Ther Rev.* 2015;20(3):210–224.
148. Batty L, Feller J, Hartwig T, Devitt B, Webster K. Single-leg squat performance and its relationship to extensor mechanism strength after anterior cruciate ligament reconstruction. *Am J Sports Med.* 2019;47(14):3423–3428.
149. Gee S, Tennent D, Cameron K, Posner M. The burden of meniscus injury in young and physically active populations. *Clin Sports Med.* 2020;39(1):13–27.
150. Feucht MJ, Bigdon S, Bode G, et al. Associated tears of the lateral meniscus in anterior cruciate ligament injuries: risk factors for different tear patterns. *J Orthop Surg Res.* 2015;10:34–34.
151. Arastu M, Grange S, Twyman R. Prevalence and consequences of delayed diagnosis of anterior cruciate ligament ruptures. *Knee Surg Sports Traumatol Arthrosc.* 2015;23(4):1201–1205.
152. Markes A, Hodax J, Ma C. Meniscus form and function. *Clin Sports Med.* 2020;39(1):1–12.
153. Sherman S, DiPaolo Z, Ray T, Sachs B, Oladeji L. Meniscus injuries: a review of rehabilitation and return to play. *Clin Sports Med.* 2020;39(1):165–183.
154. Smoak JB, Matthews JR, Vinod AV, Kluczynski MA, Bisson LJ. An up-to-date review of the meniscus literature: a systematic summary of systematic reviews and meta-analyses. *Orthop J Sport Med.* 2020;8(9):1–14.
155. Brady MP, Weiss W. Clinical assessment versus MRI diagnosis of meniscus tears. *J Sport Rehabil.* 2015;24(4):423–427.
156. Beals C, Magnussen R, Graham W, Flanigan D. The prevalence of meniscal pathology in asymptomatic athletes. *Sports Med.* 2016;46(10):1517–1524.
157. Englund M, Guermazi A, Gale D, et al. Incidental meniscal findings on knee MRI in middle-aged and elderly persons. *N Eng J Med.* 2008;359(11):1108–1115.
158. Ma J, Chen H, Liu A, Cui Y, Ma X. Medical exercise therapy alone versus arthroscopic partial meniscectomy followed by medical exercise therapy for degenerative meniscal tear: a systematic review and meta-analysis of randomized controlled trials. *J Orthop Surg Res.* 2020;15(1):1–11.
159. Wolf B, Gulbrandsen T. Degenerative meniscus tear in older athletes. *Clin Sports Med.* 2020;39(1):197–209.
160. Kise N, Risberg M, Stensrud S, Ranstam J, Engebreten L, Roos EM. Exercise therapy versus arthroscopic partial meniscectomy for degenerative meniscal tears in middle aged patients. *Br J Sports Med.* 2016;50(23):1473–1480.
161. Pihl K, Ensor J, Peat G, et al. Wild goose chase—no predictable patient subgroups benefit from meniscal surgery: patient-reported outcomes of 641 patients 1 year after surgery. *Br J Sports Med.* 2020;54(1):13–22.
162. Doral M, Bilge O, Huri G, Turhan E, Verdonk R. Modern treatment of meniscal tears. *EFORT Open Rev.* 2018;3(5):260–268.
163. Safran-Norton CE, Sullivan JK, Irrgang JJ, et al. A consensus-based process identifying physical therapy and exercise treatments for patients with degenerative meniscal tears and knee OA: the TeMPO physical therapy interventions and home exercise program. *BMC Musculoskel Disord.* 2019;20(1).
164. Katz JN, Brophy RH, Chaisson CE, et al. Surgery versus physical therapy for a meniscal tear and osteoarthritis. *N Engl J Med.* 2013;368(18):1675–1684.
165. Brelin A, Rue J. Return to play following meniscus surgery. *Clin Sports Med.* 2016;35(4):669–678.
166. Wiley T, Lemme N, Marcaccio S, et al. Return to play following meniscal repair. *Clin Sports Med.* 2020;39(1):185–196.
167. Harput G, Guney-Deniz H, Nyland J, Kocabey Y. Postoperative rehabilitation and outcomes following arthroscopic isolated meniscus repairs: a systematic review. *Phys Ther Sport.* 2020;45:76–85.
168. Spalding T, Damasena I, Lawton R. Meniscal repair techniques. *Clin Sports Med.* 2020;39(1):37–56.
169. Eberbach H, Zwingmann J, Hohloch L, et al. Sport-specific outcomes after isolated meniscal repair: a systematic review. *Knee Surg Sports Traumatol Arthrosc.* 2018;26(3):762–771.
170. Griffin L, Albohm M, Arendt E, et al. Understanding and preventing noncontact anterior cruciate ligament injuries: a review of the Hunt Valley II meeting, January 2005. *Am J Sports Med.* 2006;34(9):1512–1532.
171. Mai H, Chun D, Schneider A, et al. Performance-based outcomes after anterior cruciate ligament reconstruction in professional athletes differ between sports. *Am J Sports Med.* 2016;45(10):2226–2232.
172. Paterno MV. Incidence and predictors of second anterior cruciate ligament injury after primary reconstruction and return to sport. *J Athl Train.* 2015;50(10):1097–1099.
173. Lindanger L, Strand T, Molster A, Solheim E, Inderhaug E. Return to play and long-term participation in pivoting sports after anterior cruciate ligament reconstruction. *Am J Sports Med.* 2019;47(14):3339–3346.
174. Kiappour A, Demetropoulos C, Kiapour A, et al. Strain response of the anterior cruciate ligament to uniplanar and multiplanar loads during simulated landings. *Am J Sports Med.* 2016;44(8):2087–2096.
175. Powers CM. The influence of abnormal hip mechanics on knee injury: a mechanical perspective. *J Orthop Sports Phys Ther.* 2010;40(2):42–51.
176. Fox A. Change-of-direction biomechanics: is what's best for anterior cruciate ligament injury prevention also best for performance? *Sports Med.* 2018;48(8):1799–1807.
177. Keyhani S, Esmailiejah AA, Mirhoseini MS, Hosseininejad S-M, Ghanbari N. The prevalence, zone, and type of the meniscus tear in patients with anterior cruciate ligament (ACL) injury; Does delayed ACL reconstruction affects the meniscal injury? *Arch Bone Jt Surg.* 2020;8(3):432–438.
178. Papalia R, Torre G, Vasta S, et al. Bone bruises in anterior cruciate ligament injured knee and long-term outcomes. A review of the evidence. *Open Access J Sports Med.* 2015;6:37–48.
179. Patel SA, Hageman J, Quatman CE, Wordeman SC, Hewett TE. Prevalence and location of bone bruises associated with anterior cruciate ligament injury and implications for mechanism of injury: a systematic review. *Sports Med.* 2014;44(2):281–293.
180. van Melick N, van Rijn L, Nijhuis-van der Sanden MWG, Hoogeboom TJ, van Cingel REH. Fatigue affects quality of movement more in ACL-reconstructed soccer players than in healthy soccer players. *Knee Surg Sports Traumatol Arthrosc.* 2019;27(2):549–555.

181. Gornitzky AL, Lott A, Yellin JL, Fabricant PD, Lawrence JT, Ganley TJ. Sport-specific yearly risk and incidence of anterior cruciate ligament tears in high school athletes: a systematic review and meta-analysis. *Am J Sports Med.* 2016;44(10):2716–2723.
182. Goodwillie AD, Shah SS, McHugh MP, Nicholas SJ. The effect of postoperativeKT-1000 arthrometer score on long-term outcome after anterior cruciate ligament reconstruction. *Am J Sports Med.* 2017;45(7):1522–1528.
183. Myer G, Paterno M, Ford K, Hewett T. Neuromuscular training techniques to target deficits before return to sport after anterior cruciate ligament reconstruction. *J Strength Cond Res.* 2008;22(3):987–1014.
184. Klyne D, Keays S, Bullock-Saxton J, Newcombe P. The effect of anterior cruciate ligament rupture on the timing and amplitude of gastrocnemius muscle activation: a study of alterations in EMG measures and their relationship to knee joint stability. *J Electromyogr Kinesiol.* 2012;22(3):446–455.
185. Kaplan Y. Identifying individuals with an anterior cruciate ligament-deficient knee as copers and noncopers: a narrative literature review. *J Orthop Sports Phys Ther.* 2011;41(10):758–766.
186. Grindem H, Wellsandt E, Failla M, Snyder-Mackler L, Risberg MA. Anterior cruciate ligament injury-who succeeds without reconstructive surgery? The Delaware-Oslo ACL cohort study. *Orthop J Sports Med.* 2018;6(5):2325967118774255.
187. Wellsandt E, Failla MJ, Axe MJ, Snyder-Mackler L. Does anterior cruciate ligament reconstruction improve functional and radiographic outcomes over nonoperative management 5 years after injury? *Am J Sports Med.* 2018;46(9):2103–2112.
188. Adams D, Logerstedt D, Hunter-Giordano A, Axe M, Snyder-Mackler L. Current concepts for anterior cruciate ligament reconstruction: a criterion-based rehabilitation progression. *J Orthop Sports Phys Ther.* 2012;42(7):601–614.
189. Failla MJ, Logerstedt DS, Grindem H, et al. Does extended preoperative rehabilitation influence outcomes 2 years after ACL reconstruction? *Am J Sports Med.* 2016;44(10):2608–2614.
190. Wilk K, Macrina L, Cain E, Dugas J, Andrews J. Recent advances in the rehabilitation of anterior cruciate ligament injuries. *J Orthop Sports Phys Ther.* 2012;42(3):153–171.
191. Spindler KP, Kuhn JE, Freedman KB, Matthews CE, Dittus RS, Harrell FE Jr. Anterior cruciate ligament reconstruction autograft choice: bone-tendon-bone versus hamstring: does it really matter? A systematic review. *Am J Sports Med.* 2004;32(8):1986–1995.
192. Rogowski I, Vigne G, Blache Y, et al. Does the graft used for ACL reconstruction affect the knee muscular strength ratio at six months postoperatively? *Int J Sports Phys Ther.* 2019;14(4):546–553.
193. Lynch JR, Okoroha KR, Lizzio V, Yu CC, Jildeh TR, Moutzouros V. Adductor canal block versus femoral nerve block for pain control after anterior cruciate ligament reconstruction: a prospective randomized trial. *Am J Sports Med.* 2019;47(2):355–363.
194. Björnsson H, Samuelsson K, Sundemo D, et al. A randomized controlled trial with mean 16-year follow-up comparing hamstring and patellar tendon autografts in anterior cruciate ligament reconstruction. *Am J Sports Med.* 2016;44(9):2304–2313.
195. Joreitz R, Lynch A, Rabuck S, Lynch B, Davin S, Irrgang J. Patient-specific and surgery-specific factors that affect return to sport after ACL reconstruction. *Int J Sports Phys Ther.* 2016;11(2):264–278.
196. Morris R, Hulstyn M, Fleming B, Owens BD, Fadale PD. Return to play following anterior cruciate ligament reconstruction. *Clin Sports Med.* 2016;35:655–668.
197. Chmielewski T, Jones D, Day T, Tillman S, Lentz T, George S. The association of pain and fear of movement/reinjury with function during anterior cruciate ligament reconstruction rehabilitation. *J Orthop Sports Phys Ther.* 2008;38(12):746–753.
198. Biggs-Kinzer A, Murphy B, Shelbourne K, Urch S. Perioperative rehabilitation using a knee extension device and arthroscopic debridement in treatment of arthrofibrosis. *Sports Health.* 2010;2(5):417–424.
199. Delaloye J, Murar J, Vieira T, et al. Knee extension deficit in the early postoperative period predisposes to cyclops syndrome after anterior cruciate ligament reconstruction: a risk factor analysis in 3633 patients from the SANTI study group database. *Am J Sports Med.* 2020;48(3):565–572.
200. van Melick N, van Cingel R, Neeter C, van Tienen T, Hullegie W, Nijhuis-van der Sanden MW. Practice guidelines for anterior cruciate ligament rehabilitation based on a systematic review and multidisciplinary consensus. *Br J Sports Med.* 2016;50(24):1506–1515.
201. Kline PW, Noehren B, Burnham J, Yonz M, Johnson D, Ireland ML. Hip external rotation strength predicts hop performance after anterior cruciate ligament reconstruction. *Knee Surg Sports Traumatol Arthrosc.* 2018;26(4):1137–1144.
202. Khayambashi K, Ghoddosi N, Straub RK, Powers CM. Hip muscle strength predicts noncontact anterior cruciate ligament injury in male and female athletes. *Am J Sports Med.* 2016;44(2):355–361.
203. Tsai L-C, Powers CM. Increased hip and knee flexion during landing decreases tibiofemoral compressive forces in women who have undergone anterior cruciate ligament reconstruction. *Am J Sports Med.* 2013;41(2):423–429.
204. Buckthorpe M, Pirotti E, Della Villa F. Benefits and use of aquatic therapy during rehabilitation after ACL reconstruction—a clinical commentary. *Int J Sports Phys Ther.* 2019;14(6):979–993.
205. DeFrancesco CJ, Lebrun DG, Molony JT, Heath MR, Fabricant PD. Safer and cheaper: an enhanced milestone-based return to play program after anterior cruciate ligament reconstruction in young athletes is cost-effective compared with standard time-based return to play criteria. *Am J Sports Med.* 2020;48(5):1100–1107.
206. Rambaud A, Ardern C, Thoreux P, Regnaux J, Edouard P. Criteria for return to running after anterior cruciate ligament reconstruction: a scoping review. *Br J Sports Med.* 2017;52:1437–1444.
207. Buckthorpe M. Optimising the late-stage rehabilitation and return-to-sport training and testing process after ACL reconstruction. *Sports Med.* 2019;49(7):1043–1058.
208. Clark N, Forshey T, Mulligan I, Kindel C. Knee mechanics during a change of direction movement in division I athletes following full return to sport from anterior cruciate ligament reconstruction. *Phys Ther Sport.* 2019;35:75–78.
209. Grooms D, Appelbaum G, Onate J. Neuroplasticity following anterior cruciate ligament injury: a framework for visual-motor training approaches in rehabilitation. *J Orthop Sports Phys Ther.* 2015;45(5):381–393.
210. Webster KE, Hewett TE. What is the evidence for and validity of return-to-sport testing after anterior cruciate ligament reconstruction surgery? A systematic review and meta-analysis. *Sports Med.* 2019;49(6):917–929.
211. Marques JB, Paul DJ, Graham-Smith P, Read PJ. Change of direction assessment following anterior cruciate ligament reconstruction: a review of current practice and

considerations to enhance practical application. *Sports Med.* 2020;50(1):55–72.
212. Kaplan Y, Witvrouw E. When is it safe to return to sport after ACL reconstruction? Reviewing the criteria. *Sports Health.* 2019;11(4):301–305.
213. Grindem H, Snyder-Mackler L, Moksnes H, Engebretsen L, Risberg MA. Simple decision rules can reduce reinjury risk by 84% after ACL reconstruction: the Delaware-Oslo ACL cohort study. *Br J Sports Med.* 2016;50(13):804–808.
214. Müller U, Krüger-Franke M, Schmidt M, Rosemeyer B, Müller U, Krüger-Franke M. Predictive parameters for return to pre-injury level of sport 6 months following anterior cruciate ligament reconstruction surgery. *Knee Surg Sports Traumatol Arthrosc.* 2015;23(12):3623–3631.
215. Losciale JM, Zdeb RM, Ledbetter L, Reiman MP, Sell TC. The association between passing return-to-sport criteria and second anterior cruciate ligament injury risk: a systematic review with meta-analysis. *J Orthop Sports Phys Ther.* 2019;49(2):43–54.
216. Buckthorpe M, Della Villa F, Della Villa S, Roi GS. On-field rehabilitation part 2: a 5-stage program for the soccer player focused on linear movements, multidirectional movements, soccer-specific skills, soccer-specific movements, and modified practice. *J Orthop Sports Phys Ther.* 2019;49(8):570–575.
217. Xergia SA, Pappas E, Georgoulis AD. Association of the single-limb hop test with isokinetic, kinematic, and kinetic asymmetries in patients after anterior cruciate ligament reconstruction. *Sports Health.* 2015;7(3):217–223.
218. Rohman E, Steub JT, Tompkins M. Changes in involved and uninvolved limb function during rehabilitation after anterior cruciate ligament reconstruction: implications for limb symmetry index measures. *Am J Sports Med.* 2015;43(6):1391–1397.
219. Wren TAL, Mueske NM, Brophy CH, et al. Hop distance symmetry does not indicate normal landing biomechanics in adolescent athletes with recent anterior cruciate ligament reconstruction. *J Orthop Sports Phys Ther.* 2018;48(8):622–629.
220. Wellsandt E, Failla MJ, Snyder-Mackler L. Limb symmetry indexes can overestimate knee function after anterior cruciate ligament injury. *J Orthop Sports Phys Ther.* 2017;47(5):334–338.
221. Myers BA, Jenkins WL, Killian C, Rundquist P. Normative data for hop tests in high school and collegiate basketball and soccer players. *Int J Sports Phys Ther.* 2014;9(5):596–603.
222. Pairot de Fontenay B, Argaud S, Blache Y, Monteil K. Contralateral limb deficit seven months after ACL-reconstruction: an analysis of single-leg hop tests. *The Knee.* 2015;22(4):309–312.
223. Grassi A, Macchiarola L, Lucidi GA, et al. More than a 2-fold risk of contralateral anterior cruciate ligament injuries compared with ipsilateral graft failure 10 years after primary reconstruction. *Am J Sports Med.* 2020;48(2):310–317.
224. Schilaty ND, Nagelli C, Bates NA, et al. incidence of second anterior cruciate ligament tears and identification of associated risk factors from 2001 to 2010 using a geographic database. *Orthop J Sports Med.* 2017;5(8):2325967117724196.
225. Beischer S, Gustavsson L, Senorski EH, et al. Young athletes who return to sport before 9 months after anterior cruciate ligament reconstruction have a rate of new injury 7 times that of those who delay return. *J Orthop Sports Phys Ther.* 2020;50(2):83–90.
226. Arundale AJH, Bizzini M, Giordano A, et al. Exercise-based knee and anterior cruciate ligament injury prevention. *J Orthop Sports Phys Ther.* 2018;48(9):A1–A42.
227. Shizuka S, Eiichi T, Yuji Y, et al. Core-muscle training and neuromuscular control of the lower limb and trunk. *J Athl Train.* 2019;54(9):959–969.
228. Willadsen EM, Zahn AB, Durall CJ. What is the most effective training approach for preventing noncontact ACL injuries in high school–aged female athletes? *J Sports Rehabil.* 2019;28(1):94–98.
229. Jeong J, Choi D-H, Shin CS. Core strength training can alter neuromuscular and biomechanical risk factors for anterior cruciate ligament injury. *Am J Sports Med.* 2020;49(1):183–192.
230. Huang Y-L, Jung J, Mulligan CMS, Oh J, Norcross MF. A majority of anterior cruciate ligament injuries can be prevented by injury prevention programs: a systematic review of randomized controlled trials and cluster-randomized controlled trials with meta-analysis. *Am J Sports Med.* 2020;48(6):1505–1515.
231. Ekstrand J, Spreco A, Windt J, Khan K. Are elite soccer teams' preseason training sessions associated with fewer in-season injuries? A 15 year analysis from the Union of European Football Associations (UEFA) Elite Club Injury Study. *Am J Sports Med.* 2020;48(3):723–729.
232. Silvers-Granelli HJ, Bizzini M, Arundale A, Mandelbaum BR, Snyder-Mackler L. Does the FIFA 11+ injury prevention program reduce the incidence of ACL injury in male soccer players? *Clin Orthop Relat Res.* 2017;475(10):2447–2455.
233. Sadigursky D, Braid JA, De Lira DNL, Machado BAB, Carneiro RJF, Colavolpe PO. The FIFA 11+ injury prevention program for soccer players: a systematic review. *BMC Sports Sci Med Rehabil.* 2017;9:18.
234. Neto M, Conceição C, de Lima Brasileiro A, de Sousa C, Carvalho V, de Jesus F. Effects of the FIFA 11 training program on injury prevention and performance in football players: a systematic review and meta-analysis. *Clin Rehabil.* 2017;31(5):651–659.
235. Kim C, Chasse P, Taylor D. Return to play after medial collateral ligament injury. *Clin Sports Med.* 2016;35(4):679–696.
236. Hwang K-T, Sung I-H, Choi J-H, Lee JK. A higher association of medial collateral ligament injury of the knee in pronation injuries of the ankle. *Arch Orthop Trauma Surg.* 2018;138(6):771–776.
237. Petrie RS, Harner CD. Evaluation and management of the posterior cruciate injured knee. *Oper Tech Sports Med.* 1999;7(3):93–103.
238. Larson R. Clinical evaluation of posterior cruciate ligament and posterolateral corner insufficiency. *Oper Tech Sports Med.* 2001;9(2):39–46.
239. Logan M, Williams A, Lavelle J, Gedroyc W, Freeman M. The effect of posterior cruciate ligament deficiency on knee kinematics. *Am J Sports Med.* 2004;32(8):1915–1922.
240. Wilk KE, Andrews JR, Clancy WG. Nonoperative and postoperative rehabilitation of the collateral ligaments of the knee. *Oper Tech Sports Med.* 1996;4(3):192–201.
241. Ishibashi Y, Kimura Y, Sasaki E, Sasaki S, Yamamoto Y, Tsuda E. Acute primary repair of extra-articular ligaments and staged surgery in multiple ligament knee injuries. *J Orthop Traumatol.* 2020;21(1).
242. Reinking MF. Current concepts in the treatment of patellar tendinopathy. *Int J Sports Phys Ther.* 2016;11(6):854–866.
243. Cook JL, Purdam C. Is compressive load a factor in the development of tendinopathy? *Br J Sports Med.* 2012;46(3):163–168.
244. Vicenzino B. Tendinopathy: evidence-informed physical therapy clinical reasoning. *J Orthop Sports Phys Ther.* 2015;45(11):816–818.
245. Malliaras P, Cook J, Purdam C, Rio E. Patellar tendinopathy: clinical diagnosis, load management, and advice for

challenging case presentations. *J Orthop Sports Phys Ther.* 2015;45(11):887–898.
246. Plinsinga ML, Brink MS, Vicenzino B, Van Wilgen CP. Evidence of nervous system sensitization in commonly presenting and persistent painful tendinopathies: a systematic review. *J Orthop Sports Phys Ther.* 2015;45(11):864–875.
247. Scattone Silva R, Nakagawa TH, Ferreira ALG, Garcia LC, Santos JEM, Serrão FV. Lower limb strength and flexibility in athletes with and without patellar tendinopathy. *Phys Ther Sport.* 2016;20:19–25.
248. Rio E, Moseley L, Purdam C, et al. The pain of tendinopathy: physiological or pathophysiological? *Sports Med.* 2014;44(1):9–23.
249. Rio E, Purdam C, Girdwood M, Cook J. Isometric exercise to reduce pain in patellar tendinopathy in-season: Is it effective "on the road"? *Clin J Sport Med.* 2019;29(3):188–192.
250. van Ark M, Cook JL, Docking SI, et al. Do isometric and isotonic exercise programs reduce pain in athletes with patellar tendinopathy in-season? A randomised clinical trial. *J Sci Med Sport.* 2016;19(9):702–706.
251. Scattone Silva R, Ferreira ALG, Nakagawa TH, Santos JEM, Serrão FV. Rehabilitation of patellar tendinopathy using hip extensor strengthening and landing-strategy modification: case report with 6-month follow-up. *J Orthop Sports Phys Ther.* 2015;45(11):899–909.
252. Scattone Silva R, Purdam CR, Fearon AM, et al. Effects of altering trunk position during landings on patellar tendon force and pain. *Med Sci Sports Exerc.* 2017;49(12):2517–2527.
253. Zwerver J, Bredeweg S, Hof A. Biomechanical analysis of the single-leg decline squat. *Br J Sports Med.* 2007;41(4):264–268; discussion 268.
254. Melvin J, Mehta S. Patellar fractures in adults. *J Am Acad Orhtop Surg.* 2011;19(4):198–207.
255. Henrichsen JL, Wilhem SK, Siljander MP, Kalma JJ, Karadsheh MS. Treatment of patella fractures. *Orthopedics.* 2018;41(6):e747–e755.
256. Shabat S, Folman Y, Mann G, Gepstein R, Fredman B, Nyska M. Rehabilitation after knee immobilization in octogenarians with patellar fractures. *J Knee Surg.* 2004;17(2):109–112.
257. Shabat S, Mann G, Kish B, Stern A, Sagiv P, Nyska M. Functional results after patellar fractures in elderly patients. *Arch Gerontol Geriatr.* 2003;37(1):93–98.
258. Huber C, Zhang Q, Taylor W, Amis A, Smith C, Hosseini Nasab S. Properties and function of the medial patellofemoral ligament: a systematic review. *Am J Sports Med.* 2020;48(3):754–766.
259. Chen H, Zhao D, Xie J, et al. The outcomes of the modified Fulkerson osteotomy procedure to treat habitual patellar dislocation associated with high-grade trochlear dysplasia. *BMC Musculoskelet Disord.* 2017;18(1):73.
260. Powers CM. The influence of altered lower-extremity kinematics on patellofemoral joint dysfunction: a theoretical perspective. *J Orthop Sports Phys Ther.* 2003;33(11):639–646.
261. Ferber R, Bolgal L, Earl-Boehm J, Emery CA, Hamstra-Wright K. Strengthening of the hip and core versus knee muscles for the treatment of patellofemoral pain: a multicenter randomized controlled trial. *J Athl Train.* 2015;50(4):366–377.
262. Sanchis-Alfonso V, Dye SF. How to deal with anterior knee pain in the active young patient. *Sports Health.* 2017;9(4):346–351.
263. Mullaney M, Fukunaga T. Current concepts and treatment of patellofemoral compressive issues. *Int J Sports Phys Ther.* 2016;11(6):891–902.
264. Rathleff MS, Winiarski L, Krommes K, et al. Pain, sports participation, and physical function in adolescents with patellofemoral pain and Osgood-Schlatter disease: a matched cross-sectional study. *J Orthop Sports Phys Ther.* 2020;50(3):149–157.
265. Ibrahim MM, Alayat MS, Shousha TM. Evaluation of postural stability in patellofemoral pain syndrome patients. *Indian J Physiother Occup Ther.* 2014;8(2):100–104.
266. Fick C, Grant C, Sheehan F. Patellofemoral pain in adolescents: understanding patellofemoral morphology and its relationship to maltracking. *Am J Sports Med.* 2020;48(2):341–350.
267. Bolgla L, Boling M, Mace K, DiStefano M, Fithian D, Powers C. National Athletic Trainers' Association position statement: management of individuals with patellofemoral pain. *J Athl Train.* 2018;53(9):820–836.
268. Herrington L, Al-Sherhi A. A controlled trial of weight-bearing versus nonweightbearing exercises for patellofemoral pain. *J Orthop Sports Phys Ther.* 2007;37(4):155–160.
269. Lee TQ, Morris G, Csintalan RP. The influence of tibial and femoral rotation on patellofemoral contact area and pressure. *J Orthop Sports Phys Ther.* 2003;33(11):686–693.
270. Powers CM, Ward SR, Fredericson M, Guillet M, Shellock FG. Patellofemoral kinematics during weight-bearing and non-weight-bearing knee extension in persons with lateral subluxation of the patella: a preliminary study. *J Orthop Sports Phys Ther.* 2003;33(11):677–685.
271. Clijsen R, Fuchs J, Taeymans J. Effectiveness of exercise therapy in treatment of patients with patellofemoral pain syndrome: systematic review and meta-analysis. *Phys Ther.* 2014;94(12):1697–1708.
272. Smith TO, Drew BT, Meek TH, Clark AB, Smith TO. Knee orthoses for treating patellofemoral pain syndrome. *Cochrane Database Syst Rev.* 2015;(12):CD010513.
273. Macri E, Hart H, Thwaites D, et al. Medical interventions for patellofemoral pain and patellofemoral osteoarthritis: a systematic review. *J Clin Med.* 2020;9(11):3397.
274. Martel-Pelletier J, Maheu E, Pelletier J-P, et al. A new decision tree for diagnosis of osteoarthritis in primary care: international consensus of experts. *Aging Clin Exp Res.* 2019;31(1):19–30.
275. Lankhorst NE, Damen J, Oei EH, et al. Incidence, prevalence, natural course and prognosis of patellofemoral osteoarthritis: the Cohort Hip and Cohort Knee study. *Osteoarthritis Cartilage.* 2017;25(5):647–653.
276. Timmins KA, Leech RD, Batt ME, Edwards KL. Running and knee osteoarthritis: a systematic review and meta-analysis. *Am J Sports Med.* 2017;45(6):1447–1457.
277. Driban JB, Hootman JM, Sitler MR, Harris KP, Cattano NM. Is participation in certain sports associated with knee osteoarthritis? A systematic review. *J Athl Train.* 2017;52(6):497–506.
278. Stefanik JJ, Duncan R, Felson DT, Peat G. Use of diagnostic performance of clinical examination measures and pain presentation to identify patellofemoral joint osteoarthritis. *Arthritis Care Res (Hoboken).* 2018;70(1):157–161.
279. van Doormaal MCM, Meerhoff GA, Vliet Vlieland TPM, Peter WF. A clinical practice guideline for physical therapy in patients with hip or knee osteoarthritis. *Musculoskeletal Care.* 2020;18(4):575–595.
280. Ersoz M, Ergun S. Relationship between knee range of motion and Kellgren-Lawrence radiographic scores in knee osteoarthritis. *Am J Phys Med Rehabil.* 2003;82(2):110–115.
281. Schiphof D, van Middelkoop M, de Klerk BM, et al. Crepitus is a first indication of patellofemoral osteoarthritis (and not of tibiofemoral osteoarthritis). *Osteoarthritis Cartilage.* 2014;22(5):631–638.
282. Iversen MD, Price LL, Von Heideken J, Harvey WF, Chenchen W, Wang C. Physical examination findings and

their relationship with performance-based function in adults with knee osteoarthritis. *BMC Musculoskelet Disord.* 2016;17:1–12.
283. Cliborne AV, Wainner RS, Rhon DI, et al. Clinical hip tests and a functional squat test in patients with knee osteoarthritis: reliability, prevalence of positive test findings, and short-term response to hip mobilization. *J Orthop Sports Phys Ther.* 2004;34(11):676–685.
284. Bcikley LS. *Bates' Guide to Physical Examination and History Taking.* 13th ed. Wolters Kluwer; 2021.
285. Teo PL, Hinman RS, Egerton T, Dziedzic KS, Bennell KL. Identifying and prioritizing clinical guideline recommendations most relevant to physical therapy practice for hip and/or knee osteoarthritis. *J Orthop Sports Phys Ther.* 2019;49(7):501–512.
286. Kolasinski SL, Neogi T, Hochberg MC, et al. 2019 American College of Rheumatology/Arthritis Foundation guideline for the management of osteoarthritis of the hand, hip, and knee. *Arthritis Rheumatol.* 2020;72(2):220–233.
287. Brosseau L, Wells G, Tugwell P, et al. Ottawa panel evidence-based clinical practice guidelines for therapeutic exercises and manual therapy in the management of osteoarthritis. *Phys Ther.* 2005;85(9):907–971.
288. Duivenvoorden T, Brouwer RW, van Raaij TM, et al. Braces and orthoses for treating osteoarthritis of the knee. *Cochrane Database Syst Rev.* 2015(3):CD004020.
289. Gohal C, Shanmugaraj A, Tate P, et al. Effectiveness of valgus offloading knee braces in the treatment of medial compartment knee osteoarthritis: a systematic review. *Sports Health.* 2018;10(6):500–514.
290. Hurley M, Dickson K, Hallett R, et al. Exercise interventions and patient beliefs for people with hip, knee or hip and knee osteoarthritis: a mixed methods review. *Cochrane Database Syst Rev.* 2018;4(4):CD010842.
291. McAlindon TE, Bannuru RR, Sullivan MC, et al. OARSI guidelines for the non-surgical management of knee osteoarthritis. *Osteoarthritis Cartilage.* 2014;22(3):363–388.
292. Bartels EM, Juhl CB, Christensen R, et al. Aquatic exercise for the treatment of knee and hip osteoarthritis. *Cochrane Database Syst Rev.* 2016;3:CD005523.
293. Brosseau L, Davis J, Drouin H, et al. Continuous passive motion following total knee arthroplasty. *Cochrane Library.* 2005;2.
294. Young JL, Rhon DI, Cleland JA, Snodgrass SJ. The influence of exercise dosing on outcomes in patients with knee disorders: a systematic review. *J Orthop Sports Phys Ther.* 2018;48(3):146–161.
295. Regnaux J-P, Lefevre-Colau M-M, Trinquart L, et al. High-intensity versus low-intensity physical activity or exercise in people with hip or knee osteoarthritis. *Cochrane Database Syst Rev.* 2015;(10):CD010203.
296. Fransen M, McConnell S, Harmer AR, et al. Exercise for osteoarthritis of the knee. *Cochrane Database Syst Rev.* 2015;(1):CD004376.
297. Bove AM, Smith KJ, Bise CG, et al. Exercise, manual therapy, and booster sessions in knee osteoarthritis: cost-effectiveness analysis from a multicenter randomized controlled trial. *Phys Ther.* 2018;98(1):16–27.
298. Vincent K, Vasilopoulos T, Montero C, Vincent H. Eccentric and concentric resistance exercise comparison for knee osteoarthritis. *Med Sci Sports Exerc.* 2019;51(10):1977–1986.
299. Christensen D, Klement M, Moschetti W, Fillingham Y. Current evidence-based indications for modern noncemented total knee arthroplasty. *J Am Acad Orthop Surg.* 2020;28(20):823–829.
300. Clark C. Clinical Summary: Total Knee Arthroplasty (TKA) Rehabilitation. *J Bone Joint Surg.* 2018.
301. Jette D, Hunter S, Burkett L, et al. Physical therapist management of total knee arthroplasty. *Phys Ther.* 2020;100(9):1603–1631.
302. Dávila Castrodad I, Recai T, Abraham M, et al. Rehabilitation protocols following total knee arthroplasty: a review of study designs and outcome measures. *Ann Transl Med.* 2019;7(Suppl 7):S255.
303. Curry A, Goehring M, Bell J, Jette D. Effect of physical therapy interventions in the acute care setting on function, activity, and participation after total knee arthroplasty: a systematic review. *J Acute Care Phys Ther.* 2018;9(3):93–106.
304. Bistolfi A, Zanovello J, Ferracini R, et al. Evaluation of the effectiveness of neuromuscular electrical stimulation after total knee arthroplasty: a meta-analysis. *Am J Phys Med Rehabil.* 2018;97(2):123–130.
305. Cheuy VA, Foran JRH, Paxton RJ, Bade MJ, Zeni JA, Stevens-Lapsley JE. Arthrofibrosis associated with total knee arthroplasty. *J Arthroplasty.* 2017;32(8):2604–2611.
306. Kornuijt A, Das D, Sijbesma T, de Vries L, van der Weegen W. Manipulation under anesthesia following total knee arthroplasty: a comprehensive review of literature. *Musculoskelet Surg.* 2018;102(3):223–230.
307. Groen J, Stevens M, Kersten R, Reininga I, van den Akker-Scheek I. After total knee arthroplasty, many people are not active enough to maintain their health and fitness: an observational study. *J Physiother.* 2012;58:113–116.
308. Beaupre LA, Davies DM, Jones CA, Cinats JG. Exercise combined with continuous passive motion or slider board therapy compared with exercise only: a randomized controlled trial of patients following total knee arthroplasty. *Phys Ther.* 2001;81(4):1029–1037.
309. Ethgen O, Bruyere O, Richy F, Dardennes C, Reginster J. Health-related quality of life in total hip and total knee arthroplasty: a qualitative and systematic review of the literature. *J Bone Joint Surg Am.* 2004;86A(5):963–974.
310. Evans JT, Walker RW, Evans JP, Blom AW, Sayers A, Whitehouse MR. How long does a knee replacement last? A systematic review and meta-analysis of case series and national registry reports with more than 15 years of follow-up. *Lancet.* 2019;393(10172):655–663.
311. Charles D, Rodgers C. A literature review and clinical commentary on the development of iliotibial band syndrome in runners. *Int J Sports Phys Ther.* 2020;15(3):460–470.
312. Ménard M, Lacouture P, Domalain M. Iliotibial band syndrome in cycling: a combined experimental-simulation approach for assessing the effect of saddle setback. *Int J Sports Phys Ther.* 2020;15(6):958–966.
313. Balachandar V, Hampton M, Riaz O, Woods S. Iliotibial band friction syndrome: a systematic review and meta-analysis to evaluate lower-limb biomechanics and conservative treatment. *Muscle Ligament Tendon J.* 2019;9(2):181–193.
314. Everhart JS, Di Bartola A, Chaudhari AMW, Flanigan DC. Iliotibial band syndrome: can the lateral femoral epicondyle play a role? An anatomic study of individual variation in epicondyle prominence. *Muscle Ligament Tendon J.* 2019;9(1):49–54.
315. Stickley CD, Presuto MM, Radzak KN, Bourbeau CM, Hetzler RK. Dynamic varus and the development of iliotibial band syndrome. *J Athl Train.* 2018;53(2):128–134.
316. Aderem J, Louw QA. Biomechanical risk factors associated with iliotibial band syndrome in runners: a systematic review. *BMC Musculoskelet Disord.* 2015;16:1–16.
317. Baruah S, Vijayakumar RV. Cross-sectional study to identify iliotibial band syndrome causes among treadmill runners and its impact on functional activities. *Indian J Phys Occup Ther.* 2020;14(1):265–270.

318. Baker RL, Souza RB, Rauh MJ, Fredericson M, Rosenthal MD. Differences in knee and hip adduction and hip muscle activation in runners with and without iliotibial band syndrome. *PM R*. 2018;10(10):1032–1039.
319. Brown AM, Zifchock RA, Lenhoff M, Song J, Hillstrom HJ. Hip muscle response to a fatiguing run in females with iliotibial band syndrome. *Hum Move Sci*. 2019;64:181–190.
320. Foch E, Aubol K, Milner CE. Relationship between iliotibial band syndrome and hip neuromechanics in women runners. *Gait Posture*. 2020;77:64–68.
321. Ladenhauf HN, Seitlinger G, Green DW. Osgood-Schlatter disease: a 2020 update of a common knee condition in children. *Curr Opin Pediatr*. 2020;32(1):107–112.
322. Wilson JC, Rodenberg RE Jr. "Growing" pains: apophysitis of the lower extremities. *Contempt Pediatr*. 2011;28(6):38–46.
323. Circi E, Atalay Y, Beyzadeoglu T. Treatment of Osgood-Schlatter disease: review of the literature. *Musculoskelet Surg*. 2017;101(3):195–200.
324. Blanke F, Oehler N, Al Aidarous H, Tischer T, Vogt S, Lenz R. Predictors for an unsuccessful conservative treatment of patients with medial patellar plica syndrome. *Arch Orthop Trauma Surg*. 2021;141(1):93–98.
325. Keller J. What is plica syndrome? This irritating knee issue can be hard to pinpoint but fairly simple to manage. *IDEA Fit J*. 2017;14(1):88–88.
326. Boyd CR, Eakin C, Matheson GO. Infrapatellar plica as a cause of anterior knee pain. *Clin J Sport Med*. 2005;15(2):98–103.
327. Kosaka M, Nakase J, Kitaoka K, Tsuchiya H. Arthroscopic treatment of symptomatic lateral synovial plica of the knee. *J Orthop Surg*. 2019;27(1):1–1.
328. Crosby LA, Davick JP. Managing common football injuries on the field: ankle and knee sprains most common; knees more problematic. *J Musculoskelet Med*. 2000;17(11):651–664.
329. Ryan JB, Wheeler JH, Hopkinson WJ, Arciero RA, Kolakowski KR. Quadriceps contusions: west point update. *Am J Sports Med*. 1991;19(3):299–304.
330. Torrance DA, deGraauw C. Treatment of post-traumatic myositis ossificans of the anterior thigh with extracorporeal shock wave therapy. *J Can Chiropr Assoc*. 2011;55(4):240–246.
331. Devilbiss Z, Hess M, Ho GWK. Myositis ossificans in sport: a review. *Curr Sports Med*. 2018;17(9):290–295.
332. Rossettini G, Ristori D, Testa M. Myositis ossificans: delayed complication of severe muscle contusion. *J Orthop Sports Phys Ther*. 2018;48(5):420–420.
333. Saxena SK, Dentlinger R, Siedlik E, Spangler M. Occupational prepatellar bursitis. *Consultant*. 2013;53(11):820–820.
334. Pompan DC. Pes anserine bursitis: an underdiagnosed cause of knee pain in overweight women. *Am Fam Physician*. 2016;93(3):170.
335. Baumbach S, Lobo C, Badyine I, Mutschler W, Kanz K-G. Prepatellar and olecranon bursitis: literature review and development of a treatment algorithm. *Arch Orthop Trauma Surg*. 2014;134(3):359–370.
336. Mouarbes D, Menetrey J, Marot V, Courtot L, Berard E, Cavaignac E. Anterior cruciate ligament reconstruction: a systematic review and meta-analysis of outcomes for quadriceps tendon autograft versus bone-patellar tendon-bone and hamstring-tendon autografts. *Am J Sports Med*. 2019;47(14):3531–3540.
337. Salem HS, Varzhapetyan V, Patel N, Dodson CC, Tjoumakaris FP, Freedman KB. Anterior cruciate ligament reconstruction in young female athletes: patellar versus hamstring tendon autografts. *Am J Sports Med*. 2019;47(9):2086–2092.
338. Dempsey IJ, Norte GE, Hall M, et al. Relationship between physical therapy characteristics, surgical procedure, and clinical outcomes in patients after ACL reconstruction. *J Sport Rehabil*. 2019;28(2):171–179.

11 | Hip

Betsy Myers and June Hanks

> **CHAPTER OBJECTIVES**
> After reading this chapter, you will be able to:
> 1. Describe the anatomy of the hip joint.
> 2. Describe the biomechanics of the hip joint.
> 3. Tailor the basic history of a patient with hip pathology.
> 4. Describe the components of the physical examination for a patient with hip pathology.
> 5. Describe the pathology, history, key examination findings, rehabilitation focus, and expected outcomes of common hip pathologies.
> 6. Hypothesize differential diagnoses of hip symptoms based on location, patient complaint, and onset.
> 7. Organize the physical examination of a patient with hip pathology to maximize efficiency.

FUNCTIONAL ANATOMY

The hip joint, one of the most stable joints in the body, is a ball-and-socket joint formed by the articulation of the acetabulum of the pelvis and the head of the femur. A wide range of motion is available at the hip joint: flexion/extension in the sagittal plane, abduction/adduction in the frontal plane, and medial/lateral rotation in the transverse plane. Unlike the ball-and-socket–shaped shoulder joint that functions primarily to provide a stable base for movement of the upper extremity in open-chain activities, the hip joint functions primarily as a weight-bearing joint and as a support for the head, arms, and trunk (HAT) in static and dynamic activity. Therefore, hip function should be considered when the foot is and is not in contact with the surface. During weight bearing, forces are transmitted through the foot, ankle, and knee to the hip joint. Pathology in any of these joints can impact the hip and vice versa.

Osteology

Acetabulum The acetabulum of the pelvis is formed by contributions from the ilium, ischium, and pubic bones, creating a deep socket on the lateral side of the hip bone. The acetabulum faces anteroinferiorly and is incomplete in the inferior portion at the acetabular notch. The acetabular fossa forms the central and deepest portion of the acetabulum and is nonarticular. The periphery of the acetabulum forms the lunate surface, which is covered with hyaline cartilage and articulates with the head of the femur. The acetabular labrum is a fibrocartilaginous rim attached to the outer portion of the acetabulum, serving to deepen the acetabulum.[1] Spanning the acetabular notch is the transverse acetabular ligament. More than 50% of the femoral head fits within the acetabular rim and labrum.[2,3] See Figure 11-1 for acetabulum bony structures.

Femur The proximal femur is composed of a head, neck, and shaft. The head, nearly spherical in shape, articulates with the acetabulum. Except for a small depression (fovea) for the ligament of the head of the femur, the head is covered with thick articular cartilage of varied thickness. The acetabulum and femoral head are nearly, but not completely, congruent in their articulation. The femoral neck, located between the head and the shaft, is composed of thick cortical bone, with trabecular (cancellous) bone extending from the shaft in a bundled arrangement that increases the ability of the neck to sustain bending, tensile, and compressive forces.

The proximal femoral shaft has two large bony prominences, the greater and lesser trochanters, that serve as muscular attachments. Between the trochanters is the intertrochanteric line anteriorly and the intertrochanteric crest posteriorly. The gluteal tuberosity, pectineal line, linea aspera, and quadrate tubercle are roughened areas of bone to which muscles attach to produce movement. See Figure 11-2 for bony landmarks.

Angle of Inclination

As shown in Figure 11-3, the femoral neck is angled superiorly at approximately 125° relative to the femoral shaft in the frontal plane, forming the "angle of inclination." An angle of inclination greater or less than normal is named coxa valga and coxa vara, respectively.

Angle of Femoral Neck Torsion

The femoral neck torsion angle describes the orientation of the femoral neck relative to the femoral condyles in the transverse plane.[4] Normally, the femoral

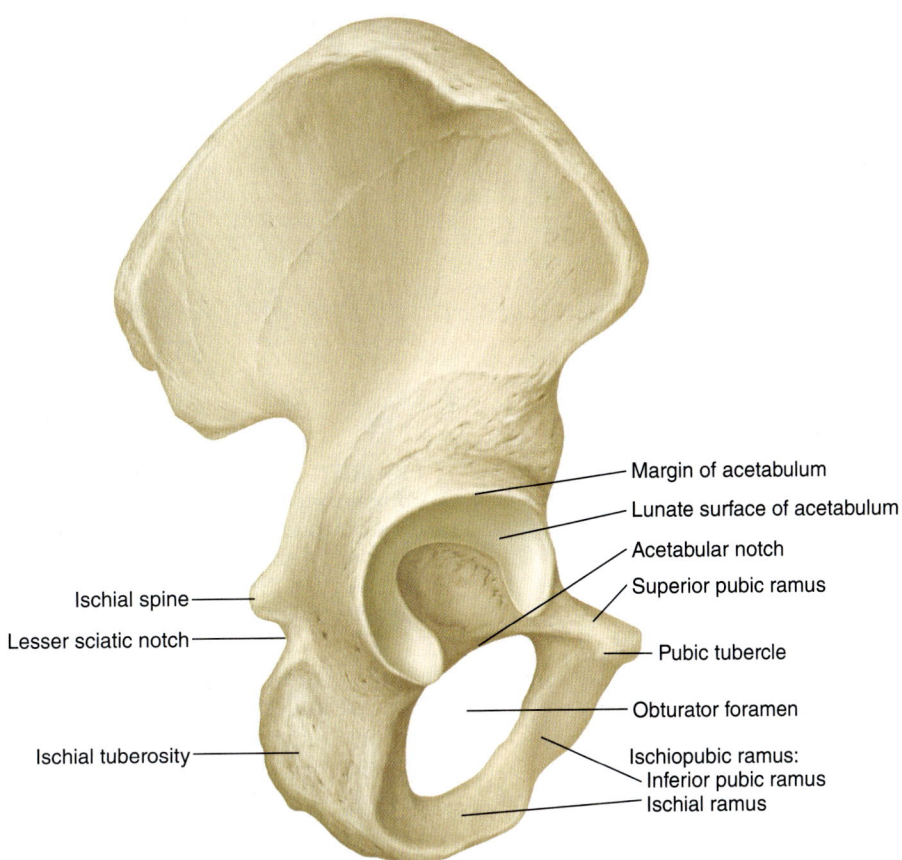

FIGURE 11-1 Bony landmarks of acetabulum. Lateral view. (Gest TR. *Lippincott Atlas of Anatomy*. 2nd ed. Wolters Kluwer; 2020: Plate 3-04.)

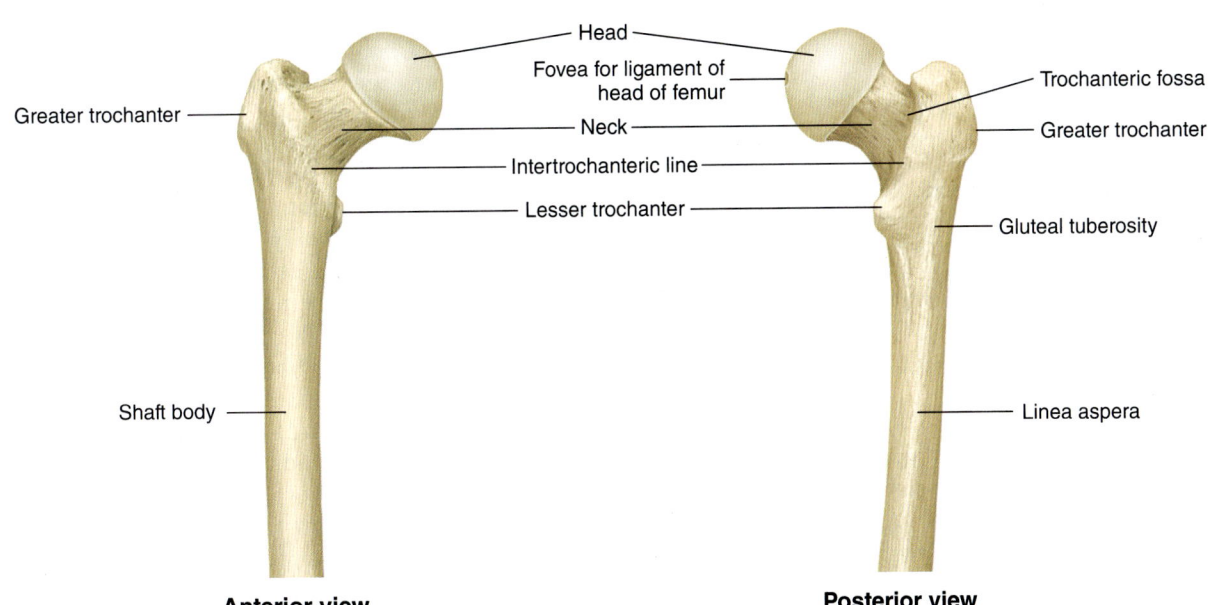

Anterior view **Posterior view**

FIGURE 11-2 Bony landmarks on proximal femur. Anterior and posterior views. (Wingerd BD. *The Human Body: Concepts of Anatomy and Physiology*. 3rd ed. Lippincott Williams & Wilkins; 2014: Figure 6.28.)

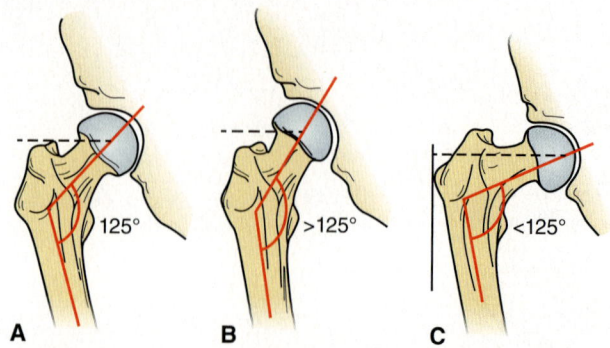

FIGURE 11-3 Orientation of femoral head and neck relative to femoral shaft, called the *angle of inclination*. **A.** The normal angle of inclination is approximately 125°. **B.** In coxa valga, the angle of inclination is greater than normal. **C.** In coxa vara, the angle of inclination is less than normal. (Adapted from Oatis CA. *Kinesiology: The Mechanics and Pathomechanics of Human Movement.* 3rd ed. Wolters Kluwer; 2017: Figures 38.16 and 38.17.)

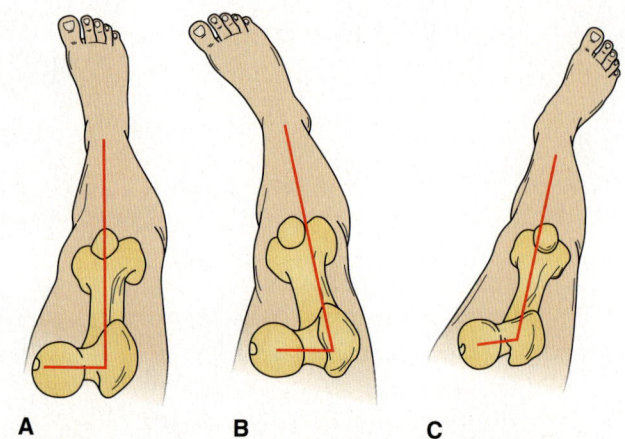

FIGURE 11-5 Craig's test. **A.** Normal hip anteversion. **B.** Uncompensated excessive anteversion resulting in an in-toed (pigeon-toed) posture. **C.** Uncompensated retroversion resulting in an out-toed posture. (Adapted from Hamill J, Knutzen KM, Derrick TR. *Biomechanical Basis of Human Movement.* 5th ed. Wolters Kluwer; 2022: Figure 6-11.)

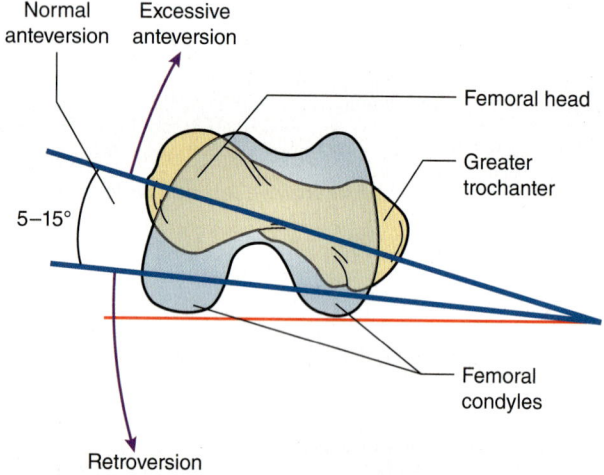

FIGURE 11-4 Superior view of the head and neck of femur with outline of femoral condyles demonstrating the normal angle of femoral torsion (anteversion of 5–15°), excessive anteversion, and retroversion. (Adapted from Oatis CA. *Kinesiology: The Mechanics and Pathomechanics of Human Movement.* 3rd ed. Wolters Kluwer; 2017: Figure 38.19.)

neck angles anteriorly at approximately 15° from the frontal plane of the shaft and is described as anteversion. The degree of anteversion decreases from approximately 30° at birth to approximately 15° in adulthood. An angle greater than 15° is described as excessive anteversion, whereas an angle less than 5° is described as retroversion (Fig. 11-4). Normal anteversion is shown in Figure 11-5A. In the case of uncompensated excessive anteversion, the head of the femur would lie anterior and outside the acetabulum, and the knees and feet would point laterally. Compensation at the hip for excessive anteversion includes medial rotation to place the femoral head in a more normal position within the acetabulum. If no additional compensation occurs, the knees face medially and the feet will adopt an in-toed (pigeon-toed) posture (Fig. 11-5B). To compensate for excessive medial hip rotation, a lateral torsion of the tibia may occur so that, in standing, the feet are pointed forward. In such a case, the knees continue to face medially, and excessive hip medial rotation and an associated reduction in hip lateral rotation will be demonstrated (refer to Craig's test).[5] Uncompensated femoral neck retroversion results in excessive lateral rotation of the femur and excessive out-toeing (Fig. 11-5C).

Joint Capsule and Ligaments

The capsule of the hip joint is attached along the bony acetabular rim proximally and to the femoral intertrochanteric line and crest distally, encapsulating the head and neck of the femur. The trochanters lie outside the joint capsule. The capsule fibers primarily run in a spiral manner, with fibers being thickest anterosuperiorly and thinnest posteroinferiorly. The thick portions of the capsule form strong intrinsic ligaments. Extension of the hip winds the capsule and ligaments tightly, drawing the femoral head into the acetabulum. The iliofemoral ligament (also called the *Y ligament*) passes anteriorly and superiorly across the hip joint and contributes most to hip joint stability by resisting hyperextension. The pubofemoral ligament runs anteroinferiorly, blending with part of the iliofemoral ligament to limit extension and abduction of the hip. The ischiofemoral ligament is located posteriorly and is the weakest of the hip ligaments.[1] Figure 11-6 illustrates hip ligaments. Deep capsular fibers pass circularly around the neck of the femur, forming a ring called the *zona orbicularis*. This orbicular ring resists distractive forces, adding to the stability of the hip joint. Multiple muscles cross the hip joint, adding to the stability.

The synovial membrane lines the interior of the capsule. Arising from the medial and lateral femoral circumflex arteries are reticular arteries that run within folds of the synovial membrane, providing blood supply to the capsule and the femoral head and neck. Though variations exist, the reticular contributions from the medial circumflex artery provide the majority of blood flow to the femoral head and neck (Fig. 11-7). Multiple branches from other arteries in the region also supply the capsule.[6] A fold in the synovium forms the ligament to the head of the femur, which attaches to the fovea of the head of the femur distally and the margins of the acetabular notch and transverse ligament proximally. The ligament transmits a small arterial branch of the obturator artery to the head of the femur. The role of the ligament in hip stability is controversial[7]; the ligament may contribute to secondary stability of the joint.[8] A malleable fat pad located within the acetabular fossa fills the remainder of the hip joint space. The fat pad deforms with movement of the hip joint to promote congruency between the acetabulum and the femoral head (Fig. 11-8).

Multiple bursae are located around the hip joint. Some bursae, such as the bursae associated with the iliopsoas and obturator externus tendons, communicate with the hip joint.[9-11] The three major bursae associated with the greater trochanteric area are greater trochanteric bursa (between the iliotibial tract and the gluteus medius and minimus), subgluteus minimus bursa (between the gluteus minimus tendon and the femur), and the subgluteus medius bursa (between the gluteus medius tendon and the femur) (Fig. 11-9).[12]

Muscles

Muscles that move the hip joint (Figs. 11-10 and 11-11) include one-joint and two-joint muscles that flex, extend, abduct, adduct, and rotate the hip. Many of the one-joint muscles crossing the hip can be divided into compartments, allowing them to participate in multiple actions. For example, the gluteus maximus is the primary extensor of the hip; however, the superior portion of the muscle also contributes to hip abduction. Along with the powerful iliacus and psoas major muscles that flex the hip, the fiber orientation of the pectineus allows contribution to hip medial rotation (along with the tensor facia latae and sartorius) and hip adduction (along with the adductor brevis, longus and magnus, and the gracilis). Although these muscles can adduct the hip, the most functional role of the adductor muscles is to stabilize the pelvis and leg during the stance and swing phases of gait. The main hip abductors are the gluteus

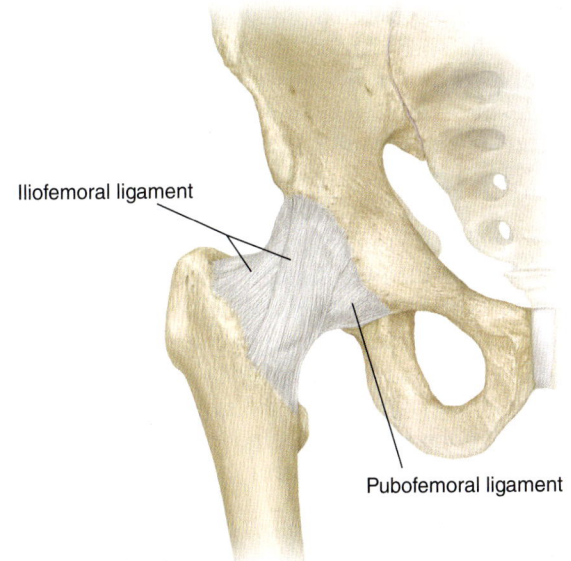
Anterior view

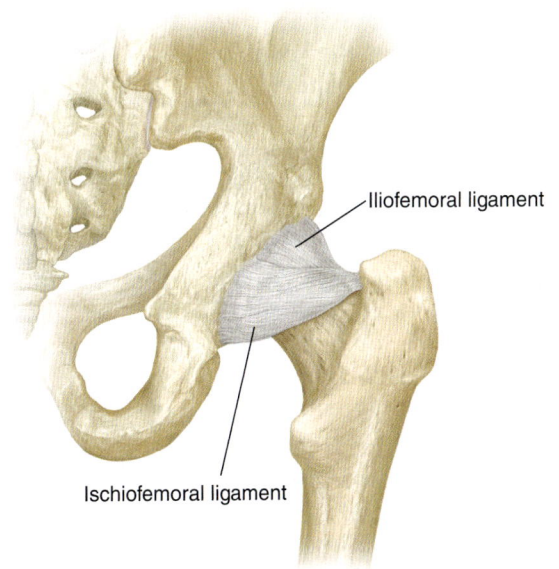
Posterior view

FIGURE 11-6 Ligaments of the hip reinforcing the hip joint capsule. (Gest TR. *Lippincott Atlas of Anatomy*. 2nd ed. Wolters Kluwer; 2020: Plate 3-54.)

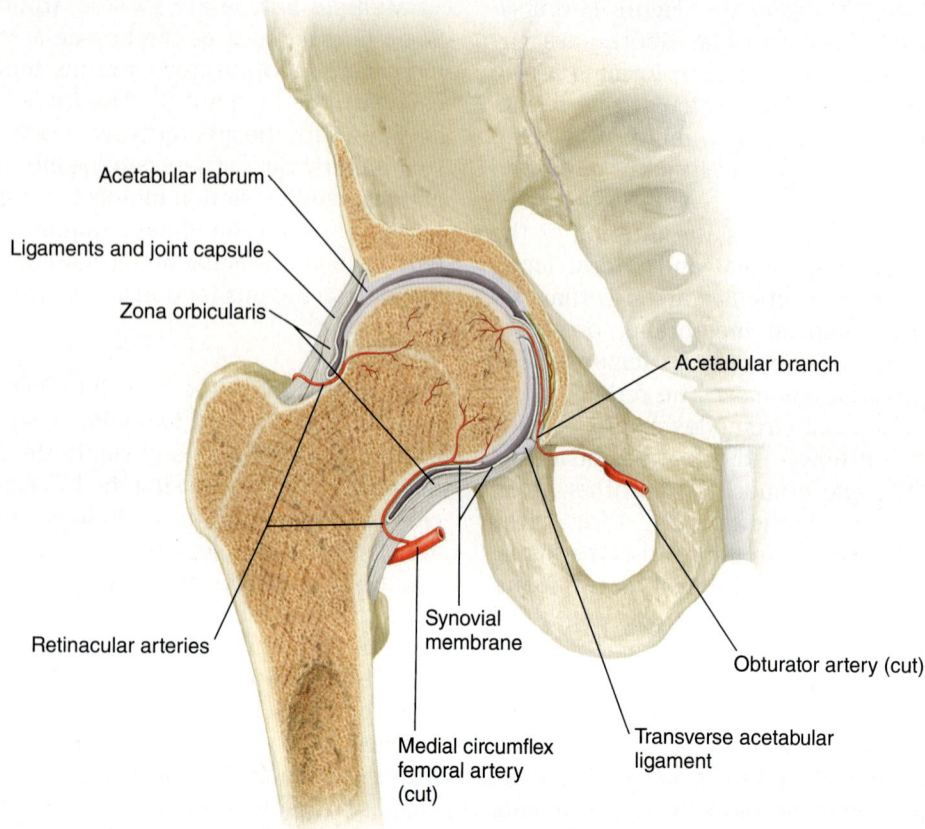

FIGURE 11-7 Joint capsule and blood supply to hip joint. (Gest TR. *Lippincott Atlas of Anatomy*. 2nd ed. Wolters Kluwer; 2020: Plate 3-55B.)

medius and minimus and the two-joint muscles, tensor facia latae, and sartorius. See Table 11-1 for details on actions of muscles on the hip. Several muscles around the hip have a different action or strength of contribution to action when they contract from a position other than the anatomic position.

Palpation

Bony palpation of the hip region includes the identification of major landmarks on the pelvis and proximal femur to include the following:

- Pelvis (anterior aspect): iliac crest, iliac tubercle, anterior superior iliac spine (ASIS), pubic tubercle
- Pelvis (posterior aspect): posterior superior iliac spine (PSIS), ischial tuberosity
- Proximal femur: greater trochanter

During palpation, the patient may either lie down or stand, with some portion of the palpation occurring in standing to allow for assessment of the impact of weight bearing. The description here is of anterior palpation during standing. While facing the patient, the clinician should place the hands on either side of the patient's waist and slide the hands downward so that the fingers are wrapped around the iliac crest and the thumbs are on the anterior portion of the iliac crests. The widest portion of the anterior part of the iliac crest is the iliac tubercle. Sliding the thumbs downward along the iliac crest just distal to the iliac tubercle, the ASIS can be felt, particularly in thin individuals. While the thumbs are in place on the ASIS on each side, the clinician moves the fingers inferiorly from the iliac crest and iliac tubercles to the proximal femur. The posterior aspect of the large greater trochanter on the proximal femur can be felt. With the fingers on the greater trochanter, the clinician moves the thumbs medially and slightly inferiorly to palpate the pubic tubercles located on the lateral sides of the pubic crest. For examination of the posterior aspect of the hip region, the patient may stand facing away from the clinician or may be in sidelying with the hip flexed. The PSISs are easily palpated under the dimples just above the patient's buttocks. Moving the fingers from the PSIS anteriorly and superiorly, the edge of the iliac crest can be felt. With the thumb on the PSIS, the fingers can be moved laterally along the proximal femur to palpate the posterior aspect of the greater trochanter. The ischial tuberosity is located in the middle of the buttock and can be palpated as the clinician

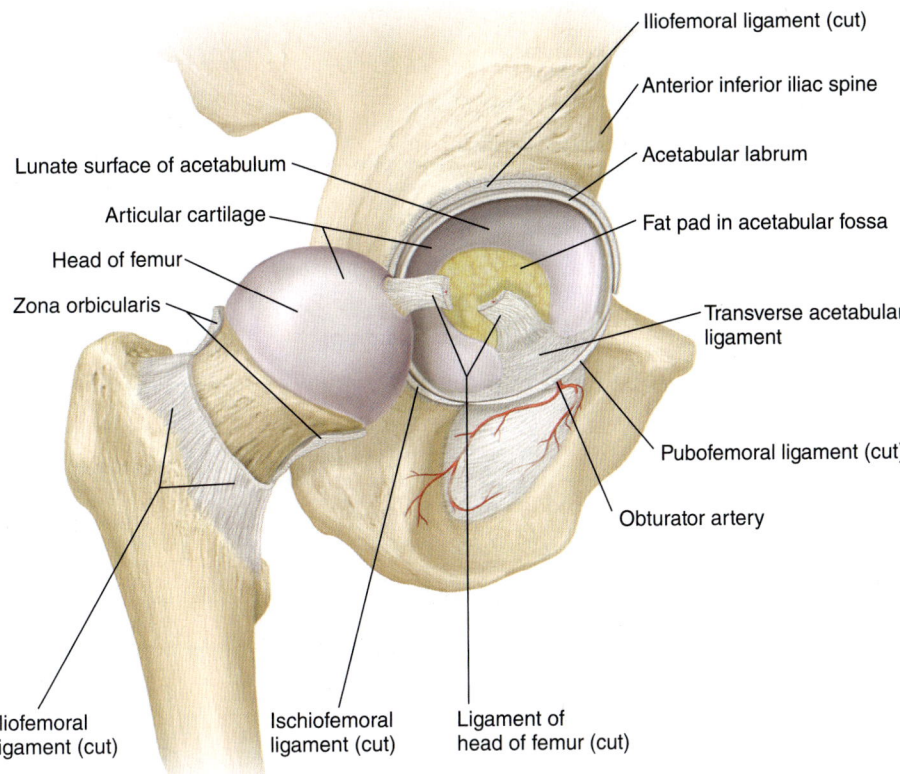

FIGURE 11-8 Internal view of hip joint with ligaments cut and femur rotated laterally to expose the ligament to the head of the femur, the acetabulum, and fat pad of the acetabular fossa. (Gest TR. *Lippincott Atlas of Anatomy*. 2nd ed. Wolters Kluwer; 2020: Plate 3-55A.)

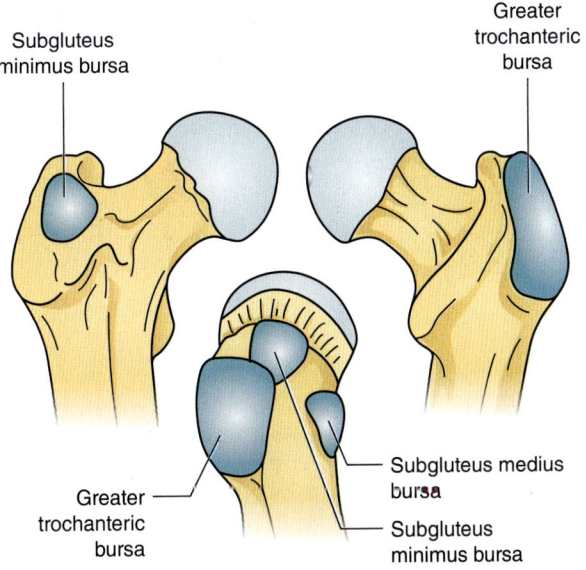

FIGURE 11-9 Major bursae of the greater trochanteric area of the hip joint. (Adapted from Oatis CA. *Kinesiology: The Mechanics and Pathomechanics of Human Movement*. 3rd ed. Wolters Kluwer; 2017:Figure 38.16.)

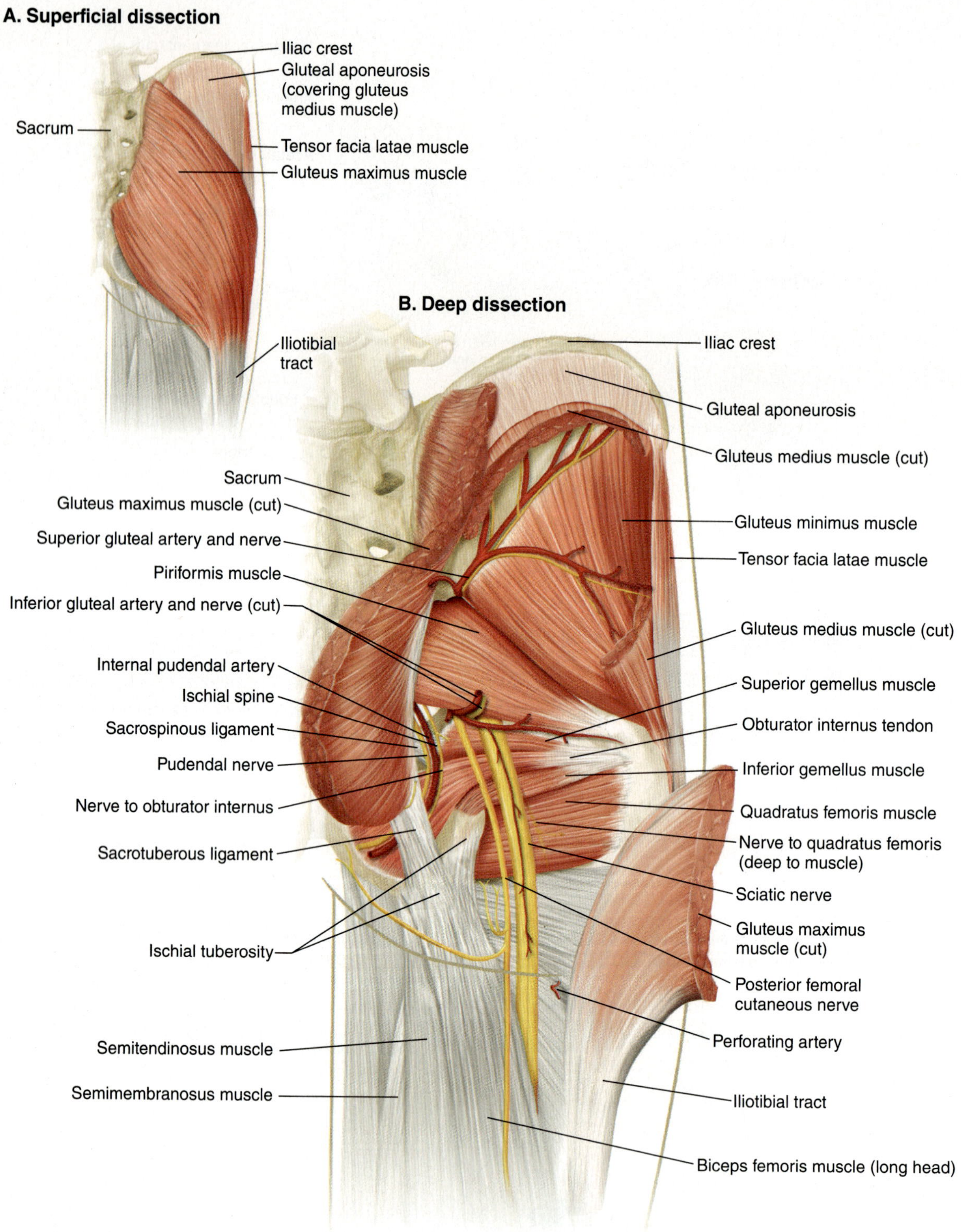

FIGURE 11-10 Muscles contributing to movement of the hip joint. Posterior view. **A.** Superficial. **B.** Deep. (Gest TR. *Lippincott Atlas of Anatomy*. 2nd ed. Wolters Kluwer; 2020: Plate 3-26A, B.)

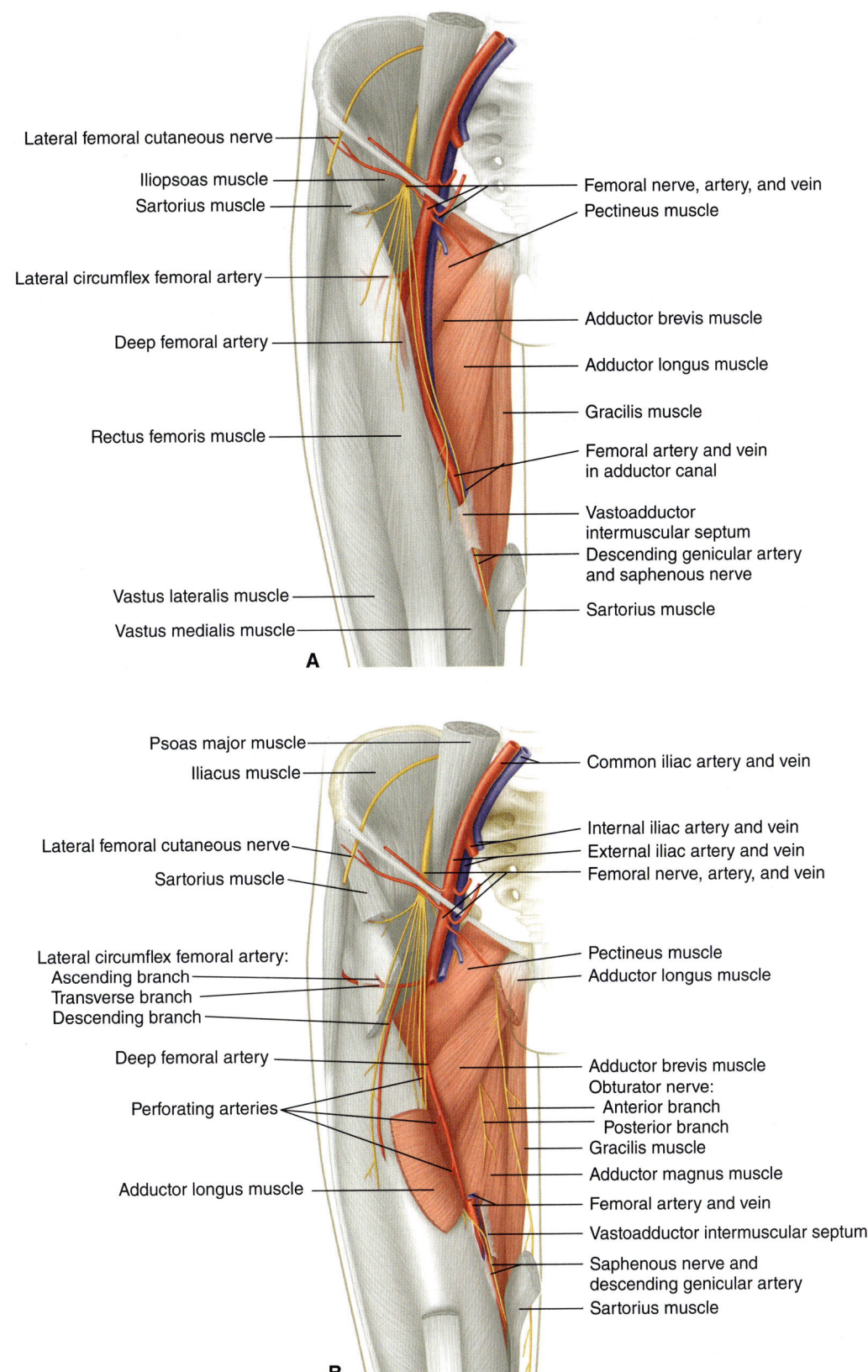

FIGURE 11-11 Muscles contributing to movement of the hip joint. Anterior view. **A.** Superficial. **B.** Intermediate. (Gest TR. *Lippincott Atlas of Anatomy*. 2nd ed. Wolters Kluwer; 2020: Plates 3-19 and 3-20.)

TABLE 11-1 ACTIONS OF MUSCLES OF THE HIP

Action	Muscles
Flexion of hip	Psoas major Iliacus Pectineus Rectus femoris Sartorius Adductor brevis Adductor magnus (anterior [adductor part]) Gracilis Gluteus minimus (anterior fibers)
Extension of hip	Gluteus maximus Biceps femoris (long head) Semimembranosus Semitendinosus Gluteus medius (posterior part) Adductor magnus (posterior [hamstrings] part)
Abductors of hip	Gluteus medius Gluteus minimus Tensor facia latae Sartorius Gluteus maximus (superior part) Piriformis Obturator internus Superior and inferior gemelli
Adductors of hip	Adductor longus Adductor brevis Adductor magnus (adductor part) Gracilis Pectineus
Medial rotation of hip	Tensor facia latae Pectineus Gracilis Adductor longus Adductor brevis Adductor magnus Gluteus medius (anterior part) Gluteus minimus (anterior part)

Modified from Neuman DA. *Kinesology of the Musculoskeletal System: Foundations for Rehabilitation*. 3rd ed. Elsevier; 2017; Moore KL, Dalley AF, Agur AMR. *Clinically Oriented Anatomy*. 8th ed. Wolters Kluwer; 2018; Magee DJ. *Orthopedic Physical Assessment*. 5th ed. Saunders/Elsevier; 2008.

keeps the fingers on the greater trochanter and moves the thumbs toward the middle of the buttocks while the patient flexes the hip. In this position of hip flexion, the ischial tuberosity is more easily identified.

From this posterior position, the clinician can begin palpation of the muscle groups surrounding the hip joint. The gluteus maximus can be felt posteriorly as a large muscle mass between the attachments on the sacrum, coccyx, and ischial tuberosity to the femur. The gluteus maximum is most prominent and easy to identify when the patient is prone and squeezes the buttocks together. The hamstrings (HSs) can be palpated at their attachment to the ischial tuberosity. The hip abductors, primarily the gluteus medius, can be felt with the patient in sidelying with the uppermost leg raised in slight abduction. With the patient supine, the adductor muscle group can be palpated on the medial thigh. The most superficial and easily palpable of this group is the adductor longus that passes from the pubic bone to the femur. With the leg positioned in abduction and external rotation, the adductor longus forms a distinct cordlike ridge near the proximal attachment to the pubic bone. The sartorius can be palpated near its proximal attachment to the ASIS. The iliopsoas and rectus femoris muscles are not easily palpated.

BIOMECHANICS
Hip Joint Stability

The hip joint is one of the most stable joints in the body due to the orientation of bony structures, spiraling arrangement of ligaments, deep acetabular socket, and the negative pressure within the joint.[13] The head of the femur has substantially more articular surface area than the acetabulum. In standing, the femoral articular surface area is exposed anteriorly and slightly superiorly. The articular contact between the femur and the acetabulum is increased in a position of flexion, abduction, and slight lateral rotation. The close-packed position of the hip is one of combined full extension, slight abduction, and slight medial rotation. There is very minimal joint play in this position, and the combined movements constituting this close-packed position can be used to stretch most of the joint capsule at once.[14] The open-packed position of the hip joint (flexion, abduction, and lateral rotation) is, unlike other joints, the position in which the articular surfaces are most congruent (rather than least congruent). The joint capsule and ligamentous structures are the most lax in this open-packed position, and such a posture is commonly assumed when trauma or inflammation is present.[15]

The hip joint is at highest risk of traumatic dislocation when in a position of flexion (ligaments lax), abduction, and internal rotation. For example, when the knees strike the dashboard in a vehicle accident, force exerted through the femoral shaft may cause dislocation as the head of the femur is forced out of the acetabulum inferiorly and posteriorly where the capsule is weakest. Anterior dislocation of the hip is not common but may occur when the hip joint is forced into extension, abduction, and lateral rotation. Commonly, a fracture of the acetabulum occurs with hip dislocations, producing a fracture dislocation.[3]

Osteokinematics

Hip joint motions of flexion/extension, abduction/adduction, and medial/lateral rotation can be viewed as movement of the femur on the pelvis or movement of the pelvis on the femur, depending on whether the proximal or distal lever arm moves. When the concave femoral head rotates within the relatively fixed acetabulum of the pelvis (i.e., the distal lever moves), the femur can move into flexion to at least 120° with additional flexion gained as the deep fibers of the posterior and inferior capsular ligaments are stretched. A small degree of posterior tilting of the pelvis occurs along with flexion of the lumbar spine at the extreme of full passive hip flexion. With the knee extended, the hip can be passively flexed to approximately 70 to 80° depending on the flexibility of the HSs muscle group. The hip can be extended approximately 20° beyond a neutral position. Hip extension is reduced with the knee flexed due to tension in the rectus femoris that crosses both the hip and the knee. Abduction of the hip is limited to approximately 40° by the length of the adductor muscles and the inferior joint ligaments. Hip adduction is limited to about 25° by passive tension in the abductors of the hip and the iliotibial band (ITB). Hip rotation varies considerably among individuals, but is generally 35 to 45° in medial rotation[16] and 45° in lateral rotation.[17]

Arthrokinematics

The constrained articulation between the nearly spherical femoral head in the acetabulum allows for minimal translation between the articular forces. The hip arthrokinematics follow the concave-convex pattern of movement with some spin throughout movement.

Motion of the Hip Joint

In weight bearing, the femur is relatively fixed, and motion at the hip joint occurs through movement of the pelvis on the femur. As such, the distal segment is fixed, and the proximal segment moves. In many other joints, the reversal of motion created by movement of the distal versus proximal segment is easily understood. For example, in sitting with the foot free to move, knee extension occurs as the tibia (distal segment) moves on the fixed femur (proximal segment). Knee extension also occurs with movement of the femur on the tibia when one moves from a seated position to upright standing. However, to describe movement of the pelvis on the fixed femur, terms relating to tilt and rotation of the pelvis are required. In addition, the head and trunk will move relative to the motion of the pelvis, with compensatory motions occurring at the lumbar spine. Terms and definitions are provided as follows:

- **Anterior/posterior pelvic tilt**: motion of the pelvis in the sagittal plane about a frontal plane axis; associated with hip flexion/extension and lumbar extension/flexion, respectively
- **Lateral pelvic tilt (pelvic hike/pelvic drop)**: motion of the pelvis in the frontal plane about an anteroposterior axis. In right limb stance, as pelvis drops on the left, the right hip adducts and lumbar spine moves in right lateral flexion; as pelvis hikes on the left, the right hip abducts and lumbar spine moves in left lateral flexion.
- **Pelvic rotation (translation)**: Motion of the pelvis in the transverse plane about a vertical axis

Anterior/Posterior Pelvic Tilt ASISs of the pelvis lie on a vertical line with the pubic symphysis. The movements of an anterior and posterior pelvic tilt occur as the pelvis moves in the sagittal plane on the fixed femur, producing hip flexion and extension, respectively. In an anterior pelvic tilt, the ASIS of the pelvis moves inferiorly and posteriorly, moving the sacrum farther away from the femur, causing hip flexion. Hip extension through posterior pelvic tilting occurs as the pubic symphysis is moved superiorly and the sacrum moves closer to the femur. The lumbar spine moves in a compensatory extension with an anterior pelvic tilt and compensatory flexion with a posterior pelvic tilt.

Lateral Pelvic Tilt A lateral pelvic tilt occurs in the frontal plane as one side of the pelvis drops inferiorly whereas the other side moves upward (pelvic hike). In unilateral stance, hiking of the opposite pelvis produces hip abduction on the stance limb side, whereas dropping of the opposite pelvis produces hip adduction on the stance limb side. Note that in the naming convention of levers, the motion of the end of the lever farthest from the joint is referenced. For example, in right leg standing, hiking of the pelvis is a movement in which the left pelvis rises; likewise, dropping of the pelvis is a movement in which the left pelvis drops. Compensatory lumbar spine movement is one of right lateral flexion with left pelvis drop and left lateral flexion with left pelvis hike. In bilateral weight bearing, a lateral tilt of the pelvis to one side or the other results in pelvic shifting. While maintaining weight bearing through both limbs, the pelvis cannot hike but rather can only drop. Shifting the pelvis to the right results in a drop of the left side of the pelvis, abduction of the left hip, and adduction of the right hip. The opposite is observed in bilateral stance when the pelvis is shifted to the left.

Pelvic Rotation Forward-and-backward rotation of the pelvis occurs in the transverse plane. In bilateral stance, the pelvic rotation occurs around a vertical axis through the middle of the pelvis. In single limb stance, the pelvic rotation occurs around the vertical axis of the stance side hip. In forward pelvic rotation, the side of the pelvis opposite the stance side hip moves forward (anteriorly) through space. This movement produces medial rotation at the stance side hip. Backward rotation occurs when the side of the pelvis opposite the stance side hip moves backward (posteriorly), creating lateral rotation at the stance side hip. In describing pelvic rotation in bilateral stance, care must be taken to clearly describe movements while referencing a specific side. For example, consider observation of walking from a side view, using the right limb as the reference limb. During swing phase on the right (as a person is in left limb stance), the pelvis moves anteriorly on the right, demonstrating right forward rotation. During right limb stance, the left pelvis will be in forward rotation (though some may erroneously describe the right pelvis as rotating backward). The meticulous choice of appropriate terms will help minimize confusion and inaccurate interpretations.

Closed-Chain Movement

As noted previously, the femur, pelvis, and spine move in a coordinated manner and are thereby able to produce a larger motion than is available by one component alone. In closed-chain activities, both ends of a movement segment are fixed, whereas in open-chain movement, one end of the segment is free to move. During weight bearing in which both feet are in contact with the supporting surface, a "closed chain" is described as being formed from one foot, up through the pelvis, and down through the other foot. The chain is closed because both feet are fixed; movement at any one segment of the chain affects movement at another. It should be noted that weight bearing and the term "closed chain" should not be used interchangeably. When one is in standing and bends forward to touch the toes, the feet are "fixed" and coordinated and related movement occurs between the pelvis, femurs, knees, and feet. However, to be a "true closed chain," the head would need to be "fixed" because the head and trunk can move. In this case, the head is often considered "functionally fixed" rather than "structurally fixed" because the head can move in space but more commonly remains upright and vertical during upright tasks. The neurologic system drives this functional fixation of the head, keeping the head relatively oriented over the sacrum. With these considerations, a "functional closed chain" is formed in which movement of a joint in the chain is accompanied by a counteracting movement in another part of the chain to keep the body stable over the base of support. Motions of the pelvis and hip joint are accompanied by compensatory motions of the lumbar spine to assist with the maintenance of balance within the functional closed chain.[18]

Hip Joint Forces

When standing with equal weight bearing through the lower extremities, weight is evenly distributed between both legs and the superimposed weight of the HAT is transmitted to the hips through the sacroiliac joints and the pelvis. The weight of the HAT is approximately two-thirds of total body weight, whereas the lower extremities contribute roughly one-third of body weight. The weight of the HAT is distributed such that each femoral head receives approximately half of the superimposed weight. The joint axis of each femoral head is of equal distance from the line of gravity; thus, the gravitational moment for each hip is the same. The rotary force around each hip is the same but in opposite directions, and the pelvis is maintained in a relatively level position (Fig. 11-12A). In unilateral stance, the weight of HAT and nonstance limb is superimposed on the weight-bearing hip; that is, the magnitude of body weight compressing the stance side hip significantly increases as one moves from bilateral to unilateral stance. In addition, the stance side hip is subjected to significant rotary forces, with a tendency for the nonstance side pelvis to drop. To keep the pelvis level, this rotary moment must be countered by the hip abductors on the weight-bearing side (Fig. 11-12B). Owing to the changing in lever arm, the hip abductors must act with a force that is approximately two to three times the body weight. Thus, during the stance phase of the normal gait cycle, the vertical forces acting at the femoral head are substantial. If the abductors are not strong enough to counter the forces tending to rotate or tilt the pelvis downward to the opposite side, this often results in one of two abnormal gait patterns. In one case, described as a Trendelenburg gait pattern, the pelvis will drop noticeably to the side opposite of the weakness, usually resulting in a short swing phase on the side to which the pelvis is dropping. Alternately, the person may walk with a "compensated" Trendelenburg gait pattern that involves leaning the trunk laterally toward the side of weakness during stance phase on that side. Such compensation shifts the center of gravity toward the femoral head of the weight-bearing side (fulcrum), reducing the moment arm about which the forces from the body weight may act and thereby reducing the necessary force required by the abductors. Such a gait pattern is often seen in patients with painful hip conditions, such as degenerative joint disease, in which there is some weakness of the abductors and for which it is desirable to reduce compressive forces acting at the joint for relief of pain. A cane may be used in the hand opposite to the side of weakness or pain to decrease the need for a lateral trunk lean (Fig. 11-12C). For example, if the right hip is painful, the use of a cane on the left side provides support for the left side such that compressive forces

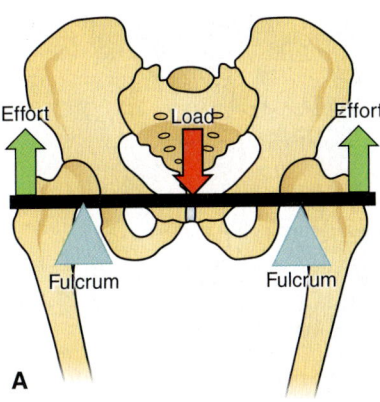
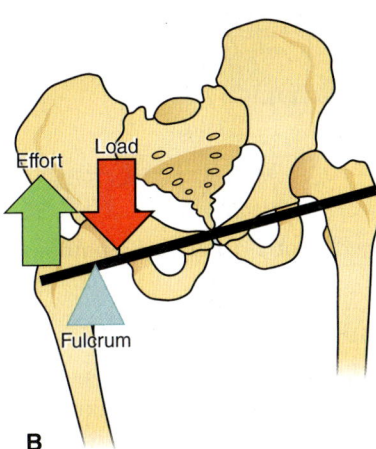
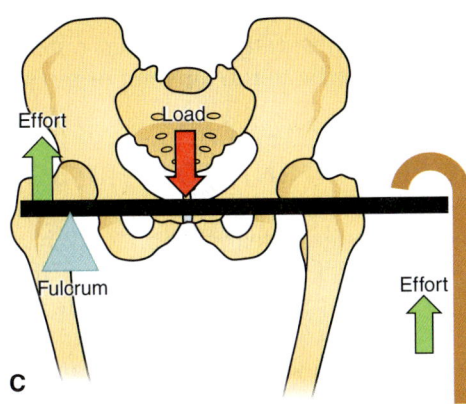

FIGURE 11-12 Forces at the hip during bilateral, unilateral, and supported stance (with a cane). The effort of the abductor musculature is demonstrated in *green*, the fulcrum is *blue*, the lever arm is *black*, and the load is *red*. **A.** Bilateral stance with equal weight bearing through the hips. **B.** Unilateral stance on the right side. Note increased load through right hip with higher force production required by hip abductors. The increased compressive load causing pain is associated with hip pathology. **C.** A cane placed in the hand opposite the painful weight-bearing hip allows weight and compressive forces passing through the painful hip to be reduced. In this example, the right hip is the painful or weak hip; the cane provides support throughout weight bearing on the right side. (Adapted from Nordin M, Frankel VH. *Basic Biomechanics of the Musculoskeletal System.* 5th ed. Wolters Kluwer; 2022: Figure 8-15.)

acting through the right hip are decreased, thereby reducing pain.

INTRODUCTION TO THE EXAMINATION OF THE HIP

The hip joint is derived from segments L2–S1. However, pain of hip joint origin is predominantly perceived in the L3 segment. Therefore, hip joint pain may be perceived in the hip joint, the groin, anterior thigh, or even the knee. Interestingly, nearly half of patients with hip osteoarthritis (OA) report not only local hip pain but also their pain extends below the knee, following the distribution pattern of the saphenous nerve.[19]

PATIENT HISTORY: HIP JOINT

A patient interview designed to elicit specific information related to the patient's health history and demographics, symptoms, and review of systems should be conducted (refer to Chapter 6, Patient History). The clinician must understand the patient's symptoms and determine the acuity, severity, irritability, stability, and functional implications of the patient's condition. The general concepts that apply to information that may be elicited when interviewing patients with common hip disorders are explained in the subsequent section. Additional questions may be required based on the nature of the specific disorder. Limb dominance may be applicable for athletes.

History of Back or Lower Extremity Pathology

As noted previously, patients should be asked if they have had prior ankle, knee, or hip injuries or surgeries on either lower extremity because of the effect each joint in a kinetic chain can have on the others. The hip is also biomechanically linked to the spine. Therefore, clinicians must also ask the patient about any current or prior back pathology. Low back disorders may mimic hip disease and vice versa because of the segmental relationships. Hip dysfunction often leads to back problems, and the reverse can also occur because of the biomechanical relationships between the two-joint complexes. Therefore, clinicians must determine whether a patient has hip pathology or back pathology or both.[20] When hip and spine pathologies co-mingle, this is referred to as *hip-spine syndrome* and is discussed further in Chapter 12, Lumbar Spine and Sacroiliac Joint.

Review of Systems

The review of symptoms is particularly important when performing a history on patients with suspected hip or spine pathology because of the potential for visceral pathology to create symptoms in the hip and trunk region. Clinicians should ask patients with suspected hip pathology questions regarding constitutional symptoms and the gastrointestinal and genitourinary systems (see Table 6.11 in Chapter 6, Patient History).[21] Given the anatomic connection between the deep hip external rotators and the pelvic floor, clinicians should specifically query patients with hip pathology about urinary continence.[22]

Onset

Understanding the mechanism of onset of hip symptoms can help with developing diagnostic hypotheses. Fracture may need to be considered in patients who report a history of a fall. Similarly, an onset of symptoms after a twisting motion increases the likelihood of a labral injury. In contrast, a nontraumatic onset, particularly in an older individual, would be more suggestive of OA. Overuse injuries, strains, and sprains should be considered in individuals who are active in recreational or sports activities.

Location of Symptoms

Patients should be asked if they can point to the location of symptoms using one finger. Lateral hip pain near the greater trochanter is suggestive of greater trochanteric pain syndrome (GTPS).[17] Patients with intra-articular hip pathology, such as osteoarthritis or labral pathology, generally note their pain is "in their hip" and use what is commonly referred to as a "C" sign (Fig. 11-13). Groin pain is common in individuals with degenerative joint disease, femoroacetabular impingement syndrome (FAIS), and labral tears.[21] Muscle strains and tendinopathy are common in the hip region and are generally easy to identify based on the location and onset of symptoms. In some instances, such as **slipped capital femoral epiphysis (SCFE)**, a disorder in which the growth plate of the femoral head moves ("slips") relative to the rest of the femur, the pain may be felt primarily in the knee.[23] Pain felt in the buttock, particularly if it spreads to the lateral or posterior thigh, is more suggestive of pain of spinal origin.[21] Although sacroiliac and pelvic dysfunction are far less common than either back or hip pathology, clinicians should keep in mind that pathology in these regions may also refer pain to the hip region.

Chief Complaint

Honing down the patient's symptoms helps clinicians develop preliminary hypotheses to test during the physical examination. Patients with hip pathology may report symptoms such as pain, stiffness, catching, snapping, instability, or weakness. Morning stiffness and difficulty donning/doffing socks and shoes are common complaints for individuals with degenerative joint disease,[24] whereas catching or locking is more common with labral pathology.[21]

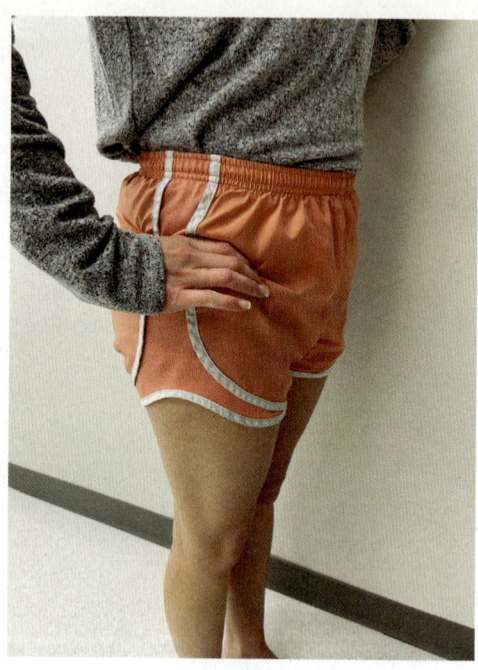

FIGURE 11-13 C sign for intra-articular hip pathology.

Outcome Measures

The Patient-Specific Function Scale (see Chapter 6, Patient History), Lower Extremity Function Scale (see Chapter 9, Ankle and Foot), and the WOMAC (see Chapter 10, Knee) introduced previously might be applicable for patients with hip pathology. The clinician should also consider patient-reported outcome measures that are specific to the hip joint or hip pathology (Table 11-2).

PHYSICAL EXAMINATION: HIP JOINT

The physical examination is composed of the systems review, quarter screen, clearing examination, and joint-specific examination. The examination of the patient with suspected hip pathology must include a complete lower quarter neurologic screen to clear the lumbar spine or determine whether the lumbar spine may also be involved in the patient's condition. However, the clinician must first consider if there are any red flags, such as potential proximal femur ("hip") fracture. There is no standard, such as the Ottawa ankle rules, to guide clinicians in identifying which patients would benefit from imaging. However, clinical practice and expert opinion suggest screening for hip fracture considering the following:

- Presence of a high-risk event (e.g., fall, bike accident)
- Patient risk factors for fracture (e.g., older, osteoporetic, taking corticosteroids)
- Constant pain that increases with weight bearing and typically require an assistive device to walk
- Limb appears shortened and/or externally rotated
- Positive log roll test (see Fig. 11-26)

TABLE 11-2
COMMON OUTCOME TOOLS FOR PATIENTS WITH HIP PATHOLOGY

Tool	Tool Basics
WOMAC	• Addresses lower level global lower extremity function • Scoring: 0–96 • 24 items rated 0–4, with higher scores indicating worse pain/function • 3 scales: pain (5 questions), stiffness (2 questions), and function (17 questions) • Points are summed and converted to a percentage • MCID varies based on population, for hip pathology ranging from 8 to 11[130] • Common diagnoses: hip/knee degenerative joint disease, total knee/hip replacement, rheumatoid arthritis
Harris Hip Score and Modified Harris Hip Score	• Addresses lower level global lower extremity function • Scoring: 1–100 points • Higher scores represent higher quality of life • 10 items for pain, functional activities, and motion • MCID: 2.44 points[131] • Scores < 70 are considered fair, >90 excellent • Ceiling effects likely with younger populations and common with patients with hip arthroplasty[132] • Common diagnoses: hip degenerative joint disease, hip fracture, total hip replacement
Hip Outcome Score	• Addresses a variety of weight-bearing activities • Scoring: items rated 0–4, with greater scores indicating higher function • ADL subscale has 19 items addressing things such as sitting and donning socks • Sports subscale has 9 items including running, rotational tasks, and jumping • MCID: 9 points for the ADL subscale, 6 points for the sports subscale • Common diagnoses: labral tear, hip arthroscopy, conservatively treated hip pain
SF-36	• Holistic survey of patient's healthy, function, and roles • 36 items rated 0–100, with higher scores indicating greater function • 7 domains: pain, function, role limitation, general health, mental health, vitality, social function • An abbreviated version, the SF-12, is less precise but more efficient to use • Common diagnoses: hip/knee replacement, arthritis
HAOGS (Hip and Groin Outcome Score)	• Addresses higher level lower extremity function • Scoring: 0–100 • 6 subscales related to pain, symptoms, daily activities, sport and recreation, participation, and quality of life • MDC: 18–34 points[133] • Common diagnoses: young adults with hip and groin pain, labral tears, femoroacetabular impingement

ADL, activities of daily living; *MCID*, minimal clinically important difference; *MDC*, minimal detectable change.

The knee should be cleared by performing overpressure to passive knee flexion and extension as well as manual muscle testing (MMT) of the quadriceps and HSs.

Structure

The clinician should observe the patient's general structure and posture in standing (see Table 8-1 in Chapter 8, Lower Quarter Screen) and sitting. Effusion in the hip is neither visible nor palpable. However, local edema can be seen and palpated in the case of trochanteric bursitis. Gluteal muscular atrophy is common in patients with hip OA[25] and may be visible.

Leg Length Discrepancy Several methods to determine leg length discrepancy have been proposed. Historically, the most common being the supine tape measure method, which has been found to be highly unreliable and, therefore, is no longer recommended.[26] The clinician can assess leg length in standing by comparing the left and right iliac crest heights and popliteal angles. If a discrepancy is noted, the clinician can place shims (or blocks) of known heights under the patient's shorter side. The shim method (Fig. 11-14) is the most functional position and reliable clinical assessment for limb length.[27,28] The shim method also takes into account the functional compensations for

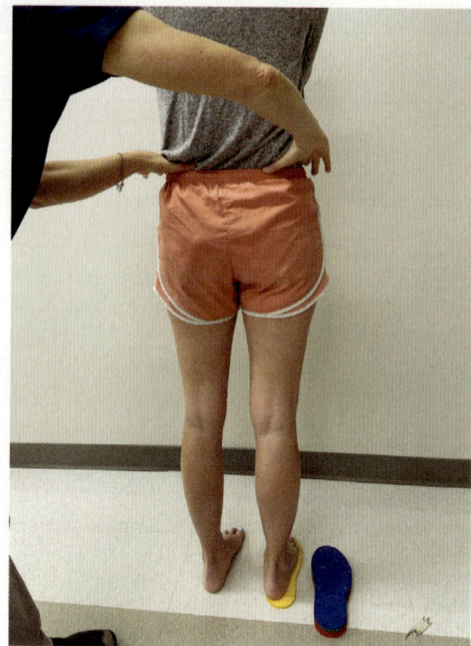

FIGURE 11-14 Shim method to assess leg length discrepancy.

leg length inequalities that may appear over time, with the patient pronating the longer side and/or supinating the shorter side. Because the shim method relies on palpation of landmarks, the test is likely to be less accurate on individuals with significant amounts of soft tissue. Leg length inequalities more than 1 cm are more likely to be identified[26] and functionally relevant.

Femoral Torsion The clinician should use Craig's test to assess femoral torsion (Fig. 11-15).

Interpretation: Normal femoral torsion is 8 to 15° of internal rotation.
Anteversion is if the hip angle is greater than 15°.
Retroversion is if the hip angle is less than 8°.

Patients with femoral anteversion will generally have excessive hip internal rotation and limited hip external rotation, leaving the total arc of motion the same. Conversely, patients with femoral retroversion will generally have excessive hip external rotation and limited hip internal rotation. It is important to identify this structural deviation and respect the patient's structural differences. For example, when standing, a patient with femoral anteversion would naturally stand with the patella and feet facing inward as this coincides with the neutral hip position. Requesting this patient perform barbell squats, for example, with toes facing forward would actually place the hip in suboptimal alignment and may cause symptoms immediately or later on.

Tibia and Femur Length If it is important to identify where the limb length inequality stems from, assessment of the relative lengths of the femurs and tibias can be performed in hooklying supine (Fig. 11-16). This may also be important in narrow cases such as a cyclist where having differing femurs or tibias lengths can create knee pain due to the inability to obtain an appropriate seat height for both limbs without changing the bike geometry (such as crank arm length).

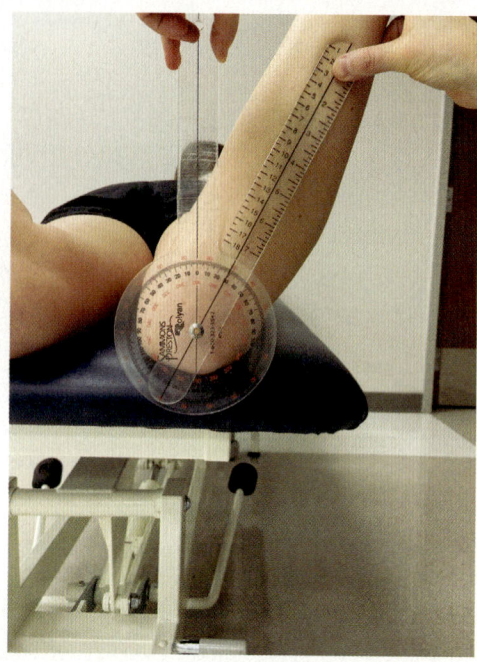

FIGURE 11-15 Assessment of femoral torsion (Craig's test). With the greater trochanter positioned most laterally, the patient's hip is 28° internally rotated indicating femoral anteversion.

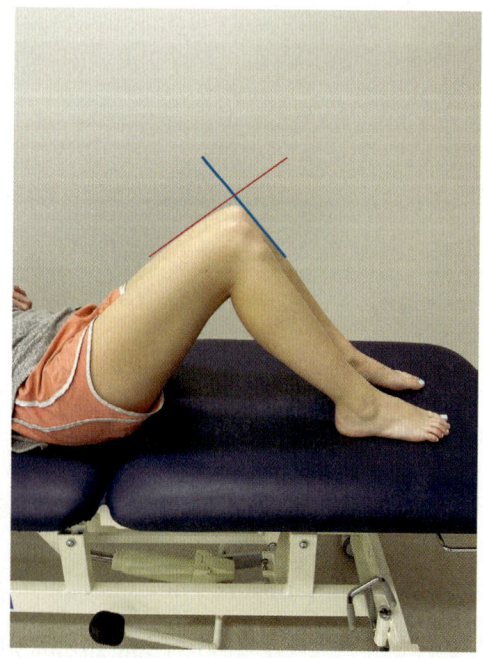

FIGURE 11-16 Assessment of relative lengths of the tibia and femur is performed by comparing the heights of the distal femurs (red line) and patellar position (blue line), respectively.

Skin

The integumentary scan of patients with hip pathology is generally noncontributory. However, because local or deep space infection can occur after hip surgery, all incisions and scars should be inspected for signs of infection, such as redness, drainage, local edema or fluctuance, and increased temperature.

Range of Motion

Active and passive hip motions should be assessed and compared with the American Academy of Orthopaedic Surgeons (AAOS) normative values (Table 11-3).[29,30] Hip rotation should also be measured in prone because this is a more functional position for gait. The clinician should note the end feel and any changes in patient symptoms. Normal hip end feels are capsular. However, the end feel for hip flexion may be soft-tissue approximation for patients who are obese or bony for those who are underweight. A firm end feel to flexion or abduction may indicate the presence of a bony block, such as a cam or pincer lesion. A labral tear may create a springy end feel.

A capsular pattern of restriction for the hip is as follows:

- Limitation of flexion/internal rotation > limitation of abduction/extension
- No or little limitation of remaining motions

Combined loss of hip motion in several planes is seen in degenerative joint disease, which can limit activities of daily living such as donning socks and tying shoes. The loss of hip extension can be quite functionally limiting, affecting step length and gait speed early on. Continued loss of motion may lead to low back pain due to compensatory lumbar hyperextension or increased quadriceps demand for gait due to the resulting increase in stance-phase knee flexion.

Muscle Length

There are several multi-joint muscles that cross the hip. In addition, shortness of the gastrocnemius can lead to compensation at the hip. The clinician should compare the patient's affected side with normative values and the nonaffected side. Table 10-6 in Chapter 10, Knee, provides normative values for the gastrocnemius, HSs, iliopsoas, rectus femoris, and ITB/tensor facia latae. Decreased hip flexor length appears to be correlated with decreased activation of the gluteal muscles and hip extensor weakness.[31]

Muscle Performance

The strength of the hip flexors, extensors, abductors, adductors, and the external and internal rotators should be assessed using MMT.[32] Hip extensor strength can be assessed as a group with the knee extended, or the gluteus maximus can be targeted by flexing the knee to 90° to create active insufficiency within the HSs.[32] Strength testing targeting individual muscles or muscle groups is likely to be painful in the case of muscle strains and tendinopathy. For athletes or higher functioning individuals, it is appropriate to assess hip external rotation strength not only in the traditional MMT position of short sitting but also in prone, as the external rotators function to control pronation and valgus collapse in a more extended position. The Trendelenburg test can be used to assess the ability of gluteus medius to control the pelvis in the frontal plane (see Fig. 11-22). It should be noted that muscle performance of both the hip external rotators and the hip abductors has been shown to be significantly impaired in women with stress incontinence.[22] Clinicians should use caution when assessing hip flexor strength in supine via the straight leg raise for patients with weight-bearing restrictions on the hip, as this test has been shown to create significant hip joint compressive forces that are greater than body weight.

Sensory Tests

Light touch sensation should be performed in all patients with suspected hip pathology. Knowledge of the cutaneous distribution of nerve roots (dermatomes) and peripheral nerves, as well as considering other supporting assessments, enables the clinician to distinguish sensory loss caused by a root lesion from that caused by a peripheral nerve lesion.

Reflexes

The clinician should routinely assess the Achilles and patellar reflexes in patients with suspected hip or lumbar pathology. Positive findings require a closer examination of spinal structures.

Neurodynamic Testing

Neurodynamic testing, including the straight leg raise and prone knee flexion, should be performed on all patients with suspected hip pathology. Positive neural tension tests are indicative of lower lumbosacral (straight leg raise) or upper lumbar (prone knee flexion) pathology. Positive findings require a closer examination of spinal structures.

TABLE 11-3
PASSIVE HIP RANGE OF MOTION NORMATIVE VALUES

Motion	Normative Value (degrees)
Flexion	0–120
Extension	0–30
Abduction	0–45
Adduction	0–30
Internal rotation	0–45
External rotation	0–45

Accessory Motion

The hip joint should be assessed for hypermobility or hypomobility and the presence or absence of pain. The four primary accessory motions to be assessed are inferior glide (Fig. 11-17), anterior glide (Fig. 11-18), posterior (Fig. 11-19) glide, and distraction (Fig. 11-20). These mobilizations can be used for both assessment and treatment purposes. For a quick assessment, all of these mobilizations can be performed in supine with the hip in the open-packed position of about 30° of flexion, 30° abduction, and slight external rotation. When used for treatment, positioning is usually changed to optimize clinician body mechanics.

Inferior Glide of Femur

Purpose: To assess joint play movement necessary for hip flexion and abduction.
Patient: Supine with the hip flexed 30 to 90°.
Clinician: Supports the lower leg by letting it rest on the shoulder. The clinician grasps the anterior aspect of the proximal femur as far proximally as possible, using both hands with the fingers interlaced.
Mobilization: An inferior glide is imparted with the hands by shifting body weight from the superior to the inferior leg. This may also be performed as a mobilization with movement by simultaneously rocking the thigh into flexion (Fig. 11-17).

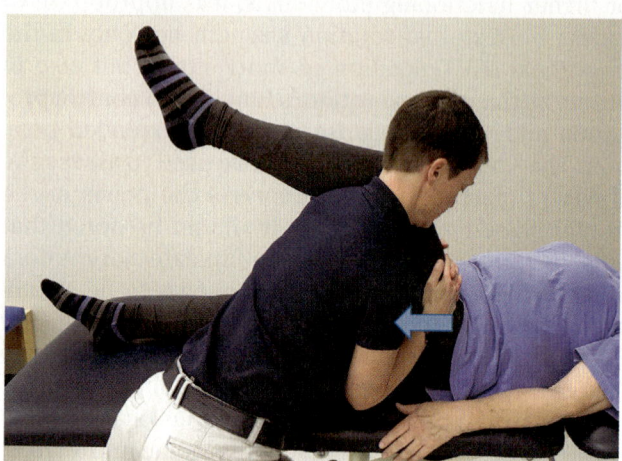

FIGURE 11-17 Inferior glide of femur.

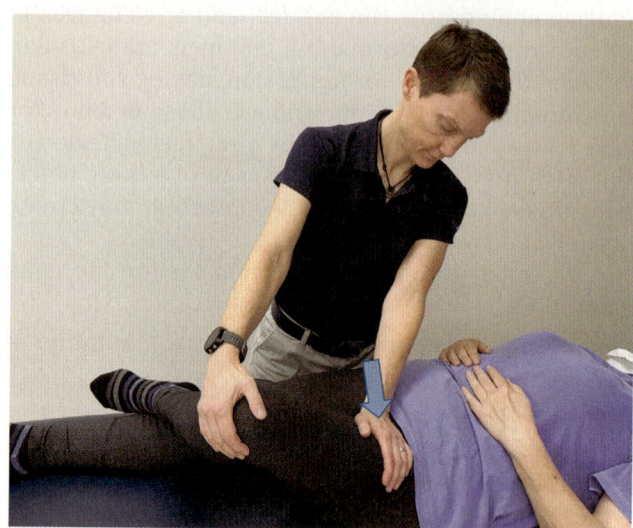

FIGURE 11-19 Posterior glide of femur.

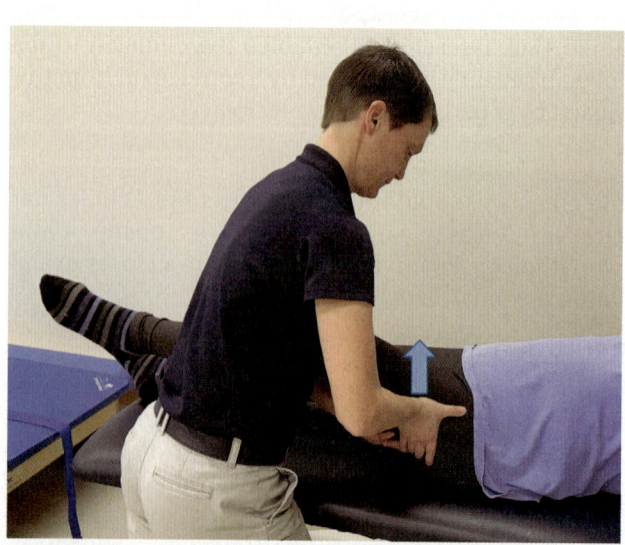

FIGURE 11-18 Anterior glide of femur.

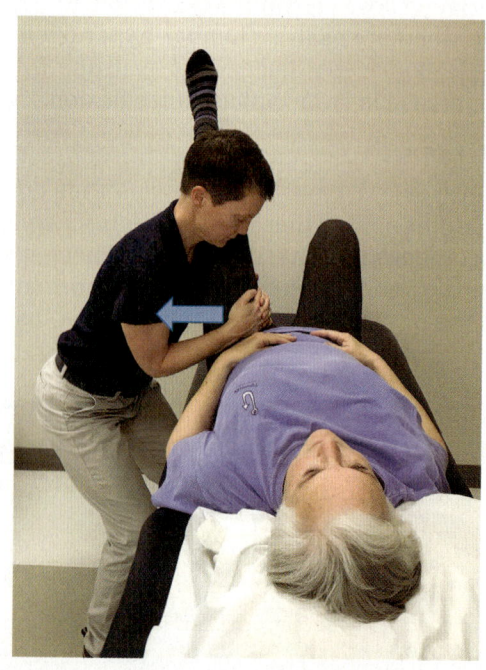

FIGURE 11-20 Lateral distraction of femur.

Anterior Glide of Femur

Purpose: To assess joint play movement necessary for hip extension and external rotation.

Patient: Supine with the hip in about 30° of flexion, 30° abduction, and slight external rotation.

Clinician: Grasps around posteriorly with both hands on the posterior aspect of the proximal femur, level with the greater trochanter. The fingers are interlaced or overlapping.

Mobilization: The slack is taken up, and an anterior glide of the proximal femur is imparted with the hands (Fig. 11-18). Because the clinician is at a biomechanical disadvantage when performing this technique, it is generally only used for assessment purposes.

Posterior Glide of Femur

Purpose: To assess joint play movement necessary for hip internal rotation.

Patient: Supine in a figure-of-four position, with ankle of the leg to be treated crossed over the opposite knee.

Clinician: Supports the knee with the inferior hand. The clinician's superior hand contacts the anterior aspect of the patient's proximal thigh and imparts a posterolateral glide by leaning forward at the trunk.

Mobilization: Mobilization force is applied by leaning laterally and distally (Fig. 11-19).

Lateral Distraction of Femur

Purpose: To assess global hip joint mobility and facilitate global hip mobility as well as flexion, internal rotation, and adduction.

Patient: Supine, hip and knee flexed, leg positioned against the clinician's trunk.

Clinician: Both hands grasp the proximal medial thigh with clasped hands.

Mobilization: Mobilization force is applied by leaning laterally and inferiorly (Fig. 11-20).

Special Tests/Provocative Testing

Clinicians should choose which special/provocative tests to perform based on the patient's history and physical examination to this point in order to help rule in and rule out competing differential diagnoses. For hip pathology, these tests may be loosely grouped into tests for contractile tissue, range of motion and stability, or intra-articular pathology (Fig. 11-21).

Special Tests for Contractile Tissue
Special tests for contractile tissue include the Trendelenburg test, resisted external rotation derotation test, and adductor test.

Trendelenburg Test

Purpose: To test for gluteus medius weakness.[21,33]

Method: The patient stands on one limb with finger tips for balance and is instructed to try to maintain a neutral posture (Fig. 11-22).

Interpretation: A positive test is (A) contralateral pelvic drop (uncompensated Trendelenburg) or (B) ipsilateral trunk lean (compensated Trendelenburg).

Resisted External Derotation Test

Purpose: To test for gluteus maximus tendinopathy as part of greater trochanteric syndrome.[34]

Method: With the patient supine, the clinician brings the patient's hip into 90° hip flexion and near-full external rotation. The patient is then asked to rotate the hip back to neutral, "derotating" the hip, against the clinician's resistance.

The modified external derotation test is performed similarly, but with the addition of hip adduction to the start position (90° hip flexion, hip adduction, then externally rotated to near end range). This increases gluteus maximus tendon compression over the greater trochanter, further stressing the tendon (Fig. 11-23).[34]

Interpretation: A positive test is reproduction of the patient's lateral hip pain with the test motion.

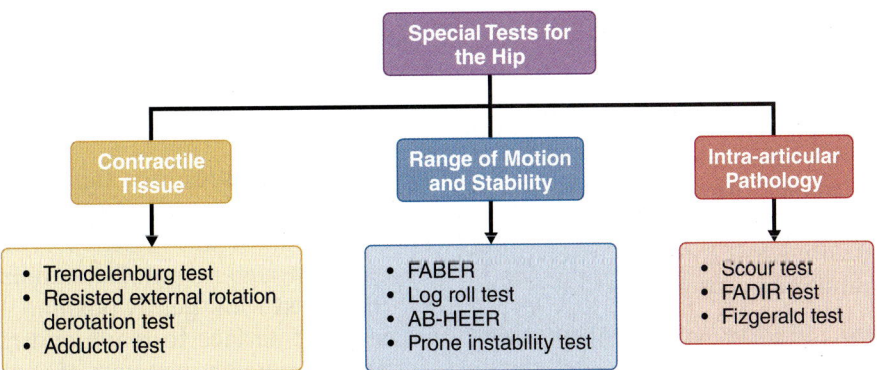

FIGURE 11-21 Special tests of hip pathology. AB-HEER, abduction-hyperextension-external rotation test.

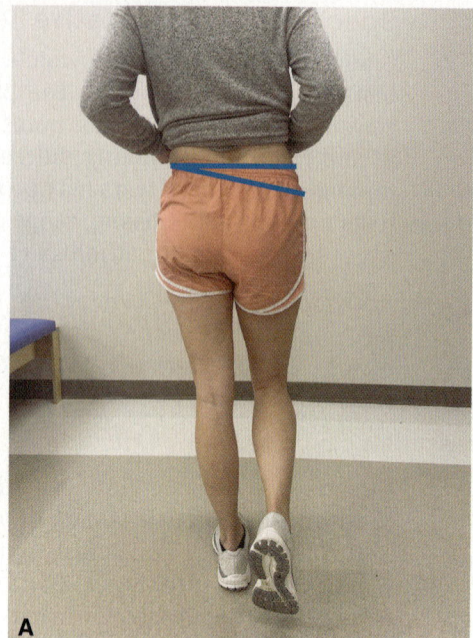
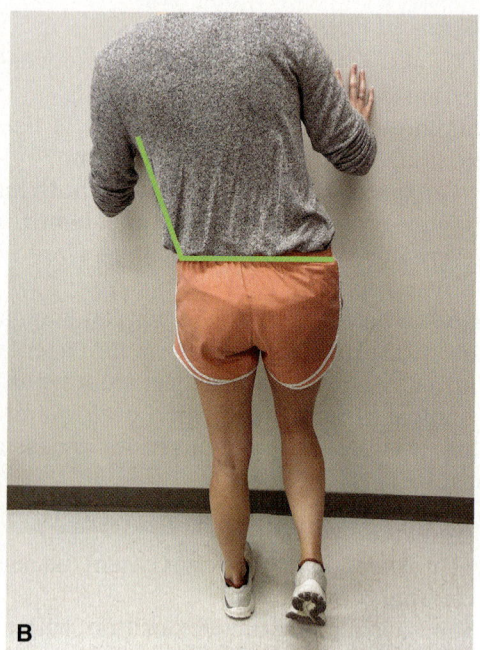

FIGURE 11-22 Trendelenburg test. A positive test is: **A.** contralateral pelvic drop (uncompensated Trendelenburg) or **B.** Ipsilateral trunk lean (commensated Trendelenburg).

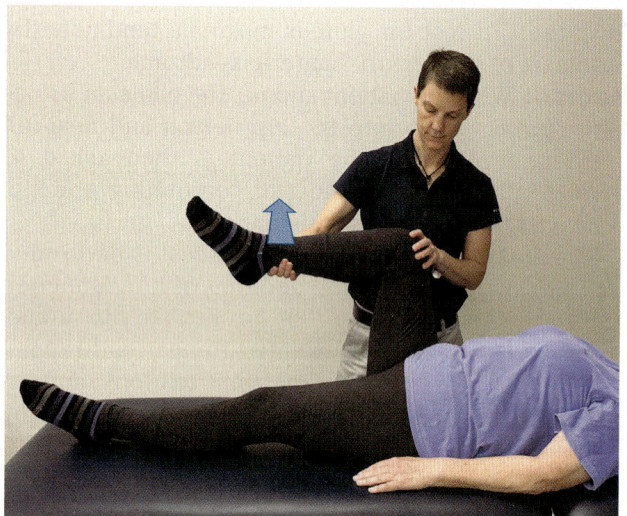

FIGURE 11-23 Resisted external derotation test.

Adductor Test

Purpose: To test for adductor pathology.[21,35]

Method: With the patient supine, the clinician brings the patient's hip into 45° hip flexion with the knees straight. The patient is then asked to perform bilateral hip adduction against the clinician's resistance (Fig. 11-24).

Interpretation: A positive test is reproduction of the patient's groin pain during contraction.

Special Tests for Range of Motion and Stability Special tests for range of motion include the FABER test and the log roll test.

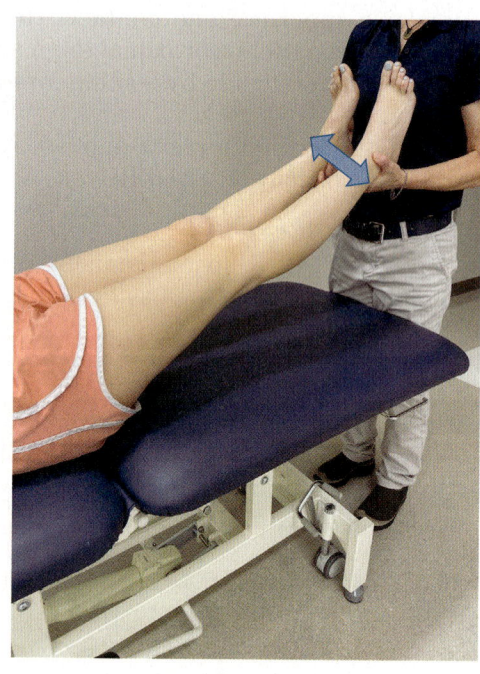

FIGURE 11-24 Adductor test.

FABER Test (aka the Figure Four or Patrick Test)

Purpose: To assess for hip capsular tightness, hip joint pathology, and sacroiliac joint pathology.[21]

Method: Cross the patient's ankle just proximal to the contralateral patella. Stabilize the contralateral iliac crest while gently pushing the knee toward the support surface to reach end range. The clinician should note the amount of motion, any pain produced, and pain location (Fig. 11-25).

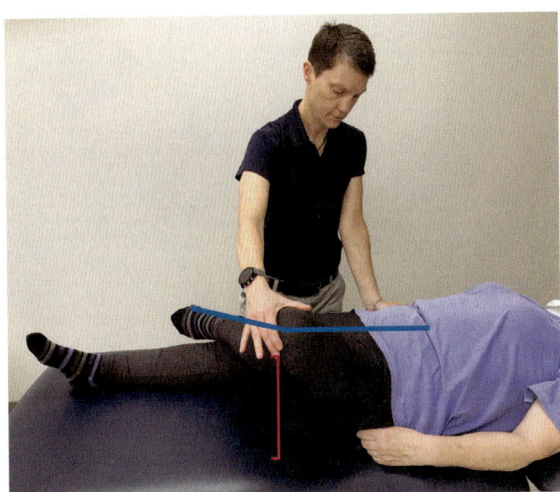

FIGURE 11-25 FABER test.

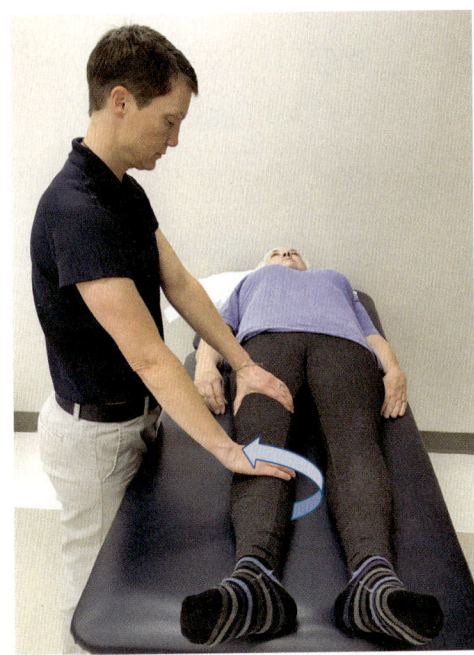

FIGURE 11-26 Log roll test.

Interpretation: With normal range of motion, the tibia should be parallel with support surface. Restriction in range indicates hip capsule tightness and can be quantified by measuring the angle of the tibia above the horizontal or the distance from the lateral knee joint line to the support surface. If the test produces hip joint pain, this indicates possible intra-articular pathology, such as degenerative joint disease or labral pathology. If the test produces pain in the region of the PSIS, this indicates possible sacroiliac joint pathology. Lateral hip pain with testing is suggestive of GTPS.

Log Roll Test

Purpose: To assess for hypermobility or intra-articular pathology, such as proximal femur fracture.[36]

Method: With the patient supine, the clinician externally rotates the femur (Fig. 11-26).

Interpretation: A positive test for hypermobility is excessive external rotation. This test is particularly relevant because it stresses the anterior hip capsule more than when rotation is assessed in the standard short sitting position and is more likely to replicate the functional position where patients report instability symptoms. A positive test for suspicion of fracture is limited motion due to pain.

Abduction-Hyperextension-External Rotation Test

Purpose: To assess for hypermobility.[37]

Method: With the patient sidelying on the unaffected hip, the clinician abducts the patients' hip approximately 30 to 45°, then extends and externally rotates the hip. The clinician then uses the superior hand to provide an anterior glide of the femur (Fig. 11-27).

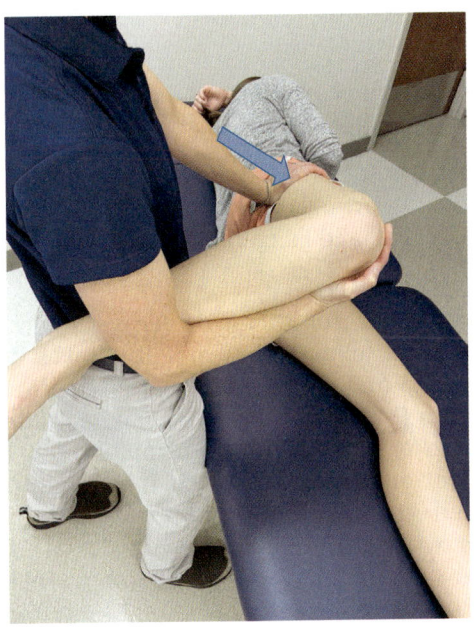

FIGURE 11-27 Abduction-hyperextension-external rotation test.

Interpretation: A positive test is if the test reproduces the patient's hip pain.

Prone Hip Instability Test

Purpose: To assess for hypermobility.[37]

Method: With the patient prone, the clinician provides an anterior glide of the femur with the superior hand while externally rotating the patient's hip (Fig. 11-28).

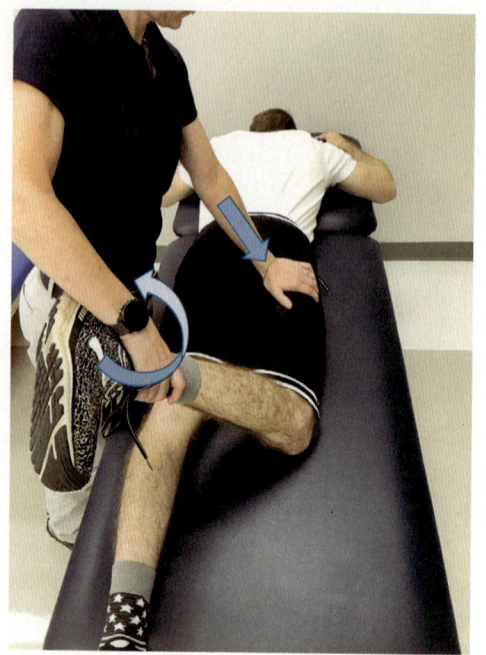

FIGURE 11-28 Prone hip instability test.

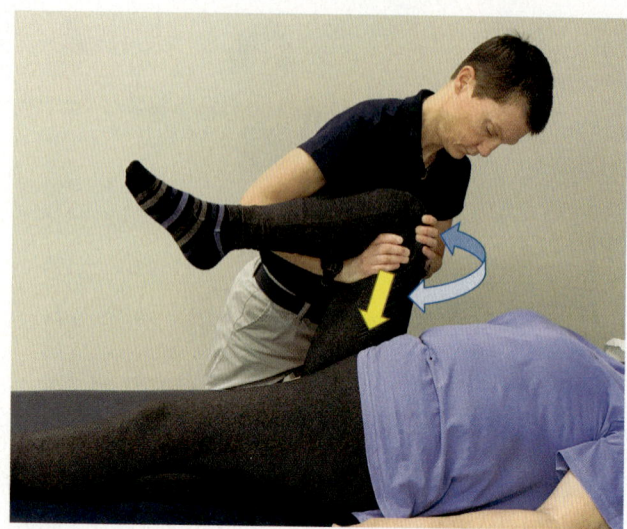

FIGURE 11-29 Scour test.

Interpretation: A positive test is if the test reproduces the patient's hip pain.

Special Tests for Intra-Articular Pathology Special tests for intra-articular pathology include the scour test, FADIR test, and Fitzgerald test, and Fulcrum test.

Scour Test
Purpose: To test for intra-articular pathology.[38]
Method: The clinician maximally flexes the patient's hip and then moves the femur through an arc from 9 to 3 o'clock, with maximal adduction and maximal abduction while maintaining flexion. The motion is repeated twice. If no symptoms are created, the test motion is repeated one to two times, while the clinician provides axial compression to the femur throughout the arc of motion (Fig. 11-29).
Interpretation: A positive test is reproduction of symptoms in the hip. The patient should rate pain with testing on a 0 to 10 scale.

FADIR Test (Hip Flexion, Adduction, Internal Rotation Impingement Test)
Purpose: To test for hip impingement or labral pathology.[39]
Method: The clinician flexes the patient's hip and knee to 90°, then internally rotates and adducts the hip (Fig. 11-30).
Interpretation: A positive test is reproduction of symptoms in the hip.

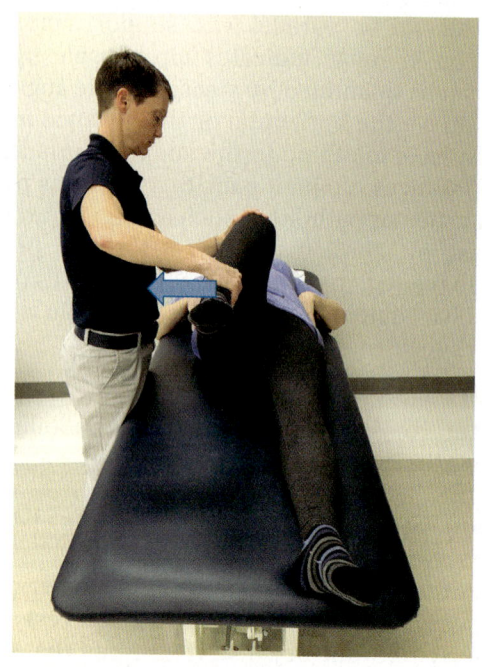

FIGURE 11-30 FADIR test.

Fitzgerald Test
Purpose: To test for labral pathology.[38,40]
Method: To assess the anterior labrum, with the knee comfortably flexed, the clinician moves patient's hip from maximal flexion, abduction and external rotation into extension (Fig. 11-31A), adduction, and internal rotation (Fig. 11-31B). To assess the posterior labrum, the clinician moves the patient's hip from maximal flexion, internal rotation, and adduction into extension (Fig. 11-31C), external rotation, and abduction (Fig. 11-31D).

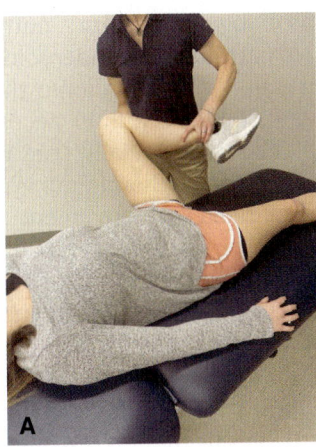 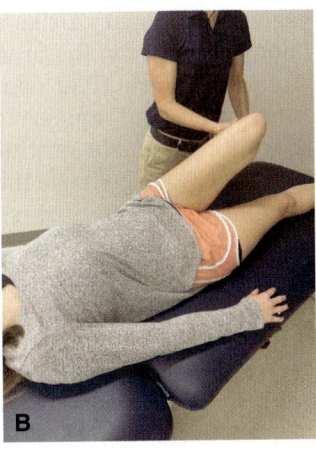 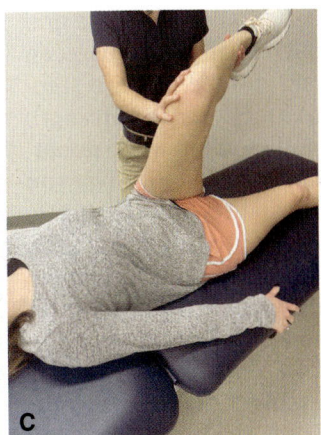 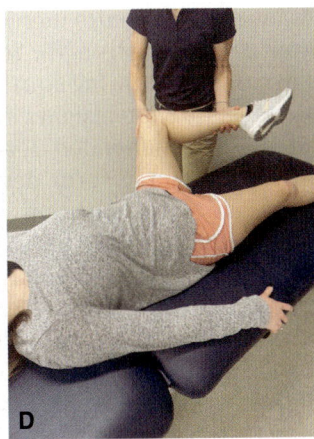

FIGURE 11-31 Fitzgerald test. Assessment of anterior labrum: start position (**A**), end position (**B**). Assessment of posterior labrum: start position (**C**), end position (**D**).

Interpretation: A positive test is reproduction of the patient's hip symptoms.

Fulcrum Test

Purpose: To test for a femoral stress fracture.[33]

Method: With the patient in short sitting, the clinician places a forearm under the patient's thigh to act as a fulcrum. The clinician presses down on the patient's knee with the other hand (Fig. 11-32).

Interpretation: A positive test is sharp hip pain or reproduction of the patient's hip symptoms. The stress fracture may be intra-articular but may also involve extracapsular portions of the femur. Note that a positive test is best for ruling in a stress fracture, but a negative test does not rule out a stress fracture.

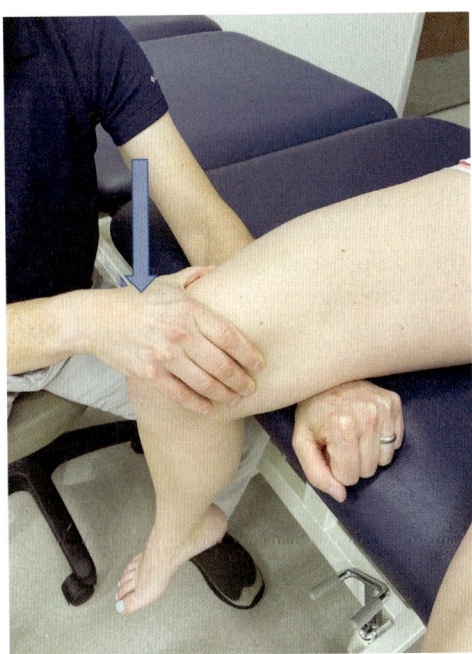

FIGURE 11-32 Fulcrum test.

Palpation

The region should be palpated for tenderness and temperature. Scar mobility should be assessed. Clinicians should methodically palpate for muscle spasm or tenderness. Tenderness at the point of attachment is common for patients with proximal HS tendinopathy.[41] Tenderness near the greater trochanter is characteristic of GTPS.[42] Trigger points (local hyperirritable spots associated with a taut band) can reflect muscle overuse or be referred from related spinal segments.[43]

Gait

The patient's gait should be assessed with and without footwear, noting any deviations of symptoms. Footwear and any assistive device used should be inspected. As noted in Chapter 5, Gait and Footwear, several gait deviations may result from a lack of hip strength or range. A compensated or uncompensated Trendelenburg gait may be due to ipsilateral hip abductor weakness or hip joint pain. A posterior trunk lean may be due to hip extensor weakness, whereas an anterior lean may be due to quadriceps weakness. Excessive lordosis during late stance may be the result of hip flexor tightness. Having the patient assume alternate gait patterns, such as longer strides or slower speeds, may amplify hip flexor tightness or balance deficits, respectively, making them easier to identify. A treadmill and video analysis may be useful in identifying more subtle deviations or deficits when moving at higher speeds.

Functional Testing

The clinician should assess functional activities, in addition to gait, that stress the hip. For example, loss of hip motion will make donning shoes and socks difficult. Single leg balance (with eyes open and then closed if able) should be assessed. Assess the patient's ability to perform a deep squat and rise from a low surface, because these require increased hip flexion range and lower extremity strength. Squatting and stair use can be assessed. Single leg squatting and the forward step-down test provide insights into functional hip strength and are recommended for individuals with nonarthritic hip pain.[44] Form deviations, specifically genu valgus and pelvic position, correlate with hip muscle strength, particularly hip abductor/rotator[44] but also hip/knee extensor strength. In addition to helping identify strength impairments, recall from Chapter 10, Knee, that these tests also help detect deficits in balance, functional dorsiflexion, and neuromuscular control.[45] Clinician visual assessment of deviations for these tests has proven to be reliable and may be improved with the use of a simple mobile phone video.[46] The Functional Reach Test, Berg Balance Scale, Timed Up and Go (TUG), 6-Minute Walk Test, and the Dynamic Gait Index (see Table 5-3 in Chapter 5, Gait and Footwear) may be beneficial. Table 11-4 provides additional functional assessments, including the Five Times Sit-to-Stand Test and the 30-Second Sit-to-Stand Test.[47]

COMMON HIP PATHOLOGIES

This section contains the most common or most problematic musculoskeletal hip pathologies, including hip OA and total hip arthroplasty (THA), hip fracture, FAIS, instability, GTPS, groin pain, proximal HS tendinopathy, SCFE, and Legg-Calvé-Perthes disease.

Hip Osteoarthritis

Pathology
Hip OA, similar to knee OA, is a chronic degenerative condition and the most common hip disorder.[48] Radiographic evidence of joint space narrowing and/or osteophytes[49] may be present before patients seeking treatment.[50] Progressive joint space narrowing is related to worse function.[24]

Major risk factors for hip OA are increased age,[48] hip dysplasia, and obesity.[50,51] Hip OA is a disease of older persons, particularly those over 50 years, because it takes a long time to cause the fatigue of tissue, such as fibrillation of articular cartilage, characteristic of the disease. The asymptomatic changes occurring with normal aging of articular cartilage probably result from a nutritional deficiency; the areas of cartilage not undergoing frequent intermittent compression do not undergo the absorption and squeezing out of synovial fluid necessary for adequate nutrition. This is especially true in older persons because they tend to use their joints less frequently and through smaller ranges of movement. If one accepts that in many, if not most, cases of OA the pathogenesis is closely related to increased stress to joint tissues with time (or fatigue), then conditions that may predispose the joint to increased stresses must be considered as the possible contributors to the cause of OA. Perhaps, the most important condition at the hip to consider in this regard is congenital hip dysplasia. Hip dysplasia can result in a deficient acetabular roof, abnormal femoral torsion, and/or an abnormally shaped femoral head. The resultant decrease in effective weight-bearing surface area at the joint predisposes the hip to early degenerative changes.

Obesity increases articular cartilage and bony stress.[52] Individuals who are obese are more likely to have muscle strength deficits. To compensate for these strength deficits, patients may adopt altered gait patterns, resulting in altered hip joint loading,[52] further stressing the joint. More severe obesity forces individuals into a larger base of support due to soft-tissue approximation, further altering hip joint stress. Lastly, obesity results in low-grade systemic inflammation, which may contribute to pain and functional limitations.[52] Individuals with prior hip injury, including surgery for FAIS, appear to be more likely to have hip OA. There may also be a genetic component to hip OA.[49,51]

Prior hip injury and prior hip surgery may increase the long-term risk of hip OA. Individuals with occupations that require heavy lifting may be more likely to develop hip OA.[49] There is increasing evidence that femoral cam lesions are associated with hip OA.[50] Leg length discrepancies and limb malalignment are more common in individuals with hip OA; however, it is unclear if this is a causative factor.[49]

Symptoms during weight bearing may be the result of both the compressive forces of body weight and the strain to capsuloligamentous structures. The hip, unlike

TABLE 11-4	
DYNAMIC BALANCE ASSESSMENTS WITH A STRENGTH COMPONENT	
Tool	Tool Basics
Five Times Sit-to-Stand Test	• Time required for the patient to move from sitting in a standard chair to standing five times • >15 seconds is considered the cutoff score for increased risk for falls
30-Second Sit-to-Stand Test	• Dynamic balance assessment with a strength component • Number of times the patient is able to move from sitting in a standard chair to standing in 30 seconds • <15 repetitions is considered the cutoff score for increased risk for falls

the shoulder, is continually moved close to its close-packed position during gait. With every step, at terminal stance, the hip is brought into extension, twisting the joint capsule and taking up most of the slack. Although capsular tightness may be considered the result of the hip OA, one must also consider the role of capsular tightness in accelerating, or even initiating the degenerative process, given the additional joint compressive forces created by a tight capsule during terminal stance. Capsular pain may be enhanced by the low-grade capsular inflammation present during OA flare-ups as the capsule is pulled prematurely tight with each step.

History Patients with hip OA are likely to report a gradual onset of hip or groin pain with ambulation, stairs, and squatting.[46] Symptoms may initially only be present at the end of the day or after prolonged activities loading the hip. Patients typically report morning stiffness lasting less than 1 hour.[45] Limitations in hip motion make it difficult for patients to don socks and shoes[51] or rise off low surfaces. Patients may report hip crepitus,[47] locking, or catching. Patients with more advanced hip OA may report rest pain[47] or pain[47] and night pain, which can reduce sleep quality.[52]

Key Examination Findings The primary diagnostic criteria for hip OA are hip pain along with:[27,45]

- Hip internal rotation 24° or below
- Hip flexion 15° less than the nonpainful side or less than 115° if bilateral
- Pain with passive hip internal rotation
- Morning stiffness lasting less than an hour

There is typically a loss of motion in multiple directions that may be in a capsular pattern.

- Limitation of flexion/internal rotation > limitation of abduction/extension
- No or little limitation of remaining motions

However, the absence of this pattern should not be used to rule out hip OA.[45,53,54]

Key physical examination findings include a loss of motion, as noted earlier. Passive range of motion may be limited by pain and spasm during acute flare-ups, but for chronic hip OA, there may be a bony or capsular end feel. Hip flexor length is typically reduced; however, clinicians should also assess HS and gastrocnemius length. Accessory motions will be limited and may be painful. Hip OA can lead to strength deficits of the gluteal muscles along with the quadriceps and HSs.[19] Gait deviations are common in patients with hip OA. Loss of hip extension range of motion can alter gait, including decreased step length, decreased push off, and decreased pace. Weakness of the gluteus medius[46] can result in a Trendelenburg gait, whereas pain with weight bearing can result in a compensated Trendelenburg gait. The lack of push off at terminal stance due to the loss of hip extension range can lead to secondary weakness of ankle plantarflexors.

The patient is likely to have positive scour and FADIR tests. FABER test will be positive for loss of motion with or without hip/groin pain. Balance is likely to be decreased.[43,45] The 6-Minute Walk test is a reliable assessment of function for patients with hip OA.[55]

Differential Diagnoses Differential diagnosis includes hip dysplasia without OA,[44] labral pathology,[44] and rheumatoid arthritis (RA). Refer to Table 10-14 in Chapter 10, Knee, for distinguishing factors between OA and RA.

Rehabilitation Focus and Key Points Physical therapy is the cornerstone of care for hip OA. As with knee OA, education is critical for patients with hip OA[44] (see Table 10-15 in Chapter 10, Knee). It is postulated that a 10-pound reduction in body weight would result in 60-pound decrease in hip joint stress.[56] Diet, exercise, and weight loss are strongly recommended to assist with reducing pain and increasing function in individuals with hip OA who are overweight or obese.[45,47,57] Stretching[45] and manual therapy[57] to improve capsular mobility can assist with improving motion, thereby improving gait deviations and functional activities, such as dressing.

An assistive device may be needed short term or long term to unload the hip joint and/or to assist with balance. Footwear should be assessed for both safety and the ability to absorb shock.[57] Balance exercises should be included and can progress to group or individual exercise programs, such as tai chi.[57] Strengthening exercises, particularly for the gluteals and quadriceps, can also lead to improved function.[19,58] Aquatic therapy may be beneficial early on for individuals with low exercise tolerance or high pain levels. In addition, aquatic exercise may be an enjoyable and safe long-term exercise program for patients with hip OA. Non–weight-bearing and low-impact aerobic exercises, such as stationary cycling, swimming, and walking, should be encouraged as part of long-term healthy lifestyle. Nonsteroidal anti-inflammatory drug (NSAID) and COX-2 inhibitors may be a useful adjunct to physical therapy.[47,59] Intra-articular corticosteroid injections may be beneficial for individuals with moderate-to-severe pain.[57,59]

Expected Outcomes Improvement in pain, range, strength, balance, gait, and function can be expected. However, hip OA is a progressive condition. Patients who fail conservative management should be referred to an orthopaedist for additional interventions.

Total Hip Arthroplasty

Nearly three-quarters of a million THAs are performed annually in the United States.[60] THA is a mainstay for the treatment of end-stage hip OA, end-stage hip RA, and on younger individuals with severe hip dysplasia. THA is the resection of the femoral head acetabulum and replacement with metal or polyethylene components. A THA or hemiarthroplasty, where only the femoral component is replaced, may also be performed after certain types of proximal femur fractures. The vast majority of THA are cemented in place, allowing for immediate full weight bearing. However, muscle inhibition, pain, and balance deficits make use of an assistive device recommended for all patients initially. The assistive device can be discontinued once the patient demonstrates satisfactory balance and gait form.[61] A 10-year survival rate for a THA implant is 95%,[61] whereas a 25-year survival rate is 78%.[62] The most common reason for the failure of THA is aseptic loosening of the components.[63]

Traditionally, THAs were performed using a large incision and a posterolateral or lateral approach, dislocating the hip posteriorly. Using these approaches damages the gluteus medius muscle,[64] potentially affecting balance and stability. In addition, because the hip is dislocated posteriorly to gain access to the head of the femur, postoperative precautions included limiting motions that would stress the posterior capsule to prevent dislocation (Table 11-5). The anterior approach is a more technically demanding approach for THA. However, this spares direct trauma to the gluteus medius. The anterior approach allows the femur to be dislocated anteriorly. Therefore, the anterior capsule must be protected short term by limiting aggressive movement into hip extension and external rotation. While some studies demonstrate that using a lateral approach results in decreased hip abductor strength, lower functional scores, and higher pain levels,[65] a recent systematic review and meta-analysis failed to show a difference in outcomes based on surgical approach.[66]

Postoperative precautions are typically in place between 4 and 12 weeks after surgery to allow the hip joint capsule to heal. However, the need for such vigorous protection is now in question as a large systematic review found similar rates of dislocation (~2%) between patients whose postoperative protocol included these restrictions and those patients whose motions were unrestricted. It may be that, for the posterolateral approach, patients need only be careful of the combined motions of hip flexion, adduction, and internal rotation in conjunction with weight-bearing forces, such as may occur during transfers with valgus positioning. Similarly for the anterior approach, patients may only need to avoid stretching into extension or external rotation and not avoid all motion in these ranges. Individual patient tissue tolerance may differ. In addition, the fit and orientation of the implant may need to be considered on an individual basis. Therefore, clinicians should clearly communicate with each patient's surgeon to best understand the postoperative precautions for a given patient.

Three advances in THA include the use of mini-open techniques, joint resurfacing, and outpatient hip replacements. A mini-open technique is when the surgeon uses a smaller incision, thus creating less tissue damage, presumably resulting in decreased pain and decreased strength deficits. Joint resurfacing is a technique where, rather than resecting the proximal femur and implanting a component with a large femoral stem, the surgeon carefully cuts around the femoral head and places an artificial cap on to create a new joint surface. Joint resurfacing is generally used on younger patients because it allows for an easier revision surgery to convert to a traditional total hip replacement when aseptic loosening occurs over time. Using a less invasive surgery that preserves the patient's femoral bone stock, it is easier for the surgeon to perform a revision. Lastly, outpatient surgery is now a safe option for certain individuals. Patients who are younger and have few or no comorbidities are now able to go home the same day as their procedure, akin to less invasive surgical procedures like rotator cuff repairs or anterior cruciate ligament reconstruction surgeries. Outpatient THAs account for about 3% of all hip replacements today, and there has not been an increase complication rate by allowing these carefully selected patients to leave the hospital on the same day.[60,67,68]

Preoperative physical therapy for patients undergoing a planned THA should include education, expected postoperative outcomes, and information regarding the recovery process.[61] For example, patients should be educated in any postoperative precautions and their functional implications, how to use an assistive device,[43] the expected functional recovery and time frame, and simple, beginning postoperative exercises.[43] Patients should also be taught exercises to help prevent deep vein thrombosis and pneumonia.

Postoperative physical therapy on the day of surgery and should include early mobilization with an assistive device.[61] Unlike with a total knee replacement, restoring range of motion is seldom a problem after THA. Anecdotally, compared with patients who have had total knee arthroplasty (TKA), patients after THA appear to have less problems with pain but more difficulty

TABLE 11-5
TRADITIONAL TOTAL HIP ARTHROPLASTY POSTOPERATIVE PRECAUTIONS

Posterolateral Approach	Anterior Approach
No hip flexion >90° No hip adduction No hip internal rotation	Limit hip extension

with regaining hip strength. This may be due to muscle damage from surgery, preoperative weakness, and/or learned nonuse. Strengthening of the gluteals and quadriceps has shown to reverse the preoperative atrophy seen in patients with hip OA.[19] Therefore, strengthening of the hip and entire lower extremity should be emphasized throughout rehabilitation. Neuromuscular electrical stimulation to the quadriceps may be beneficial[69] for patients with poor quadriceps control. Strength training should include weight-bearing and non–weight-bearing exercises for the entire lower extremity, including heel raises, squats, sit-to-stands, and step-ups as able. Exercises should progress to the use of resistance bands, cuff weights, and machine weights, such as the leg press and leg extension machines. Clinicians in the past have tended to under-strength train patients with OA and after joint replacements. Therefore, it is important to note that heavy strength training, working up to loads of 85 to 90% of 1RM (1 repetition maximum) (sets of 4–6 repetitions), is well tolerated and does improve lower extremity strength deficits.[70] However, clinicians may choose to work up to an exercise volume closer to 3 sets of 8 repetitions[69] for most patients, and slightly lighter loads for individuals with other joint-related problems. Progressive balance training should be included as patients after THA have been shown to continue to have balance deficits compared with the nonarthritic population.[69]

Gait training should progress as able to include a progressive walking program and use of the least restrictive (or no) assistive device. It should be noted that patients may have OA in multiple joints or other comorbidities that may affect strength, balance, and mobility gains. However, those patients without additional comorbidities who were not using an assistive device before surgery are generally able to walk without an assistive device within 4 to 6 weeks after surgery. Therefore, clinicians must individually titrate exercise dosing. Long-term aerobic exercise options may include walking, stationary cycling, the elliptical machine, or aquatics.

THA results in a predictable decrease in hip pain. Rehabilitation after THA results in improved strength, balance, gait,[71] and function.[61,69]

Hip Fracture

Pathology

Hip fractures are one of the most common fractures. The diagnostic term "hip fracture" is a bit of a misnomer, as the term specifically only refers to proximal femur fractures and not to acetabular fractures or femoral head fractures. Because of poor local blood supply, femoral head fractures have an increased risk of **avascular necrosis** (bone death due to lack of blood supply), making arthroplasty a likely treatment option.[72] Hip (proximal femur) fractures have a high mortality rate,[73] making integrated, holistic care paramount. Proximal femur fractures may be intracapsular or extracapsular (Fig. 11-33). Intracapsular fractures involve the femoral neck. Because the femoral neck has a more tenuous blood supply and these fractures are bathed in synovial fluid that inhibits angiogenesis, nonoperative treatment is seldom possible.[73] Operative treatment may include closed or open reduction with internal fixation, hemiarthroplasty, or, when combined with preexisting hip OA, THA.[73] Extracapsular fractures include intertrochanteric and subtrochanteric fractures. The majority of proximal femur fractures are intertrochanteric. Because the blood supply to these regions is better, most extracapsular femur fractures are treated with open or closed reduction with internal fixation using implants such as compression screws and intramedullary nails,[72,74] with or without a plate.[74]

There are several risk factors for hip fracture, including:[74]

- Older age
- Osteoporosis
- Decreased balance
- Decreased mobility
- Prior hip fracture
- Diabetes mellitus
- Dementia
- Polypharmacy
- Use of sedatives
- Excessive intake of alcohol or caffeine
- Not living at home
- Female gender
- Smoking
- Postmenopausal

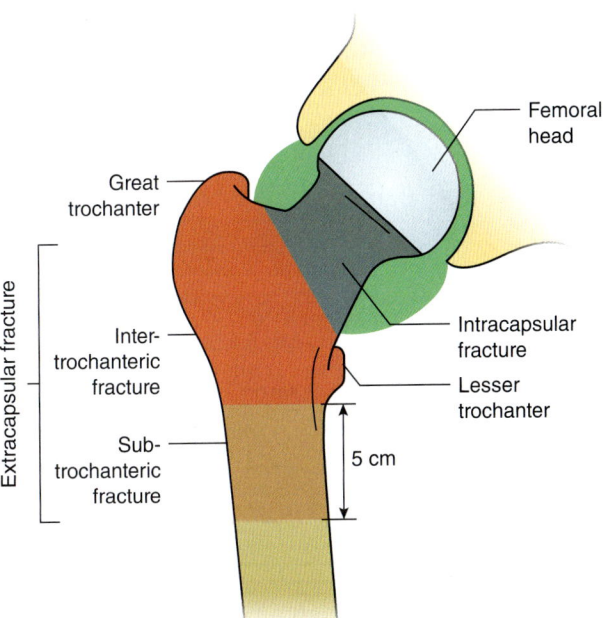

FIGURE 11-33 Types of proximal femur fractures.

Postoperative Course It is important to gather information regarding the patient's prior functional status, the use of assistive device, and fall history. Figure 11-34 represents the many possible trajectories for patients after hip fracture.[74,75] Generally speaking, those with dementia and/or more complex medical histories may be discharged to a skilled nursing facility or a long-term-care facility. Individuals with higher cognitive levels who have limited assistance at home may be discharged to inpatient rehabilitation where they receive up to 3 hours of therapy per day. Patients with help at home or who are more mobile may be discharged to home-based rehabilitation, whereas those who are more mobile immediately after surgery may be discharged to outpatient rehabilitation. Some patients may move from one setting to another as their condition changes. Hand-off communication between clinicians in the various settings is imperative to maximizing patient outcomes.

Early rehabilitation, as may occur in the acute care setting, should focus on pain management, early mobilization, and prevention of secondary impairments,[74] such as pressure ulcer, pneumonia, deep vein thrombosis, and falls. Because delirium is not uncommon after hip fracture, clinicians should assess cognitive function across all setting[75] and appropriate referrals made. Postacute care clinicians should assess patient strength, mobility, balance, gait, and functional abilities. It is logical that after hip fracture, patients will have limited hip strength, particularly of the functionally important hip extensors and abductors. Knee extension strength has also been found to sharply decline after fracture.[76] Therefore, strength training should include at least these key muscle groups. Neuromuscular electrical stimulation may be beneficial[74] for patients with significant quadriceps deficits or for those in whom quadriceps strength is slow to return.

Progressive strength and functional training should be included.[77] Electrical stimulation may be beneficial as part of multimodal pain management[74] and decrease the use of medications known to increase the risk of falls. Functional assessments, such as the Five Times Sit-to-Stand test, Berg Balance Scale, TUG, and 6-Minute Walk, should be included based on the patient's abilities. Clinicians may use the Falls Efficacy Scale – International (FES-I) to identify patients with a fear of falling,[74] as this may both limit patient mobility and increase the risk of falls.

Historically, rehabilitation has under-trained patients with hip fracture, using only minimal resistance and discontinuing care too quickly.[78–80] However, it is now known that these patients not only tolerate a progressive resistance training program that works up to 75% of 1-RM, they have greater functional gains with these programs as well.[74,77,81] Weight-bearing and non–weight-bearing exercises should be included to provide adequate muscle strengthening and decrease osteoporetic bone loss. Progressive balance exercises, including dual tasking, should be incorporated as soon as possible. In addition, aerobic exercise[74] should be a part of a holistic rehabilitation program to maximize patient outcomes. When possible, patients should be transitioned from rehabilitation to community-based fitness programs[74] to assist with adhering to a healthy lifestyle and make continued gains upon discharge from formal rehabilitation. Some patients may be ideal candidates for group exercise classes, including tai chi, chair yoga, aquatic exercise classes, and Silver Sneakers. Clinicians should discuss any needed modification for safe participation with individual patients, such as rest breaks, performing exercises next to a secure handrail, and seated alternatives.

Rehabilitation using this progressive approach over a period of up to 3 months predictably leads to improvements in balance, strength, walking endurance, patient-reported functional activities, and patient confidence.[74,78,82] Patients who were community dwelling before fracture, who lacked cognitive or visual impairments, had good nutritional status, and had surgery soon after fracture had better outcomes.[83]

Femoroacetabular Impingement Syndrome

Pathology

FAIS is hip-related pain in combination with
- Abnormal bony morphology
- Vigorous, repetitive end range hip motion
- Soft-tissue damage

In FAIS, there are two bony changes that can occur (Fig. 11-35). Most commonly, bone is deposited at the edge of the femoral head, creating a cam lesion. This lesion prevents normal femur motion within the

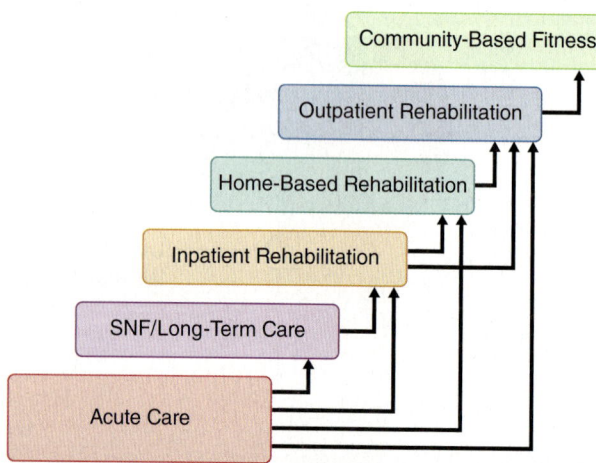

FIGURE 11-34 Possible progressive trajectories after hip fracture.

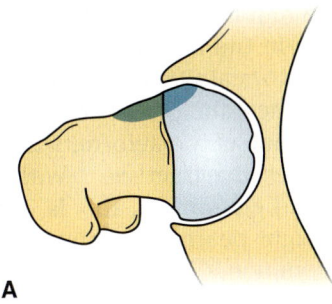

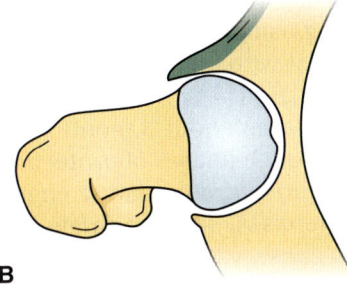

FIGURE 11-35 Cam (**A**) and pincer (**B**) lesions.

acetabulum. A pincer lesion is a bony overgrowth of the lip of the acetabulum. Cam and pincer lesions can occur either in isolation or in combination[84] and are identified via radiograph or diagnostic ultrasound.[85] The result of these bony changes is the potential to pinch, crush, or grind the labrum[33] and/or articular cartilage when the abnormal surfaces make bony contact at end ranges. Because soccer, dance, baseball, and ice hockey are sports requiring excessive and/or repeated end range hip flexion, internal rotation, and/or abduction, individuals who participate in these sports are more likely to have FAIS.[86,87] Cam and pincer lesions may be more likely to develop if skeletally immature individuals participate at a higher level in these sports.[87] It is important to note that these lesions are not rare, and the mere presence of abnormal bony morphology does not mean an individual will have hip symptoms, even if one participates in sports with high hip motion demands.[88] Because bony changes are relatively common in the asymptomatic population, it is believed that conservative treatment should be the first line of interventions for symptomatic patients.[89,90] In addition, prophylactic surgery to reshape the bony structure should not be performed in asymptomatic individuals with cam or pincer lesions. Currently, it is unclear if articular cartilage lesions resulting from FAIS may change over time and f they may lead to early-onset hip OA.[87]

History Individuals with FAIS report a slow progressive onset of anterior hip or groin pain[33,91] and may demonstrate the location of pain using the "C" sign.[84] However, pain may also be located in the back, buttock, or thigh.[50] They will report stiffness or a loss of motion. Pain is generally intermittent,[84] occurring at end range hip pain, and the patients are likely to have pain with sitting as this may place them close to their end range hip flexion. Patients are likely to report catching, pinching, and locking and may participate in the higher risk sports noted previously.[50]

Key Examination Findings One of the most important examination findings for FAIS is the presence of a painful limitation of hip passive range of motion[84] in one or more direction: flexion, internal rotation, and/or abduction, due to the early contact of the abnormally shaped bony surfaces. Less than 20° of hip internal rotation when assessed in the 90° of hip flexion but greater motion with the hip in prone with neutral hip flexion/extension is strongly suggestive of FAIS[50] because the flexed hip position is more likely to lead to premature bony contact due to cam or pincer lesions. Likewise, patients with FAIS may have pain with resisted hip internal rotation when performed in the standard MMT position but less pain when tested in prone. Patients with FAIS will commonly have pain with several special tests: FADIR, FABER, scour, and Fitzgerald tests.[91] However, these tests are not specific to FAIS. A negative FADIR test should be used to rule out FAIS.[33,84,92] Clinicians should assess hip flexor length using the Thomas test.[92]

Several functional tests should be performed to assess functional hip range and neuromuscular control. For example, when a patient with FAIS performs a deep squat, they are likely to have less depth and altered lumbopelvic control.[93] Similar impairments are typically seen when having the patient perform a single leg squat or step down. Common deviations include altered trunk position (ipsilateral sidebend and/or anterior lean), pelvis position (contralateral drop and/or rotation), hip position (adduction and/or internal rotation), knee position (valgus), decreased depth, or muscle tremor.[39] These form deficits correlate with hip and quadriceps strength deficits.[39]

Differential Diagnoses Differential diagnosis should include groin pain,[84,86] hip OA, the presence of loose bodies, avascular necrosis, and radiculopathy.[33]

Rehabilitation Focus and Key Points Current guidelines recommend physical therapy as the first choice of treatment for patients with FAIS.[89] The focus of rehabilitation should be on activity modification, strengthening, and neuromuscular control.[50,89,94] Patients should be taught to limit end range motion and avoid impinging positions.[95] For example, patients with painful end range flexion should limit sitting and interrupt sitting frequently with a short walk or backward bending.[94] Other methods to avoid bony impingement include performing squats in a smaller range of motion and/or slightly externally rotating the hips. NSAID may be prescribed for 2 to 4 weeks for individuals with higher pain or greater irritability.[94,95]

Strengthening exercises should emphasize the quadriceps as well as hip abductors, extensors, and external rotators.[94] Strength training alone is likely to yield suboptimal results.[96] Neuromuscular control exercises for hip control and pelvic stability should focus on improving abnormal movement patterns, such as genu valgus, pelvic drop, or anterior pelvic tilting, to prevent premature bony contact.[97] Neutral spine core strengthening should be included to assist with pelvic stability.[94] Balance training should be considered if deficits are noted.

It is unclear what role hip range of motion, stretching, and joint mobilization should play in the conservative treatment of FAIS.[98] Stretching tight hip flexors is likely to be beneficial.[94] Lateral distraction of the hip[95] and inferior femoral glides may be used to reduce pain and improve capsular mobility. However, pushing into passive end ranges with a painful or bony end feels is likely to exacerbate patient symptoms.[98] Therefore, stretching into restricted hip flexion, internal rotation, and abduction should be performed with caution.[95]

Expected Outcomes Physical therapy consistently results in improvements in pain and function.[98] Some patients with high initial pain or irritability may benefit from an intra-articular corticosteroid injection to calm symptoms.[50] Despite the significant rise in arthroscopic hip surgery for FAIS, physical therapy alone appears to result in equivalent gains to physical therapy plus surgical resection of cam/pincer lesions.[99] Up to 12 weeks of rehabilitation may be needed to reach optimal results.[94–96]

Rehabilitation After Surgery for Femoroacetabular Impingement Syndrome For the small percentage of patients with FAIS who have continued symptoms despite conservative care, arthroscopic surgery tends to provide significant improvements in pain and function.[90] Surgery may entail acetabuloplasty and/or femoroplasty to reshape bony morphology.[100] Chondral lesions may be treated with microfracture.[101] Frayed labrum may be debrided,[100] whereas torn labrums are typically repaired[100] in order to preserve the labrum's functional role in weight bearing and hip stability.[84] There is also conflicting information in the literature and in clinical practice as to the degree of anterior capsule protection needed after hip arthroscopy.

Perhaps because of the variety of surgical procedures that may be required to manage FAIS, there are no clear guidelines in the literature for rehabilitation after surgery.[101] Historically, patients were limited in weight bearing after acetabuloplasty and femoroplasty because overcorrection of the deformity increased the likelihood of postoperative fracture.[102] With newer surgical techniques and equipment, this is less of an issue. Restricted weight bearing after labral repair and microfracture is common,[87,103] yet not universal.[104] The most consensus appears to be with the recommendations for ice, limiting repeated or resisted hip flexor activity in the early postoperative period to lessen the chance of hip flexor tendinitis, and prone lying to decrease the risk of a hip flexion contracture.[102,104] Stationary cycling using no resistance[102] is commonly prescribed to assist with joint nutrition while minimizing hip flexor activation.

Rehabilitation takes about 3 months[102] and generally progresses through phases of protection and early motion exercises, stabilization and strengthening, and sport-specific exercises, if appropriate.[89] Rehabilitation is similar to conservative management, except for the early postoperative period. Nearly 90% of athletes are able to return to sport, mostly at the same level of participation.[87,105] Five years after FAIS surgery, although athlete satisfaction remains high, a longer term follow-up is needed as the number of athletes who continue to participate in sport declines.[104]

Hip Instability

Pathology Hip stability is provided by a delicate balance between the bony architecture of the hip joint, passive soft-tissue restraints, and dynamic stabilizers.[103] As such, there are numerous causes of hip instability (Fig. 11-36).[106] The osseous structure of the femoral head and acetabulum normally provide a deep, stable ball-and-socket joint. Hip dysplasia is a congenital malformation of either the femoral head or the acetabulum in which they may be smaller, shallower, flatter, or altered in orientation that can be confirmed with radiographs. Mild hip dysplasia allows for greater hip range of motion and may, in part, be the reason that some athletes are successful in their sport. Hip dysplasia places greater stress on the remaining stabilizers and may lead to hip instability.[103,107]

The hip capsule, capsular ligaments, and labrum provide static support to the hip joint. The capsule and ligaments are noticeably thicker anteriorly, where there is less bony stability. Laxity in these structures can lead to hip instability. Capsular laxity may be genetic, as in individuals with systemic hypermobility, such as Ehlers-Danlos syndrome, and those scoring 4 or more on the Beighton scale.[106,108] Capsular laxity

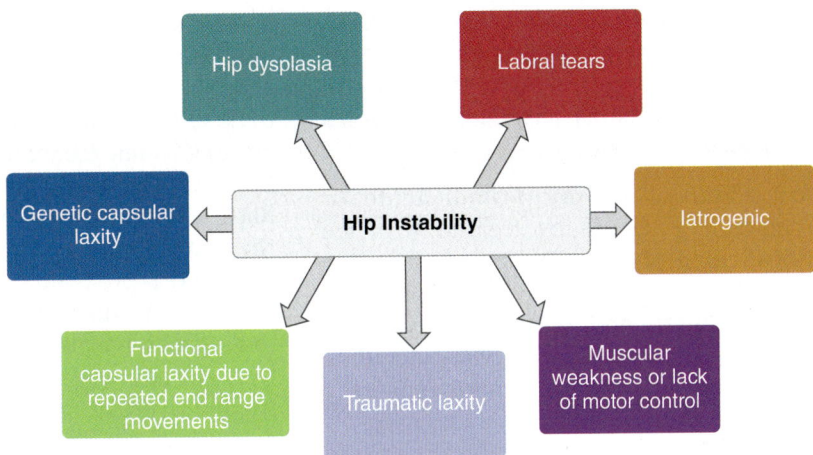

FIGURE 11-36 Causes of hip instability.

may be local, and the result of repeated end range of movement occurs in certain sports, such as dancers attempting to improve their toe out. Lastly, capsular laxity can be caused by trauma,[106] such as traumatic hip dislocation or capsular sprain, such as being forced into end range hip abduction when a ski catches in the snow. Unlike with the glenohumeral joint, instability after hip dislocation is relatively rare.[106]

The labrum and negative intra-articular pressure created by the labral fluid seal provide additional hip stability. Capsular hypermobility and labral tears[109] place greater stress on the hip musculature to provide dynamic hip stability. Muscular weakness, poor neuromuscular control, or muscular fatigue can reduce hip dynamic stability by placing increased stress on the static stabilizers. In this way, labral tears can be both the cause and the result of hip instability. FAIS can lead to hip instability. For example, an anterior cam lesion may act as a fulcrum, resulting in posterolateral hip instability.[106] Hip instability may also be iatrogenic,[106] resulting from labral debridement, overaggressive osteotomies for FAIS, or poorly/unrepaired capsulotomy. Hip instability may cause pain due to damage to nociceptive tissue, such as the labrum[109]; increased altered joint loads; and overuse of the dynamic stabilizers.

History Patients with hip instability frequently report the hip "gives way"[103] pops, locks, or catches. Pain, if present, may be in the anterior hip or groin but is typically noted by the patient using the "C" sign.[109] Patients may report a one-time traumatic event forcing the hip into an extreme range of motion. More often, the symptoms of instability are gradual and progressive in onset in individuals who participate in sports requiring significant hip range, such as dance, soccer, and ice hockey, or sports that may subject the hip to repetitive microtraumas, such as skiing.[103] Patients who must over rely on the dynamic hip stabilizers may report symptoms occur later within an activity as these stabilizers begin to fatigue.

Key Examination Findings The key objective finding for instability is the presence of excessive hip range of motion in at least one direction. It is important to assess hip external rotation both in the traditional test position of 90° of hip flexion and in neutral hip flexion, as the traditional test position may not capture acquired hip hypermobility. External rotation range may be assessed in supine. However, prone assessment allows more precise measurement and may be more likely to recreate the patient's sense of instability. The patient may have excessive external rotation with the log roll test or overt systemic hypermobility, scoring 4 or more on the Beighton scale.[103] A positive prone instability test or positive abduction-hyperextension-external rotation test[32] help to rule in instability. If the labrum is torn, the patient may have a positive scour, FADIR, or Fitzgerald test. If irritable, the patient may have spasming of the hip flexors or adductors. A positive Thomas test may be due to this protective spasming but may also be due to muscle hyperactivity in an attempt to control anterior hip instability. Hip flexor tightness may lead to decreased gluteal muscle activation.[24] Patients with instability are likely to have reduced hip and abdominal strength and may have poor neuromuscular control with functional testing, such as a single leg squat. Muscular endurance should be assessed in individuals whose symptoms arise after prolonged activity. Patients may have decreased balance or poor neuromuscular control with functional tasks, such as a single leg squat or jump landing.

Differential Diagnoses Differential diagnosis for hip instability includes FAIS and OA. Imaging noting bony dysplasia and/or pathologic labral changes may help rule in hip instability. However, these pathologic changes may also be seen in asymptomatic individuals.[92] Therefore, the clinician must be careful to match the patient's complaint with the physical examination findings as well as any imaging studies that may have been performed.

Rehabilitation Focus and Key Points Acute or irritable hip instability should be treated with ice and NSAIDs. Stretching of tight structures, including the iliopsoas, rectus femoris, and adductors, can be beneficial.[109] Strength and endurance exercises should target identified areas of weakness, including the hip abductors, external rotators, and extensors[109] as well as the abdominals and trunk extensors.[103] Neuromuscular control exercises should work on hip/pelvic and trunk control.[109] A progressive balance program should also be provided.

Expected Outcomes Conservative management of hip instability of all causes, including FAIS and labral tears, can lead to lasting resolution of pain and full return to function.[110] An intra-articular corticosteroid injection may result in long-term resolution of patient pain complaint and confirms an intra-articular cause of patient symptoms, such as a torn labrum.[111] The small portion of patients who fail to make satisfactory gains after 12 or more weeks of rehabilitation may benefit from a surgical consult.[109]

Surgical Options for Hip Instability Similar to patellar instability, surgery for hip dysplasia involves osteotomies to improve the bony stability of the hip.[107] Capsular plication may be appropriate for patients with capsular hypermobility.[108] Because capsular hypermobility tends to be anterior, the anterior capsule is typically tightened and, therefore, requires short-term protection from excessive loading. These patients may be braced to limit excessive hip extension and external rotation for about 6 weeks until the tissue strength has improved.[103] For older individuals, debridement of a torn labrum is indicated. However, labral repair may be more appropriate for younger individuals, as it preserves the labral function. As with FAIS surgery, clinicians must know the surgical procedure(s) performed, protect healing tissue, and prevent hip flexor tendinitis. A progressive program of strength, neuromuscular control, and balance training should be part of postoperative rehabilitation for hip instability. Patients generally report a high degree of satisfaction with surgical outcomes, including decreased pain, improved function, and the ability to return to sport.[106,109]

Greater Trochanteric Pain Syndrome

Pathology Greater trochanteric pain syndrome is a term used for pain in the region of the greater trochanter and lateral thigh that appears to be originating from the lateral structures of the hip, including the tendon and bursae.[112] The term includes gluteus medius/minimus tendinopathy, trochanteric bursitis, and external snapping hip.[113] Historically, symptoms were believed to be solely the result of trochanteric bursitis. However, although some trochanteric edema is present,[112] bursitis is rarely noted on magnetic resonance imaging.[114] Rather, tendinopathy, including degenerative tears of the gluteus medius, minimus, short hip external rotators, and ITB, is the most common finding.[114,115] Tendinopathy is likely the result of biomechanical deficits (e.g., excessive hip adduction during stance), structural deviations (anteversion), poor tendon vascularity, and overuse.[115] External snapping hip (also known as *external coxa saltans*) is a snapping, or flipping, of the ITB over the greater trochanter during hip flexion and extension. External snapping hip is believed to be mostly due to thickening of the posterior portion of the ITB and the anterior portion of the gluteus maximus.[115] GTPS is more common in women than in men and in 30- to 50-year-olds.[114] Younger, active individuals are more likely to have GTPS due to external snapping hip.[114] GTPS is also seen after THA with a lateral or posterior approach. This is most likely because these methods damage the gluteus medius, gluteus minimus, and short external rotators, which can lead to scarring, fatty degeneration, and bursal irritation.[115]

History Individuals with GTPS report dull, aching lateral hip pain that increases with stairs, transfers, and active hip abduction.[27] Occasionally, symptoms may also be described as a burning pain in the posterior/posterolateral hip.[27] Sidelying on the affected side causes pain[51] due to direct compression of the involved tissues against the support surface. However, sidelying on the contralateral side[116] can also cause discomfort due to compression of the tissues against the greater trochanter that occurs with hip adduction.

True acute bursitis, inflammation of a bursa around the greater trochanter, can occur from an acute blow to the side of the hip, such as falling on the side of the leg or being hit with a lacrosse ball in the region of the greater trochanter.

Key Examination Findings GTPS should be suspected with the following examination findings:[29,51,114,116,117]

- Tenderness upon palpation of the greater trochanter
- Pain with resisted hip abduction
- Positive external rotation derotation test
- Pain with the modified external derotation test
- Positive Trendelenburg test for lateral hip pain or weakness
- Lateral hip pain with 30″ single leg stance
- Palpable or audible snapping of the ITB over the greater trochanter with hip flexion and extension that recreates the patient's complaint

While a hallmark of GTPS is pain upon palpation of the greater trochanter,[51,114] this has some degree of error, with about 15-mm differences between examiners.[118] However, it is important to note that several tissues, not just the tissue directly over the bony trochanter, are involved with GTPS. Patients with GTPS may have pain with hip adduction and Ober's test[113] due to compression of the involved tissues. Likewise, they may have lateral hip pain with a FABER test.[116] If snapping is noted with hip flexion and extension, the clinician can manually compress the ITB proximal to the greater trochanter or externally rotate the hip to see if symptoms during these hip motions resolve.[114]

Differential Diagnoses The presence of morning hip stiffness and/or difficulty donning socks and shoes is more indicative of hip OA.[51] A positive straight leg raise or the presence of pain more distal in the thigh or radiating pain is more indicative of lumbar spine pathology.[116] Concurrent low back pain is not uncommon.[112,119] Rheumatologic conditions may also coexist with GTPS[115] and, if present, would benefit from collaboration with a rheumatologist or skilled primary care provider.

Rehabilitation Focus and Key Points Rehabilitation should focus on relative rest, education, and exercise.[93,112,114] Active individuals with external snapping hip should avoid modifying activities short term to avoid the range of hip flexion that elicits symptoms. Avoiding sidelying (or contralateral sidelying without a pillow between one's legs) and hip adduction, such as crossing one's legs or standing with a contralateral pelvic drop, also allows the tissue time to recover. Ice may also be beneficial to all patients with GTPS because of its analgesic effects. Runners may benefit from avoiding running on a sloped surface (such as roads that are banked toward the curb).[112] Patients with a Trendelenburg sign may benefit from gait training or an assistive device to decrease pain and/or improve gait form. Progressive core and gluteal strengthening are critical. Core strengthening can assist with pelvic control. Hip abductor and extensor strengthening should include non–weight-bearing and weight-bearing exercises.[114] Gluteal strengthening should initially avoid hip adduction and clamshell exercises[93] (see Fig. 11-49) because these exercises create combined loading on the tendon, tension due to muscle contraction with simultaneous compression against the grater trochanter. Soft-tissue restrictions of the hip abductors benefit from stretching and manual therapy.[93,112] Extracorporeal shock wave therapy or corticosteroid injection may be beneficial for those who are progressing slowly.[112,114]

Expected Outcomes More than 90% of patients will improve and be able to return to daily activities/work/sport without restriction using conservative treatment alone. For recalcitrant cases, gluteal tendon repair appears to have good results, whereas the impact of ITB release with bursectomy is unknown.[37]

Groin Pain

Groin pain is common cause of pain in athletes. Hip joint–related groin pain is generally accompanied by reports of catching, locking, or giving way as well as positive FADIR and/or FABER test. The four main nonarticular causes of groin pain are listed in Table 11-6.[105] Treatment of groin pain includes ice, controlled rest, and symptom-modulated rehabilitation that puts gradual progressive stress on the involved tissue. For example, progressive exercises for a soccer player with adductor-related groin pain may begin with small arc supine hip adduction/abduction and small arc sidelying hip abduction. As the patient improves, adduction is progressed to ipsilateral sidelying active range of motion, then standing resisted range of motion, then versions of an adduction plank (Fig. 11-37). Likewise, gradual adductor lengthening is performed. Given that adductors function as both hip flexors and hip extensors pending the angle of the hip, strengthening should include the hip flexors and extensors as well. Closed-chain progressions of single leg squats can be progressed to small and then larger, forward, and side lunges. Sport-specific activities such as running, jumping, passing, and cutting should be added as the patient tolerates greater stress to the adductors. Cardiovascular fitness can be maintained acutely with stationary bicycling and progressed to an elliptical and, eventually, to running. Soft-tissue mobilization to the involved tissue may be beneficial. Clinicians may use the adductor test as a means of tracking progress over time and titrating exercise. If the patient's pain with the adductor test is less than 2/10, exercise is

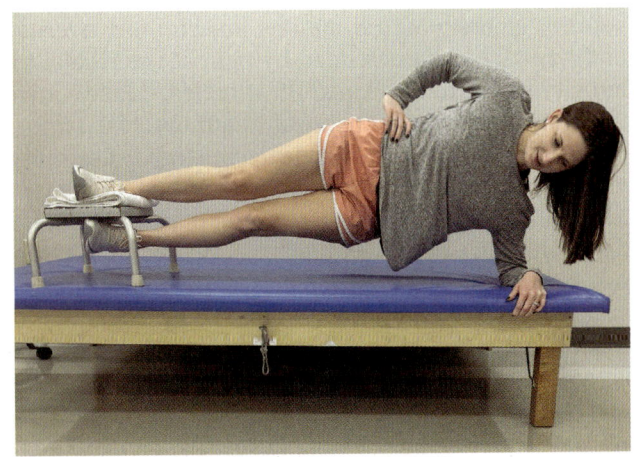

FIGURE 11-37 Adduction plank.

TABLE 11-6
NONARTICULAR CAUSES OF GROIN PAIN

Type	Characteristics
Adductor related	Tenderness to palpation of the adductors Pain with hip adductor test
Iliopsoas related	Pain with active or resisted hip flexion Pain with hip extension Tenderness to palpation of the iliopsoas
Inguinal related	Tenderness in the inguinal canal without the presence of a hernia Pain increased with abdominal contraction, such as coughing, sneezing, or trunk curl
Pubic related	Local tenderness to palpation of the pubic symphysis

progressing at an appropriate level. If pain is higher, exercise stressing the adductors should be reduced.

The clinician must consider multiple other structures and systems for the differential diagnosis of groin pain. Groin pain may be due to a hernia, nerve entrapment, lumbar or sacroiliac dysfunction, apophysitis, as well as an avulsion or stress fracture.[105] Groin pain may also be caused by diverticulitis, appendicitis, urinary tract infection, or kidney stones.[105]

Proximal Hamstring Tendinopathy

Pathology

Proximal HS injuries include rupture, avulsion, acute strain, and chronic tendinopathy. Surgical repair is recommended for young athletes who have an avulsion along with proximal retraction of the HS.[120] Open or endoscopic repair results in high patient satisfaction and the ability to return to preinjury activities in most cases.[120] Acute strains may occur in both the nonathletic population (slip on the ice leading to sudden lengthening of the HS) and the athletic population (first baseman reaching for a low throw). However, the majority of proximal HS injuries are chronic, overuse tendinopathies characterized by pain at the ischial tuberosity where the proximal HS attaches. Conservative rehabilitation is the mainstay of treatment. Risk factors for proximal HS injuries include decreased HS flexibility, decreased HS strength, poor HS endurance, decreased core stability, lack of a proper warm-up and other training errors, and prior HS injury.[120,121] The proximal HS tendon may be subject to combined loading in two ways. First, the attachment of the semimembranosus crosses under the semitendinosis and biceps femoris, leading to shear forces during tendon loading.[122] Second, compression against the ischial tuberosity can occur when the hip is flexed, as occurs when performing a lunge. Proximal HS tendinopathy has a high degree of recurrence.

History Patients with proximal HS tendinopathy will report proximal HS pain that increases in proportion to the degree of HS loading. So, patients may report jogging is pain free, running is painful, and sprinting is not possible due to significant pain. For athletes, symptoms may be present during warm-up and then resolve. However, as the condition worsens, pain may continue or even increase.

Key Examination Findings Patients with proximal HS tendinopathy will report pain with active or passive stretching of the HS and limited HS length is to be expected.[27] Resisted knee flexion and, if severe or irritable, resisted hip extension will be painful.[27,120] A single leg deadlift will also be painful as it creates significant HS load.[121] Local tenderness at the ischial tuberosity and proximal tendon should be expected.[27] Given the potential for central sensitization with tendinopathies, pain may be more diffuse and/or disproportionate to the extent of the injury.[121]

Differential Diagnoses Differential diagnosis of proximal HS tendinopathy includes avulsion fracture, apophysitis, and sciatic nerve irritation.

Rehabilitation Focus and Key Points Treatment for chronic proximal HS tendinopathy should include progressive loading of the HS tendon, similar to that described for patellar tendinopathy (see Chapter 10, Knee): isometrics, heavy slow resistance, energy storage, and sport-specific training. To limit combined compressive and shear loading, HS exercises should be performed in a more neutral hip angle initially, before progressing to a more flexed position.[123] So, for example, isotonic knee flexion should be performed in prone before using the seated knee flexion machine. In this way, HS strengthening also progresses from midrange strengthening to strengthening at increased HS length, such as with the Nordic HS curl (Fig. 11-38).[123,124] Energy storage exercises might include alternate leg split squat jumps or kettlebell swings. Sport-specific training should then be to replicate the HS load at various hip flexion ranges, such as cutting, uphill running, and HS lengthening at speed, as occurs with sprinting. Finally, the volume of proximal HS loading is increased to meet sport-specific demands. Rehabilitation must also work to remediate risk factors, such as limited HS flexibility and poor core strength. Quadriceps and hip strengthening and neuromuscular control exercises are recommended as higher levels of gluteus maximus and core activation during activities such as sprinting are associated with a decreased risk of reinjury.[125]

Expected Outcomes The vast majority of athletes and nonathletes recover with conservative interventions.[123,124]

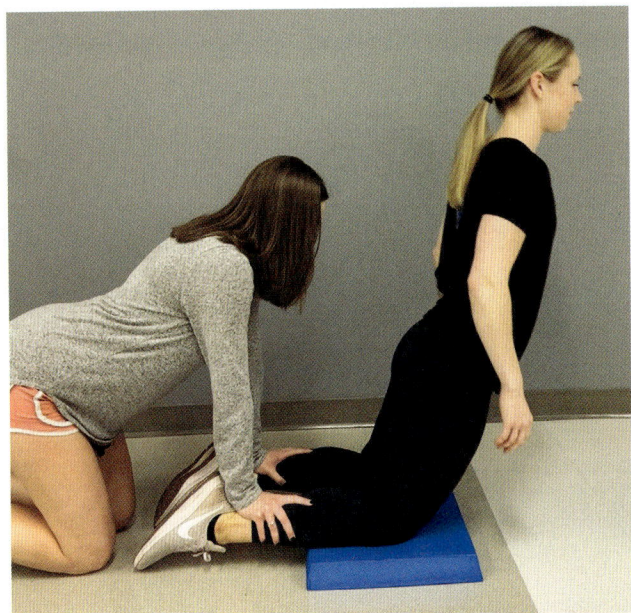

FIGURE 11-38 Nordic hamstring curl.

Slipped Capital Femoral Epiphysis

SCFE is a hip disorder that occurs in children aged 8 to 15 years.[126] It is not fully understood why the femoral head slides backward off the femoral neck at the epiphyseal plate. The majority of individuals with an SCFE are overweight,[126] placing increased stress on the epiphyseal plate. SCFE is also more prevalent during growth spurts, in individuals with endocrine disorders, and after radiation therapy to the region.[126,127] Males are more commonly affected than females.[126]

Children with an SCFE most often present with complaints of poorly localized hip, groin, or thigh pain. They may also have a limp. Unfortunately, SCFE is frequently missed initially and may be misdiagnosed as a groin pull. About 12% of patients will present with only knee pain,[126] which can further delay diagnosis. Delayed diagnosis is problematic because this can lead to early-onset hip degenerative joint disease and a possible need for a hip arthroplasty due to osteonecrosis of the femoral head.

Very rarely, an SCFE occurs due to trauma. Therefore, it is critical for clinicians to thoroughly examine hip motion in children with hip, groin, thigh, or knee pain and should consider the possibility of SCFE in a child aged 8 to 15 years who presents with atraumatic limping. The physical examination will present with limited hip internal rotation, and there will be obligatory hip external rotation with passive hip flexion due to the abnormal position of the femoral head.[127] Patients with suspected SCFE should be made non–weight bearing and referred immediately to an orthopaedist. An SCFE is treated surgically with internal fixation realigning the femoral head. At times, this condition may occur bilaterally, and the literature is not conclusive as to the value of prophylactic surgery on an asymptomatic limb.[127]

Legg-Calvé-Perthes Disease

Legg-Calvé-Perthes disease is a hip condition affecting children aged 4 to 10 years; it occurs when the blood supply to the femoral head is spontaneously, temporarily disrupted. If not protected from weight-bearing forces during this time, the femoral head is likely to collapse (avascular necrosis). Legg-Calvé-Perthes disease is more common in males, and up to 15% of cases are bilateral. Legg-Calvé-Perthes disease is less prevalent than SCFE but should be considered for children of this age with reports of vague hip, groin, or thigh pain along with limited hip internal rotation.[127] If Legg-Calvé-Perthes disease is suspected, the patient should be referred immediately to an orthopaedist. Mild cases of Legg-Calvé-Perthes disease are typically treated nonoperatively with observation, serial imaging, and limiting impact activities such as running.[128] Moderate cases may require partial weight bearing, casting, or bracing to help with femoral head remodeling. Older children or more severe cases may require surgery and have a higher risk for hip degenerative joint disease later in life. Physical therapy is often required to assist with hip range of motion[128]; however, long-term outcomes even for those requiring surgical intervention are generally good.[129]

DIFFERENTIAL DIAGNOSIS

Clinicians can begin to narrow down differential diagnosis of patients with hip pathology by symptom location (Fig. 11-39), patient symptoms (Table 11-7), and onset (Fig. 11-40).

ADDITIONAL JOINT MOBILIZATION TREATMENT TECHNIQUES

When performing hip joint mobilizations to improve range of motion, a mobilization belt can reduce the amount of effort required by the clinician and the patient may be able to relax better.

Inferior Glide of Femur with Belt

Purpose: To increase joint play movement necessary for hip flexion and abduction.
Patient: Supine with the hip flexed, angled slightly on the table so that the hips are closer to the edge and shoulders are further away.
Clinician: The clinician stands at the side of the table facing the patient's head, and a belt encircles the clinician's buttock and the patient's proximal femur close to the joint line.
Mobilization: An inferior glide is imparted through the belt by shifting hips backward, while the hands

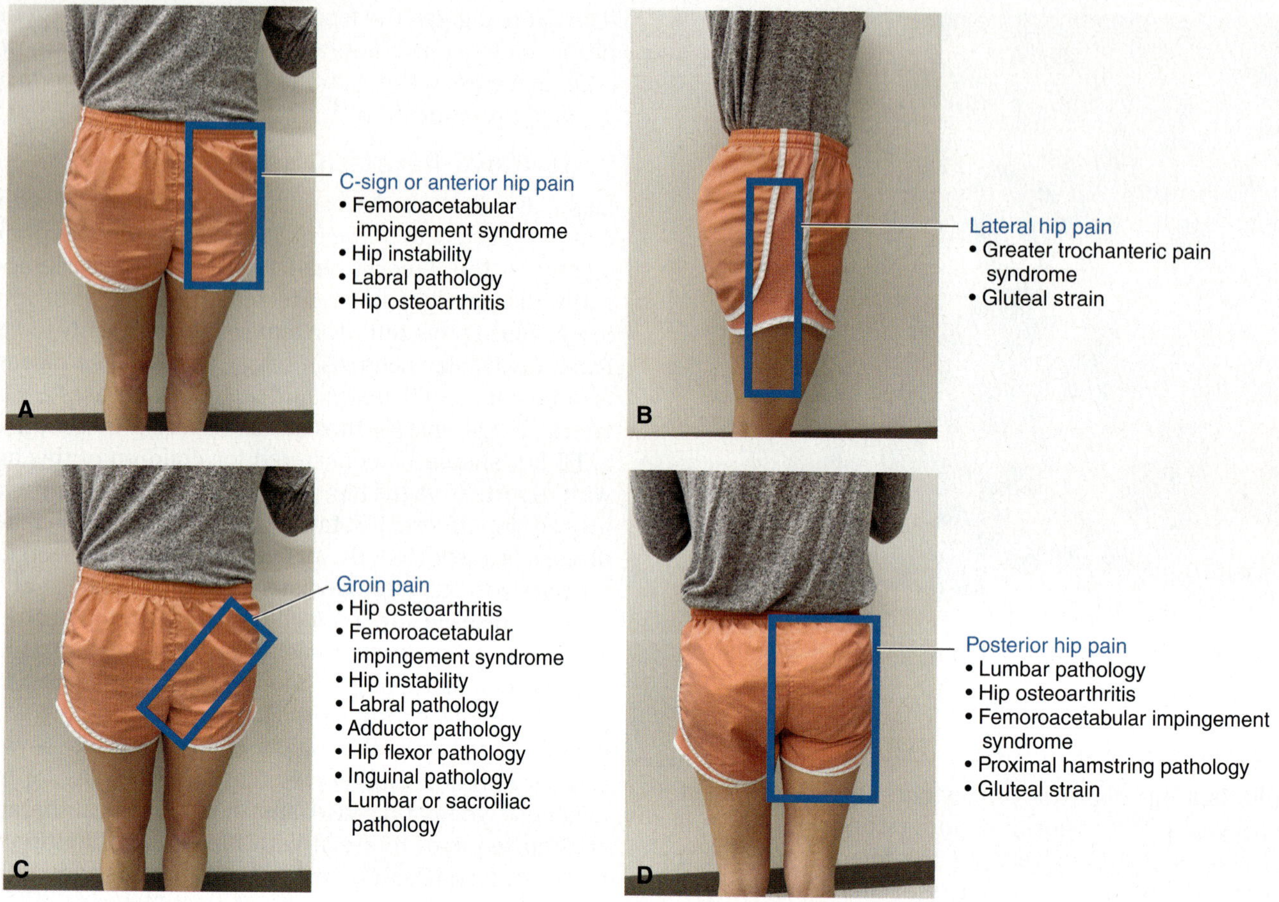

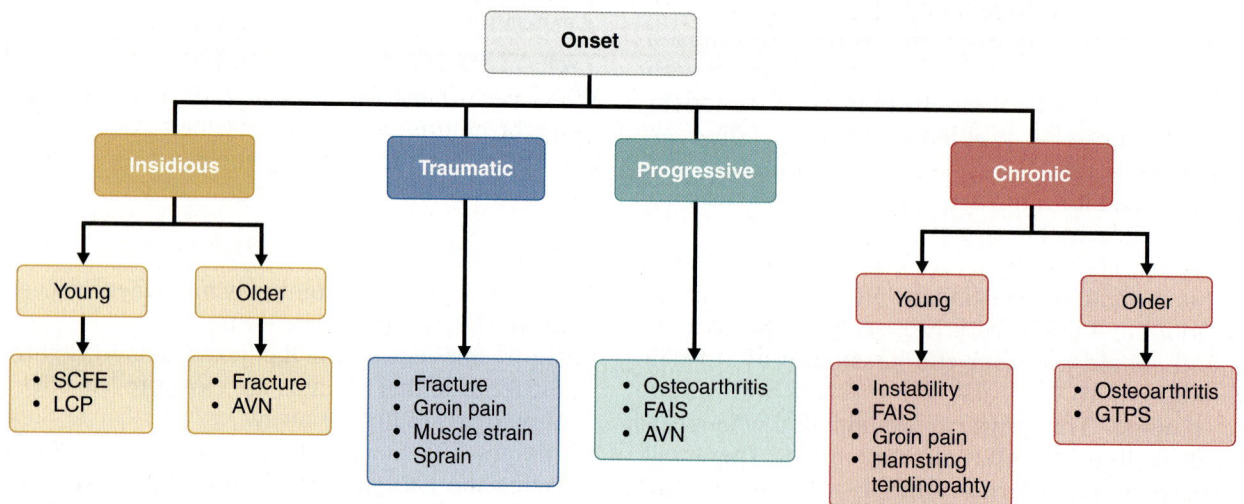

FIGURE 11-39 Hip pathology by symptom location. **A.** C-sign or anterior hip pain. **B.** Lateral hip pain. **C.** Groin pain. **D.** Posterior hip pain.

FIGURE 11-40 Hip pathology based on typical onset. *AVN*, avascular necrosis; *FAIS*, femoroacetabular impingement syndrome; *GTPS*, greater trochanteric pain syndrome; *LCP*, Legg-Calvé-Perthes; *SCFE*, slipped capital femoral epiphysis.

TABLE 11-7
DIFFERENTIAL DIAGNOSIS OF HIP PATHOLOGY BY COMPLAINT

Complaint	Differential Diagnoses
Paresthesias: numbness, tingling, burning	Proximal structure (e.g., lumbar spine, sciatic nerve)
Difficulty with donning shoes/socks	Osteoarthritis
Stiffness or loss of motion	Osteoarthritis Femoroacetabular impingement syndrome
Giving way or instability	Hip instability
Clicking, locking, catching	Osteoarthritis Labral pathology Femoroacetabular impingement syndrome
Pain with active movement or resistance activities	Greater trochanteric pain syndrome Hamstring tendinopathy Adductor pathology Hip flexor pathology Inguinal-related pathology
Pain with weight bearing	Osteoarthritis Greater trochanteric pain syndrome Hip fracture Slipped capital femoral epiphysis Legg-Calvé-Perthes

hold the distal thigh stable. This may also be performed as a mobilization with movement by simultaneously rocking the thigh into flexion (Fig. 11-41).

Anterior Glide of Femur in Prone Figure-of-Four Position

Purpose: To increase joint play movement necessary for hip extension and external rotation.
Patient: Prone with hip to be mobilized in a figure-of-four position: slightly flexed, abducted, and externally rotated.
Clinician: Standing on the contralateral side to be mobilized, the superior hand stabilizes the pelvis by holding the anterior pelvis. A towel roll can be placed for additional stabilization. The inferior hand contacts the proximal femur at the level of the greater trochanter.
Mobilization: An anterior, lateral, and slightly superior glide of the proximal femur is imparted with the inferior hand (Fig. 11-42). To perform as a mobilization with movement, the clinician can rely on the toweling for stabilizing the pelvis. The superior hand performs the mobilization, and the inferior hand holds the patient's ankle to move the hip into external rotation during the glide.

Anterior Glide of Femur in Prone with Belt

Purpose: To increase joint play movement necessary for hip extension and external rotation.
Patient: Prone with the knee flexed.
Clinician: Standing on the side to be mobilized, a belt encircles the clinician's inferior shoulder and the patient's distal femur to support the patient's femur near end range hip extension. The clinician's

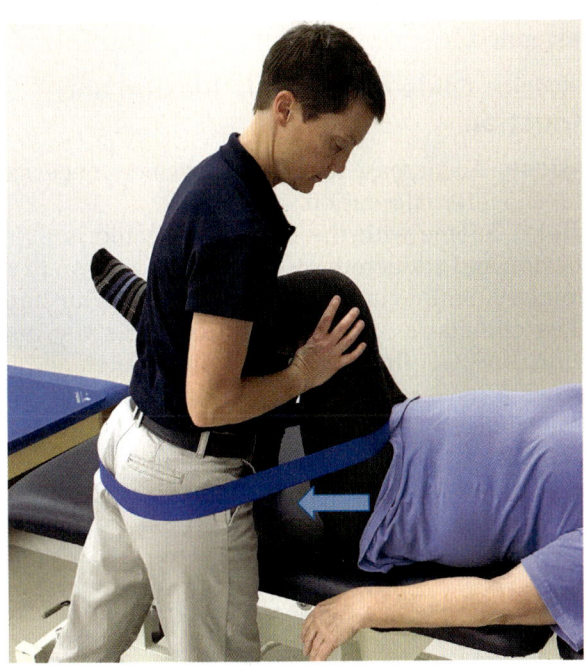

FIGURE 11-41 Inferior glide of femur with belt.

inferior hand holds the patient's distal femur, with the forearm supporting the patient's tibia. The superior hand contacts the proximal femur at the level of the greater trochanter.
Mobilization: An anterior, lateral, and slightly superior glide of the proximal femur is imparted with the superior hand (Fig. 11-43). This may also be performed as a mobilization with movement by simultaneously extending the thigh using tension in the belt while performing the anterior glide. If the patient's recuts femoris is tight, the mobilization

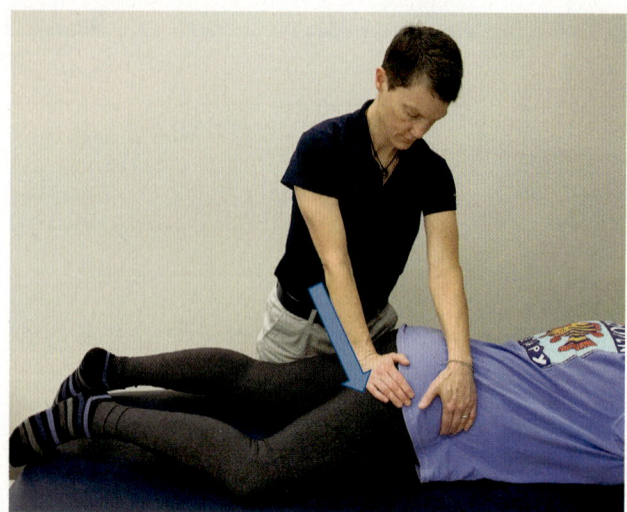

FIGURE 11-42 Anterior glide of femur in prone figure-of-four position.

should be performed with the patient's knee more extended.

Posterior Glide of Femur in Flexion and Adduction

Purpose: To increase joint play movement necessary for hip internal rotation.
Patient: Supine with the hip to be treated in 90° of flexion and adducted.
Clinician: Supports the knee with the inferior hand. The clinician's superior hand contacts the anterior aspect of the patient's proximal thigh and imparts a posterolateral glide by leaning forward at the trunk.
Mobilization: Mobilization force is applied by leaning laterally and distally (Fig. 11-44).

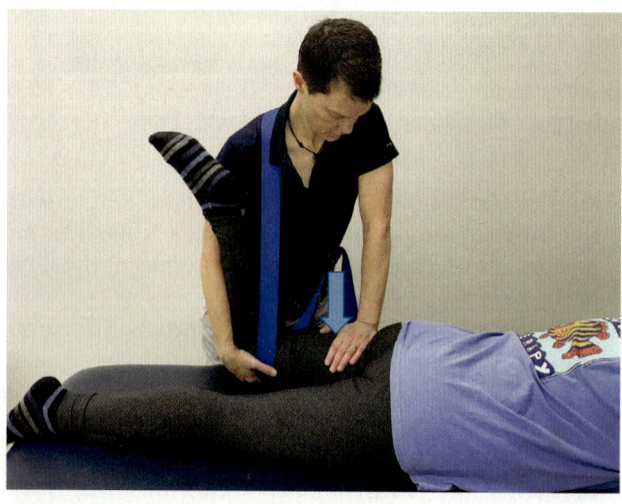

FIGURE 11-43 Anterior glide of femur in prone with belt.

Lateral Distraction of Femur with Belt

Purpose: To facilitate global hip mobility as well as flexion, internal rotation, and adduction.
Patient: Supine, hip and knee flexed, angled slightly on the table so that the hips are closer to the edge and shoulders are further away.
Clinician: The clinician stands at the side of the table facing the patient, and a belt encircles the clinician's buttock and the patient's proximal femur close to the joint line. The superior hand stabilizes the distal femur.
Mobilization: A lateral distracting force is applied through the belt by shifting hips backward, while the proximal hand stabilizes the distal femur (Fig. 11-45). This can be performed as a

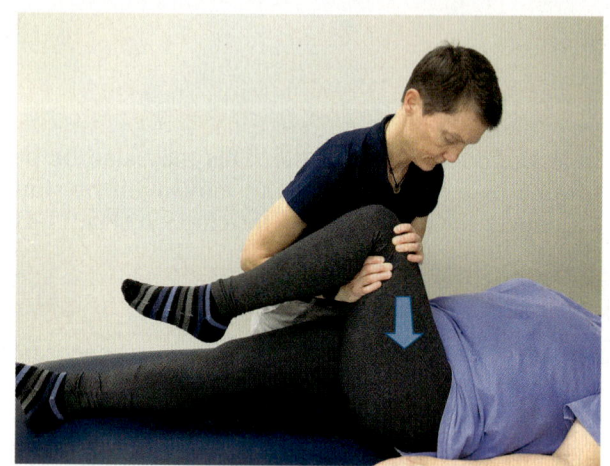

FIGURE 11-44 Posterior glide of femur in flexion and adduction.

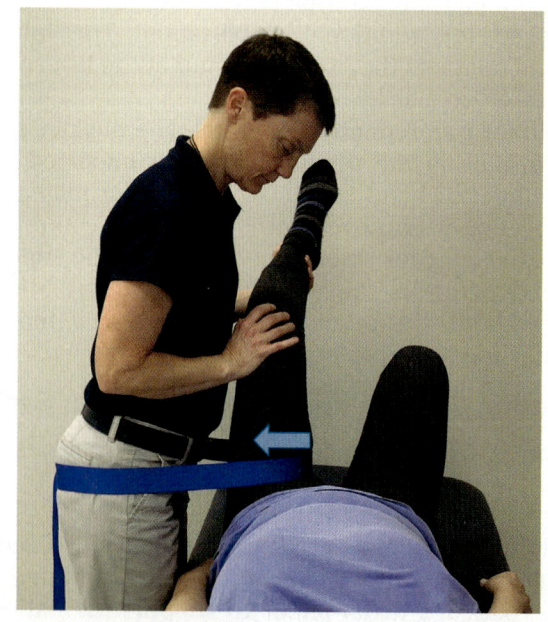

FIGURE 11-45 Lateral distraction of femur with belt.

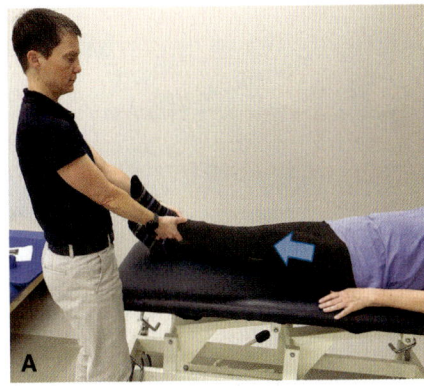 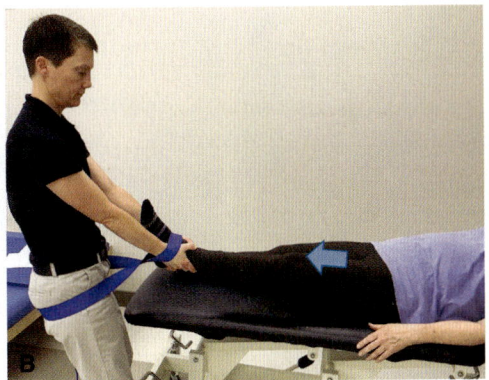 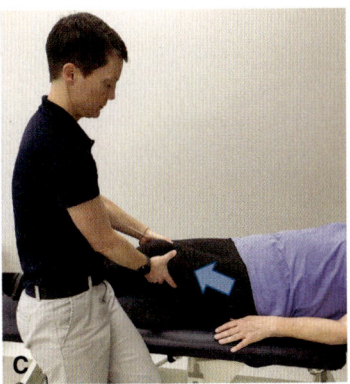

FIGURE 11-46 Long-axis distraction of femur. **A.** Using a long lever arm. **B.** Using a belt. **C.** Using a short lever arm.

mobilization with movement with the clinician's inferior hand moving the femur into various degrees of internal rotation.

Long-Axis Distraction of Femur

Purpose: To increase general joint mobility as well as flexion and abduction.
Patient: Supine with the hip to be treated in 30° flexion, 30° abduction, and slight external rotation.
Clinician: A. The clinician encircles the patient's lower leg, just proximal to the malleoli, with both hands (Fig. 11-46A).
  B. The clinician makes a figure-of-eight with a belt, encircling the clinician's buttock and the patient's lower leg to help clamp the hands more comfortably around the patient's lower leg (Fig. 11-46B).
  C. The clinician's hands encircle the distal femur. This method should be used for patients with coexisting knee dysfunction as the mobilizing force no longer does through the knee joint (Fig. 11-46C).
Mobilization: Mobilization force is applied by leaning inferiorly (Fig. 11-46).

ADDITIONAL THERAPEUTIC EXERCISES

A primary goal of hip rehabilitation is improvement in hip strength and motor control. The following section provides examples of common strengthening exercises. Hip extensor strengthening can begin with a bridge or a squat and progress to a single leg bridge (Fig. 11-47) or a single leg squat. Hip extensor exercises can be performed in standing (or prone) with or without additional resistance of bands or cuff weights.

Hip abductor strength can be performed unilaterally in sidelying (Fig. 11-48A) and progressed with the addition of a cuff weight, resistance band, or manual resistance. Standing hip abduction requires isometric contraction of the stance limb while simultaneously challenging the moving limb (Fig. 11-48B). For a greater challenge that requires more core stabilization, the

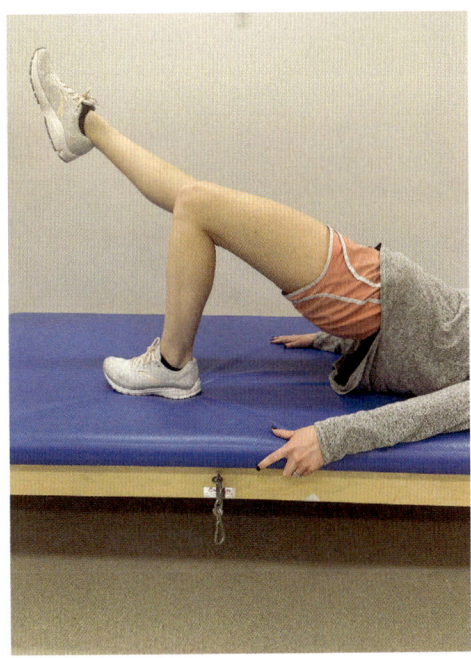

FIGURE 11-47 Single leg bridge.

patient can perform a side plank (Fig. 11-48C). Progressing to a side plank with hip abduction (Fig. 11-48D), the patient no longer has the hip adductors of the top limb to assist with holding the position. In addition, the hip abductors of the top limb must now work against gravity to hold the limb in place.

A common hip external rotator and abductor strengthening program is the sidelying clam progression (Fig. 11-49). These exercises progress in intensity for the gluteus maximus, gluteus medius, and small hip external rotators. The clinician may choose the hardest exercise a patient is able to perform for 8 to 10 repetitions as a strengthening progression or the exercises can be performed in sequence for more of a challenge to muscular endurance. Prone resisted hip external rotation strengthens the hip external

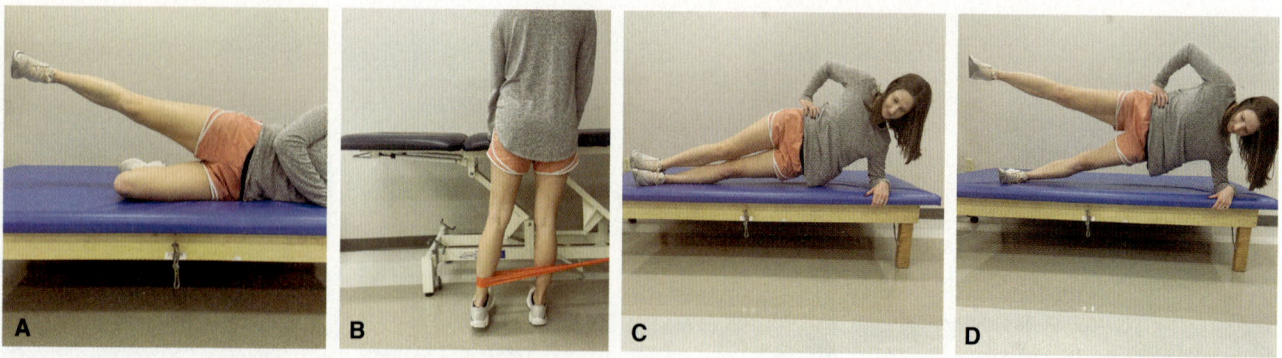

FIGURE 11-48 Hip abductor progression. **A.** Sidelying hip abduction. **B.** Standing hip abduction with resistance band. **C.** Side plank. **D.** Side plank with hip abduction.

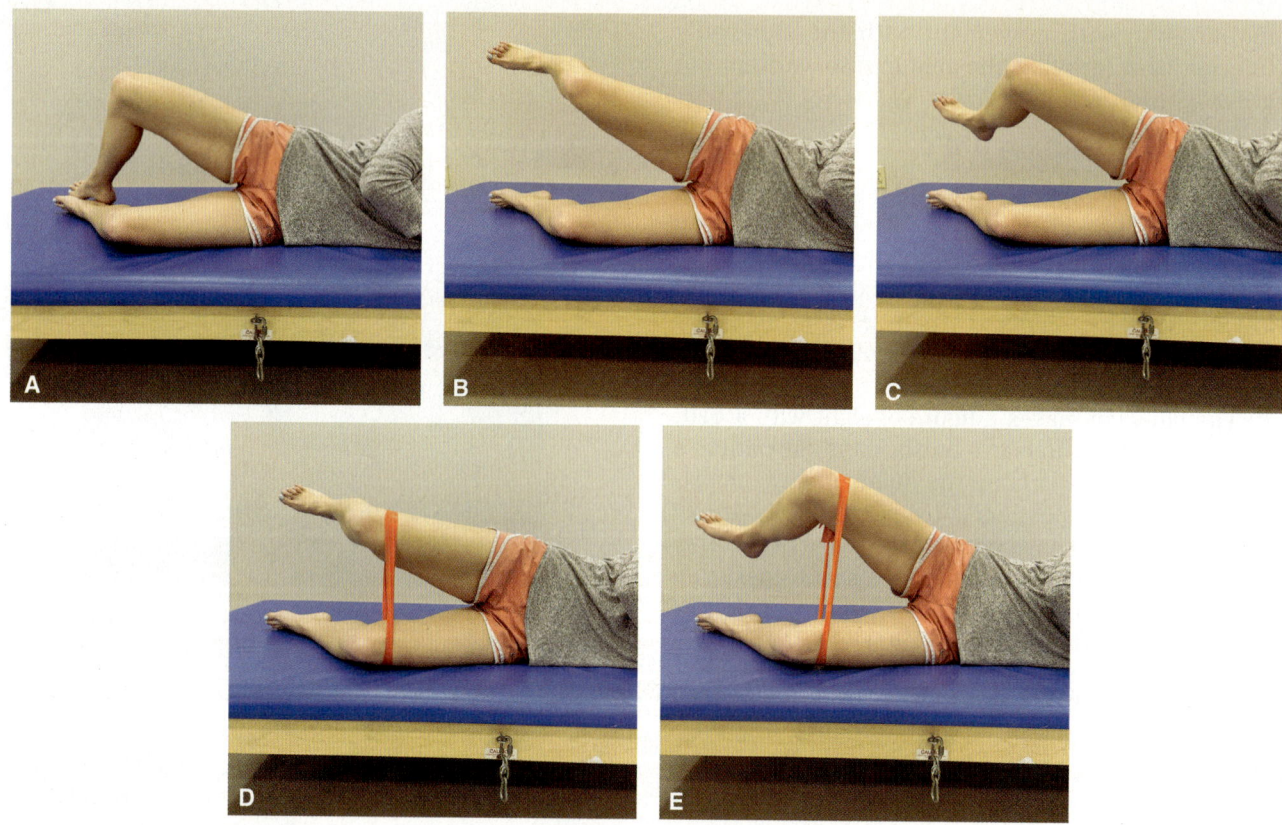

FIGURE 11-49 Sidelying clam progression. **A.** Hip external rotation. **B.** Hip abduction. **C.** Hip external rotation in abduction. **D.** Band resisted hip abduction. **E.** Band resisted hip external rotation in abduction.

rotators at a more functional angle of hip flexion/extension (Fig. 11-50).

Stretching in combination with manual therapy can help improve hip motion. Hip extension range of motion and hip flexor length can be achieved by stretching in the Thomas test position. For individuals who are less mobile, they can be positioned supine in hooklying diagonally across the plinth with the leg to be stretched hanging off the edge of the support surface. Hip flexion can be facilitated by bringing one knee up to the chest. However, many times, patients prefer a gentle rocking into flexion from a quadruped position (Fig. 11-51). External rotation can be facilitated in sitting or supine with a figure-of-four position in which the ankle of the leg to be stretched is crossed over the opposite knee. The stretch can be intensified by moving into a more flexed position. For internal rotation, patients can be taught to self-stretch (Fig. 11-52).

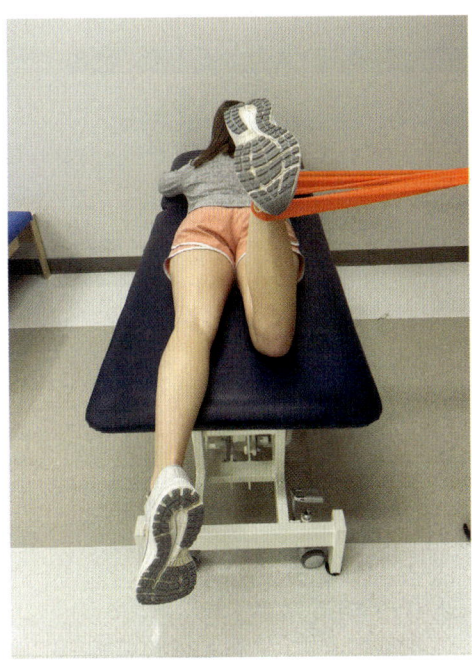

FIGURE 11-50 Prone hip external rotation with resistance band.

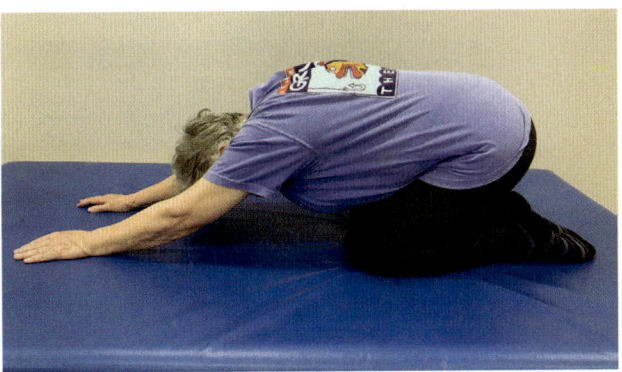

FIGURE 11-51 Quadruped rocking into hip flexion.

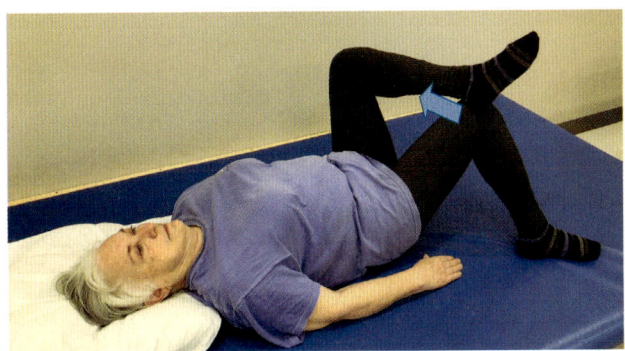

FIGURE 11-52 Patient self-stretch into right hip internal rotation.

CASE STUDY 11-1

Monica: Patient with Left Hip Fracture

Monica is a 71-year-old woman grandmother who fell in the yard while gardening, fracturing her left hip. Because of her preexisting hip OA, she and her surgeon decided she would be best served with a left THA using an anterior approach. The surgery was performed the day after fracture, and she was discharged home 2 days after surgery WBAT on the left lower extremity. Upon arrival at outpatient physical therapy 4 days after surgery, Monica reports only minimal pain and that she has been doing ankle pumps and taking small walks in the house. All tests begin with the uninvolved (right) side unless otherwise noted. As noted previously, the examination should be organized by position, begin away and progress toward the involved area, and provide increasing stress to injured or potentially involved structures. Table 11-8 provides an example of how an experienced clinician might organize the physical examination after performing the history and systems review.

The clinician chose not to perform trunk range of motion but did perform myotome, sensation, and reflex testing to assess lower quarter neurologic function after fall and surgery with spinal anesthesia. Note that sensation testing was not simply an assessment of dermatomal sensation for nerve root pathology, as the surgery might have injured a lower extremity peripheral nerve. The examination began in the seated position, starting with the distal lower extremity and working proximally. HS length was not specifically assessed but was observed during knee extension strength testing. The clinician did not assess hip external rotation or extension range of motion, specifically due to the anterior approach for THA. However, the clinician did assess that the hip went to at least neutral in supine and would note any loss of functional hip extension during gait assessment. Functional assessment of hip

TABLE 11-8
SAMPLE HIP EXAMINATION

Monica: a 71-year-old female 4 days after a left total hip arthroplasty for a proximal femur fracture sustained from a fall

Position	Assessments
Observation	Continues from history
Seated	Great toe extension (A, OP, MMT) Ankle dorsiflexion (A, OP, MMT) Ankle plantarflexion (A, OP, MMT) Knee extension (A, OP, MMT) Knee flexion (MMT with knee at 90°) Hip internal rotation (A, OP) Hip external rotation (isometric resisted testing in neutral) Sensory testing bilateral lower extremity Reflexes: Achilles, patellar
Supine	Knee flexion (P) Knee extension (P) Hip flexion: heel slide and straight leg with assist if needed Hip abduction (A, P, resistance if able) Hip adduction (A from abducted to neutral, resistance if able) Bridge to assess hip extensor strength Muscle length: gastrocnemius Integument including incision inspection and edema assessment
Standing	Footwear inspection Structure/posture screen including leg length Weight shift right ↔ left Single leg balance: eyes open, eyes closed as able MMT: plantarflexion right, left if able to full WB Function: gait Functional testing: Five Times Sit-to-Stand, Timed Up and Go, Berg Balance Test

A, active; *MMT*, manual muscle test; *OP*, overpressure; *P*, passive range of motion.

extensor strength was performed in safe ranges using both the bridge and sit-to-stand rather than attempting prone hip extension or modifying hip extensor testing in standing bent over a plinth. In addition, sidelying hip abduction and adduction strength was not attempted as the patient was unlikely to have greater than 3+/5 strength at this time. The incision was inspected to assess tissue healing. The clinician did assess Monica's leg length during the structural examination as leg length discrepancies can occur after THA. However, finer details, such as femoral torsion, were not required. Balance and functional testing was performed in a progressive manner, beginning with simple weight shifting, progressing to single leg stance as able. During single leg stance, the clinician observed not only balance but also pelvic position (Trendelenburg test). Functional strength testing was performed via the Five Times Sit-to-Stand test. The Berg Balance test was performed to provide additional understanding of the patient's current fall risk, which is particularly crucial given Monica's recent fall. The 6-Minute Walk test was deemed to be too difficult for Monica at this time, so the shorter TUG was used to get a baseline of her walking speed.

In a different scenario, trunk active range of motion, quadrant testing, hip accessory motions, and hip joint–specific special tests may have been performed to assist with determining a differential diagnosis. Core strength may have been performed, but this did not appear to be relevant to Monica's balance and function as a 71-year-old gardener and grandmother.

CHAPTER SUMMARY

The examination and treatment of patients with pain in the region of the hip begins with a thorough history and must include questions regarding potential nonmusculoskeletal causes of hip pain, such as the gastrointestinal and genitourinary systems. In addition, a lower quarter neurologic screen should be performed to clear the lumbar spine or determine whether the lumbar spine may be involved in the patient's condition. This is particularly true if the patient reports the presence of paresthesias. Age can assist with differential diagnosis of hip pathology: with younger individuals more likely to have an SCFE or Legg-Calvé-Perthes disease, whereas older patients are more likely to have OA or GTPS. Patients with hip pain may have bony impingement or instability or a combination of both. Musculotendinous tissue can also be the source of both acute and chronic pain in the hip region. Rehabilitation may need to address range of motion, flexibility, strength, motor control, balance of the involved lower extremity, the uninvolved lower extremity, and trunk.

REFERENCES

1. Polkowski G, Clohisy J. Hip biomechanics. *Sports Med Arthrosc Rev*. 2010;18(2):56–62. doi:10.1097/JSA.0b013e3181dc5774
2. Williams PL. *Gray's Anatomy: The Anatomical Basis of Medicine and Surgery*. 38th ed. Churchill Livingstone; 1995.
3. Moore KM, Dalley AF, Agur AMR. *Clinically Oriented Anatomy*. 8th ed. Wolters Kluwer; 2018.
4. Mesgarzadeh M, Revesz G, Bonakdarpour A. Femoral neck torsion angle measurement by computed tomography. *J Comput Assist Tomogr*. 1987;11(5):799–803. doi:10.1097/00004728-198709000-00011
5. Staheli L. Rotational problems of the lower extremities. *Orthop Clin North Am*. 1987;18(4):503–512.
6. Kalhor M, Beck M, Huff T, Ganz R. Capsular and pericapsular contributions to acetabular and femoral head perfusion. *J Bone Joint Surg Am*. 2009;91(2):409–418. doi:10.2106/jbjs.G.01679
7. Jo S, Hooke A, An K, Trousdale R, Sierra R. Contribution of the ligamentum teres to hip stability in the presence of an intact capsule: a cadaveric study. *Arthroscopy*. 2018;34(5):1480–1487. doi:10.1016/j.arthro.2017.12.002
8. O'Donnell J, Devitt B, Arora M. The role of the ligamentum teres in the adult hip: redundant or relevant? A review. *J Hip Preserv Surg*. 2018;5(1):15–22. doi:10.1093/jhps/hnx046
9. Varma D, Richli W, Charnsangavej C, Samuels B, Kim E, Wallace S. MR appearance of the distended iliopsoas bursa. *AJR Am J Roentgenol*. 1991;156(5):1025–1028. doi:10.2214/ajr.156.5.2017926
10. Omoumi P, Vande Berg B. Hip imaging: normal variants and asymptomatic findings. *Semin Musculoskelet Radiol*. 2017;21(5):507–517. doi:10.1055/s-0037-1606136
11. Kassarjian A, Llopis E, Schwartz R, Bencardino J. Obturator externus bursa: prevalence of communication with the hip joint and associated intra-articular findings in 200 consecutive hip MR arthrograms. *Eur Radiol*. 2009;19(11):2779–2782. doi:10.1007/s00330-009-1476-5
12. Chowdhury R, Naaseri S, Lee J, Rajeswaran G. Imaging and management of greater trochanteric pain syndrome. *Postgrad Med J*. 2014;90(1068):576–581. doi:10.1136/postgradmedj-2013-131828
13. Hertling D, Kessler RM. *Management of Common Musculoskeletal Disorders: Physical Therapy Principles and Methods*. 4th ed. Lippincott Williams & Wilkins; 2006.
14. Neumann DA. *Kinesiology of the Musculoskeletal System: Foundations for Rehabilitation*. 3rd ed. Elsevier; 2017.
15. Wingstrand H, Wingstrand A, Krantz P. Intracapsular and atmospheric pressure in the dynamics and stability of the hip. A biomechanical study. *Acta Orthop Scand*. 1990;61(3):231–235. doi:10.3109/17453679008993506
16. Hoppenfeld S. *Physical Examination of the Spine and Extremities*. Prentice-Hall; 1976.
17. Clarkson, HM. *Musculoskeletal Assessment: Joint Range of Motion, Muscle Testing and Function*. 4th ed. Wolters Kluwer; 2021.
18. Levangie PK, Norkin CC. *Joint Structure and Function: A Comprehensive Analysis*. 5th ed. F.A. Davis; 2011.
19. Uemura K, Takao M, Sakai T, Nishii T, Sugano N. Volume increases of the gluteus maximus, gluteus medius, and thigh muscles after hip arthroplasty. *J Arthroplasty*. 2016;31(4):906–912.e1. doi:10.1016/j.arth.2015.10.036
20. Gibbons P, Dumper C, Gosling C. Inter-examiner and intra-examiner agreement for assessing simulated leg length inequality using palpation and observation during a standing assessment. *J Osteopath Med*. 2002;5(2):53–58. doi:10.1016/S1443-8461(02)80002-8
21. Sabharwal SMD, Kumar AMD. Methods for assessing leg length discrepancy. *Clin Orthop Relat Res*. 2008;466(12):2910–2922. doi:10.1007/s11999-008-0524-9
22. Badii M, Wade A, Collins D, Nicolaou S, Kobza J, Kopec JA. Comparison of lifts versus tape measure in determining leg length discrepancy. *J Rheumatol*. 2014;41:1689–1694.
23. American Academy of Orthopedic Surgeons. *Joint Motion: Method of Measuring and Recording*. AAOS; 1965.
24. Mills M, Frank B, Goto S, et al. Effect of restricted hip flexor muscle length on hip extensor muscle activity and lower extremity biomechanics in college-aged female soccer players. *Int J Sports Phys Ther*. 2015;10(7):946–954.
25. Kendall FP, McCreary EK, Provance PG, Rogers MM, Romani WA. *Muscles: Testing and Function with Posture and Pain*. 5th ed. Lippincott Williams & Wilkins; 2005.
26. Hartigan E, McAuley A, Lawrence M, et al. Pelvic floor muscle performance, hip mobility, and hip strength in women with and without self-reported stress urinary incontinence. *J Women Health Phys Ther*. 2019;43(4):160–170. doi:10.1097/jwh.0000000000000141
27. Battaglia PJ, D'Angelo K, Kettner NW. Posterior, lateral, and anterior hip pain due to musculoskeletal origin: a narrative literature review of history, physical examination, and diagnostic imaging. *J Acad Chiropr Orthop*. 2019;16(1):1–2.
28. Reiman MP, Mather RC, Cook CE. Physical examination tests for hip dysfunction and injury. *Br J Sports Med*. 2015;49(6):357–361. doi:10.1136/bjsports-2012-091929
29. Ganderton C, Cook J, Pizzari T, Semciw A. Demystifying the clinical diagnosis of greater trochanteric pain syndrome in women. *J Women Health*. 2017;26(6):633–643. doi:10.1089/jwh.2016.5889
30. Verrall GM, Slavotinek JP, Barnes PG, Fon GT. Description of pain provocation tests used for the diagnosis of sports-related chronic groin pain: relationship of tests to defined clinical (pain and tenderness) and MRI (pubic bone marrow oedema) criteria. *Scand J Med Sci Sports*. 2005;15(1):36–42.
31. Byrd JW. Evaluation of the hip: history and physical examination. *N Am J Sports Phys Ther*. 2007;2(4):231–240.
32. Hoppe DJ, Truntzer JN, Shapiro LM, Abrams GD, Safran MR. Diagnostic accuracy of 3 physical examination tests in the assessment of hip microinstability. *Orthop J Sports Med*. 2017;5(11). doi:10.1177/2325967117740121
33. Leibold MR, Huijbregts PA, Jensen R. Concurrent criterion-related validity of physical examination tests for hip labral lesions: a systematic review. *J Man Manip Ther*. 2008;16(2):E24–E41. doi:10.1179/jmt.2008.16.2.24E
34. Reiman MP, Goode AP, Cook CE, Holmich P, Thorborg K. Diagnostic accuracy of clinical tests for the diagnosis of hip femoroacetabular impingement/labral tear: a systematic review with meta-analysis. *Br J Sports Med*. 2015;49(12):811.
35. Springer BA, Gill NW, Freedman BA, Ross AE, Javernick MA, Murphy KP. Acetabular labral tears: diagnostic accuracy of

36. Robinson KA. Tendinopathy and application to hamstring strain injuries. *Orthop Phys Ther Pract*. 2013;25(4):207–214.
37. Reid D. The management of greater trochanteric pain syndrome: a systematic literature review. *J Orthop*. 2016;13(1):15–28. doi:10.1016/j.jor.2015.12.006
38. Simons DG, Travell JG, Simons LS. *Travell & Simons' Myofascial Pain and Dysfunction: The Trigger Points Manual. Volume 1: Upper Half of Body*. 2nd ed. Williams & Wilkins; 1999.
39. McGovern RP, Kivlan BR, Martin RL, Christoforetti JJ. Evidence-based procedures for performing the single leg squat and step-down tests in evaluation of non-arthritic hip pain: a literature review. *Int J Sports Phys Ther*. 2018;13(3):526–536.
40. Lenzlinger-Asprion R, Keller N, Meichtry A, Luomajoki H. Intertester and intratester reliability of movement control tests on the hip for patients with hip osteoarthritis. *BMC Musculoskelet Disord*. 2017;18:1–10. doi:10.1186/s12891-017-1388-5
41. Whatman C, Hume P, Hing W. The reliability and validity of visual rating of dynamic alignment during lower extremity functional screening tests: a review of the literature. *Phys Ther Rev*. 2015;20(3):210–224.
42. Kisner C, Colby LA, Borstad J. *Therapeutic Exercise: Foundations and Techniques*. 7th ed. F.A. Davis; 2018.
43. van Doormaal MCM, Meerhoff GA, Vliet Vlieland TPM, Peter WF. A clinical practice guideline for physical therapy in patients with hip or knee osteoarthritis. *Musculoskeletal Care*. 2020;18(4):575–595. doi:10.1002/msc.1492
44. Martel-Pelletier J, Maheu E, Pelletier J-P, et al. A new decision tree for diagnosis of osteoarthritis in primary care: international consensus of experts. *Aging Clin Exp Res*. 2019;31(1):19–30. doi:10.1007/s40520-018-1077-8
45. Cibulka M, Bloom M, Enseki KR, Macdonald C, Woehrle J, McDonough C. Hip pain and mobility deficits—hip osteoarthritis: revision 2017. *J Orthop Sports Phys Ther*. 2017;47(6):A1–A37.
46. Metcalfe D, Perry DC, Claireaux HA, Simel DL, Zogg CK, Costa ML. Does this patient have hip osteoarthritis?: The rational clinical examination systematic review. *JAMA*. 2019;322(23):2323–2333. doi:10.1001/jama.2019.19413
47. Ariani A, Manara M, Fioravanti A, et al. The Italian Society for Rheumatology clinical practice guidelines for the diagnosis and management of knee, hip and hand osteoarthritis. *Reumatismo*. 2019;71(S1):5–21. doi:10.4081/reumatismo.2019.1188
48. Vincent HK, Heywood K, Connelly J, Hurley RW. Obesity and weight loss in the treatment and prevention of osteoarthritis. *PM R*. 2012;4(5 suppl):S59–S67. doi:10.1016/j.pmrj.2012.01.005
49. O'Sullivan S, Schmitz T, Fulk G. *Physical Rehabilitation* 6th ed. F.A. Davis; 2014.
50. Griffin DR, Dickenson EJ, Donnell J, et al. The Warwick Agreement on femoroacetabular impingement syndrome (FAI syndrome): an international consensus statement. *Br J Sports Med*. 2016;50(19):1169. doi:10.1136/bjsports-2016-096743
51. Fearon A. You can clinically diagnose 'bursitis': you probably don't need to order that ultrasound or MRI to do it. *J Womens Health (Larchmt)*. 2017;26(6):602–604. doi:10.1089/jwh.2017.6417
52. Martinez R, Reddy N, Mulligan EP, Hynan LS, Wells J. Sleep quality and nocturnal pain in patients with hip osteoarthritis. *Medicine (Baltimore)*. 2019;98(41):1–5. doi:10.1097/MD.0000000000017464
53. Hayes KW, Petersen C, Falconer J. An examination of Cyriax's passive motion tests with patients having osteoarthritis of the knee. *Phys Ther*. 1994;74(8):697–708.
54. Klässbo M, Harms-Ringdahl K. Examination of passive ROM and capsular patterns in the hip. *Physiother Res Int*. 2003;8(1):1–12. doi:10.1002/pri.267
55. Dobson F, Hinman RS, Hall M, et al. Reliability and measurement error of the Osteoarthritis Research Society International (OARSI) recommended performance-based tests of physical function in people with hip and knee osteoarthritis. *Osteoarthritis Cartilage*. 2017;25(11):1792–1796. doi:10.1016/j.joca.2017.06.006
56. Lespasio MJ, Sultan AA, Piuzzi NS, et al. Hip osteoarthritis: a primer. *Perm J*. 2018;22. doi:10.7812/TPP/17-084
57. Kolasinski SL, Neogi T, Hochberg MC, et al. 2019 American College of Rheumatology/Arthritis Foundation guideline for the management of osteoarthritis of the hand, hip, and knee. *Arthritis Rheumatol*. 2020;72(2):220–233. doi:10.1002/art.41142
58. Brosseau L, Wells GA, Pugh AG, et al. Ottawa Panel evidence-based clinical practice guidelines for therapeutic exercise in the management of hip osteoarthritis. *Clinical Rehabilitation*. 2016;30(10):935–946. doi:10.1177/0269215515606198
59. American Academy of Orthopaedic Surgeons. *Management of Osteoarthritis of the Hip: Evidence-Based Clinical Practice Guideline*. March 13, 2017. https://www.aaos.org/globalassets/quality-and-practice-resources/osteoarthritis-of-the-hip/oa-hip-cpg_6-11-19.pdf
60. Arshi A, Leong NL, Wang C, Buser Z, Wang JC, SooHoo NF. Outpatient total hip arthroplasty in the United States: a population-based comparative analysis of complication rates. *J Am Acad Orthop Surg*. 2019;27(2):61–67. doi:10.5435/jaaos-d-17-00210
61. Colibazzi V, Coladonato A, Zanazzo M, Romanini E. Evidence based rehabilitation after hip arthroplasty. *Hip Int*. 2020;30:20–29. doi:10.1177/1120700020971314
62. Evans JT, Evans JP, Walker RW, Blom AW, Whitehouse MR, Sayers A. How long does a hip replacement last? A systematic review and meta-analysis of case series and national registry reports with more than 15 years of follow-up. *Lancet*. 2019;393(10172):647–654. doi:10.1016/S0140-6736(18)31665-9
63. Kenney C, Dick S, Lea J, Jiayong L, Ebraheim NA. A systematic review of the causes of failure of revision total hip arthroplasty. *J Orthop*. 2019;16(5):393–395. doi:10.1016/j.jor.2019.04.011
64. Damm P, Zonneveld J, Brackertz S, Streitparth F, Winkler T. Gluteal muscle damage leads to higher in vivo hip joint loads 3 months after total hip arthroplasty. *PloS One*. 2018;13(1):e0190626. doi:10.1371/journal.pone.0190626
65. Winther SB, Foss OA, Husby OS, Wik TS, Klaksvik J, Husby VS. Muscular strength and function after total hip arthroplasty performed with three different surgical approaches: one-year follow-up study. *Hip Int*. 2019;29(4):405–411. doi:10.1177/1120700018810673
66. Peng L, Zeng Y, Wu Y, Zeng J, Liu Y, Shen B. Clinical, functional and radiographic outcomes of primary total hip arthroplasty between direct anterior approach and posterior approach: a systematic review and meta-analysis. *BMC Musculoskelet Disord*. 2020;21(1):1–13. doi:10.1186/s12891-020-03318-x
67. Shapira J, Chen SL, Rosinsky PJ, Maldonado DR, Lall AC, Domb BG. Outcomes of outpatient total hip arthroplasty: a systematic review. *Hip Int*. 2021;31(1):4–11. doi:10.1177/1120700020911639
68. Xu J, Cao JY, Chaggar GS, Negus JJ. Comparison of outpatient versus inpatient total hip and knee arthroplasty: a systematic review and meta-analysis of complications. *J Orthop*. 2020;17:38–43. doi:10.1016/j.jor.2019.08.022
69. Madara KC, Marmon A, Aljehani M, Hunter-Giordano A, Zeni J Jr, Raisis L. Progressive rehabilitation after total hip

70. Winther SB, Foss OA, Husby OS, Wik TS, Klaksvik J, Husby VS. A randomized controlled trial on maximal strength training in 60 patients undergoing total hip arthroplasty. *Acta Orthop.* 2018;89(3):295–301. doi:10.1080/17453674.2018.1441362
71. Yoo J-I, Cha Y-H, Kim K-J, Kim H-Y, Choy W-S, Hwang S-C. Gait analysis after total hip arthroplasty using direct anterior approach versus anterolateral approach: a systematic review and meta-analysis. *BMC Musculoskelet Disord.* 2019;20(1):1–10. doi:10.1186/s12891-019-2450-2
72. Sheehan SE, Shyu JY, Weaver MJ, Sodickson AD, Khurana B. Proximal femoral fractures: what the orthopedic surgeon wants to know. *Radiographics.* 2015;35(5):1563–1584. doi:10.1148/rg.2015140301
73. Kim DC, Honeycutt MW, Riehl JT. Hip fractures: current review of treatment and management. *Curr Orthop Pract.* 2019;30(4):385-394.
74. McDonough CM, Harris-Hayes M, Kristensen MT, et al. Physical therapy management of older adults with hip fracture. *J Orthop Sports Phys Ther.* 2021;51(2):CPG1–CPG81. doi:10.2519/jospt.2021.0301
75. Sheehan KJ, Smith TO, Martin FC, et al. Conceptual framework for an episode of rehabilitative care after surgical repair of hip fracture. *Phys Ther.* 2019;99(3):276–285. doi:10.1093/ptj/pzy145
76. Mitchell SL, Stott DJ, Martin BJ, Grant SJ. Randomized controlled trial of quadriceps training after proximal femoral fracture. *Clin Rehabil.* 2001;15(3):282–290. doi:10.1191/026921501676849095
77. Hauer K, Specht N, Schuler M, Bartsch P, Oster P. Intensive physical training in geriatric patients after severe falls and hip surgery. *Age Aging.* 2002;31:49–57.
78. Host HH, Sinacore DR, Bohnert KL, Steger-May K, Brown M, Binder EF. Training-induced strength and functional adaptations after hip fracture. *Phys Ther.* 2007;87(3):292–303.
79. Mangione KK, Lopopolo RB, Neff NP, Craik RL, Palombaro KM. Interventions used by physical therapists in home care for people after hip fracture. *Phys Ther.* 2008;88(2):199–210.
80. Binder EF, Brown M, Sinacore DR, Steger-May K, Yarasheski KE, Schechtman KB. Effects of extended outpatient rehabilitation after hip fracture: a randomized controlled trial. *JAMA.* 2004;292(7):837–846.
81. Mangione KK, Craik RL, Tomlinson SS, Palombaro KM. Can elderly patients who have had a hip fracture perform moderate-to high-intensity exercise at home? *Phys Ther.* 2005;85(8):727–739.
82. Mangione KK, Palombaro KM. Exercise prescription for a patient 3 months after hip fracture. *Phys Ther.* 2005;85(7):676–687.
83. Rodriguez-Fernandez P, Adarraga-Cansino D, Carpintero P. Effects of delayed hip fracture surgery on mortality and morbidity in elderly patients. *Clin Orthop Relat Res.* 2011;469(11):3218–3221. doi:10.1007/s11999-010-1756-z
84. O'Shea A, Crowley C, Crowley D. Diagnosis and management of femoroacetabular impingement: a review of the literature. *Physiother Pract Res.* 2018;39(1):5–13. doi:10.3233/PPR-170101
85. Lerch S, Kasperczyk A, Berndt T, Rühmann O. Ultrasound is as reliable as plain radiographs in the diagnosis of cam-type femoroacetabular impingement. *Arch Orthop Trauma Surg.* 2016;136(10):1437–1443. doi:10.1007/s00402-016-2509-6
86. de Sa D, Hölmich P, Phillips M, et al. Athletic groin pain: a systematic review of surgical diagnoses, investigations and treatment. *Br J Sports Med.* 2016;50(19):1181–1186. doi:10.1136/bjsports-2015-095137
87. Lee S, Kuhn A, Draovitch P, Bedi A. Return to play following hip arthroscopy. *Clin Sports Med.* 2016;35(4):637–654. doi:10.1016/j.csm.2016.05.008
88. Jung KA, Restrepo C, Hellman M, AbdelSalam H, Morrison W, Parvizi J. The prevalence of cam-type femoroacetabular deformity in asymptomatic adults. *J Bone Joint Surg Br.* 2011;93(10):1303–1307. doi:10.1302/0301-620x.93b10.26433
89. Lynch TS, Minkara A, Aoki S, et al. Best practice guidelines for hip arthroscopy in femoroacetabular impingement: results of a Delphi process. *J Am Acad Orthop Surg.* 2020;28(2):81–89.
90. Clapp IM, Nwachukwu BU, Beck EC, Jan K, Gowd AK, Nho SJ. Comparing outcomes of competitive athletes versus nonathletes undergoing hip arthroscopy for treatment of femoroacetabular impingement syndrome. *Am J Sports Med.* 2020;48(1):159–166. doi:10.1177/0363546519885359
91. Tijssen M, Cingel REH, Visser E, Hölmich P, Nijhuis-van der Sanden MWG. Hip joint pathology: relationship between patient history, physical tests, and arthroscopy findings in clinical practice. *Scand J Med Sci Sports.* 2017;27(3):342–350. doi:10.1111/sms.12651
92. Reiman MP, Agricola R, Kemp JL, et al. Consensus recommendations on the classification, definition and diagnostic criteria of hip-related pain in young and middle-aged active adults from the International Hip-related Pain Research Network, Zurich 2018. *Br J Sports Med.* 2020;54(11):631–641. doi:10.1136/bjsports-2019-101453
93. Kivlan BR, Martin RL. Functional performance testing of the hip in athletes: a systematic review for reliability and validity. *Int J Sports Phys Ther.* 2012;7(4):402–412.
94. McGovern RP, Martin RL, Kivlan BR, Christoforetti JJ. Nonoperative management of individuals with non-arthritic hip pain: a literature review. *Int J Sports Phys Ther.* 2019;14(1):135–147.
95. Wall PDH, Dickenson EJ, Robinson D, et al. Personalised hip therapy: development of a non-operative protocol to treat femoroacetabular impingement syndrome in the FASHIoN randomised controlled trial. *Br J Sports Med.* 2016;50(19):1217–1223. doi:10.1136/bjsports-2016-096368
96. Kemp JL, May Arna R, Mosler A, et al. Physiotherapist-led treatment for young to middle-aged active adults with hip-related pain: consensus recommendations from the International Hip-related Pain Research Network, Zurich 2018. *Br J Sports Med.* 2020;54(9):504–511. doi:10.1136/bjsports-2019-101458
97. Philippon MJ, Decker MJ, Giphart JE, Torry MR, Wahoff MS, LaPrade RF. Rehabilitation exercise progression for the gluteus medius muscle with consideration for iliopsoas tendinitis: an in vivo electromyography study. *Am J Sports Med.* 2011;39(8):1777–1785. doi:10.1177/0363546511406848
98. Mallets E, Turner A, Durbin J, Bader A, Murray L. Short-term outcomes of conservative treatment for femoroacetabular impingement: a systematic review and meta-analysis. *Int J Sports Phys Ther.* 2019;14(4):514–524.
99. Mansell NS, Rhon DI, Meyer J, Slevin JM, Marchant BG. Arthroscopic surgery or physical therapy for patients with femoroacetabular impingement syndrome: a randomized controlled trial with 2-year follow-up. *Am J Sports Med.* 2018;46(6):1306–1314. doi:10.1177/0363546517751912
100. Maldonado DR, Diulus SC, Shapira J, et al. Hip arthroscopic surgery in the context of femoroacetabular impingement syndrome, labral tear, and acetabular overcoverage: minimum 5-year outcomes with a subanalysis against patients without overcoverage. *Am J Sports Med.* 2021;49(1):55–65. doi:10.1177/0363546520969985
101. Cvetanovich GL, Lizzio V, Meta F, et al. Variability and comprehensiveness of North American online available physical therapy protocols following hip arthroscopy for

102. Kuhns BD, Weber AE, Batko B, Nho SJ, Stegemann C. A four-phase physical therapy regimen for returning athletes to sport following hip arthroscopy for femoroacetabular impingement with routine capsular closure. *Int J Sports Phys Ther*. 2017;12(4):683–696.
103. Bolia I, Chahla J, Locks R, Briggs K, Philippon MJ. Microinstability of the hip: a previously unrecognized pathology. *Muscles Ligaments Tendons J*. 2016;6(3):354–360.
104. Lindman I, Öhlin A, Desai N, et al. Five-year outcomes after arthroscopic surgery for femoroacetabular impingement syndrome in elite athletes. *Am J Sports Med*. 2020;48(6):1416–1422. doi:10.1177/0363546520908840
105. Weir A, Brukner P, Delahunt E, et al. Doha agreement meeting on terminology and definitions in groin pain in athletes. *Br J Sports Med*. 2015;49(12):768–774. doi:10.1136/bjsports-2015-094869
106. Parvaresh KC, Rasio J, Azua E, Nho SJ. Hip instability in the athlete: anatomy, etiology, and management. *Clin Sports Med*. 2021;40(2):289–300. doi:10.1016/j.csm.2020.11.005
107. Nepple J CJ. The dysplastic and unstable hip: a responsible balance of arthroscopic and open approaches. *Sports Med Arthrosc Rev*. 2015;23(4):180–186. doi:10.1097/JSA.0000000000000096
108. Saadat A, Lall A, Battaglia M, Mohr M, Maldonado D, Domb B. Prevalence of generalized ligamentous laxity in patients undergoing hip arthroscopy: a prospective study of patients' clinical presentation, physical examination, intraoperative findings, and surgical procedures. *Am J Sports Med*. 2019;47(4):885–893. doi:10.1177/0363546518825246
109. Harris JD. Hip labral repair: options and outcomes. *Curr Rev Musculoskelet Med*. 2016;9(4):361–367. doi:10.1007/s12178-016-9360-9
110. Quinlan NJ, Alpaugh K, Upadhyaya S, Conaway WK, Martin SD. Improvement in functional outcome scores despite persistent pain with 1 year of nonsurgical management for acetabular labral tears with or without femoroacetabular impingement. *Am J Sports Med*. 2019;47(3):536–542. doi:10.1177/0363546518814484
111. Byrd JWT. The role of hip arthroscopy in the athletic hip. *Clin Sports Med*. 2006;25(2):255–278.
112. Torres A, Fernández-Fairen M, Sueiro-Fernández J. Greater trochanteric pain syndrome and gluteus medius and minimus tendinosis: nonsurgical treatment. *Pain Manag*. 2018;8(1):45–55. doi:10.2217/pmt-2017-0033
113. Redmond J, Chen A, Domb B. Greater trochanteric pain syndrome. *J Am Acad Orthop Surg*. 2016;24:231–240.
114. Mulligan E, Middleton E, Brunette M. Evaluation and management of greater trochanter pain syndrome. *Phys Ther Sport*. 2015;16(3):205–214. doi:10.1016/j.ptsp.2014.11.002
115. Hirschmann A, Falkowski AL, Kovacs B. Greater trochanteric pain syndrome: abductors, external rotators. *Semin Musculoskelet Radiol*. 2017;21(5):539–546. doi:10.1055/s-0037-1606139
116. Speers C, Bhogal G, Speers C. Greater trochanteric pain syndrome: a review of diagnosis and management in general practice. *Br J Gen Pract*. 2017;67(663):479–480. doi:10.3399/bjgp17X693041
117. Ebert JR, Retheesh T, Mutreja R, Janes GC. The clinical, functional and biomechanical presentation of patients with symptomatic hip abductor tendon tears. *Int J Sports Phys Ther*. 2016;11(5):725–737.
118. Moriguchi CS, Carnaz L, Silva LC, et al. Reliability of intra- and inter-rater palpation discrepancy and estimation of its effects on joint angle measurements. *Man Ther*. 2009;14(3):299–305. doi:10.1016/j.math.2008.04.002
119. Tortolani PJ, Carbone JJ, Quartararo LG. Greater trochanteric pain syndrome in patients referred to orthopedic spine specialists. *Spine J*. 2002;2(4):251–254. doi:10.1016/s1529-9430(02)00198-5
120. Fletcher AN, Cheah JW, Nho SJ, Mather RC. Proximal hamstring injuries. *Clin Sports Med*. 2021;40(2):339–361. doi:10.1016/j.csm.2021.01.003
121. Goom T, Malliaras M, Reiman M, Purdam C. Proximal hamstring tendinopathy: clinical aspects of assessment and management. *J Orthop Sports Phys Ther*. 2016;46(6):483–493. doi:10.2519/jospt.2016.5986
122. Feucht MJ, Plath JE, Seppel G, Hinterwimmer S, Imhoff AB, Brucker PU. Gross anatomical and dimensional characteristics of the proximal hamstring origin. *Knee Surg Sports Traumatol Arthrosc*. 2015;23(9):2576–2582. doi:10.1007/s00167-014-3124-0
123. Askling CM, Tengvar M, Tarassova O, Thorstensson A. Acute hamstring injuries in Swedish elite sprinters and jumpers: a prospective randomised controlled clinical trial comparing two rehabilitation protocols. *Br J Sports Med*. 2014;48(7):532–539. doi:10.1136/bjsports-2013-093214
124. Schmitt B, Tim T, McHugh M. Hamstring injury rehabilitation and prevention of reinjury using lengthened state eccentric training: a new concept. *Int J Sports Phys Ther*. 2012;7(3):333–341.
125. Schuermans J, Danneels L, Van Tiggelen D, Palmans T, Witvrouw E. Proximal neuromuscular control protects against hamstring injuries in male soccer players: a prospective study with electromyography time-series analysis during maximal sprinting. *Am J Sports Med*. 2017;45(6):1315–1325. doi:10.1177/0363546516687750
126. Herngren B, Stenmarker M, Vavruch L, Hagglund G. Slipped capital femoral epiphysis: a population-based study. *BMC Musculoskelet Disord*. 2017;18(1):304. doi:10.1186/s12891-017-1665-3
127. Peck DM, Voss LM, Voss TT. Slipped capital femoral epiphysis: diagnosis and management. *Am Fam Physician*. 2017;95(12):779–784.
128. Lyons R. Acute limping in a young child: evaluation and management review. *J Nurs Pract*. 2015;11(10):1004–1010. doi:10.1016/j.nurpra.2015.08.023
129. Shohat N, Copeliovitch L, Smorgick Y, et al. The long-term outcome after varus derotational osteotomy for Legg-Calvé-Perthes Disease: a mean follow-up of 42 years. *J Bone Joint Surg*. 2016;98(15):1277–1285. doi:10.2106/JBJS.15.01349
130. Weick JW, Bullard J, Green JH, Gagnier JJ. Measures of hip function and symptoms. *Arthritis Care Res*. 2020;72:200–218. doi:10.1002/acr.24231
131. Wright A, Johnson J, Cook C. Do the reported estimates of minimal clinically important difference scores amongst hip-related patient-reported outcome measures support their use? *Phys Ther Rev*. 2014;19(3):186–195. doi:10.1179/1743288X14Y.0000000134
132. Wamper KE, Sierevelt IN, Poolman RW, Bhandari M, Haverkamp D. The Harris hip score: do ceiling effects limit its usefulness in orthopedics? *Acta Orthop*. 2010;81(6):703–707. doi:10.3109/17453674.2010.537808
133. Thorborg K, Holmich P, Christensen R, Petersen J, Roos E. The Copenhagen Hip and Groin Outcome Score (HAGOS): development and validation according to the COSMIN checklist. *Br J Sports Med*. 2011;45(6):478–491.

12 | Lumbar Spine and Sacroiliac Joint

Betsy Myers and June Hanks

CHAPTER OBJECTIVES
After reading this chapter, you will be able to:
1. Tailor the basic history to a patient with lumbosacral pathology.
2. Describe the components of the physical examination for a patient with lumbosacral pathology.
3. Describe the pathology, history, key examination findings, rehabilitation focus, and expected outcomes of common lumbosacral pathologies.
4. Describe interventions for patients with non-specific low back pain and low back pain presumed to be from pathoanatomic causes.
5. Organize the physical examination of a patient with lumbosacral pathology to maximize efficiency.

INTRODUCTION TO THE EXAMINATION OF LUMBAR SPINE AND SACROILIAC JOINT

Low back pain (LBP) is a leading cause of pain disability worldwide.[1] Although many people with LBP do not seek care, the direct cost of medical care for individuals with LBP has been noted to be billions of dollars annually.[2] Most patients with acute LBP can expect a complete recovery within 4 to 6 weeks, but recurrence is common.[2] However, some patients will experience a prolonged or incomplete recovery. Despite significant improvements in medical imaging, laboratory studies, pharmaceuticals, and surgical techniques, the incidence and burden of LBP continues to rise.[3]

Chapter 4, Spine Osteology and Arthrology, provides detailed anatomy and biomechanics of the lumbar spine and sacroiliac joints (SIJs). The complexity of the spine, the lack of a clear anatomic cause to many cases of LBP, and the numerous approaches to examination and treatment can be overwhelming. This chapter adapts the history and physical examination to patients with suspected pathology of the lumbar spine and SIJ to provide clear guidance for the clinician when managing patients with back pain.

PATIENT HISTORY: LUMBAR SPINE AND SACROILIAC JOINT

A thorough and efficient patient history is imperative to optimize patient care, given the complexity of the lumbar region. A detailed history may implicate symptoms referred from a non-neuromusculoskeletal source or coexisting pathologies that require further investigation. Once these potential sources of symptoms are ruled out, the clinician should investigate spine-specific questions to help guide the physical examination.

Review of Systems

As noted in Chapter 6, Patient History, the clinician must review systems that can refer symptoms to the patient's area of complaint, systems that can cause the symptoms described by the patient, as well as all systems involved in the patient's past medical history.[4] Therefore, when evaluating each patient with LBP, clinicians should review, at minimum, the cardiovascular, pulmonary, gastrointestinal, genitourinary, endocrine, and psychiatric systems.

Cardiovascular and Pulmonary Systems While the cardiovascular system generally refers pain to the chest, left arm, and left jaw, an abdominal aortic aneurysm (AAA) can cause abdominal or back pain.[4,5] An AAA is more likely in older males with a history of smoking or a family history of AAA.[2,6] Hypertension is a frequently comorbidity. Symptoms related to an AAA are seldom changed by positioning and do not appear to be mechanical in nature. Screening for an AAA includes asking if the patient notices a pulsing sensation in the abdomen or back and palpating for an abdominal aorta width that is greater than 4.0 cm.[6] Abdominal aorta diameter is the largest predictor of potential rupture, with a substantial increase in risk with diameter greater than 5.5 cm.[7]

Clinicians should consider the possibility that buttock or lower extremity symptoms during walking may be vascular induced and not just neurogenic. For example, patients with lumbar stenosis and peripheral arterial disease are likely to have pain that develops with ambulation. For patients with stenosis, these symptoms are lessened by assuming a more flexed trunk posture; however, trunk flexion has no effect on symptoms caused by arterial insufficiency. The section "Lumbar Stenosis" in this chapter provides additional details on differentiating between vascular and neurogenic claudication.

Pleuritic pain and pneumothorax can create upper lumbar/lateral costal pain and abdominal pain, respectively. In addition, metastatic lung cancer frequently affects the spine and may be the cause of a patient's back pain.

Gastrointestinal and Genitourinary Systems The gastrointestinal and genitourinary systems can refer pain to the low back, costovertebral angle, groin, and abdominal regions.[6] Mechanical back pain and back pain due to visceral origin may be distinct, or they may coexist. Three scenarios may help elucidate these concepts. First, patients may come to physical therapy with back pain that is made worse by the nonsteroidal anti-inflammatory drugs (NSAIDs) prescribed to manage their back pain. This would be consistent with a patient with musculoskeletal-related back pain and an exacerbation, or new onset, of a gastric ulcer. Gastric ulcers are the most common intra-abdominal condition referring pain to the musculoskeletal system.[6] Second, patients may believe the pain from a gastric ulcer or kidney stone is musculoskeletal in origin and seek physical therapy for these visceral complaints.[4] Lastly, patients may have mechanical back pain that is causing some of their symptoms, but have coexisting visceral pathology, such as cholecystitis, that is responsible for other symptoms.[8] Patients reporting their pain is affected by food or worsened by NSAIDs should be referred for further assessment. Additional signs and symptoms may include heartburn, nausea, vomiting, or melena.

Clinicians should ask about incontinence and changes in bowel or bladder habits. **Cauda equina syndrome** is a collection of symptoms related to damage to the cauda equina,[2,6] which consists of 20 nerve roots that comprise the terminal portion of the spinal cord. Symptoms of cauda equina may include LBP along with

- new bowel or bladder dysfunction
- saddle anesthesia
- decreased lower extremity reflexes
- persistent or increasing lower extremity weakness
- sexual dysfunction

If cauda equina syndrome is identified, urgent referral is warranted.

Urinary incontinence is an underreported and underrecognized problem, affecting roughly 14% of men and half of women.[9] Incontinence increases the risk of falls,[10] possibly due to urinary urgency and rushing to get to the bathroom. Although more common in individuals over the age of 50, incontinence is also prevalent in young female athletes, women after childbirth, men after prostate surgery, smokers, and individuals who are obese or have diabetes.[9,11] Regularly asking patients about continence not only improves detection of serious pathologies, such as cauda equina syndrome, it can help provide the necessary referrals to help manage a significant social, psychological, and functional problem.

Kidney or ureteral stones can create pain at the costovertebral angle and low back that may be intermittent or spasmodic in nature. The pain may change locations, traveling more anteriorly and inferiorly if the stone is mobile, but is unaffected by changes in trunk motion. Nausea, vomiting, fever, and/or chills are commonly noted.[6] Patients with a history of stones, urinary tract infections, autoimmune diseases, and those over 60 years of age are at increased risk for stones.[6]

Endocrine System For patients with paresthesias or symptoms in the feet, the endocrine system should be reviewed. Peripheral neuropathy from diabetes may be the cause of, or contribute to, these symptoms. Peripheral neuropathy from diabetes is typically symmetrical following a stocking pattern and may be identified with Semmes-Weinstein monofilaments testing. In contrast, nerve root lesions follow a dermatomal pattern and may be accompanied by weakness and reflex changes of the involved nerve root.

Psychiatric System Given the well-established association between chronic LBP and depression,[12] a psychiatric system review should include screening for depression, but may also involve assessing for kinesiophobia, catastrophizing, and perceived life stressors. See Chapter 19, Pain Management: A Mechanism-Centered Approach, for additional information.

Constitutional Symptoms Clinicians should screen for constitutional symptoms, such as unexplained weight changes, nighttime pain, fever, night sweats, and lack of symptom response to changes in loading. The presence of constitutional symptoms requires referral because they may represent a systemic disorder or be warning signs of cancer. A paraspinal abscess[13] or infection, such as osteomyelitis,[14] may also produce pain in the back.[4] Those at risk for infection include individuals who are immunosuppressed and have a history of drug use, recent infection, or recent spinal procedure.[2]

Patient Demographics

Basic patient demographics, such as age, gender, height, and weight, are the first information most clinicians have access to and are useful in beginning to form diagnostic hypotheses. Radiculopathy is more common among individuals between 25 and 55 years of age.[15] Women over the age of 65 and men over the age of 75 are at increased risk of osteoporotic vertebral fracture.[2] Loss of height with aging is indicative of degenerative kyphoscoliosis or compression fractures. Obesity is associated with LBP.[16] Therefore, clinicians should consider how this basic information may relate to the patient's condition.

General Medical Information

Clinicians should thoroughly review the patient's general medical history. A patient with a new onset of LBP and a prior history of cancer should be referred for further evaluation, as bone metastases to the spine are common, particularly with breast, lung, and prostate cancers.[2]

Medication reconciliation is important, as many patients with LBP may be seeing multiple medical providers and may have been prescribed multiple types of medications. For example, a typical practice pattern for pharmacologic management of patients with LBP includes prescribing NSAIDs, muscle relaxers, and anticonvulsant medications.[17,18] In addition, despite the dangers of addiction and the lack of evidence to support their use, many patients may also be prescribed opioid medications. Clinicians should learn if, and when, the patient is taking the medication, the dosage, and the patient's perception of effect.[19] For example, a patient may have been prescribed an NSAID, but may also note that 20 minutes after taking this medication, the back pain symptoms worsen. This would be consistent with a potential gastric ulcer.[6] Alternatively, the NSAID may consistently reduce the patient's back pain, confirming an inflammatory component to the condition, but the patient may now have a blood pressure of 180/96 mm Hg and ankle edema, consistent with a different adverse drug reaction to the NSAID. Muscle relaxers and anticonvulsant medications, along with polypharmacy, also affect balance, increasing the risk of falls.[6,19]

The clinician should determine whether any imaging has been performed as well as the results. While imaging can be useful, particularly to rule out a fracture, it can also be misleading. Degenerative changes have not been found to be correlated with symptoms of LBP.[20] Abnormal magnetic resonance imaging (MRI) findings have been noted in more than one-third of asymptomatic 20-year-olds and almost all asymptomatic 80-year-olds.[21] In addition, when examining individuals with radicular pain, the clinical examination matched the MRI findings only one-third of the time.[22]

Nevertheless, if imaging was performed and the results are known, it is important to ask the patient's perspective on the findings. For example, a 32-year-old reporting "I have the spine of a 90-year-old" or "my discs are blown" appears to be catastrophizing and may benefit from further assessment of psychosocial factors that may be contributing to the patient's condition.

Lifestyle and Occupation

Clinicians should inquire about work, exercise, and leisure activities to best understand the physical demands of patients' daily lives and identify potential predisposing or exacerbating factors as well as any repetitive stresses that may be related to their chief complaint. Any recent changes, such as transfer to a new job, increase in work hours, or increase in training intensity or playing time, should be noted. Health habits, such as smoking and exercise, affect patient healing potential and injury risks. Smoking not only increases the risk of cancer[23] but is also associated with delayed healing after lumbar surgery.[24] Physical activity has a host of beneficial effects for older adults, including improving bone density, decreasing fall risk, and reducing risk factors for chronic diseases, such as diabetes and cardiovascular disease. In contrast, sedentary behavior[25] and occupations requiring heavy lifting[26] increase the risk of LBP. Participation in sports requiring repeated trunk extension, such as gymnastics, increases the risk of spondylolysis in adolescents.[27,28]

History of Neck Pathology

Patients should be asked about prior or current neck pathology because lower extremity paresthesia or weakness may be due to more proximal central cord compression.

History of Back Pathology

Clinicians should inquire about prior back surgery. Patients having more than one surgery are at increased risk of developing chronic back pain.[29] Patients who have had a spinal fusion are likely to have increased intervertebral motion at the levels above and below the fusion, which may play a role in the patient's current chief complaint. Patients should be asked if they have had prior episodes of back or leg pain. If so, a series of follow-up questions might include what brought the symptoms on, how long did they last, what was done that improved the symptoms, how often did the symptoms occur, and if any imaging or laboratory work was performed. For example, a patient may report a history of intermittent LBP occurring twice a year and lasting for several days. If the episodes are occurring more frequently, the pain is more severe, or the patient is now experiencing leg symptoms, the condition appears to be gradually worsening.

Learning what interventions were tried in the past can provide insights into both pathology and future treatment. Symptoms that improve with heat may be related to muscle hypertonicity, stress, or degenerative arthritis. If prior symptoms resolved with exercise, the patient should be asked what type of exercise and if these exercises have been attempted for the current exacerbation. A patient who recounts several weeks of manipulation with only transient symptom relief is unlikely to benefit from additional attempts of mobilization or manipulation.

Chief Complaint

While pain may be one of the leading reasons for patients to seek treatment, it is important to clarify the patient's chief complaint. Stiffness from ankylosing spondylitis may be limiting a patient's ability to dress. A patient may report tripping and decreased balance due to an L4 nerve root lesion causing foot drop. A patient may have mild back pain, but be more concerned about the "annoying tingling sensation in my leg."

Onset

Patients should be asked about possible causes of their back symptoms. An insidious onset of LBP is not uncommon. However, many times careful questioning may lead the patient to acknowledge a seemingly inconsequential 8-hour car ride the day before symptoms began. Back pain of muscular origin may begin after a weekend of rigorous household chores. Patients reporting the onset of back and leg symptoms after a sudden twisting motion may be experiencing symptoms from a herniated disc or muscular strain.

Location and Intensity of Symptoms

Clinicians should thoroughly investigate the location of current and prior symptoms and whether the current symptoms are central, bilateral, or unilateral. Local symptoms near the posterior superior iliac spine (PSIS) are commonly seen with sacroiliac dysfunction. Unilateral back symptoms may indicate facet pathology or muscular strain. Symptoms localized to the buttock may represent a gluteal or hip external rotator strain, but if tingling and numbness are also felt in the leg, deep gluteal syndrome (DGS) or nerve root pathology is more likely. Symptoms that are felt in bilateral lower extremities when walking through the grocery store but that are absent when pushing a cart raise the suspicion for lumbar stenosis.

The patient should be asked if symptoms are constant or intermittent. Intermittent symptoms are likely to be mechanical in nature, whereas constant symptoms may represent inflammation or an acute injury. Putting these two pieces of information together along with symptom intensity provides significant information about diagnostic hypotheses. A patient who currently has moderate back pain, but previously had mild back pain and severe leg symptoms, would be considered to be improving, as the symptoms are **centralizing** (Fig. 12-1). In contrast, a patient whose

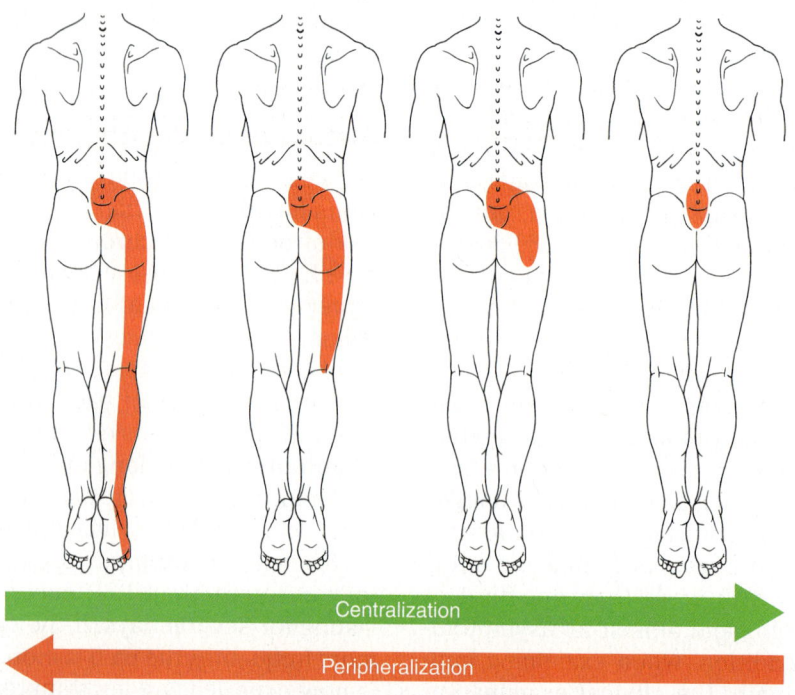

FIGURE 12-1 Centralization and peripheralization.

symptoms began in the low back, but now are felt in the lower leg and lateral aspect of the foot, is experiencing **peripheralization** and, hence, worsening of the condition. Patients who exhibit centralization or peripheralization of symptoms are classified as having a **derangement** in the mechanical diagnosis and therapy (MDT) approach to back pain assessment and treatment.[30] The term *derangement* is used for its conciseness at times in the remainder of this chapter.

Symptom Quality

Patients should be asked about the quality of their symptoms. Pain that is dull and aching is consistent with muscular or ligament pathology,[31] whereas pain that is sharp and shooting or tingling and numb is indicative of nerve involvement. A pinching pain may represent facet pathology.[31] Pulsing or throbbing pain should make the clinician consider the possibility of an AAA. Patients reporting pain that is exhausting or frightening appear to have a psychoemotional component to their condition, which warrants further exploration.

Symptom Behavior

Patients should be questioned about aggravating and remitting factors. The patient history can provide valuable insights into a patient's **directional preference**. Directional preference is the direction of mechanical loading that reduces, centralizes, and/or abolishes patient symptoms.[32,33] For example, patients reporting that sitting (an activity typified by static lumbar flexion and high disc loading) worsens symptoms but standing and walking (more extended lumbar postures) improves symptoms has a directional preference for lumbar extension. Up to 70% of patients with nonspecific LBP have been found to have a directional preference to movement.[34] Identification of a patient's directional preference helps to classify the patient's condition and provides guidance for interventions.

Patients should specifically be asked about the effect of various positions and activities, including bending, sitting, rising, standing, walking, stairs, and lying (Table 12-1). Symptoms that are noticed during transitional movements may represent spinal instability or lumbar derangement. Symptoms that worsen with bending may represent a compression fracture, herniated disc, instability, or derangement. Symptoms that worsen with more extended postures may be due to stenosis or spondylolisthesis. Pain that occurs with unilateral activities, such as stairs, may be caused by DGS or SIJ pathology. Back pain symptoms that worsened with coughing or sneezing may represent a muscular strain or compression fracture. However, if leg symptoms are produced or worsened with these activities, the clinician should consider possible nerve root or disc pathology.

TABLE 12-1
TRUNK LOADING WITH ACTIVITY

Activity	Directional Preference if Symptoms Are Reduced	Type of Loading
Sitting	Flexion	Static
Bending	Flexion	Dynamic
Standing	Extension	Static
Walking	Extension	Dynamic
Rising	Transitional from flexion to extension	Dynamic
Lying: prone	Extended	Static, unloaded
Lying: hooklying or sidelying	Flexed	Static, unloaded

Patients should be asked about quality, postures, and surface of sleep. It is common for patients with LBP to report that pain wakes them at night. However, patients who are unable to return to sleep due to pain, or unable to find a position that reduces pain, may be experiencing pain from non-neuromusculoskeletal sources that warrant referral. The clinician should determine the effects of various sleep postures. Prone lying is a more extended position, particularly when lying on a soft or sagging mattress, and may be poorly tolerated by patients with degenerative disc disease (DDD). In contrast, sidelying may exacerbate radicular symptoms or SIJ dysfunction, but may feel better for patients with lumbar stenosis. Symptoms that are noted when sleeping at home but that are absent when sleeping on vacation may be due to the home mattress or life stressors.

Clinicians should try to understand the 24-hour pattern of the patient's symptoms. Stiffness present for the first 30 minutes of the morning are consistent with osteoarthritis, whereas stiffness that lasts for the morning may be more consistent with inflammatory conditions such as ankylosing spondylitis.[4] The clinician should learn how easy it is to provoke the patient's symptoms. Is the patient able to sit for 2 hours before symptoms being provoked or merely 5 minutes? Similarly, the clinician should ask how long it takes for symptoms to resolve. Lower extremity symptoms from lumbar stenosis that are provoked by ambulation generally resolve within 3 minutes of sitting. Radicular symptoms may be fleeting, occurring during motion, or may be constantly present once triggered.

Tracking Patients Symptoms

Patients should be asked about variation in symptoms. Does the location of symptoms change? Are the symptoms only in the back or only in the leg or both? Are symptoms in only one leg or are both legs affected symmetrically? It can be challenging for clinicians to follow symptoms in multiple locations. However, this is necessary to get the full picture of the patient's condition. The clinician may want to use the body diagram

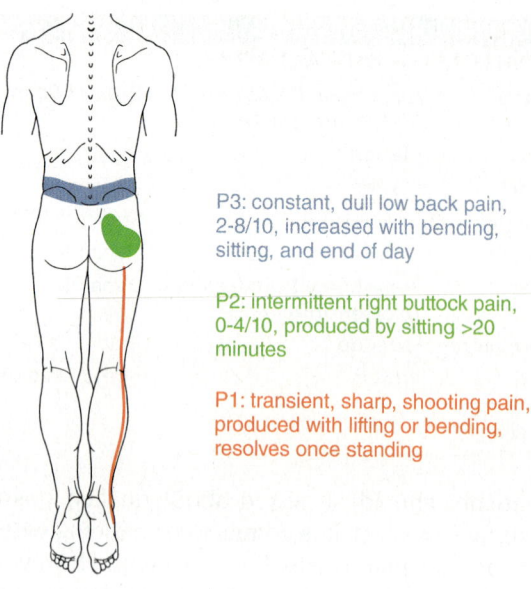

FIGURE 12-2 Tracking symptom location and intensity.

P3: constant, dull low back pain, 2-8/10, increased with bending, sitting, and end of day

P2: intermittent right buttock pain, 0-4/10, produced by sitting >20 minutes

P1: transient, sharp, shooting pain, produced with lifting or bending, resolves once standing

to track symptoms (Fig. 12-2). The clinician may want to start by asking about the most infrequent or most distal symptoms and understand this behavior fully before moving on to the next region of symptoms.

Outcome Measures

Chapter 6, Patient History, introduced common general outcome measures, such as the Patient-Specific Functional Scale and the Global Rating of Change. The Roland-Morris Disability Questionnaire[20] and the Oswestry Disability Index[20,35] are common region-specific patient-reported outcome measures used for patients with back pain (Table 12-2).[36] The STarT Back Screening Tool[37,38] and the Fear Avoidance Beliefs Questionnaire (FABQ) help address psychosocial risk factors that may help identify patients who would benefit from a biopsychosocial approach to patient care.[39] The Pain Catastrophizing Scale (PCS)[40] and the Tampa Scale for Kinesiophobia (TSK) may be beneficial for patients exhibiting avoidance behaviors or catastrophizing.[36,41]

TABLE 12-2	
COMMON OUTCOME TOOLS FOR PATIENTS WITH LOW BACK PAIN	
Tool	**Tool Basics**
Roland-Morris Disability Questionnaire	• 24 items scored 0 (disagree) or 1 (agree), with higher scores indicating worse function • Assesses the influence of back pain on common lower level functional tasks • MCID: 5 points or 30% from baseline

Oswestry Disability Index	• 10 items rated on a 0–5 scale, with higher scores indicating worse function
	• Total score is converted to a percentage
	  • 0–20% thought to indicate minimal disability
	  • 21–40% moderate disability
	  • 41–60% severe disability
	• MCID: 10 points or 30% of baseline

STarT back Screening Tool	• Screening tool for patients with back pain meant to identify patients at risk for persistent back-related disability
	• 9 items scored 0 (disagree) or 1 (agree), with higher scores indicating greater risk
	• Scoring: 0–9
	  • Low risk = 0–3
	  • Medium risk = 4–9
	  • High risk = scoring >3 on the last 5 items (distress scale)
	• Patients deemed at high risk may benefit from psychologically informed care

Fear Avoidance Beliefs Questionnaire (FABQ)	• Screening tool to detect individuals with high pain avoidance behaviors • Two subscales: work (7 items) and physical activity (4 items) • Items are scored 0–6, with higher scores indicating greater fear avoidance • Higher scores on the work subscale may represent poorer outcomes, but there is insufficient data to provide relevant cut scores • Patients with high fear avoidance may benefit from psychologically informed care
Pain Catastrophizing Scale (PCS)	• 13 items rated 0–4, with higher scores indicative of greater tendency to magnify the threat of pain or feel helpless to control pain • Scores of 30 or more represent a clinically relevant level of catastrophizing
Tampa Scale for Kinesiophobia (TSK)	• Two subscales: activity avoidance and somatic focus • Original scale included 17 items scored on a 4-point Likert scale (strongly disagree to strongly agree), with higher scores indicating greater fear of movement • Modified scales include the TSK-13 and TSK-11 making cutoff scores difficult to compare • Common diagnoses: chronic pain, low back pain, neck pain, fibromyalgia syndrome, post-anterior cruciate ligament reconstruction

MCID, minimum clinically important difference.

PHYSICAL EXAMINATION: LUMBAR SPINE AND SACROILIAC JOINT

The physical examination of patients with suspected spinal pathology includes the systems review, a lower quarter screen including a thorough lower quarter neurologic screen, a clearing examination, and a joint-specific examination.[42] The clearing examination for patients with LBP is slightly different from other joints. First, the lumbar spine does not function in isolation from the pelvis, hip, and thoracic spine. Second, muscles cross multiple joints, both within the spine and across the hip and pelvis. The latissimus dorsi provides substantial stability to the thoracolumbar fascia and is also influenced by a distal attachment on the upper extremity. Third, it is not uncommon to have pathology in the hip or thoracic spine concurrent with lumbar spine pathology.[43-45] These considerations indicate the phrase "clearing examination" is somewhat of a misnomer. All components of the physical examination need not be performed on every patient. As with other joint complexes, the experienced clinician will titrate the examination based on the patient history, presentation, and goals. In practice, the physical examination is organized by position and should proceed from uninvolved (or less involved) to involved side, but is presented here by category to aide conceptualization.

Serious pathologies are extremely rare in patients with LBP, occurring in less than 1% of all cases.[46] However, the clinician must consider if there are any potential red flags that warrant investigation, such as an AAA or fracture. If an AAA is suspected, the clinician should palpate for the abdominal aorta pulse width along the left parasternal line, just superior and lateral to the umbilicus. A pulse width greater than 4.0 cm should be reported to the patient's primary care provider. The clinician can safely continue the remainder of the physical examination to determine whether the patient's symptoms have a mechanical response,[5] although it would be wise to defer assessments such as spinal accessory motion or the prone instability test. Should a neuromusculoskeletal condition be found, interventions should not be initiated before medical clearance. If cauda equina syndrome is suspected, the clinician should perform the necessary portions of the physical examination (lower quarter neurologic screen) and contact the referring practitioner or the patient's primary care provider immediately to discuss any positive findings.

Lumbar fractures are rarely seen by rehabilitation professionals such as primary care providers, and there are no reliable clinical prediction rules, such as the Ottawa Ankle Rules of the Canadian C-Spine Rules, available for the back. A history of trauma is the strongest predictor of fracture.[5] Clinicians should have a high degree of suspicion for thoracolumbar fracture in patients with a history of trauma who are over 75 years of age, have a history of osteoporosis, and back pain rated greater than 6/10 on a visual analog scale.[5] The most likely type of fracture is a vertebral body compression fracture (see Fig. 4-5, in Chapter 4, Spine Osteology and Arthrology). Because these fractures are generally stable, the clinician may proceed with caution with the physical examination and report suspicious findings to the patient's primary care provider.

Observation

Observation begins when first meeting the patient and continues throughout the session. A patient with disc pathology may choose to stand rather than sit in the waiting room. Observe the patient during transitional movements, such as supine to sitting and rising from a chair. Difficulty may represent overall deconditioning, whereas a "hitch" or pause while rising may indicate a transient increase in pain caused by instability. During the history, the patient may sit, but frequently shift positions. While taking the patient's history, the clinician should unobtrusively observe the patient's overall sitting posture. Observe if the patient's shoulders appear level or if one is higher than the other, potentially indicating the presence of a scoliosis. Note if the patient holds the trunk rigidly, as if guarding, or if the patient slumps into excessive trunk flexion.

Neurologic Examination of the Lumbar Spine

Lower extremity strength and paresthesias from lumbar spine pathology can change as a result of changes in trunk loading.[47] Therefore, the examination of the neurologic status of the lumbar nerve roots is performed in the seated position before assessment of trunk range of motion (ROM) (Fig. 12-3). Functional screening for patients can include toe walking (S1,2), heel walking (L4), bilateral or single leg squat (L3), and the Trendelenburg test, which includes hip abduction muscle performance and mild increase in SIJ stress. However, these tests may not be as sensitive as manual muscle testing and can be difficult for patients with higher pain levels or without adequate balance. Repeat testing after trunk ROM testing can be performed as needed. Assessment of upper extremity reflexes is sometimes helpful, as it provides the clinician with a comparison point in case of pathology proximal to the L3 level. For example, a patient may present with symmetrical bilateral lower extremity reflexes. However, when assessing the upper extremity reflexes, all lower extremity reflexes and the triceps reflex are hyperreflexic and the Hoffman reflex is positive. This would be consistent with cervical myelopathy at the level of C6-7. (See Fig. 7-5 in Chapter 7, The Physical Examination, for illustrations of the lower extremity dermatomes.)

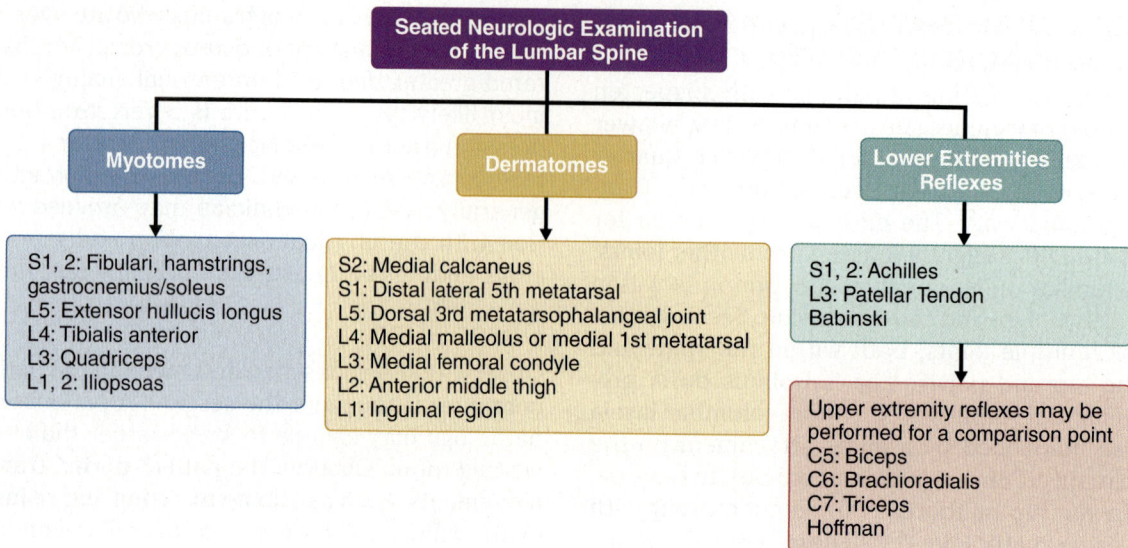

FIGURE 12-3 Seated neurologic examination of the lumbar spine.

Structure and Posture

Before assessing trunk ROM, it is helpful to first focus on the patient's overall structure and posture with the patient standing barefoot.[42] Ideally, male patients are shirtless and female patients are in a gown opened to the back or sports bra to maximize visualization of the entire region. Particular attention should be paid to the angle of the pelvis and spine. The clinician should palpate the iliac crests, inferior scapular borders, and superior shoulder girdle to determine whether they appear to be level. Gently follow the course of the patient's spinal curvature with one or two fingers noticing if the curves are smooth and neither excessive nor reduced. Note if a step deformity is present, which may represent a spondylolisthesis. To identify a step deformity, patient should be standing, while the clinician palpates adjacent spinous processes with the index, middle, and ring fingers. Beginning with the sacrum, the clinician should note the position of each vertebra relative to one another.[48] The clinician then moves the fingers up to simultaneously palpate L5, L4, L3, and so on. Normally, a smooth and gentle lordosis should be noted. A step deformity is anterior displacement of one vertebra, and all vertebrae superior to it, relative to the vertebra below. From a lateral view, observe the lumbar lordosis and pelvic tilt (formed by the line between the anterior superior iliac spine [ASIS] and the PSIS). There are no normative values for lumbar lordosis or pelvic tilt; therefore, clinicians should obtain a general impression of the patient's preferred static alignment. Most individuals present with a slight anterior pelvic tilt.[49]

Observe for the presence of scoliosis (see Fig. 4-3E in Chapter 4, Spine Osteology and Arthrology), a lateral spinal curvature that may be accompanied by a posterior rib hump, or a lateral shift (Fig. 12-4) in which the patient's shoulders are shifted laterally relative to the pelvis. A leg length discrepancy may be a contributing factor in the development of scoliosis or SIJ-related pain.[50] Note the general muscular contour for atrophy, hypertrophy, or hypertonicity of the paraspinals. Examine the lower extremity alignment and muscular development. Patients with a chronic S1–S2 radiculopathy may present with ipsilateral calf atrophy.

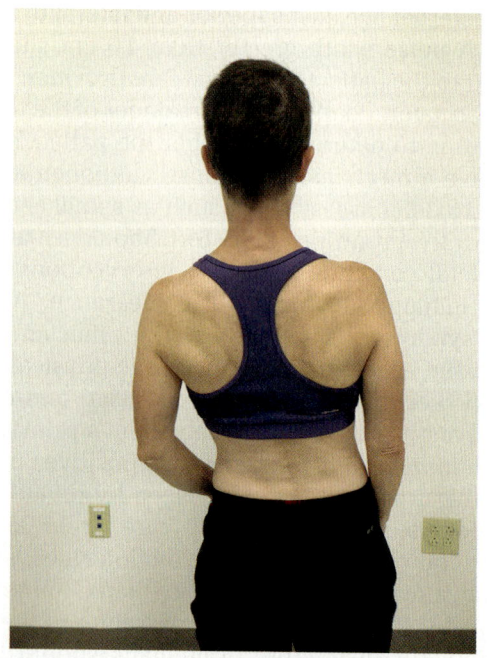

FIGURE 12-4 Lateral shift.

Trunk Range of Motion

Motions to Assess Trunk active range of motion (AROM) should be assessed and may include flexion, extension, side glide or lateral flexion, and rotation. Trunk motion is typically measured with a goniometer or via visual observation (Table 12-3). Alternatively, measurement can be made using one or two inclinometers or a tape measure. While quantification beyond visual observation of lumbar motion provides a means of more reliably tracking changes over time, lumbar ROM has not been shown to be consistently related to function.[51-53] Many clinicians prefer to visually assess side gliding (translocation of the pelvis laterally while maintaining the position of the shoulder girdle and upper trunk) rather than lateral flexion.[30] Biomechanically, these two maneuvers appear to have identical effects.[54] However, side gliding may be preferred to lateral flexion for three reasons. First, side gliding is an easier motion for the patient to control and may produce less load to the vertebral segments than lateral flexion. Second, side gliding more closely replicates the lateral shift seen in some patients with lumbar pathology. Third, it is used as an intervention strategy for individuals who respond to frontal plane loading. Because lumbar rotation ROM is limited, some clinicians do not specifically assess this motion when examining for lumbar spine pathology.

Passive trunk ROM by a clinician is not generally performed for several reasons. If performed in sitting, passive ROM continues to load the vertebral bodies, lumbar discs, and stretch the facet joints. In addition, a patient's ability to be truly passive is extremely doubtful. Assessment of trunk motion with the patient in sidelying is an extremely difficult maneuver for the clinician. Lastly, passive testing does not appear to be able to accurately identify segmental passive motion.[31,55] Rather, patient-generated spine motion in supine (knees to chest) and prone (extension in lying; aka a prone press up) are performed later in the examination.

Clinicians should note range, symmetry, quality of motion, and symptoms during trunk AROM in standing.[36] Normal lumbopelvic rhythm is when trunk flexion is initiated from the lumbar spine followed by anterior tilting of the pelvis and hip flexion. When returning from a flexed position, this rhythm is reversed: motion is initiated by posterior tilting of the pelvis and hip extension, followed by trunk extension. Aberrant movement patterns include abnormal lumbopelvic rhythm or the need to use the upper extremities on the thighs to raise back to standing.

The clinician should ask the patient about the location and intensity of all current symptoms before trunk AROM testing. Patients should be asked to note any changes in these symptoms during motion, at end range, and upon return to the neutral position. A painful arc during movement may represent motor control issues or a derangement, whereas end-range pain may indicate a soft-tissue lesion, such as an interspinous ligament sprain.

Systematic Approach to Trunk Loading Strategies One-time and repeated trunk ROM are performed to determine the effects of various loading strategies on patient symptoms and motion. This loading strategy was first described by McKenzie and is part of the MDT approach to back pain assessment and treatment.[30] The goal of exploring trunk loading strategies is to identify a directional preference. The identification of directional preference, and treatment using these loading strategies, consistently leads to better outcomes than other interventions, such as manual therapy and stabilization exercises.[33] Because the majority of patients with nonspecific LBP have a directional preference,[34,56-59] this examination strategy is an important first step in the management of patients with LBP.[60] Based on the patient history, the clinician is likely to have an idea as to the patient's directional preference. However, following the systematic process is likely to provide better results than a more haphazard approach. Figure 12-5 provides basic terminology and outlines a traffic light system to help the new clinician. Patients with a directional preference will have a rapid change in symptoms or ROM as a result of trunk loading strategies.[34]

Patient symptoms are noted before, during, and after each test motion. One-time motion testing provides a baseline for future comparison. Repeated movements are performed to try to find a direction that decreases or abolishes symptoms (green light). Each motion is performed for at least one set of 10 repetitions or until there is a response to loading. As with one-time motion testing, patient symptoms are noted before, during, and after each repeated movement. The loading strategy is stopped (red light) if, after any repetition of the test movement, symptoms remain peripheralized, increased, or worse. If symptoms are produced or increased during testing but do not remain worse, the

TABLE 12-3
PASSIVE RANGE OF MOTION NORMATIVE VALUES FOR THE THORACOLUMBAR SPINE

Motion	Normative Value (Degrees)
Flexion	0-80°
Extension	0-30°
Lateral flexion	0-35°
Rotation	0-45°

American Academy of Orthopaedic Surgeons. *Joint Motion: Method of Measuring and Recording.* Churchill Livingstone; 1965.

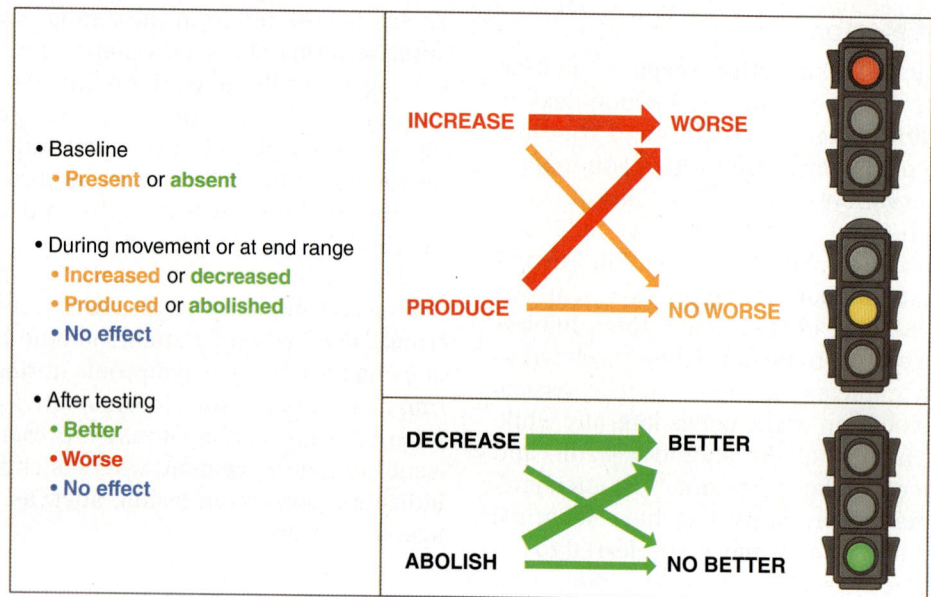

FIGURE 12-5 Symptom response to trunk loading.

loading strategy may be continued with caution (yellow light).

In addition to symptom monitoring, the clinician should note the mechanical response to repeated movements. Changes in ROM may occur before changes in symptoms.[34] ROM may increase with repetition because the tissue is "loosening up," as the patient may not have moved to full range recently. ROM may also increase if the movement coincides with the patient's directional preference. Figure 12-6 provides a flowchart for repeated movement assessment.

Most patients with a directional preference respond to movement in the sagittal plane.[61] For this reason, these strategies are performed in a loaded (standing) and then an unloaded position (lying) first. If no directional preference is found, the frontal plane is then explored. Anecdotally, patients who respond to frontal plane motion are likely to present with asymmetrical symptoms and asymmetrical side glide ROM. Should repeated movements in the frontal plane fail to detect a directional preference, then static positioning is explored. If no movements or positions reduce or centralize symptoms, or improve ROM, the patient does not have a directional preference.

Hip Range of Motion and Muscle Performance

The influence of the hip on the lumbar spine cannot be overstated. Patients with reduced hip ROM may attempt to compensate for this motion loss by moving more through the lumbar spine. A loss of hip extension ROM will lead to compensatory lumbar hyperextension during gait, and, if the motion loss is significant, during

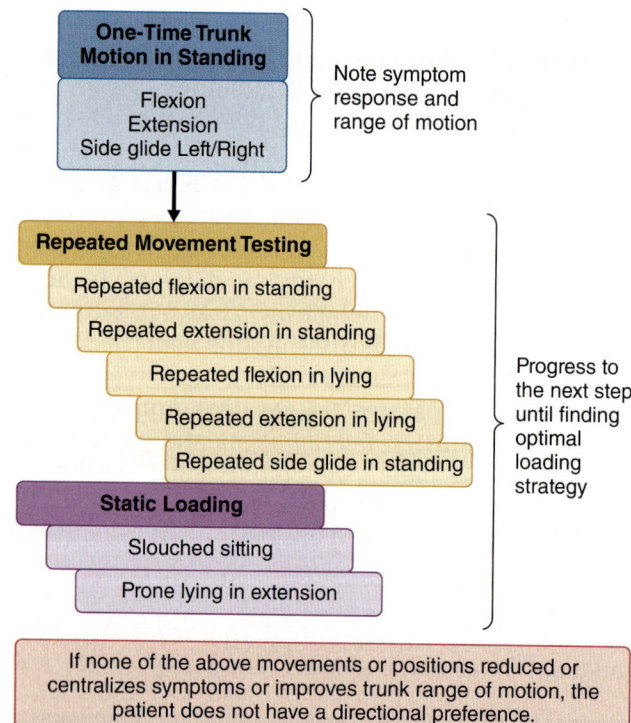

FIGURE 12-6 Flowchart for trunk loading strategies.

standing as well. A loss of hip flexion ROM will require excessive lumbar flexion to perform basic tasks, such as donning socks, squatting, or sitting. Hip muscle performance also has an effect on the lumbar spine. Pain with hip rotation may indicate DGS.[62,63] Weakness of the hip extensors will require greater hip flexion to rise from a chair. Weakness of the hip abductors can lead to a Trendelenburg gait. The hip and lumbar spine have overlapping referral patterns: both can cause buttock, groin, and thigh pain.[43,44] Therefore, clinicians must thoroughly assess hip ROM and muscle performance in patients with lumbar pathology.[36,43,44] It may also be necessary to perform a hip-specific examination on patients with LBP.[42] A more thorough discussion of hip-spine syndrome is presented later in this chapter.

Trunk Muscle Performance

The clinician should assess the muscle performance of the trunk flexors, extensors, and lateral flexors. Muscle performance tests can be roughly grouped into strength-biased tests and activation/movement control–biased tests.

Strength-Biased Tests Clinicians may choose to perform the trunk curl (straight or diagonal partial sit-up) and prone trunk raise tests to assess concentric and eccentric trunk musculature.[64] Patients demonstrating weakness in these assessments may benefit from strengthening interventions. The trunk curl assessment and exercise should be used with caution in patients with (or suspected of having) osteoporosis, given the increased stress to the vertebral bodies. Similarly, caution should also be used with patients with suspected disc pathology.

Activation/Movement Control–Biased Tests Activation/movement control assessments should be performed to help identify patients who might benefit from exercises targeting these impairments (Table 12-4). Specific muscle activation exercises focus on activation and co-contraction of key stabilizing muscles.[65] Movement control exercises focus on the ability to coordinate movements of the trunk and extremities to maintain alignment within a neutral zone, a small ROM surrounding the anatomic neutral position. Assessments of muscle activation and movement control may include the ability to attain and maintain a position with or without the addition of distal movement.

The leg-lowering abdominal test provides a good assessment of the anterior trunk musculature, whereas the Sorenson test is biased toward the posterior trunk musculature. To perform the leg-lowering abdominal test (Fig. 12-7), the clinician judges how far the patient is able to lower the legs while maintaining a neutral lumbar spine and pelvis.[36,64] To perform the Sorenson test (Fig. 12-8), the patient must maintain a neutral spine and pelvis as long as possible while the legs are stabilized by the clinician or straps.[20,36] The ability of a patient to attain and maintain a side plank (on the knee or feet) provides an assessment of the lateral trunk muscles.[36] A patient's ability to perform a timed front plank or bridge can also be examined.[36] Performing a bridge or standing hip hinge is an example of exercise that can help identify a patient's ability to disassociate hip motion from spine motion.

Muscle Length

Decreased length of multi-joint hip muscles can alter lumbopelvic motion. Loss of hip flexor length has already been discussed. Decreased hamstring (HS) length promotes a posterior pelvic tilt and lumbar flexion. Decreased gastrocnemius length may indirectly affect the lumbar spine pathology by causing increased hip internal rotation. Table 10-5, in Chapter 10, Knee, provides normative values for the gastrocnemius, HS, iliopsoas, rectus femoris, and iliotibial band/tensor facia latae. Latissimus dorsi length testing (see Chapter 14, Shoulder Complex, Table 14-11) may be appropriate, given its vast attachment into the thoracolumbar fascia.[66]

Neurodynamic Testing

Neurodynamic testing, including the straight leg raise (SLR) and prone knee flexion, should be performed.[42] If the SLR test is negative, greater neural stress can be applied using the slump test.

Straight Leg Raise
Purpose: To identify lumbar herniated disc at the L4–S1 levels.[36,41,67]

TABLE 12-4
EXERCISE TYPES

	Specific Muscle Activation	Movement Control	Strengthening	Endurance
Description	Focus on activation and co-contraction of the transversus abdominis, multifidus, diaphragm, and pelvic floor. Also referred to as stabilization exercises.	Focus on the ability to co-ordinate movements of the trunk and extremities to maintain alignment within a neutral zone.[a]	Focus on improving maximal muscle force production	Focus on the ability of a muscle to contract repeatedly or sustain a contraction. Postural exercises are typically prescribed as endurance exercises.
Example	Abdominal drawing in maneuver	Sit-to-stand	Sit-up	Sorenson test

[a]Small range of motion surrounding the anatomic neutral position.

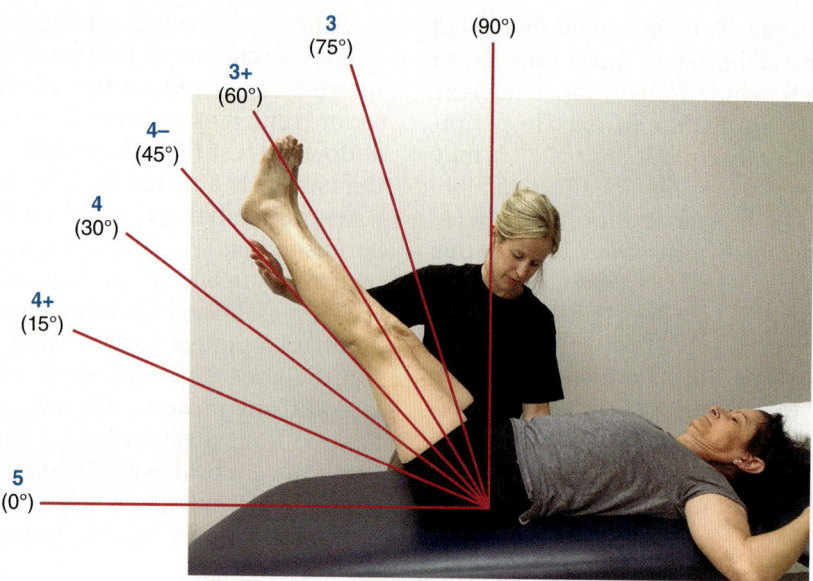

FIGURE 12-7 The leg-lowering abdominal test.

Method: With the patient supine and the knee in full extension, the clinician slowly flexes the hip (Fig. 12-9).
Interpretation: A positive test is reproduction of the patient's lower extremity neurologic symptoms below 45° of hip flexion. The test can be sensitized by flexing the hip until symptoms develop, then decreasing hip flexion slightly and dorsiflexing the patient's ankle.[68] If symptoms are reproduced with dorsiflexion, the test is positive. For patients with limited HS length, adding dorsiflexion to the SLR may help identify positive neural tension.

Prone Knee Flexion (aka Ely Test)
Purpose: To identify lumbar herniated disc at the L1–L3 levels.[66,67]
Method: With the patient prone, the clinician slowly flexes the knee.
Interpretation: A positive test is reproduction of the patient's neurologic symptoms in the anterior thigh.

Slump Test
Purpose: To identify neuropathic pain, most commonly a herniated disc at the L4–S1 levels.[36,67,69]

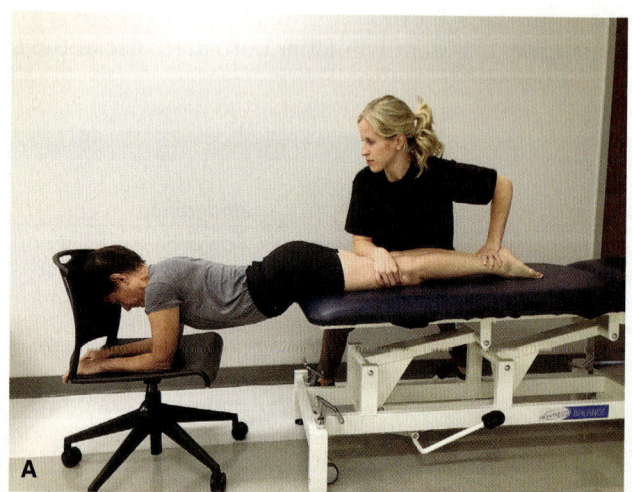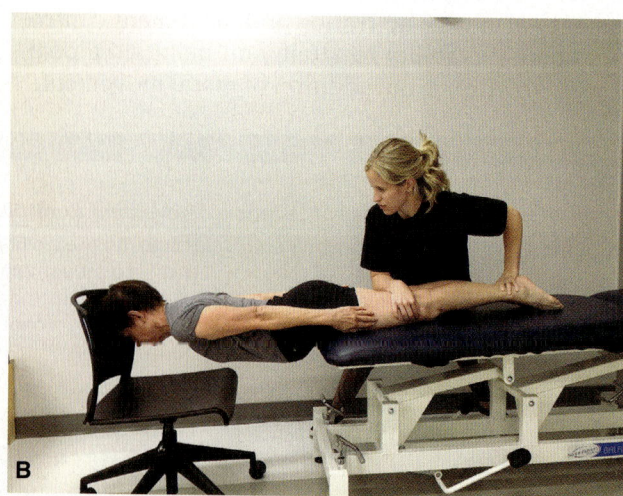

FIGURE 12-8 The Sorenson test. **A.** Setup position. **B.** Test position.

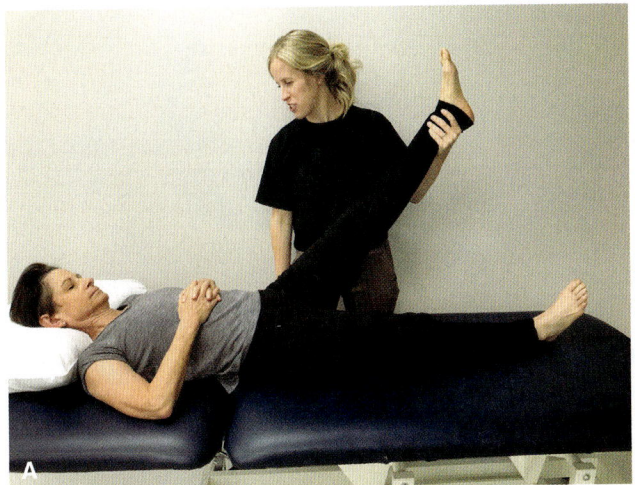
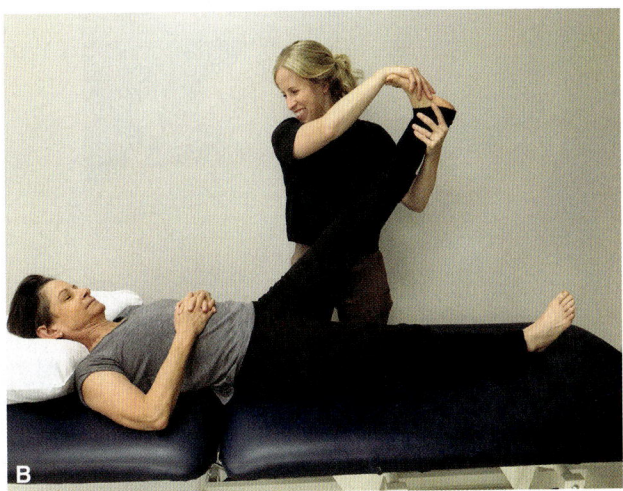

FIGURE 12-9 **A.** Straight leg raise. **B.** Sensitized straight leg raise.

Method: With the patient seated, the patient slumps into trunk flexion. The clinician maintains cervical flexion while extending the patient's knee to the point of symptom reproduction. The patient is then allowed to extend the cervical spine (Fig. 12-10).

Interpretation: A positive test is if symptoms are created with knee extension and abolished with cervical extension.

Passive Accessory Intervertebral Movements

Accessory motion of the intervertebral joints of the lumbar and lower thoracic spine can be assessed using posteroanterior pressures and transverse pressures.

Central Posteroanterior Pressure

Purpose: To assess general intervertebral joint-play movement with an emphasis on sagittal plane motion.[70] When applying grade I and II mobilizations, this technique may be used to help decrease pain.[70] When applying grade III and IV mobilizations, this technique may be used to treat local joint hypomobility and improve trunk extension ROM.[70] For a more aggressive technique, the patient can be positioned in greater amount of lumbar extension.

Patient: Prone.

Clinician: The clinician places the hypothenar eminence of the nondominant hand on the spinous process of the vertebra to be mobilized. The clinician's dominant hand is placed on top of the contact hand.

Mobilization: The clinician uses body weight to create a force perpendicular to the angle of the spine (Fig. 12-11).

Interpretation: The clinician should note if any symptoms are created or increased and attempt to judge the amount of motion (hypomobile, normal, or hypermobile). A positive test for instability is if symptoms are provoked or increased,[31,55] or if accessory motion is believed to be hypermobile. Note inter-rater reliability is somewhat limited[71] and hypermobility may be asymptomatic.[72]

Unilateral Posteroanterior Pressure

Purpose: To assess facet joint mobility with an emphasis on rotation.[70] When applying grade III and IV mobilizations, this technique may be used to treat local joint hypomobility.[70]

Patient: Prone.

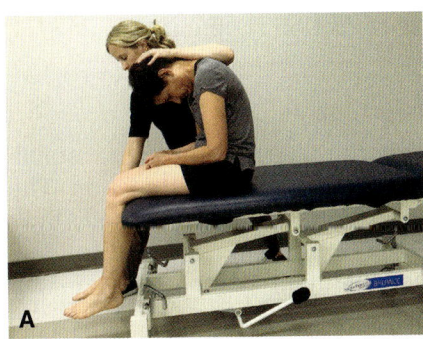
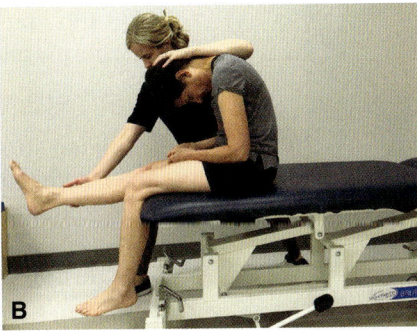
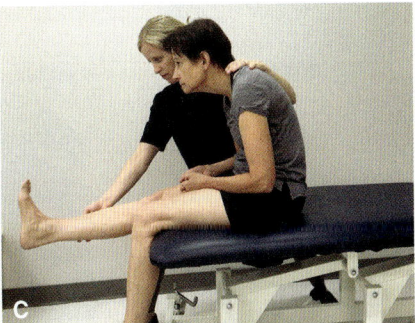

FIGURE 12-10 Slump test: **A.** With the patient in a slumped position, the clinician flexes the cervical spine. **B.** The patient extends the knee until symptoms are felt. **C.** The patient is allowed to extend the cervical spine to see if symptoms are abolished.

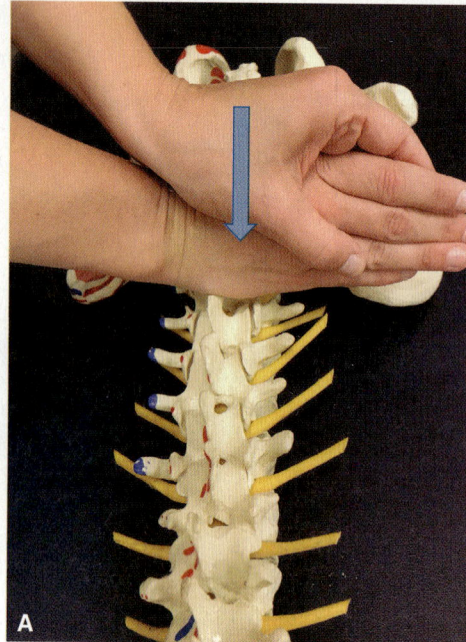
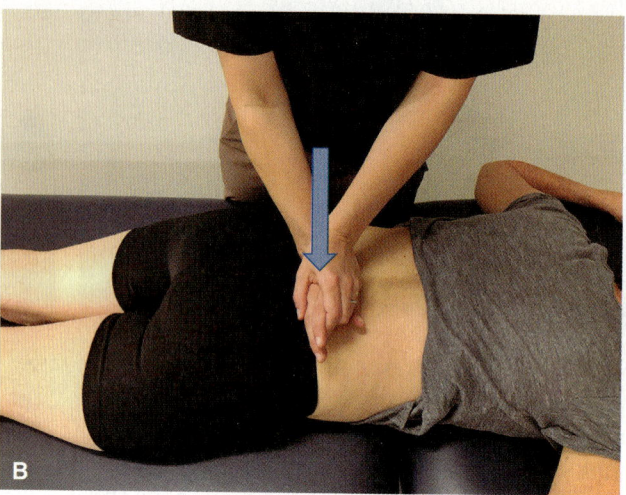

FIGURE 12-11 Central posteroanterior pressure. **A.** Performed on a skeleton. **B.** Performed on a patient.

Clinician: The thumb of the nondominant hand is placed on the articular pillar of the vertebra to be mobilized. The thumb of the dominant hand (mobilizing thumb) is placed over the other thumb. Alternately, the clinician may use the hand position noted for the central posteroanterior pressure.

Mobilization: The mobilizing thumb imparts a downward force perpendicular to the angle of the spine (Fig. 12-12).

Interpretation: The tests interpreted the same as central posteroanterior pressure assessment.

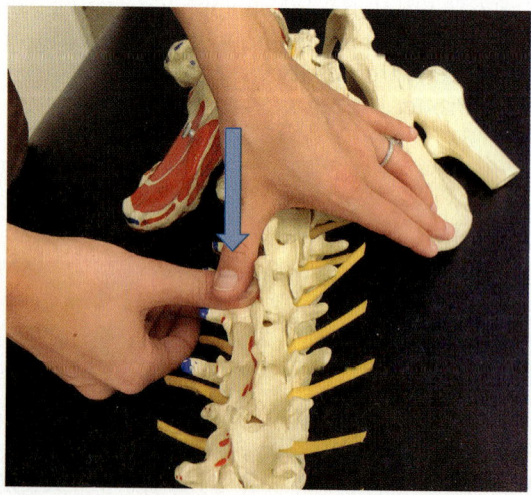

FIGURE 12-12 Unilateral posteroanterior pressure performed on a skeleton.

Transverse Pressure

Purpose: To assess facet joint mobility with an emphasis on rotation.[70] When applying grade I and II mobilizations, this technique may be used to help decrease pain.[70] When applying grade III and IV mobilizations, this technique may be used to treat local joint hypomobility.[70] For a more aggressive technique, the patient can be positioned in greater amount of lumbar extension.

Patient: Prone.

Clinician: The thumb of the nondominant hand is placed on the spinous process of the vertebra to be mobilized. The thumb of the dominant hand (mobilizing thumb) is placed over the other thumb.

Mobilization: The clinician imparts a transverse force to the spinous process (Fig. 12-13).

Interpretation: The clinician should note if any symptoms are created or increased and attempt to judge the amount of motion (hypomobile, normal, or hypermobile).

Special Tests/Provocative Testing

The clinician should perform special tests for instability, facet arthropathy, DGS, and SIJ dysfunction. The clinician should also consider performing the FABER, FADIR, and scour tests (see Chapter 11, Hip) to identify, or rule out, concomitant hip pathology.

Instability Tests To identify instability, clinicians should perform the prone instability test and assess spinal accessory motion.

CHAPTER 12 | LUMBAR SPINE AND SACROILIAC JOINT

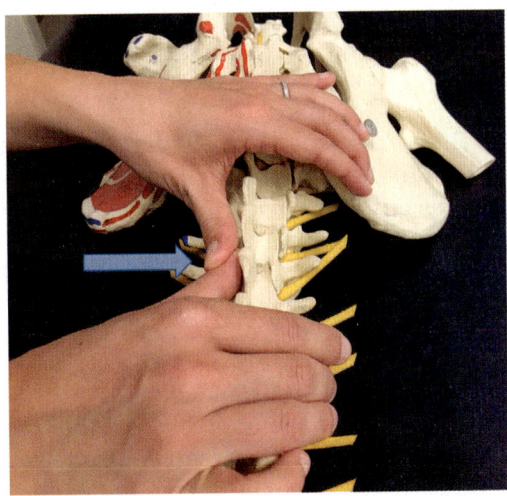

FIGURE 12-13 Transverse pressure.

Method: The clinician guides the patient into trunk extension, lateral flexion, and ipsilateral rotation to maximally approximate the facet joints on the side to be tested (Fig. 12-15).

Interpretation: A positive test is recreation of the patient's local lateral lumbar pain or radicular symptoms. The combination of negative myotomal, dermatomal, and reflex testing along with symptom-free trunk AROM and quadrant test is used to rule out the lumbar spine as a symptom generator.

Special Tests for Deep Gluteal Syndrome Special tests for DGS include the seated piriformis stretch and active piriformis test.

Prone Instability Test
Purpose: To identify instability or muscle activation/movement control deficits.
Method: The patient stands facing the end of the plinth and places the trunk on the plinth. The patient then raises both legs off the ground (Fig. 12-14A). The amount of pain is noted. The test is repeated, while the clinician applies an anterior force to the patient's sacrum (Fig. 12-14B).
Interpretation: A positive test is if pain was present on first test and substantially reduced on repeat test with clinician applied pressure.[20,36]

Facet Arthropathy Test/Quadrant Test The quadrant test can be used to identify facet arthropathy.

Quadrant Test
Purpose: To identify facet arthropathy[20] or assist with ruling out the lumbar spine as a source of patient symptoms.

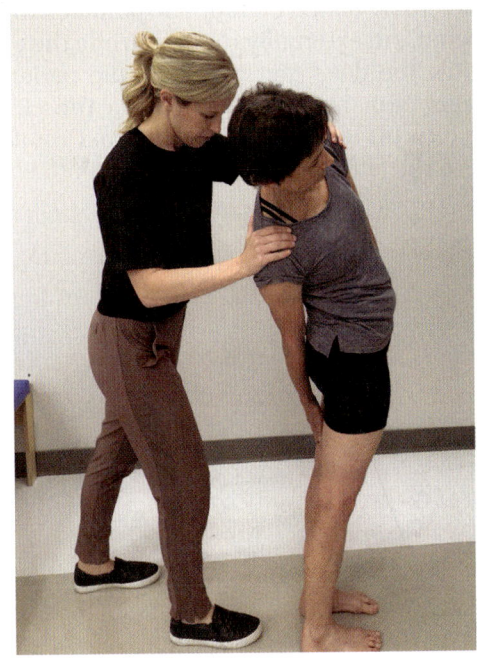

FIGURE 12-15 Quadrant test.

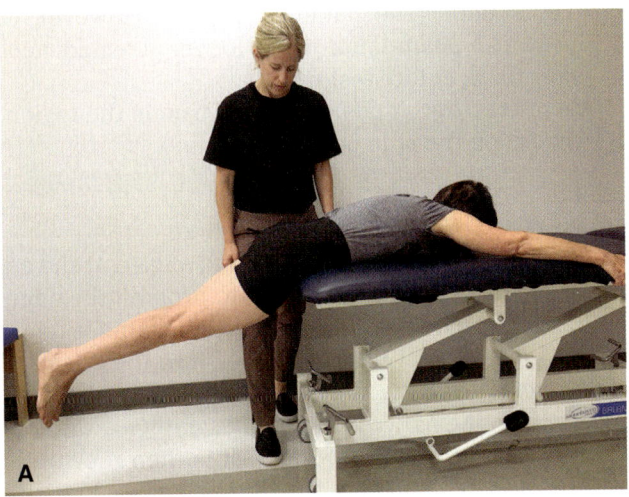
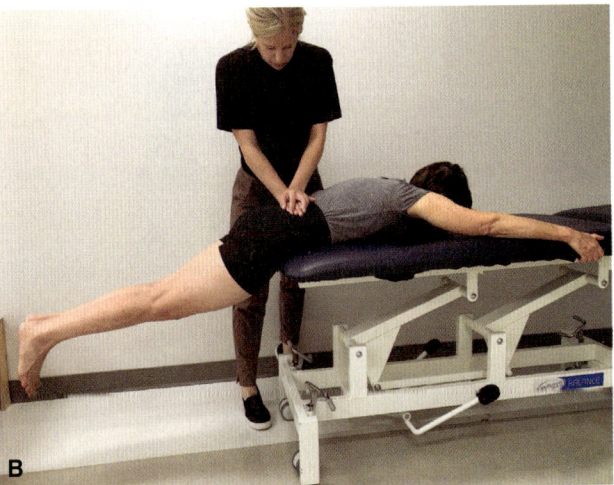

FIGURE 12-14 Prone instability Test. **A.** The patient raises both legs off the floor. **B.** The test is repeated while the clinician applies an anterior force to the patient's sacrum.

Seated Piriformis Stretch

Purpose: To identify sciatic nerve entrapment due to DGS.

Method: With the patient seated, the clinician extends the patient's knee, then passively adducts and internally rotates the hip while palpating the deep gluteal space (Fig. 12-16).

Interpretation: A positive test is reproduction of symptoms in the buttock or sciatic nerve distribution.

Active Piriformis Test

Purpose: To identify sciatic nerve entrapment due to DGS.

Method: The patient is hooklying in sidelying with the side to be tested on top. The patient's top hip is abducted and externally rotated. While the clinician palpates the deep gluteal space, the patient pulls the heel into the table and resists the clinician's force into hip adduction and internal rotation applied to the lateral knee (Fig. 12-17).[62,63,73]

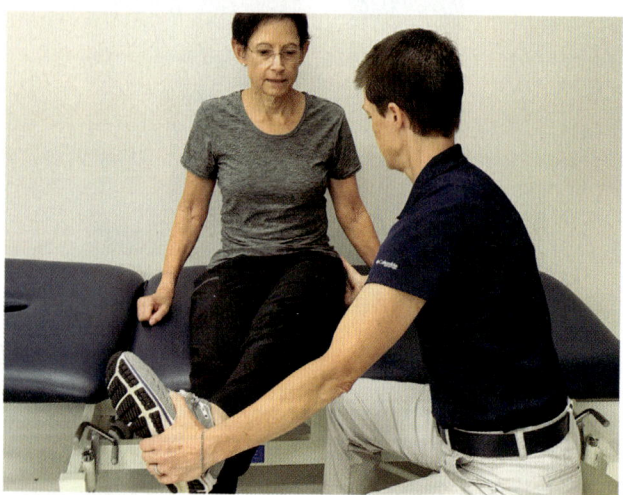

FIGURE 12-16 Seated piriformis stretch.

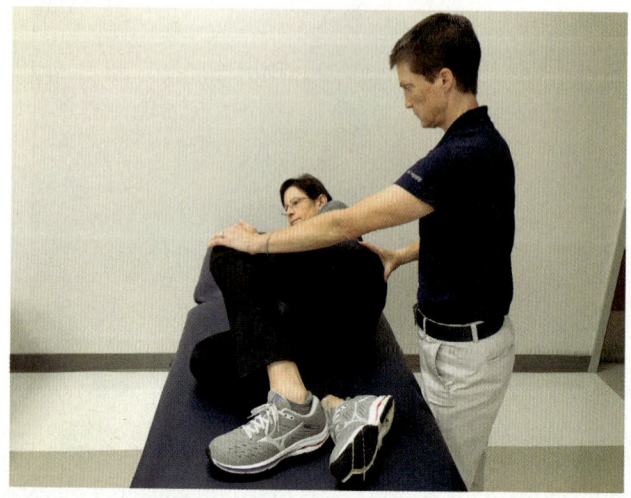

FIGURE 12-17 Active piriformis test.

Interpretation: A positive test is reproduction of symptoms in the buttock or sciatic nerve root distribution.

Special Tests for Sacroiliac Dysfunction

A cluster of tests used to diagnosis SIJ dysfunction (sometimes referred to as *Laslett cluster*[74]) include sacroiliac (anterior) compression, sacroiliac (anterior) gapping, posterior thigh thrust, Gaenslen test, and the FABER test (see Fig. 11-25 in Chapter 11, Hip).[75]

Sacroiliac (Anterior) Compression

Purpose: To identify SIJ dysfunction.

Method: With the patient sidelying, the clinician places both hands on the lateral ilium and provides a downward force compressing the anterior SIJ (Fig. 12-18A).[76,77]

Interpretation: A positive test is pain in the region of the SIJ.

Sacroiliac (Anterior) Gap

Purpose: To identify SIJ dysfunction.

Method: With the patient supine, the clinician places opposite hands on the medial aspect of the patient's anterior ilium and applies lateral force with both hands gapping the anterior SIJ (Fig. 12-18B).[76,77]

Interpretation: A positive test is pain in the region of the SIJ.

Posterior Thigh Thrust

Purpose: To identify SIJ dysfunction.

Method: With the patient supine, the clinician places the patient's thigh in 90° of hip flexion and slight adduction. The clinician then applies a downward force along the shaft of the femur, creating a shearing force to the SIJ (Fig. 12-18C).[77] The test is then repeated on the opposite side. Note this test was previously performed with one of the clinician's hands under the patient's sacrum. However, this awkward positioning is no longer deemed necessary for accurate test results.[77]

Interpretation: A positive test is pain in the region of the SIJ on the side being tested.

Gaenslen Test

Purpose: To identify SIJ dysfunction.

Method: The patient is supine and angled at the edge of the bed allowing one thigh to drop off the edge of the table. The patient and clinician stabilize one hip into flexion by pulling the knee into the chest. The clinician uses the lateral hand to apply a downward force on the patient's thigh, thus applying torsion to the SIJ (Fig. 12-18D).[77] The test is then repeated on the opposite side.

Interpretation: A positive test is pain in the region of the SIJ of the extended side.

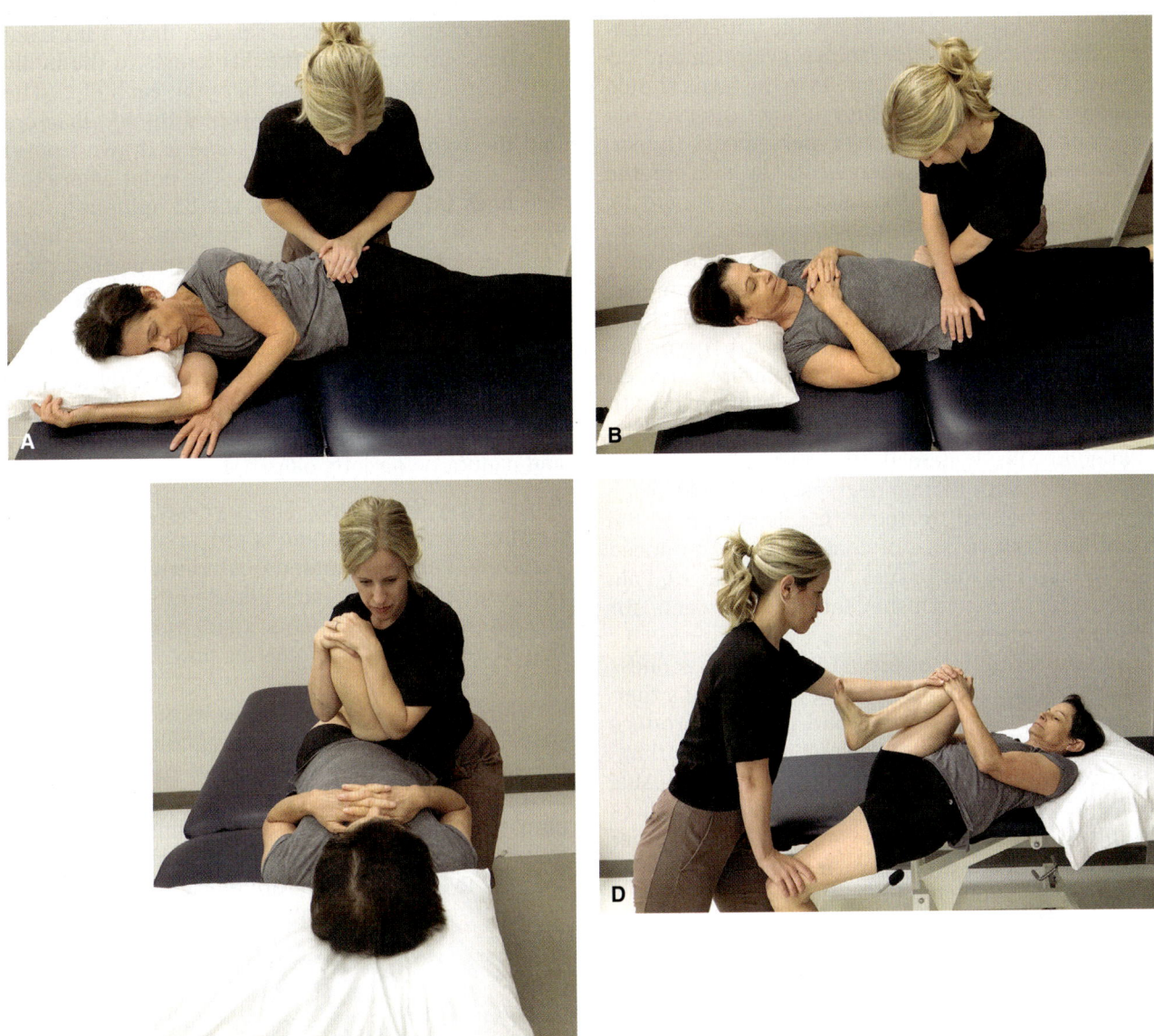

FIGURE 12-18 Special test cluster for sacroiliac (SI) dysfunction. **A.** SI compression. **B.** SI gap. **C.** Posterior thigh. **D.** Gaenslen test.

Palpation

The skin, soft tissue and bone of the entire lower thoracic, and lumbar and gluteal region may be palpated. The location and extent of abnormalities should be documented and investigated as appropriate.

Starting Position To palpate the back, the patient is preferably in the prone position. The positions of unsupported sitting and sidelying may be utilized, if necessary, but may impact palpation findings because of preliminary tension on the skin from the pull of gravity and the impact on the musculature and spinal curvatures. If possible, the patient should be prone on the treatment table, with the head in a neutral position and the nose place in the face hole of the table. The arms should be placed in the position of comfort for the patient, preferably by the side at the level of the pelvis or over the side of the treatment table. The lower legs may rest on a pillow or foot roll, to ensure relaxation of the muscles of the leg and back. If necessary, the midportion of the treatment table may be adjusted or a pillow placed under the patient's abdomen or chest to assure a relaxed starting position.

Skin Observation and Palpation The purpose of skin observation and palpation is to determine the presence of redness, unusual skin marking indicating patchy redness from infection compliance of tissue, moisture, and temperature. Sensory deficits are rare in the trunk. If an area of decreased or lost sensation is identified, the clinician should ask the patient to clarify whether that is a new or familiar symptom and determine the cause. Sensory deficits in the trunk should be monitored carefully, as they impact intervention choice and dosage. Likewise, hyperesthesia (hypersensitivity to touch) or hyperalgesia (an exaggerated response to a normally painful stimulus) should be identified, as patients with such abnormalities may develop with chronic pain. During palpation, allodynia, a painful response to a normally nonpainful stimulus, may be identified. The types of allodynia are mechanical allodynia (pain response to light touch), thermal allodynia (pain response to mild temperature variation in affected area), and movement allodynia (pain with normal movement of muscles or joints).[78]

Patients with hyperesthesia may perceive pain when touched with certain degrees of pressure. Such patients may be best treated with adjustments to the amount of pressure, size of contact area, and speed of mobilization of soft tissues.[79] See Chapter 19, Pain Management: A Mechanism-Centered Approach, for additional information.

The skin should be observed for areas of redness that may indicate infection or long-term use of a thermal device such as a heating pad that can produce patchy areas of red/white discoloration (mottling) of the skin. Lipomas (soft, fatty masses) or unusual patches of hair may indicate a spinal defect such as spina bifida, a nonunion of the vertebral arch, or other bony defects. Skin tags indicate neurofibromatosis tumors that may impinge on the spinal cord and nerve roots. Birth marks or excessive skin markings should be investigated as they suggest the presence of underlying bony pathology.

Bony Palpation The line between the top of the iliac crests indicates the position of the lower edge of L3 spinous process.[79] To palpate this location, the index fingers of the clinician can be placed on the iliac crests of the patient, with the clinician thumbs meeting in the midline of the lumbar spine. The thumbs should fall in the interspace between the spinous processes of the L4 and L5 vertebrae. At the point where the gluteal and lumbar fascia connect with deeper fascial layers, an indentation (dimple) is created. The posterior inferior iliac spine (PIIS) is located approximately 2 cm inferior and lateral to these indentations. After locating the L4/L5 interspace, the clinician can palpate inferiorly along the posterior iliac crest to assure palpation of the PSIS. A line drawn between the right and left PSIS falls at the S2 spinous process. Palpating superiorly from the L4/L5 interspace, the clinician can identify the L4, L3, L2, L1, and lower thoracic spinous processes. Palpating inferiorly from the L4/L5 interspace, the L5 spinous process and base of the sacrum can be felt. Alternatively, the clinician can draw a horizontal line between the top of the iliac crests to the midline and another horizontal line between each PSIS. Then, a line is drawn between the top of the left iliac crest and the right PSIS; likewise, a line is drawn from the right iliac crest to the left PSIS. The point where these two lines intersect indicates the L5 spinous process (Fig. 12-19). The transverse processes of the lumbar spine vertebrae are covered by the transversospinalis muscles (particularly, the multifidus) and are not easily palpated.

The posterior inferior portion of SIJ can be palpated just inferior to the PSIS and slightly medial to the PIIS. The PIIS is located at the level of S3. The main portion of the SIJ is located superior to the S3 level and cannot be directly palpated.

Soft-Tissue Palpation The supraspinous ligaments passing between the spinous processes of the lumbar vertebrae can be palpated posteriorly. Although it is not possible to distinguish between the supraspinous and interspinous ligaments, tenderness to palpation between the spinous processes may represent a ligament sprain.

The lumbar multifidus muscle belly can be palpated just lateral to the vertebral column from L3 to the sacrum. The multifidus is most prominent on the posterior sacrum, just lateral to the midline. To palpate, the clinician places the palpating fingers next to the posterior sacral midline and asks the patient to increase the lordotic curvature of the spine. The fibers

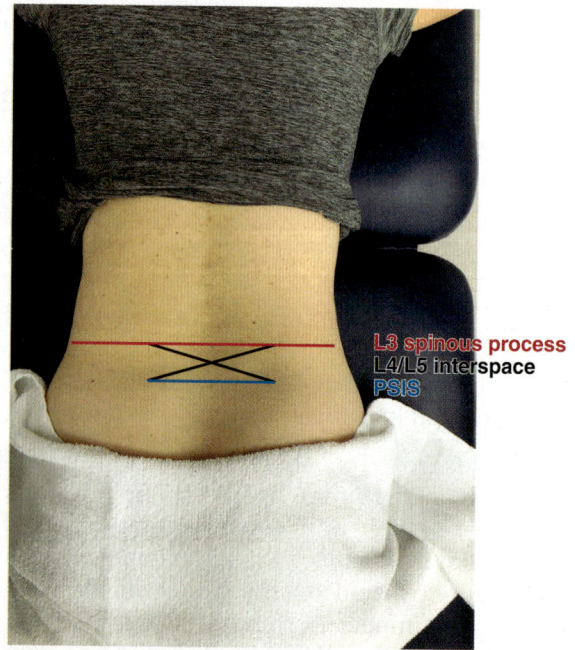

FIGURE 12-19 Palpation of iliac crest, posterior superior iliac spine, and L5 spinous process.

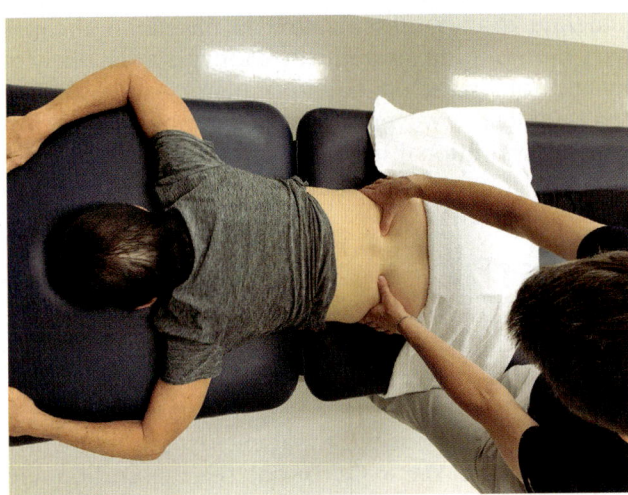

FIGURE 12-20 Palpation of the lumbar multifidus.

of the multifidus will tighten within the enveloping fascial layers and can be differentiated from surrounding tissue (Fig. 12-20). The superficial erector spinae musculature (see Table 4-5 and Fig. 4-35 in Chapter 4, Spine Osteology and Arthrology) in the lumbar region is located just lateral to the lumbar multifidus. The individual erector spinae muscles are not palpable individually, but can be palpated as a unit and made easier by asking the patient to raise part of the upper body to activate the muscles. The erector spinae muscles may feel especially prominent if they are in spasm. If in spasm on one side, the contraction of the muscles may cause the patient to shift to one side.

The gluteal muscles originate from the ilium, just below the iliac crest. Most notably, the large gluteus maximus, a primary hip extensor muscle, can be palpated along its course by visualizing the proximal-medial attachment as a vertical line passing from the PSIS to the coccyx; the upper border passing along an imaginary line from the PSIS to slightly above the greater trochanter of the femur; and the inferior line passing from the coccyx to the ischial tuberosity and continuing on to the iliotibial band and lateral border of the femur. The gluteus maximus can be palpated with the patient prone with the buttocks squeezed together or with an attempt to extend the hip while the knee is flexed. The superior aspect of the gluteus medius can be palpated just superior to the upper margin of the gluteus maximus muscle. The gluteus minimus is deep to the gluteus medius and is not directly palpable. The piriformis is deep to the gluteus maximus, but can be indirectly palpated along the midportion of a line between the sacrum and the greater trochanter. The sciatic nerve may split or remain united to pass superior to, through, or inferior to the piriformis muscle. Tenderness to palpation of the piriformis suggests possible involvement of the piriformis muscle or the sciatic nerve in pathology in the region. The obturator internus and gemelli muscles are located just inferior to the piriformis.

The sacrotuberous ligament can be palpated between the inferolateral sacrum and the ischial tuberosity. To palpate the ischial tuberosity, the clinician should palpate at the midportion of the gluteal fold and press superiorly until the large posterior portion of the ischial tuberosity is felt. Direct pressure can be applied to the sacrotuberous ligament to appreciate the elasticity of the structure along its course. The long posterior sacroiliac ligament passes between the PSIS and the lateral edge of the sacrum on the same side. The ligament is approximately one finger-width wide, merges with the sacrotuberous ligament, and provides attachment for the multifidus.[79] The proximal HSs are palpated at their attachment to the ischial tuberosity. The anteriorly located iliopsoas is deep and not easily palpable.

Gait

The patient's gait should be assessed with and without footwear, noting any deviations of symptoms. Patients with LBP or kinesiophobia may ambulate with reduced trunk rotation due to guarding.[80] Patients with an L4 nerve root lesion may have a foot drop or foot slap. Reduced hip extension ROM may cause lumbar hyperextension during terminal stance. This may cause back pain due to increased facet joint compression or may cause neurogenic symptoms due to lumbar stenosis. Common gait abnormalities and their causes are discussed in Chapter 5, Gait and Footwear.

Functional Testing

Functional testing may include observing the patient perform squatting, lifting, and/or carrying. Back pathology can affect balance, and several tests can be used to assess patient capability, including the single leg balance test with eyes open and eyes closed.[81,82] Standardized tests such as the Timed Up and Go and Five Times Sit-to-Stand (see Chapter 11, Hip) can be performed.

DIAGNOSIS OF LUMBAR SPINE AND SACROILIAC JOINT PATHOLOGY

LBP appears to be a heterogeneous condition. A specific pathoanatomic cause can be found for some cases of back pain.[83] However, most cases of chronic back pain have no definitive pathoanatomic source and are commonly referred to as "nonspecific low back pain." Subgrouping or classifying patients with back pain is generally thought to be needed guide interventions and attain optimal outcomes. LBP may be defined in terms of acuity or recurrence as follows[36,65]:

- Acute pain has been present for less than 1 month.
- Subacute pain has been present for 2 to 3 months.
- Chronic pain has been present for greater than 3 months.
- Recurrent back pain is pain that returns after resolution of an episode.

Chronic and recurrent back pain are considered problematic due to the high degree of disability and both individual and societal cost. Risk factors for chronic back pain include psychological factors such as depression and kinesiophobia and passive coping style, high pain intensity, and the presence of symptoms below the knee.[36] Risk factors for recurrent back pain include history of prior back pain and excessive spinal mobility.[36]

The 2012 LBP clinical practice guideline from the American Physical Therapy Association[36] further subdivides LBP:

- Mobility deficits
- Movement coordination impairments
- Radiating pain
- LBP with cognitive of affective tendencies
- Chronic LBP with related generalized pain

These subgroups are loosely defined, have significant overlap, and remain insufficient to guide interventions. The updated clinical practice guideline draft focuses on physical therapist interventions for LBP by subgrouping patients into four groups[65]:

- Acute or chronic LBP
- LBP with leg pain
- LBP in older adults
- Postoperative LBP

Although globally useful, each grouping continues to encompass a heterogeneous population, making clinical implementation of recommendations problematic.

Several clinical prediction rules have been developed in an attempt to combine information from the patient history and physical examination to help guide interventions and predict prognosis. However, most diagnostic clinical prediction rules are in their infancy and remain unvalidated.[84] Although some classification systems, such as lumbar derangement,[30] appear to have more concrete definitions and greater support than others,[85] at this time, there is still no universally agreed-upon classification system for LBP.

Recognizing the challenges of diagnosing LBP, the following two sections are roughly divided into nonspecific and pathoanatomic LBP.

NONSPECIFIC LOW BACK PAIN

This section reviews three subgroups of nonspecific LBP: mobility deficits, LBP associated with centralization, and muscle activation and movement control deficits. Akin to the 2021 LBP intervention practice guideline draft,[65] classification is based on the primary intervention strategy the patient is most likely to benefit from based on individual history and examination findings. However, this does not preclude performance of additional interventions. In fact, it appears that a multimodal intervention strategy may lead to improved results.[2,65,86]

Low Back Pain Associated with Mobility Deficits

The key finding of patients with LBP with mobility deficit is restricted trunk or segmental ROM. Symptoms are intermittent and produced at, or near, end range.[36] When acute or more severe, patient symptoms are provoked earlier in the ROM. During the maturation and remodeling phase, symptoms are only felt at an early end range. Symptoms may include stiffness or aching pain. Using the terminology of MDT, the patient would be classified as having a dysfunction.[30] Although the term "dysfunction" is well defined within the MDT system, other health care providers utilize the term differently. Therefore, the use of the more universally understood "mobility deficits" is preferred. Although a pathoanatomic cause may be present, many times, it is not possible to determine a single structure that is limiting motion. In addition, the primary focus of interventions, to improve motion and mobility, does not vary based on involved structure(s). For example, multilevel DDD may lead to a global reduction in trunk motion with end-range pain. Treatment would focus on improving the patient's functionally limiting motion deficits.

History Patients with mobility deficits complain of stiffness and limited trunk motion. While patients typically report difficulty related to a loss of trunk flexion, such as donning shoes or picking objects off the floor, some patients may report difficulty attaining an upright posture or that their relatives notice they have become "stooped over." Patients may report difficulty with rotational motions, such as difficulty swinging a golf club or reaching for the seat belt in the front seat. Pain may be present, but is intermittent and occurring at or near end ranges.

Patients may report a gradual loss of motion over time. Patients may also note a one-time event that produced LBP, such as lifting or carrying. The patient then may have avoided aggravating activities and now finds that motion is reduced. Patients may report significant restrictions in their activity after an episode of back pain due to fear of injury or fear of exacerbating the condition.

Key Examination Findings The key examination finding is loss of trunk AROM. Motion loss may be in one direction or may be more globally affected. Back or buttock pain may be present at or near end range. Repeated movement testing does not change symptom location, and other ROMs are unaffected by the repeated motion (Fig. 12-21).[30] Using the example in Figure 12-21, because repeated trunk flexion in standing and in lying produced end-range back pain that was not worse as a result (an orange light), the clinician could have performed another set or two of each flexion test movements to ensure that, with increased stress, the result was the same: a static, restrictive lesion into trunk flexion. Spinal accessory motion may be reduced or guarded at one or more segments.[36] Lower extremity symptoms, if present, are intermittent and produced at, or near, end range.[30,36] Muscular spasm or guarding may be present. Symptoms do not centralize or peripheralize.[30,36] Myotomal weakness is not present, and reflexes are normal.[30,36] Anecdotally, repeated movement testing in some patients might result in a *minor* improvement in ROM as the tissue "loosens up," but there will not be the rapid change in range that can occur with a derangement.

Differential Diagnoses Differential diagnosis should include lumbar derangement, stenosis, spondylolisthesis, hip-spine syndrome, and facet arthropathy.

Rehabilitation Focus and Key Points The primary focus of rehabilitation for patients with mobility deficits is exercise that improves the restricted motion(s). Patients who are acute or guarded may benefit from beginning with gentle on-off motions in an unloaded position. Exercise may begin with midrange motions and work into end range with increasing repetitions. Exercises should be performed multiple times per day to gradually remodel the tissue and reduce pain. Patients with restricted motion with little or no end-range pain may benefit from holding end ranges for a stretch of 10 to 30 seconds and performing fewer repetitions.[87] Patients should also be prescribed exercises to use the new ROM gained.

To prevent movement imbalances, it may be important to perform an exercise in the opposite direction to that creating the stretch. Using the example from Figure 12-21, the patient might be prescribed two sets of 10 repetitions of bilateral knee to chest in lying (Fig. 12-22) to emphasize gaining lower lumbar mobility, as flexion in standing would be more biased toward the thoracic and upper lumbar spine before affecting the lower lumbar region. The patient would also be instructed in a convenient exercise to maintain her current extension ROM, such as performing five repetitions of extension in lying (see Fig. 12-25B). For patients with a mobility deficit into extension, a lower trunk rotation exercise may be performed (Fig. 12-23A). For patients with high irritability, this may be performed as a midrange on-off exercise, whereas patients with symptom free but limited motion may perform to end range using the contralateral upper extremity to help stabilize the thoracic spine and hold for a sustained stretch (Fig. 12-23B). Additional exercises, such as trunk muscle strengthening, trunk stabilization, lower extremity flexibility, lower extremity strengthening, balance, or aerobic exercises, may also be prescribed

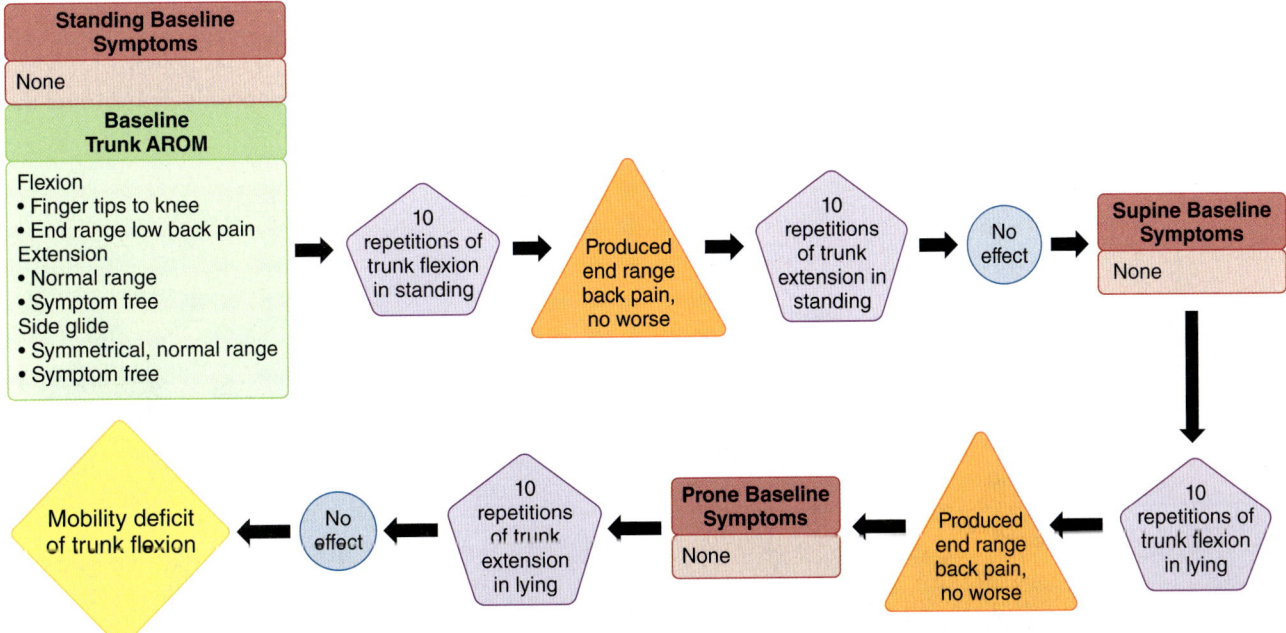

FIGURE 12-21 Example of the response to repeated trunk movements in a patient with mobility deficits. *AROM*, active range of motion.

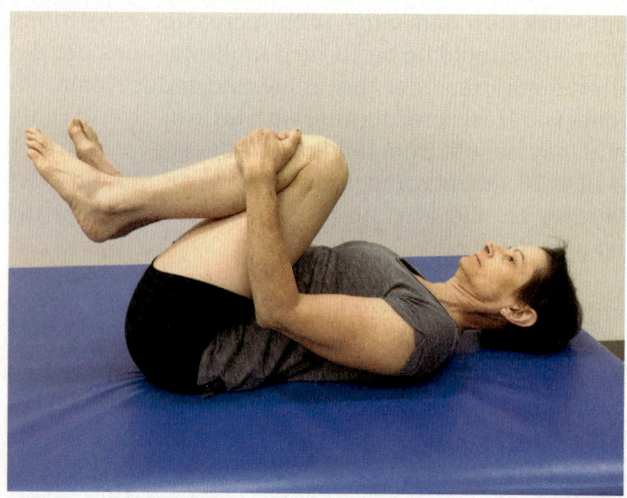

FIGURE 12-22 Double knee to chest exercise to improve lumbar flexion.

based on the patient examination findings, but do not address the patient's specific mobility deficit.

Manual therapy may be incorporated into the plan of care.[65] Soft-tissue mobilization may reduce muscle guarding or address trigger points. Joint mobilizations may improve local restrictions in motion. Manipulation may assist with pain modulation or mobility but should not be the sole intervention.

Patients with high fear avoidance may benefit from graded exposure to fearful movements, activities, and positions. Patient education may include pain neuroscience education,[65] including the differences between stretching, stretching pain, and harm. Patients should also be educated in specific methods to maintain rehabilitation gains and prevent recurrence.

Expected Outcomes Patients with mobility deficits generally respond well to progressive mechanical loading. The longer a mobility deficit has been present, the longer it will take to be regained.[87] Older patients may be expected to take longer to recover, and ROM may not be fully restored. Improvements in motion will be noted over days to weeks because tissue remodeling requires time.[30,87]

Low Back Pain Associated with Centralization

The key finding of patients with LBP associated with centralization is the centralization and/or peripheralization of back, buttock, or leg symptoms as a result of spinal loading. In addition, lumbar ROM may change rapidly (improve or worsen) in response to repeated motions or sustained positions. This concept was first identified by McKenzie as part of MDT and defined as a lumbar derangement.[30] This system has been found to be reliable for classifying patients and directing interventions.[88] Centralization occurs in about 60% of patients with LBP.[59] Because centralization is strongly associated with positive outcomes, clinicians should strive to identify a centralizing loading strategy.[60]

History Patients with an LBP associated with centralization report constant or intermittent back, buttock, or lower extremity pain or paresthesias. Symptoms may follow a dermatomal pattern. Symptoms may be sharp and shooting, or dull and achy, and are affected by position changes. Symptoms may result from a trivial motion (e.g., picking up a slipper or unloading the dishwasher), from a sudden movement (e.g., swinging a tennis racquet or performing a barbell squat), or after prolonged activity or rest (e.g., several hours gardening or riding a car). Patients may go to sleep symptom free, yet wake with symptoms. Symptoms may progress gradually from back pain to back and leg symptoms or solely leg symptoms. Symptoms may

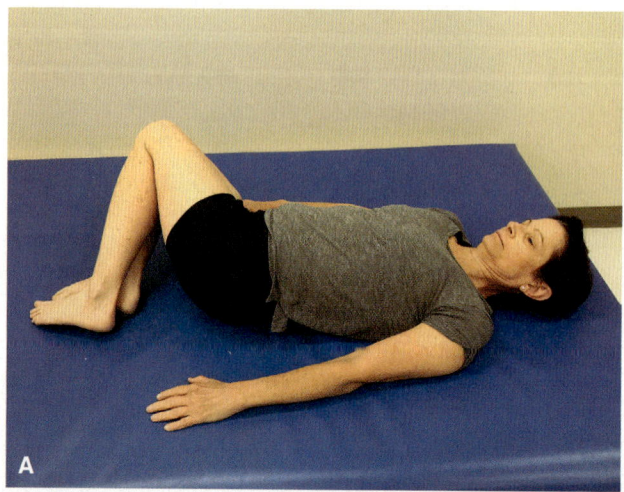
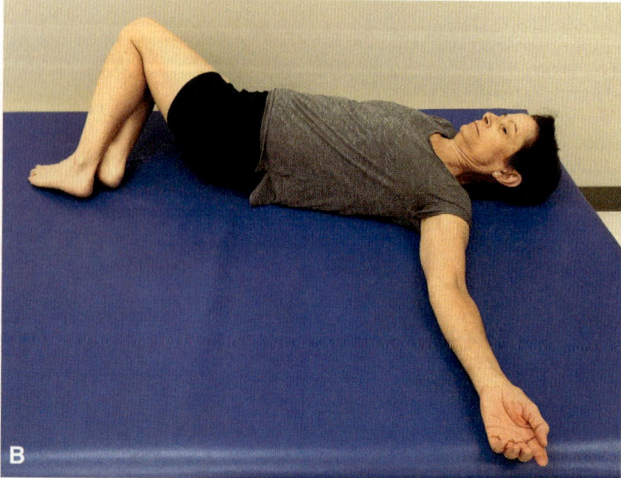

FIGURE 12-23 Lower trunk rotation. **A.** Midrange. **B.** End range.

also begin in the leg rather than the back. Patients may report the inability to stand fully upright due to back or leg pain. Occasionally, patients will report they are shifted laterally and cannot move their trunk back to center. Frequently, patients will note difficulty sitting and lifting. Patients may note pain or a "catch" when rising from a chair.

Key Examination Findings Patients may have positive testing for nerve root pathology, including decreased sensation in a dermatomal pattern with corresponding myotomal weakness and reflex changes. Postural examination may reveal changes to the lumbar lordosis or a lateral shift. Patients with LBP associated with centralization present with a painful loss of trunk ROM in one or more directions. They may have pain during movement or end-range pain. Careful monitoring of symptom location, symptom intensity, and trunk motion during systematically applied trunk loading strategies will reveal a directional preference and centralization/peripheralization of symptoms (Fig. 12-24). For this patient example, flexion in standing peripheralized symptoms, but repeated trunk flexion in lying (lower disc load position) only transiently increased symptoms. Note that there was an improvement in trunk extension ROM as a result of repeated movements that were consistent with the patient's directional preference (extension). For some patients, there will be a decrease in motion when symptoms peripheralize. Using the example in Figure 12-24, the first repetition of extension in standing may have been reduced compared to baseline trunk extension ROM.

Frontal plane repeated motions were not needed in this example, as the patient's directional preference was identified. The figure demonstrates a hallmark of LBP associated with centralization: symptoms and/or motion change rather quickly in response to loading.

Differential Diagnoses Differential diagnosis should include spondylolisthesis, stenosis, hip-spine syndrome, and DGS.

Rehabilitation Focus and Key Points The primary focus of rehabilitation for patients with LBP associated with centralization is repeated movements or end-range positioning in the direction that centralizes, reduces, or abolishes symptoms. In addition, patients should avoid or limit motions, positions, and activities that peripheralize symptoms as much as possible. Centralization is an actively changing condition that requires constant reassessment of patient symptoms and mechanical effects. Patients may initially centralize with a given loading strategy and then fail to respond after days of the same exercise (plateau). Before progressing a loading strategy, the clinician should determine whether the patient is performing the prescribed centralizing exercise correctly, the effect of the exercise when performed at home, and the frequency of performance. This can help determine whether the exercise was correct and if the instructions were followed. Next, it should be determined whether there are other factors that might be delaying or precluding improvement. For example, consider a patient whose symptoms peripheralize with sitting who had to sit on

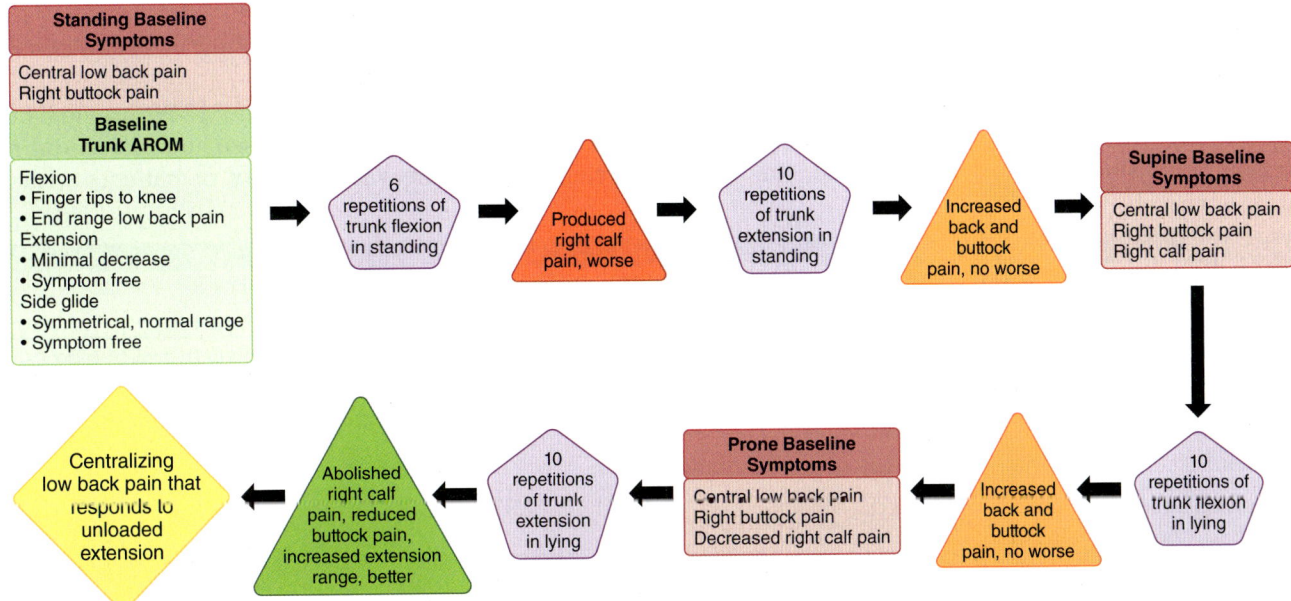

FIGURE 12-24 Example of the response to repeated trunk movements in a patient with low back pain associated with centralization. *AROM*, active range of motion.

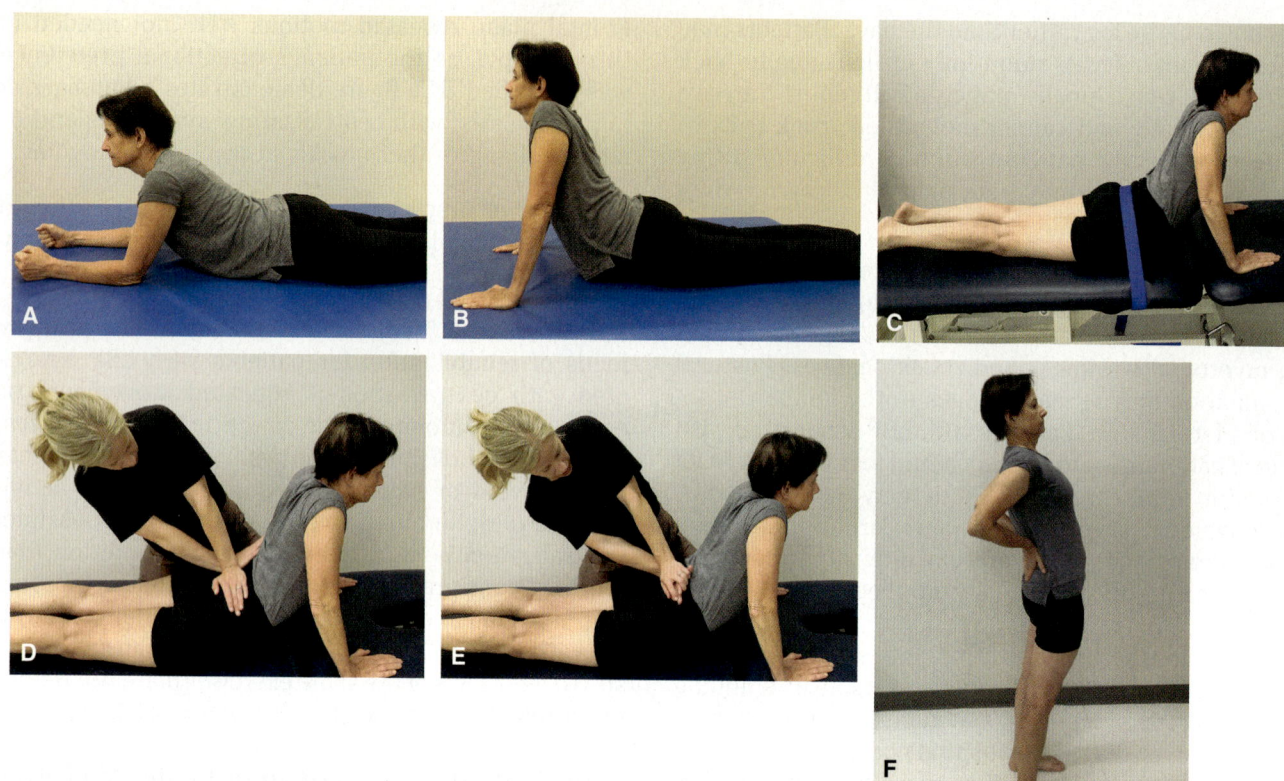

FIGURE 12-25 Examples of force progressions for patients with a directional preference of extension. **A–D.** Prone lying can be progressed as follows: prone prop (**A**), extension in lying (**B**), extension in lying with belt fixation (**C**), and extension in lying with global clinician overpressure (**D**). **E.** Extension in lying with overpressure to a specific lumbar segment. **F.** Extension in standing.

a plane for 4 hours for a work-related trip. A lack of symptom improvement (or worsening of symptoms) as a result of this trip would be an expected result and not indicative of an incorrectly identified and implemented loading strategy.

If this investigation reveals no reason for the lack of improvement, the patient should be reassessed: beginning with clarifying the patient's current symptoms and the response to one-time trunk AROM in standing (flexion, extension, and side glide). Then, the trunk loading examination strategy outlined previously is followed. A progression of trunk force is indicated if the clinician has identified the patient's directional preference and

- the patient's response plateaus
- improvements are slow
- improvements are transient

Table 12-5 and Figures 12-25 and 12-26 provide potential force progressions based on direction of preference.[30,89] The vast majority of patients with a

TABLE 12-5		
FORCE PROGRESSIONS BASED ON DIRECTION OF PREFERENCE		
Extension Progression	*Flexion Progression*	*Frontal Plane Progression*
• Prone lying • Prone prop • Ext. in lying • Ext. in lying with belt fixation or clinician overpressure • Sustained ext. • Ext. in standing[a] • Posteroanterior mobilization	• Double knees to chest • Flex. in standing • Flex. in sitting	• Self-correction with arm by side • Self-correction with arm abducted • Clinician correction

Ext., extension; *Flex.,* flexion.

[a]Extension in standing represents a progression from unloaded to loaded lumbar extension. However, this exercise may also be placed earlier in the force progression, given it only involves patient-generated forces. In addition, extension in standing may be prescribed instead of an exercise in lying owing to its relative convenience and lack of upper body strength requirement as long as the exercise still has the desired effect.

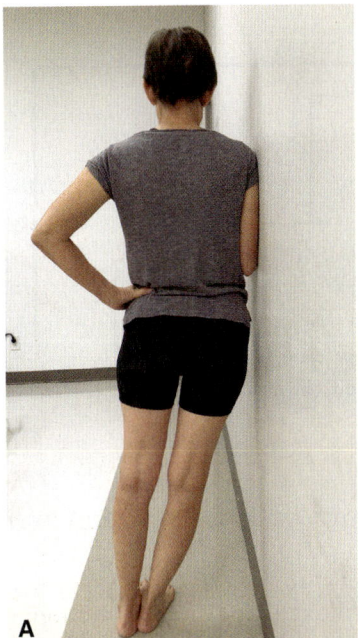 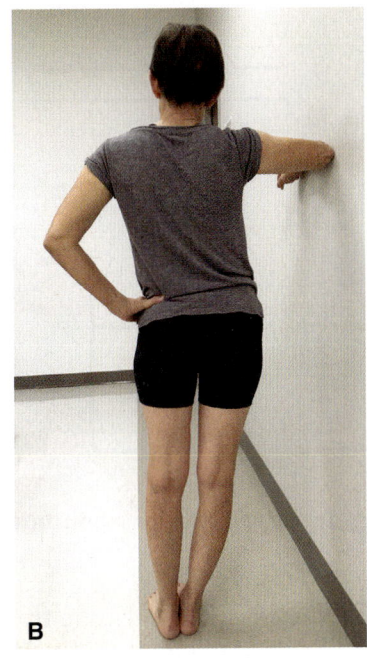 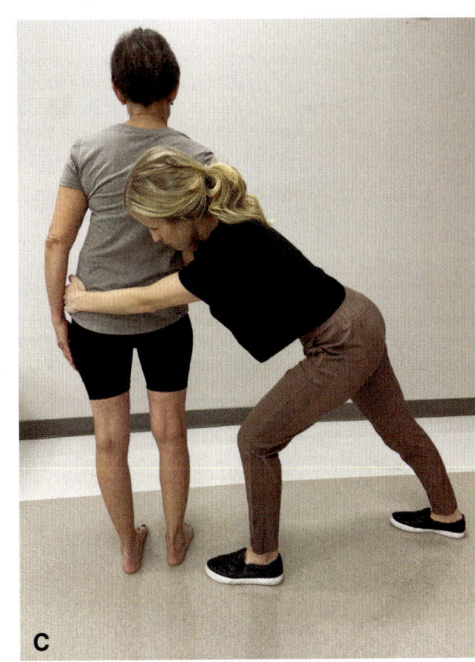

FIGURE 12-26 Examples of force progressions for patients with a directional preference in the frontal plane. **A.** Midrange left side glide in standing with arm by side. **B.** End-range left side glide in standing with arm abducted 90°. **C.** Clinician manual left side glide for correction of a right lateral shift.

directional preference respond trunk loading strategies into extension.[61]

Once symptoms have resolved and the condition is stable, it is important to reintroduce the previously peripheralizing movements in a controlled manner. This progression can assist with reducing kinesiophobia and restore normal, safe movement patterns.

Patients with LBP associated with centralization are likely to benefit from additional types of exercise, such as functional training and stretching, strengthening, muscular endurance, and aerobic exercise. However, these exercises must not create or increase peripheral symptoms. For example, core activation and stabilization exercises may be indicated. However, if performing abdominal bracing, abdominal hollowing maneuver, or rhythmic stabilization in quadruped produces leg symptoms, such exercises are not currently appropriate and should be delayed until the patient's symptoms are consistently centralized or abolished. Progression from exercises that produce centralization to core activation and stabilization exercises is consistent with standard of care.[90]

Expected Outcomes The performance of repeated movements or holding sustained positions that are consistent with a patient's directional preference can reduce symptoms and improvement mobility for individuals with acute, subacute, and chronic LBP.[1,36,65] Patients with LBP associated with centralization have better outcomes than patients with other types of nonspecific LBP.[57,58] For these patients, treatment using repeated movements has been shown to be more effective than manual therapy.[33,91–93] Significant improvements in pain, motion, and disability can be expected within 2 to 4 weeks,[47,61,88] although patients with a lateral shift may require more time to achieve optimal results.[30]

Muscle Activation and Movement Control Deficits

Impaired muscle performance is a key finding of patients with muscle activation and movement control deficits. Altered muscle performance may include:

- Decreased muscle activation
- Abnormal muscle recruitment
- Decreased coordination among muscles

Injury, acute pain, and nociceptive stimulation can affect trunk muscle function. Specifically, pain seems to change muscle activation,[80] particularly the multifidi.[94] Reflex inhibition of the multifidi may be an attempt to unload the spine.[80] Decreased and delayed activation of the transversus abdominis (TrAb) may also be present.[85] Together, this reduction in dynamic support may result in increased intervertebral motion[80] and stress to local ligaments and capsules.[95] Many patients with LBP have increased activation of the erector spinae, rectus abdominis (RA), and obliques.[94,96] This may be the result of pain, an attempt to provide spinal stabilization, or may be the result of psychological factors, such as kinesiophobia. However, increased erector spinae activity also increases spinal joint loading[80] and may lead to faster

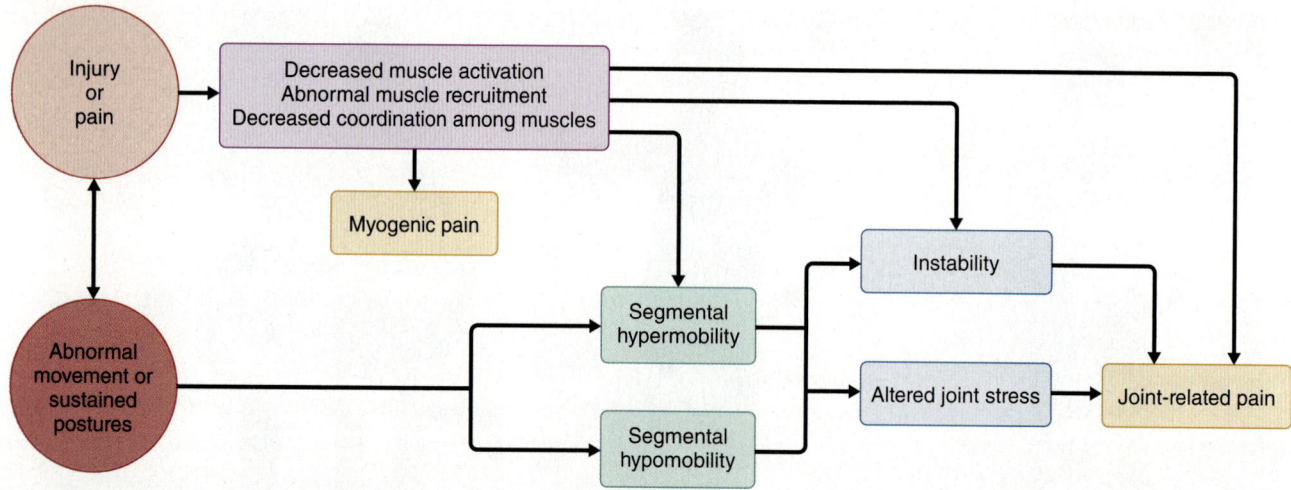

FIGURE 12-27 Potential relationships between nonspecific low back pain and muscle activation and movement control deficits.

muscle fatigue. Muscular hyper-recruitment may lead to an articular or a myogenic source of LBP.[80] Studies have shown morphologic changes after injury, including a transition from slow- to fast-twitch muscle fibers, along with fatty infiltration within the multifidi, leading to inflammatory muscle fibrosis.[80,94] Chronically, this results in muscle unloading and atrophy. Muscle disuse can lead to further muscle atrophy in patients on "bed rest" or among those with psychosocial factors, such as kinesiophobia or catastrophization.

While the previous argument is based on the body's response to injury or the perception of the potential for injury, it is also possible that repeated movements or sustained positioning can create pathology.[60] This type of kinesiopathologic approach, known as the *movement system impairment*, was first developed by Sahrmann.[97] This system is based on the concept that repeated movements and sustained postures can create changes in relative flexibility. Patients may move more readily from one joint than another, and body movement takes the path of least resistance. Over time, tissue adaptations can develop, resulting in hypermobility in one area and hypomobility in another.[83] This may cause tissue microtrauma and, eventually, macrotrauma[85,97] if the patient is unable to adequately control lumbar segments during movements in one or more directions.

Changes in trunk muscle activation, function, morphology, and movement patterns may be a *cause* of LBP, the *result* of LBP, or *contribute* to the recurrence of LBP.[80,94] While once believed to be solely a problem of structural instability, LBP associated with muscle activation and movement control deficits is much more nuanced. Recall that osseous structures including the facet joints, ligaments, joint capsules, muscle stiffness, and neuromuscular control all contribute to spinal stability.[95] Figure 12-27 provides an example of the complex relationships between nonspecific LBP and deficits in muscle activation and movement control. Therefore, exercises that help recruit inhibited muscles and restore normal muscle recruitment patterns are appropriate in these patients.[94] Once normal muscle activation and recruitment has been restored, strength and endurance exercises may help resolve muscle atrophy and reverse morphologic changes.

Debate exists regarding the best way to perform and teach muscle activation and stabilization exercises. The TrAb and internal oblique (IO) are thought to play a greater role in lumbar stability than either the RA or external oblique (EO). Therefore, exercises that preferentially activate the TrAb and IO are desirable for improving lumbopelvic stability. Abdominal bracing and abdominal hollowing (aka the abdominal drawing in maneuver) are two different exercise methods described in the literature (Table 12-6). Abdominal

TABLE 12-6		
ABDOMINAL BRACING AND ABDOMINAL HOLLOWING		
Training Method	Abdominal Bracing	Abdominal Hollowing (aka Abdominal Drawing in Maneuver)
Description	Contraction of the entire abdominal wall without changing the lumbopelvic alignment	Hollowing the lower abdomen by pulling the umbilicus up and in toward the spine while maintaining lumbopelvic alignment

bracing has been used in the field of strength and conditioning, whereas abdominal hollowing has gained favor in the field of rehabilitation. Studies consistently demonstrate that both abdominal bracing and abdominal hollowing preferentially activate the TrAb and IO,[98–100] and several studies have found no difference between these two exercises.[101,102] Abdominal bracing creates a larger increase in intra-abdominal pressure[103] and allows for greater force generation from the limbs[104] and better trunk stabilization.[105] It is possible that muscle activation is both population (healthy versus injured or painful) and task specific (exercise in a certain position or during a certain activity). Given the current evidence, it would seem that for rehabilitation purposes, clinicians can choose either method, perhaps adapting based on the patient's ability to perform each exercise as well as the effect each maneuver has on patient symptoms. It also appears that, for higher level patients, such as athletes performing heavy lifting such as squats and deadlifts, abdominal bracing is more appropriate.

History Symptoms may be constant or intermittent and are most commonly noted in the back and buttock. Patients may report catching, locking, or giving way.[31] Patients may also report muscle spasms and tightness, fatigue, or pain with joint loading. There may be a history of trauma, or the onset of symptoms may be insidious and gradually progressive. Patients may report pain with activities that require the trunk to be a stable base from which the extremities should function, such as lifting, climbing stairs, or getting out of bed. Patients may report a prior history of similar symptoms.

Key Examination Findings The key examination findings for patients with muscle activation and movement control deficits are pain that is concurrent with abnormal movement patterns or functional instability. Patients may have abnormal postural alignment due to local hypomobility or abnormal muscular activation. For example, a patient may have LBP as a result of prolonged standing with an anterior pelvic tilt and lumbar hyperextension. If, during the examination, correction of the static posture, either manually or with cueing, improves the patient's symptoms, this is a positive finding and, therefore, interventions would involve addressing the cause(s) of the abnormal alignment, such as reduced hip flexor length, decreased abdominal activation, or hyperactive erector spinae. Trunk AROM may be excessive.[106] Examination of muscle performance may reveal decreased muscle activation or hyper-recruitment. Muscle spasms or trigger points may be present.

Patients may demonstrate aberrant movement patterns, such as a reverse lumbosacral rhythm with trunk AROM,[31] or exhibit a pause or "catch" with transfers and bed mobility. The examination should include assessment for abnormal movement patterns with various motions.[107] For example, the following motions require the patient to be able to disassociate hip movement and spine motion, that is, maintain the spine in a neutral zone while moving the hip in various planes:

- Standing hip hinge
- Sidelying hip abduction
- Prone hip extension
- Prone knee flexion
- Prone hip rotation
- Seated knee extension
- Seated hip hinge
- Supine SLR
- Supine hip abduction and external rotation (Fig. 12-28)
- Supine knee to chest
- Quadruped rocking forward and backward (Fig. 12-29)
- Quadruped arm lift

If a motion creates symptoms and the patient is unable to maintain a neutral lumbar spine and pelvis when performing them, the motions are repeated with stabilization and the effect on symptoms is reassessed. If symptoms are resolved with proper form, the patient is taught to do exercises to restore normal movement patterns.[108] This approach is similar to the scapular assistance test described in Chapter 14, Shoulder Complex.

The prone instability test may be positive.[31,55] Patients may have findings consistent with hypermobility, such as increased posteroanterior pressure accessory motion or a positive Beighton test for systemic hypermobility.[31] However, the clinician must recall that, as with ankle sprains, the presence of hypermobility need not equate to functional instability.[106] This is particularly true for the spine, as the assessment

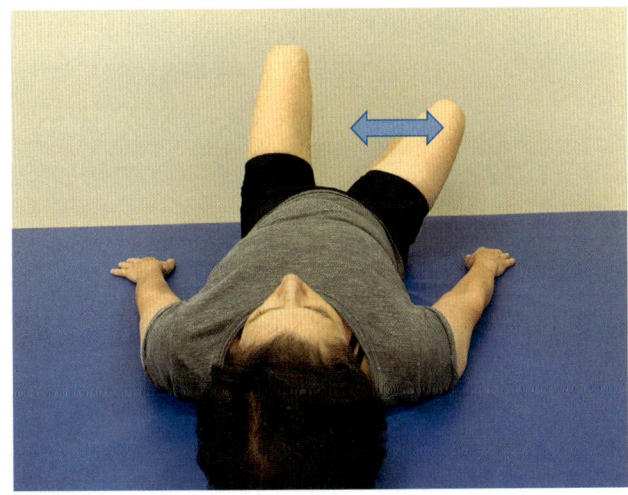

FIGURE 12-28 Supine hip abduction and external rotation.

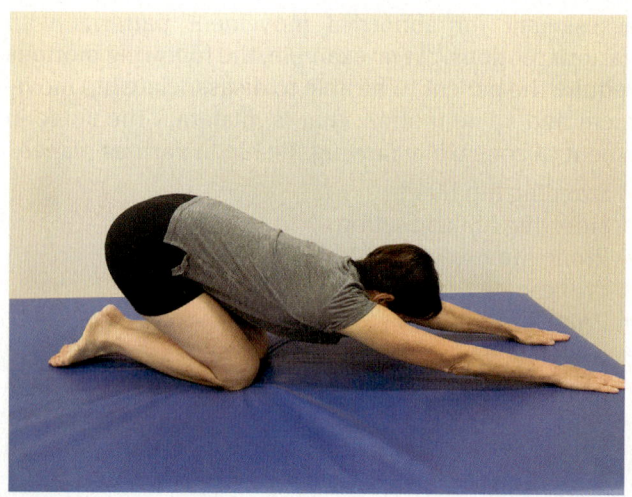

FIGURE 12-29 Quadruped rocking forward and backward.

of accessory motion is performed unloaded in lying without concomitant muscular contraction, which is known to contribute to both static and dynamic stability.[109] Patients may also present with areas of hypomobility or decreased muscle length, most commonly shortness of the hip flexors.

Differential Diagnoses Differential diagnosis should include myofascial pain syndrome (MFPS), hip-spine syndrome, DGS, and facet arthropathy.

Rehabilitation Focus and Key Points The clinician must attempt to identify symptoms related to abnormal movement and provide exercises to rectify this. If patient movement is aberrant, but symptoms are unchanged, stabilization exercises may be prescribed based on the assumption that abnormal movement patterns are maladaptive and that correction to a more normal movement pattern will lead to improvement in symptoms over time.[85] It is important to note that exercises may be needed not only to increase muscle activation but also to modulate muscle activation. For example, maintaining a neutral spinal alignment requires very little muscular activation, approximately 2% of maximal voluntary isometric contraction (MVIC),[109] and muscle contractions of greater than 5% MVIC have been shown to lead to muscular fatigue[110] and pain.[111] Relaxation exercises may be useful to reduce hypertonicity in patients with psychological distress.

Muscle activation and movement coordination exercises are the mainstay of treatment, and exercise prescription should begin with low-level contractions performed for multiple repetitions throughout the day. A potential progression would be to first train core stabilizer activation to attain and maintain a neutral spine while limiting recruitment of global trunk extensors or hip musculature. Training may be easiest to begin in supported positions, such as supine (Fig. 12-30) and

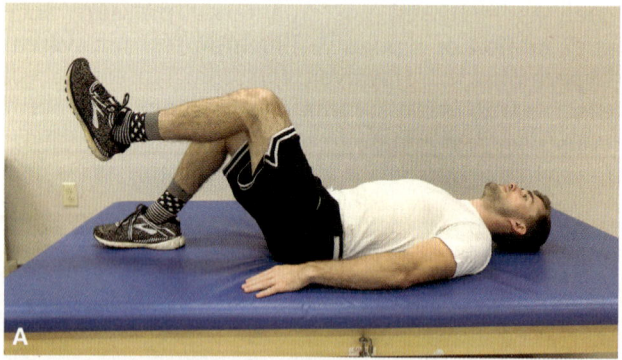
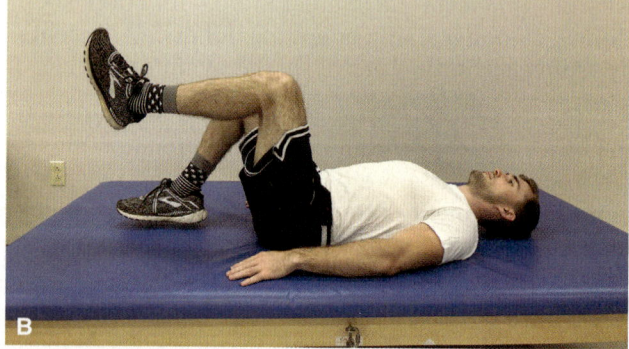
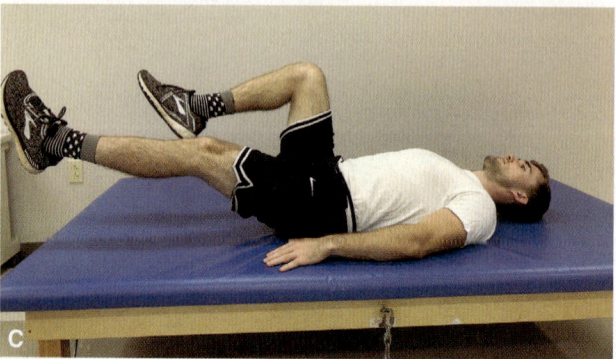
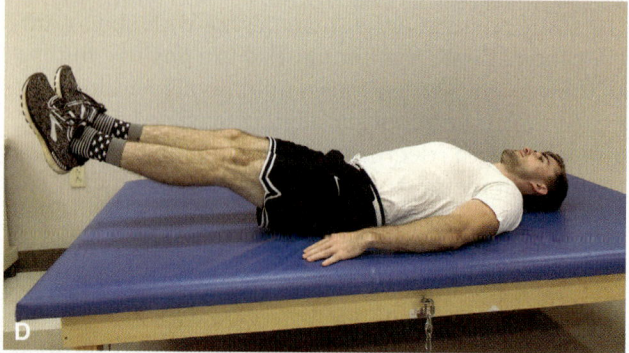

FIGURE 12-30 Dead bug progression. **A.** Hooklying alternate march. **B.** Alternate hip extension with a start position of 90° of hip flexion. **C.** Alternate hip and knee extension. **D.** Bilateral hip and knee extension.

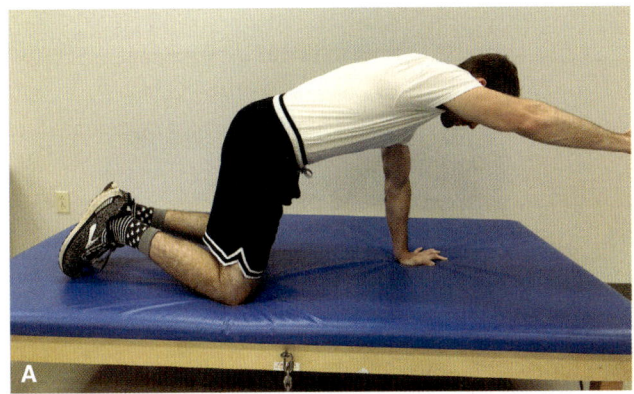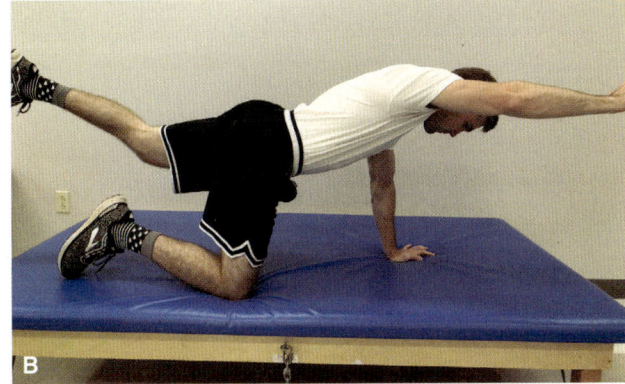

FIGURE 12-31 Examples of quadruped stabilization exercises. **A.** Alternate shoulder flexion. **B.** Alternate hip extension with shoulder flexion.

seated in a chair with a back, and progress to unsupported positions, such as quadruped (Fig. 12-31). Exercises may add challenges by adding upper extremity motion (smaller load without a direct connection to the pelvis and lumbar spine), followed by lower extremity motion (heavier load with a direct connection to the pelvis and lumbar spine). Exercise may begin moving in a single plane, then progress to multiple planes, across planes, or rhythmic stabilization (Fig. 12-32).

Some functional activities, such as using optimal alignment with bed mobility and transfers, should begin as early as possible. However, higher level functional activities should be incorporated after the patient has mastered muscle activation and movement control.[112] As the patient's neuromuscular control and irritability improve, exercises can be progressed from this midrange toward more challenging positions in an expanded neutral spine zone (Fig. 12-33). For example, a tennis player must be able to control excessive trunk hyperextension with overhead serves and rotational forces of hitting a powerful backhand. Without incorporating muscle performance into function, the potential for symptom resolution will be limited.[66]

Interventions must also include stretching exercises to correct adaptive tissue shortening.[97] Postural endurance exercises to improve the ability to maintain more neutral postures and strengthening exercises to address adaptive muscle weakness should also be considered.[97] Manual therapy such as joint mobilizations helps improve areas of hypomobility.[65] Soft-tissue mobilization may help reduce muscle tone or assist with regaining ROM.

Expected Outcomes Muscle activation and movement control are effective at reducing pain and improving function.[1] Most studies note symptom improvement or resolution within 4 to 6 weeks.[71] Addressing patient-specific muscle activation and movement control deficits has led to superior results when compared with education,[113] stretching,[114] or general strengthening exercises.[60,115,116] When compared, muscle activation exercises and movement control exercises appear to result in similar improvements in symptoms.[117] Given that they have also been shown to result in similar improvements in muscle activation, there is little evidence to support the use of one exercise type over the other for the management of nonspecific LBP.

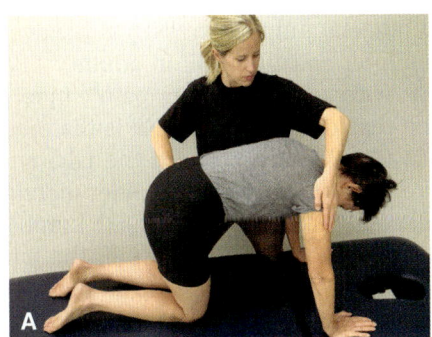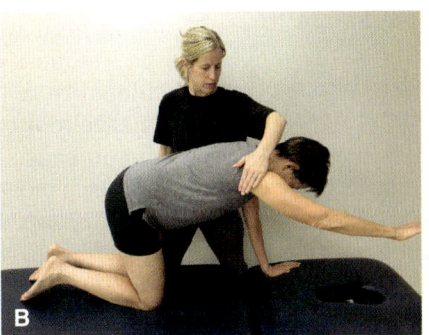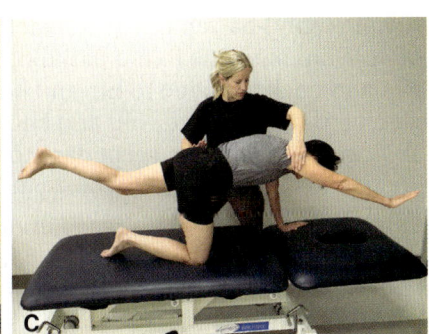

FIGURE 12-32 Rhythmic stabilization. **A.** Quadruped. **B.** Shoulder flexion. **C.** Shoulder flexion and hip extension.

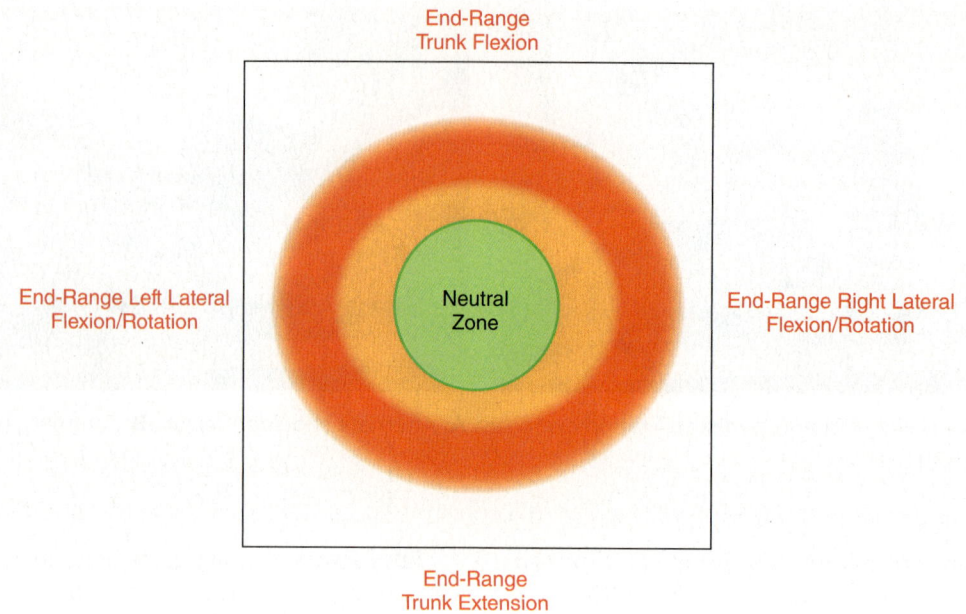

FIGURE 12-33 Neutral zone for spine function.

PATHOANATOMIC CLASSIFICATIONS OF LOW BACK PAIN

Pathoanatomic classifications of LBP can sometimes provide guidance for interventions. For example, LBP in the presence of vertebral body fracture would support providing an optimal environment for fracture healing via the avoidance of trunk flexion activities. This section reviews the following pathoanatomic conditions: hip-spine syndrome, pelvic floor dysfunction, disc pathology, stenosis, spondylolisthesis, spondylolysis and stress reactions, facet arthropathy, fracture, strains, MFPS, DGS, and SIJ dysfunction.

Hip-Spine Syndrome

The intimate relationship between the lumbar spine, pelvis, and hip has been discussed earlier and in Chapter 11, Hip. The hip and spine have overlapping pain distributions, which can make it difficult to identify the source of a patient's symptoms.[45] The clinician must utilize the information from the patient history and examination to determine whether a patient has:

- Simple (only) back pain due to back pathology
- Simple hip pain due to hip pathology
- Hip and back pain due to hip and back pathology
- Complex (interrelated) hip and back pain where pathology of one joint is secondary to the other.

Hip spine syndrome was first described in 1983 by Offierski and MacNab[118] as a recognition that there can be coexisting hip and lumbar spine pathology.[44] Nearly one-third of patients presenting with LBP had positive hip provocation tests.[43] Patients with LBP frequently have reduced hip ROM and routinely improve after surgical intervention for hip disease.[119] For example, a total hip arthroplasty (THA) resolved a patient's back and calf pain (a pain pattern more typical of lumbar pathology).[120] Hip osteoarthritis can lead to spine osteoarthritis.[45] Another patient had a THA but continued to have persistent posterior hip pain that only resolved with treatment of the lumbar spine.[120] Even with complex imaging and direct observation from surgery, it is not always easy to identify the source(s) of patient symptoms.[121] Therefore, clinicians should meticulously consider the hip as a potential source of pathology or a contributor to spine pathology. Examination should seek concordant symptom reproduction and an impairment-based approach to treatment.[122] Interventions for hip-spine syndrome often involve a combination of mobility and movement control exercises for both joints. Failure of the clinician to recognize concurrent pathology at the hip and spine is likely to lead to suboptimal results.

Lumbar Herniated Disc

Lumbar herniated nucleus pulposus (HNP) is believed to be the most common cause of LBP in adults.[123] Radiculopathy is LBP with associated leg pain[89] involving nerve root compression.[20] Lumbar HNP is the most common cause of radiculopathy,[2,18] with the L4-5 and L5-S1 discs most frequently affected.[124] In older individuals, more superior segments may be involved. Lumbar HNPs are generally posterolateral because of the narrower posterior longitudinal ligament and thinner annulus in this region. Symptoms of Lumbar HNP may be related to a combination of nerve compression and inflammatory changes.[18] Computed tomography (CT), myelography, and MRI appear to have equivalent diagnostic accuracy in identifying a lumbar HNP.[125] However, MRI is the imaging of choice because of the lower exposure to radiation.[126] Nerve conduction study results are weakly associated with history and examination findings.[127] Routine imaging should not be performed.[1,18,65]

History Patients with a lumbar HNP report constant or intermittent, central or asymmetrical back pain. Symptoms may extend into the buttock, thigh, calf, or foot. They may report throbbing, aching, numbness, tingling, or burning in a dermatomal pattern.[126,127] Leg symptoms are typically unilateral. If bilateral, symptoms are asymmetrical and may alternate between the left and right legs. Patients will report increased pain with coughing and sneezing due to increased disc loading.[18] Likewise, sitting and activities requiring lumbar flexion typically exacerbate patient symptoms. Patients may report a history of injury, including twisting or lifting, or prolonged sitting before the onset of symptoms. However, many times, the onset is insidious.

Key Examination Findings Patients with a lumbar HNP with radiculopathy may present with the following positive findings[1,18,126]:

- Myotomal weakness
- Dermatomal paresthesia
- Reflex changes
- Positive SLR
- Positive prone knee flexion test if upper lumbar segments are involved

Trunk motion is generally limited and may peripheralize or centralize symptoms.[127] Lateral flexion may be asymmetrical, and a lateral shift may be present.[127] Patients may have a directional preference and centralize with repeated movements or sustained positioning. Patients may ambulate with decreased speed and decreased trunk rotation due to guarding. Bed mobility and transfers may be slow, guarded, and aggravate symptoms. Patient's frequently have posterior trunk muscle spasms.

Differential Diagnoses Differential diagnosis should include nonspecific LBP, stenosis, spondylolisthesis, and DGS.

Rehabilitation Focus and Key Points Patients with lumbar HNP who exhibit signs of centralization should be treated as same for patients with nonspecific LBP associated with centralization.[18,89] Patients should be instructed in short-term activity modification and advised to stay active.[18,128] As symptoms are centralized, reduced, or abolished, patients should be progressed to stretching, muscle activation and movement control,[18] and strengthening exercises as able.[90] Aquatic exercise may be beneficial[129] and may be a good long-term method of meeting recommended physical activity guidelines.

Patients with subacute or chronic LBP with leg pain may benefit from neural mobilization.[18,36,65] Biomechanically, leg symptoms are thought to be related to adhesions around peripheral nerve tissue. These adhesions may prevent the nerve's ability to freely glide during ROM and reduce the nerve's tolerance to mechanical tension.[41] Two types of neural glides have been recommended: tensioning and sliding techniques. For the sciatic nerve, nerve tensioning can be performed in the following manner:

1. Perform an SLR to the point of neural symptoms.
2. Decrease hip flexion slightly.
3. Perform on-off repetitions of active or passive ankle dorsiflexion.
4. Each repetition should create symptoms with dorsiflexion (elongation), and symptoms should abate with plantarflexion (slackening).

For the femoral nerve, the patient could perform prone knee flexion in a similar manner.

Neural sliding, sometimes referred to as *nerve flossing*, is purported to have improved results when compared with tensioning techniques.[130] A common sciatic nerve sliding technique can be performed in the following manner[62]:

1. Have the seated patient extend the knee, dorsiflex the ankle, and extend the neck.
2. Hold for 5 seconds.
3. Have the patient flex the knee, plantarflex the ankle, and flex the neck.

Extension is purported to pull the nerve and dura distally, whereas flexion pulls it proximally.[62] Nerve sliding may also reduce nerve edema.[20]

Current practice guidelines suggest manual therapy could be considered in addition to exercise.[18] There is conflicting evidence as to the benefit of traction added to traditional care.[65,89,131] Should other methods fail to centralize symptoms, manual traction can be attempted in supine or prone (Fig. 12-34). If symptoms are reduced, mechanical traction can be added to the plan of care.

Some patients may benefit from concomitant pharmacologic management, including NSAID, antidepressants, and muscle relaxers.[17,18] Anticonvulsants may help reduce neuropathic pain,[128] and short-term use of corticosteroids may also be beneficial. As with all cases of LBP, opioid prescription should be rare, short term, and only for severe intractable pain[128] owing to the likelihood of addiction and limited effect.[18]

Expected Outcomes Six to eight weeks of conservative care appears to result in significant improvements

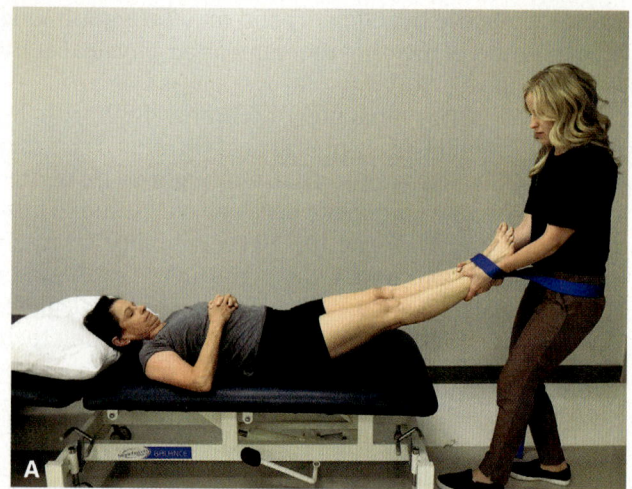
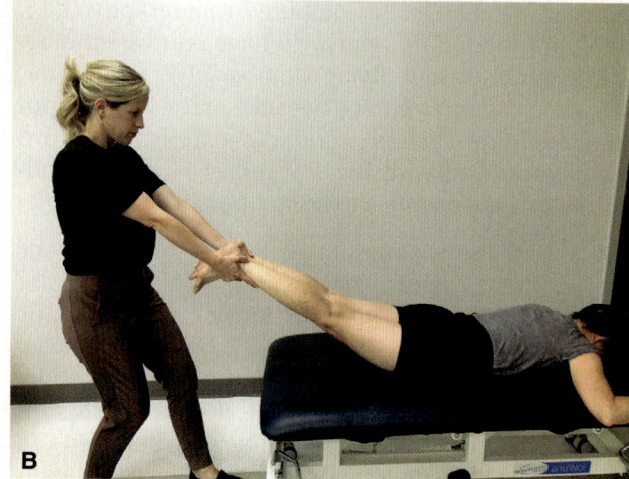

FIGURE 12-34 Manual lumbar traction. **A.** Supine with belt. **B.** Prone.

in pain, trunk endurance, function, and disability.[90,129] These gains appear to be maintained over time.[89] Fluoroscopy-guided steroid injections appear to provide at least short-term (<6 months) symptom reduction.[132]

The absence of centralization is associated with worse outcomes,[59] as are depression, kinesiophobia, and poor coping strategies.[133] Although there may be a subgroup of patients who do better with surgery,[123] there appears to be no difference in long-term outcomes between patients with lumbar HNP who are treated surgically or conservatively.[134] In addition, patients who received preoperative physical therapy had better postoperative outcomes.[135] Therefore, a trial of up to 12 weeks of conservative care should be considered before contemplating surgery, unless there is a progressive loss of neurologic function.[128] Regardless of conservative care or surgery, patients who smoke, have a higher body mass index, have a history of diabetes or other joint conditions, are receiving workers compensation, or who have disc herniations that are not posterolateral have worse outcomes.[134,136]

Surgical Options There are multiple surgical options for patients with lumbar HNP who fail conservative care, including discectomy or microdiscectomy, with or without decompression. Lumbar total disc arthroplasty and lumbar fusion may also be appropriate and appear to have similar outcomes.[137–139] Preoperative physical activity levels, gait speed, and quadriceps strength were positively correlated with postoperative function,[135] but comorbid psychiatric conditions are associated with worse outcomes.[126,140]

Postoperative care should include early mobilization and a walking program. Patients may be prescribed a postoperative lumbar corset or thoracolumbosacral orthosis (TLSO) during the immediate postoperative period (Fig. 12-35). The addition of physical therapy 4 to 6 weeks after surgery appears to improve patient outcomes.[18] Rehabilitation should include core stabilization exercise, graded activity, and stretching. General exercise is also appropriate and may reduce pain and improve disability.[65] Because neural adhesions may develop after surgery,[20] neural mobilizations may be indicated postoperatively.[65]

Pelvic Floor Muscle Dysfunction

Pelvic floor muscle (PFM) dysfunction is generally defined as weakness, decreased coordination, and tenderness of the pelvic floor.[141] PFMs perform the dual functions of assisting with continence and providing

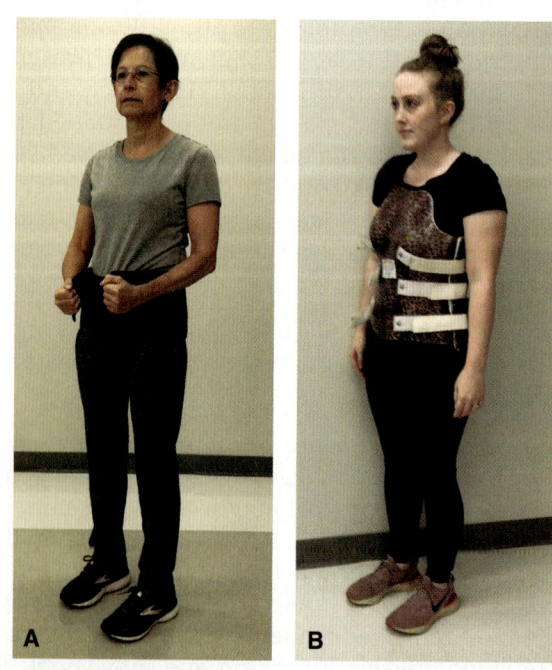

FIGURE 12-35 Orthoses for patients with lumbar pathology. **A.** Lumbar corset. **B.** Thoracolumbosacral orthosis.

TABLE 12-7
COMMON TYPES OF PELVIC FLOOR DYSFUNCTION

Dysfunction	Description	Pelvic Floor Muscle Activation
Stress incontinence	Involuntary urine leakage with effort or exertion	Hypoactive
Urge incontinence	Involuntary urine leakage associated with urgency	Poorly timed muscle activation
Voiding dysfunction	Hesitancy initiating or continuing urine flow, incomplete bladder emptying	Hyperactive
Dyspareunia	Painful vaginal penetration	Hyperactive
Muscle pain or low back pain	Pain from sustained high levels of muscular activity	Hyperactive

trunk stability (see Chapter 4, Spine Osteology and Arthrology). Many patients with LBP have altered PFM activation.[142,143] Therefore, improving the synergy between PFMs and other trunk stabilizers, such as the diaphragm, multifidi, and TrAb, may lead to restoring continence as well as improvements in back pain.

PFMs are recruited along with the TrAb and diaphragm to increase intra-abdominal pressure during functional activities such as lifting, carrying, and vacuuming and with coughing, sneezing, and laughing.[144] Continence requires carefully modulated PFM contraction. The PFM must have a resting level of contraction to maintain urethral closing pressure. Hypoactivity can lead to trunk instability and stress or urge incontinence.[144] Hyperactivity can lead to muscle pain, decreased bladder emptying, and dyspareunia.[144] Abnormalities in PFM activation can lead to various types of dysfunction (Table 12-7).

Only about half of women may be able to adequately contract PFM.[145] A basic muscle synergy training program may be easiest for patients to learn in supine. First, patients should be taught to diaphragmatic breathing. Next, patients combine diaphragmatic breathing with low levels of TrAb activation.[146] A study involving women with stress incontinence found that abdominal bracing and abdominal hollowing were equally effective in preferentially activating the TrAb.[101] Once the patient has mastered this, the exercise is progressed to adding a gentle pelvic floor contraction, with an attempt to raise the PFMs upward and inward. To assist with identifying and properly activating PFM, the patient may be instructed to imagine trying to hold the flow of urine. Alternatively, if performed in sitting, the patient can imagine sitting on a marble and trying to contract the PFMs to lift the marble up. The patient should feel a slight lift in the pelvic floor if performing the exercise correctly. The emphasis is not on strong contraction, but rather, to train prolonged low level of activation. It is important to emphasize that the PFM and other trunk stabilizers require a prolonged, but not high, level of contraction. Strong holds may contribute to pain and continence problems. Patients should try to maintain this gentle co-contraction for holds increasing to 30 seconds or a minute.

Patients with hypoactive PFM may notice urinary leakage during activities that increase intra-abdominal pressure, such as carrying groceries, gardening, or running. For these patients, the preceding series of exercises can be modified to attempting to increase the lift of the pelvic floor without co-contracting additional stabilizers. The patient should try to hold this more targeted contraction of the PFM for about 5 seconds while breathing normally. This will then be repeated for several repetitions. The patient should then progress to contracting the PFM while lifting or performing other tasks. Patients should be trained to increase PFM activation before coughing or sneezing.

Patients with LBP who perform pelvic floor exercises along with traditional stabilization exercises have better relief of back pain and lower levels of disability than patients who only perform trunk stabilization exercises.[143] Teaching PFM activation has also been found to improve TrAb muscle activation and timing.[147] Therefore, clinicians should strongly consider including PFM training for patients with LBP. This section provides an introduction to pelvic floor dysfunction. Clinicians interested in improving knowledge and skills in the examination and treatment of patients with pelvic floor dysfunction are encouraged to pursue additional training.

Lumbar Degenerative Disc Disease

Lumbar DDD is believed to be a common cause of LBP in individuals over the age of 40.[148] As with lumbar HNP, the most common levels affected are L4–L5 and L5–S1. Posterior osteophytes may also be present, and multidisc involvement occurs in more than one-third of patients.[149] Loss of disc height may lead to increased stress to the facet joints and vertebral bodies, increased intersegmental motion, and contribute to lateral foraminal stenosis.[148] Although imaging studies may support the presence of lumbar DDD, many individuals are asymptomatic.

Symptomatic patients with positive imaging findings for DDD may report back, buttock, or thigh pain. Symptoms are likely to be intermittent. Patients may report stiffness and limited motion that is worse in the morning. Pain is typically increased with standing and walking or after activity. Common physical examination findings include decreased trunk ROM, painful end-range trunk extension, reduced trunk strength and movement control, lower extremity and cardiovascular deconditioning, and reduced balance. Hip ROM and lower extremity muscle length are commonly globally reduced from deconditioning rather than a myotomal weakness. The neurologic examination will be negative.

Clinicians should follow an impairment-based approach to rehabilitation. After a thorough history and physical examination, interventions should address key impairments and primarily consist of education and therapeutic exercise.[65] Manual therapy may be incorporated as an adjunct to assist with ROM and symptom management. The majority of patients are managed conservatively with a combination of rehabilitation and pharmacologic management, and significant improvements are noted over the course of 1 to 3 months.[148] About a quarter of patients not responding to conservative care are managed surgically via decompression, fusion, or total disc arthroplasty with generally positive results.[148,150]

Lumbar Stenosis

Pathology Stenosis, or narrowing, of the central canal or lateral foramen may occur at any area of the spine. Lumbar stenosis is primarily a degenerative disorder in which the central canal size is reduced by osteophytes, decreased intervertebral disc height, hypertrophy of the ligamentum flavum, or hypertrophy of the facet.[151] This space reduction leads to **neurogenic claudication**, tingling, numbness, and/or pain in the buttocks and bilateral lower extremities due to compression of the nerves of the lumbar spine. Lumbar stenosis is most common in the lower lumbar spine, particularly at L4-5, and may occur at more than one level. The condition may be congenital or inherited. Most people over the age of 65 have some degree of spinal stenosis. However, lumbar stenosis is usually asymptomatic until narrowing reaches a critical level. Therefore, conservative interventions are normally the first line of treatment.

History Patients with lumbar stenosis report central back, buttock or bilateral lower extremity paresthesias, and pain. Because the lumbar spinal canal size is reduced with lumbar extension and increased with lumbar flexion, patients report symptoms worsen with walking, particularly with an increase in time or distance. They may report walking through the grocery store is symptom free if pushing a shopping cart compared with walking in a more upright posture. Symptoms also occur while standing in line, but not with prolonged standing such as when washing dishes, which tends to be performed in a more flexed posture. Importantly, patients report no pain with flexion. Sitting commonly reduces symptoms from standing and walking.[152] Functionally, patients will report limited walking and standing tolerance. Over time, this leads to avoidance of walking, restricted participation in many functional activities, general deconditioning, and a loss of lower extremity strength.[153] Therefore, many times, patients will report functional limitations, such as difficulty rising from a chair, squatting, or climbing stairs.

Key Examination Findings Static and dynamic posture examination is likely to reveal trunk flexion and a posterior pelvic tilt. This may lead to compensatory hip and knee flexion. Lumbar ROM is likely to be limited owing to age-related changes. However, with lumbar stenosis, there is a greater loss of trunk extension, possibly because patients avoid this symptom-provoking position and gradually lose motion over time. Muscle performance deficits due to disuse are common in the lower extremity,[151,153] particularly the gluteals, quadriceps, and plantarflexors. Single limb balance is also typically reduced.[151,153]

Gait speed is generally reduced,[42] with patients demonstrating small step lengths. A self-selected walking test, treadmill test, or two-stage treadmill test (Table 12-8) can be useful for diagnostic purposes and for tracking changes over time.[154,155] Lower extremity weakness may occur with testing,[156] helping to rule in lumbar stenosis,[152] and may be assessed by comparing the patient's strength immediately after stopping with the patient's prewalking assessment. Alternatively, the Six-Minute Walk Test (see Chapter 11, Hip) could be performed. Patients with very limited gait may be assessed with a bicycle test.[157] The time the patient is able to bike is compared with the time the patient is able to walk before symptom-limited stopping. Although suboptimal, given the differing workloads between walking and biking, patients with lumbar stenosis should be able to cycle without symptoms, given the flexed posture. For both the walking tests and the bike tests, clinicians must consider that symptoms may not just be neurogenic, but may be vascular in origin. Performing pulse palpation and an ankle-brachial index (ABI) before and after testing helps differentiate between the two pathologies. Standardized tests such as the Timed Up and Go and Five Times Sit-to-Stand (see Chapter 11, Hip) should be performed. Table 12-9 provides proposed cutoff values to discriminate between

TABLE 12-8
WALKING TESTS FOR PATIENTS WITH LUMBAR STENOSIS

Test	Self-Selected Walking Test	Treadmill Test	Two-Stage Treadmill Test
Method	Patient walks over ground at self-selected pace.	Patient walks on a treadmill at a self-selected speed.	Patient walks on a treadmill on a 0° incline for up to 12 minutes at a self-selected pace. The patient then sits for 10-15 minutes until symptoms have fully resolved. The test is repeated at the same speed with the treadmill on a 15° incline.
End of Test	Patient reports inability to continue (reason noted).	Patient reports inability to continue (reason noted).	Patient reports inability to continue (reason noted).
Documentation	• Time and distance when symptoms began. • Total time and distance covered. • Symptom location.	• Patient selected walking speed. • Time and distance when symptoms began. • Total time and distance covered. • Symptom location.	• Patient selected walking speed. • Total time and distance covered. • Symptom location.
Key points	Many older patients may be more comfortable walking over ground than on a treadmill. Patients with orthopaedic comorbidities may not be safe to ambulate on a treadmill. Can be used for patients with assistive devices.	Re-testing can be performed using the same speed as initial test for ease of comparison.	If the patient is able to walk further on the inclined treadmill, lumbar stenosis is confirmed. Requires longer testing time, making it less optimal for patients with lower functional levels.
Vascular claudication	Patients with symptoms due to peripheral arterial disease may have an abnormal ankle-brachial index (ABI) at rest (ankle systolic pressure/arm systolic pressure <0.9). If walking tests are stopped due to vascular pain, repeat ABI testing immediately upon test cessation will reveal a decrease from resting levels along with >20% drop in ankle systolic pressure.[a]		

Data from Myers B. *Wound Management: Principles and Practice*. 4th ed. Pearson; 2020.

patients with lumbar stenosis on the Five Times Sit-to-Stand Test.[157]

Differential Diagnoses Differential diagnosis includes hip pathology, DGS, and spondylolisthesis. Clinicians must also rule out arterial insufficiency by assessing pedal pulses and performing an ABI.[42] The clinicians should perform a cervical examination, including upper extremity reflexes, to rule out cervical myelopathy.[42]

Rehabilitation Focus and Key Points Figure 12-36 provide an overview of rehabilitation for patients with lumbar stenosis.[154,158–160] Interventions should initially focus on a flexion-based program to reduce symptoms by increasing spinal canal size. Improving hip extension ROM and hip flexor length will reduce the need for compensatory lumbar hyperextension during standing and walking. Joint and soft-tissue mobilization can assist with gaining range. Strengthening should be designed to improve functional abilities lost due to deconditioning, such as rising from a chair or climbing stairs, as well as to improve the patient's ability to maintain a less lordotic posture when upright. Aerobic exercise begins in a flexed posture for reconditioning progressing as able to more extended and loaded postures. Balance exercises are needed to decrease the risk of falls, particularly given that most patients with lumbar stenosis are older and at risk for osteoporosis.

Patient education should include methods for reducing lumbar hyperextension with functional activities. For patients with severe stenosis, this may mean changing some activities, such as cutting fruits and vegetables for meal preparation, from standing to sitting. For less severe patients, it may be teaching patients to perform a slight posterior pelvic tilt during prolonged standing in line. Patients can place one foot up in a split stance position to discourage anterior pelvic tilt and lumbar extension: when at the grocery

TABLE 12-9
FIVE TIMES SIT-TO-STAND TEST FOR LUMBAR STENOSIS

Time (Seconds)	Interpretation
≤10.4	No lumbar stenosis
10.5–15.2	Mild lumbar stenosis
15.3–22.0	Moderate lumbar stenosis
>22.0	Severe lumbar stenosis

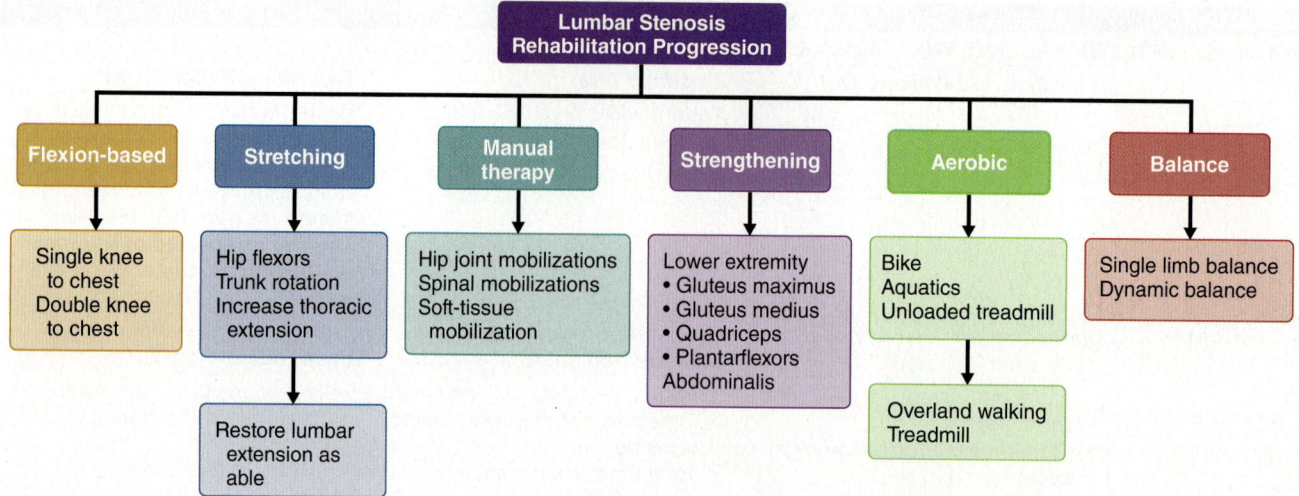

FIGURE 12-36 Lumbar stenosis rehabilitation progression.

store, place one foot up on the rung of the cart; or when washing dishes, place one foot up on the cabinet under the sink. Patients should be educated on the importance of performing a maintenance program[161] to assist with symptom modulation as well as to maintain or improve function.

Expected Outcomes Over the course of 6 weeks of rehabilitation, patients can be expected to have lasting improvements[162] in symptoms, pain-free walking, physical function, and strength,[135,160,161,163–165] despite lumbar stenosis being a degenerative, progressive condition. A structured, individualized rehabilitation program along with a home exercise program appears to be superior to a home program alone.[158] In one study,[154] patients who had consented to, and been scheduled for, surgery participated in 6 weeks of physical therapy following the general principles noted earlier. Forty-three percent of these patients improved in that they chose not to have surgery and remained surgery free even at the 2-year follow-up, demonstrating that even patients with significant stenosis, severe symptoms, or functional limitations can improve with conservative interventions. For patients with severe stenosis or who are slow to respond to conservative measures, fluoroscopy-guided epidural corticosteroid or lidocaine injections can lead to positive short-term results,[166,167] allowing improved participation in rehabilitation. Individuals with depression, who are receiving workers' compensation, or who have had prior spine surgery are less likely to have positive outcomes.[168]

Surgical Interventions Surgery was once considered the standard of care for patients with lumbar stenosis, but recent reviews have found that outcomes from surgery are either worse or the same as a 6-week course of conservative care.[158] Approximately 10% of patients will have significant surgical complications or a second surgery.[169] In contrast, there have been no negative side effects for conservative interventions.[151] Despite this, lumbar spinal stenosis remains the most common reason for spine surgery in the older adult.[154,162] Surgery may include spinal decompression such as a laminectomy, where the posterior elements are removed, with or without fusion of adjacent spinal segments. Current evidence supports similar results[170,171] but lower costs and shorter hospitalizations with simple decompression.[172]

Postoperative rehabilitation begins immediately after surgery with a basic walking program, lower extremity strengthening, and core stabilization. Deficits in lower extremity flexibility, such as a lack of hip extension range, can also be addressed. Gentle supine nerve glides are performed with the patient supine using a symptom-free range of knee flexion/extension with the hip in 90° flexion. Anterior/posterior pelvic tilts and single knee to chest should be delayed if a lumbar fusion was performed.

After spinal stenosis surgery, people report significant improvements as early as 3 months postsurgery,[173] including an increase in balance, gait speed, and ambulation distance. Despite having increased functional capacity, they do not increase their physical activity and most still do not meet basic physical activity recommendations.[174] Soon after surgery, patients note mild-to-moderate levels of disability.[173] Therefore, it is important for clinicians to help patients change learned habits of decreased activity and educate them on the importance of physical fitness/activity so that increased capacity leads to increased real-life performance of physical activity.

Spondylolisthesis

Pathology Spondylolisthesis is a pathologic anterior slippage of one vertebral body on another (Fig. 4-6).[175] In childhood, the incidence of spondylolisthesis is about 4% and is most common at L5 on S1 due to a bilateral defect in the pars interarticularis.[48,176] Spondylolisthesis is slightly more common in adulthood where it is usually degenerative and occurs at the L4/L5 level.[176] Spondylolisthesis is more common in women, and there is at least some genetic component.[176] Spondylolisthesis is classified based on the degree of vertebral slippage noted on a lateral radiograph using the Meyerding classification system (Table 12-10). While grade I spondylolisthesis is not progressive, higher grades may worsen over time.[176] Larger amounts of anterior vertebral slippage result in narrowing of the spinal canal and, to a lesser extent, the lateral foramen at that level.

History Spondylolisthesis may be asymptomatic; however, symptomatic patients report central LBP or buttock pain that worsens with trunk extension. Radiculopathy or neurogenic claudication may occur with walking and tend to be bilateral. Symptoms are relieved with sitting.[176] Severe spondylolisthesis can cause cauda equina syndrome and requires immediate referral.

Key Examination Findings The most specific clinical examination finding for spondylolisthesis is a positive step deformity.[48] Examination of trunk AROM often yields pain with one-time, repeated, or sustained extension. Because spondylolisthesis causes instability, patients may exhibit aberrant movement patterns during trunk flexion or when returning to an upright posture from a flexed position. A wide spectrum of neurologic signs and symptoms may be present based on the location and grade of pathology. An L5 radiculopathy is most common because this would occur with an L5–S1 spondylolisthesis. Signs of neurogenic claudication may be noted when performing the self-selected walking test or treadmill test. In patients with grade II or higher spondylolisthesis, a posterior pelvic tilt and spinal flexion increase central canal size; therefore, subtle positional changes, such as standing in less anterior pelvic tilt, using a rolling walker, or pushing a grocery cart, may improve or resolve patient symptoms. Abdominal weakness is typical, and patients often complain of HS tightness as these muscles may be tonically active to reduce anterior pelvic tilting.

Differential Diagnoses Differential diagnosis includes spinal stenosis and cauda equina syndrome.

Rehabilitation Focus and Key Points Patients with spondylolisthesis should be educated to temporarily refrain from trunk extension and extended activities until symptoms resolve, after which these can be gradually resumed.[176] Patients with tight hip flexors or loss of hip extension range might benefit from stretching to reduce compensatory lumbar hyperextension. Posterior pelvic tilting and more supported, flexion-based stabilization exercises, such as the dead bug sequence, are generally well tolerated, even acutely. Stabilization exercises are advanced to bridging and quadruped progressions to train co-contraction of the multifidi to provide dynamic spinal stability.[177] Functional activities with core stabilization are incorporated as motor control and symptoms allow.[178] General abdominal strengthening exercises, such as trunk curls or diagonal curl-ups, may also be included for patients without osteopenia. Stabilization exercise parameters should focus on muscular endurance training. Lower extremity strengthening, aerobic exercise, and balance training should be included based on individual patient presentation.

Patients with high irritability or higher grades may benefit from lumbar bracing and NSAID.[176] Spinal injections may also provide short-term relief to allow participation in rehabilitation and improve function.[176]

Expected Outcomes Most patients with grade I spondylolisthesis can expect a reduction of symptoms, decreased kinesiophobia, and improved function within 8 weeks.[177,178] However, conservative interventions do not appear to change the degree of vertebral slippage.[178]

Surgical Interventions Patients not responding to 6 months of conservative care, with progressive neurologic deficit, or with more than one grade of slippage progression should be referred for further evaluation. Surgical management includes decompression or fusion based on the degree of slippage, age, and the degree of degeneration.[176] Surgical treatment for patients with degenerative spondylolisthesis appears to result in lasting improvements in back pain and functional abilities.[179]

Spondylolysis and Stress Reactions

Spondylolysis is a defect of the pars interarticularis in the lumbar spine and the leading cause of acute

TABLE 12-10	
MEYERDING CLASSIFICATION OF SPONDYLOLISTHESIS	
Grade	Percentage of Vertebral Body Slippage
I	0–25
II	25–50
III	50–75
IV	75–100
V	>100

LBP in adolescent athletes.[180] However, like spondylolisthesis, spondylolysis may be asymptomatic.[48] The gold standard for diagnosis is a CT scan, but MRI poses less radiation risk, making it more appealing.[27] Initial screening via radiographs may also detect spondylolysis.[27] The condition can occur unilaterally or bilaterally and is most common at L5. Bilateral defects may lead to spondylolisthesis because the lack of posterior restraint can allow progressive anterior translation of the superior vertebra on the inferior vertebra. The pars injury is multifactorial. There seems to be a genetic component to a pars defect. It may also be a spectrum of stress reaction caused by repeated hyperextension[181] and rotational maneuvers in athletes who participate in overhead sports such as tennis and volleyball as well as gymnastics, wrestling, and diving.

Spondylolysis or a stress reaction should be considered in adolescent athletes with LBP who participate in high-risk sports. Back pain worsens with extension, but flexion is usually symptom free. The lower quarter neurologic screen is normal, and there is no peripheralization or centralization. If either condition is suspected, the patient should be sent for imaging.

Stress reactions are treated with 6 to 12 weeks of activity restriction to limit stress to the posterior elements of the spine.[27] The literature is inconclusive on the benefits of bracing to limit lumbar hyperextension. Aerobic exercises that do not load the posterior elements, such as stationary cycling, are permitted during this time. Once symptoms are controlled, the athlete begins a spinal stabilization program followed by progressive resistance exercises loading the lumbar spine. A running program can also be initiated as tolerated. Exercises are progressed to include sport-specific ranges and speeds. The athlete is gradually advanced to full activity as long as symptoms continue to be resolved,[182] with most athletes returning to sport in about 5 to 6 months.[27]

Spondylolysis is treated similar to stress reactions with a few exceptions. First, 12 weeks of restriction from sporting activities is more common and appears to lead to better results than shorter rest periods.[180,182] Second, most patients are prescribed either a lumbar corset or a TLSO to limit lumbar extension.[180,182] Third, at least one study notes that athletes who do not begin rehabilitation until after 12 weeks of immobilization required nearly an additional month of rehabilitation before returning to sport.[180] Therefore, it may be wise to begin formal rehabilitation and neutral spine stabilization exercises after about 6 to 8 weeks of immobilization. Full return to play can be expected in 5 to 7 months.[180] Conservative interventions for spondylolysis are successful in 70 to 90% of patients.[182]

Facet Joint Arthropathy

Pathology Facet, or zygapophyseal, joint dysfunction is a possible pathoanatomic cause of LBP.[183] It is estimated that 15 to 30% of back pain may involve the facet joints.[184] Degenerative changes are common with aging and are not always symptomatic. Facet arthropathy may be more common with age because DDD results in increased facet joint stress.[181] Joint dysfunction may also occur from repetitive joint stress, such as overhead throwing, volleyball, and tennis.

History Patients with facet pathology report dull, unilateral back pain that worsens with extension and is relieved by flexion. They may also have intermittent, sharp, catching pain.[184]

Key Examination Findings The gold standard for diagnosis of facet arthropathy is relief of symptoms with a facet block. Clinical findings suggestive of facet arthropathy are presented in Table 12-11.[41,183–185]

Differential Diagnoses Differential diagnosis includes chronic back pain and DDD.

Rehabilitation Focus and Key Points Rehabilitation of facet arthropathy includes exercise and manual therapy. Stretching into flexion may reduce pain, whereas targeting the facet joint more specifically may involve adding contralateral lateral flexion. Stabilization exercises targeting the multifidi, TrAb, and pelvic floor have also proven to be effective.[183,185] However, this may be due to the pain-modulating effect of exercise rather than a purely mechanical effect. Manual therapy may include soft-tissue mobilization to reduce muscle spasms and abolish trigger points.[186] Unilateral posteroanterior joint mobilizations or joint manipulations may also be effective.[185]

Medical management may include oral NSAIDs, facet injections, and radiofrequency ablation.

Expected Outcomes Patients can expect a reduction in pain and improvement in motion within 4 to 5

TABLE 12-11
FINDINGS CONSISTENT WITH FACET ARTHROPATHY

Present	Absent
• Unilateral, dull back pain that may refer to the buttock or proximal thigh • Pain with extension and quadrant test • Unilateral, local muscle spasms • Reduced unilateral posteroanterior pressures that may be painful • Possible intermittent, sharp catching pain	• Neurologic signs and symptoms • Pain with flexion • Centralization/peripheralization

weeks.[185,186] While injections may provide short-term relief, the combination of exercise and manual therapy appear to provide more lasting improvements.[186]

Lumbar and Pelvic Fractures

Lumbar fractures are far less common than thoracic fractures. Lumbar vertebral fractures are usually caused by trauma, such as a fall from a height or motor vehicle accident. Lumbar fractures are diagnosed by radiograph or CT. (The majority of compression fractures affect the thoracic vertebrae and are discussed in Chapter 17, Cervical and Thoracic Spine.) A burst fracture is a specific type of high-energy vertebral body fracture that may damage the spinal cord. Fracture management is dependent upon fracture location, stability, neurologic deficit, the degree of central canal compromise, and the patient's general health. Surgical management may include decompression (removal of bone or disc that is compressing neural tissue) or fusion with hardware, such as rods and screws. Nonoperative management includes bracing, generally using a TLSO and pharmacologic management for pain. The orthosis prevents trunk flexion, thus reducing, but not eliminating, vertebral body stress and intervertebral motion.

Acute postfracture rehabilitation emphasizes early mobility and restoring the ability to perform activities of daily living to prevent the deleterious effects bed rest can have on the integument, cardiovascular, pulmonary, and musculoskeletal systems. Deep breathing, abdominal setting exercises, gentle extremity AROM, and a walking program are encouraged. Static balance exercises should be incorporated as able. Once the fracture is healed, rehabilitation may not be needed. However, rehabilitation may assist with resolving deficits such as postimmobilization stiffness, muscular weakness or reduced endurance—particularly of the trunk musculature, or decreased balance.

Pelvic fractures are rare. Rehabilitation after pelvic fracture varies based on the patient age, onset, fracture location, and stability. Stress fracture of the pubic rami or sacrum may occur as a result of relative energy deficiency syndrome or repetitive stresses of gymnastics and running. For these individuals, treatment involves ensuring adequate nutrition availability and relative rest from sporting activities. Patients with stress fractures who are at high risk for progression may require a period of limited weight bearing. Most fractures respond well to rest, and athletes are able to return to competition in 7 to 12 weeks after rami stress fractures and 4 to 6 weeks after sacral stress fractures.[187]

Older adults may sustain a pelvic fracture from a fall. An assistive device may be required even with stable fractures because gait may be limited by pain and reduced balance increases the risk of additional falls. Rehabilitation mirrors that of proximal femur fractures (see Chapter 11, Hip): prevention of secondary impairments, mobility training, and balance training. Decreasing the fear of falling and improving balance confidence may lead to improved outcomes.[188,189] Lower extremity strengthening and aerobic exercise are added as tolerated.

Pelvic fractures in younger individuals are generally the result of trauma, such as motor vehicle accidents, and frequently require open reduction and internal fixation or placement of an external fixator.[190] Pelvic fracture is generally only one of many injuries sustained. Limited unilateral or bilateral weight bearing may be prescribed based on fracture location and fixation. Post-acute care evaluation should include a thorough assessment to identify any neurologic deficits. Once the surgeon has determined adequate fracture healing, the clinicians should examine lower extremity strength, mobility, balance, gait, and function and address any deficits noted.

Acute Lumbar Strains

Muscle strains in this region most commonly involve the erector spinae, multifidi, quadratus lumborum, and abdominal muscles.[20] Acute lumbar strains may be more common in certain settings, such as industrial rehabilitation and athletics. Acute work-related lumbar strains may result from overwork during staffing shortages, poor ergonomics, and worker deconditioning.[191] In health care, an additional cause of injury is caring for patients who are obese or lack of proper equipment, or training, to safely move these patients.[191] The presentation of patients with strains varies based on the involved tissue but may include stiffness, loss of motion, difficulty with transitional movements, and muscle spasms.[20] Strains generally heal quickly, given the excellent blood supply of muscles. Two major goals of rehabilitation include preventing the condition from becoming chronic and preventing recurrence. Rehabilitation should encourage active rest along with short-term modifications of job-related tasks. For the athlete, interventions may involve a reduction in playing or practice time or scheduled day(s) off.

Although the use of progressive exercise is theoretically sound, there are limited data to base exercise prescription. Gentle midrange AROM exercises in a symptom-modulated ROM, such as single knee to chest, lower trunk rotation, and extension in lying or standing along with a walking program, can begin immediately. These general back exercises are then progressed to exercises that target the affected muscle. For example, exercise progression for a patient with an erector spinae strain may progress to bridging or quadruped alternate upper extremity flexion, then to unilateral bridging and quadruped alternate lower extremity extension, before transitioning to active trunk extension with the arms by the side. Problems can arise when trying to return to high levels of activity without properly restoring muscle strength, endurance, and power. Therefore, clinicians should strive to advance muscular workload until the patient is able to perform work or sport-specific tasks, including simulation of repetitions, time, planes of motion, and speed.

Myofascial Pain Syndrome

MFPS is a regional condition characterized by muscle pain due to the presence of one or more (myofascial) trigger points that is thought to affect about 9 million Americans.[192] MFPS can affect any region, but most commonly involves the back and neck. Common locations for trigger points within the lower spine include the iliocostalis lumborum, longissimus thoracis, multifidi, quadratus lumborum, and gluteus medius.[20] Diagnostic criteria continue to be based on the work of Simons and Travell[193] who define a trigger point as a hyperirritable region within a muscle that can be identified by the presence of point tenderness within a taut band of muscle.[194] There may be a local twitch response, where the muscle "jumps" when palpating perpendicular to the band.[194] Trigger points have a typical pattern of referred pain[195] and can also cause decreased motion of the affected muscle(s), tingling, weakness, early fatigue, abnormal movement patterns, and muscular imbalances.[196] Trigger points may be active (causing symptoms at rest) or passive (symptomatic upon provocation, such as palpation or compression). Trigger points can also create satellite (new) trigger points in the region to which they refer pain.

Trigger points may occur as a result of overuse, trauma, persistent muscular contraction (such as stress, repetitive activity, abnormal positioning), or prolonged immobilization of a muscle in a shortened position.[194] Systemic causes of trigger points include deficiencies of B12, magnesium, or iron.[194] While our understanding of trigger points continues to evolve, trigger points appear to be related to an excessive release of acetylcholine and resulting increase in electrical activity at the motor endplate. Persistent sarcomere contraction may lead to a local energy crisis and the release of inflammatory mediators.[193,194] Central sensitization, including hyperalgesia and allodynia, may also play a role in MFPS.[192]

The primary interventions for trigger points include exercise and manual therapy. Overall, exercise appears to reduce pain intensity and pain pressure threshold of individuals with MFPS.[195,197] Stretching may help reduce trigger point hyperirritability, restoring motion and reducing pain. Strengthening, postural, and stabilization exercises may help improve the affected muscle(s) ability to handle daily stresses. Aerobic exercise, including walking, cycling, and aquatic exercise, tends to improve chronic pain.[198] Ischemic compression (maintaining manual pressure on the taut band) is thought to reduce pain via the gate control theory and eliminate the taut band. This manual technique appears to be equally effective to dry needling in the management of MFPS.[199]

Electrical stimulation, such as transcutaneous electrical nerve stimulation, may assist with pain reduction.[200,201] Some patients with MFPS have comorbidities, such as depression, anxiety, and fear. Patients with these psychological factors may benefit from an interdisciplinary, biopsychosocial approach. Multiple types of pharmacologic interventions have been prescribed for MFPS. Current evidence appears to support the use of ibuprofen as well as benzodiazepine and tricyclic antidepressants, such as clonazepam and amitriptyline, respectively.[201]

Deep Gluteal Syndrome

Pathology DGS is an entrapment of the sciatic nerve in the deep gluteal space from nondiscogenic causes[202] and is responsible for 6 to 17% of all cases of sciatica.[203] The deep gluteal space is defined by the following borders[62,63]:

- Superiorly: the inferior sciatic notch
- Inferiorly: the HS attachment at the ischial tuberosity
- Posteriorly: the gluteus maximus
- Anteriorly: the proximal femur and hip joint capsule
- Medially: the sacrotuberous ligament
- Laterally: the linea aspera and gluteal tuberosity

DGS was initially called *piriformis* syndrome, as the original pathology was believed to be due to either piriformis hypertrophy, contracture, trigger points compressing the sciatic nerve, or anatomic variations in the sciatic nerve in which the nerve passes through or above the piriformis (Fig. 12-37).[73,203] While the majority of cases have been shown to be due to this,[204] many other structures are now known to be potentially involved, including the quadratus femoris, gemelli, obturator internus, fibrous bands,[73] HS, or gluteal muscles.[204]

History Patients with DGS report pain in the buttock or radicular pain. Many report limping due to pain as well as difficulty sitting on for more than 20 to 30 minutes due to pain.[202]

Key Examination Findings On observation, patients with DGS may sit unloading the involved side.[73] For example, patients with right-sided DGS may sit leaning to the left to unload the right buttock. Passive internal rotation performed in the standard seated position may reproduce symptoms or be limited. Resisted hip external rotation may be weak or symptomatic in sitting or in prone with the hip in neutral flexion. The clinician

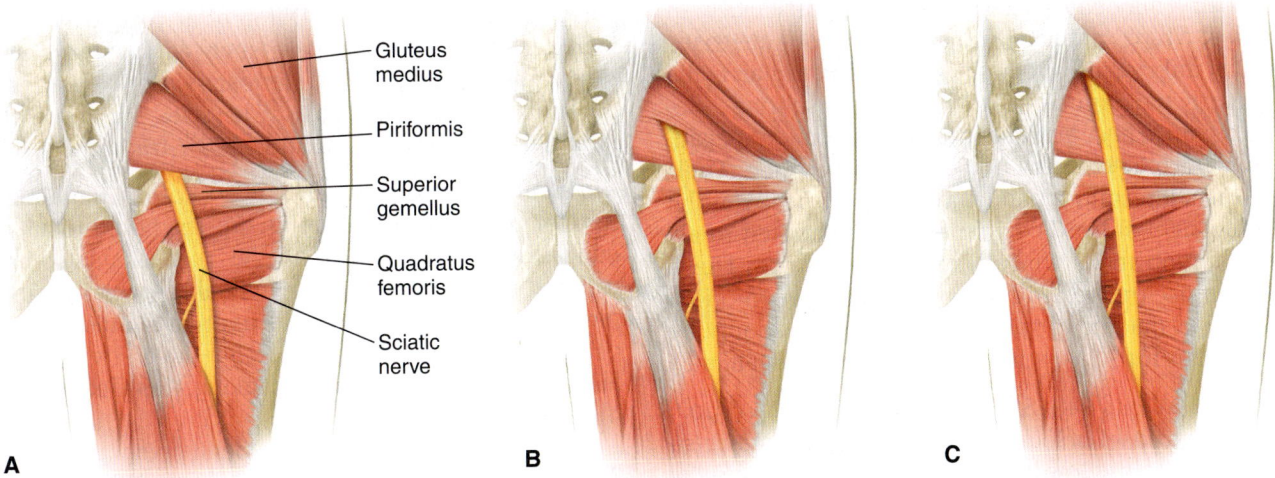

FIGURE 12-37 Relationship of the sciatic nerve to the piriformis. **A.** Usual anatomic structure. **B** and **C.** Known anatomic variations. (Modified from Lee GK, Chung KC. *Operative Techniques in Lower Limb Reconstruction and Amputation*. Wolters Kluwer; 2020: Figure 41.1.)

should assess muscle performance of the gluteus maximus and gluteus medius. Weakness of these muscles can help identify the reason for potential overload of the muscles within the deep gluteal space. Likewise, assessment of the amount of pronation during gait and tibialis posterior strength may also lead the clinician to additional interventions, which may help with controlling symptoms via preventing excessive pronation.

The patient will have tenderness upon palpation of the deep gluteal space that reproduces their familiar symptoms.[45] Trigger points may be noted within any of the hip rotators or the gluteus maximus. The seated piriformis stretch and active piriformis test[62,63] will reproduce the patient's familiar symptoms as well.[202]

Differential Diagnoses Differential diagnosis includes lumbar HNP or a space-occupying lesion, such as a tumor or abscess.

Rehabilitation and Key Points Rehabilitation generally involves manual stretching and soft-tissue mobilization of the hip rotators. Patients can perform a seated rotator stretch by crossing the affected ankle over the contralateral knee, then passively moving the hip into adduction and internal rotation by pulling the knee of the side to be stretched toward the contralateral shoulder. Variations of stretches may be required based on the structures involved; for example, stretching into pure internal rotation may also be beneficial when the deep rotators are involved. Hip or core weakness that may be contributing to overload of muscles within the deep gluteal space should be gradually strengthening. Gentle sciatic nerve mobilizations in a range that does not produce symptoms can be initiated in patients with low irritability. At times, patients may benefit from NSAIDs.

Expected Outcomes Rarely, conservative interventions fail to lead to symptom resolution. In such cases, the patient should be referred for further examination. Surgical management generally involves the release of fibrotic bands.[62,63]

Sacroiliac Joint Dysfunction

Pathology SIJ dysfunction is an area of controversy. Once thought to be a common generator of low back or leg symptoms, current evidence suggests that SIJ dysfunction may account for only about 10% of all cases.[205] Some authors contend that SIJ dysfunction is a result of SIJ instability and recommend palpation of pelvic landmarks, including the PSIS, sacral sulcus, ASIS, and pubic symphysis, for symmetry to determine whether pathology exists and to classify SIJ instability. However, palpation of these landmarks has proven highly imprecise,[206,207] making the use of palpation for the purpose of diagnosis questionable. The SIJ, as noted in Chapter 4, Spine Osteology and Arthrology, is an inherently stable joint. The roughened, reciprocal sacral and iliac joint surfaces; the dense, fibrous anterior, posterior, and interosseous sacroiliac ligaments; the robust sacrotuberous, sacrospinous, and iliolumbar ligaments; and the sacrum's wedged shape render it essentially immobile, allowing just 0.8° to 3° of motion.[208] Therefore, SIJ-related pain is unlikely to be related to excessive movement at the SIJ, but may be related to excessive stress to the SIJ or its supporting structures.[209]

There appears to be consensus on three main causes of SIJ-related pain.[4] First, the hormonal changes of pregnancy lead to ligamentous laxity, which may cause SIJ pain or dysfunction. Second, asymmetrical trauma, such as a hard landing on one ischial tuberosity, may cause SIJ-related pain, particularly in females. Third, patients with inflammatory diseases such as ankylosing spondylitis and psoriatic arthritis frequently have spondyloarthropathy presenting as local SIJ pain. These patients are typically middle aged, report morning stiffness that eases with motion. Their SIJ pain is intermittent and may alternate between the left and right sides. The pain may be unrelated to activity/motion and is typically referred vertically. These patients also present with a progressive loss of motion. Patients suspected of spondyloarthropathy should be referred for further testing and medical management.

History Patients with SIJ-related pain typically report a traumatic onset of local SIJ pain. Symptoms may also be referred to the low back, buttock, and occasionally to the groin or thigh.[50] Symptoms are worsened by asymmetrical activities, such as climbing stairs, carrying a child on one hip, or getting into or out of a car. Pregnancy-related complaints of SIJ or pubic pain generally occur later in the pregnancy and may continue into the postpartum period.

Key Examination Findings There are no valid and reliable imaging studies to detect SIJ dysfunction.[50] The gold standard for diagnosis of SIJ dysfunction is relief of symptoms with fluoroscopy-guided anesthetic injection to the SIJ.[50,210] In some cases, this may also provide lasting symptom relief.[77]

A recognized cluster of tests is used to diagnosis SIJ dysfunction (sometimes referred to as Laslett cluster[74]) including provocation of local SIJ pain with sacroiliac (anterior) gapping, sacroiliac (anterior) compression, posterior thigh thrust,[75] Gaenslen test, and the FABER test[75] (see Fig. 11-25 in Chapter 11, Hip). Importantly, none of these tests assess SIJ motion or relative motion. Rather, the tests stress the SIJ in various ways: compression, gapping, shearing, and torsion. If three or more of these tests are positive, there is a high likelihood that SIJ dysfunction is present.[210,211] More recently, Nejati et al.[77] found the combination of a positive FABER with either a positive posterior thigh thrust or positive Gaenslen test appears to be more accurate in diagnosing SIJ dysfunction. Local tenderness to palpation of the SIJ (aka Fortin sign) or ipsilateral SIJ pain with the Trendelenburg test may also be present,[211] but should not be used as a sole indicator of SIJ dysfunction.[77]

The lower quarter neurologic screen will be normal. Hip strength testing and the Trendelenburg test may be painful due to the asymmetrical SIJ loading. Patients with SIJ-related pain have been noted to have poor activation and motor control of trunk musculature.[212,213] Because SIJ dysfunction during pregnancy appears to be related to instability, clinicians may want to assess the patient's Beighton score to obtain a sense of the patient's systemic hypermobility.

Differential Diagnoses Differential diagnosis must include lumbar pathologies, such as facet dysfunction, radiculopathy, spinal stenosis, spondylolisthesis, chronic back pain, and DGS.[210] In cases of trauma, differential diagnosis may include pelvic fracture.

Rehabilitation Focus and Key Points Rehabilitation for patients with SIJ-related pain should focus on education and exercise. However, there may also be a role for sacroiliac belts and manual therapy for some patients. Patients with SIJ dysfunction should be educated on activity modification to reduce stress to the SIJ (Table 12-12). Generally speaking, this means using more symmetrical postures.

Two types of exercise have been shown to reduce SIJ-related pain: progressive core stabilization exercises[205,214] and repeated movements. Core exercises, beginning with symmetrical exercises, such as bridging and trunk curls, can be progressed to exercises that are more asymmetrical, such as the dead bug and quadruped progressions. Exercises are then progressed to weight-bearing positions, with the patient first mastering symmetrical activities without symptoms before attempting more asymmetrical activities. Activity modification and stabilization exercises have also been shown to be effective for patients with SIJ dysfunction during pregnancy and postpartum.[214]

The MDT approach using repeated movements has been used successfully to reduce SIJ-related pain using the test, treat, reassess method.[215] A benefit of repeated

TABLE 12-12

MODIFICATIONS TO ACTIVITIES OF DAILY LIVING FOR PATIENTS WITH SACROILIAC JOINT PAIN.

Activity	Recommendations
Sitting	• If crossing legs, cross at the ankle and not the knee • Avoid side-sitting (leaning to one side or the other)
Transfers	• Move from sitting and standing with equal weight on both feet • Getting into the car, sit first, then bring both legs into the vehicle • Getting out of the car, bring both legs out of the vehicle, then rise
Standing	• Stand with equal weight on both feet • Place one foot up on a small step or box if it feels better
Walking	• Take small steps • Walk at slower speeds
Lifting and carrying	• Carry equal loads in both hands • Hold children with both hands close to the body or use a front or back carrier
Stairs	• Do not take two steps at a time • Avoid during period of high irritability if possible

movements is that the clinician need not rely on palpation to classify SIJ pathology. Using the MDT approach, the patient would perform a provocative activity, such as walking with long strides, and rate the intensity of symptoms. For patients with suspected SIJ pathology that is reduced in posteriorly rotated positions or worsened in more anteriorly rotated SIJ positions, the patient would perform about 10 repetitions of a posterior SIJ rotating exercise, such as bringing the affected knee to chest.[216] The patient would then repeat the provocative activity. If symptoms were improved, the exercise is deemed appropriate and would be incorporated into a home program. Multiple sets of the exercise can be performed if additional gains are made with each set. For patients who appear to respond to (improve with) anterior SIJ rotation stresses, the patient would perform a trial of a half kneeling lunge on the affected side.[216]

An SIJ belt may be effective,[212,217] particularly in pregnant or postpartum women or those who report a decrease in symptoms with manual SIJ (anterior) compression test. The belt is worn snugly below the iliac crests and PSIS and generally has a small, wedge-shaped pad that overlies the sacrum. An SIJ belt may be effective for three main reasons. First, it may provide proprioceptive feedback. Second, by compressing the SIJ anteriorly, the belt is also gapping, or unloading, the joint posteriorly. Third, if instability is part of the pain-generating pathology, the belt may provide a degree of stabilization. However, a randomized controlled trial comparing core stabilization exercises with core stabilization exercises and an SIJ belt in nonpregnant and non-postpartum patients found no benefit to adding the SIJ belt.[212]

Manual therapy, including mobilization, manipulation, and muscle energy techniques, may be useful adjuncts for patients with SIJ-related pain. Muscle energy techniques utilize muscle contractions that are thought to provide a mobilizing force to a malaligned joint. The use of these techniques on SIJ dysfunction is based on the concept that innominate malpositioning occurs and that clinicians can accurately identify the direction the innominate moved.[205] Table 12-13 describes three basic muscle energy techniques, including their originally defined palpation findings and one manipulation that may provide symptom relief to some patients with SIJ dysfunction. Resisted hip adduction utilizes the hip adductors to try to pull the SIJ back into realignment (Fig. 12-38). It is a general technique that does not rely on confirmatory palpation findings and, therefore, a good first choice. Muscle energy techniques are performed with the patient holding an isometric contraction with an intensity of about 30% MVIC that is held for 6 to 10 seconds.[75] The isometric contraction is usually repeated for four to six repetitions. At times, the patient may report or hear a small cavitation or "pop." Improvement in symptoms is considered a positive result. Patients who report their SIJ frequently "goes out" may be taught how to perform the hip adductor muscle energy technique at home using a yoga block or similar object.

A posteriorly rotated innominate is treated by having the patient contract the hip flexors on the

TABLE 12-13
MANUAL INTERVENTIONS FOR SACROILIAC DYSFUNCTION

Suspected Condition	Proposed Palpation Findings	Recommended Treatment Technique
Sacroiliac dysfunction	Global technique for instability regardless of findings	• Muscle energy using hip adductors • With the patient hooklying supine, the clinician places the forearm between the patient's knees. The patients then isometrically contract the hip adductors.
Posteriorly rotated innominate	• PSIS of the painful side appears posterior and inferior • ASIS and pubic symphysis on the painful side appear superior	• Muscle energy using hip flexors • With the patient in a Thomas stretch position with the uninvolved knee to chest, the clinician resists hip flexion of the affected side.
Anteriorly rotated innominate	• PSIS of the painful side appears anterior and superior • ASIS and pubic symphysis on the painful side appear inferior	• Muscle energy using gluteus maximus • With the patient supine and the involved hip flexed to midrange, the clinician resists hip extension of the affected side.
Sacroiliac dysfunction or innominate upslip	• Global technique to unload the SIJ • ASIS, PSIS, and pubic symphysis of the involved side appear higher	• Mobilization/manipulation • With the patient supine, the clinician moves the involved leg into internal rotation and 10–15° of hip adduction. The clinician then slowly provides longitudinal traction to the leg for a sustained mobilization. To perform a manipulation, the clinician provides a quick inferior thrust after taking up all the slack with longitudinal traction.

ASIS, anterior superior iliac spine; *PSIS*, posterior superior iliac spine; *SIJ*, sacroiliac joint.

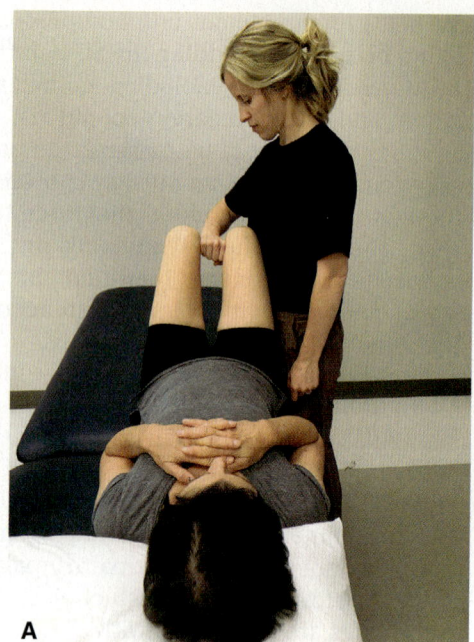
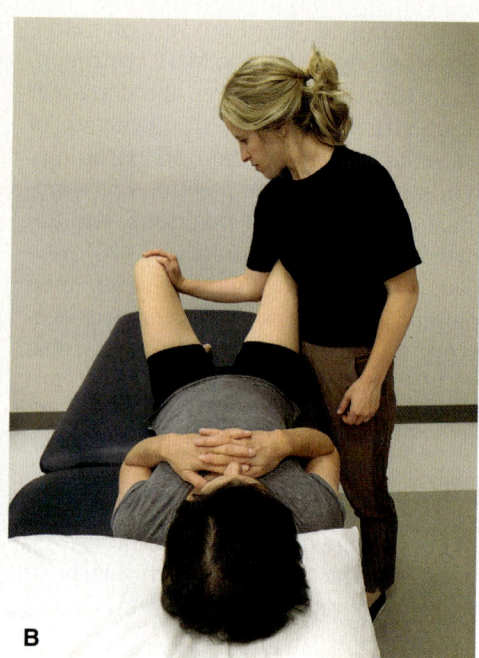

FIGURE 12-38 General muscle energy technique for sacroiliac dysfunction using hip adductors. **A.** Fist bracing for smaller patients. **B.** Forearm bracing for larger patients.

hypermobile, symptomatic side.[215] According to muscle energy technique theory, the hip flexors will pull a posteriorly rotated innominate back to its neutral position (anteriorly) by pulling the proximal attachment toward the stabilized distal attachment. Biomechanically, this technique is likely to unload the anterior portion of the SIJ. Treatment for an anteriorly rotated innominate is simply reversed by using the gluteus maximus.[215,218] Biomechanically, this technique is likely to unload the posterior portion of the SIJ. Self-treatment can be taught by having the patient grasp the posterior thigh to maintain hip flexion while isometrically trying to extend the hip. An inferior mobilization or manipulation may successfully resolve SIJ-related pain by realigning an innominate that has been driven superiorly from a fall (an upslip) or by unloading the SIJ (Fig. 12-39).[205,219] The positive effects of these manual techniques may also be explained by their ability to modulate nociplastic pain (see Chapter 19, Pain Management: A Mechanism-Centered Approach).

The addition of manual therapy to an exercise program does not appear to yield additional benefit.[75] A recent randomized controlled trial demonstrated no difference between patients treated with stabilization exercises compared with patients treated with manual therapy.[205] Given these data and the limited accuracy of palpation as a diagnostic tool for which to base SIJ dysfunction manual therapy techniques,[206,207] clinicians should consider adding manual therapy for patients noting limited improvements with stabilization exercises and repeated movements.

Expected Outcomes Patients with SIJ-related pain can expect improvements in pain, muscle performance, and function within 1 to 2 months of conservative interventions outlined earlier. Patients with systemic hypermobility may have episodes of recurrence until age-related reductions in motion occur. The SIJ-related symptoms of patients who are pregnant and postpartum can be reduced, but may not fully resolve until after delivery and hormone levels return to prepregnancy levels.[214] Rarely, open reduction and internal fixation is required for non–high-velocity SIJ dysfunction.

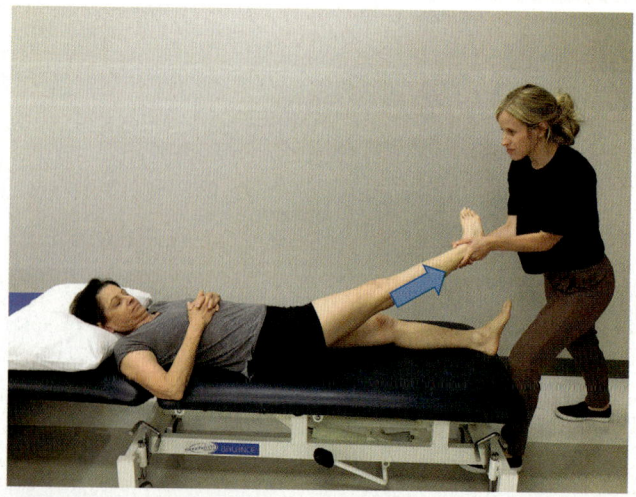

FIGURE 12-39 Inferior sacroiliac mobilization/manipulation.

CASE STUDY 12-1
Fahad: Patient with Right Low Back and Buttock Pain

Fahad is a 42-year-old carpenter who reports a sudden onset of right LBP and buttock pain 9 days ago after twisting suddenly to try to prevent a piece of lumbar from falling. Fahad reports his symptoms became worse the following day when he had difficulty getting out of bed and standing upright. All tests begin with the uninvolved (left) side first unless otherwise noted. The physical examination of a patient with lumbar spine pathology should be methodical to ensure all necessary information needed to guide clinical decision-making is obtained. Table 12-14 provides an example of how an experienced clinician might perform and interpret the physical examination after performing the history and systems review.

TABLE 12-14
SAMPLE LUMBAR EXAMINATION

Fahad, 42-year-old carpenter with 6/10 right low back and buttock pain.

Position	Assessments	Positive Findings
Observation	Continues from history	
Seated	L5: Great toe extension (A, OP, MMT) L4: Ankle dorsiflexion (A, OP, MMT) S1/2: Ankle eversion (A, OP, MMT) L3: Knee extension (A, OP, MMT) L1/2: Hip flexion (A, OP, MMT) Hip external rotation (A, OP, MMT) Hip internal rotation (A, OP, MMT) Dermatomes L1-S2 Reflexes: patellar, Achilles, Babinski, biceps, brachioradialis, triceps	Reduced strength right great toe extension Reduced sensation right dorsal 3rd metatarsophalangeal joint and L5 region.
Standing	Structure/posture screen Single leg balance Standing PF MMT Baseline trunk AROM flexion, extension, side glide Repeated trunk flexion Repeated trunk extension x 10 Repeated trunk extension x 10	Lumbar paraspinal hypertonicity Baseline trunk flex, side glide all increased back and buttock pain, no worse. Major loss of trunk flexion. Moderate loss of trunk extension. Repeated trunk flexion increased back and buttock symptoms, no worse. Repeated trunk extension • Set 1: Decreased back and buttock pain, no better. • Set 2: Abolished buttock symptoms, reduced back pain, better. Mild increase in trunk extension motion.
Supine	Hip PROM: flexion, abduction Hip: scour, FADIR, FABER SLR (also assesses hamstring length) Trunk flexion in lying	Positive R SLR Trunk flexion in lying increased back symptoms, no worse
Right sidelying	MMT: L hip abduction	
Prone	Prone knee flexion test Hip extension (P) MMT: gluteus maximus Extension in lying	Extension in lying increased back pain, produced buttock pain, worse
Left sidelying	MMT: R hip abduction	
Supine	Abdominal drawing in maneuver Abdominal drawing in maneuver with alternate hip flexion Bridge	Bridge and abdominal drawing in maneuver with hip flexion produced buttock pain, no worse

A, active; *L*, left; *MMT*, manual muscle test; *OP*, overpressure; *P*, passive; *R*, right.

(continued)

> **CASE STUDY 12-1 (continued)**
>
> Based on the history, there are no red flags and no signs of psychological distress. The patient's history of a sudden onset of pain with a twisting motion makes the clinician have initial hypotheses of strain, herniated disc, hip labral tear, and nonspecific back pain. The positive findings from the seated examination are consistent with an L5 radiculopathy. The standing examination reveals guarding. Baseline trunk motion demonstrates significant motion loss. Repeated motion testing reveals a directional preference for extension loading and centralization of symptoms. Supine examination does not reveal hip pathology, but does reveal positive neural tension testing and peripheralization of symptoms with increased intra-abdominal pressure. The clinician attempted unloaded trunk extension in lying to see if this would reveal superior results to extension in standing, but one repetition peripheralized symptoms. The clinician deferred accessory motion testing because a directional preference was determined, and the results of this assessment would not change the intervention strategy. The clinician concluded that the patient had an L5 radiculopathy that centralized with repeated trunk extension in standing. The condition was deemed highly irritable, given the ease of centralization and peripheralization. Note that the clinician could have reassessed great toe extension strength and sensation after the repeated movement examination or performed additional repetitions of repeated trunk in standing.

CHAPTER SUMMARY

The lumbar spine and SIJ are common sources of pain and disability. A thorough systems review must be performed to rule out referred sources of patient symptoms. Because hip and spine pathology has overlapping symptoms and may coexist, the hip should be examined as a potential symptom generator. A methodical examination tracking patient signs and symptoms is pivotal to determining an optimal course of action. The clinician must consider pathoanatomic causes of LBP but also recognize that nonspecific LBP is common. Interventions should focus on education and exercise but may also include manual therapy.

REFERENCES

1. Bitenc-Jasiejko A, Konior K, Lietz-Kijak D. Meta-analysis of integrated therapeutic methods in noninvasive lower back pain therapy (LBP): the role of interdisciplinary functional diagnostics. *Pain Res Manag.* 2020;2020:1–17.
2. Maher C, Underwood M, Buchbinder R. Non-specific low back pain. *Lancet.* 2017;389:736–747.
3. US Burden of Disease Collaborators, Mokdad AH, Ballestros K, et al. The state of US health, 1990–2016: burden of diseases, injuries, and risk factors among US states. *JAMA.* 2018;319(14):1444–1472.
4. Davenport D, Colaco HB, Kavarthapu V. Examination of the adult spine. *Br J Hosp Med (Lond).* 2015;76(12):C182–C185.
5. Mechelli F, Preboski Z, Boissonault W. Differential diagnosis of a patient referred to physical therapy with low back pain: abdominal aortic aneurysm. *J Orthop Sports Phys Ther.* 2008;38(9):551–557.
6. Goodman CC, Fuller KS. *Pathology: Implications for the Physical Therapist.* 5th ed. Elsevier; 2021.
7. Glimåker H, Holmberg L, Elvin A, et al. Natural history of patients with abdominal aortic aneurysm. *Eur J Vasc Surg.* 1991;5(2):125–130.
8. Petersen EJ, Thurmond SM. Differential diagnosis in a patient presenting with both systemic and neuromusculoskeletal pathology: resident's case problem. *J Orthop Sports Phys Ther.* 2018;48(6):496–503.
9. Markland AD, Richter HE, Fwu CW, Eggers P, Kusek JW. Prevalence and trends of urinary incontinence in adults in the United States, 2001 to 2008. *J Urol.* 2011;186(2):589–593.
10. Soliman Y, Meyer R, Baum N. Falls in the elderly secondary to urinary symptoms. *Rev Urol.* 2016;18(1):28–32.
11. Danforth KN, Townsend MK, Lifford K, Curhan GC, Resnick NM, Grodstein F. Risk factors for urinary incontinence among middle-aged women. *Am J Obstet Gynecol.* 2006;194(2):339–345.
12. Kao Y-C, Chen J-Y, Chen H-H, Liao K-W, Huang S-S. The association between depression and chronic lower back pain from disc degeneration and herniation of the lumbar spine. *Int J Psychiatry Med.* 2021:912174211003760. doi:10.1177/00912174211003760
13. Harris KK, Delic JA, Nelson EO. Epidural and paraspinal abscess presenting as acute low back pain. *J Orthop Sports Phys Ther.* 2019;49(6):482.
14. Wall CM, Paterno MV, Sturm PF. Lumbar spine osteomyelitis in an adolescent girl with nonspecific low back pain. *J Orthop Sports Phys Ther.* 2017;47(10):814.
15. Jordan J, Konstantinou K, O'Dowd J. Herniated lumbar disc. *BMJ Clin Evid.* 2009;2009:1118.
16. Su CA, Kusin DJ, Li SQ, Ahn UM, Ahn NU. The association between body mass index and the prevalence, severity, and frequency of low back pain: data from the osteoarthritis initiative. *Spine (Phila Pa 1976).* 2018;43(12):848–852.
17. Qaseem A, Wilt TJ, McLean RM, et al. Noninvasive treatments for acute, subacute, and chronic low back pain: a clinical practice guideline from the American College of Physicians. *Ann Intern Med.* 2017;166(7):514–530.
18. Ostelo RW. Physiotherapy management of sciatica. *J Physiother.* 2020;66(2):83–88.
19. Osborne J, Osborne R, Nielsen L, Rowe RH. Low back pain in the geriatric population (28.3.4). In: *The Lumbopelvic Complex: Advances in Evaluation and Treatment.* Academy of Orthopaedic Physical Therapy; 2018:1–33.

20. Rowe R, Langer L, Malaman F, Salvatori N, Shreve T. Acute and subacute low back pain with radiating pain (28.3.3). In: *The Lumbopelvic Complex: Advances in Evaluation and Treatment.* Academy of Orthopaedic Physical Therapy; 2018:1–45.
21. Brinjikji W, Luetmer PH, Comstock B, et al. Systematic literature review of imaging features of spinal degeneration in asymptomatic populations. *AJNR Am J Neuroradiol.* 2015;36(4):811–816.
22. van Rijn JC, Klemetso N, Reitsma JB, et al. Symptomatic and asymptomatic abnormalities in patients with lumbosacral radicular syndrome: clinical examination compared with MRI. *Clin Neurol Neurosurg.* 2006;108(6):553–557.
23. Goodman CC, Heick J, Lazaro R. *Differential Diagnosis for Physical Therapists: Screening for Referral.* 6h ed. Elsevier Science; 2018.
24. Hermann PC, Webler M, Bornemann R, et al. Influence of smoking on spinal fusion after spondylodesis surgery: a comparative clinical study. *Technol Health Care.* 2016;24(5):737–744.
25. Aweto HA, Aiyejusunle CB, Egbunah IV. Age-related musculoskeletal disorders associated with sedentary lifestyles among the elderly. *Ind J Physiother Occup Ther.* 2016;10(1):145–150.
26. Karahan A, Kav S, Abbasoglu A, Dogan N. Low back pain: prevalence and associated risk factors among hospital staff. *J Adv Nurs.* 2009;65(3):516–524.
27. Chung CC, Shimer AL. Lumbosacral spondylolysis and spondylolisthesis. *Clin Sports Med.* 2021;40(3):471–490.
28. Carroll A, Dreger M, O'Rourke P, Manal T. Adolescent spine (28.3.5). In: *The Lumbopelvic Complex: Advances in Evaluation and Treatment.* Academy of Orthopaedic Physical Therapy; 2018:1–33.
29. Daniell JR, Osti OL. Failed back surgery syndrome: a review article. *Asian Spine J.* 2018;12(2):372–379.
30. McKenzie R, May S. *The Lumbar Spine: Mechanical Diagnosis and Therapy.* Vol 1. Spinal Publications; 2013.
31. Alqarni AM, Schneiders AG, Hendrick PA. Clinical tests to diagnose lumbar segmental instability: a systematic review. *J Orthop Sports Phys Ther.* 2011;41(3):130–140.
32. Halliday MH, Pappas E, Hancock MJ, et al. A randomized controlled trial comparing the McKenzie method to motor control exercises in people with chronic low back pain and a directional preference. *J Orthop Sports Phys Ther.* 2016;46(7):514–522.
33. Surkitt LD, Ford JJ, Hahne AJ, Pizzari T, McMeeken JM. Efficacy of directional preference management for low back pain: a systematic review. *Phys Ther.* 2012;92(5):652–665.
34. Apeldoorn AT, van Helvoirt H, Meihuizen H, et al. The influence of centralization and directional preference on spinal control in patients with nonspecific low back pain. *J Orthop Sports Phys Ther.* 2016;46(4):258–269.
35. Fairbank JC, Pynsent PB. The Oswestry Disability Index. *Spine.* 2000;25(22):2940–2952; discussion 2952.
36. Delitto A, George SZ, van Dillen L, et al. Low back pain clinical practice guidelines linked to the International Classification of Functioning, Disability, and Health from the Orthopaedic Section of the American Physical Therapy Association. *J Orthop Sports Phys Ther.* 2012;42(4):A1–A57.
37. Robinson HS, Dagfinrud H. Reliability and screening ability of the StarT Back screening tool in patients with low back pain in physiotherapy practice, a cohort study. *BMC Musculoskelet Disord.* 2017;18(1):232.
38. Hill JC, Whitehurst DG, Lewis M, et al. Comparison of stratified primary care management for low back pain with current best practice (STarT Back): a randomised controlled trial. *Lancet.* 2011;378(9802):1560–1571.
39. Cleland JA, Fritz JM, Brennan GP. Predictive validity of initial fear avoidance beliefs in patients with low back pain receiving physical therapy: is the FABQ a useful screening tool for identifying patients at risk for a poor recovery? *Eur Spine J.* 2008;17(1):70–79.
40. Sullivan MJL, Bishop SR, Pivik J. The pain catastrophizing scale: development and validation. *Psychol Assess.* 1995;7(4):524–532.
41. Alrwaily M, Timko M. Acute and subacute low back pain with mobility deficits: lumbosacral segmental/somatic dysfunction (28.3.1). In: *The Lumbopelvic Complex: Advances in Evaluation and Treatment.* Academy of Orthopaedic Physical Therapy; 2018:1–49.
42. Tomkins-Lane C, Melloh M, Wong A. Diagnostic tests in the clinical diagnosis of lumbar spinal stenosis: consensus and results of an International Delphi Study. *Eur Spine J.* 2020;29(9):2188–2197.
43. Prather H, Cheng A, Steger-May K, Maheshwari V, Van Dillen L. Hip and lumbar spine physical examination findings in people presenting with low back pain, with or without lower extremity pain. *J Orthop Sports Phys Ther.* 2017;47(3):163–172.
44. Prather H, van Dillen L. Links between the hip and the lumbar spine (hip spine syndrome) as they relate to clinical decision making for patients with lumbopelvic pain. *PM R.* 2019;11(Suppl 1):S64–S72.
45. Buckland AJ, Miyamoto R, Patel RD, Slover J, Razi AE. Differentiating hip pathology from lumbar spine pathology: key points of evaluation and management. *J Am Acad Orthop Surg.* 2017;25(2):e23–e34.
46. Finucane L, Downie A, Mercer C, et al. International framework for red flags for potential serious spinal pathologies. *J Orthop Sports Phys Ther.* 2020;50(7):350–372.
47. Favaro L, Boggs RG, Geraci J, Michael C. Conservative management of a foraminal lumbar disc herniation. *JOSPT Cases.* 2021;1(1):49–50.
48. Alqarni AM, Schneiders AG, Cook CE, Hendrick PA. Clinical tests to diagnose lumbar spondylolysis and spondylolisthesis: a systematic review. *Phys Ther Sport.* 2015;16(3):268–275.
49. Herrington L. Assessment of the degree of pelvic tilt within a normal asymptomatic population. *Man Ther.* 2011;16(6):646–648.
50. Thawrani DP, Agabegi SS, Asghar F. Diagnosing sacroiliac joint pain. *J Am Acad Orthop Surg.* 2019;27(3):85–93.
51. Nattrass CL, Nitschke JE, Disler PB, Chou MJ, Ooi KT. Lumbar spine range of motion as a measure of physical and functional impairment: An investigation of validity. *Clin Rehabil.* 1999;13(3):211–218.
52. Riddle DL. *Relationships between Disability and Physical Impairment in Patients with Low Back Pain*, Virginia Commonwealth University; 1997.
53. Wernli K, Tan JS, O'Sullivan P, Smith A, Campbell A, Kent P. Does movement change when low back pain changes? A systematic review. *J Orthop Sports Phys Ther.* 2020;50(12):664–670.
54. Takasaki H. Comparable effect of simulated side bending and side gliding positions on the direction and magnitude of lumbar disc hydration shift: in vivo MRI mechanistic study. *J Man Manip Ther.* 2015;23(2):101–108.
55. Abbott JH, McCane B, Herbison P, Moginie G, Chapple C, Hogarty T. Lumbar segmental instability: a criterion-related validity study of manual therapy assessment. *BMC Musculoskelet Disord.* 2005;6(1):56.
56. Aina A, May S, Clare H. The centralization phenomenon of spinal symptoms—a systematic review. *Man Ther.* 2004;9(3):134–143.

57. Werneke MW, Hart DL, Cutrone G, et al. Association between directional preference and centralization in patients with low back pain. *J Orthop Sports Phys Ther.* 2011;41(1):22–31.
58. May S, Aina A. Centralization and directional preference: a systematic review. *Man Ther.* 2012;17(6):497–506.
59. Albert HB, Hauge E, Manniche C. Centralization in patients with sciatica: are pain responses to repeated movement and positioning associated with outcome or types of disc lesions? *Eur Spine J.* 2012;21(4):630–636.
60. Hides JA, Donelson R, Lee D, Prather H, Sahrmann SA, Hodges PW. Convergence and divergence of exercise-based approaches that incorporate motor control for the management of low back pain. *J Orthop Sports Phys Ther.* 2019;49(6):437–452.
61. Long A, May S, Fung T. Specific directional exercises for patients with low back pain: a case series. *Physiother Can.* 2008;60(4):307–317.
62. Martin HD, Reddy M, Gómez-Hoyos J. Deep gluteal syndrome. *J Hip Preserv Surg.* 2015;2(2):99–107.
63. Perez Carro L, Fernandez Hernando M, Cerezal L, Saenz Navarro I, Alfonso Fernandez A, Ortiz Castillo A. Deep gluteal space problems: piriformis syndrome, ischiofemoral impingement and sciatic nerve release. *Muscles Ligaments Tendons J.* 2016;6(3):384–396.
64. Kendall FP, McCreary EK, Provance PG, Rogers MM, Romani WA. *Muscles: Testing and Function with Posture and Pain.* 5th ed. Lippincott Williams & Wilkins; 2005.
65. George SZ, Fritz JM, Selfies SP, et al. Physical therapist interventions for low back pain: low back pain revision 2021: clinical practice guidelines from the Academy of Orthopedic Physical Therapy of the American Physical Therapy Association. *J Orthop Sports Phys Ther.* 2021;51:A1–A57.
66. Alrwaily M, Timko M, Schneiider M, et al. Treatment-based classification system for low back pain: revision and update. *Phys Ther.* 2016;96(7):1057–1066.
67. Ekedahl H, Jönsson B, Annertz M, Frobell RB. Accuracy of clinical tests in detecting disk herniation and nerve root compression in subjects with lumbar radicular symptoms. *Arch Phys Med Rehabil.* 2018;99(4):726–735.
68. Scaia V, Baxter D, Cook C. The pain provocation-based straight leg raise test for diagnosis of lumbar disc herniation, lumbar radiculopathy, and/or sciatica: a systematic review of clinical utility. *J Back Musculoskelet Rehabil.* 2012;25(4):215–223.
69. Urban LM, MacNeil BJ. Diagnostic accuracy of the slump test for identifying neuropathic pain in the lower limb. *J Orthop Sports Phys Ther.* 2015;45(8):596–603.
70. Hengeveld E, Banks K. *Maitland's Vertebral Manipulation.* Vol 1. 8th ed. Churchill Livingstone Elsevier; 2014.
71. Fritz JM, Whitman JM, Childs JD. Lumbar spine segmental mobility assessment: an examination of validity for determining intervention strategies in patients with low back pain. *Arch Phys Med Rehabil.* 2005;86(9):1745–1752.
72. Hayes MA, Howard TC, Gruel CR, Kopta JA. Roentgenographic evaluation of lumbar spine flexion-extension in asymptomatic individuals. *Spine.* 1989;14(3):327–331.
73. Hernando MF, Cerezal L, Pérez-Carro L, Abascal F, Canga A. Deep gluteal syndrome: Anatomy, imaging, and management of sciatic nerve entrapments in the subgluteal space. *Skeletal Radiol.* 2015;44(7):919–934.
74. Laslett M, Aprill CN, McDonald B, Young SB. Diagnosis of sacroiliac joint pain: validity of individual provocation tests and composites of tests. *Man Ther.* 2005;10(3):207–218.
75. Mathew R, Srivastava N, Joshi S. A study to compare the effectiveness of met and joint mobilization along with conventional physiotherapy in the management of SIJ joint dysfunction in young adults. *Ind J Physiother Occup Ther.* 2015;9(3):203–208.
76. Konin J, Lebscak D, Snyder Valier A. *Special Tests for Orthopaedic Examination.* SLACK Incorporated; 2016.
77. Nejati P, Sartaj E, Imani F, Moeineddin R, Nejati L, Safavi M. Accuracy of the diagnostic tests of sacroiliac joint dysfunction. *J Chiropr Med.* 2020;19(1):28–37.
78. Sanzarello I, Merlini L, Rosa M, et al. Central sensitization in chronic low back pain: a narrative review. *J Back Musculoskelet Rehabil.* 2016;29:625–633.
79. Reichert B. *Palpation Techniques: Surface Anatomy for Physical Therapists.* Thieme; 2011.
80. van Dieën JH, Reeves NP, Kawchuk G, van Dillen LR, Hodges PW. Motor control changes in low back pain: divergence in presentations and mechanisms. *J Orthop Sports Phys Ther.* 2019;49(6):370–379.
81. Hooper TL, James CR, Brismée J-M, et al. Dynamic balance as measured by the Y-Balance Test is reduced in individuals with low back pain: a cross-sectional comparative study. *Phys Ther Sport.* 2016;22:29–34.
82. Tsigkanos C, Gaskell L, Smirniotou A, Tsigkanos G. Static and dynamic balance deficiencies in chronic low back pain. *J Musculoskelet Rehabil.* 2016;29:887–893.
83. O'Sullivan P. Diagnosis and classification of chronic low back pain disorders: maladaptive movement and motor control impairments as underlying mechanism. *Man Ther.* 2005;10(4):242–255.
84. Haskins R, Osmotherly PG, Rivett DA. Diagnostic clinical prediction rules for specific subtypes of low back pain: a systematic review. *J Orthop Sports Phys Ther.* 2015;45(2):61–76.
85. van Dieën JH, Reeves NP, Kawchuk G, van Dillen LR, Hodges PW. Analysis of motor control in patients with low back pain: a key to personalized care? *J Orthop Sports Phys Ther.* 2019;49(6):380–388.
86. Hahne AJ, Ford JJ, Hinman RS, et al. Individualized functional restoration as an adjunct to advice for lumbar disc herniation with associated radiculopathy. A preplanned subgroup analysis of a randomized controlled trial. *Spine J.* 2017;17(3):346–359.
87. Kisner C, Colby LA. *Therapeutic Exercise: Foundations and Techniques.* 7th ed. F.A. Davis; 2018.
88. Garcia AN, Costa LdCM, de Souza FS, et al. Reliability of the Mechanical Diagnosis and Therapy system in patients with spinal pain: a systematic review. *J Orthop Sports Phys Ther.* 2018;48(12):923–933.
89. Thackeray A, Fritz JM, Childs JD, Brennan GP. The effectiveness of mechanical traction among subgroups of patients with low back pain and leg pain: a randomized trial. *J Orthop Sports Phys Ther.* 2016;46(3):144–154.
90. Thackeray A, Fritz JM, Brennan GP, Zaman FM, Willick SE. A pilot study examining the effectiveness of physical therapy as an adjunct to selective nerve root block in the treatment of lumbar radicular pain from disk herniation: a randomized controlled trial. *Phys Ther.* 2010;90(12):1717–1729.
91. Petersen T, Larsen K, Nordsteen J, Olsen S, Fournier G, Jacobsen S. The McKenzie method compared with manipulation when used adjunctive to information and advice in low back pain patients presenting with centralization or peripheralization: a randomized controlled trial. *Spine.* 2011;36(24):1999–2010.
92. Petersen T, Christensen R, Juhl C. Predicting a clinically important outcome in patients with low back pain following McKenzie therapy or spinal manipulation: a stratified

analysis in a randomized controlled trial. *BMC Musculoskelet Disord.* 2015;16:74.
93. Shah SG, Kage V. Effect of seven sessions of posterior-to-anterior spinal mobilisation versus prone press-ups in non-specific low back pain—randomized clinical trial. *J Clin Diagn Res.* 2016;10(3):Yc10–Yc13.
94. Hodges PW, Danneels L. Changes in structure and function of the back muscles in low back pain: different time points, observations, and mechanisms. *J Orthop Sports Phys Ther.* 2019;49(6):464–476.
95. Reeves NP, Cholewicki J, van Dieën JH, Kawchuk G, Hodges PW. Are stability and instability relevant concepts for back pain? *J Orthop Sports Phys Ther.* 2019;49(6):415–424.
96. Sung W, Jeblonski E. Acute, subacute, and recurrent low back pain with movement coordination impairments (28.3.2). In: *The Lumbopelvic Complex: Advances in Evaluation and Treatment.* Academy of Orthopaedic Physical Therapy; 2018:1–43.
97. Sahrmann S, Azevedo DC, Dillen LV. Diagnosis and treatment of movement system impairment syndromes. *Braz J Phys Ther.* 2017;21(6):391–399.
98. Drysdale CL, Earl JE, Hertel J. Surface electromyographic activity of the abdominal muscles during pelvic-tilt and abdominal-hollowing exercises. *J Athl Train.* 2004;39(1):32–36.
99. Beith ID, Synnott RE, Newman SA. Abdominal muscle activity during the abdominal hollowing manoeuvre in the four point kneeling and prone positions. *Man Ther.* 2001;6(2):82–87.
100. Sumiaki M, Takumi T, Yohei T, Hiroaki K. Trunk muscle activities during abdominal bracing: comparison among muscles and exercises. *J Sports Sci Med.* 2013;12(3):467–474.
101. Arab AM, Chehrehrazi M. Ultrasound measurement of abdominal muscles activity during abdominal hollowing and bracing in women with and without stress urinary incontinence. *Man Ther.* 2011;16(6):596–601.
102. Suehiro T, Mizutani M, Watanabe S, Ishida H, Kobara K, Osaka H. Comparison of spine motion and trunk muscle activity between abdominal hollowing and abdominal bracing maneuvers during prone hip extension. *J Bodyw Mov Ther.* 2014;18(3):482–488.
103. Tayashiki K, Takai Y, Maeo S, Kanehisa H. Intra-abdominal pressure and trunk muscular activities during abdominal bracing and hollowing. *Int J Sports Med.* 2016;37(2):134–143.
104. Ji-Hun H, Kwan-Sik S, Chung-Hwi Y. Effects of abdominal hollowing and bracing maneuvers on hip extension strength in prone standing position. *Isokinet Exerc Sci.* 2020;28(2):161–169.
105. Grenier SG, McGill SM. Quantification of lumbar stability by using 2 different abdominal activation strategies. *Arch Phys Med Rehabil.* 2007;88(1):54–62.
106. Fritz JM, Erhard RE, Hagen BF. Segmental instability of the lumbar spine. *Phys Ther.* 1998;78(8):889–896.
107. Van Dillen LR, Sahrmann SA, Wagner JM. Classification, intervention, and outcomes for a person with lumbar rotation with flexion syndrome. *Phys Ther.* 2005;85(4):336–351.
108. Azevedo DC, Van Dillen LR, Santos Hde O, Oliveira DR, Ferreira PH, Costa LO. Movement system impairment-based classification versus general exercise for chronic low back pain: protocol of a randomized controlled trial. *Phys Ther.* 2015;95(9):1287–1294.
109. Cholewicki J, Panjabi MM, Khachatryan A. Stabilizing function of trunk flexor-extensor muscles around a neutral spine posture. *Spine.* 1997;22(19):2207–2212.
110. van Dieën JH, Westebring-van der Putten EP, Kingma I, de Looze MP. Low-level activity of the trunk extensor muscles causes electromyographic manifestations of fatigue in absence of decreased oxygenation. *J Electromyogr Kinesiol.* 2009;19(3):398–406.
111. Caldwell LS, Smith RP. Pain and endurance of isometric muscle contractions. *J Eng Psychol.* 1966;5(1):25–32.
112. Alrwaily M, Timko M, Schneider M, et al. Treatment-based classification system for patients with low back pain: the movement control approach. *Phys Ther.* 2017;97(12):1147–1157.
113. Areeudomwong P, Wongrat W, Neammesri N, Thongsakul T. A randomized controlled trial on the long-term effects of proprioceptive neuromuscular facilitation training, on pain-related outcomes and back muscle activity, in patients with chronic low back pain. *Musculoskeletal Care.* 2017;15(3):218–229.
114. Park K-N, Kwon O-Y, Yi C-H, et al. Effects of motor control exercise vs muscle stretching exercise on reducing compensatory lumbopelvic motions and low back pain: A randomized trial. *J Manipulative Physiol Ther.* 2016;39(8):576–585.
115. Hodges PW. Hybrid approach to treatment tailoring for low back pain: a proposed model of care. *J Orthop Sports Phys Ther.* 2019;49(6):453–463.
116. Areeudomwong P, Buttagat V. Proprioceptive neuromuscular facilitation training improves pain-related and balance outcomes in working-age patients with chronic low back pain: a randomized controlled trial. *Braz J Phys Ther.* 2019;23(5):428–436.
117. Areeudomwong P, Vitsarut B. Comparison of core stabilisation exercise and proprioceptive neuromuscular facilitation training on pain-related and neuromuscular response outcomes for chronic low back pain: a randomised controlled trial. *Malays J Med Sci.* 2019;26(6):77–89.
118. Offierski CM, MacNab I. Hip-spine syndrome. *Spine.* 1983;8(3):316–321.
119. Redmond JM, Gupta A, Hammarstedt JE, Stake CE, Domb BG. The hip-spine syndrome: how does back pain impact the indications and outcomes of hip arthroscopy? *Arthroscopy.* 2014;30(7):872–881.
120. Harris JD. Editorial commentary: the hip bone's connected to the spine bone-but correlation does not equal causation. *Arthroscopy.* 2016;32(11):2249–2250.
121. Devin CJ, McCullough KA, Morris BJ, et al. Hip-spine syndrome. *J Am Acad Orthop Surg.* 2012;20(7):434–442.
122. Burns SA, Mintken PE, Austin GP. Clinical decision making in a patient with secondary hip-spine syndrome. *Physiother Theory Pract.* 2011;27(5):384–397.
123. Chen B-L, Guo J-B, Zhang H-W, et al. Surgical versus non-operative treatment for lumbar disc herniation: a systematic review and meta-analysis. *Clin Rehabil.* 2018;32(2):146–160.
124. Koes BW, van Tulder MW, Thomas S. Diagnosis and treatment of low back pain. *BMJ.* 2006;332(7555):1430–1434.
125. Kim J-H, van Rijn RM, van Tulder MW, et al. Diagnostic accuracy of diagnostic imaging for lumbar disc herniation in adults with low back pain or sciatica is unknown; a systematic review. *Chiropr Man Therap.* 2018;26(1):37.
126. Kreiner DS, Hwang SW, Easa JE, et al. An evidence-based clinical guideline for the diagnosis and treatment of lumbar disc herniation with radiculopathy. *Spine J.* 2014;14(1):180–191.
127. Savage NJ, Fritz JM, Thackeray A. The relationship between history and physical examination findings and the outcome of electrodiagnostic testing in patients with sciatica referred to physical therapy. *J Orthop Sports Phys Ther.* 2014;44(7):508–517.

128. Wong JJ, Côté P, Sutton DA, et al. Clinical practice guidelines for the noninvasive management of low back pain: a systematic review by the Ontario Protocol for Traffic Injury Management (OPTIMa) Collaboration. *Eur J Pain.* 2017;21(2):201–216.
129. Bayraktar D, Guclu-Gunduz A, Lambeck J, Yazici G, Aykol S, Demirci H. A comparison of water-based and land-based core stability exercises in patients with lumbar disc herniation: a pilot study. *Disabil Rehabil.* 2016;38(12):1163–1171.
130. Pallipamula K, Singaravelan RM. Efficacy of nerve flossing technique on improving sciatic nerve function in patients with sciatica—a randomized controlled trial. *Rom J Phys Ther.* 2012;18(30):13–22.
131. Isner-Horobeti M-E, Dufour SP, Schaeffer M, et al. High-force versus low-force lumbar traction in acute lumbar sciatica due to disc herniation: a preliminary randomized trial. *J Manipulative Physiol Ther.* 2016;39(9):645–654.
132. Manchikanti L, Benyamin RM, Falco FJE, Kaye AD, Hirsch JA. Do epidural injections provide short-and long-term relief for lumbar disc herniation? A systematic review. *Clin Orthop Relat Res.* 2015;473(6):1940–1956.
133. Quack V, Boecker M, Mueller CA, et al. Psychological factors outmatched morphological markers in predicting limitations in activities of daily living and participation in patients with lumbar stenosis. *BMC Musculoskelet Disord.* 2019;20(1):557.
134. Kerr D, Zhao W, Lurie JD. What are long-term predictors of outcomes for lumbar disc herniation? A randomized and observational study. *Clin Orthop Relat Res.* 2015;473(6):1920–1930.
135. Fors M, Enthoven P, Abbott A, Öberg B. Effects of pre-surgery physiotherapy on walking ability and lower extremity strength in patients with degenerative lumbar spine disorder: secondary outcomes of the PREPARE randomised controlled trial. *BMC Musculoskelet Disord.* 2019;20(1):1–11.
136. Koerner JD, Glaser J, Radcliff K. Which variables are associated with patient-reported outcomes after discectomy? review of SPORT disc herniation studies. *Clin Orthop Relat Res.* 2015;473(6):2000–2006.
137. Eliasberg CD, Kelly MP, Ajiboye RM, SooHoo NF. Complications and rates of subsequent lumbar surgery following lumbar total disc arthroplasty and lumbar fusion. *Spine.* 2016;41(2):173–181.
138. Yue JJ, Garcia R, Blumenthal S, et al. Five-year results of a randomized controlled trial for lumbar artificial discs in single-level degenerative disc disease. *Spine.* 2019;44(24):1685–1696.
139. Ding F, Jia Z, Zhao Z, et al. Total disc replacement versus fusion for lumbar degenerative disc disease: a systematic review of overlapping meta-analyses. *Eur Spine J.* 2017;26(3):806–815.
140. Kalakoti P, Sciubba DM, Pugely AJ, et al. Impact of psychiatric comorbidities on short-term outcomes following intervention for lumbar degenerative disc disease. *Spine.* 2018;43(19):1363–1371.
141. Keizer A, Vandyken B, Vandyken C, et al. Predictors of pelvic floor muscle dysfunction among women with lumbopelvic pain. *Phys Ther.* 2019;99(12):1703–1711.
142. Arab AM, Behbahani RB, Lorestani L, Azari A. Assessment of pelvic floor muscle function in women with and without low back pain using transabdominal ultrasound. *Man Ther.* 2010;15(3):235–239.
143. Bhatnagar G, Sahu M. Comparison of pelvic floor exercises and conventional regimen in patients with chronic low back pain. *Indian J Physiother Occup Ther.* 2017;11(3):38–42.
144. Sapsford R. Rehabilitation of pelvic floor muscles utilizing trunk stabilization. *Man Ther.* 2004;9(1):3–12.
145. Bump RC, Hurt WG, Fantl JA, Wyman JF. Assessment of Kegel pelvic muscle exercise performance after brief verbal instruction. *Am J Obstet Gynecol.* 1991;165(2):322–327; discussion 327–329.
146. Sung-min H, Oh-yun K, Su-jung K, Sung-dae C. The importance of a normal breathing pattern for an effective abdominal-hollowing maneuver in healthy people: an experimental study. *J Sport Rehabil.* 2014;23(1):12–17.
147. Critchley D. Instructing pelvic floor contraction facilitates transversus abdominis thickness increase during low-abdominal hollowing. *Physiother Res Int.* 2002;7(2):65–75.
148. Ajiboye LO, Alimi M, Gbadegesin SA, Oboirien M. Treatment outcome of quality of life and clinical symptoms in patients with symptomatic lumbar degenerative disc diseases: which treatment modality is superior? *Int Orthop.* 2019;43(4):875–881.
149. Ravikanth R. Magnetic resonance evaluation of lumbar disc degenerative disease as an implication of low back pain: a prospective analysis. *Neurol India.* 2020;68(6):1378–1384.
150. Bai D-Y, Liang L, Zhang B-B, et al. Total disc replacement versus fusion for lumbar degenerative diseases—a meta-analysis of randomized controlled trials. *Medicine (Baltimore).* 2019;98(29):e16460-e16460.
151. Zaina F, Tomkins-Lane C, Carragee E, Negrini S. Surgical versus nonsurgical treatment for lumbar spinal stenosis. *Spine.* 2016;41(14):E857–E868.
152. Cook CJ, Cook CE, Reiman MP, Joshi AB, Richardson W, Garcia AN. Systematic review of diagnostic accuracy of patient history, clinical findings, and physical tests in the diagnosis of lumbar spinal stenosis. *Eur Spine J.* 2020;29(1):93–112.
153. Thornes E, Robinson HS, Vøllestad NK. Degenerative lumbar spinal stenosis and physical functioning: an exploration of associations between self-reported measures and physical performance tests. *Disabil Rehabil.* 2018;40(2):232–237.
154. Delitto A, Piva SR, Moore CG, et al. Surgery versus nonsurgical treatment of lumbar spinal stenosis: a randomized trial. *Ann Intern Med.* 2015;162(7):465–473.
155. Fritz JM, Erhard RE, Delitto A, Welch WC, Nowakowski PE. Preliminary results of the use of a two-stage treadmill test as a clinical diagnostic tool in the differential diagnosis of lumbar spinal stenosis. *J Spinal Disord.* 1997;10(5):410–416.
156. Tanishima S, Fukada S, Ishii H, Dokai T, Morio Y, Nagashima H. Comparison between walking test and treadmill test for intermittent claudication associated with lumbar spinal canal stenosis. *Eur Spine J.* 2015;24(2):327–332.
157. Stienen MN, Ho AL, Staartjes VE, et al. Objective measures of functional impairment for degenerative diseases of the lumbar spine: a systematic review of the literature. *Spine J.* 2019;19(3):1276–1293.
158. Minetama M, Kawakami M, Teraguchi M, et al. Supervised physical therapy vs. home exercise for patients with lumbar spinal stenosis: a randomized controlled trial. *Spine J.* 2019;19(8):1310–1318.
159. Marchand A-A, Suitner M, O'Shaughnessy J, Châtillon C-É, Cantin V, Descarreaux M. Effects of a prehabilitation program on patients' recovery following spinal stenosis surgery: study protocol for a randomized controlled trial. *Trials.* 2015;16(1):483.
160. Minetama M, Kawakami M, Nakagawa M, et al. A comparative study of 2-year follow-up outcomes in lumbar spinal stenosis patients treated with physical therapy alone and those with surgical intervention after less successful physical therapy. *J Orthop Sci.* 2018;23(3):470–476.

161. Masakazu M, Mamoru K, Masatoshi T, et al. Therapeutic advantages of frequent physical therapy sessions for patients with lumbar spinal stenosis. *Spine.* 2020;45(11):E639–E646.
162. Schneider MJ, Ammendolia C, Murphy DR, et al. Comparative clinical effectiveness of nonsurgical treatment methods in patients with lumbar spinal stenosis: a randomized clinical trial. *JAMA Netw Open.* 2019;2(1):e186828–e186828.
163. Hammerich A, Whitman J, Mintken P, et al. Effectiveness of physical therapy combined with epidural steroid injection for individuals with lumbar spinal stenosis: a randomized parallel-group trial. *Arch Phys Med Rehabil.* 2019;100(5):797–810.
164. Beyer F, Geier F, Bredow J, et al. Non-operative treatment of lumbar spinal stenosis. *Technol Health Care.* 2016;24(4):551–557.
165. Chow NW, Southerst D, Wong JJ, Kopansky-Giles D, Ammendolia C. Clinical outcomes in neurogenic claudication using a multimodal program for lumbar spinal stenosis: a study of 49 patients with prospective long-term follow-up. *J Manipulative Physiol Ther.* 2019;42(3):203–209.
166. Sharma AK, Vorobeychik Y, Wasserman R, et al. The effectiveness and risks of fluoroscopically guided lumbar interlaminar epidural steroid injections: a systematic review with comprehensive analysis of the published data. *Pain Med.* 2017;18(2):239–251.
167. Zhao W, Wang Y, Wu J, et al. Long-term outcomes of epidurals with lidocaine with or without steroids for lumbar disc herniation and spinal stenosis: a meta-analysis. *Pain Phys.* 2020;23(4):365–374.
168. Hébert JJ, Abraham E, Wedderkopp N, et al. Preoperative factors predict postoperative trajectories of pain and disability following surgery for degenerative lumbar spinal stenosis. *Spine.* 2020;45(21):E1421–E1430.
169. Ma X-L, Zhao X-W, Ma J-X, Li F, Wang Y, Lu B. Effectiveness of surgery versus conservative treatment for lumbar spinal stenosis: a system review and meta-analysis of randomized controlled trials. *Int J Surg.* 2017;44:329–338.
170. Bo C, Yao L, Zhi-Cui W, et al. Decompression with fusion versus decompression in the treatment of lumbar spinal stenosis: a systematic review and meta-analysis. *Medicine (Baltimore).* 2020;99(38):1–8.
171. Shuai X, Jinyu W, Yan L, et al. Decompression with fusion is not in superiority to decompression alone in lumbar stenosis based on randomized controlled trials: a PRISMA-compliant meta-analysis. *Medicine (Baltimore).* 2019;98(46):1–11.
172. Li-Hui Y, Wei L, Jian L, et al. Lumbar decompression and lumbar interbody fusion in the treatment of lumbar spinal stenosis: a systematic review and meta-analysis. *Medicine (Baltimore).* 2020;99(27):1–11.
173. Fritsch C, Ferreira M, Maher C, et al. The clinical course of pain and disability following surgery for spinal stenosis: a systematic review and meta-analysis of cohort studies. *Eur Spine J.* 2017;26(2):324–335.
174. Smuck M, Muaremi A, Zheng P, et al. Objective measurement of function following lumbar spinal stenosis decompression reveals improved functional capacity with stagnant real-life physical activity. *Spine J.* 2018;18(1):15–21.
175. Matz PG, Meagher RJ, Lamer T, et al. Guideline summary review: an evidence-based clinical guideline for the diagnosis and treatment of degenerative lumbar spondylolisthesis. *Spine J.* 2016;16(3):439–448.
176. Koslosky E, Gendelberg D. Classification in brief: the Meyerding classification system of spondylolisthesis. *Clin Orthop Relat Res.* 2020;478(5):1125–1130.
177. Ferrari S, Villafañe JH, Berjano P, Vanti C, Monticone M. How many physical therapy sessions are required to reach a good outcome in symptomatic lumbar spondylolisthesis? A retrospective study. *J Bodyw Mov Ther.* 2018;22(1):18–23.
178. Mohammadimajd E, Lotfinia I, Salahzadeh Z, et al. Comparison of lumbar segmental stabilization and general exercises on clinical and radiologic criteria in grade-I spondylolisthesis patients: a double-blind randomized controlled trial. *Physiother Res Int.* 2020;25(3):1–10.
179. Oster BA, Kikanloo SR, Levine NL, Lian J, Woojin C, Cho W. Systematic review of outcomes following 10-year mark of Spine Patient Outcomes Research Trial (SPORT) for degenerative spondylolisthesis. *Spine.* 2020;45(12):820–824.
180. Selhorst M, Fischer A, Graft K, et al. Timing of physical therapy referral in adolescent athletes with acute spondylolysis: a retrospective chart review. *Clin J Sport Med.* 2017;27(3):296–301.
181. Mo AZ, Gjolaj JP. Axial low back pain in elite athletes. *Clin Sports Med.* 2021;40(3):491–499.
182. Fryhofer GW, Smith HE. Return to play for cervical and lumbar spine conditions. *Clin Sports Med.* 2021;40(3):555–569.
183. Wahyuddin W, Mantana V, Keerin M, Sunee B, Rachaneewan A. Immediate effects of muscle energy technique and stabilization exercise in patients with chronic low back pain with suspected facet joint origin: a pilot study. *Hong Kong Physiother J.* 2020;40(2):109–119.
184. Wilde VE, Ford JJ, McMeeken JM. Indicators of lumbar zygapophyseal joint pain: survey of an expert panel with the Delphi technique. *Phys Ther.* 2007;87(10):1348–1361.
185. Ford JJ, Slater SL, Richards MC, et al. Individualised manual therapy plus guideline-based advice vs advice alone for people with clinical features of lumbar zygapophyseal joint pain: a randomised controlled trial. *Physiotherapy.* 2019;105(1):53–64.
186. Chambers H. Physiotherapy and lumbar facet joint injections as a combination treatment for chronic low back pain. A narrative review of lumbar facet joint injections, lumbar spinal mobilizations, soft tissue massage and lower back mobility exercises. *Musculoskeletal Care.* 2013;11(2):106–120.
187. Kahanov L, Eberman LE, Games KE, Wasik M. Diagnosis, treatment, and rehabilitation of stress fractures in the lower extremity in runners. *Open Access J Sports Med.* 2015;6:87–95.
188. Kampe K, Kohler M, Albrecht D, et al. Hip and pelvic fracture patients with fear of falling: development and description of the "Step by Step" treatment protocol. *Clin Rehabil.* 2017;31(5):571–581.
189. Pfeiffer K, Kampe K, Klenk J, et al. Effects of an intervention to reduce fear of falling and increase physical activity during hip and pelvic fracture rehabilitation. *Age Ageing.* 2020;49(5):771–778.
190. Idrissi M, Ibrahimi A. Tile type C pelvic fractures: initial management, surgery and rehabilitation results of 12 cases with literature review. *J Phys Med Rehabil Stud Rep.* 2021;3(1):1–8.
191. Choi SD, Brings K. Work-related musculoskeletal risks associated with nurses and nursing assistants handling overweight and obese patients: a literature review. *Work.* 2016;53(2):439–448.
192. Bourgaize S, Newton G, Kumbhare D, Srbely J. A comparison of the clinical manifestation and pathophysiology of myofascial pain syndrome and fibromyalgia: implications for differential diagnosis and management. *J Can Chiropr Assoc.* 2018;62(1):26–41.

193. Bourgaize S, Janjua I, Murnaghan K, Mior S, Srbely J, Newton G. Fibromyalgia and myofascial pain syndrome: two sides of the same coin? A scoping review to determine the lexicon of the current diagnostic criteria. *Musculoskeletal Care*. 2019;17(1):3–12.
194. Simons DG, Travell JG, Simons LS. *Travell & Simons' Myofascial Pain and Dysfunction: The Trigger Points Manual (Vol 1: Upper Half of Body)*. 2nd ed. Lippincott Williams & Wilkins, 1999.
195. Guzmán-Pavón MJ, Cavero-Redondo I, Martínez-Vizcaíno V, Fernández-Rodríguez R, Reina-Gutierrez S, Álvarez-Bueno C. Effect of physical exercise programs on myofascial trigger points–related dysfunctions: a systematic review and meta-analysis. *Pain Med*. 2020;21(11):2986–2996.
196. Sergienko S, Kalichman L. Myofascial origin of shoulder pain: a literature review. *J Bodyw Mov Ther*. 2015;19(1):91–101.
197. Mata Diz JB, de Souza JRLM, Leopoldino AAO, Oliveira VC. Exercise, especially combined stretching and strengthening exercise, reduces myofascial pain: a systematic review. *J Physiother*. 2017;63(1):17–22.
198. Ambrose KR, Golightly YM. Physical exercise as non-pharmacological treatment of chronic pain: why and when. *Best Pract Res Clin Rheumatol*. 2015;29(1):120–130.
199. Lew J, Kim J, Nair P. Comparison of dry needling and trigger point manual therapy in patients with neck and upper back myofascial pain syndrome: a systematic review and meta-analysis. *J Man Manip Ther*. 2021;29(3):136–146.
200. Ahmed S, Haddad C, Subramaniam S, Khattab S, Kumbhare D. The effect of electric stimulation techniques on pain and tenderness at the myofascial trigger point: a systematic review. *Pain Med*. 2019;20(9):1774–1788.
201. Annaswamy TM, De Luigi AJ, O'Neill BJ, Keole N, Berbrayer D. Emerging concepts in the treatment of myofascial pain: a review of medications, modalities, and needle-based interventions. *PM R*. 2011;3(10):940–961.
202. Kizaki K, Uchida S, Shanmugaraj A, et al. Deep gluteal syndrome is defined as a non-discogenic sciatic nerve disorder with entrapment in the deep gluteal space: a systematic review. *Knee Surg Sports Traumatol Arthrosc*. 2020;28(10):3354–3364.
203. Hopayian K, Heathcote J. Deep gluteal syndrome: an overlooked cause of sciatica. *Br J Gen Pract*. 2019;69(687):485–486.
204. Vassalou EE, Katonis P, Karantanas AH. Piriformis muscle syndrome: a cross-sectional imaging study in 116 patients and evaluation of therapeutic outcome. *Eur Radiol*. 2018;28(2):447–458.
205. Kamali F, Zamanlou M, Ghanbari A, Alipour A, Bervis S. Comparison of manipulation and stabilization exercises in patients with sacroiliac joint dysfunction patients: a randomized clinical trial. *J Bodyw Mov Ther*. 2019;23(1):177–182.
206. O'Haire C, Gibbons P. Inter-examiner and intra-examiner agreement for assessing sacroiliac anatomical landmarks using palpation and observation: pilot study. *Man Ther*. 2000;5(1):13–20.
207. van Deursen LLJM, Patijn J, Ockhuysen AL, Vortman BL. The value of some clinical tests of the sacroiliac joint. *J Man Med*. 1990;5:96–99.
208. Kiapour A, Joukar A, Elgafy H, Erbulut DU, Agarwal AK, Goel VK. Biomechanics of the sacroiliac joint: anatomy, function, biomechanics, sexual dimorphism, and causes of pain. *Int J Spine Surg*. 2020;14(Suppl 1):3–13.
209. Palsson TS, Gibson W, Darlow B, et al. Changing the narrative in diagnosis and management of pain in the sacroiliac joint area. *Phys Ther*. 2019;99(11):1511–1519.
210. Gusfa D, Bashir DA, Saffarian MR. Diagnosing and managing sacroiliac joint pain. *Am J Phys Med Rehabil*. 2021;100(4):e40-e42.
211. Polly DW, Jr. The sacroiliac joint. *Neurosurg Clin N Am*. 2017;28(3):301–312.
212. Brizzolara KJ, Wang-Price S, Roddey TS, Medley A. Effectiveness of adding a pelvic compression belt to lumbopelvic stabilization exercises for women with sacroiliac joint pain: a feasibility randomized clinical trial. *J Women Health Phys Ther*. 2018;42(2):76–86.
213. Edgar K, Appel A, Clay N, et al. Influence of sacroiliac bracing on muscle activation strategies during 2 functional tasks in standing-tolerant and standing-intolerant individuals. *J Appl Biomech*. 2019;35(2):107–115.
214. Stuge B, Laerum E, Kirkesola G, Vøllestad N. The efficacy of a treatment program focusing on specific stabilizing exercises for pelvic girdle pain after pregnancy: a randomized controlled trial. *Spine*. 2004;29(4):351–359.
215. Srivastava S, Kumar K U D, Mittal H, Dixit S, Nair A. Short-term effect of muscle energy technique and mechanical diagnosis and therapy in sacroiliac joint dysfunction: a pilot randomized clinical trial. *J Bodyw Mov Ther*. 2020;24(3):63–70.
216. Horton SJ, Franz A. Mechanical Diagnosis and Therapy approach to assessment and treatment of derangement of the sacro-iliac joint. *Man Ther*. 2007;12(2):126–132.
217. Dolunay ET, Can F. The results of exercise and sacroiliac orthosis application in sacroiliac joint dysfunction. *Turk J Physiother Rehabil*. 2005;16(3):113–119.
218. Sanika V, Prem V, Karvannan H. Comparison of gluteus maximus activation to flexion bias exercises along with met technique in subjects with anterior rotated sacroiliac joint dysfunction—a randomised control trial. *Int J Ther Massage Bodywork*. 2021;14(1):30–38.
219. Srivastava S, K. U DK, Mittal H. Effect of muscle energy technique on upslip and inflare dysfunction of sacroiliac joint: a case report. *Ind J Physiother Occup Ther*. 2017;11(4):190–194.

PART IV

Upper Quarter

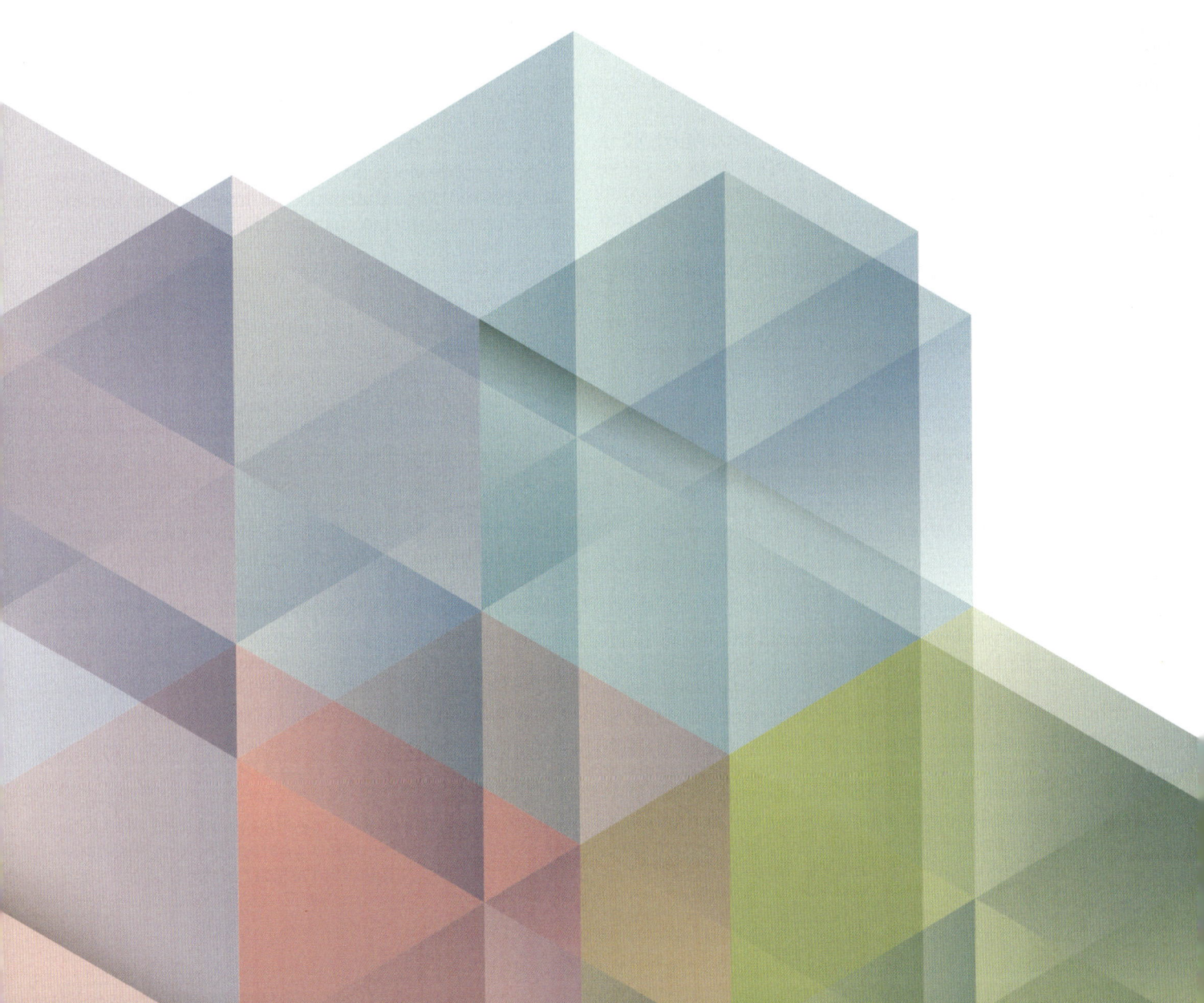

13 | Upper Quarter Screen

Betsy Myers

CHAPTER OBJECTIVES

After reading this chapter, you will be able to:
1. Describe the elements of an upper quarter screen.
2. Describe reasons for performing an upper quarter screen.
3. Identify key anatomic landmarks to screen upper quarter structural alignment.
4. Describe the components of an upper quarter neurologic screen.
5. Adapt the upper quarter screen based on patient presentation.

PURPOSE OF THE UPPER QUARTER SCREEN

The upper quarter screen (UQS) is performed when a patient has symptoms in the upper body or cervical/thoracic region. The UQS helps narrow the working hypotheses generated from the patient history and interview. The UQS screen includes observation, gross assessment of structure and posture, an **upper quarter neurologic screen (UQNS)**, assessment of upper extremity motion and strength, and functional testing.

The four main purposes for the lower quarter screen (LQS) and UQS are as follows:
- Rule out sources of patient symptoms
- Identify relevant deviation and impairments within the kinetic chain
- Identify issues that might alter rehabilitation interventions, precautions, or patient prognosis
- Expedite referral and consultation when needed

These purposes are reviewed in depth in Chapter 8, Lower Quarter Screen.

The effect of the kinetic chain is, perhaps, more obvious in the lower quarter than in the upper quarter, as the lower extremity regularly functions in the closed kinetic chain linking joints with limited degrees of freedom. However, consider a patient with limited shoulder elevation who reports difficulty with overhead reaching. This requires complex interactions at the glenohumeral joint, acromioclavicular joint, sternoclavicular joint, scapulothoracic joint, and thoracic spine. To provide the most efficient and effective care, the clinician must perform a thorough assessment of the kinetic chain in order to know where to direct treatment. A middle-aged patient with restricted shoulder motion after a distal humerus fracture would likely benefit from mobilizations that emphasize the glenohumeral joint, whereas an older individual with increased kyphosis would likely benefit, at least in part, from thoracic mobilizations.[1] Likewise, a patient with lateral epicondylalgia will have symptoms in the elbow region. However, neglecting to address wrist positioning will lead to subpar outcomes.[2]

GENERAL RULES FOR UPPER QUARTER SCREENING

Before performing the UQS, the clinician must have performed a thorough history including medical history, symptom investigation, and the review of systems and must also have concluded that it was safe to proceed to the physical examination. As with the LQS, the clinician must then determine whether there are any red flags that must be investigated. For example, if the clinician suspects the patient might have a scaphoid fracture, then the next step would be for the clinician to perform key tests (such as scaphoid compression test, snuff box tenderness, scaphoid tubercle tenderness, and active thumb range of motion)[3–5] in an attempt to determine whether imaging is warranted (see Chapter 16, Wrist and Hand Complex, for additional details). If these tests are positive, the examination should be halted and the patient should be referred for radiographs. The UQS is organized by patient position and proceeds with examination of the uninvolved side to the involved side. Clinicians should use traditional test positions to allow immediate and reproducible measurements and abnormalities should be noted. During testing, the clinician should ask the patient to note if any new symptoms arise or if there are any changes in existing symptoms. Recall that the experienced clinician will eliminate portions of the UQS that are not believed to be indicated based on the patient's history and area of chief complaint.

COMPONENTS OF THE UPPER QUARTER SCREEN

Figure 13-1 contains the key components of the UQS. Although part of the upper quarter, the temporomandibular joint is not included as part of the UQS because

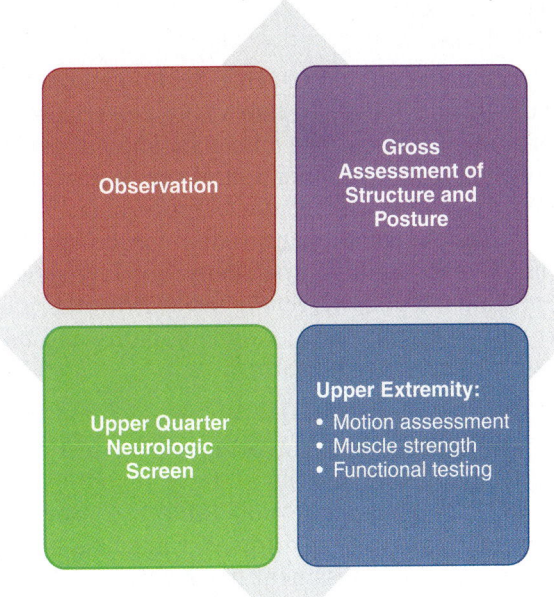

FIGURE 13-1 Components of the upper quarter screen.

it does not refer to symptoms outside the head and neck region. This joint would, of course, require further investigation in patients with cervical, neck, or facial complaints and is discussed further in Chapter 18, Temporomandibular Joint.

Observation

The UQS begins upon first observation of the patient and continues throughout the patient encounter. How did the patient complete any paperwork in the waiting room? Does the patient have reciprocal arm swing while walking to the examination room? What is the patient's positioning during the history? Does the patient maintain eye contact during the interview?

Structure and Posture

The clinician should take a cursory view of the patient's overall structure and posture. To maximize exposure of the affected region, male patients should be shirtless and female patients should wear a sports bra or a gown that is open in the back. It is useful to assess the patient both in standing and in sitting as the position of the upper quarter may change. Starting with this big picture approach, the clinician should then proceed from either a top-down or bottom-up approach observing the patient from posterior, anterior, and lateral views. The clinician should make a visual and palpatory examination of bony landmarks, symmetry, atrophy, edema, scars, and skin lesions. Table 13-1 provides key alignments the clinician should observe along with a description of optimal

TABLE 13-1

EXAMINATION OF PATIENT STRUCTURE AND POSTURE IN STANDING

Landmark	Optimal Alignment
Posterior View	
Calcaneal alignment	In the relaxed calcaneal stance position, the calcaneus should be close to vertical.
Popliteal crease height	Popliteal crease heights should be even.
Iliac crest height	Iliac crest heights should be even.
Shoulders	Shoulder heights should be even.
Scapulae	Medial borders should be flush with the thorax. Inferior angles should be level.
Cubital fossa and hand	Observe the resting position of the patient's hand. While patient's rarely stand in anatomic alignment, observe for excessive shoulder internal rotation causing palms to face posteriorly.
Anterior View	
Patellae	Patellae should be facing anteriorly.
Shoulders	Shoulder heights should be symmetrical.
Lateral View	
Knee alignment	Knees should be in neutral extension.
Spine	The lumbar and cervical spine should have a small lordosis. The thoracic spine should have a small kyphosis.
Jaw	Mouth should be relaxed in a closed position.
Line of gravity	The line of gravity should fall through or near the following structures: external auditory meatus, acromioclavicular joint, 7th cervical vertebra, 3rd lumbar vertebra, and hip joint. The line of gravity should fall slightly posterior to the hip joint but anterior to the knee and ankle joints.

alignment. From posterior and anterior views, the patient should appear symmetrical from left to right with the line of gravity running through the vertebrae and falling equally between the patient's base of support. From a lateral view, an imaginary vertical line should pass through the external auditory meatus, the acromioclavicular joint, and body of 3rd lumbar vertebra, just posterior to the hip joint, slightly anterior to the knee joint, and the lateral malleolus (see Fig. 8-2 in Chapter 8, Lower Quarter Screen).[6] The pelvis, trunk, and upper quarter posture should be the same in both standing and sitting.

This big picture assessment should be used to begin to understand the patients' overall structure. However, the clinician should be wary of making firm conclusions based on this one-time, static observation. The presence of postural deviations of suboptimal alignment may or may not relate to pain and dysfunction. For example, a forward head position is associated with subacromial pain syndrome,[7] and improving neck position (craniovertebral angle) appears to result in reduced pain.[8] However, when considering thoracic posture, there does not appear to be a direct relationship between increased kyphosis and shoulder pain, despite the immediate effect increased kyphosis has on reducing shoulder range.[9]

Likewise, the absence of structural deviations also does not guarantee normal posture or function. A patient who is able to attain optimal alignment during observation may not be able to maintain this alignment for a functional length of time. Repeated movements or sustained postures can lead to tissue changes and altered movement patterns. Consider a patient who habitually maintains a position of increased kyphosis, scapular protraction, and forward head. This patient's lower trapezius, middle trapezius, and thoracic extensors are maintained in a lengthened position, creating a potential stretch weakness.[10,11] Simultaneously, the patient's pectoralis muscles are maintained in a shortened position, creating the propensity for tightness.[10,11] The individual may be able to sit in a neutral postural alignment when observed by a clinician. However, the patient may quickly fatigue because the altered length-tension relationships make it harder to maintain a more neutral alignment.

Clinicians should remember that structural and postural deviations may be relevant to the patient's chief complaint and warrant further investigation. However, these deviations may not be contributory to the patient's current (or future) pathology. The structural assessment is just one data point that must be put into context with the patient history and remainder of the physical examination. Additional details on structural and postural assessments, as well as the implications of deviations from typical alignment, are covered in the appropriate joint-specific chapters.

Upper Quarter Neurologic Screen

A UQNS is required when the patient reports any upper extremity neurologic symptoms (e.g., tingling, numbness, burning pain, shooting pain). The UQNS consists of four parts: cervical active range of motion (AROM), myotomes, dermatomes, and reflexes (Fig. 13-2). The UQNS is not an examination of the cervical spine but rather a quick screen. If positive, a detailed examination of the spine should follow (see Chapter 17, Cervical and Thoracic Spine).

Cervical Screen To screen the cervical spine, the clinician should assess AROM for the following:
- Cervical flexion and extension
- Cervical sidebending
- Cervical rotation
- Spurling test

The clinician should provide gentle manual overpressure at end range. To maximally close lateral intervertebral foramen, the clinician should perform the Spurling test: a combination of cervical sidebending and extension with gentle overpressure.[12] If this is symptom-free, axial compression can be applied.[13] Spurling's test has high specificity but low sensitivity,[12] making it a poor screening test.[13] However, it can assist with ruling in cervical radiculopathy and takes only a few seconds to perform.[12]

Myotome Screen The purpose of a myotome screen is to identify neurologic involvement by testing the strength of specific muscles that are *primarily* innervated by one spinal nerve root. Table 13-2 provides a list of upper extremity myotomes. Clinicians need to only perform one assessment per myotome. Strength can be assessed using traditional manual muscle testing.

Dermatome Screen A dermatome screen is used to identify neurologic involvement by testing specific areas of cutaneous sensation that are innervated by one spinal nerve root. To perform a dermatomal assessment, the clinician should assess for the presence of light touch sensation using a wisp of cotton or light contact with a fingertip.[14] Testing should be performed directly on the patient's skin and may be performed simultaneously on both sides. The clinician should ask the patient, "Do these feel the same and normal?" Patient response options include normal, absent, hypoesthesia (reduced light touch sensation), or hyperesthesia (increased sensitivity to light touch).

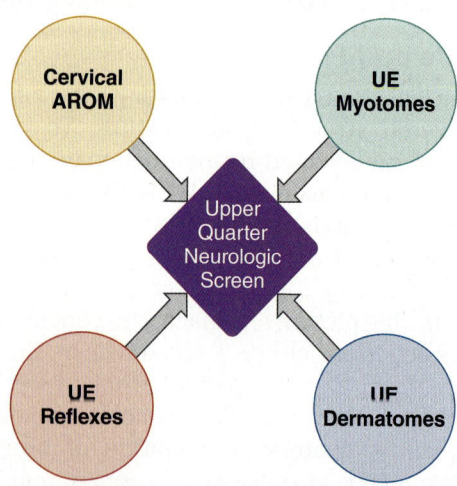

FIGURE 13-2 Components of the upper quarter neurologic screen. *AROM,* active range of motion; *UE,* upper extremity.

TABLE 13-2
UPPER EXTREMITY MYOTOMAL SCREEN

Spinal Nerve Root	Muscle
C5	Deltoid
C6	Biceps, wrist extensors
C7	Triceps, wrist flexors
C8	Extensor pollicis longus, flexor digitorum profundus
T1	Interossei

The clinician may touch specific landmarks or sweep across the general dermatomal region (Fig. 13-3).

Reflex Screen The clinician should assess the biceps (C5), brachioradialis (C6), and triceps (C7) reflexes (Table 13-3). Reflexes should be graded normal, hyperreflexive, diminished, or absent. The Hoffmann test is a sensitive but nonspecific test for upper motor neuron lesion, such as cervical myelopathy.[15] It is performed with the patient in a relaxed seated position. The clinician holds the patient's middle phalanx of 3rd digit and flicks the distal phalanx into flexion. An abnormal response (positive Hoffman sign) is involuntary flexion of the thumb and index finger.

Upper Extremity Motion and Strength

The UQS includes range of motion and strength assessment of all the major joints of the upper quarter (Table 13-4). These tests are designed to provide stress to the contractile and noncontractile tissues for the purposes of identifying a possible source of the patient's symptoms. These also provide an overall understanding of the patient's upper quarter motion, ability to move, and muscle performance. The patient should perform AROM of each joint for each direction. The clinician should note the quantity and quality of movement as well as any change in symptoms. If the motion is pain-free, the clinician should add gentle overpressure to each motion. The clinician should assess passive range of motion of each joint for each direction, noting quantity, end feel, and any crepitus or changes in movement quality. Manual muscle testing should be performed for each motion. Note, unlike the LQS, the assessment of muscle length is not a standard portion of the UQS. This information, when needed, is gathered during the joint-specific examination.

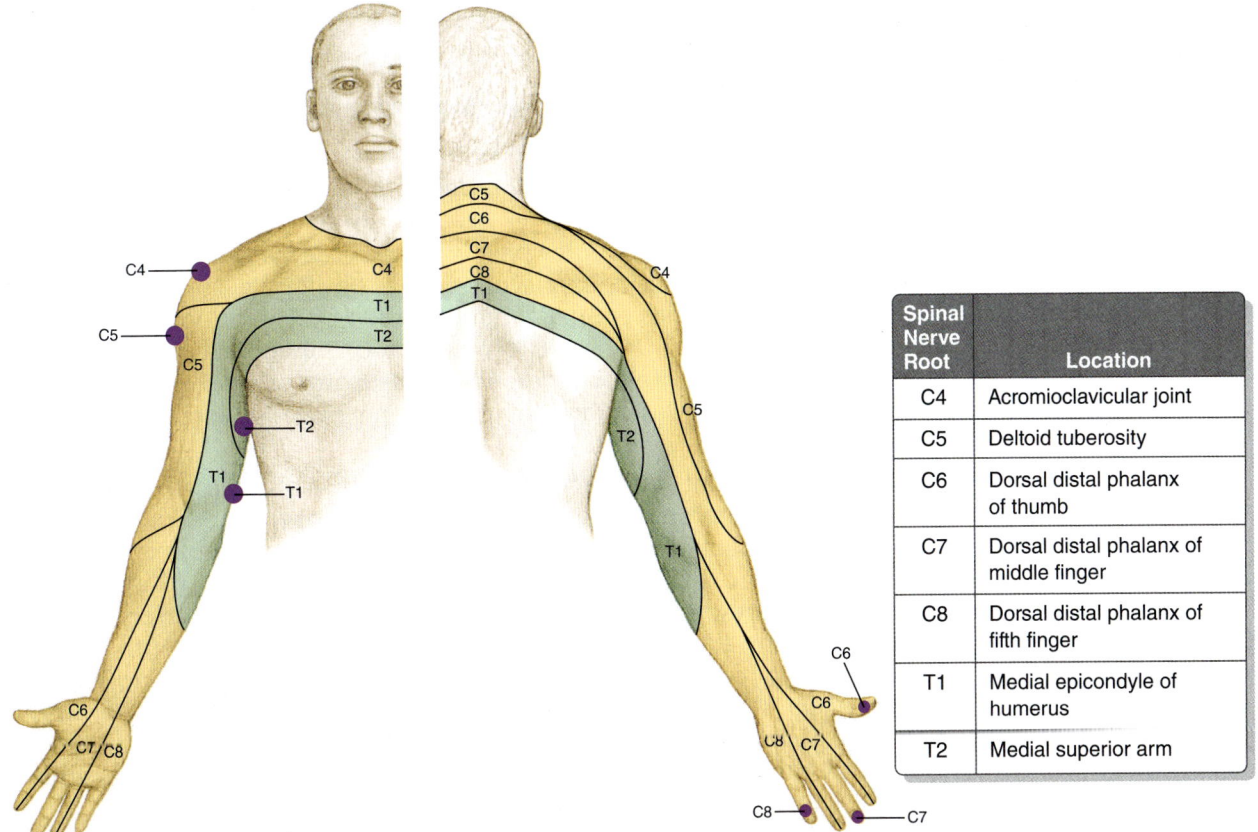

Spinal Nerve Root	Location
C4	Acromioclavicular joint
C5	Deltoid tuberosity
C6	Dorsal distal phalanx of thumb
C7	Dorsal distal phalanx of middle finger
C8	Dorsal distal phalanx of fifth finger
T1	Medial epicondyle of humerus
T2	Medial superior arm

FIGURE 13-3 Upper extremity dermatomal screen. (Modified from Gest TR. *Lippincott Atlas of Anatomy*. 2nd ed. Wolters Kluwer; 2020: Plate 2-54.)

TABLE 13-3
UPPER QUARTER REFLEX SCREEN

Spinal Nerve Root	Tendon Reflex
C5	Biceps
C6	Brachioradialis
C7	Triceps
Upper motor neuron	Hoffman test

TABLE 13-4
UPPER QUARTER SCREEN FOR MOTION AND STRENGTH

Active and Passive Range and Strength

Joint	Motions
Fingers	Flexion, extension
Wrist	Flexion, extension Radial and ulnar deviation
Elbow/forearm	Flexion, extension Pronation, supination
Shoulder	Flexion, extension Abduction, adduction Internal rotation, external rotation Horizontal abduction, horizontal adduction
Cervical	Flexor endurance test*

*Note cervical range of motion was assessed as part of the upper quarter neurologic screen.

Functional Testing

Functional testing during the UQS might include reaching behind the head, behind the back, or overhead. While this concludes the basic UQS functional examination, other functional tasks might include dressing, grooming, opening a jar, writing, and keyboarding. Upper extremity functional tasks related to sport might include having the patient perform a push-up, pull-up, or throw a ball. Grip and pinch assessment using a handheld dynamometer or pinch gauge can provide objective measures of strength that can be compared with normative values.

Integument

Although technically a part of the systems review, assessment of the integument should be performed as part of the UQS. The integumentary screen includes observing the skin color, integrity, pliability, and for abnormalities such as scars, calluses, and nail changes such as staining, splitting, and increased thickness.

Vasculature

Although technically a part of the systems review, assessment of the vasculature, including palpation of the radial, ulnar, and brachial arteries, can be performed as part of the UQS.

CASE STUDY 13-1
Kerwin: Patient With Left Shoulder Pain

Kerwin is a 62-year-old patient who reports left shoulder pain with overhead activities and dressing. Tia is a 25-year-old patient who reports left wrist pain and occasional tingling in her hand after gardening. Neither patient had any contraindications for examination based on the patient interview. All tests begin with the uninvolved (right) side first unless otherwise noted. Similar to the LQS, the UQS should be organized by position, include a progressive increase in tissue stress, and progress toward the area of chief complaint. Table 13-5 provides examples of how an experienced clinician might choose to organize the UQS for two different patients.

The basic framework of the UQS is present for both patients, but there are subtle differences in both content and rationale. For both patients, the clinician began with observation during the history, an overall structural screen, and inspection of the integument. A UQNS was performed on both patients. Even though Kerwin did not report any neurologic symptoms, a thorough investigation of the joint proximal to the shoulder (i.e., the cervical spine) required the clinician to perform a UQNS. This also required the clinician to perform the cervical flexion endurance test and strength testing of scapular muscles. A UQNS was required for Tia because the patient reported hand tingling. However, a more in-depth evaluation of cervical, scapular, or shoulder strength was not necessary. For Kerwin, the clinician chose to use elbow flexion and extension for testing the C6 and C7 myotome rather than the wrist flexors and extensors. This choice was made because assessment of the elbow was required,

TABLE 13-5
SAMPLE UPPER QUARTER SCREENS

	Kerwin: 62-Year-Old Patient Who Reports Left Shoulder Pain With Overhead Activities and Dressing		Tia: 25-Year-Old Patient Who Reports Left Wrist Pain and Occasional Tingling in Her Hand After Gardening
Position	**Assessments**	**Position**	**Assessments**
Observation	Continues from history	Observation	Continues from history
Standing and seated	Structure/posture screen Integument		
Seated	Dermatomes C4-T1 Reflexes: brachialis, biceps, triceps, Hoffman test Cervical AROM with OP: flex, ext, SB, rot Spurling test Finger add (A, MMT) Thumb ext (A, MMT) Elbow flex (A, OP, MMT) Elbow ext (A, OP, MMT) MMT: upper trapezius Shoulder flex (A, OP, MMT) Shoulder abd (A, OP, MMT) Shoulder H abd (A) Shoulder H add (A) Function: reaching, hand behind head, hand behind back	Seated	Structure/posture screen Integument Dermatomes C4-T1 Reflexes: brachialis, biceps, triceps, Hoffman test Cervical AROM with OP: flex, ext, SB, rot Spurling test Finger add (A, MMT) Finger flexion (A, OP, MMT) Finger ext (A, OP, MMT) Thumb flex (A, OP, MMT) Thumb ext (A, OP, MMT) Thumb opposition (A, OP, MMT) Elbow flex (A, OP, P*, MMT) Elbow ext (A, OP, P*, MMT) Forearm pronation (A, OP, P, MMT) Forearm supination (A, OP, P, MMT) Wrist flex (A, OP, P) MMT: FCR, FCU Wrist ext (A, OP, P) MMT: ECRB, ECRL, ECU Wrist radial deviation (A, P) Wrist ulnar deviation (A, P) Function: handheld dynamometer and pinch gauge: grip, pinch
Supine	Elbow PROM: flexion, ext Cervical endurance test Shoulder PROM: flex, ext, abd, ER, IR, H abd, H Add MMT: pectoralis major, serratus anterior	Supine*	Elbow PROM: flex, ext
Prone	MMT: rhomboids, lower trapezius, middle trapezius Shoulder ER (A, OP, MMT) Shoulder IR (A, OP, MMT)	Seated	Transition to wrist-specific examination
Supine	Transition to shoulder-specific examination		

A, active range of motion (AROM); *abd*, abduction; *add*, adduction; *ECRB*, extensor carpi radialis brevis; *ECRL*, extensor carpi radialis longus; *ECU*, extensor carpi ulnaris; *ER*, external rotation; *ext*, extension; *FCR*, flexor carpi radialis; *FCU*, flexor carpi ulnaris; *flex*, flexion; *H Abd*, horizontal abduction; *H Add*, horizontal adduction; *IR*, internal rotation; *L*, left; *MMT*, manual muscle test; *OP*, overpressure; *R*, right; *rot*, rotation; *SB*, side bend.
*For efficiency, passive elbow flexion and extension are screened in the seated position. If limited or painful, they are reassessed in the supine test position.

given the elbow joint is adjacent to the shoulder and, therefore, is also part of the clearing examination for the shoulder whereas the wrist musculature is not. The majority of Tia's evaluation can be performed in the seated position. Therefore, to maximize efficiency, passive elbow flexion and extension are screened in the seated position. If either motion is found to be limited or painful, they will be reassessed in supine for accurate measurements.

There are many acceptable ways to organize the basic upper extremity screen. Clinicians should determine an efficient and inclusive flow that works best for them. Once mastering this basic framework, clinicians should consider modifications based on individual patient presentation. For example, it might be useful for the new clinician to map how the examination flow might be adapted for a patient with elbow pain or a patient who has postoperative restrictions on shoulder motion.

CHAPTER SUMMARY

The UQS includes observation; gross assessment of structure and posture, a UQNS, assessment of upper extremity motion and strength, and functional testing. The UQS helps rule out areas as sources of a patient's complaint, identify relevant impairments within the kinetic chain, elucidate issues that might alter the plan of care, and expedite referral when needed. Clinicians should adapt the basic UQS based on the patient's history, chief complaint, and presentation. Finally, clinicians should organize the screen to maximize efficiency.

REFERENCES

1. Ludewig PM, Kamonseki DH, Staker JL, Lawrence RL, Camargo PR, Braman JP. Changing our diagnostic paradigm: movement system diagnostic classification. *Int J Sports Phys Ther.* 2017;12(6):884–893.
2. Coombes BK, Bisset L, Vicenzino B. Management of lateral elbow tendinopathy: one size does not fit all. *J Orthop Sports Phys Ther.* 2015;45(11):938–949.
3. Urch EY, Lee SK. Carpal fractures other than scaphoid. *Clin Sports Med.* 2015;34(1):51–67.
4. Burrows B, Moreira P, Murphy C, Sadi J, Walton DM. Scaphoid fractures: a higher order analysis of clinical tests and application of clinical reasoning strategies. *Man Ther.* 2014;19(5):372–378.
5. Tsyrulnik A. Emergency department evaluation and treatment of wrist injuries. *Emerg Med Clin North Am.* 2015;33(2):283–296.
6. Kendall FP, McCreary EK, Provance PG, Rogers MM, Romani WZ. *Muscles: Testing and Function with Posture and Pain.* 5th ed. Lippincott Williams & Wilkins; 2005.
7. Land H, Gordon S. Clinical assessment of factors associated with subacromial shoulder impingement: a systematic review. *Phys Ther Rev.* 2016;21(3–6):192–206.
8. Sheikhhoseini R, Shahrbanian S, Sayyadi P, O'Sullivan K. Effectiveness of therapeutic exercise on forward head posture: a systematic review and meta-analysis. *J Manipulative Physiol Ther.* 2018;41(6):530–539.
9. Barrett E, O'Keeffe M, O'Sullivan K, Lewis J, McCreesh K. Is thoracic spine posture associated with shoulder pain, range of motion and function? a systematic review. *Man Ther.* 2016;26:38–46.
10. Sahrmann S. *Diagnosis and Treatment of Movement Impairment Syndromes.* Mosby/Elsevier; 2002.
11. Page P, Frank CC, Lardner R. *Assessment and Treatment of Muscle Imbalance: The Janda Approach.* Human Kinetics; 2010.
12. Bier JD, Scholten-Peeters WGM, Staal JB, et al. Clinical practice guideline for physical therapy assessment and treatment in patients with nonspecific neck pain. *Phys Ther.* 2018;98(3):162–171.
13. Tong HC, Haig AJ, Yamakawa K, Tong HC, Haig AJ, Yamakawa K. The Spurling test and cervical radiculopathy. *Spine.* 2002;27(2):156–159.
14. Leighton RD, Sheldon MR. Model for teaching clinical decision making in a physical therapy professional curriculum. *J Phys Ther Educ.* 1997;11(2):23–30.
15. Grijalva R, Hsu F, Wycliffe N, et al. Hoffman sign. *Spine.* 2015;40(7):475–479.

14 | Shoulder Complex

Betsy Myers and June Hanks

CHAPTER OBJECTIVES

After reading this chapter, you will be able to:
1. Describe the anatomy of the joints forming the shoulder complex to include osteologic ligamentous, capsular, and muscular features.
2. Describe the biomechanics of the articulations of the shoulder complex to include the glenohumeral, acromioclavicular, and sternoclavicular joints.
3. Tailor the basic history to a patient with shoulder pathology.
4. Describe the components of the physical examination for a patient with shoulder pathology.
5. Describe the pathology, history, key examination findings, rehabilitation focus, and expected outcomes of common shoulder pathologies.
6. Hypothesize differential diagnoses of shoulder symptoms based on location, patient complaint, and onset.
7. Organize the physical examination of a patient with shoulder pathology to maximize efficiency.

FUNCTIONAL ANATOMY

The shoulder complex is composed of three bony articulations forming three synovial joints: the glenohumeral (GH) joint, acromioclavicular (AC) joint, and sternoclavicular (SC) joint (Fig. 14-1). Although there is no bony articulation of the scapula directly with the thorax, a "physiologic" scapulothoracic (ST) joint is sometimes described, because the scapula is stabilized to the thorax by musculature attaching to the thorax. The manubrium, along with the clavicles and scapulae on each side, forms an "incomplete girdle" around the superior thorax, referred to as the *shoulder girdle*. The components of the shoulder complex interrelate functionally to provide coordinated movement of the entire upper extremity. The bony, capsular, ligamentous, and muscular anatomy of the associated joints provides an example of a compromise between joint mobility and stability.[1] The shoulder complex allows a tremendous amount of mobility necessary to place the hand in space for the performance of tasks, such as throwing a baseball or placing a box on an overhead shelf. Stability and mobility provided by the bony shapes, joint capsules, ligaments, and muscles surrounding the shoulder complex allows for daily activities, such as reaching to change a lightbulb overhead, mopping the floor with sweeping motions, or reaching to put on a seatbelt. The transferring of forces

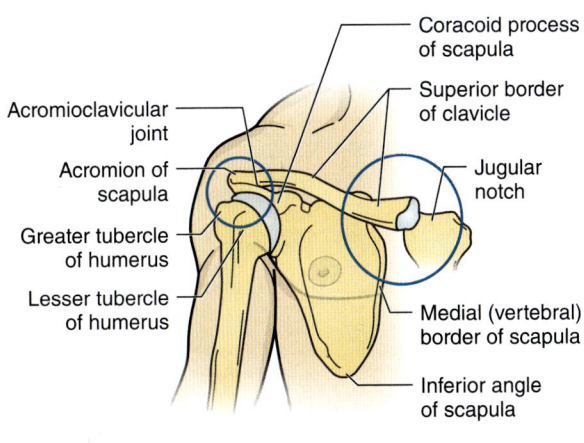

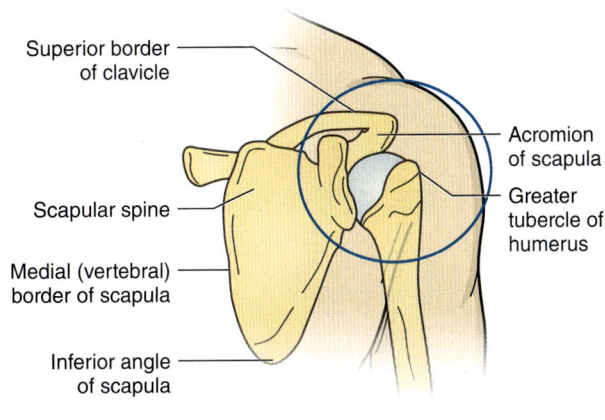

FIGURE 14-1 Major joints of the shoulder girdle. Half of the right shoulder girdle is depicted here. **A.** Anterior view **B.** Posterior view. Note that there is no direct bony articulation of the scapula with the thorax. (Adapted from Gest TR. *Lippincott Atlas of Anatomy*. 2nd ed. Wolters Kluwer; 2020: Plate 2-42.)

to and from the trunk, as occurs with activities such as splitting wood with an axe, hitting a softball, or serving a tennis ball, occurs through the shoulder joint.

The shoulder complex is subjected to a high level of overuse stresses in many manual occupations and sporting activities. Muscle imbalance, direct trauma, repetitive microtrauma, postural adaptations, and degenerative processes lead to a broad spectrum of pathologies. Diagnosing and treating shoulder motion abnormalities is ultimately dependent upon a strong understanding of movement at all portions of the shoulder complex.

Osteology

This section provides an overview of osteology and discusses the functional anatomy of each joint composing the shoulder complex. The bones of the shoulder complex include the clavicle, scapula, and humerus. The manubrium of the sternum is part of the axial skeleton and is discussed in this section as part of the SC joint. The upper thoracic and cervical vertebrae and superior ribs provide attachment for muscles of the shoulder complex. Therefore, the shape and stability of the spine influences function of the shoulder complex.

Clavicle The clavicle (collar bone) is a double-curved, angulated bone that lies primarily in the transverse plane. The medial half of the clavicle is convex anteriorly, following the convexity of the thorax, and the lateral half is concave anteriorly. The large triangularly shaped medial articulating end of the clavicle articulates with the manubrium of the sternum. The lateral end of the clavicle articulates with the acromial facet of the scapula (Fig. 14-2). The conoid tubercle

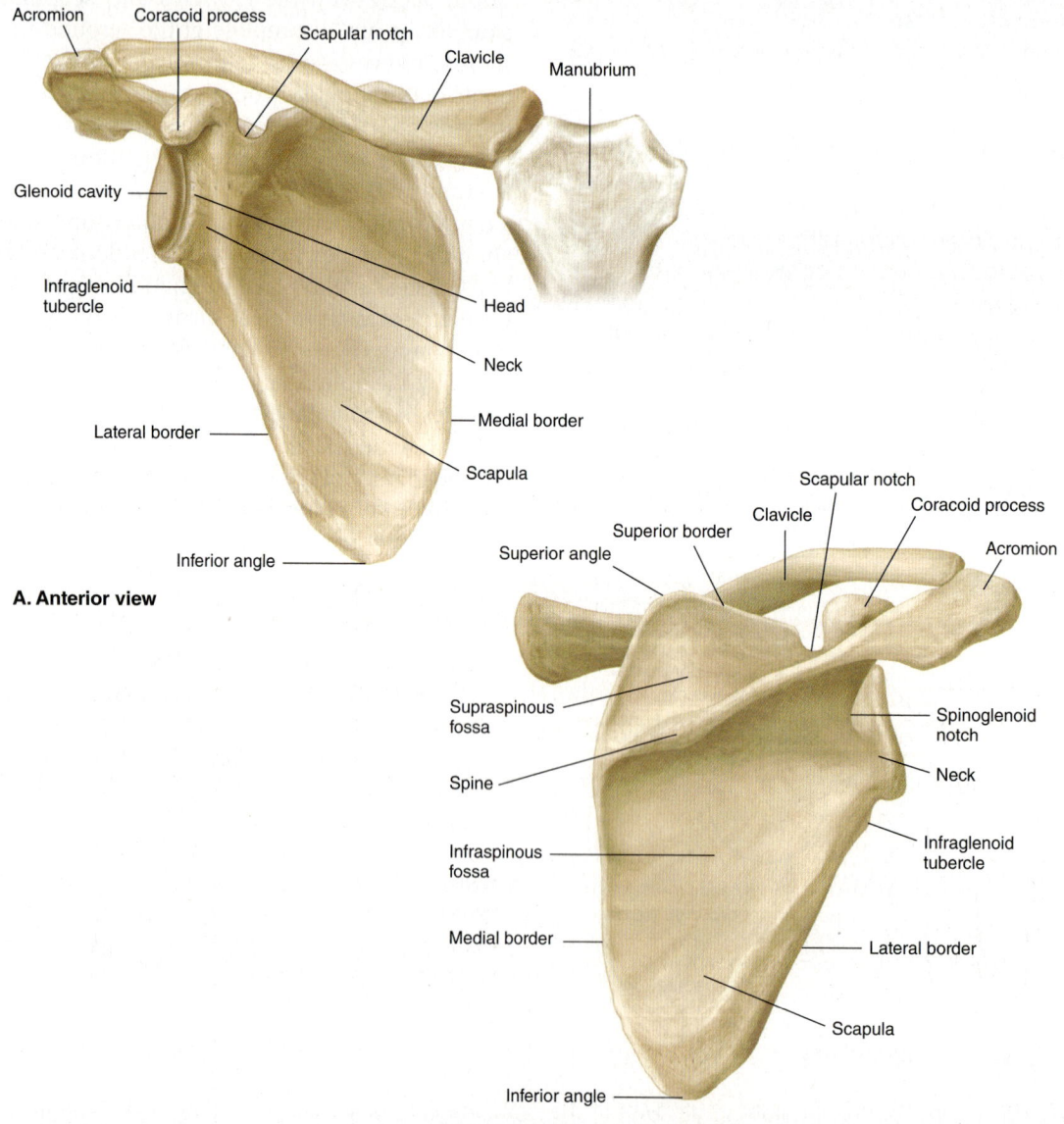

FIGURE 14-2 Manubrium, clavicle, and scapula with major landmarks. **A.** Anterior view **B.** Posterior view. (Modified from Gest TR. *Lippincott Atlas of Anatomy*. 2nd ed. Wolters Kluwer; 2020: Plate 2-03.)

and trapezoid line on the inferolateral aspect of the clavicle provide attachment sites for ligaments that suspend the scapula on the clavicle and stabilize the AC joint. The clavicle protects the underlying blood vessels and nerves and contributes to shoulder range of motion.

Scapula The flat scapula (shoulder blade) is a triangularly shaped bone with a thin body and thickened superior, medial (vertebral), and lateral (axillary) borders. The scapula lies over ribs 2 to 7 on the posterolateral portion of the upper thorax. The posterior surface is convexly curved and divided into a superior and inferior portion by the spine of the scapula, a thick bony ridge that creates two fossae: the supraspinatus fossa and the more shallow and larger infraspinatus fossa. The concave-shaped costal (anterior) surface of the scapula forms the subscapular fossa. The body of the scapula is thin, whereas the borders are thick, providing attachment for muscles of the shoulder girdle. Beginning on the posterior medial scapular border as the root, the spine of the scapula passes laterally and superiorly, ending as a large projection called the *acromion* process. The acromion forms a large partially curved surface of varied shape and slope,[2] providing a roof over the humerus. The shape of the acromion may contribute to impingement problems of the GH joint. The anteromedial portion of the acromion bears a facet for articulation with the clavicle. The lateral border of the scapula passes from the inferior angle toward the axilla, with the thickest portion forming the head of the scapula, whose primary feature is the glenoid cavity (fossa). The glenoid cavity is a shallow, concave surface facing anterolaterally and slightly superiorly from the lateral scapula. Superior and medial to the glenoid cavity is the coracoid process, a beaklike projection with the tip pointing toward the shoulder joint. Along the superior border of the scapula near the base of the coracoid process is the depression named the suprascapular notch. The superior transverse scapular ligament passes to either side of the notch, creating a tunnel for passage of the suprascapular nerve. Between the lateral base of the scapular spine and the scapular head is the spinoglenoid fossa (notch), around which the suprascapular nerve passes, bounded by the inferior transverse scapular ligament (spinoglenoid ligament), on its course to innervate the infraspinatus. Figure 14-2 shows key bony landmarks on the scapula.

Proximal Humerus The humerus is the largest bone of the upper extremity. The convex-shaped humeral head articulates with the concave-shaped glenoid cavity of the scapula, forming the GH joint. The head of the humerus is inclined 135° in the frontal plane (Fig. 14-3A) and angled posteriorly in the transverse

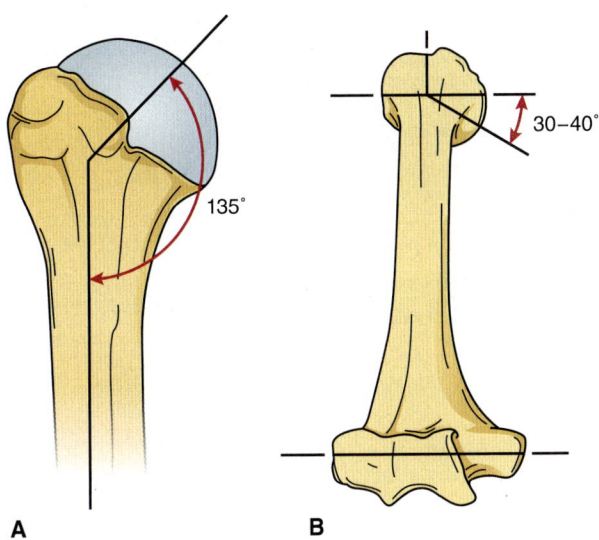

FIGURE 14-3 Orientation of the head of the humerus. **A.** In the frontal plane, the humeral head is inclined approximately 135° with the humeral shaft. **B.** The humeral head is retroverted 30 to 40° in the transverse plane relative to the distal aspect of the humerus. (From Itoi E, Morrey BF, An KN. Biomechanics of the shoulder. In: Rockwood CA, Matsen FA, eds. *The Shoulder, Volume 1.* W.B. Saunders Co; 1990. Used with permission of Mayo Foundation for Medical Education and Research. All rights reserved.)

plane approximately 30 to 40° relative to the distal condyle of the humerus (Fig. 14-3B), allowing the humerus to align with the glenoid fossa of the scapula while maintaining the elbow alignment. The joint capsule of the GH joint extends from the neck of the humerus to the glenoid cavity of the scapula.[3] The greater tubercle projects laterally as a prominence just distal to the neck of the humerus. The greater tubercle bears three facets: the superior, middle, and inferior facet. Each facet serves as a muscular attachment for the supraspinatus, infraspinatus, and teres minor, respectively. Distal to the humeral neck and projecting anteriorly is the lesser tubercle that serves as a muscular attachment for the subscapularis muscle. Located between the greater and lesser tubercles is the intertubercular groove that follows along the anterior portion of the proximal humerus. The intertubercular groove is also known as the *bicipital* groove that houses the long head of the biceps brachii before the tendon reaches its proximal attachment of the supraglenoid tubercle of the scapula. Distal to the intertubercular groove on the anterolateral aspect of the humeral shaft is the deltoid tuberosity that serves as the distal attachment of the deltoid muscle. Along the shaft of the humerus is the radial groove that runs obliquely along the posterior aspect of the bone, guiding the radial nerve as it passes from behind the proximal humerus to the anterior distal humerus (see Fig. 14-4 for major bony landmarks).

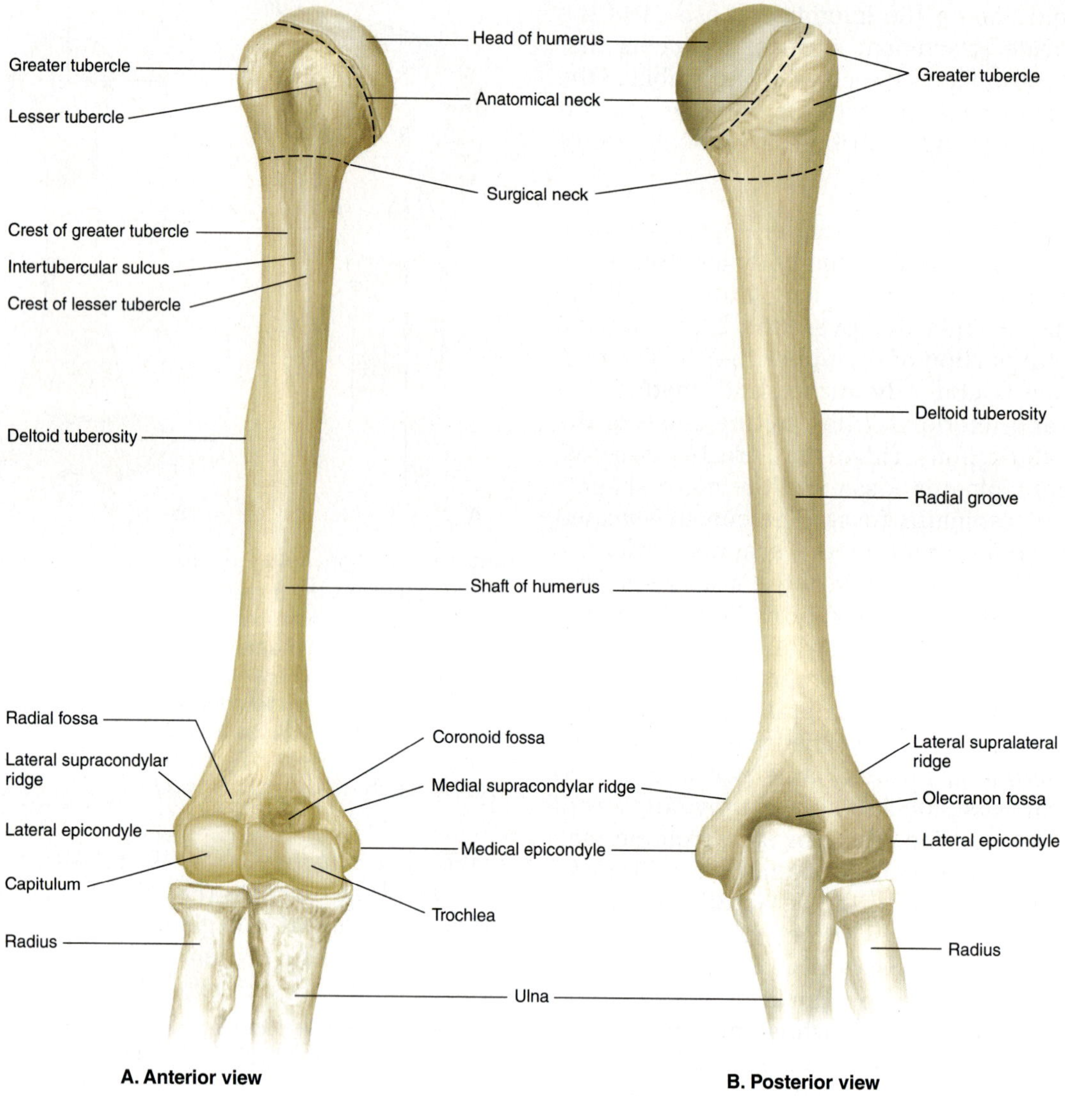

FIGURE 14-4 Humerus with major bony landmarks. **A.** Anterior view **B.** Posterior view. (Modified from Gest TR. *Lippincott Atlas of Anatomy*. 2nd ed. Wolters Kluwer; 2020: Plate 2-03.)

JOINTS OF THE SHOULDER COMPLEX

Before considering the joints of the shoulder complex, the resting position of the scapula on the thorax should be clarified. The scapula is internally rotated approximately 30 to 40° from the frontal plane, described as the "plane of the scapula," as illustrated in Figure 14-5. The scapula is anteriorly tilted 10 to 15° from vertical and is upwardly rotated 5 to 10° (Fig. 14-6).[4] The resting position of the scapula varies greatly even among healthy individuals.

Motions of the scapula from the resting position include elevation/depression (Fig. 14-7A), adduction/abduction (also called *protraction/retraction*) (Fig. 14-7B), anterior/posterior tilting (Fig. 14-7C), upward/downward rotation (Fig. 14-7D), and internal/external rotation (Fig. 14-7E). Scapular motions occur as combined simultaneous motions. For example, when the arm is abducted, the scapula normally moves into a position of upward rotation, external rotation, and posterior

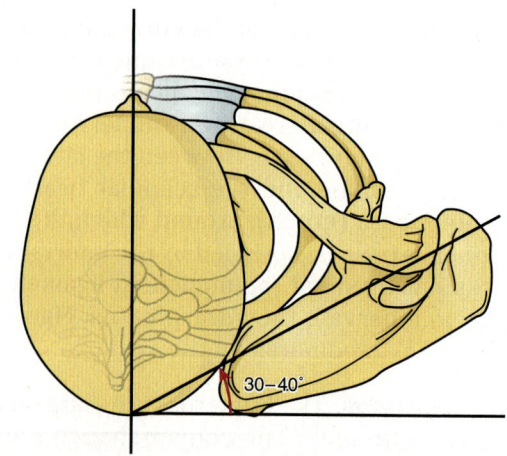

FIGURE 14-5 Plane of the scapula. (Warner JP. The gross anatomy of the joint surfaces, ligaments, labrum, and capsule. In: Matsen FA, Fu FH, Hawkins RJ, eds. *The Shoulder: A Balance of Mobility and Stability*. American Academy of Orthopaedic Surgeons; 1993:9.)

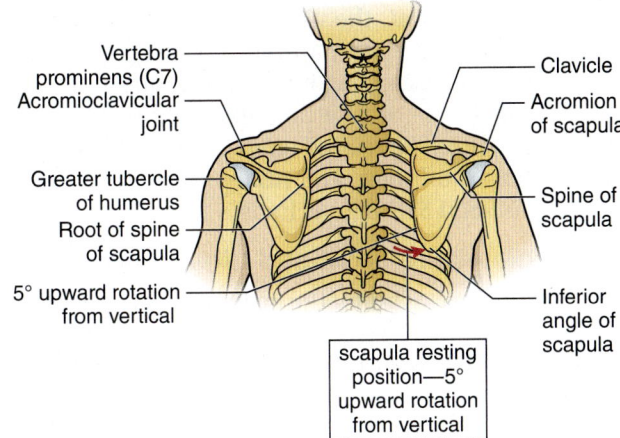

FIGURE 14-6 Posterior view of scapula demonstrating resting position on the thorax. Note the slight upward rotation from vertical. (Adapted from Gest TR. *Lippincott Atlas of Anatomy*. 2nd ed. Wolters Kluwer; 2020: Plate 1-02.)

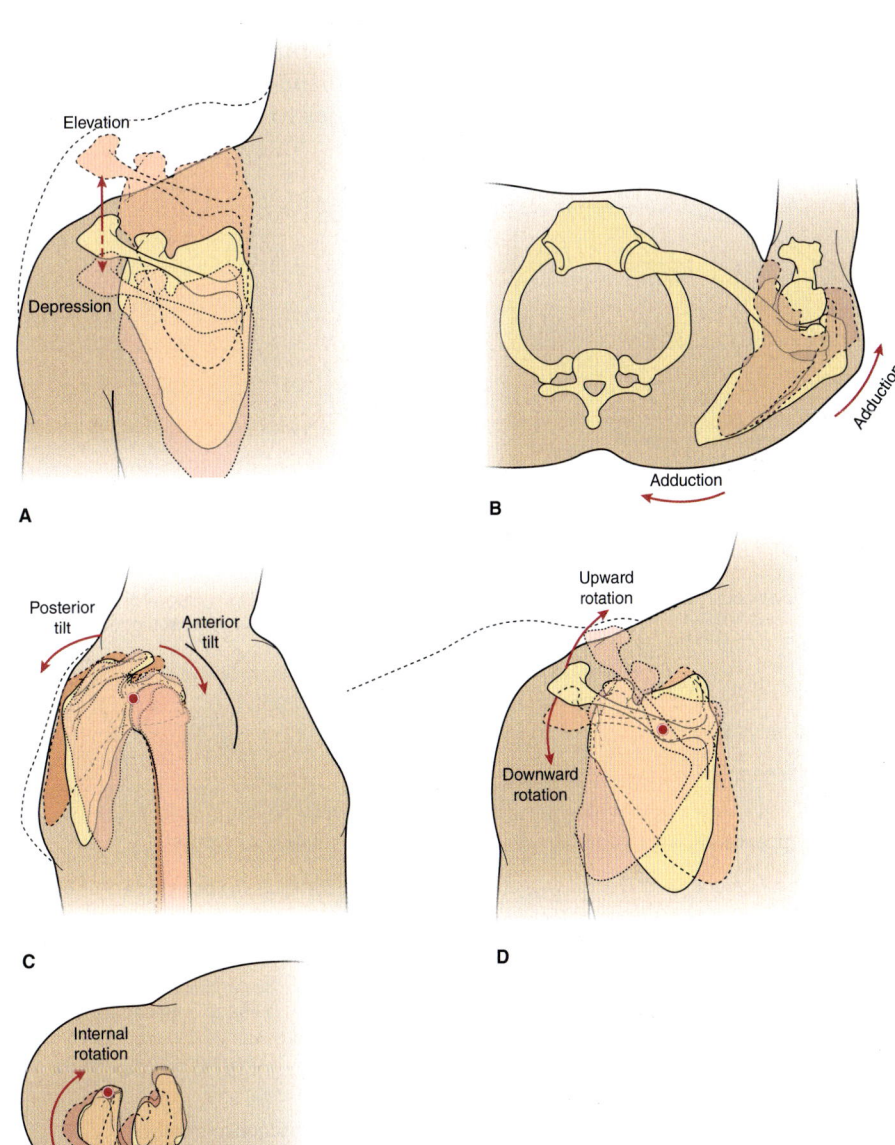

FIGURE 14-7 Movements of the scapula. **A.** Elevation/depression. **B.** Abduction/adduction (protraction/retraction). **C.** Anterior/posterior tilt. **D.** Upward/downward rotation. **E.** internal/external rotation. (Adapted from Oatis, CA. *Kinesiology: The Mechanics and Pathomechanics of Human Movement*. 3rd ed. Wolters Kluwer; 2017: Figure 8.22.)

tilting. Scapular motion is linked to motions allowed by, and occurring at, the AC and SC joints. During active elevation of the arm, upward rotation is the most easily observed scapular motion. Motions at the AC and SC joints are not as easily observed and are difficult to measure. The related movements of the scapula on the thorax, SC joint, and AC joint are described in the AC joint and ST joint sections.

Sternoclavicular Joint and Ligaments

The SC joint is formed by the articulation between the medial end of the clavicle with the manubrium of the sternum and the first costal cartilage (Fig. 14-8). The SC joint relies heavily on capsuloligamentous structures for stability[5] owing to the inherent instability from the sellar-shaped joint surfaces.[6] A fibrocartilaginous articular disc lies between the bony structures, attaching superiorly and posteriorly to the clavicle and to the interclavicular ligament that passes between the clavicles. Inferiorly, the disc attaches to the manubrium (Fig. 14-9). The outer rim of the disc attaches to

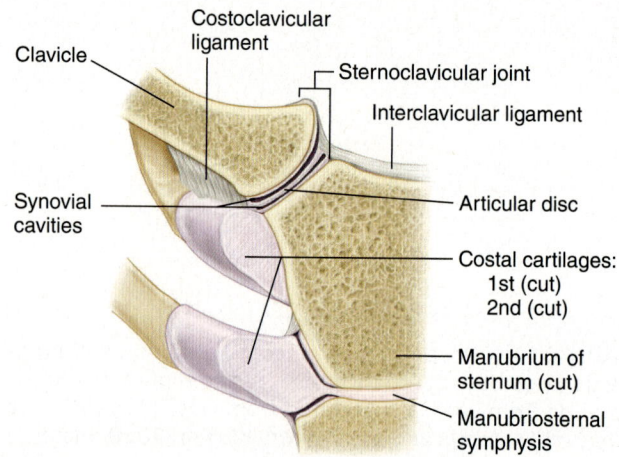

FIGURE 14-9 Coronal view of sternoclavicular joint with disc and ligaments. (Gest TR. *Lippincott Atlas of Anatomy*. 2nd ed. Wolters Kluwer; 2020: Plate 2-42C.)

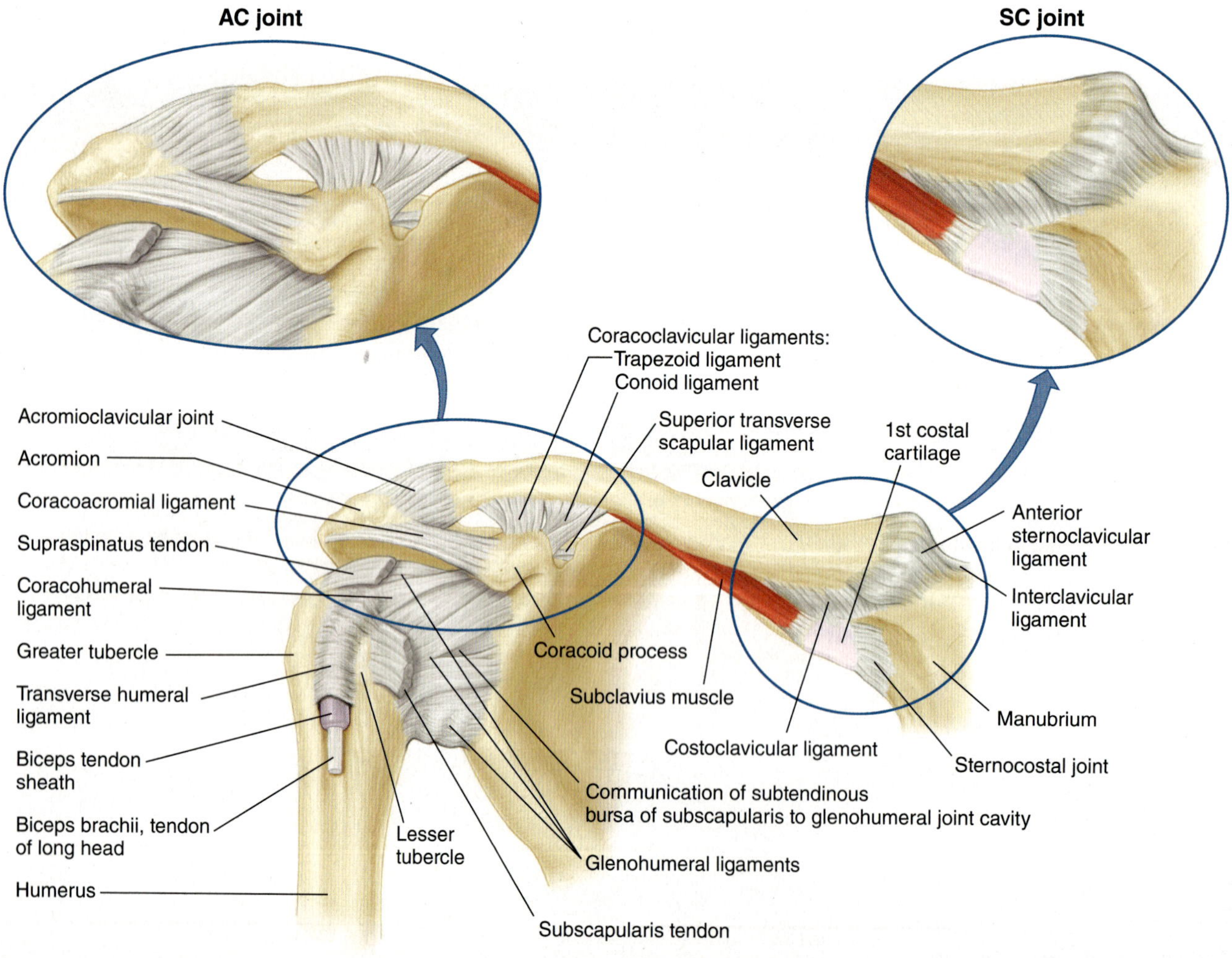

FIGURE 14-8 Sternoclavicular (SC) and acromioclavicular (AC) joints with associated ligaments. (Modified from Gest TR. *Lippincott Atlas of Anatomy*. 2nd ed. Wolters Kluwer; 2020: Plate 2-42A.)

the surrounding joint capsule, dividing the joint into two compartments,[7,8] which adds to resistance to medial displacement of the clavicle on the sternum,[6] as could occur with a blow to the lateral shoulder. This section provides an overview of osteology and discusses the functional anatomy of each joint composing the shoulder complex.

Thickenings of the joint capsule form the stabilizing anterior and posterior SC ligaments that limit anterior and posterior gliding of the medial clavicle on the sternum. The interclavicular ligament, another thickening of the capsule, passes between the superior medial clavicles and the restricting superior and lateral movement of the clavicle on the sternum. The costoclavicular ligament lies outside the joint capsule and attaches to the clavicle and the first rib. The fibers of the costoclavicular ligament run in multiple directions, providing significant stabilization to the clavicle during scapular movement (see Fig. 14-7).[9] The strong stabilization of the clavicle at and near the ends of the bone limits movement in all directions, rendering the clavicle more vulnerable to traumatic fracture than dislocation.[10] Clavicle fractures are common, constituting 5 to 10% of all upper limb fractures,[11] with the majority occurring in the middle third portion of the bone.[10,12] Most clavicle fractures are closed fractures, with a first rib fracture being the most common concomitant fracture along with clavicle fractures.[13]

Movement at the SC joint allows for large amounts of clavicular and scapular motion. The movements of elevation and depression occur in the frontal plane about an anteroposterior (AP) axis. With elevation and depression, the lateral clavicle moves upward and downward, respectively. In this movement, the medial articular surface of the ST joint glides on the disc.[14] Posterior and anterior (long-axis) rotation runs longitudinally throughout the clavicle occurring about a mediolateral (ML) axis. Movement is between a portion of the disc over the first rib and the anteroinferior edge of the medial clavicle articular surface.[15] With posterior clavicle rotation, the inferior portion of the clavicle moves to face anteriorly in a motion some refer to as upward or backward rotation.[14] From this upwardly rotated position, the clavicle can anteriorly rotate, returning to the neutral position. Figure 14-10 demonstrates axes of rotation for the SC joint.

Acromioclavicular Joint and Ligaments

The AC joint is a plane synovial joint formed by the acromion of the scapula and the lateral end of the clavicle. The articulating ends are covered with fibrocartilage and are reciprocally slightly concave and convex to varying degrees, but are essentially flat.[16] The articulating facets are small and allow limited motion. Joint surfaces are separated by a partial or complete wedge-shaped articular disc[17] that degenerates

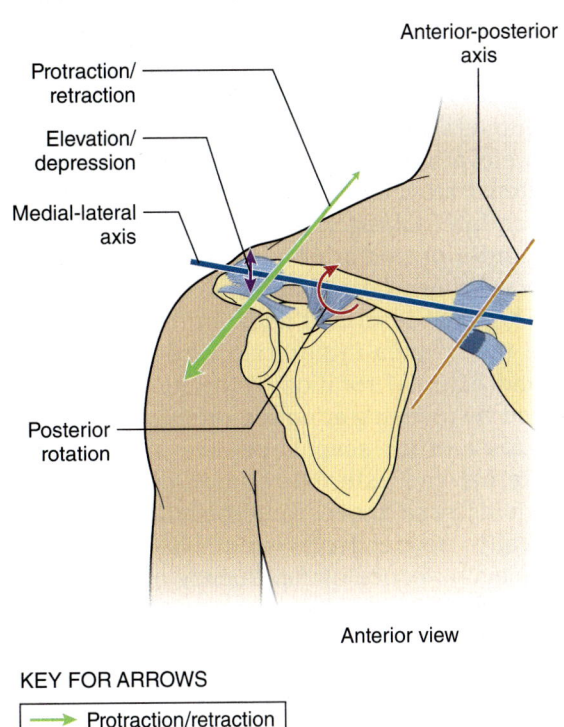

FIGURE 14-10 Axis of rotation and movements for sternoclavicular joint demonstrating elevation/depression, protraction/retraction, and posterior/anterior rotation. (Gest TR. *Lippincott Atlas of Anatomy*. 2nd ed. Wolters Kluwer; 2020: Plate 2-42A.)

significantly by the fourth decade.[7,18] The joint capsule is relatively thin and weak, but has heavy ligamentous support through the AC ligaments, particularly superiorly where the superior AC ligament is thickest.[19,20] The two extracapsular coracoclavicular ligaments, the trapezoid and coracoid ligaments, are important stabilizers of the joint and help maintain the relationship between the clavicle and the scapula[21,22] through the orientation of the ligamentous fibers (see Fig. 14-8). The oblique orientation of the trapezoid ligament resists longitudinal compressive forces that could move the acromion inferior to and medially along the clavicle,[23] such as could occur with a blow to or fall onto the shoulder. The conoid ligament is more vertically aligned and constrains most other directions of loading, especially as displacement and loading increases.[18,21,23] The coracoacromial ligament attaches to the acromion and coracoid processes of the scapula, forming a roof over the humeral head and providing fibers that blend with the inferior AC ligament.

Terminology describing motion at the AC joint and movement of the scapula varies. Motion at the AC joint allows for motion between the scapula and the clavicle and influences the mobility of the scapula on the thorax. AC joint movement is more subtle than that of the SC joint, allowing for minor adjustments in movement of the scapula on the thorax and keeping the humeral head aligned in the glenoid fossa during arm elevation. Although plane joints allow only translational movement, some authors describe AC motion as internal/external rotation around a vertical axis, anterior/posterior tilting around an ML axis, and upward/downward rotation occurring around an AP axis.[4,24] The described axes are oriented to the plane of the scapula rather than cardinal planes. Internal and external rotation of the AC joint may be visualized by focusing attention on movement of the glenoid fossa of the scapula relative to the clavicle. With internal and external rotation of the scapula, the glenoid fossa moves anteromedially and posterolaterally, respectively, orienting the glenoid fossa for maintenance of congruency of the humeral head to maximize stability and movement at the GH joint.[8] The motion of anterior and posterior tilting of the scapula occurs in the sagittal plane relative to the plane of the scapula, with anterior tilting of the scapula superior scapula whereas the inferior angle of the scapula tilts backward, resulting in forward tilting of the acromion. With posterior tilting of the scapula, the acromion moves backward whereas the inferior angle of the scapula moves forward. Upward and downward rotation tilts the glenoid fossa superiorly and inferiorly, respectively, about an AP axis oriented perpendicular to the plane of the scapula. The motion is limited by tension in the coracoclavicular ligaments. The range of motion at the AC joint is difficult to assess and is reported with a wide range of variability among studies.[14,25,26] The upward rotation motion is dependent, in part, on rotation of the SC joint on the ML axis. Posterior rotation of the clavicle reduces tension in the coracoclavicular ligaments, allowing more upward rotation of the scapula.

Scapulothoracic Joint

As previously described, the lack of bony articulation between the scapula and the thorax renders the ST "joint" as a functional rather than true anatomic joint. Muscle separates the scapula from the thorax and guides movement of the scapula. The shoulder complex requires "coupled" scapular and clavicular motion. In other words, ST motion occurs due to SC and AC joint motions occurring together.[27] The ST muscles function through the SC and AC joints, though motions at these joints are not as easily observed on clinical examination as are the majority of scapular motions. Coordinated movement among all joints of the shoulder girdle is critical to normal movement of the scapula on the curved thorax.

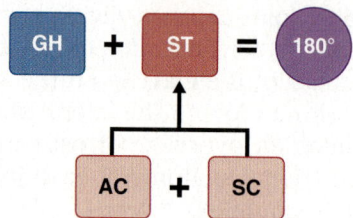

FIGURE 14-11 Components of shoulder motion. *AC*, acromioclavicular joint; *GH*, glenohumeral joint; *SC*, sternoclavicular joint; *ST*, scapulothoracic joint.

Specifically, during elevation of the arm, the scapula upwardly rotates approximately 60° with concurrent and varied degrees of movement at both the SC and AC joints (Fig. 14-11). Typically, scapular upward/downward rotation results from a combination of SC joint posterior/anterior rotation, SC joint elevation/depression, and AC joint upward/downward rotation.[25] The more obvious movements of the scapula on the thorax are produced by movement of the SC joint and the adjusted movement of the AC joint. That is, the SC joint movement proportionately contributes more to the overall scapular movement with the "fine-tuning" of the movement occurring at the AC joint as an "adjusted" movement. For example, SC joint elevation with posterior rotation is coupled with ST joint upward rotation[25] and an adjusted movement of upward rotation at the AC joint. Elevation and depression of the scapula occurs through shrugging of the shoulders up and down. During a shoulder shrug upward, the clavicle is elevated at the SC joint, with more subtle adjusted rotations (anterior/posterior tilting and internal/external rotation) at the AC joint.[8] During protraction of the scapula, the glenoid fossa faces somewhat anteriorly, whereas the SC joint is protracted and the AC joint is internally rotated.

The coordinated movement among the SC and AC joints allows the scapula to maintain contact with the thorax during movement of the arm. Excessive internal rotation of the scapula occurs primarily at the AC joint and will be observed clinically as "scapular winging" in which the vertebral border of the scapula loses contact with the thorax as the arm is elevated. Anterior/posterior tilting of the scapula on the thorax occurs primarily at the AC joint[4] and may occur as a coupled movement with elevation/depression at the SC joint.[25] Excessive scapula internal rotation or anterior tilting may be the result of poor neuromuscular control or tightness of the ST muscles.

The muscles attaching to the thorax and shoulder girdle maintain contact between the clavicle and the scapula and produce movements of the scapula. In addition, these ST muscles help stabilize the scapula to the thorax to provide a stable base for movement at the GH joint. These muscular associations are discussed later in this chapter.

Subacromial Space

The coracoid process, acromion and coracoacromial ligament, and inferior AC joint form an osseoligamentous arch over the humeral head (see Fig. 14-8) with the intervening region called the *subacromial space*. Occupying a portion of this space are fluid-filled bursal sacs that reduce friction between structures. The subacromial and subdeltoid bursae may be separate or continuous with each other and are collectively referred to as the *subacromial bursa* (Fig. 14-12). Normally, the bursae have a thin layer of fluid, but may become inflamed, thus reducing the subacromial space. Inflammation of the bursa may occur due to pathology of the rotator cuff or, in some cases, occurs as the primary problem. Other bursae around the GH include the subscapular bursa, which may communicate with the GH joint cavity.

Glenohumeral Joint and Ligaments

The GH joint, formed by the articulation of the proximal humeral head and the glenoid fossa of the scapula, lacks inherent bony stability[28] and is the most mobile joints in the body.[29] Both articular surfaces are ovoid shaped (nearly spherical) with differing, but similar curvatures, allowing a relatively congruent fit between the surfaces. The size of the convex-shaped humeral articular surface is nearly twice that of the concave-shaped glenoid fossa, with only a small portion of its surface contacting the glenoid fossa. The difference in size of the joint surfaces affords a great amount of mobility, but offers limited stability.

Static Stabilization of Glenohumeral Joint Stabilization of the GH joint occurs through various static and dynamic mechanisms (Table 14-1). Factors contributing to the stability of the GH joint include the static restraints of bony configuration, glenoid labrum, joint capsule, ligaments, and deep surrounding muscles. The coracoid, acromion, and distal clavicle restrain proximal migration of the humeral head.[30] The glenoid fossa is of varying depth, being deeper superoinferiorly than anteroposteriorly.[31] The glenoid labrum, a fibrocartilaginous rim around the glenoid fossa, further increases the depth of the fossa and provides an anchor for the joint capsule, GH ligaments, and biceps tendon long head (Fig. 14-13).[32] The glenoid labrum is more loosely attached in the anterior and anterosuperior aspects and more firmly attached inferiorly. Superiorly, the labrum is loosely attached and envelops the tendon of the long head of the biceps. The contact between the humerus and glenoid surfaces help maintain a relatively constant ligamentous tension and capsule volume.[28] Even a small disruption of bone from either the glenoid fossa or humeral head results in instability.[28,33–35] The capsule and ligaments around the GH joint form a capsuloligamentous complex (see Fig. 14-8). The GH

TABLE 14-1
MECHANISMS CONTRIBUTING TO STABILIZATION OF GLENOHUMERAL JOINT

Dynamic	Static
Rotator cuff	Glenoid labrum
Long head of biceps	Glenohumeral joint capsule
Proprioception	Ligaments
Neuromuscular control	Negative intra-articular pressure

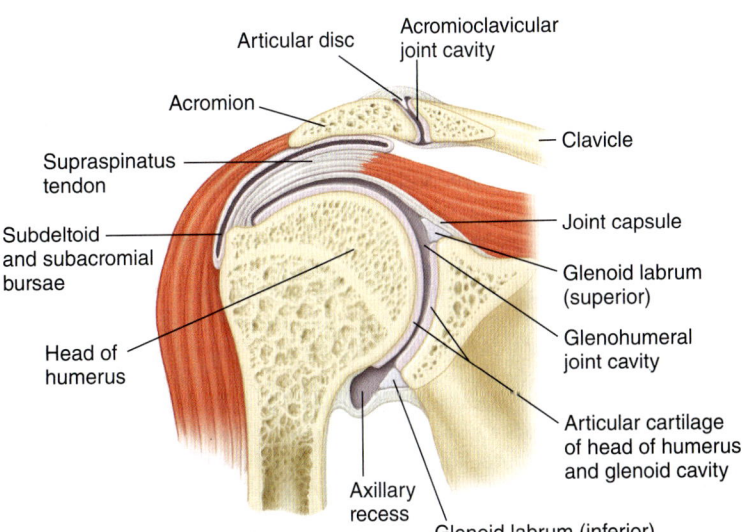

FIGURE 14-12 Coronal section of glenohumeral joint. (Gest TR. *Lippincott Atlas of Anatomy*. 2nd ed. Wolters Kluwer; 2020: Plate 2-42B.)

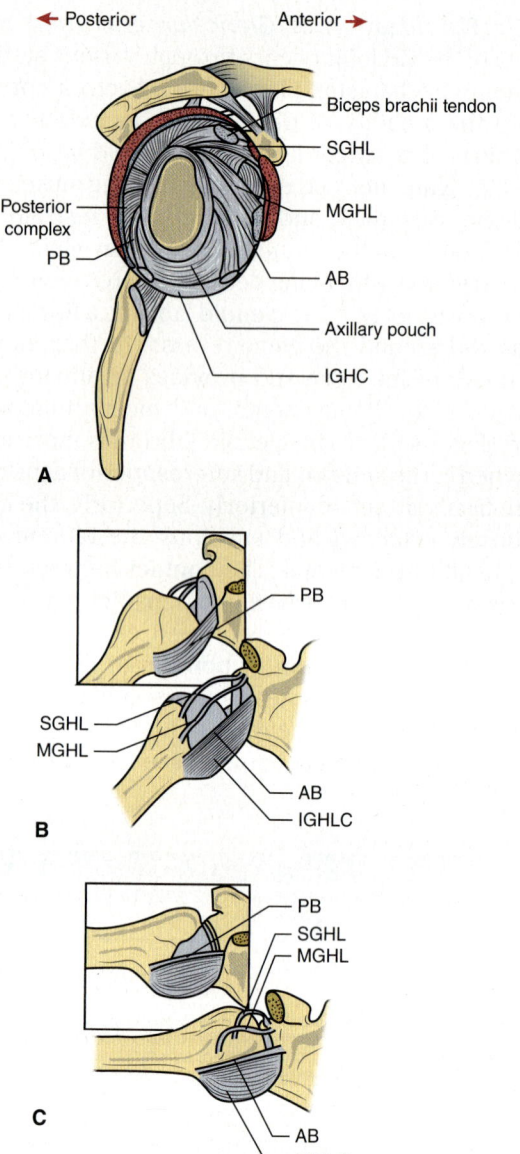

FIGURE 14-13 Glenoid fossa, labrum with associated ligaments. **A.** Lateral view of glenoid fossa showing superior glenohumeral ligament (SGHL) and middle glenohumeral ligament (MGHL) and the larger inferior glenohumeral ligament, referred to as the inferior glenohumeral ligament complex (IGHLC). **B.** Glenohumeral ligaments with shoulder in slight abduction. The upper image shows a posterior view illustrating the narrow SGHL and MGHL and delineation of the posterior band (PB) component of the IGHLC. The lower image shows the same ligaments from the anterior view, with the IGHLC anterior band (AB) component delineated. **C.** Glenohumeral ligaments with shoulder 90° abduction. The upper image shows a posterior view with the visible PB component of the IGHLC delineated. The lower image shows the same ligaments from the anterior view, with the IGHLC AB component delineated. (**A:** O'Brien SJ, Neves MC, Arnoczky SP, et al. The anatomy and histology of the inferior glenohumeral ligament complex of the shoulder. *Am J Sports Med*. 1990;18:579–584. Copyright © 1990 SAGE Publications. **B, C:** Warner JJ, Deng XH, Warren RF, et al. Static capsuloligamentous restraints to superior-inferior translation of the glenohumeral joint. *Am J Sports Med*. 1992;20:675–685. Copyright © 1992 SAGE Publications.)

joint capsule attaches to the anatomic neck of the humerus and to the periphery of the glenoid fossa and labrum. The capsule is taut superiorly and loose inferiorly, forming folds (axillary recesses) that open or unfold during GH joint elevation (see Fig. 14-12). The capsule as a whole is tightest when the humerus is abducted and laterally rotated.

The capsule is reinforced by GH ligaments anteriorly and by the coracohumeral ligament (CHL) superiorly. The GH ligaments (superior, anterior, and inferior) are thickenings of the joint capsule, with each contributing to stability of the joint. The inferior glenohumeral ligament (IGHL) is hammock-like with multiple components (anterior and posterior band with intervening axillary pouch) and is sometimes referred to as the *IGHL complex* (IGHLC). The bands of the IGHLC become taut in varying degrees of GH abduction (Fig. 14-13). The inferior glide of the humeral head created by the weight of the upper extremity in upright posture is resisted by the CHL,[29] whereas the resistance of the superior GH ligament (SGHL) and IGHL is debated when the arm is in this position.[29,36] The three GH ligaments limit excessive anterior movement of the humeral head on the glenoid fossa, particularly during external rotation,[37] with the IGHL playing a greater role as the magnitude of external rotation increases.[38] Similarly, these ligaments limit excessive lateral rotation, with the IGHL providing more of the resistance to motion as abduction increases.[39] Table 14-2 provides a description of the ligaments of the GH joint.

Dynamic Stabilization of the Glenohumeral Joint

The rotator cuff muscles are major contributors to dynamic stabilization of the GH joint.[40–42] Coordinated contractions of the rotator cuff muscles create a compressive force that maintains the humeral head centered within the shallow glenoid fossa. The rotator cuff muscles are intimately blended with the joint capsule[43]; thus, contraction also increases tension within the capsule and GH ligaments, further increasing joint stability. The lines of pull of the infraspinatus, teres minor, and subscapularis create a compressive force on GH joint. The long head of the biceps may assist with joint stability[44,45] through its attachment with the glenoid labrum, by increasing joint compression forces, and by acting as a barrier to humeral head translation. Dynamic stability is also improved by proper firing of the muscles of the shoulder girdle,[43] such as the latissimus dorsi, pectoralis major, serratus anterior, and rhomboids, which allow the scapula to follow the humeral head during elevation.[46] Joint proprioception also improves GH stability.[46] Sensory fibers within the capsule and ligaments provide feedback about joint position sense, allowing more precise neuromuscular control.

The negative intra-articular pressure and compression of the humeral head into the glenoid fossa via the capsuloligamentous complex and rotator cuff muscles

TABLE 14-2
GLENOHUMERAL LIGAMENTS

Glenohumeral Ligament	Attachments	Function
Superior glenohumeral ligament	Supraglenoid tubercle, anterior to the origin of the long head of the biceps, to proximal tip of lesser tuberosity of humerus	Resists inferior translation with the arm in neutral abduction. Limits external rotation of the adducted shoulder (with coracohumeral ligament)
Middle glenohumeral ligament	Anterosuperior portion of labrum to lesser tuberosity of humerus, blending with fibers of the subscapularis tendon	Stabilizes anterior shoulder with arm in neutral and up to 30–45° abduction
Inferior glenohumeral ligament (complex)	Anterior and inferior portion of glenoid labrum and rim to anatomic neck of humerus; three components: anterior and posterior bands with axillary pouch between; sometimes anterior or posterior band is missing	Resists anteroinferior humeral head translation, particularly when arm in external rotation, abduction, and extension
Coracohumeral ligament	Lateral border of coracoid process of scapula to anterior aspect of greater tubercle of humerus and possibly second band attaching to less tubercle of humerus	Resists posterior and inferior translation in the suspended shoulder; stabilizes inferiorly with the arm in neutral abduction; taut with external rotation

Modified from Lugo R, Kung P, Ma CB. Shoulder biomechanics. *Eur J Radiol.* 2008;68(1):16-24; Houglum P, Burtoti D. *Brunnstrom's Clinical Kinesiology.* 6th ed. F.A. Davis; 2012.

provide GH joint stability. The capsuloligamentous complex contributes to compression primarily near end ranges of movement and rotator cuff muscles during midrange motions.[28,47–49]

Glenohumeral Joint Osteokinematics The motions of the GH joint are flexion/extension, abduction/adduction, and medial/lateral rotation. See Table 14-3 for the reported range of these motions varied

TABLE 14-3
SHOULDER COMPLEX MOTIONS

Motion	Normative Values	Arthrokinematics (Humeral Head Motion)	Prime Movers
Flexion	0–180°	Inferior glide and internal spin	Anterior deltoid Coracobrachialis Pectoralis major—clavicular Long head of biceps
Extension	0–60°	Inferior glide	Posterior deltoid Latissimus dorsi Pectoralis major—sternal Teres major Long head of triceps
Abduction	0–180°	Inferior glide and external spin	Deltoid Supraspinatus Long head of biceps
Adduction			Pectoralis major Latissimus dorsi Teres major Long head of triceps
External rotation	0–90°	Anterior glide	Infraspinatus Teres minor Posterior deltoid
Internal rotation	0–70°	Posterior glide	Subscapularis Anterior deltoid Pectoralis major Latissimus dorsi Teres major
Horizontal adduction	0–135°	Posterior glide	Pectoralis major Anterior deltoid
Horizontal abduction	0–45°	Anterior glide	Posterior deltoid Teres major Teres minor Infraspinatus

Adapted from Houglum P, Burtoti D. *Brunnstrom's Clinical Kinesiology.* 6th ed. F.A. Davis; 2012; Dutton M. *Dutton's Orthopedic Examination: Evaluation and Intervention.* 5th ed. McGraw Hill; 2020.

considerably among studies. Generally, the GH joint motion is described as a portion of total shoulder complex motion. Of the 180° of shoulder complex flexion and abduction, GH flexion and abduction are approximately 100 to 120°, with the remainder of total shoulder complex movement occurring at the SC and AC joints (Fig. 14-14). While the terms *arm-trunk* and *shoulder elevation* are often used interchangeably, a distinction should be made between shoulder elevation, which involves movement of the shoulder complex, and scapular elevation, in which the scapula moves superiorly indirectly elevating the clavicle, but not moving the GH joint.

Medial and lateral rotation motion occurs solely at the GH joint, although SC protraction and ST joint abduction and medial rotation of the shoulder cause the humerus to face medially without true rotation at the GH joint. The term "elevation" may refer to flexion or abduction occurring in the sagittal or frontal planes, respectively, or may be distinguished as movement in the plane of the scapula, sometimes referred to clinically as the movement of "scaption." In two-dimensional analyses, medial and lateral rotation of the humerus occurs concurrently with shoulder flexion and abduction, respectively,[50,51] whereas little to no rotation occurs with elevation in the plane of the scapula.[51]

Glenohumeral Joint Arthrokinematics The GH joint surfaces are reciprocally ovoid shaped rather than true spheres and are not completely congruent. This factor, along with the pull of the capsuloligamentous complex and dynamic muscle activation, results in a variety of rotational and sliding motions of the humeral head on the glenoid fossa. Humeral head translation in the superior, inferior, anterior, posterior, medial, and lateral directions is minimal,[1] with the reported magnitude of movement varying among studies.[47,52–54] However, studies consistently indicate less translational motion with active than passive movement,[53] supporting the concept that dynamic muscle activation helps to stabilize and center the humeral head in the glenoid fossa.[8,55] The rotation of the humeral head occurs about a moving axis, demonstrating an instant center of rotation (ICR). During elevation of the GH joint, the humeral head slides inferiorly[53] and thereby minimizes upward rolling of the humeral head under the coracoacromial arch. The ICR of the humeral head translates slightly upward on the glenoid fossa during this inferior slide until approximately 60° of active elevation. With further elevation, the humeral head remains relatively stable and centered on the glenoid fossa.[53,54,56–58] In persons with rotator cuff pathology, excessive upward slide has been observed.[29,56,58,59] The observed joint surface translation movements accompanying GH motions indicate the importance of glide mobilizations in restoring full GH movement.[60]

Scapulohumeral Rhythm

During shoulder elevation, the scapula upwardly rotates and, to a lesser extent, posteriorly tilts and laterally rotates. The working relationship between the two is known as the *scapulohumeral rhythm*. The arm can move through only 30° of abduction and 45 to 60° of flexion with minimal scapular movements. Past these points, scapular movements occur concomitantly with the arm movements. For 180° of flexion or abduction, approximately 120° of motion occurs in the GH joint and 60° of motion occurs as a result of scapular movement on the thorax.

The classic description of scapulohumeral rhythm with shoulder elevation in the sagittal and frontal planes is that an approximate 2° of GH motion occurs for every 1° of ST motion (i.e., 2:1 ratio), with individual variation during the initial stage of movement.[61,62] With shoulder elevation in the plane of the scapula, slightly lower ratios of GH to ST motion are

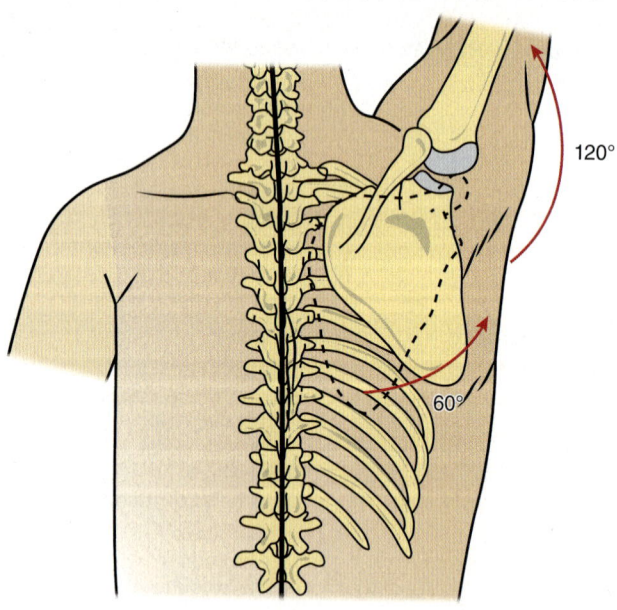

FIGURE 14-14 Movement of the shoulder complex. With 180° of shoulder elevation, approximately 120° is attributed to movement at the glenohumeral joint and 60° of motion to movement of the scapula on the thorax by associated movement at the sternoclavicular and acromioclavicular joints. The movements occur concomitantly rather than sequentially. (Adapted from Hamill J, Knutzen KM, Derrick TR. *Biomechanical Basis of Human Movement.* 5th ed. Wolters Kluwer; 2022: Figure 5-8.)

reported, ranging from 1.25:1 to 1.7:1.[53,54,62,63] Some authors report a variable ratio as opposed to a constant ratio.[37,64,65] Although there is a lack of agreement on the actual ratio with shoulder elevation in any plane, most report a less contribution from the ST joint in early and midrange motion than in late range motion. Variations in study outcomes may depend on methodological differences, such as reference angles, landmarks, and two-dimensional or three-dimensional analysis. Regardless of the reported differences in the exact ratio, it is clear that a greater contribution to full elevation is provided by the GH joint than ST joint and that the scapula and humerus move in a systematic and coordinated manner (Fig. 14-14).

The normal scapulohumeral rhythm is important to allow distribution of shoulder motion over more than one joint, allowing a larger total arc of motion while minimizing joint instability. To maintain GH joint congruency, the scapula upwardly rotates, posteriorly tilts, and laterally rotates as the scapula glides along the thorax to follow the humerus. The upward rotation and posterior tilt elevate the acromion preventing impingement of the subacromial structures, such as the rotator cuff and subacromial bursa, between the humeral head and the underside of the acromion.[66] A normal scapulohumeral rhythm maintains an ideal length-tension relationship of the deltoid, preventing active insufficiency during shoulder elevation.[43,46]

Movement of the ST articulation is linked with movement at the SC and AC joints. As the arm elevates, the scapula upwardly rotates and the clavicle elevates and posteriorly rotates through movement occurring at the SC and AC joints. The unique crank-like shape of the clavicle along with the vertical orientation and attachments of the conoid ligament serves to limit excursion of the scapula and clavicle away from each other as arm elevation progresses, allowing the clavicle to posteriorly rotate without reaching the limit of available motion at the SC joint.[61] The spine can contribute to shoulder elevation as well. During bilateral shoulder flexion, the thoracic spine extends to enable the individual to elevate the arm higher, whereas thoracic sidebending occurs with unilateral shoulder flexion.

MUSCLES

The three major muscle groups acting on the shoulder complex are the scapulohumeral muscles (Table 14-4), ST muscles (Table 14-5), and axiohumeral muscles (Table 14-6). Most of these muscles are primarily innervated by nerves arising from the C5–C6 spinal segments. Table 14-7 provides a summary of prime movers associated with specific ST motions.

Scapulohumeral Muscles

The scapulohumeral muscles include the four muscles of the rotator cuff: supraspinatus, infraspinatus, teres

TABLE 14-4			
SCAPULOHUMERAL MUSCLES			
Muscle	Motion/Action	Peripheral Nerve	Spinal Segments
Supraspinatus	Glenohumeral joint stability Shoulder abduction	Suprascapular nerve	C4, C5, C6
Infraspinatus	Shoulder external rotation Humeral head depression/glenohumeral joint compression	Suprascapular nerve	C5, C6
Teres minor	Shoulder external rotation Humeral head depression/glenohumeral joint compression	Axillary nerve	C5, C6
Subscapularis	Shoulder internal rotation Humeral head depression/glenohumeral joint compression	Subscapular nerve	C5, C6, C7
Biceps brachii	Elbow flexion Forearm supination Shoulder flexion	Musculocutaneous nerve	C5, C6
Deltoid • Anterior • Middle • Posterior	• Shoulder flexion and internal rotation • Shoulder abduction • Shoulder extension and external rotation	Axillary nerve	C5, C6
Coracobrachialis	Shoulder flexion and adduction	Musculocutaneous nerve	C5, C6, C7
Teres major	Shoulder adduction and internal rotation	Lower subscapular nerve	C5, C6, C7

Adapted from Moore KL, Dalley AF, Agur AMR. *Clinically Oriented Anatomy*. 8th ed. Wolters Kluwer; 2018:Table 3.6.

TABLE 14-5
SCAPULOTHORACIC MUSCLES

Muscle	Motion/Action	Peripheral Nerve	Spinal Segments
Trapezius • Upper • Middle • Lower	• Scapular elevation and upward rotation • Scapular retraction • Scapular depression and upward rotation	Spinal accessory nerve, C3 and C4	CN XI, C3, and C4
Rhomboid major	Scapular retraction and downward rotation	Dorsal scapular nerve	C4, C5
Rhomboid minor	Scapular retraction and downward rotation	Dorsal scapular nerve	C4, C5
Levator scapulae	Scapular elevation and downward rotation	Dorsal scapular nerve	C5, and C3, C4
Serratus anterior	Upward scapular rotation, holds medial scapular border against thorax	Long thoracic nerve	C5, C6, C7, C8
Pectoralis minor	Downward scapular rotation, scapular depression and protraction	Medial pectoral nerve	C7, C8, T1

Adapted from Moore KL, Dalley AF, Agur AMR. *Clinically Oriented Anatomy*. 8th ed. Wolters Kluwer; 2018.

TABLE 14-6
AXIOHUMERAL MUSCLES

Muscle	Motion/Action	Peripheral Nerve	Spinal Segments
Latissimus dorsi	Shoulder extension, adduction, and internal rotation Scapular depression	Thoracodorsal nerve	C6, C7, C8
Pectoralis major • Clavicular • Sternal	• Shoulder flexion, internal rotation, and horizontal adduction • Shoulder girdle depression, horizontal adduction	Medial and lateral pectoral nerves	C5, C6, C7, C8, T1

Adapted from Moore KL, Dalley AF, Agur AMR. *Clinically Oriented Anatomy*. 8th ed. Wolters Kluwer; 2018.

TABLE 14-7
SCAPULOTHORACIC MOTIONS AND MUSCLE WORKING AS PRIME MOVERS

Motion	Prime Movers
Elevation	Trapezius—upper Levator Rhomboid major Rhomboid minor
Depression	Pectoralis major Pectoralis minor
Upward rotation	Serratus anterior Trapezius—upper/lower
Downward rotation	Latissimus dorsi Pectoralis minor Rhomboid major Rhomboid minor Levator scapulae
Protraction	Pectoralis major—clavicular Pectoralis minor Serratus anterior
Retraction	Rhomboid major Rhomboid minor Trapezius—middle

minor, and subscapularis (Fig. 14-15). To optimize the distance between the acromion and humeral head during shoulder elevation, coordinated activity must occur among the rotator cuff, deltoid, and trapezius muscles (Fig. 14-16).[67] The deltoid muscle has an anterior, middle, and posterior part, and the trapezius has an upper, middle, and lower part. As the arm elevates, the orientation of the scapulohumeral muscle fibers varies, affecting their contribution to movement.[68] During humeral abduction, the rotator cuff muscles and capsuloligamentous complex help stabilize the humeral head in the glenoid fossa.[43] Unopposed action of the deltoid muscle may lead to excessive superior translation of the humeral head, resulting rotator cuff pathology.[48,54] The supraspinatus assists with shoulder abduction, with activation of the muscle along with the middle trapezius and middle deltoid, before actual abduction movement.[69] The supraspinatus is at a mechanical disadvantage to create much force, especially when compared to the prime mover for abduction, the deltoid. While the anterior and posterior components of the deltoid contribute to humeral abduction, the middle deltoid plays a significant role, particularly in midrange abduction.[70] With the arm by the side, the line of pull of the supraspinatus causes a superior translation of the humeral head and pulls the humeral head medially into the glenoid, providing GH joint compression.[43] With the arm at 90° of elevation, the line of pull of the supraspinatus produces even greater joint compression helping to stabilize the humerus and minimize shear on the glenoid fossa in concert with other rotator cuff muscles.[43,71] The infraspinatus and the smaller teres minor provide the majority of the strength for shoulder external rotation.[45] Due to their line of pull and larger size, these two muscles contribute more to dynamic GH joint stability than the supraspinatus. The subscapularis is

CHAPTER 14 | SHOULDER COMPLEX   449

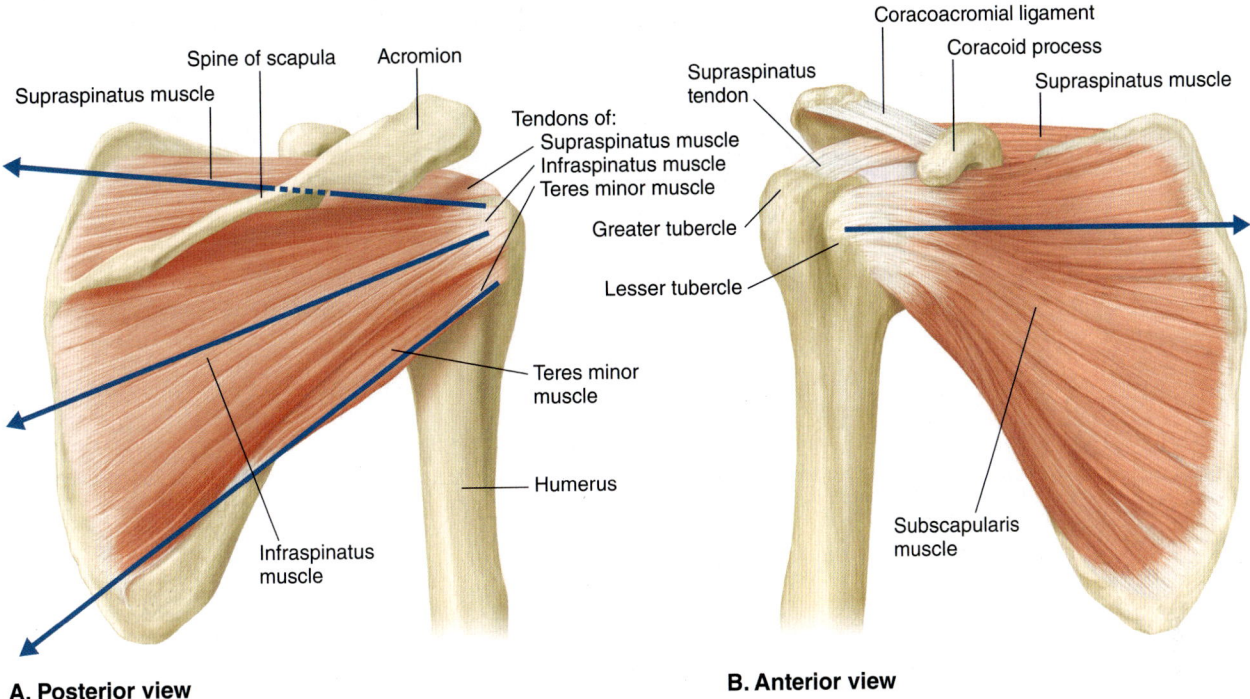

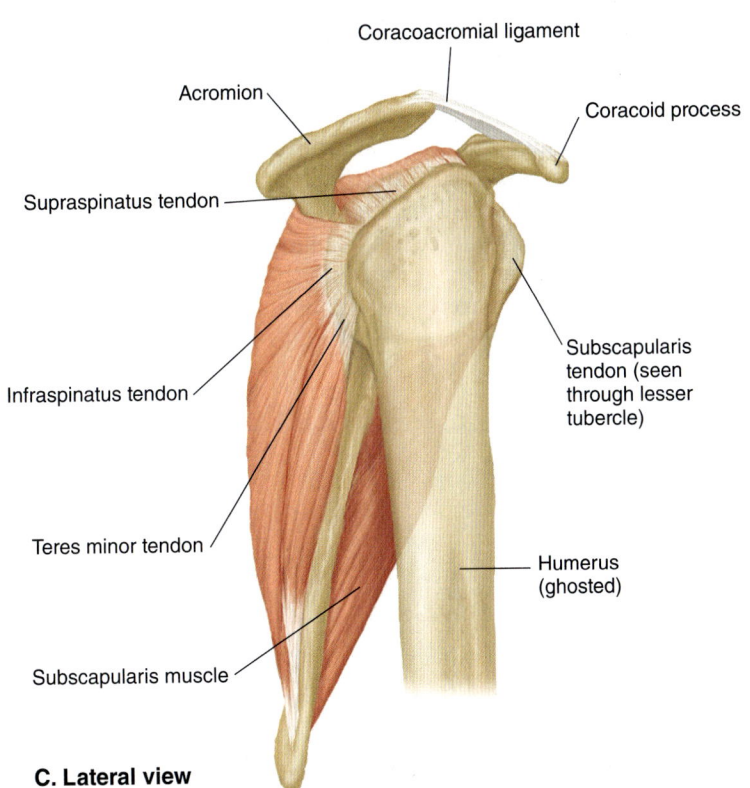

FIGURE 14-15 Rotator cuff muscles. **A.** Posterior view. **B.** Anterior view **C.** Lateral view. Blue lines denote lines of action on humerus. (Gest TR. *Lippincott Atlas of Anatomy*. 2nd ed. Wolters Kluwer; 2020: Plate 2-16.)

the prime mover for shoulder internal rotation and is the largest of the rotator cuff muscles, comprising more than 50% of the total volume.[43] The subscapularis provides anterior GH joint stability by adhering to the anterior capsule[72] and acting as a buttress to limit anterior humeral excursion. In addition, the line of pull of the subscapularis assists the infraspinatus and teres minor with humeral head stabilization.[73]

The rotator cuff maintains humeral head depression throughout shoulder elevation in order to

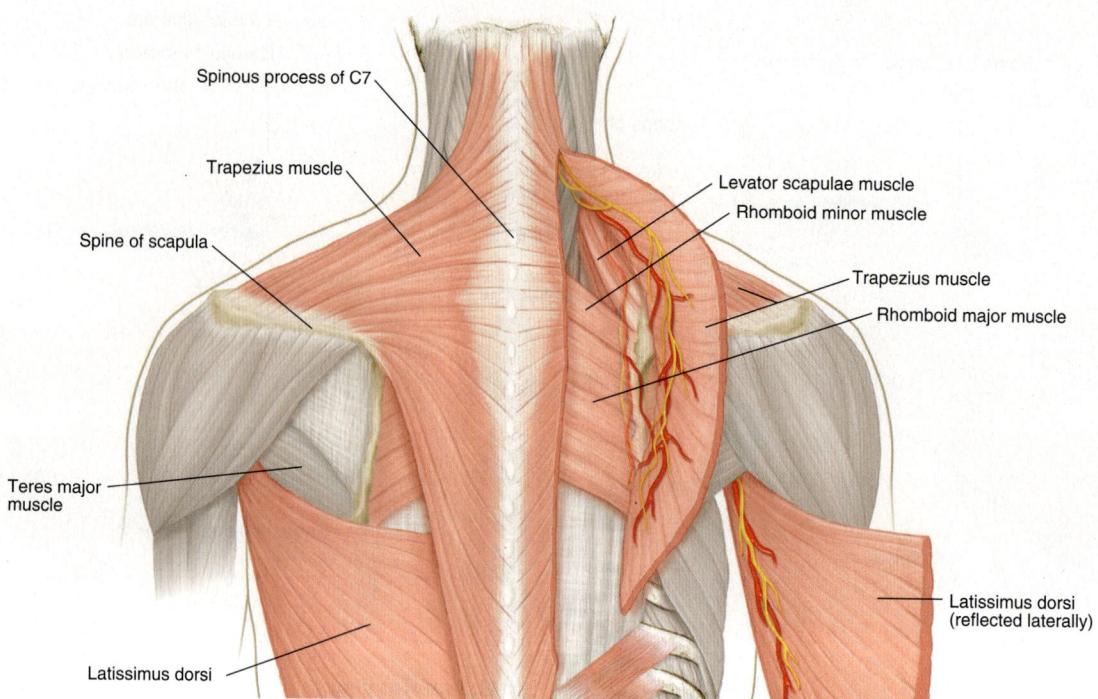

FIGURE 14-16 Scapulohumeral muscles, posterior view. Note the fiber orientation of the parts of the deltoid and trapezius. (Gest TR. *Lippincott Atlas of Anatomy*. 2nd ed. Wolters Kluwer; 2020: Plate 1-14.)

maximize the subacromial space. Tears of the rotator cuff, particularly the infraspinatus, are associated with migration of the humerus proximally.[74] As rotator cuff tears increase in size, further disruption of normal GH kinematics can occur.[75] Weakness or fatigue of the rotator cuff increases the stress on the static GH joint stabilizers and may lead to capsular, ligamentous, or labral pathology.[46] If these static stabilizers begin to fail, an even greater stress is placed upon the rotator cuff to compensate.[73] Increased superior humeral head translation may cause impingement, tendinitis, and bursitis. Rotator cuff inhibition due to pain may further contribute to GH joint pathology.

The large deltoid is a prime mover for shoulder flexion, extension, and horizontal abduction and assists the pectoralis major with horizontal adduction (Fig. 14-17).

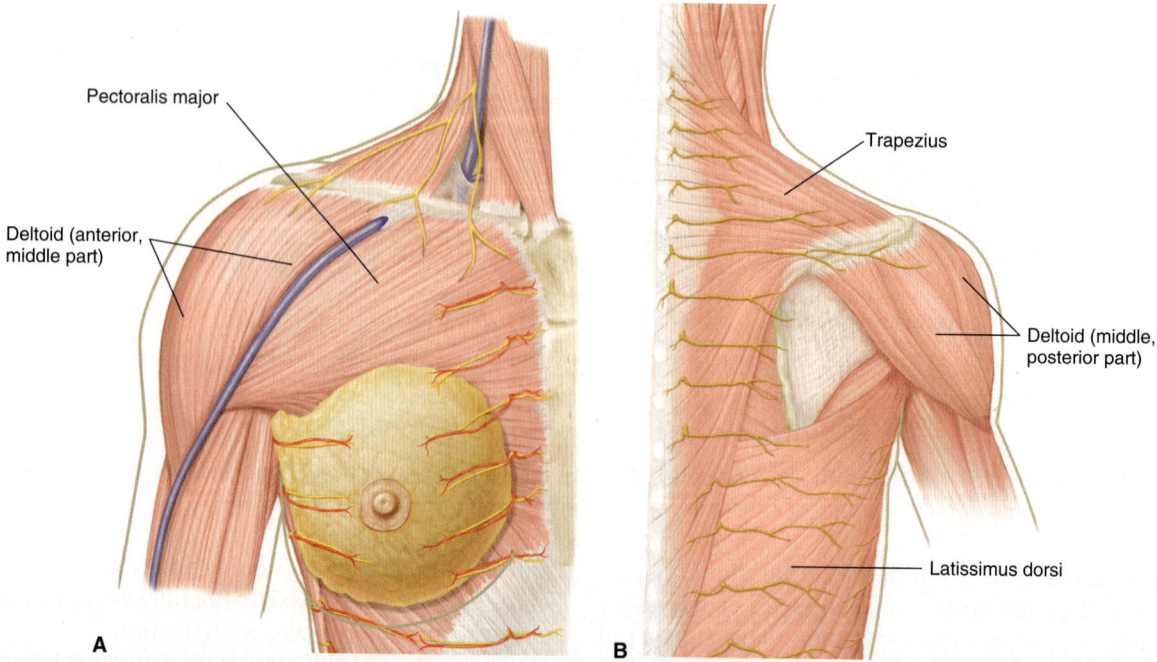

FIGURE 14-17 Large muscle groups of the shoulder. **A.** Anterior view. **B.** Posterior view. (Gest TR. *Lippincott Atlas of Anatomy*. 2nd ed. Wolters Kluwer; 2020: Plate 4-02.)

The superior humeral translation created by the deltoid is counterbalanced by the inferior glide created by the infraspinatus, teres minor, and subscapularis allowing the humeral head to remain centered within the glenoid fossa.[71] Adjacent structures in the shoulder play an interrelated role with the rotator cuff in joint stability. For example, the long head of the biceps tendon (LHBT) originates from the supraglenoid tubercle of the scapula and penetrates the joint capsule, but not the synovium, through an opening between the supraspinatus and subscapularis muscles. The LHBT courses in the bicipital groove between the greater and lesser tubercles where it is maintained by the transverse humeral ligament (Fig. 14-18).[16] The LHBT assists the rotator cuff with humeral head depression by its attachment to the supraglenoid tubercle and functions as a dynamic stabilizer of the GH joint. The teres major, pectoralis major, and latissimus dorsi act with the rotator cuff to depress the humeral head.[71] These factors suggest that general rehabilitation of the shoulder should involve training of these muscles.

Scapulothoracic Muscles

The ST muscles include the three-part trapezius muscle that serves a suspensory function and contributes to scapular elevation, upward rotation, and

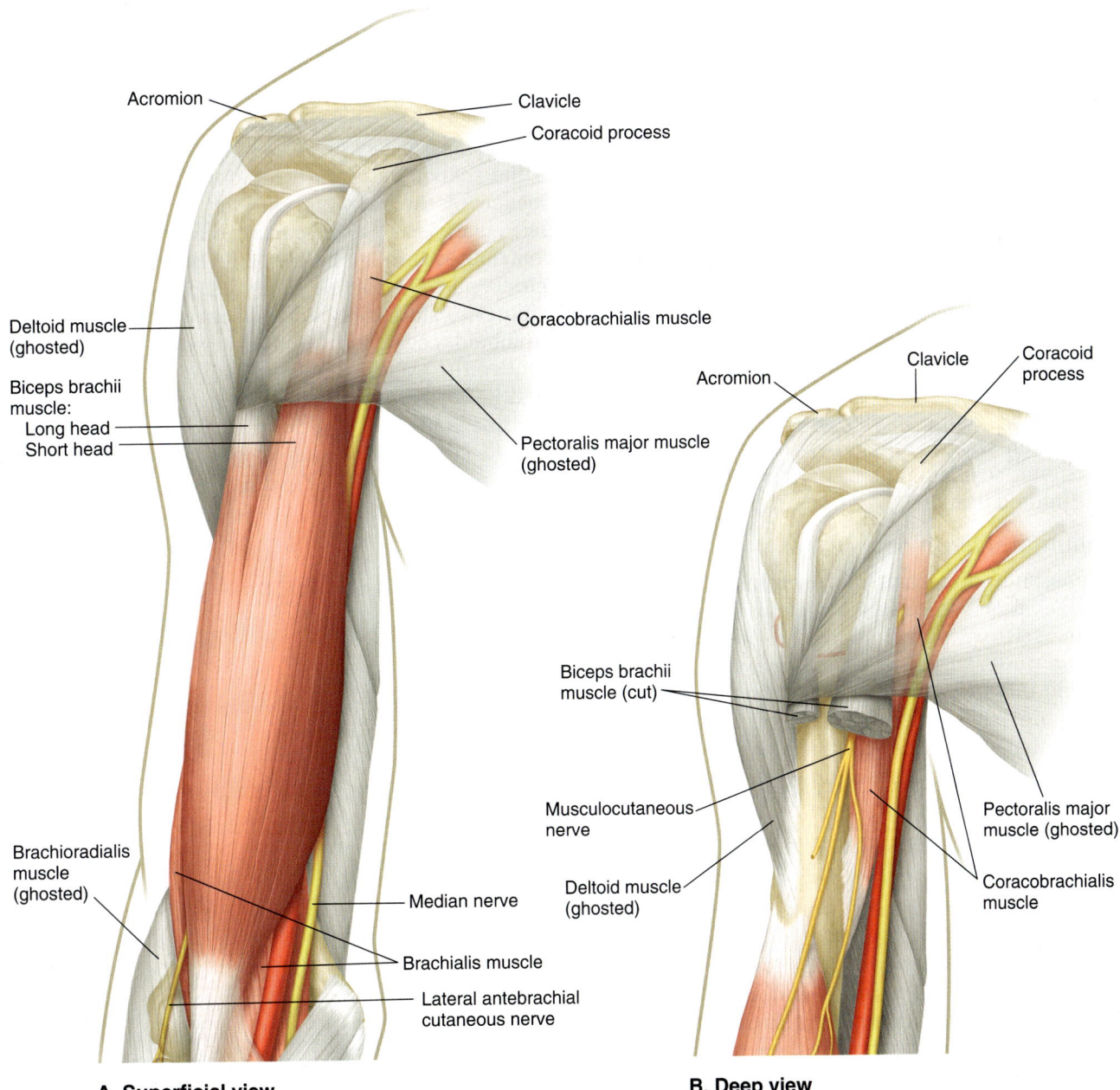

A. Superficial view **B. Deep view**

FIGURE 14-18 Biceps brachii and coracobrachialis. **A.** Superficial view. **B.** Deep view. (Gest TR. *Lippincott Atlas of Anatomy*. 2nd ed. Wolters Kluwer; 2020: Plate 2-17.)

retraction.[76] The rhomboid major and rhomboid minor retract and downwardly rotate the scapula (see Fig. 14-16). Weakness of the rhomboids results in insufficient scapular retraction, which may place increased stress on anterior shoulder structures during overhead activities. The serratus anterior upwardly rotates and protracts the scapula. Isolated injury to the serratus anterior or the long thoracic nerve decreases active shoulder flexion strength and causes scapular winging (where the medial scapular border is no longer flush with the thoracic wall).[77,78] Damage to the spinal accessory nerve or weakness of the trapezius may lead to lateral scapular winging in which the scapula droops (i.e., is depressed and protracted with the lateral projection of the inferior angle).[78,79] The pectoralis minor depresses, downwardly rotates, and protracts the scapula through its attachment on the coracoid process.[76] Lack of flexibility of the pectoralis minor increases scapular protraction and downward rotation, resulting in an abnormal scapular resting position, which limits shoulder elevation and may place the individual at risk for shoulder pathology and pain.

The ST muscles help maintain a stable base for the humerus by rotating and positioning the scapula. These muscles may be elongated and weak in patients with poor postural alignment, such as increased kyphosis or excessive scapular protraction. In addition, these muscles are at fault in patients with scapular dyskinesia.[76] The ST muscles themselves are not frequently injured, and therapeutic exercises targeting these muscles can generally be started early in the rehabilitation process to improve the scapular resting position and scapulohumeral rhythm without stressing the injured tissues.

Axiohumeral Muscles

The latissimus dorsi and the pectoralis major (see Fig. 14-17) attach to the axial skeleton and humerus and can assist with humeral head depression. These large and powerful muscles transfer power from the trunk and the lower extremities to the arm. Because they act on long lever arms and with high forces, muscle imbalances often exist between the large axiohumeral internal rotators and the relatively smaller GH external rotators.

Force Couples of the Shoulder

A **force couple** is a system in which the force of one muscle (the primary agonist) works with the antagonist muscle producing a resultant movement that differs from those muscles working independently. For example, the serratus anterior and trapezius work together to stabilize and move the scapula during upper extremity elevation, though their primary independent action on the scapula differs. Through their attachments to the scapula and clavicle, the serratus anterior and trapezius contribute significantly to scapular upward rotation and play important roles in scapular protraction/retraction (internal/external scapular rotation) and tilting. The varying fiber orientation of the upper, middle, and lower trapezius and the upper and lower portions of the serratus anterior help explain their contributions to scapular movement. Consider the components of the trapezius with the upper fibers descending, lower fibers ascending, and middle fibers passing horizontally to converge and attach to the shoulder. The upper trapezius attaches directly to the clavicle[80] and thus contributes to scapular movement through the linked kinematics between the SC and ST joints.[79] Elevation of the clavicle through activation of the upper trapezius contributes more significantly to anterior tilting than to upward rotation of the scapula.[25] Thus, the contribution of the upper trapezius to scapular upward rotation occurs through coordinated action with other muscles that attach to the scapula.

The most easily observed force couple movement of the scapula is upward rotation, created by the influence of the serratus anterior and the trapezius, particularly the lower part, though the upper part contributes through influence on the clavicle and the middle part plays a role early in elevation[81,82] and contributes to stabilization of the scapula (along with the rhomboids) against the pull of the serratus anterior.[8,83] Though the trapezius is more active during abduction than in flexion and the lower portion of the serratus anterior is more active during shoulder flexion, both muscle groups are required for full active shoulder elevation (Fig. 14-19). Posterior tilting and external

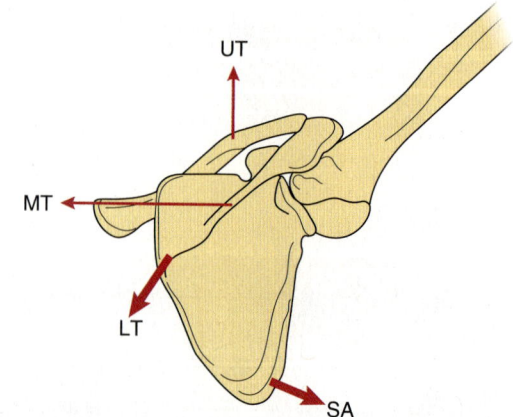

FIGURE 14-19 Upward rotation of the scapula occurs through force couple mechanics of the trapezius and serratus anterior (SA). *LT*, lower trapezius; *MT*, middle trapezius; *UT*, upper trapezius.

rotation (retraction) of the upwardly rotating scapula may occur through adjustments of the serratus anterior and trapezius. These adjustments that help hold the scapula to the thorax[83] are made through the AC joints and are most evident as the scapula nears full abduction.[84–86]

Scapular downward rotation occurs through action of the rhomboids and pectoralis minor muscles. The rhomboids may also act eccentrically during upward rotation of the scapula to control the scapular position. Acting as stabilizers, the rhomboids hold the scapula to the thorax to prevent excessive internal rotation of the scapula at the AC joint and counteract the lateral translation force of the serratus anterior on the scapula during arm elevation. In addition, the rhomboids and pectoralis minor stabilize the scapula during contraction of the teres major to allow the muscle to effectively extend and adduct the humerus.

The deltoid and the rotator cuff also act in a force coupled relationship, with the infraspinatus, teres minor, and subscapularis allowing the humeral head to remain centered and inferiorly slide within the glenoid fossa to counteract the superior humeral translation created by the deltoid during shoulder elevation (Fig. 14-20).[87,88] The supraspinatus rolls the humeral head superiorly, while compressing the humeral head to the glenoid for added stability. The infraspinatus and teres minor may externally rotate the humerus to varying degrees to provide greater clearance between the humerus and the acromion during abduction.

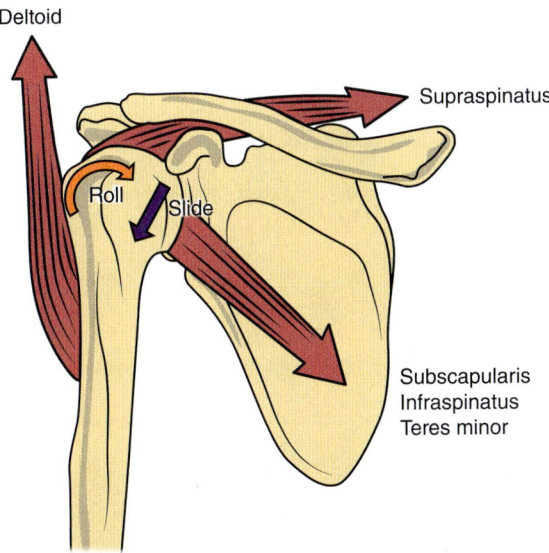

FIGURE 14-20 Anterior view of shoulder depicting actions of the rotator cuff (infraspinatus, teres minor, subscapularis) to exert a downward force counteracting upward translation of the deltoid during shoulder abduction. The supraspinatus rolls the head of the humerus toward abduction.

PALPATION

The patient should be in an upright, seated, and relaxed position with arms hanging from the sides. Palpation generally starts posteriorly on the scapula, progressing to the AC joint and clavicle and ending with palpation of the anterolateral structures. (See Fig. 14-20 for a depiction of easily palpated bony structures and Figs. 14-15, 14-16, 14-17, and 14-18 for schematics of muscles.)

Bony Palpation

Standing behind the patient, the clinician should observe and palpate the scapula. In a normal, resting position, the scapula is positioned on the thorax with the superior angle at the level of T1 spinous process, the base (root) of the scapular spine at the T3 spinous process and the inferior angle at the T7 spinous process (see Fig. 14-6).[89] The inferior angle is easiest to palpate first with the arm in the resting position. The patient is then asked to elevate the arm and the clinician palpates the inferior angle when the arm is in maximal elevation. The patient then returns the arm to the resting position. The medial border of the scapula can be palpated with the fingertips pointed perpendicular to the vertebral column, moving laterally from the T1–T7 spinous processes approximately 2 inches toward the medial scapula border. The medial border may be more easily palpated with the shoulder moved into internal rotation. The superior angle is more difficult to palpate than the inferior angle because of the overlying trapezius and the inserting levator scapulae. Palpation of the superior angle is made easier by gently palpating at the superior medial border of the scapula while passively elevating the shoulder girdle by pushing upward along the long axis of the hanging arm. Just opposite the T3 spinous on the scapula, the spine of the scapula can be palpated and followed laterally toward shoulder until reaching the lateral end, which is the acromial angle. To palpate the inferior edge of the scapular spine, the clinician should place the palpating finger pads against the skin in a position perpendicular to the scapular spine and push in against the soft tissues toward the body of the scapula in the area of the infraspinatus muscle, moving the fingers superiorly until hard resistance is felt. To palpate the superior edge of the scapular spine, the clinician places the palpating fingers perpendicular to the superior portion of the scapular spine, following the spine from medial to lateral while gently pushing into the skin and underlying muscles located just superior to the scapular spine (the deepest being the supraspinatus).[90]

Returning to the acromion, the clinician can move the fingers along the lateral edge of the acromion and anteriorly to reach the junction between the acromion and the clavicle (see Fig. 14-8). The clavicle is concave along the lateral one-third and convex along the medial one-third. Because muscles attach to the clavicle inferiorly and posteriorly, the anterosuperior aspect is easily palpated for continuity. The large medial end of the clavicle can be palpated immediately lateral to the suprasternal notch just above the manubrium of the sternum, as approximately half of the medial clavicle sits above the manubrium and sternal notch (see Fig. 14-9). The SC joint can be palpated in this region. The medial end of the clavicle and SC joints should be palpated bilaterally for symmetry. Medial clavicle dislocation typically manifests by a medial and superior displacement of the clavicle over the manubrium.

Moving laterally along the clavicle at the point of greatest concavity, the clinician can lower the fingers from the anterior edge approximately 1 inch and press posteriorly and laterally within the deltopectoral triangle to feel the tip and medial surface of the coracoid process. Returning to the clavicle and palpating laterally, the AC joint can be felt and is easier to identify during movement of arm (see Fig. 14-8).

Just inferior to the acromion's lateral edge, the greater tubercle can be felt. External rotation of the humerus exposes the bicipital groove, located between the greater and lesser tubercle of the humerus. Moving the palpating fingers just medial to the bicipital groove, the lesser tubercle can be felt.

Soft-Tissue Palpation

The supraspinatus, infraspinatus, and teres minor muscles are difficult to distinguish from each other at their insertion onto the greater tubercle because the fibers blend together and incorporate into the GH joint capsule (see Fig. 14-15). The insertion of the supraspinatus is most exposed with the patient positioned in passive shoulder extension, slight abduction, and significant internal rotation (with the hand behind the back) (Fig. 14-21).[90] The palpating finger moves along the edge of the acromion from the posterior angle to the anterior tip and then just inferior to position over the supraspinatus insertion. The superficial portion of the supraspinatus muscle belly can be palpated just anterior to the superior border of the spine of the scapula in the supraspinous fossa. To palpate the infraspinatus, the clinician can palpate below the inferior border of the scapular spine with the patient sitting (Fig. 14-22), prone, or prone on elbows with the arm in approximately 80° flexion, slight adduction, and external rotation. The teres minor muscle is just inferior to the infraspinatus. The subscapularis is difficult to palpate, but its tendon may be felt just medial to the insertion onto the lesser tubercle while the shoulder is positioned at end-range external rotation with resistance to internal rotation with the patient in the sitting position. The tendon of the long head of the biceps is most easily palpated in the bicipital groove.[89] To palpate the right bicipital groove, the clinician can stand behind the sitting patient with the clinician's index and middle fingers positioned on the anterior proximal humerus and the right hand supporting the patient's bent elbow. The clinician externally rotates the humerus, locates the lesser tubercle, moves the

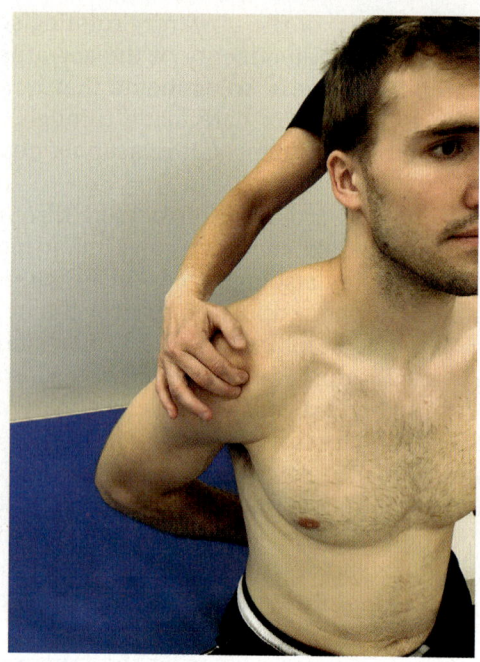

FIGURE 14-21 Positioning to maximally expose supraspinatus tendon for palpation.

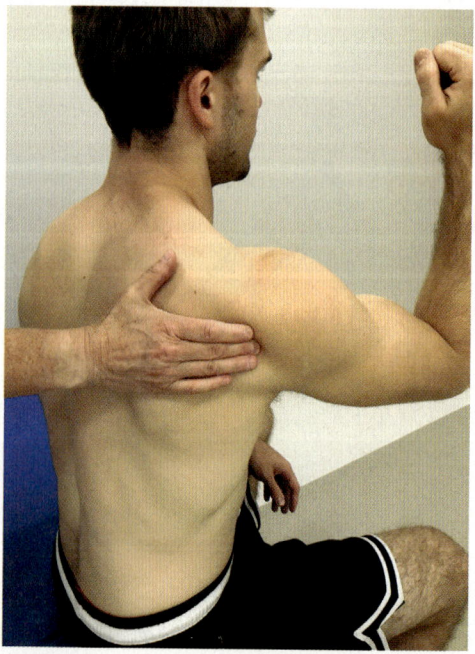

FIGURE 14-22 Position for palpating the infraspinatus (can also be palpated in prone or prone on elbows).

palpating fingers slightly laterally, and alternately internally and externally rotates the humerus, while palpating the bicipital groove and long head of biceps tendon with the groove.[90]

The larger, more superficial muscles of the shoulder girdle are more easily palpated. The anterior, middle, and posterior portions of the deltoid muscle converge together to insert onto the deltoid tuberosity of the humerus. The anterior portion can be palpated just distal to the lateral clavicle, lateral to the deltopectoral groove (junction between the anterior deltoid and pectoralis major muscle). The middle and posterior parts of the deltoid are palpated just distal to the acromion and the lateral spine of the scapula, respectively. The upper, middle, and lower trapezius can be palpated between their respective attachments. The latissimus dorsi is thin in most people, but can be palpated along the lateral edge during contraction of the muscle. The reader is referred to a textbook of anatomy, palpation, and manual muscle testing for more detail.

INTRODUCTION TO THE EXAMINATION OF THE SHOULDER COMPLEX

Shoulder pain is third most common musculoskeletal complaint in primary care.[91] The shoulder and arm are common sites of referred pain from other areas sharing the same innervation, such as the cervical region and heart. The history and upper quarter screening (UQS) examination are used to help delineate the origin of pain. Once identified as the source of pain, the shoulder-specific examination is performed. While acute and isolated pathologies such as a traumatic rotator cuff tear do occur, shoulder pain is more commonly multifactorial, requiring a thorough assessment of the entire shoulder complex.

PATIENT HISTORY: SHOULDER COMPLEX

A thorough patient history will help identify the patient's chief complaint and formulate preliminary hypotheses. The detailed history may implicate referral from another musculoskeletal region or from a nonmusculoskeletal source. Once these potential sources of symptoms are ruled out, the clinician should investigate shoulder-specific questions to help guide the physical examination.

Review of Systems

The review of symptoms is particularly important for patients with suspected shoulder or scapular pathology because of the potential for visceral pathology to create symptoms in this region.[92] Clinicians should ask patients with suspected shoulder pathology questions regarding constitutional symptoms and review the cardiovascular, pulmonary, gastrointestinal, and genitourinary/reproductive systems (see Table 6.8 in Chapter 6, Patient History).

Cardiovascular and Pulmonary Systems Right or left shoulder or scapular pain may be referred from the heart[3] (myocardial ischemia, coronary artery insufficiency, pericarditis), aorta (aortic aneurysm), or lung (pleurisy, spontaneous pneumothorax, emphysema, tuberculosis, primary or metastatic tumors).[93] Diaphragm irritation, either primary or secondary to gallbladder, liver, or lung disorders, can stimulate the phrenic nerve, causing shoulder pain.[93-95] Pancoast tumor with coincident Horner syndrome can cause shoulder pain.[93,95] Patients with the following complaints require consultation with, or referral to, a physician[93]:

- Chest pain or diaphoresis
- Shoulder pain that increases with exertion
- Persistent dry or productive cough
- Blood in the sputum
- Shoulder pain that is exacerbated with respiration or coughing
- Shoulder pain that is exacerbated with recumbency
- Concomitant nausea or vomiting or anorexia
- Uncontrolled hypertension

Because upper extremity exercises increase blood pressure more than lower extremity exercise at the same workload, clinicians should use caution and monitor cardiac response when prescribing upper body ergometry or resistive upper extremity exercise in patients with hypertension.

Gastrointestinal System Right shoulder or scapular pain may be referred from the liver (cirrhosis, abscess, hepatitis, or primary or metastatic tumors) or gall bladder (cholecystitis).[93-96] Left shoulder or scapular pain may be referred from the spleen (rupture) or pancreas.[93,95] Left shoulder pain may also be caused by a ruptured ectopic pregnancy or when free air is within the peritoneum after a laparoscopic procedure.[93] Hiatal hernias and peptic ulcers may cause shoulder pain.[94] Patients with the following complaints require consultation with, or referral to, a physician:

- Concomitant nausea or vomiting or anorexia
- Jaundice that has not been diagnosed or treated
- Symptoms that are affected by food
- Symptoms that are worsened by the use of nonsteroidal medications
- Symptoms that are alleviated with antacids

Urogenital System Kidney disease (tumor or pyelonephritis) or urinary tract infections may cause shoulder pain.[93] Left shoulder pain may also be caused by a ruptured ectopic pregnancy.[93]

Constitutional Symptoms As noted in Chapter 6, Patient History, constitutional symptoms such as weight loss and night sweats are suggestive of possible systemic disease process or pathology.[97,98] Bone metastases, particular to the thoracic spine, humerus, or ribs, are common in patients with lung and breast cancer. Because these bone metastases can cause shoulder pain, patients with a history of cancer and an insidious onset of shoulder pain may benefit from physician evaluation.[99] Breast cancer may cause shoulder pain. When examining patients with insidious onset of pain in the shoulder region who are current or former smokers, clinicians should consider the possibility of lung cancer, with or without metastatic spread.[98,100]

History of Neck Pathology

Patients should be asked about any past or current neck pathology because symptoms in the shoulder and scapular region can be referred from the cervical spine. Complaints such as tingling, numbness, or shooting pains are suggestive of nerve involvement. Symptoms that are brought on by neck active range of motion, overpressure, or Spurling test[101,102] (see Chapter 17, Cervical and Thoracic Spine) warrant a thorough examination of the cervical spine. Cervical spinal cord tumors may produce shoulder pain[93] in addition to alterations in lower extremity strength, motor control, and gait.

History of Shoulder Pathology

A prior history of shoulder problems either to the same or contralateral shoulder can be helpful in creating a potential list of differential diagnoses. Patients with rotator cuff pathology or degenerative joint disease (DJD) may report progressive cycles of exacerbation and remittance. Individuals with a prior history of adhesive capsulitis are more likely to have a recurrence in the same or contralateral shoulder.[3,103] Patients with multidirectional instability typically have bilateral shoulder complaints. Patients who have sustained a shoulder dislocation are likely to have repeat dislocations or subluxations.

Patient Characteristics

Some shoulder pathologies are more common within certain age ranges. Atraumatic and traumatic shoulder instability is more common in patients under the age of 30, although instability is still fairly common up to the age of 45. Middle-aged patients have an increased incidence of adhesive capsulitis, partial-thickness rotator cuff tears, and subacromial impingement syndrome (SIS). In contrast, older patients have an increased rate of DJD and full-thickness rotator cuff tears.[103,104]

It is important to ask about the patient's hand dominance and upper extremity functional requirements. Patients may tolerate loss of motion or strength in the nondominant upper extremity for quite some time before seeking help. However, this same loss in the dominant extremity may be less well-tolerated. For example, hammering and throwing requires primarily dominant extremity function. In contrast, some occupations and sports, such as construction and swimming, require maximal range from bilateral upper extremities.

The clinician should inquire about the patient's occupation and hobbies to identify potential predisposing or exacerbating factors as well as any repetitive stresses that may be related to the patient's chief complaint. Any recent changes, such as transfer to a new job, increase in work hours, or increase in training intensity or playing time, should be noted.

Onset

Patients should be asked about possible causes for their shoulder pain or dysfunction. At times, patients can relate the onset to a specific traumatic event, such as a fall or a direct blow to the shoulder. Common traumatic shoulder pathologies include shoulder strains, sprains, labral tears, subluxations, and tendon ruptures.[3,105] Radiographic testing may be required to rule out fractures or dislocations. Patients who sustained significant traumatic events, such as a motor vehicle accident or fall from a height, may have additional injuries, such as abdominal trauma or multiple fractures that require interventions or additional precautions. Patients may report their symptoms began gradually or insidiously. In such cases, fractures and dislocations are doubtful, and DJD and soft-tissue pathologies such as overuse injuries, adhesive capsulitis, or impingement are more likely. Patients should be asked about any changes in activity or function around the time of onset. Patients who have had recent surgical procedures, such as a mastectomy or pacemaker implantation, are more likely to have adhesive capsulitis. An increase in athletic activity or training or new job tasks may suggest an overuse injury, impingement, or instability.

Location of Symptoms

Patients should be asked about symptom location. SC and AC joints pathology generally causes only local joint complaints. Patients with rotator cuff injuries are likely to complain of lateral brachium pain. Superior shoulder pain may indicate impingement, bursitis, or labral pathology. Anterior shoulder pain may indicate labral or capsular pathology. Symptoms that extend past the elbow are less likely to originate from within the shoulder complex, but may be due to cervical pathology or thoracic outlet syndrome. Scapular pain should be considered to be derived from the cervical spine until proven otherwise.[101,106]

Chief Complaint

Many times, the primary reason patients provide for coming to physical therapy are to abolish pain. Pain may be the chief complaint after trauma, with overuse injuries, and with many different shoulder pathologies, such as sprains, strains, rotator cuff tears, and adhesive capsulitis. The astute clinician will probe the patient further to distinguish pain from other sensations to assist in making preliminary hypotheses. Complaints of stiffness may indicate adhesive capsulitis. Complaints of weakness may indicate a contractile lesion, such as a muscle strain or a rotator cuff tear. Less frequently, weakness may be the result of a neurologic impairment, such as suprascapular neuropathy or a long thoracic nerve traction injury. Complaints of instability or joint slippage may indicate capsular or labral pathology. Complaints of clicking, catching, or locking may indicate labral pathology[107] or possibly a loose body within the joint. Complaints of paresthesias may indicate transient subluxation causing a traction injury to the brachial plexus, cervical dysfunction, thoracic outlet syndrome, or a peripheral nerve injury. More regional complaints of upper extremity pain or paresthesias may warrant further examination to rule out complex regional pain syndrome.

Symptom Behavior

Patients should be questioned about aggravating and remitting factors. Specifically, patients should be asked about their abilities to reach overhead, behind the back, forward, and sideways. Clinicians should ask about patients' abilities to perform functional tasks, such as dressing, grooming, and driving, as well as work and recreational tasks, such as throwing or working overhead. Sleep may be interrupted in patients with full-thickness rotator cuff tears as well as patients with active cancer. Shoulder pain that occurs with exertion, such as walking, indicates the need to thoroughly screen the cardiovascular system.

Pain intensity and irritability helps guide the extensiveness or aggressiveness of the examination. Patients should be asked about current symptoms and response to interventions tried during this episode. Overall, is the condition getting better, worse, or staying the same? For example, symptoms responding to heat or showing gradual improvement with increase in activity may indicate DJD or adhesive capsulitis. Pain at the start of an activity that slowly goes away after warm-up, is increased with increased load on tendon, and/or is relieved with relative rest, is indicative of tendon pathology.[108]

Outcome Measures

Chapter 6, Patient History, introduced common outcome measures such as the Patient-Specific Functional Scale. Clinicians may want to use a tool designed for the upper extremity (Disabilities of Arm, Shoulder, and Hand or Upper Extremity Functional Index) or a tool that is specific for patients with shoulder dysfunction (Shoulder Pain and Disability Index). Table 14-8

TABLE 14-8
COMMON OUTCOME TOOLS FOR PATIENTS WITH SHOULDER PATHOLOGIES

Tool	Tool Basics
Disabilities of Arm, Shoulder, and Hand (DASH)	• Addresses basic activities of daily living as well as pain, weakness, and stiffness • 30 items rated 1-5, with higher scores indicating worse function • Scoring: 0-100% perceived disability • Alternate versions include the DASH-Sport, DASH-Work, and QuickDash • MCID: 10* Common diagnoses[†]: Nonspecific shoulder pain, rotator cuff pathology, osteoarthritic, rheumatoid arthritis, humeral fracture, total shoulder arthroplasty
Shoulder Pain and Disability Index (SPADI)	• Addresses very basic activities of daily living (8 items) and pain (5 items) • 13 items divided into two subscales: pain and disability • Scoring: each item is scored 0-10, with higher scores indicating worse function/pain • Total score obtained by averaging pain and disability scores • MCID: 13 Common diagnoses are the same as with the DASH[†]
Upper Extremity Functional Index	• Addresses basic activities of daily • 20 items rated 0-4, with higher scores indicating higher function • Scoring: 0-80 • MDC: 9.4 points[‡] Common diagnoses are the same as with the DASH

*Schmitt JS, Di Fabio RP. Reliable change and minimum important difference (MID) proportions facilitated group responsiveness comparisons using individual threshold criteria. *J Clin Epidemiol.* 2004;57(10):1008-1018. doi:10.1016/j.jclinepi.2004.02.007.
[†]Shirley Ryan Ability Lab. Rehabilitation measures database. Updated 2021. Accessed April 12, 2021. https://www.sralab.org/rehabilitation-measures
[‡]Stratford P, Binkley J, Stratford D. Development and initial validation of the upper extremity functional index. *Physiother Can.* 2001;53:259-267.

provides details of the three most commonly used outcome measures for patients with shoulder dysfunction.

PHYSICAL EXAMINATION: SHOULDER COMPLEX

The physical examination consists of the systems review, the quarter screen, the clearing examination, and the joint-specific examination. However, the clinician must first consider if there are any potential red flags, such as fracture or dislocation, as these require urgent orthopaedic consultation.[92,109] GH dislocation should be suspected in case of seizure or a history of trauma with resulting deformity or loss of the normal contour of the shoulder girdle along with an inability to move the shoulder.[110] Acute proximal humeral fracture should be suspected in case of significant trauma accompanied by disabling pain and loss of motion.[110] Clavicle fractures are more common in cyclists from crashes and football players due to falling on the side of the adducted shoulder.[109] Clavicle fractures are more easily identifiable by visible or palpable deformity of the shaft of the clavicle along with bony tenderness of the clavicle.[110] Acute AC joint separations are frequently the result of falling on the point (superior aspect) of the shoulder, as in martial arts, cycling, football, and skiing.[109] While minor AC sprains can be evaluated and treated by a physical therapist, severe separations, in which the lateral clavicle is displaced superiorly, posteriorly, or inferiorly, require orthopaedic evaluation.[6,109]

Once the patient has been cleared of any red flags and the history and systems review have been performed, the clinician should perform an UQS including an upper quarter neurologic screen to clear the cervical spine or determine whether there is concomitant cervical spine involvement. Next, a clearing examination of the distal joint (in this case, active and passive elbow flexion and extension) is performed to ensure that the area of pathology has been narrowed down to the shoulder complex. All components of the joint-specific examination need not be performed on every patient. Like, the UQS, the experienced clinician will titrate the joint-specific examination based on the patient history, presentation, and goals. In practice, the joint-specific examination is organized by position and should proceed from uninvolved (or less involved) to involved side but is presented here by category to aide conceptualization.

Structure

Before beginning a detailed examination, it is helpful to first focus on the patient's overall structure and posture in sitting and standing. Ideally, male patients are shirtless and female patients are in a gown opened to the back or sports bra to maximize visualization of the region. The clinician should inspect the shoulder girdle for gross deformity. Patients with an anterior GH dislocation may exhibit a fullness anteriorly and inferiorly due to the displaced humeral head.[110] Patients with an AC separation commonly have a step deformity where the clavicle has overridden the acromion.[110] Patients with AC or SC joint sprains may have localized joint edema. Observe for local areas of muscle atrophy.[3] Chronic rotator cuff pathology may lead to wasting in the suprascapular and/or infrascapular fossa, whereas suprascapular nerve entrapment can result in atrophy of the infraspinatus muscle. Hypertrophy and/or depression of the dominant shoulder girdle are not abnormal.[111] Visible scars may indicate prior surgical procedures.

Clinicians should note any protective behavior, such as holding the extremity to the side in adduction and internal rotation or guarded movements with ambulation or disrobing. Particular attention should be paid to the resting positions of the thoracic spine and scapulae. Increased kyphosis or protracted scapulae place increased stress on the rotator cuff during reaching and elevation, placing the patient at risk for impingement or other rotator cuff pathology.[112,113] A forward shoulder position may be related to shortness of the pectoralis minor.[114] The clinician should note the position of the medial and inferior scapular borders to check for scapular winging or tipping. When standing, the hands should rest by the patient's sides with the palms facing the body. If the hands face posteriorly, excessive internal rotation of the humerii is present and may be indicative of shortness of the axiohumeral internal rotators.[115]

Although significantly less common than in the lower extremity, clinicians should observe for upper extremity edema and consider the possibility of lymphedema or a deep vein thrombosis (DVT). Upper extremity lymphedema is a common side effect of cancer treatment and should be considered if the patient has swelling in the chest, axilla, or arm and a history of lymph node resection or radiation to the axilla, chest, or arm. Upper extremity lymphedema can be treated with a combination of compression, manual lymph drainage, and exercise[116] and is beyond the scope of this text. If a DVT is suspected, the clinician should utilize the upper extremity DVT clinical prediction guideline proposed by Constans et al.[117] Details are outlined in Table 14-9. Patients scoring higher than 1 should be considered to have a high probability of DVT and referred for additional medical assessment.

Skin

Assessment of the integument is typically noncontributory unless the patient has had surgery or has scars from a previously undisclosed surgery. After shoulder

TABLE 14-9
UPPER EXTREMITY DEEP VEIN THROMBOSIS CLINICAL PREDICTION GUIDELINE

	Points
One point is awarded for each of the following clinical parameters: • Venous material such as a catheter (access device in subclavian or jugular vein) or pacemaker • Localized pain • Unilateral pitting edema	
One point is deducted from this score if an alternative diagnosis is plausible	
Total score	
If total score is >1, consult physician	

Adapted from Constans J, Salmi LR, Sevestre-Pietri MA, et al. A clinical prediction score for upper extremity deep venous thrombosis. *Thromb Haemost.* 2008;99(1):202–207. doi:10.1160/th07-08-0485

surgery, the patient's incision should be inspected for signs of infection, such as redness, drainage, local edema or fluctuance, and increased temperature.

Range of Motion

Active and passive range of motion should be assessed in all planes, including flexion, extension, abduction, scaption, internal and external rotation, and horizontal abduction and adduction. The clinician should assess movement quantity, pain provocation, quality, and end feel using normative values (Table 14-10).[118,119] A **painful arc** (Fig. 14-23) with elevation may indicate impingement.[102,104,120] End-range pain may indicate adhesive capsulitis. Superior shoulder pain with end-range elevation or horizontal adduction may indicate AC joint pathology.[3] Anterior shoulder pain with external rotation may indicate labral or capsular pathology.[121]

Crepitus during movements may indicate DJD or internal derangement, such as a labral tear or Hill-Sachs lesion. Many overhead athletes develop a shift in rotational range of motion, such that there is a 10 to 15°

TABLE 14-10
PASSIVE SHOULDER RANGE OF MOTION NORMATIVE VALUES

Motion	Normative Value (Degrees)
Flexion	0–180 (shoulder girdle)
Extension	0–60
Abduction	0–180 (shoulder girdle)
Internal rotation	0–70
External rotation	0–90
Horizontal abduction	0–45
Horizontal adduction	0–135

Adapted from America Academy of Orthopedic Surgeons. *Joint Motion: Method of Measuring and Recording.* America Academy of Orthopedic Surgeons; 1965; Clarkson HM. *Musculoskeletal Assessment: Joint Range of Motion, Muscle Testing, and Function.* 4th ed. Wolters Kluwer; 2021.

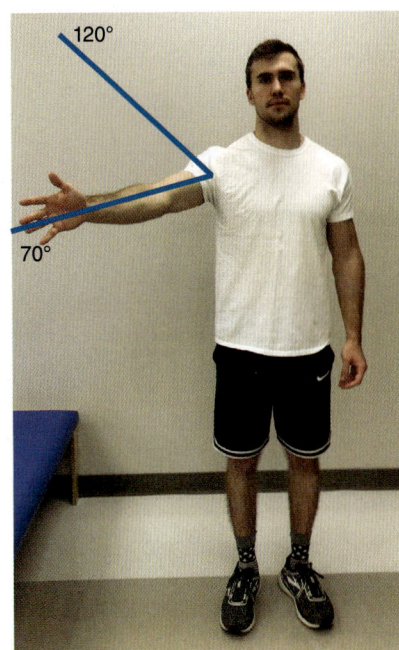

FIGURE 14-23 Painful arc.

increase in external rotation along with an equivalent decrease in internal rotation on the dominant shoulder.[122] This change appears to be the result of both an osseous adaptation (humeral retroversion) and a soft-tissue response (increase anterior GH capsule extensibility with a decrease in posterior capsule) to repeated loading, usually in throwers.[111] Many overhead athletes develop **GIRD** (glenohumeral internal rotation deficit) in which there is a loss of 20° or more of internal rotation range of motion[123] or a loss of more than 5° in the total rotational arc of motion compared to the contralateral side (Fig. 14-24).[124] GIRD appears to increase the risk for shoulder injury.[124] It should be noted that because of adaptive changes over time, many overhead throwing athletes have a 180° total arc of shoulder rotation[125] rather than the traditional normative value of 160°.

Combined movements involved in functional reaching should also be assessed (Fig. 14-25). For the behind

	Athlete A		Athlete B	
	Dom	NonDom	Dom	NonDom
ER (degrees)	105	90	105	90
IR (degrees)	55	70	40	70
Total arc (degrees)	160	160	145	160
Interpretation	No GIRD		GIRD	

FIGURE 14-24 Example of glenohumeral internal rotation deficit (GIRD). *ER,* external rotation; *IR,* internal rotation.

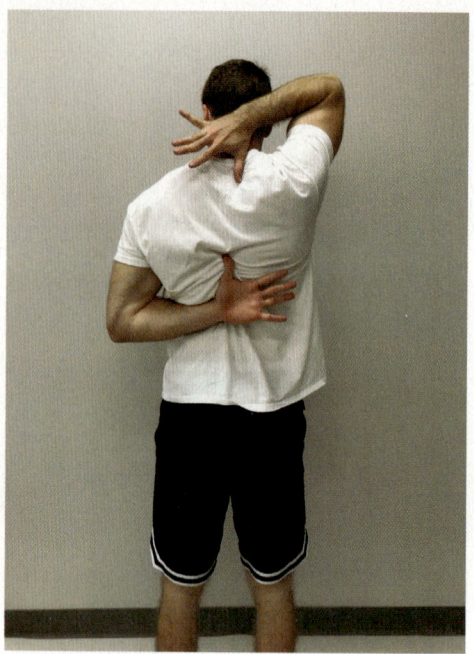

FIGURE 14-25 Combined plane shoulder motion testing.

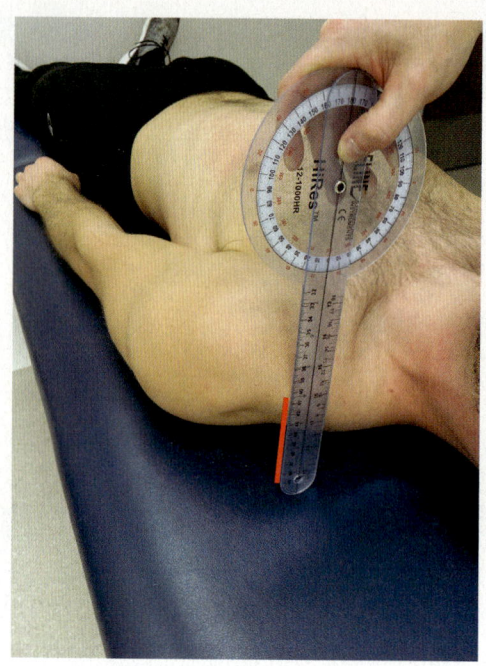

FIGURE 14-26 Assessment of pectoralis minor length.

back reach, the patient is asked to slide the thumb behind the back from the sacrum as far up the spine as possible combining extension, adduction, and internal rotation.[126] The level of the spinous process reached is recorded. Normal motion is the ability to reach between T10 and T5.[127] For the behind neck reach, the patient is asked to slide the thumb up the sternum, the midline of the face, and top of the head, then lower the thumb down the midline of the posterior head to the neck while maintaining the elbow out to the side.[126] This movement combines shoulder flexion, abduction, and external rotation. Normal motion is the ability to reach T1. The motions can be performed bilaterally simultaneously, and the distance between the thumbs can be measured.

Patients who have had recent surgical procedures or recent humeral fractures may have active or passive range of motion precautions that must be followed.

Muscle Length

Unlike the gastrocnemius or hip flexors, there is limited standardization for muscle length tests at the shoulder. The clinician should consider assessing muscle length of the latissimus dorsi, pectoralis major, pectoralis minor (Fig. 14-26), biceps, and triceps noting any differences between affected and unaffected sides, any pain with testing, as well as any large deviations from proposed norms listed in Table 14-11.[114]

TABLE 14-11		
SHOULDER GIRDLE MUSCLE LENGTH ASSESSMENT		
Muscle	*Test Position*	*Proposed Norm*
Latissimus dorsi	Hook-lying supine maintaining posterior pelvic tilt with lumbar spine flat against support surface, measure shoulder flexion	180° shoulder flexion
Pectoralis major—clavicular head	Patient lying supine, horizontally abduct the arm	90° horizontal abduction
Pectoralis major—sternal head	Patient lying supine, raise the arm to 135° abduction with the elbow extended, then lower the arm toward the support surface	Ability of the arm to rest flat on the support surface
Pectoralis minor	Patient lying supine in the anatomic position, measure the vertical distance between the AC joint and the support surface. Note the amount of resistance to overpressure into scapular retraction	No normative data available
Biceps—long head	Seated with back support, measure shoulder extension with the elbow extended	60° shoulder extension
Triceps—long head	Seated, elbow maximally flexed, measure shoulder flexion	180° shoulder flexion

AC, acromioclavicular.

Muscle Performance

The scapulohumeral, ST, and axiohumeral muscle groups should be included in the muscle performance examination of patients with shoulder dysfunction. Manual muscle testing is a convenient, practical, and efficient method to assess muscle strength. Resisted isometric midrange muscle contractions may assist with determining joint pathology.[128,129] Because joint movement is eliminated and testing is performed in a position that minimizes stretching of inert tissues, such as the joint capsule, labrum, and ligaments, these tests may be used as a quick screen of the status of shoulder contractile tissues, muscles, and tendons.

A handheld dynamometer (Fig. 14-27) or weight training equipment may be used to provide more objective information to compare affected and unaffected extremities, particularly in patients with higher levels of strength or higher functional demands. Some patients, such as overhead athletes, may benefit from an assessment of muscle power using an isokinetic device (Fig. 14-28), so comparisons can be made to normative data based on gender, age, and sport. At times, it might be useful to compare strength of one muscle group, both concentrically and eccentrically, with others within the same limb. For example, an isokinetic strength ratio of external rotator to internal rotator strength for throwing athletes is recommended to be 2:3.[130]

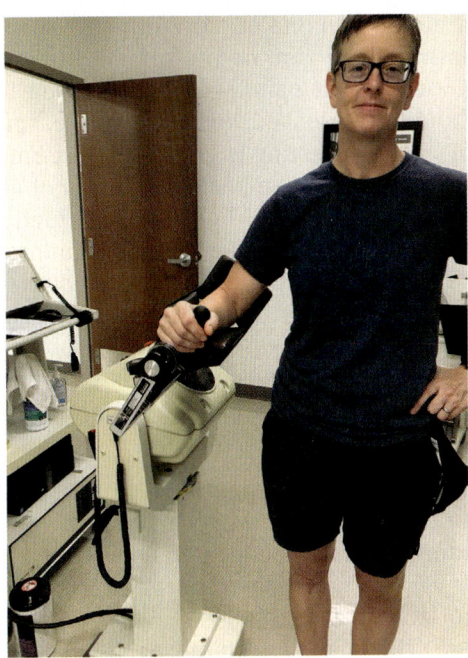

FIGURE 14-28 Isokinetic assessment and training of shoulder external rotators.

Sensory Tests

Light touch sensation should be performed in all patients with suspected shoulder pathology. Knowledge of the cutaneous distribution of nerve roots (dermatomes) and peripheral nerves, as well as considering other supporting assessments, enables the clinician to distinguish sensory loss caused by a root lesion from that caused by a peripheral nerve lesion or thoracic outlet syndrome.

Reflexes

The clinician should routinely assess the biceps (C5), brachioradialis (C6), and triceps (C7) reflexes in patients with suspected shoulder or cervical pathology. Positive findings mandate a closer examination of spinal structures.

Neurodynamic Testing

Neurodynamic testing, including the upper limb tension test described in Chapter 17, Cervical and Thoracic Spine, should be performed on patients with suspected cervical or upper thoracic pathology with symptoms into the upper extremity. Positive findings mandate a closer examination of spinal structures.

Accessory Motion

The GH joint should be assessed for hypermobility or hypomobility and the presence or absence of pain. Patients with adhesive capsulitis generally present with a global decrease in GH joint mobility. In contrast, patients with instability will present with an increase in

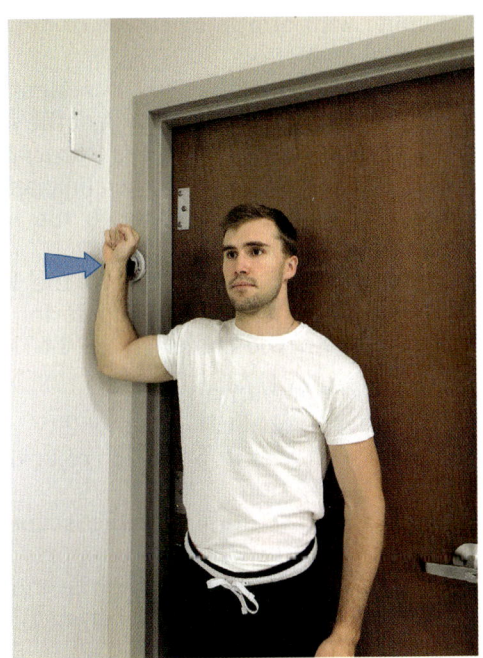

FIGURE 14-27 Handheld dynamometry for shoulder external rotation.

GH joint mobility in one or more directions. ST mobility assessment can also be performed. In the case of local AC or SC joint pain, accessory motion of these joints should be assessed. For a quick assessment, GH accessory motion testing is generally performed with the shoulder in the open-packed position of about 55 to 70° of flexion and 30° horizontal abduction. The open-packed position for the AC and SC joints is with the arm resting by the patient's side. Recall that these same mobilizations can be used fro both assessment and treatment purposes. When used for the treatment of hypomobility, positioning may be altered so the joint is near end-range and/or to optimize clinician body mechanics.

Anterior Glide of Humerus
Purpose: To assess joint-play movement necessary for external rotation and extension.
Patient: Supine with arm in 55 to 70° of flexion and 30° horizontal abduction.
Clinician: The clinician stabilizes the scapula and clavicle anteriorly. The clinician supports the patient's arm against the body using the mobilizing arm. The clinician contacts the posterior proximal humerus with the lateral hand.
Mobilization: An anteromedial glide of the humerus is imparted by mobilizing hand (Fig. 14-29).

Posterior Glide of Humerus
Purpose: To assess joint-play movement necessary for internal rotation and horizontal adduction.
Patient: Supine with arm in 55 to 70° of flexion and 30° horizontal abduction.

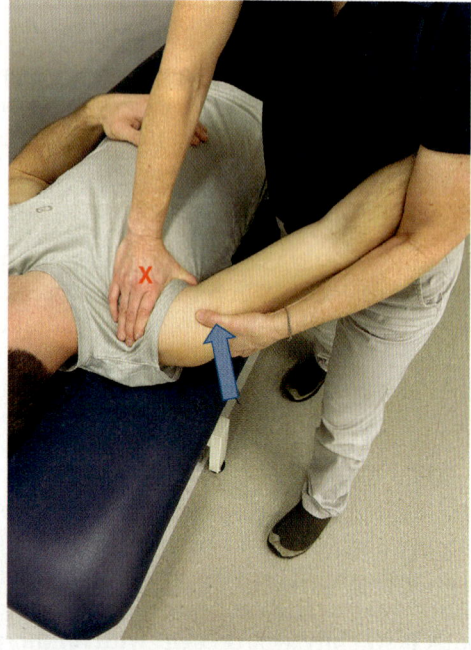

FIGURE 14-29 Anterior glide of humerus.

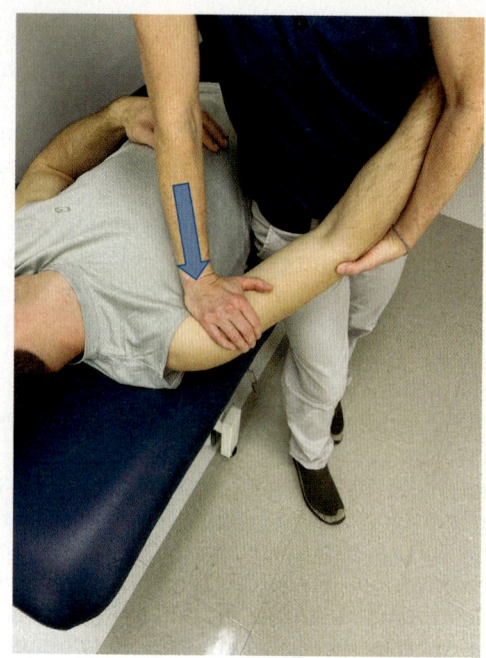

FIGURE 14-30 Posterior glide of humerus.

Clinician: The clinician supports the patient's arm against the body using the nonmobilizing arm. The clinician contacts the anterior proximal humerus with the medial hand.
Mobilization: A posterolateral glide of the humerus is imparted by mobilizing hand (Fig. 14-30).

Inferior Glide of Humerus
Purpose: To assess joint-play movement necessary for elevation (flexion, scaption, and abduction).
Patient: Supine with arm in 55 to 70° of flexion and 30° horizontal abduction.
Clinician: The clinician stabilizes the patient's scapula with the medial hand at the neck of the scapula. The clinician supports the patient's arm against the body using the mobilizing arm. The clinician grasps the distal humerus just proximal to the humeral epicondyles.
Mobilization: The clinician rotates to the left and shifts the body weight to create an inferior, lateral, and anterior glide of the humerus (Fig. 14-31).

Lateral Distraction of Humerus
Purpose: To assess global GH joint mobility.
Patient: Supine with arm in 55 to 70° of flexion and 30° horizontal abduction.
Clinician: The clinician stabilizes the scapula and clavicle anteriorly. The clinician supports the patient's arm against the body using the mobilizing arm. The clinician contacts the posteromedial proximal humerus with the inferior hand.
Mobilization: A lateral, anterior, and superior glide of the humerus is imparted by mobilizing hand by leaning in the direction of the glide (Fig. 14-32).

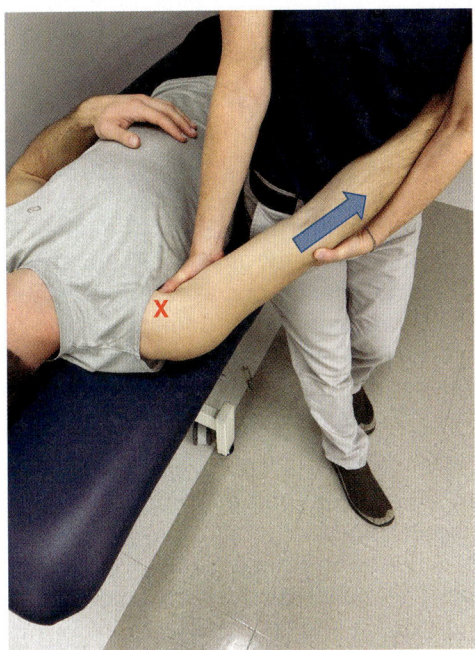

FIGURE 14-31 Inferior glide of humerus.

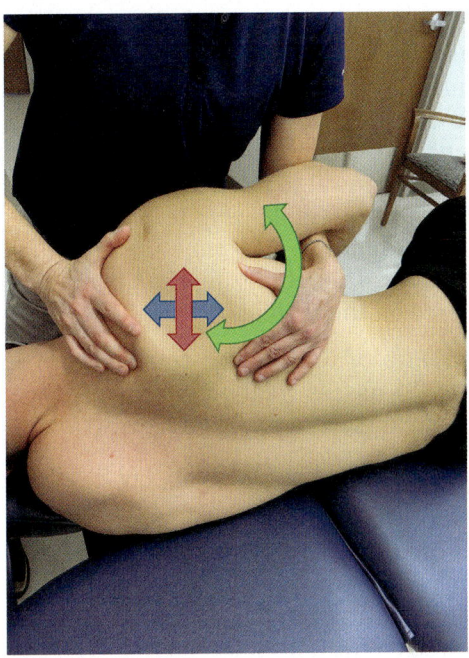

FIGURE 14-33 Scapular mobilization.

Scapular Mobilization
Purpose: To assess scapular mobility.
Patient: Side lying.
Clinician: The clinician's inferior hand gasps the inferior angle of the scapula between the thumb and the index finger whereas the superior hand holds the acromion and superior border of the scapula.
Mobilization: The clinician glides the scapula medial-laterally (blue arrows), superiorly-inferiorly (red arrows), and into upward-downward rotation (green arrows) (Fig. 14-33).

Inferior Glide of Clavicle on the Acromion
Purpose: To assess joint-play movement necessary for scapular elevation and general AC joint mobility.
Clinician: The thumb of the nondominant hand is place on the distal clavicle just medial to the AC joint. The thumb of the dominant hand (mobilizing thumb) is placed over the other thumb.
Mobilization: The mobilizing thumb imparts an inferior glide of the clavicle, creating a relative superior glide of the acromion (Fig. 14-34).

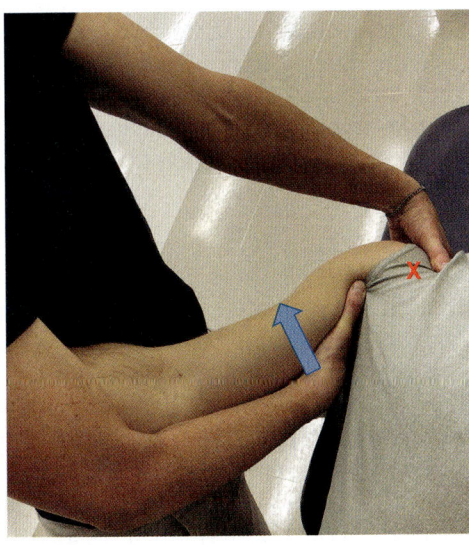

FIGURE 14-32 Lateral distraction of humerus.

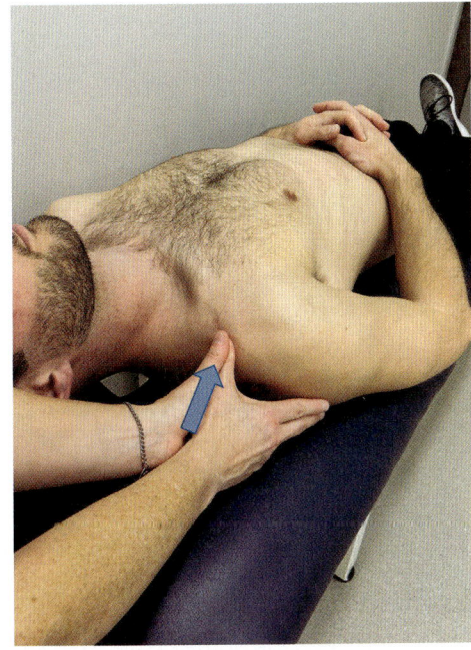

FIGURE 14-34 Inferior glide of the clavicle on the acromion.

Inferior Glide of Acromion on the Clavicle
Purpose: To assess joint-play movement necessary for scapular depression and general AC joint mobility.
Patient: Supine with arm by side.
Clinician: The thumb of the nondominant hand is placed just lateral to the AC joint. The thumb of the dominant hand (mobilizing thumb) is placed over the other thumb.
Mobilization: The mobilizing thumb imparts an inferior force on the acromion.

Inferior Glide of Clavicle on the Sternum
Purpose: To assess joint-play movement necessary for scapular elevation and general SC joint mobility.
Patient: Supine with arm by side.
Clinician: The thumb of the nondominant hand is placed on the medial clavicle just lateral to the SC joint. The thumb of the dominant hand (mobilizing thumb) is placed over the other thumb.
Mobilization: The mobilizing thumb imparts an inferior force on the acromion (Fig. 14-35).

Superior Glide of Clavicle on the Sternum
Purpose: To assess joint-play movement necessary for scapular depression and general SC joint mobility.
Patient: Supine with arm by side.
Clinician: The clinician stands at the side of the patient, facing cranially, and contacts the inferior aspect of the medial clavicle with the nondominant thumb. The thumb of the dominant hand (mobilizing thumb) is placed over the other thumb.
Mobilization: The mobilizing thumb imparts a superior force on the clavicle.

Posterior Glide of Clavicle on the Sternum
Purpose: To assess joint-play movement necessary for scapular retraction.
Patient: Supine with arm by side.
Clinician: The clinician stands at the side of the patient, facing cranially, and contacts the anterior aspect of the medial clavicle with a nondominant thumb. The thumb of the dominant hand (mobilizing thumb) is placed over the other thumb.
Mobilization: The mobilizing thumb imparts a posterior force on the clavicle.

Anterior Glide of Clavicle on the Sternum
Purpose: To assess joint-play movement necessary for scapular protraction.
Patient: Supine with arm by side.
Clinician: The clinician stands at the side of the patient, facing cranially, and contacts the posterior aspect of the medial clavicle with two to three fingers of both hands with the thumbs resting on the anterior ribs.
Mobilization: The clinician imparts an anterior force on the clavicle.

Special Tests/Provocative Testing

Clinicians should choose special/provocative tests to perform based on the patient history and the examination to this point in order to help rule in and rule out competing differential diagnoses. For shoulder pathology, these tests can be grouped into five main categories: AC joint tests, tests for contractile lesions, tests for scapular dyskinesia, tests for subacromial impingement, and tests for instability or labral pathology (Fig. 14-36).

Acromioclavicular Joint Tests Special tests for the AC joint are used to identify the presence or absence of joint hypermobility or joint irritation. There are four main special tests for the AC joint. The AC joint compression test, also known as the AC shear test, and the piano key sign are the most specific. The O'Brien active compression test for labral pathology and the horizontal adduction test for impingement are suggestive of AC joint pathology if producing local AC joint pain.

Acromioclavicular Joint Compression Test (aka the Acromioclavicular Shear Test)
Purpose: To identify an AC separation.
Method: With the patient seated or standing and the arm relaxed by the side, the clinician places one hand on the patient's anterior distal clavicle and the other on the spine of the patient's scapula. The clinician then gently compresses the hands toward each other (Fig. 14-37).
Interpretation: A positive test is if local AC joint pain or increased clavicular motion is noted.

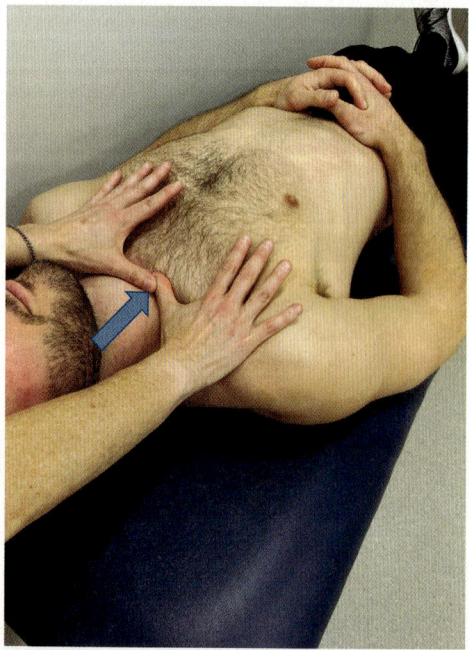

FIGURE 14-35 Inferior glide of the medial clavicle on the sternum.

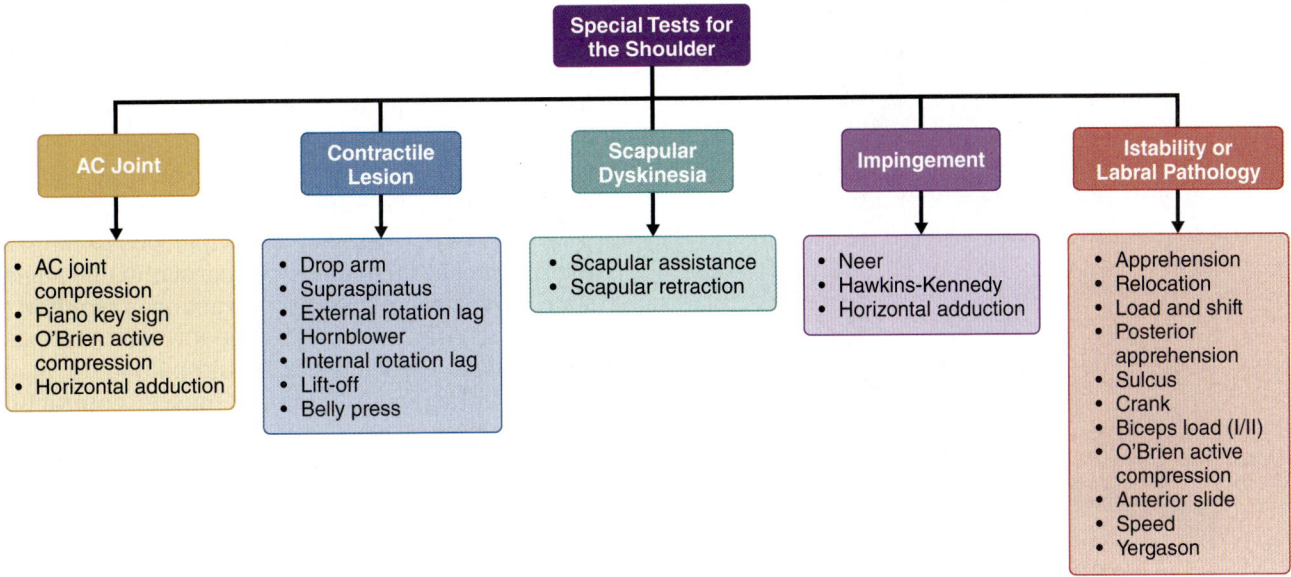

FIGURE 14-36 Special tests for shoulder pathology. *AC,* acromioclavicular.

Piano Key Sign
Purpose: To identify an AC separation.
Method: With the patient seated or standing and the arm relaxed by the side, the clinician applies an inferior force to the patient's distal clavicle.
Interpretation: A positive test is if local AC joint pain or increased clavicular motion is noted.

Special Tests for Contractile Lesions Special tests for contractile lesions are used to identify pain or weakness that may indicate a partial or complete tendon rupture. These tests should be considered for patients with pain during GH active range of motion or manual muscle testing, patients whose shoulder active motion is significantly less than passive motion, and patients demonstrating an abnormal scapulohumeral rhythm. These tests are contraindicated in patients who have had tendon repairs in the past 6 to 8 weeks or if surgical precautions preclude test positioning. Special tests involving a resisted biceps contraction should not be performed in patients who have had a labral repair in the past 6 to 8 weeks. The drop arm test and supraspinatus test assess supraspinatus integrity. The external lag sign targets the infraspinatus, whereas the hornblower test is presumed to more closely target the teres minor. The internal rotation lag sign, lift-off test, and belly press test assess for subscapularis integrity.

Drop Arm Test
Purpose: To identify potential full-thickness supraspinatus tears.[104]
Method: With the patient sitting or standing, the clinician passively places the patient's shoulder in 90° abduction. The patient is asked to hold the test position and slowly lower the arm back to his side (Fig. 14-38).
Interpretation: If the patient is unable to hold the test position or perform the test movement using a normal scapulohumeral rhythm, the test is positive for a supraspinatus lesion.

Supraspinatus Test (aka Full Can Test)
Purpose: To detect a lesion of the supraspinatus muscle. The full can test has been shown to have slightly higher specificity, sensitivity, and predictive

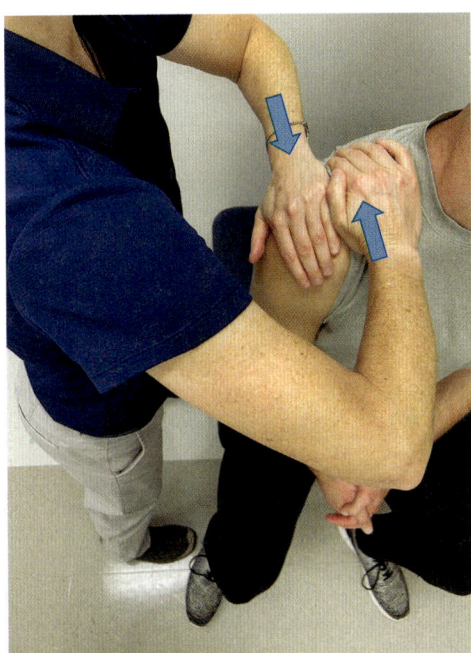

FIGURE 14-37 Acromioclavicular joint compression test.

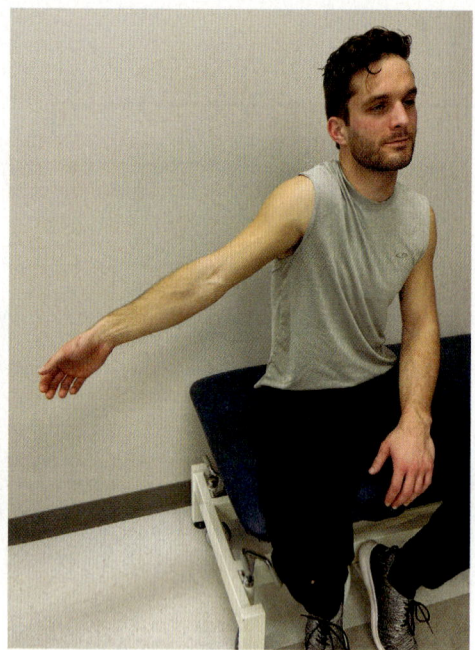

FIGURE 14-38 Drop arm test.

value than the empty can test, possibly due to decreased pain with testing.[131–133]

Method: With the patient sitting or standing, the patient places his arm in 90° of scaption with the thumb pointing upward. The clinician then applies an inferior force at the patient's distal forearm, attempting to adduct the patient's arm (Fig. 14-39).

Interpretation: Test results are documented as positive or negative for pain and for weakness. Weakness is considered a positive test for full-thickness rotator cuff tears. Pain without weakness is considered a positive test for partial-thickness rotator cuff tears or rotator cuff tendinitis.

External Rotation Lag Test
Purpose: To detect possible infraspinatus tears.[120,134–137]

Method: With the patient seated, the clinician passively flexes the patient's elbow to 90° and elevates the shoulder 20°. Holding the patient's wrist and elbow, the clinician rotates the patient's arm to within 5° of maximal external rotation. The patient tries to maintain this position after the clinician releases the patient's wrist but maintains support at the elbow (Fig. 14-40). The key to proper positioning for the test is that the patient's forearm must be angled such that external rotator contraction is required to prevent gravity from pulling the forearm into internal rotation. The clinician should palpate or monitor the infraspinous fossa for muscle contraction during testing.

Interpretation: The external rotation lag test is considered positive for a torn infraspinatus tendon if there is a lag of more than 5° toward internal rotation upon release of the patient's wrist.[135] Clinicians should be careful to ensure that the patient is not placed in maximal passive external rotation because this will create active insufficiency of the external rotators, and a false-positive test. Because the infraspinatus tendon is rarely torn in isolation, in the case of a positive test, the clinician should also assess the integrity of the supraspinatus tendon. Patients with massive rotator cuff tears and a positive external rotation lag test may also have a torn teres minor, which may be more accurately assessed using the hornblower test.

Hornblower Test
Purpose: To detect possible teres minor tears.[3,135,138]

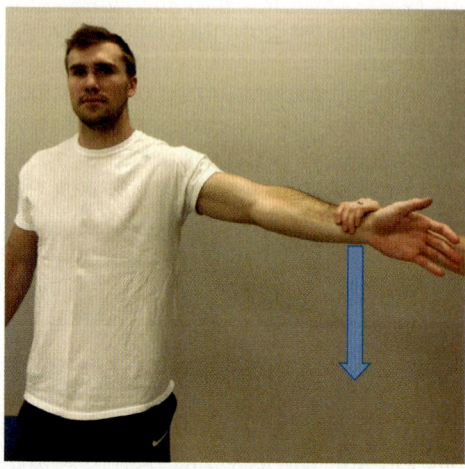

FIGURE 14-39 Supraspinatus test.

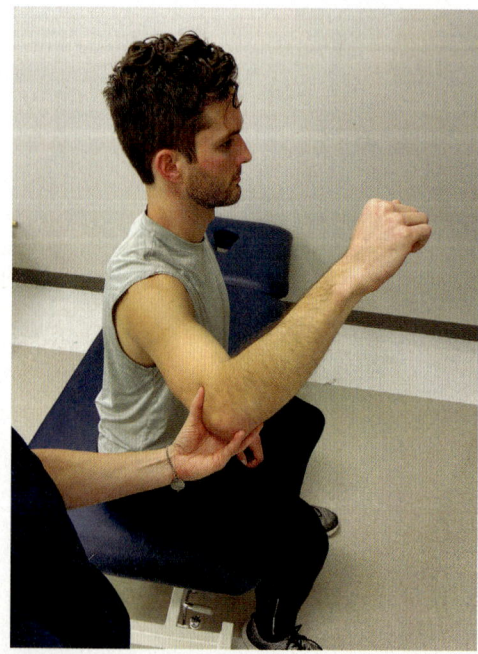

FIGURE 14-40 External rotation lag test.

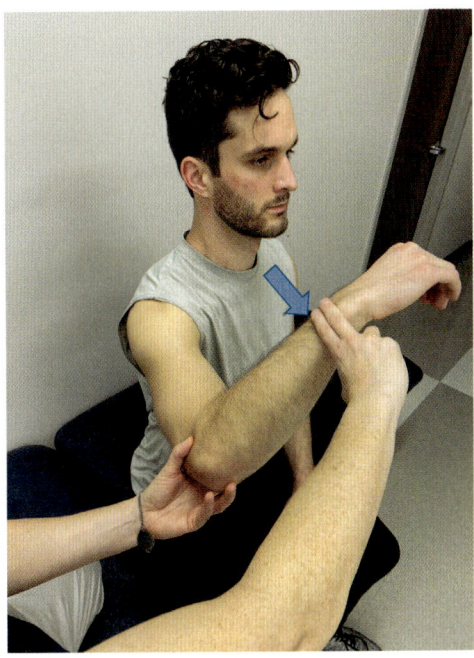

FIGURE 14-41 Hornblower test.

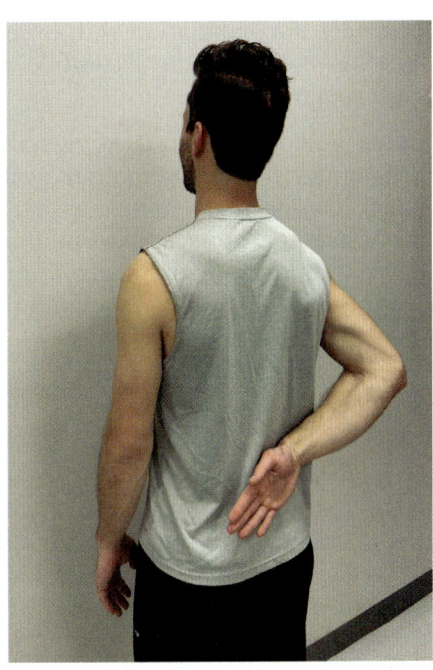

FIGURE 14-42 Lift-off test.

Method: The seated or standing patient seated is asked to bring the hands to the mouth, as in preparing to play a trumpet or horn, without elevating the elbows[135] higher than the hands (Fig. 14-41). Resistance into internal rotation can be added.

Interpretation: A positive test is the inability to do keep the hands higher than the elbows.

Internal Rotation Lag Test

Purpose: To detect a lesion of the subscapularis.[136,138,139]

Method: With the patient seated, the clinician places the patient's hand behind their back by maximally internally rotating the shoulder with the elbow flexed 90° and the shoulder in approximately 20° extension. The patient tries to maintain the hand away from the back after clinician releases their wrist. Clinicians should be careful to ensure that the patient is not placed in maximal passive internal rotation because this will create active insufficiency of the internal rotators, and a false-positive test.

Interpretation: The internal rotation lag test is considered positive for a torn subscapularis if the patient is unable to maintain the dorsal hand away from the back.

Lift-Off Test

Purpose: The lift-off test is a modification of the internal rotation lag test used to detect a lesion of the subscapularis.[134,136,139,140]

Method: The patient places their hand behind the back in extension and internal rotation and then attempts to lift the hand away from the back (Fig. 14-42).

Interpretation: The test is considered positive if the patient cannot lift the dorsum of the hand away from their back. Electromyography (EMG) analysis of the lift-off test demonstrates maximum EMG for the subscapularis and low EMG activity in other shoulder internal rotators, making the test valid and specific. A positive lift-off test in combination with excessive external rotation increases the likelihood of a ruptured subscapularis tendon.

Belly Press Test

Purpose: To detect a lesion of the subcapularis.[102,134,140]

Method: With the patient's hand pressed against their belly, the clinician resists internal rotation. The clinician must prevent the patient from substituting by extending the shoulder by allowing the elbow to move posterior to the trunk.

Interpretation: The patient's inability to maintain the hand against the belly and the elbow anterior to the trunk against maximum resistance is considered positive for a torn subscapularis. False-positive tests can occur if the patient substitutes by extending the shoulder by moving the elbow posterior to the trunk. Note the anterior deltoid, pectoralis major, latissimus dorsi, and teres major can substitute for the subscapularis. The belly press test selectively recruits the upper fibers of the subscapularis, whereas the lift-off test selectively recruits more of the lower subscapularis fibers.[140] Therefore, it may be wise to perform both test maneuvers when assessing the integrity of the subscapularis. A positive belly press test in combination with excessive external rotation increases the likelihood of a ruptured subscapularis tendon.

Special Tests for Scapular Dyskinesia Scapular dyskinesia is abnormal scapular motion during shoulder movement. During the scapular assistance test, the clinician assists upward scapular rotation. During the scapular retraction test, the clinician provides a stable base for the rotator cuff to function from.

Scapular Assistance Test
Purpose: To assess for scapular dyskinesia as a cause for shoulder pain.[102]

Method: With the patient standing, the clinician contacts the inferior medial angle of the scapula and pushes the scapula into upward rotation as the patient actively performs shoulder elevation (Fig. 14-43). The test can be modified by having the clinician's other hand on the superior scapula to provide a slight posterior tilt of the scapula.

Interpretation: A positive test for scapular dyskinesia is if pain with shoulder elevation decreases when performed with clinician assistance for scapular motion.

Scapular Retraction Test
Purpose: To identify scapular dyskinesia.[102,141]

Method: With the patient standing or sitting, the patient raises the arm to 90° in the scapular plane in internal rotation (with the thumb pointing down). The clinician then applies a downward force. If pain is produced (previously referred to as a *positive empty can test*), the test is repeated with the clinician stabilizing the patient's scapula in a retracted and posteriorly tilted position using the forearm.

Interpretation: A positive test for scapular dyskinesia is if pain or weakness occurs with the first test, but alleviated when the scapula is stabilized (Fig. 14-44). The empty can test was designed to assess for a supraspinatus lesion. However, it has been found to be inaccurate and should not be used to make clinical decisions.

Special Tests for Subacromial Impingement The Neer impingement test, Hawkins-Kennedy test, and horizontal adduction test are special tests for impingement and are used to identify the presence or absence of tissue pathology within the subacromial space, including the rotator cuff, long head of biceps, and subacromial bursa. All of the impingement tests attempt to compress, or impinge, pathologic tissue between the humeral head/greater tuberosity and the antero-inferior acromion. None of the impingement tests can correctly identify which structure is involved and, therefore, responsible for shoulder pain. Because each test compresses the subacromial space differently, clinicians should perform all three impingement tests. Impingement tests should be considered for patients with a painful arc during active range of motion, pain at the end of active range of motion, or with scapulohumeral manual muscle testing, or patients with abnormal scapulohumeral rhythm. These tests should be used with caution in patients who have had shoulder surgery in the past 6 to 8 weeks and should not be used if surgical precautions preclude test positioning.

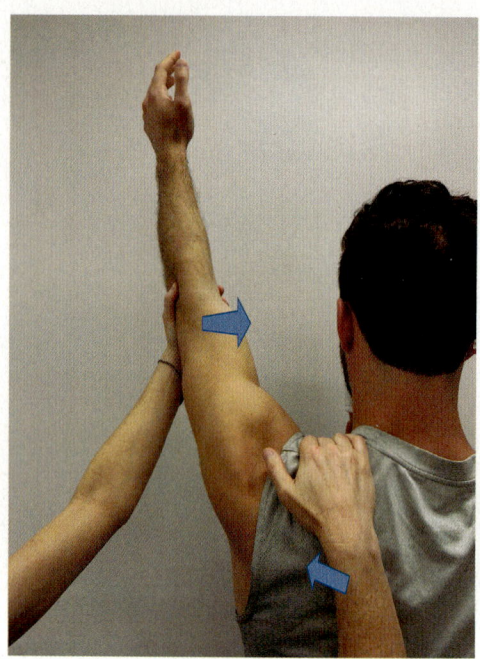

FIGURE 14-44 Scapular retraction test.

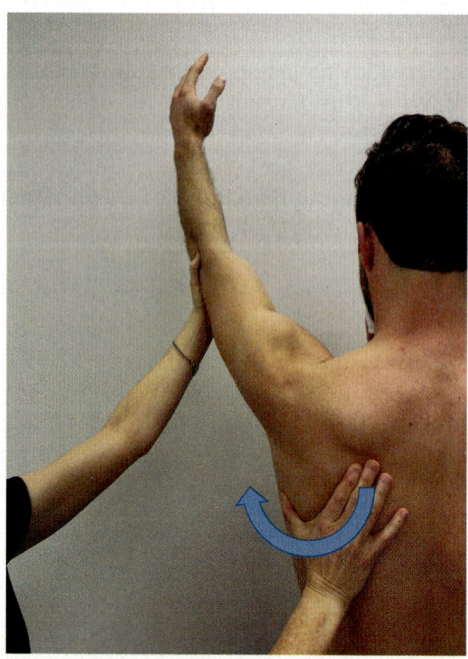

FIGURE 14-43 Scapular assistance test.

Neer Impingement Test

Purpose: To detect SIS and indicate pathology of the rotator cuff, biceps, and/or subacromial bursa.[102,120,131,134]

Method: The Neer impingement test creates subacromial impingement by applying overpressure to shoulder flexion. With the patient seated or standing, the clinician internally rotates the humerus and then fully flexes the shoulder. If excessive scapular elevation occurs, it may be helpful for the clinician to first stabilize the scapula before flexing the humerus (Fig. 14-45).

Interpretation: Shoulder pain produced with testing is considered a positive test for SIS.

Hawkins-Kennedy Impingement Test

Purpose: To detect SIS and indicate pathology of the rotator cuff, biceps, and/or subacromial bursa.[102,120,134]

Method: The Hawkins-Kennedy test creates subacromial impingement by applying overpressure to shoulder internal rotation. With the patient seated or standing, the clinician passively flexes the shoulder and elbow to 90° and then forcefully internally rotates the humerus (Fig. 14-46).

Interpretation: Shoulder pain produced with testing is considered a positive test.

Horizontal Adduction Test (aka the Clancy Impingement Test or Cross Body Test)

Purpose: To detect SIS and indicate pathology of the rotator cuff, biceps, and/or subacromial bursa.[120,134]

Method: The horizontal adduction test creates subacromial impingement by applying overpressure

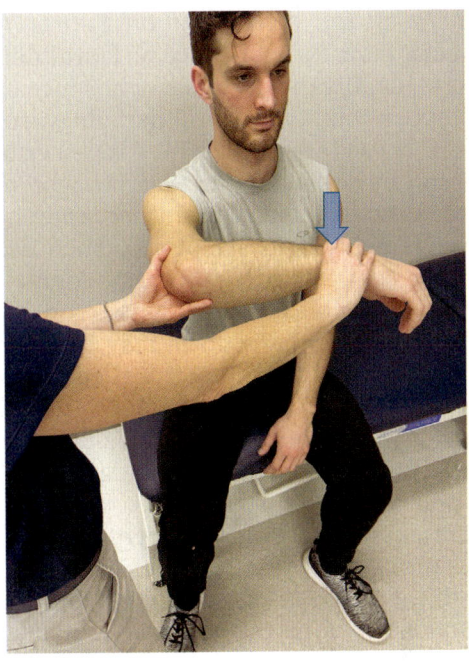

FIGURE 14-46 Hawkins-Kennedy impingement test.

to shoulder horizontal adduction. With the patient seated or standing, the clinician passively elevates the shoulder to 90° with the elbow flexed 90° and then passively, horizontally adducts the shoulder (Fig. 14-47).

Interpretation: Shoulder pain produced with testing is considered a positive test for SIS. Local AC joint pain with testing may indicate AC joint pathology[3,142] and should be followed up with the O'Brien active compression test and local palpation.[138]

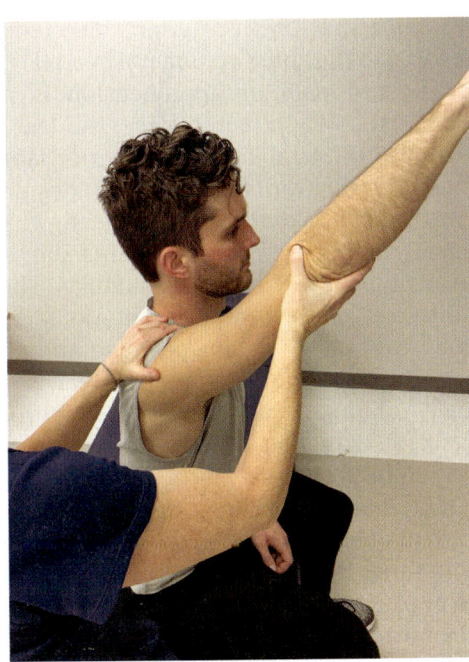

FIGURE 14-45 Neer impingement test.

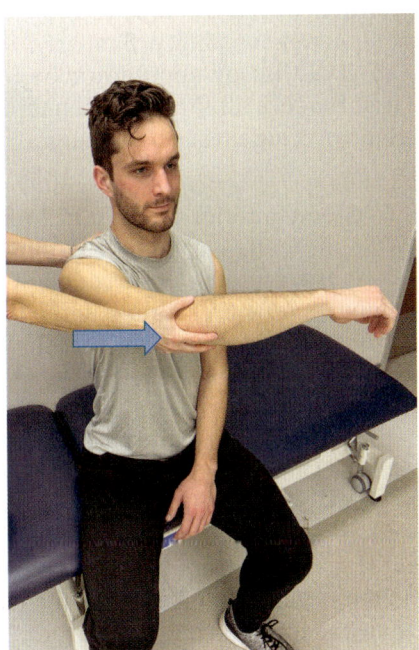

FIGURE 14-47 Horizontal adduction test.

Special Tests for Instability or Labral Pathology Special tests for instability or labral deficiency are used to identify the presence or absence of symptomatic hypermobility or labral pathology, such as a labral tear. These tests are grouped together because they should be considered in patients who report a feeling of looseness, slippage, shifting, apprehension, or transient neurologic symptoms, such as paresthesias or a "dead arm," as well as patients reporting a history of subluxation or dislocation. It should be noted that some individuals may have systemic hypermobility and the Beighton test can assist with detecting this (see Fig. 7-3 in Chapter 7, The Physical Examination). In addition, some individuals, particularly overhead athletes, may have acquired shoulder hypermobility. Clinicians must keep in mind that, as with joint mobility assessment, there are large variations of normal. For these reasons, it is important to note both the quantity of test motion and symptom reproduction in both the affected and unaffected shoulders.

When assessing for shoulder instability, clinicians should choose at least one test stressing each of the following directions: anterior (apprehension, relocation, and load-and-shift tests), posterior (load-and-shift and posterior apprehension test), and inferior (sulcus test). Because clinical tests for labral pathology lack accuracy, clinicians should choose two or three tests[107] based on research support and ability to position the patient appropriately for testing. Tests for labral pathology include crank, biceps load (I/II), O'Brien active compression test, and anterior slide test.

To protect healing tissues, instability tests should not be performed within the first 6 to 8 weeks after surgery for shoulder instability. Similarly, tests used to detect labral pathology should not be performed within the first 8 weeks after a labral repair or if surgical precautions preclude test positioning.

Apprehension Test
Purpose: To detect anterior GH joint instability.[143–146]
Method: With the patient supine, the clinician passively moves the arm into 90° abduction and then into maximum external rotation (Fig. 14-48). If there is no response to this position, the clinician may grasp the posterior humeral head and apply an anteriorly directed force to the proximal humerus to increase the strain on the anterior GH joint.
Interpretation: The apprehension test is considered positive for anterior instability if the test produces anterior shoulder pain or apprehension. The apprehension test may also produce pain in patients with superior labral tears[131] and impingement. Test accuracy may be improved if apprehension is used to determine a positive test rather than pain.

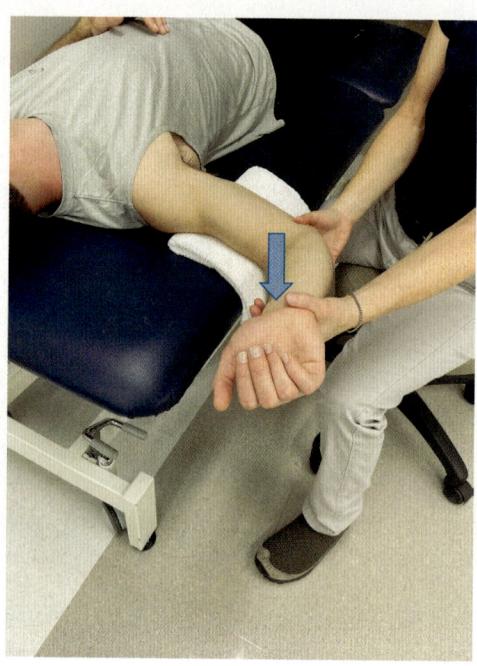

FIGURE 14-48 Apprehension test.

Relocation Test
Purpose: The relocation test is a continuation of the apprehension test that is used to detect possible type II superior labrum anterior and posterior (SLAP) lesions. It may also be used to differentiate anterior instability from posterior impingement.[3,143–148]
Method: The first part of the test is to perform the apprehension test by passively abducting the patient's shoulder to 90° and then slowly externally rotating the arm to the point of pain or apprehension. The second step is to apply a posteriorly directed, or relocating, force to the anterior humeral head (Fig. 14-49).
Interpretation: If pain or apprehension is reduced with the posteriorly directed force, the test is positive for anterior instability or a superior labral tear. Externally rotating the abducted shoulder produces anterior translation of the humeral head, which may cause pain or apprehension in patients after an anterior dislocation or with anterior instability. The posteriorly directed force recenters an anteriorly displaced humeral head, thus reducing pain and apprehension in this patient population. If a labral tear is present, externally rotating the abducted shoulder produces a peel-back phenomenon in which the posterosuperior labrum subluxes laterally.[134] The subsequent posteriorly directed force places traction on the biceps tendon, reducing the subluxed labrum back to a normal position, thus decreasing pain. If posterior shoulder pain is produced with external rotation and reduced with the posteriorly directed force, the test is positive for posterior or internal impingement.[111]

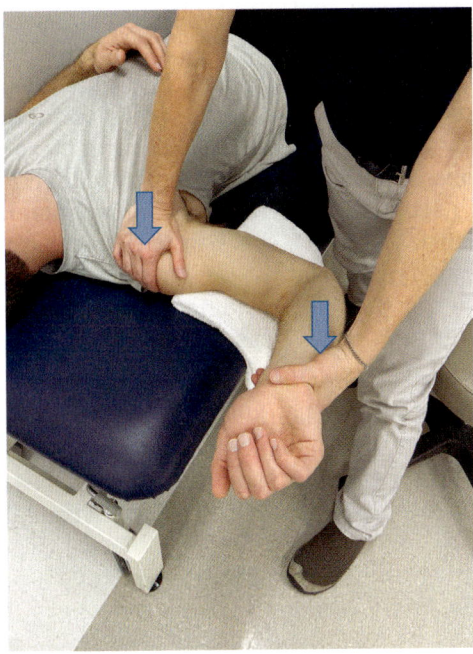

FIGURE 14-49 Relocation test.

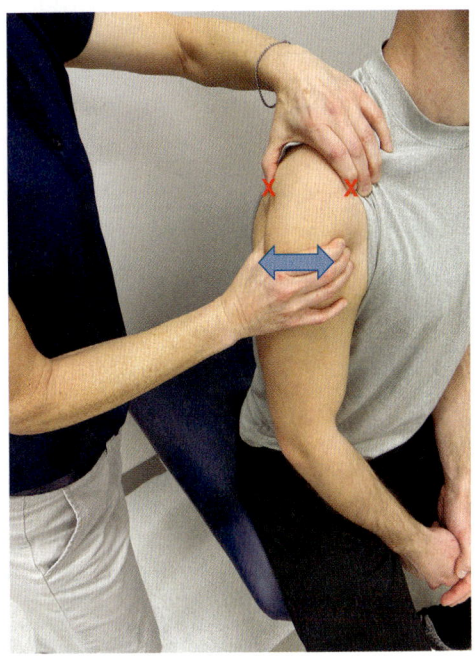

FIGURE 14-50 Load-and-shift test.

Load-and-Shift Test
Purpose: To detect anterior and posterior GH instability.[134,143,145]

Method: With the patient seated with his arm by his side, the clinician stabilizes the scapula with one hand while holding the proximal humerus with the mobilizing hand. The clinician first applies a small compressive force to the GH joint, meant to center the humeral head within the glenoid if it was originally in a subluxed position. Next, the clinician applies an anterior, and then a posterior, force to proximal humerus (Fig. 14-50).

Interpretation: The load-and-shift test is graded based on the relative movement noted between the humerus and the glenoid using the following scale:
- Normal: Humeral head translates less than 25% of the width of the humeral head in either direction.
- Grade I laxity: 25 to 50% of the humeral head translates over the glenoid rim.
- Grade II laxity: More than 50% of the humeral head translates over the glenoid rim, but the humerus does not completely sublux.
- Grade III laxity: The entire humeral head subluxes over the glenoid rim.

While patients with a positive load-and-shift test will likely also present with other positive instability tests, clinicians should be cautious of false-negative test results. Because the load-and-shift test is performed in the anatomic position, it may not stress the capsular and ligamentous structures as much as other instability tests. Therefore, the load-and-shift test should not be used as the sole indicator of instability. The advantage of the load-and-shift test is that the test position may allow the patient to relax better than with other instability tests, thus providing a more accurate result.

Posterior Apprehension Test
Purpose: To detect posterior GH instability.[149]

Method: With the patient supine, the clinician flexes the patient's elbow, then moves the shoulder into 90° of elevation, followed by horizontal adduction and internal rotation. With the lateral hand stabilizing the scapula posteriorly, the clinician uses the medial hand to apply an axial load through the patient's elbow (Fig. 14-51).

Interpretation: A positive test is patient report of instability or apprehension.

Sulcus Test
Purpose: To detect inferior capsular and ligamentous laxity.[134,150]

Method: With the patient seated or standing, the clinician grasps the patient's distal humerus with one hand and applies an inferior traction force (Fig. 14-52). The clinician's other hand is placed at the anterior border of the inferior acromion to palpate joint separation. The test can also be performed in 45 and 90° of shoulder abduction to assess different shoulder structures.

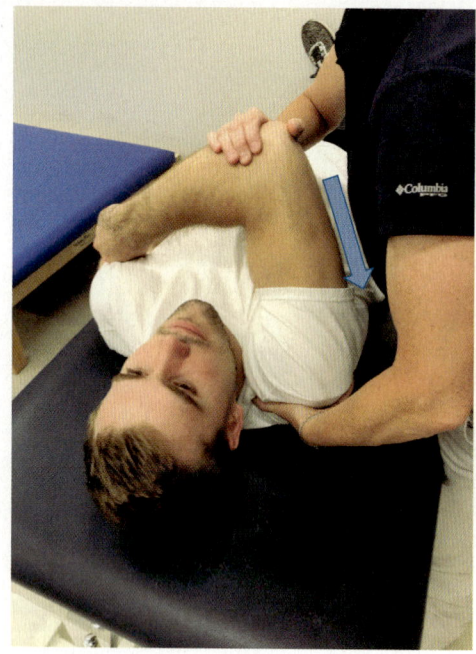

FIGURE 14-51 Posterior apprehension test.

Interpretation: The sulcus test is graded based on the estimated amount of acromiohumeral separation using the following scale:
- 1+: 0.5 to 1 cm separation
- 2+: 1 to 2 cm separation
- 3+: greater than 2 cm separation

Dimpling of the skin under the acromion may occur with an increase in joint separation. The primary restraints to the sulcus test vary based on the position tested. With the arm by the side, the SGHL, CHL, and superior capsule are the primary restraints. With the arm in 45° abduction, the primary restraint is the IGHL, with the posterior capsule and middle GH ligament (MGHL) providing secondary restraint to inferior humeral head translation. With the arm in 90° abduction, the primary restraint is the IGHL, with the MGHL and inferior capsule providing secondary restraint to inferior humeral head translation.

Crank Test
Purpose: To detect labral tears.[131,138,144,151]
Method: With the patient supine, the clinician places the arm in maximal scaption and then applies an axial load to the GH joint while passively maximally internally and externally rotating the humerus (Fig. 14-53).
Interpretation: The crank test is positive if pain or a click is noted with testing.

Biceps Load I and II Tests
Purpose: To detect long head of biceps and labral pathology.[138,144,147,152–154]
Method: With the patient supine, the elbow flexed 90°, and the forearm supinated, the clinician abducts the shoulder to 90° for the biceps load I test and 120° for the biceps load II test. The clinician externally rotates the shoulder to end-range external rotation or to the point of pain or apprehension and then resists elbow flexion with the forearm supinated (Fig. 14-54).
Interpretation: The biceps load I and II tests are positive for a SLAP lesion if the patient's symptoms are created or increased with resisted elbow flexion because biceps contraction increases tension on the biceps-labral complex.[152]

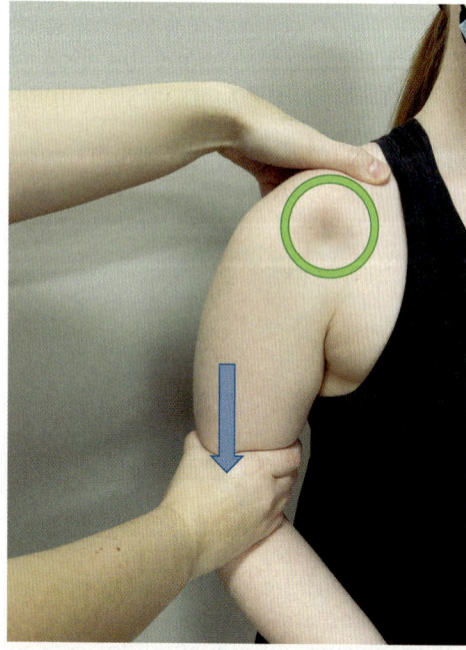

FIGURE 14-52 Sulcus test. Note void (green circle) due to inferior translation of the humeral head.

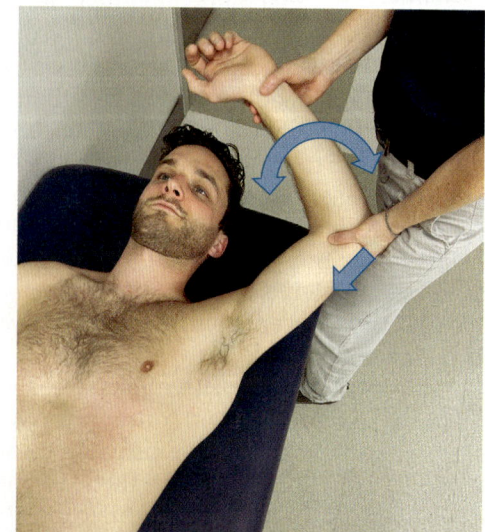

FIGURE 14-53 Crank test.

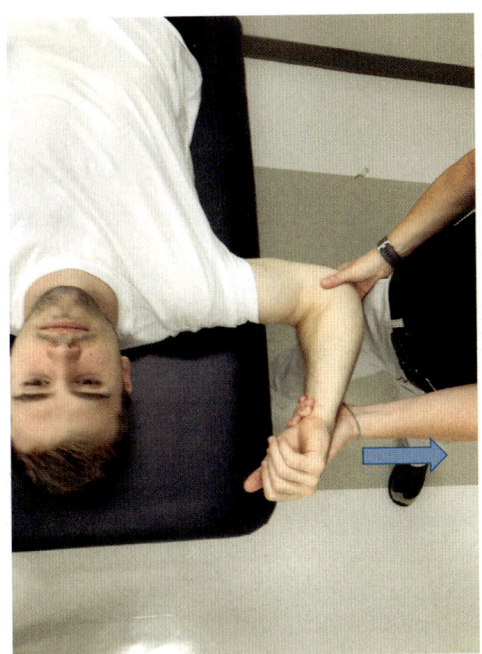

FIGURE 14-54 Biceps load I test.

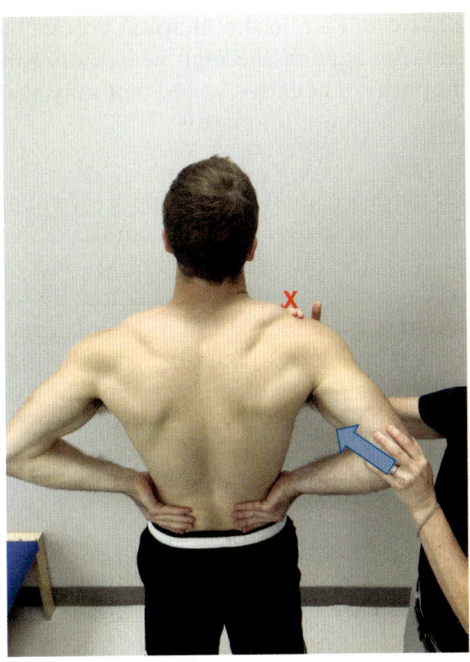

FIGURE 14-55 Anterior slide test.

O'Brien Active Compression Test (aka the Active Compression Test)
Purpose: To detect a labral tear and AC joint pathology.[134,138,142,151,155]

Method: The seated or standing patient is asked to flex the shoulder to 90° with the elbow fully extended, then adduct the shoulder approximately 10°, and maximally internally rotate the shoulder. The clinician then applies an inferior force at the patient's wrist. The test is then repeated with the patient maximally externally rotated.

Interpretation: The O'Brien active compression test is positive for labral pathology, particularly a SLAP lesion, if pain is present when tested in internal rotation but absent in the externally rotated position. Local AC joint pain provocation is indicative of AC joint pathology and should be followed up with AC joint compression test and local palpation.

Anterior Slide Test (aka the Anterior Scapular Slide Test)
Purpose: To detect anterior SLAP lesions.[107,134,156]

Method: The patient stands and places his hand on his iliac crest with his thumbs anteriorly. The clinician stabilizes the anterior shoulder with one hand and then grasps the patient's elbow applying an anterior and superiorly directed force to the GH joint (Fig. 14-55).

Interpretation: The anterior slide test is positive if the test produces deep or anterior shoulder pain or a click. Although the anterior slide test has a high specificity, it should not be used as a sole diagnostic test to detect a labral injury because of its low sensitivity.

Speed Test
Purpose: To detect possible lesions of the superior glenoid labrum or biceps tendon complex.[3,138]

Method: With the patient seated or standing, the clinician places the patient in 60 to 90° shoulder flexion with the forearm supinated and the elbow extended. The patient is asked to resist shoulder flexion, thereby putting stress on the LHBT (Fig. 14-56).

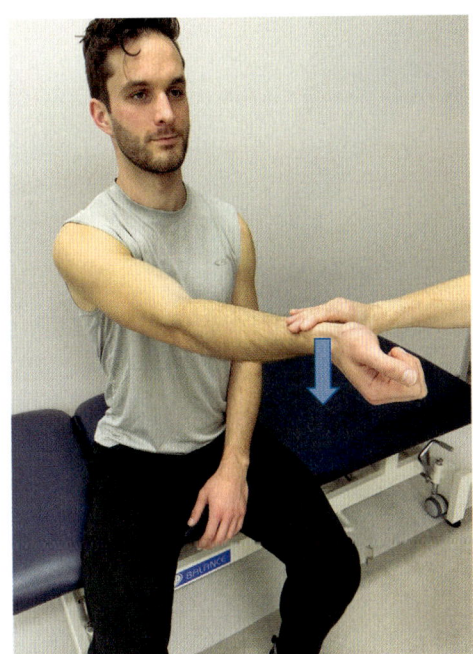

FIGURE 14-56 Speed test.

Interpretation: Pain in the bicipital groove is a positive test. Because of the high sensitivity for biceps tendinopathy, a negative speed test may essentially rule out biceps tendinopathy.

Yergason Test

Purpose: To detect possible lesions of the superior glenoid labrum or biceps tendon complex.[3,131,138,144,157]

Method: With the patient seated or standing, the clinician places the patient in pronation, 90° of elbow flexion, and shoulder adduction against thorax. The clinician resists supination, thereby placing increased stress on the biceps tendon-labral complex (Fig. 14-57).

Interpretation: Tenderness or pain in the bicipital groove is considered a positive test.

Palpation

The region should be palpated for tenderness, temperature, edema, and deformity. Bony tenderness with a history of trauma may indicate fracture.[110] After an acute sprain or strain, tenderness of the involved structure can be expected. In cases of significant superficial sprains or strains, there may be a loss of fiber continuity that can be felt as a palpable breach of gap in the involved tissue. The mobility of any scars should be assessed.

Functional Testing

While a preliminary idea of functional range of motion is obtained from active range of motion testing including moving the hand behind the back and behind the neck, the clinician should consider observing

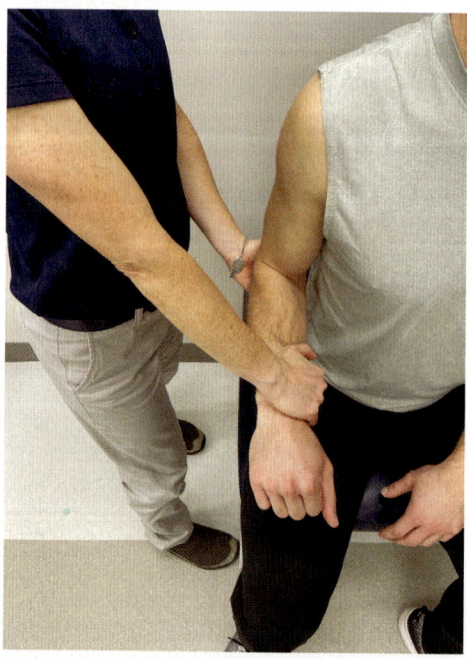

FIGURE 14-57 Yergason test.

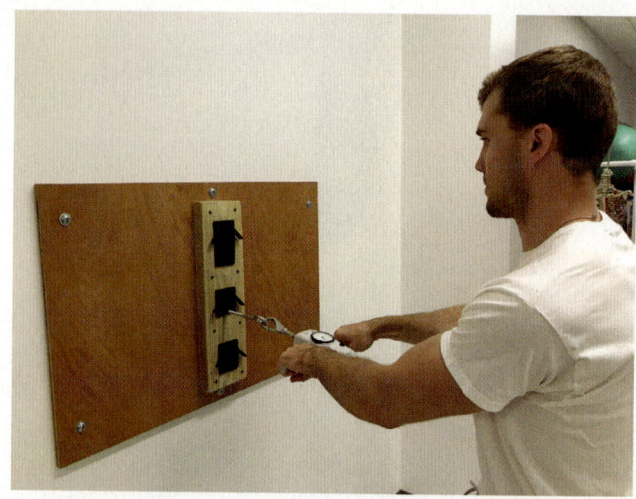

FIGURE 14-58 Horizontal pull.

the patient performing movements reported as being difficult or painful during the history or those items marked as difficult on the patient-reported outcome measure. For example, the clinician should observe the patient perform overhead activities, such as reaching or throwing, or activities that require force through the extremity, such as push-ups or lifting. A tension gauge can be used to measure the patient's ability to perform horizontal and vertical pushing or pulling (Fig. 14-58).

COMMON SHOULDER PATHOLOGIES

This section contains details on the most common or most problematic shoulder pathologies a clinician is to see in an outpatient setting, including fracture, AC and SC joint pathology, GH osteoarthritis (OA) and shoulder arthroplasty, adhesive capsulitis, rotator cuff tears, scapular dyskinesia, SIS, GH instability, labral tears, bicipital tendinopathy, and suprascapular neuropathy.

Acromioclavicular Joint Separation

Pathology Instability and degeneration are the two primary pathologies of the AC joint. AC joint sprains and dislocations (commonly referred to as *AC joint separations*) may result in instability and are classified based on tissues affected. Type I to III separations are most common (Table 14-12).[110] Higher grade AC separations, such as those with posterior or inferior displacement of the clavicle, require surgical intervention[6,110] and are not typically seen before surgery, given the obvious deformity and significant pain associated with these injuries.

History AC joint sprains are more common in younger individuals and generally result from direct contact to the acromion,[110] such as a football tackle or a fall, but may also occur indirectly from a fall landing on an

TABLE 14-12
CLASSIFICATION OF ACROMIOCLAVICULAR SEPARATIONS

Type	Ligament(s) Involved	Joint Deformity	Examination Findings
I	AC—stretched	None	AC joint is stable joint Pain with AC joint mobility testing and shear testing
II	AC—ruptured CC—stretched	Minor	Palpable joint gapping with distal clavicle superior to acromion AC joint is mildly unstable Pain and hypermobility with AC joint mobility and shear testing Moderate-to-severe pain
III	AC and CC ruptured	Dislocation with distal clavicle superior to acromion	Positive step sign AC joint is unstable Pain and hypermobility with AC joint mobility and shear testing

AC, acromioclavicular; *CC*, coracoclavicular.

outstretched arm, as might occur with ice hockey or skiing.[6,158] Individuals report an immediate onset of local AC joint pain. Active elevation may be painful or impossible pending injury severity.

Key Examination Findings The examination of patients with AC joint pathology should begin with observation of the joint for symmetry, swelling, and deformity. Patients with type III sprains will have a persistent joint deformity due to ligamentous rupture. Active shoulder elevation should be assessed with concomitant palpation at the AC joint. Patients with type I to III sprains may have limited elevation due to pain. End-range elevation and horizontal adduction will be painful. The AC joint may be tender, warm, or edematous to palpation. Patients who sustained type IV to VI sprains will be seen after surgical fixation and generally present with decreased shoulder range of motion and strength. Table 14-12 includes special test findings of patients for the various types of AC joint separation.

Differential Diagnoses Differential diagnosis includes possible fracture of the clavicle or glenoid. Fracture should be considered based on deformity, bony tenderness, and disproportionate pain.[6]

Rehabilitation Focus and Key Points Table 14-13 provides an overview of key physical therapy interventions after AC joint sprains. Sling or figure-of-eight harness immobilization is not required for patients with type I sprains, but may be used for 1 to 2 weeks for patients with a type II or III sprain.[159] To prevent secondary motion loss, active

TABLE 14-13
REHABILITATION AFTER ACROMIOCLAVICULAR SEPARATION*

	Type I	Type II	Type III
Symptom modulation	Sling: Rarely Ice Pendulum exercise AC joint taping	Sling: 0-2 weeks Ice Pendulum exercise AC joint taping	Sling: 0-2 weeks Ice Pendulum exercise AC joint taping
Distal UE AROM	Immediately	Immediately	Immediately
Shoulder isometrics	Immediately	Immediately	Immediately
Shoulder A A-AROM#	*Immediately* AROM rotation AA-AROM elevation *Progression* As tolerated	As type I except begin with AA-AROM elevation 0-90°	As type II
PRE	0-2 weeks	0-2 weeks	3-4 weeks
UECKC	2-4 weeks	4-6 weeks	6-12 weeks
Return to normal function	0-2 weeks	1-6 weeks	6-12 weeks

*Timeframes given are generalized. Progression must be individualized and symptom modulated.
AC, acromioclavicular joint; *PRE*, progressive resistive exercises for the elbow and shoulder; *UECKC*, upper extremity closed kinetic chain exercises.

distal extremity motion should be encouraged for all patients, particularly those who require a sling. Acutely, patients with AC sprains should be instructed to limit overhead lifting and overhead activities. Exercises with significant deltoid and upper trapezius activation should also be limited early on. Pain-modulated exercise can be initiated immediately after injury, including shoulder and elbow isometrics, active shoulder rotation with the arm by the side, and active assisted to active elevation beginning with ranges up to 90° elevation and increasing to higher ranges as pain decreases.[159] AC joint taping may be beneficial for patients with type I to III sprains to decrease forces through the acutely or subacutely injured AC joint while allowing an increase in range of motion.[160] Progressive resistive exercise to the elbow, shoulder, and scapular stabilizers[159] can generally be initiated in the first week for type I sprains and within the first 2 weeks for type II sprains. Patients with type III sprains can be progressed to resistive exercise as pain allows, generally in the second or third week postinjury.

Expected Outcomes Return to full function and sport can be expected within 2 to 12 weeks based on the extent of injury. Patients with type III AC joint separations who fail to improve with conservative treatment generally do well with distal clavicle excision or primary repair.[6,159] Two-year follow-up for patients undergoing surgery versus conservative treatment has shown no difference in functional recovery, including strength and the ability to perform overhead activity- or sport-specific function.[161]

Acromioclavicular Degenerative Joint Disease

In contrast to AC joint separation, patients with AC DJD report a more gradual onset of local AC joint pain that increases with overhead activities or tasks requiring horizontal adduction. Patients are generally middle aged[142] and may have concomitant tendinitis or impingement. Weight lifters may report a gradual onset of a dull ache at the AC joint that increases with bench press, military press, dips, and push-ups due to the increased AC joint weight bearing during these activities.[162,163] AC joint degeneration may occur as a delayed complication after AC separation or due to repetitive horizontal adduction or heavy weight training.[163]

Patients with AC joint DJD typically present with local AC joint pain. A positive horizontal adduction test helps to rule in the diagnosis, whereas a negative O'Brien active compression test helps to rule out AC joint DJD.[142] Positive instability testing for pain including joint mobility testing and AC shear test is suggestive of acute AC separation rather than DJD.

Patients with AC joint DJD should be educated in activity modification. Exercise should be limited to below 90° of elevation to reduce joint compression.[162] Patients should be instructed to limit weight-bearing exercises such as bench press, military press, dips, and push-ups until symptoms have resolved. Ice or iontophoresis may assist with inflammation control and pain modulation acutely. Exercise is progressed as pain allows. Patients with AC joint degeneration may benefit from nonsteroidal anti-inflammatory drugs (NSAIDs). A corticosteroid injection may be indicated for those who continue to have significant pain complaints. Although uncommon, patients who fail to improve with conservative treatment do well with distal clavicle resection.[142,162,163]

Sternoclavicular Joint Pathology

Injuries to the SC joint are rare and, due to the strong ligamentous support, require significant force.[164] The SC joint's articular disc is much thicker than that of the AC joint, increasing joint congruity and decreasing the incidence of SC joint DJD.[165] Up to one-third of the most common rheumatic diseases, such as ankylosing spondylitis and rheumatoid arthritis, may affect the SC joint.[165] Patients without a diagnosis of rheumatic disease should be asked about symptoms in other joints, and appropriate referrals should be made. In addition, the possibility of septic arthritis should be considered particularly in patients with diabetes, rheumatoid arthritis, indwelling catheters, intravenous drug use, or prior intra-articular injections.[166] If infection is suspected, the patient should be referred to a primary care provider immediately.

SC joint inflammation produces local pain. Active shoulder elevation, retraction, and protraction are likely painful in the early ranges due to clavicular elevation at the SC joint. Palpation will generally reveal local warmth, mild edema, and crepitus with range of motion. Muscle performance is rarely affected, although it may be limited by pain in very acute cases. Patients may report functional deficits in activities requiring reaching.

Physical therapy interventions should be directed toward controlling SC joint inflammation.[165] Ice and activity modification to decrease SC joint movement are beneficial. Gentle, small arc active or active-assisted motion may assist with joint nutrition without increasing the inflammatory process. Patients should be encouraged to perform distal extremity range of motion and shoulder external rotation to prevent secondary loss of motion during the acute phase. Exercise and activity are then progressed as tolerated.

If dislocation does occur, anterior dislocations are more likely and recurrent instability or post-traumatic arthritis are common sequelae.[164] Surgical management, including reconstruction or arthroplasty,[164] results in consistent improvements in pain.[167–169] However, the ability to return to the same level of sport or work, or ability to perform a push-up varies greatly, from nearly 50[168] to 90%.[167]

Glenohumeral Osteoarthritis

Pathology GH OA is a chronic degenerative condition of the shoulder that can lead to pain and functional limitation.[170] As with other joints, GH OA can be primary or secondary. Primary GH OA is the progressive joint narrowing related to aging and is more common in individuals over the age of 65.[171] Secondary GH OA may occur with avascular necrosis and dysplasia, and over time, OA is common after dislocation, shoulder surgery, or unrepaired rotator cuff tears.[171,172]

History Patients with GH OA report progressive deep shoulder pain and stiffness that are most notable with reaching overhead or activities. Patients are typically older and will report night pain. Clinicians should ask about prior shoulder injuries and surgery, particular in patients under 65 years of age.

Key Examination Findings It should be noted that GH OA can occur in combination with subacromial impingement and rotator cuff pathology. Although radiographs are the primary method of diagnosing GH OA, the clinical examination will reveal a loss of GH motion, particularly external rotation.[170,172] Fine or coarse crepitus[172] with active and/or passive motion is the norm. Clinicians should perform tests for impingement and rotator cuff pathology to help rule these in or out as well as to guide interventions.

Differential Diagnoses If pain is only felt with active or resisted motions, rotator cuff pathology, SIS, or labral pathology should be suspected.[172]

Rehabilitation Focus and Key Points Physical therapy is a mainstay of treatment for patients with GH OA[171] and should include activity modification[171] and range of motion exercises.[172,173] Passive, active-assisted, and active range of motion exercises should be performed to tolerance with progression to strengthening exercises,[173] including the scapular musculature. Manual therapy, including joint and soft-tissue mobilization, can assist to improve joint range of motion and decrease pain.[172] Modalities including ice or heat[173] may assist with symptom modulation. A home exercise program should be provided that includes stretching and strengthening exercises. Medical management of GH OA may include the use of nonsteroidal anti-inflammatories, corticosteroid injection, sodium hyaluronate injection,[170] or a short course of oral corticosteroids.[174]

Expected Outcomes Maximal improvements can be expected in pain, range, and function within 1 to 3 months[172] and have been maintained in follow-up studies lasting at least 3 years.[173] Patients with continued pain and functional deficits should be referred for possible surgical intervention.

Shoulder Arthroplasty

Total shoulder arthroplasty (TSA), reverse total shoulder arthroplasty (rTSA), and joint resurfacing are techniques used to manage end-stage shoulder OA or, in the case of rTSA, large, massive, or recurrent rotator cuff tears.[174] TSA may also be performed after severe proximal humerus fractures.[175] TSA, implanting both a humeral and glenoid component, was once deemed a salvage procedure as the result was pain relief, but a significant loss of function remained. However, improvement in surgical technique and components now leads to significant gains in shoulder motion, strength, and function. After TSA, patients can reliably attain 145° of active elevation and 40° of external rotation. rTSA is performed for patients with severe rotator cuff deficiency and reverses the joint geometry moving the center of rotation more medially to provide the deltoid with an improved moment arm for shoulder elevation (Fig. 14-59).[175] Joint resurfacing is used to provide pain relief and improved function for younger individual with intact rotator cuff function and minimal glenoid articular surface defects to allow later conversion to a TSA or rTSA.

There is limited evidence in the literature to guide interventions after TSA or rTSA, and rehabilitation is typically guided by surgeon preference. After a TSA, sling immobilization varies from 3 to 8 weeks. External rotation is generally limited to 30° for the first few weeks to protect the subscapularis, which is disrupted by the surgical approach. Rupture of the subscapularis

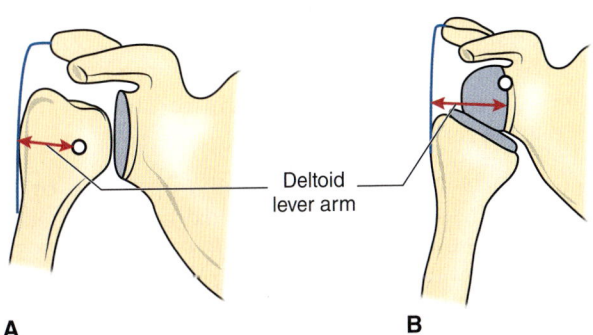

FIGURE 14-59 **A.** Normal shoulder anatomy and deltoid lever arm (*red arrow*). **B.** Larger deltoid lever arm created by a reverse total shoulder arthroplasty.

leads to anterior shoulder instability and poor results. External rotation is gradually progressed, and most surgeons allow unlimited external rotation range after 12 weeks.[176] Rehabilitation after a rTSA does not require such protection and, therefore, tends to progress more quickly. For example, many surgeons prescribe a sling may be used for comfort but may not be required, and exercises can be progressed on a faster timeline.[176] Exercises working toward functional internal rotation with the hand behind the back are limited for the first 4 to 6 weeks to prevent dislocation resulting from the surgical approach. Resisted exercise after rTSA should focus on deltoid and scapular strengthening, with many surgeons allowing resistive exercise after 6 weeks.[176] After rTSA, patients can expect substantial reductions in pain, improvements in function, and to attain 120° of active elevation and 30° of external rotation.[177,178] Although short-term lifting restrictions are the norm, some surgeons will place a lifelong restriction of not lifting more than 15 pounds (6.8 kg).[176]

Adhesive Capsulitis

Pathology Adhesive capsulitis, also known as a *frozen shoulder*, is a progressive loss of GH motion and is controversial in both pathophysiology and management. Adhesive capsulitis has a complex and varied course. Research suggests that adhesive capsulitis is an inflammatory reaction that begins with synovial inflammation. Inflammation leads to thickening of the synovium, capsular fibrosis, adhesion formation, and loss of the axillary fold of the inferior GH joint capsule.[179] Adhesive capsulitis affects 2 to 5% of the general population,[180] but nearly 10 to 20% of patients with diabetes.[181]

Primary adhesive capsulitis is historically described in terms of stages.[121,182,183] The first stage, sometimes referred to as "freezing,"[180] is characterized by painful inflammation limiting active flexion, abduction, and rotations. When examined under anesthesia, there is normal or minimal range loss. With time, inflammation is replaced by stiffness due to a progressive increase in fibrosis and loss of capsular volume ("frozen" stage).[180] Ultimately, the patient reaches the "thawing" stage, which is characterized by a gradual, progressive return in motion.[180]

History In many cases, the onset of primary or idiopathic adhesive capsulitis is insidious. Adhesive capsulitis is more common in females and patients between the ages of 40 and 65 years.[180,184,185] Women,[182] younger patients, patients with diabetes, and patients who did not receive physical therapy are more likely to develop adhesive capsulitis in the contralateral shoulder.[186] The nondominant extremity is more often affected. Individuals with diabetes and thyroid disease are at higher risk of developing primary adhesive capsulitis.[121,180,184,185]

Patients generally report a gradual and progressive loss of motion that affects reaching overhead, donning a bra or belt, hair care, and bathing due to shoulder pain, loss of shoulder motion, or both. They may report generalized shoulder or deltoid area pain. Pain may be severe and may disrupt sleep. Owing to attempts to compensate for motion loss through excessive scapular elevation, patients may report pain or spasm of the upper trapezius.[181] Many times, it is this secondary dysfunction that leads patients to seek assistance.

Secondary causes of adhesive capsulitis include patients whose loss of shoulder motion followed a recent myocardial infarction or cervical or thoracic surgery, such as pacemaker placement, breast cancer surgery,[187] or placement of a chest tube.[181,182,188] Secondary adhesive capsulitis may also develop after shoulder trauma, such as a proximal humerus fracture, tendinitis, or rotator cuff repair,[121,179] in which inflammation and pain lead to disuse and gradual, progressive loss of motion. Though infrequent, adhesive capsulitis may occur after a shoulder surgery, such as rotator cuff repair.[121]

Key Examination Findings Patients with adhesive capsulitis present with decreased active and passive range of motion in multiple planes. There is a characteristic loss of external rotation with the arm by the side as well as in varying degrees of abduction.[185] Interestingly, a capsular pattern of restriction, in which external rotation is more limited than abduction, which is more limited than flexion, which is more limited than internal rotation, is not consistently seen.[185] Acutely, patients may exhibit protective behaviors, holding the extremity in shoulder adduction and internal rotation with the forearm resting against the abdomen.[181] When attempting to raise the affected extremity, patients may exhibit a reverse scapulohumeral rhythm, increased scapular elevation, and decreased GH joint motion, to avoid pain or because of stiffness. Initially, passive motion is unaffected, but as fibrosis progresses, passive range loss equals that of active motion. Endfeels are initially empty or guarded, but become progressively more firm as fibrosis replaces inflammation.[181] Using either modified manual muscle testing positioning or midrange isometric testing, clinicians should assess muscle performance within the patient's available range of motion to ensure that adhesive capsulitis is not secondary to a rotator cuff tear.[179] Postural changes, such as increased kyphosis, increased scapular abduction, and a forward head, are common.[181] The humeral head may rest in a more anterior position. GH arthrokinematic motions are decreased,[179] particularly inferiorly and posteriorly.

TABLE 14-14			
TISSUE IRRITABILITY DEFINED			
Tissue Irritability	*Low*	*Moderate*	*High*
Pain level (0–10)	≤3	4–6	≥7
Rest/night pain	None	Intermittent	Consistent
Pain-motion relationship	Minimal pain with overpressure	Pain at end-range	Pain before end-range
Degree of disability	Low	Moderate	High
Intervention focus	Progressive interventions to address impaired range	Controlled increase in tissue stress Gradually address impaired range	Activity modification Symptom modification Midrange A/AAROM

A, active; *AAROM*, active-assisted range of motion.

The GH joint capsule may be tender to palpation. Patients may have positive impingement tests[181] owing to end-range positioning. However, these tests are nonspecific, and overall examination findings must be considered, including the key factors of insidious onset; loss of motion in multiple planes, particularly external rotation; and end-range pain.[92] Tissue irritability should be established (Table 14-14)[92] and used to guide interventions.[185]

Differential Diagnoses The clinician should consider other reasons for a loss of shoulder range of motion, such as pain, from fracture, dislocation, or positive neural tension tests. As noted previously, modified assessments for muscle performance can help to rule in or out rotator cuff pathology. Likewise, loss of motion in a single direction, such as may occur with subscapularis myofascial restrictions, rule out the possibility of adhesive capsulitis.[185]

Rehabilitation Focus and Key Points Interventions for adhesive capsulitis vary with patient presentation. For patients with high irritability, medical management,[92] including anti-inflammatory medication or corticosteroid medication, can be beneficial.[121,180] Patients should be instructed in rest and relief positions, such as propping the shoulder in the loose-packed position with the arm away from the side and simple pendulum exercises, sometimes referred to as *Codman's exercise* (Fig. 14-60). Patient education must stress the importance of posture correction to decrease impingement and activity modification, such as limiting overhead activities. Active and active-assisted midrange motion should be encouraged that either do not increase pain or increase pain only marginally. Grade I to II joint mobilizations, ice, and heat may be beneficial. Patients should be instructed to perform frequent small bouts of exercise rather than one aggressive exercise session per day. Because recovery from adhesive capsulitis may be prolonged, clinicians must educate patients in the need for adherence to a home program and activity modifications. Aquatic exercises[182] may be beneficial because the buoyancy of the water decreases muscle activation required for active motion and the warm water may promote relaxation and decrease pain. Throughout the recovery process, clinicians must emphasize a normal scapulohumeral rhythm and patients should not be allowed to elevate using poor form, so as to prevent secondary complications, such as impingement, upper trapezius overuse/trigger points, or muscle imbalances. Visual feedback using mirrors, verbal or tactile cues, limiting the arc of movement, and performing exercises bilaterally may help improve scapulohumeral rhythm.

Moderate irritability is characterized by decreased motion with pain at end-range allowing more intensive exercise. An active warm-up, such as walking or low resistance upper body ergometry, followed by active-assisted range of motion and gentle stretching is recommended. There is a direct correlation between gains in external rotation and gains

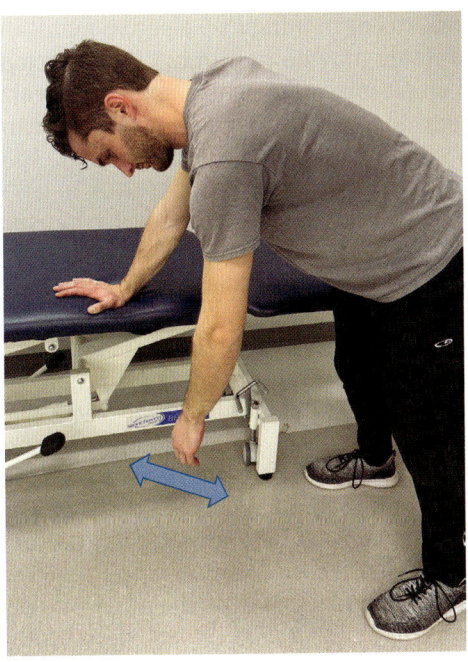

FIGURE 14-60 Pendulum exercise.

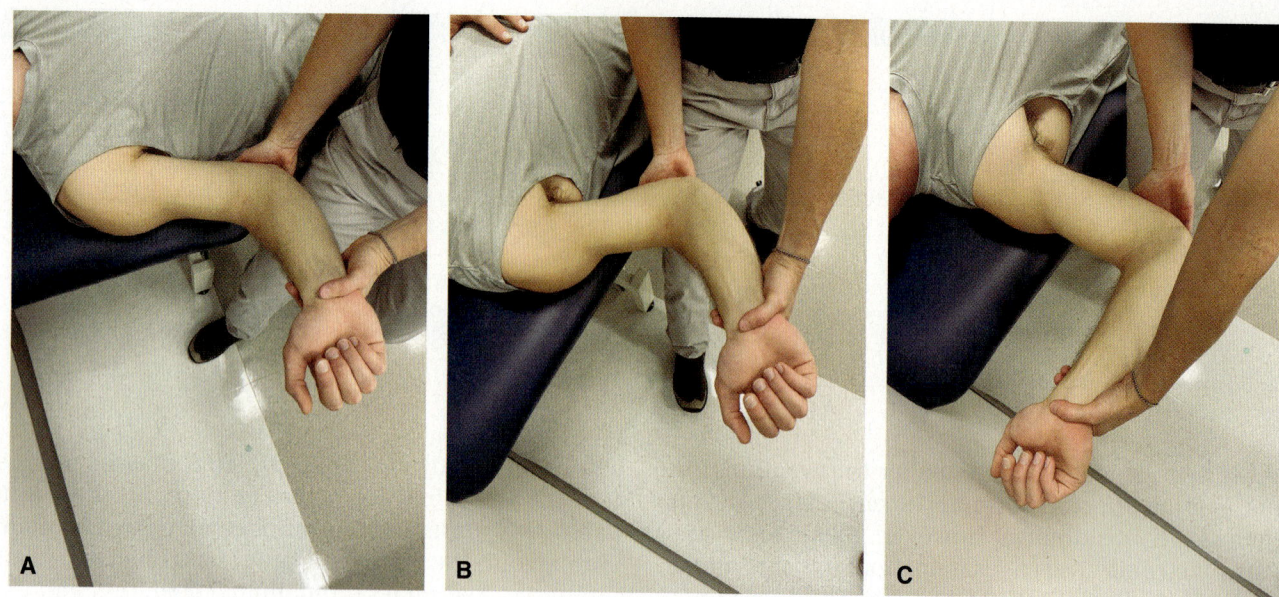

FIGURE 14-61 Shoulder external rotation passive/active-assisted range of motion progression **A.** Arm by side. **B.** Arm in 45° of scaption. **C.** Arm in 90° of scaption.

in elevation. To decrease impingement and the risk of secondary complications, external rotation range gains should be stressed over elevation gains.[181] Therefore, passive, active-assisted, and active external rotation should be initiated first with the arm by the side and progressed to 45° of abduction (or scaption) and then to 90° (Fig. 14-61). Because patients treated with mobilization have been shown to have greater gains in range and a significant decrease in pain, grade III GH joint mobilizations and self-mobilizations are indicated. As patients gain range of motion, strengthening exercises to maintain these improvements may be required. Clinicians must continue to emphasize a normal scapulohumeral rhythm and teach the patient scapular stabilization exercises, if needed. Ice after exercise may help control pain or inflammation.

Low irritability is characterized by capsular end-feels and pain after resistance. Patients may benefit from an active warm-up, moist heating pad, or even ultrasound to the GH joint capsule in elevation and external rotation, followed by more aggressive stretching,[182] such as contract-relax and low-load, long-duration stretching (Fig. 14-62). Aggressive grade III and IV GH joint mobilizations are progressed from mid- to end-range. Strengthening in newly gained ranges and proper movement patterns should be emphasized. Additional manual techniques may be indicated. The clinician should assess for myofascial restrictions or trigger points, particularly of the subscapularis, pectorals, or trapezius. Although not specifically affecting the GH capsule, manual subscapularis myofascial

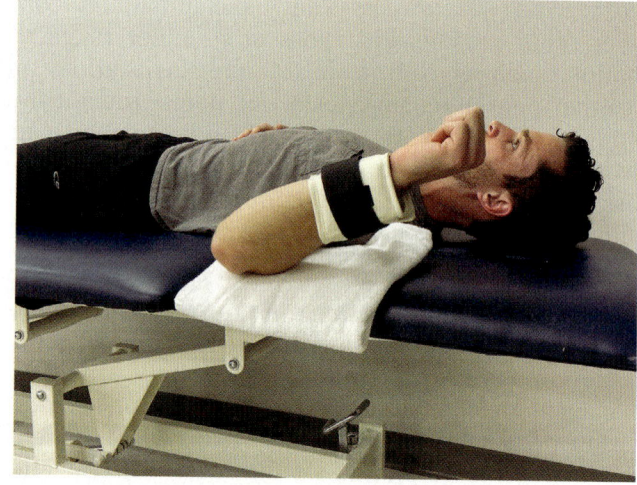

FIGURE 14-62 Low-load, long-duration stretching into shoulder external rotation.

release can help improve shoulder external rotation (Fig. 14-63). Scapular distraction may be beneficial because this technique will stretch the anterior capsule and subscapularis. Focusing stretches to the GH joint by stabilizing the scapula can be extremely beneficial in patients with low irritability (Fig. 14-64). More aggressive stretching with orthotic devices, such as those made by Joint Active Systems or Dynasplint, may be indicated in patients whose range fails to improve with more conservative methods or who cannot maintain range of motion gains.

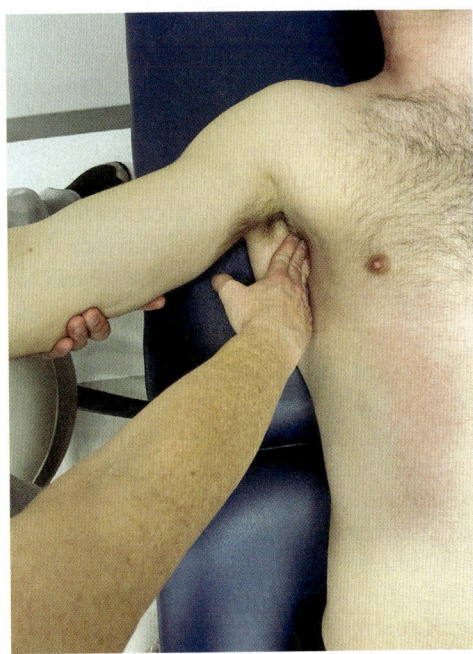

FIGURE 14-63 Subscapularis release.

Expected Outcomes Ninety percent of patients with adhesive capsulitis improve with conservative interventions.[189] Part of the controversy over adhesive capsulitis stems from studies that suggest adhesive capsulitis may be self-limiting with spontaneous resolution in 6 months to 2 years.[180,181] However, it is difficult to make a case for benign neglect given the prolonged time that may be needed for this natural progression and the successful gains noted with rehabilitation. The longer the symptoms have been present, the longer the recovery time, and early treatment appears to lead to a faster recovery.[182] Patients who are covered by worker's compensation have a higher failure rate and an increased likelihood of surgical intervention.[189] Because secondary adhesive capsulitis is identified sooner and has a known precipitating factor, symptom resolution is considerably faster than for primary adhesive capsulitis. Patients not responding after 3 months of physical therapy may benefit from surgical interventions. Women and patients with diabetes appear to be more likely to require surgery.[184]

Surgical Interventions The first choice of surgical intervention is an arthroscopic capsular release followed by shoulder manipulation under a scalene block.[121,180,190] The surgeon may choose to inject the GH joint with a corticosteroid at the time of manipulation to decrease premorbid or procedurally induced inflammation.[191] A continuous block with a portable infusion pump and/or concomitant anti-inflammatory medication are common additional interventions.[190] Surgical manipulation must be followed by intensive and aggressive physical therapy,[190] generally daily[121] for the first week or 2. Clinicians should strive to achieve and maintain the total range of motion gained in surgery. Post-manipulation, patients must be encouraged to perform frequent bouts, three to five times per day, of range of motion exercises and are frequently prescribed a home continuous passive motion machine. The vast majority of patients have good to excellent results following manipulation with intensive therapy.[190,192] It is currently unclear if there is an optimal time to consider arthroscopic interventions for adhesive capsulitis. It was once feared that performing surgery would only be successful if performed later into the disease process (during the "frozen" or even during a stalled "thawing" stage). While it appears prudent that all patients receive a trial of conservative management before surgical intervention, patients have had satisfactory outcomes when surgery is performed early in the disease process.[193]

Rotator Cuff Pathology

Pathology Rotator cuff pathology can be divided into two main categories: rupture and tendinopathy. Acute, traumatic tendon rupture can occur from falling on an outstretched arm or during heavy lifting and results in a sudden loss of shoulder function, such as the inability to raise the arm overhead. The rotator cuff may be torn after an anterior dislocation or proximal humerus fracture, particularly in middle-aged or older individuals.[194] In such cases, the damage to the rotator cuff

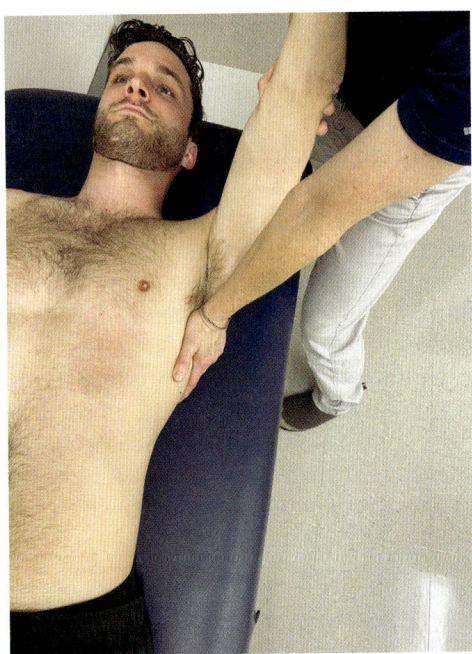

FIGURE 14-64 Stretching into glenohumeral flexion with scapular stabilization.

may initially go unnoticed as the pain and weakness the patient is experiencing are attributed to the more obvious pathology.

Rotator cuff tears are classified by extent, size, tendon involved, and the quality of the remaining tissue (Table 14-15). The supraspinatus is the most commonly torn rotator cuff tendon.[194] Full-thickness rotator cuff tears greater than 1 cm are likely to progress.[195,196] If left unrepaired, the tendon retracts and the muscle and tendon undergo fatty infiltration and degeneration. These changes are associated with poorer conservative and surgical outcomes.[197] Although most full-thickness rotator cuff tears follow a predictable pattern in which the supraspinatus is torn and the tear progressively enlarges to include the infraspinatus, then the teres minor, and rarely the subscapularis, it is possible to have isolated tears of each rotator cuff tendon.

Age-related changes to the rotator cuff are common, in part because of the poor vascularity of the rotator cuff limiting its ability to heal.[198] Thirteen percent of 50-year-old and 50% of 80-year-old persons will have an asymptomatic full-thickness rotator cuff tear.[199] In addition to age, smoking,[200] hypercholesterolemia, diabetes,[201] family history of rotator cuff disease,[202] and having an occupation that requires over-shoulder height work are linked to rotator cuff pathology.[137] Half of all large and massive tears are due to trauma, whereas the remaining are chronic, progressive tears.[203] Age- and chronicity-related decreases in tendon quality lead to a high failure rate for rotator cuff repair in those over 60 years of age or in those with long-standing tendon ruptures.[196]

In contrast to traumatic rotator cuff rupture, the histologic changes of rotator cuff tendinopathy include an increased number of cells, apoptosis, fatty infiltration, and degeneration, along with an increased number of nerves and neurotransmitters.[198] The latter may be why central sensitization plays a role in shoulder pain in some patients with rotator cuff tendinopathy.[198] There may or may not be an increase in inflammatory mediators,[198] likely due to the limited tendon vascularity.[108] Rotator cuff tendinopathy is likely the result of degenerative microtrauma and/or chronic impingement. The degenerative microtrauma theory states that repeated microtrauma overloads the tendon and exceeds the capacity of tenocytes to heal.[198] Continued stress leads to small tears within the tendon. Once a tear occurs, the remaining fibers undergo greater-than-normal loading, increasing the risk of progressive tearing. The degenerative microtrauma theory is supported by the findings that most rotator cuff tears in throwers are partial-thickness tears resulting from instability.[163,204] Because partial-thickness tears were twice as common as full-thickness tears on cadaver dissection,[205] these tears may represent a continuum of normal tendon degeneration. However, the repetitive stress of overhead athletics may accelerate normal age-related degeneration. The chronic impingement theory, originally proposed by Neer,[206] states that repeated compression of the rotator cuff against the inferior acromion and coracoacromial ligament causes tendon damage. In addition, the rotator cuff is a dynamic stabilizer of the GH joint. Preactivation of the rotator cuff provides a compressive force before activation of more global power musculature,[137] such as the latissimus dorsi, pectoralis major, and deltoid. Recall, without adequate rotator cuff contraction and timing, superior translation of the humerus is thought to occur.[196] The chronic impingement theory is also supported by the poorer outcomes for conservative management of patients with type III (hooked) acromions when compared with type I (flat) or type II (curved) acromions.[207]

History Patients with rotator cuff pathology report pain in the deltoid region and pain at night. They may report stiffness or crepitus. The dominant shoulder is more often affected than the nondominant shoulder.[137] Individuals with a rotator cuff tear are more likely to

TABLE 14-15
CLASSIFICATION OF ROTATOR CUFF TEARS

Classification	Characteristics

Extent	• Partial thickness
	  • Articular side
	  • Bursal side
	  • Intratendinous
	• Full thickness

Size and involved tendons*	• Small
	  • <1 cm
	  • Supraspinatus
	• Medium
	  • 1–3 cm
	  • Supraspinatus
	  • Infraspinatus
	  • +/− Teres minor
	• Large
	  • 3–5 cm
	  • Supraspinatus
	  • Infraspinatus
	  • Teres minor
	• Massive
	  • >5 cm
	  • Supraspinatus
	  • Infraspinatus
	  • Teres minor
	  • Possibly subscapularis

Tissue quality	• Healthy • Degenerated • Retracted

*Although generally true, the exact number of tendons involved is dependent on the size of the individual. For example, large patients may have a medium rotator cuff tear that involves only the supraspinatus.

report constant pain[196] and a sudden onset of weakness, such as the inability to raise the arm overhead. For degenerative rotator cuff ruptures, patients are likely to report a history of intermittent shoulder pain along with mild weakness and stiffness. Then, a small trauma, such as trying to start a lawnmower, results in a sudden, but significant, decrease in shoulder function.

Key Examination Findings The remainder of this section addresses rotator cuff tears, whereas rotator cuff tendinopathy is considered within the following section on subacromial impingement syndrome. Individuals with a full-thickness tear are likely to have profound weakness of that muscle group. For example, an individual with a full-thickness supraspinatus tear is likely to utilize excessive scapular elevation in attempts at active shoulder elevation and has a positive drop arm test, whereas an individual with a torn infraspinatus is likely to have a positive external rotation lag test. Individuals with chronic tears are likely to have significant atrophy of the affected muscles, whereas those with partial-thickness tears are likely to have painful weakness of the affected muscle and pain with active, but not passive, motion.[196] A painful arc, increased pain, or pain in the range of 70 to 120° of shoulder elevation may be present.

Differential Diagnoses Differential diagnoses for full-thickness rotator cuff tears include SIS, instability, or adhesive capsulitis. Fracture and dislocation should be ruled out in cases of significant trauma.

Rehabilitation Focus and Key Points A partial-thickness tear is amenable to rehabilitation and may not require surgical interventions, even for athletes or workers performing consistent overhead activities. Initial interventions should be directed toward pain modulation and regaining pain-free active range of motion. Patients should not be allowed to elevate through a painful arc or with an abnormal scapulohumeral rhythm. Activity modification to decrease stress to the affected muscle and tendon will provide an environment that is more conducive for healing. Postural deficits and weakness of the scapular muscles can be addressed early in the rehabilitation process. Isometric exercises, particularly of GH rotators and scapular musculature, in a neutral GH position can assist with symptom modulation and improved GH positioning. Active-assisted elevation by a clinician, a wand (Fig. 14-65), or the unaffected arm can assist with providing a gradual increase in stress to the deltoid and remaining rotator cuff while maintaining range of motion. Individuals who fail to improve after 6 to 12 weeks of conservative care should be referred to an orthopaedist.[208] Younger individuals with full-thickness rotator cuff tears and individuals with a traumatic onset of small and medium-sized tears are the most likely to benefit from surgical repair.

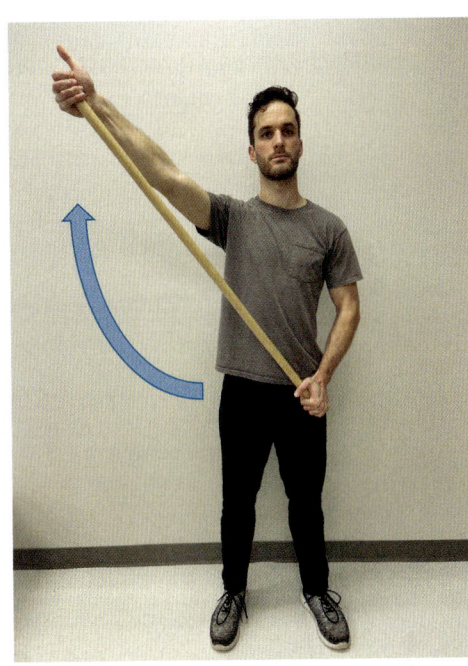

FIGURE 14-65 Active-assisted shoulder scaption with a wand.

Rehabilitation After Rotator Cuff Repair Significant variation exists in rehabilitation after rotator cuff repair. Most commonly, there is a period of immobilization in a sling with an abduction pillow and slight internal rotation to minimize static stress on the repair. Currently, there appears to be two competing guidelines for rehabilitation after rotator cuff repair: prolonged immobilization and early mobilization. Proponents of prolonged immobilization[209] point to the fact that most rotator cuff tears occur within the first 3 to 6 months after surgery. Animal model studies note the presence of Sharpey fibers occurring at 12 weeks after bilateral single-row infraspinatus repairs in sheep who were allowed unrestricted walking partial weight bearing in a sling[210] or goats in which an open procedure was performed to create and repair a simulated infraspinatus tendon rupture followed by the goats being "housed in covered pens that allowed ample walking space."[211] Prolonged immobilization is based on the fear that any stress to the repair is inherently bad. In contrast, the early mobilization supporters believe that tissue responds to controlled increases in stress, pointing to several studies[212–215] that note equivalent 1- and 2-year post-surgical outcomes when comparing early mobilization with prolonged immobilization but significantly better range of motion and function in the first 3 to 6 months in the early mobilization group.[216,217]

TABLE 14-16
SAMPLE PROGRESSION AFTER AN ARTHROSCOPIC SMALL ROTATOR CUFF REPAIR ON A HEALTHY, YOUNG ATHLETE

Time	Interventions
Post-op days 1–14	• Immediate passive ROM with limitations on shoulder internal and external rotation and elevation • Active ROM scapular muscles, elbow, wrist, and hand
Post-op week 2	• Pain-modulated active-assisted shoulder ROM* • Low-intensity elbow and shoulder isometrics
Post-op week 4	• Active ROM internal/external rotation in sitting • Resisted wrist ROM with forearm supported • Gradual progression to full shoulder range as tolerated
Post-op week 6	• Active ROM progression for shoulder flexion and scaption[†,‡] beginning with a short lever arm
Post-op week 8	• Begin resisted ROM progression for remaining muscle groups starting with low intensity and increasing repetitions, then sets, before increasing load

• Progression can be no faster than outlined above.
• Do not progress intensity without achieving previous milestone. For example, if unable to perform active shoulder flexion without pain from 0 to 90° at post-op week 8, do not add resistance to shoulder flexion.

ROM, range of motion.

*Mazzocca AD, Arciero RA, Shea KP, et al. The effect of early range of motion on quality of life, clinical outcome, and repair integrity after arthroscopic rotator cuff repair. *Arthroscopy.* 2017;33(6):1138-1148. doi:10.1016/j.arthro.2016.10.017

[†]Mollison S, Shin JJ, Glogau A, Beavis RC. Postoperative rehabilitation after rotator cuff repair: a web-based survey of AANA and AOSSM members. *Orthop J Sports Med.* 2017;5(1):2325967116684775. doi:10.1177/2325967116684775

[‡]Jancuska J, Matthews J, Miller T, Kluczynski MA, Bisson LJ. A systematic summary of systematic reviews on the topic of the rotator cuff. *Orthop J Sports Med.* 2018;6(9):2325967118797891. doi:10.1177/2325967118797891

Rather than simply choosing one or the other of these postoperative positions, a growing body of literature supports that progression after a rotator cuff repair should be based on the size of the tear, surgical approach (open versus arthroscopic), the ability to recreate the anatomic footprint of the tendons, tissue quality, the number of suture anchors, additional procedures performed, and patient-related factors, such as age, diabetes, smoking status, and goals.[137,218] The key issue for tendon repair rehabilitation is a gradual, progressive increase in tendon loading.[219] As such, a young individual with an acute supraspinatus rupture who underwent a small rotator cuff repair with good-quality tissue and double-row fixation can reasonably begin the progression noted in Table 14-16 that outlines a clear progression of load to the affected tendon. Additional guidance on exercise progression can utilize data from EMG studies (Fig. 14-66).[220] Some clinicians prefer to modify the traditional pendulum exercise to one in which the patient cradles the surgical arm with the unaffected arm to decrease rotator cuff activation early in the rehabilitation process (Fig. 14-67). Because it can be difficult to know how much assistance a patient is providing with self-assisted active range of motion exercises using a wand, clinicians can utilize a pulley to provide constant

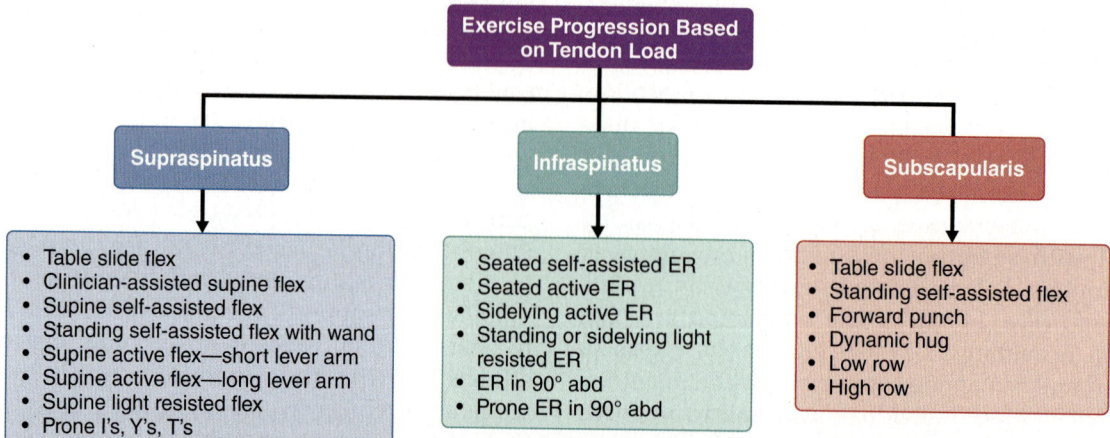

FIGURE 14-66 Exercise progression based on tendon load. *abd*, abduction; *ER*, external rotation; *flex*, flexion.

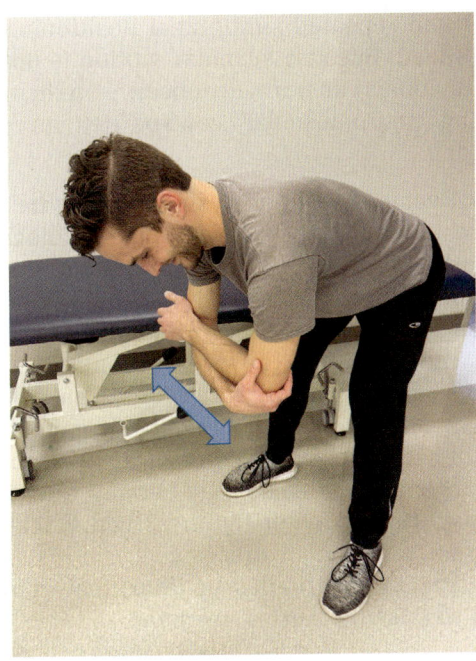

FIGURE 14-67 Modified pendulum exercise for the left shoulder.

amount of assistance (Fig. 14-68). For example, the amount of weight assisting the patient can be gradually reduced from 3, to 2, to 1 lb., and even to 0.5 lb. as the patient is able to perform the movement without an increase in symptoms or abnormal scapulohumeral rhythm. Currently, a continuous passive motion unit does not appear to provide any additional benefit.[137]

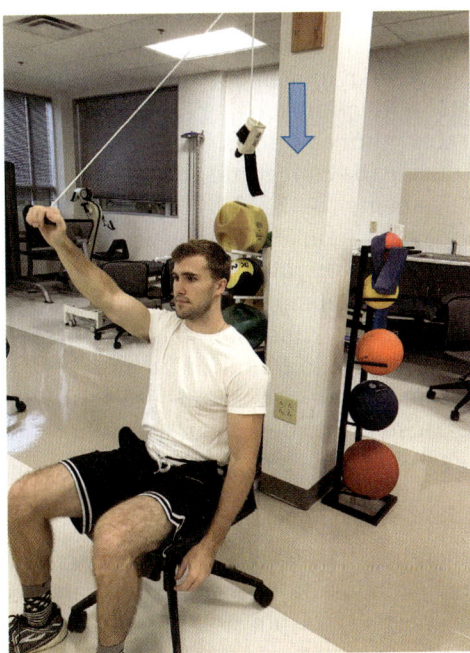

FIGURE 14-68 Active-assisted shoulder flexion with a pulley and cuff weight.

For overhead athletes, it is important to address the entire kinetic chain, including lower extremity and core strength.[221] This can be started early in the rehabilitation process. Once range of motion has been restored and the athlete is tolerating resisted exercise for all muscle groups, an interval throwing program (e.g., baseball, softball) or hitting program (e.g., tennis, golf) can be initiated. Any biomechanical errors should be addressed with the assistance of a sport-specific coach as needed.

In addition to repairing the rotator cuff, some surgeons will perform an acromioplasty, where the underside of the acromion is shaved down at the time of surgery, particularly if there is a type II acromion or the presence of osteophytes. Platelet-rich plasma, stem cell injection, or the use of biologic scaffolds may be beneficial.[222]

Outcomes after Rotator Cuff Repair Rotator cuff repair leads to decreased pain and improved function for most individuals and is most successful when performed within 3 months of an acute tendon rupture,[196] because this seems to preserve tissue quality for repair. For athletes, there is an overall 85% return to sports in 4 to 17 months.[223] While recreational athletes are likely to return to preinjury level of play, only half of professional athletes will have this degree of success.[223,224] Those who are older, smokers, have larger tears, poor tendon quality, diabetes, obesity, or preoperative motion loss[196] are more likely to experience a re-tear.[137] It should be noted that, even when there is evidence of a recurrent tendon defect, shoulder-related symptoms may still be improved postoperatively.[196]

Scapular Dyskinesia

Pathology The scapula serves as a stable base for the humerus and muscular attachments. The acromion must elevate during overhead activities to prevent impingement. Scapular retraction and posteriorly tilt is also required for overhead activities, such as cocking motion for throwing, and protracting along the thorax to maintain relationship with humeral head during follow-through. Lack of full retraction increases stress on anterior shoulder structures.[76]

Scapular dyskinesia is the lack of the normal scapular kinematics. There are many potential causes of scapular dyskinesia (Fig. 14-69). Patients with painful GH elevation, such as those with SIS, may utilize compensatory movement strategies of excessive scapular elevation and upward rotation to avoid pain. Several studies have noted scapular instability in the vast majority of patients with shoulder pain.[112,225]

Scapular dyskinesia may result from inflexibility. Patients with rotator cuff tears or adhesive capsulitis may excessively elevate the scapula to compensate for

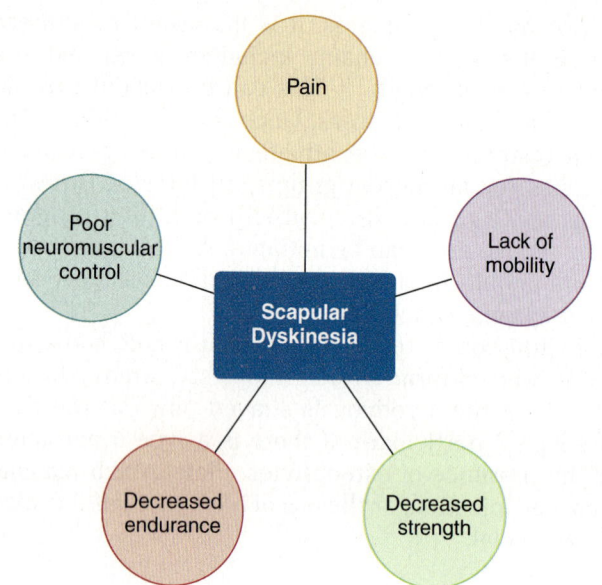

FIGURE 14-69 Causes of scapular dyskinesia.

limited GH motion. Lack of pectoralis minor or short head of biceps flexibility can create excessive anterior scapular tilt or protraction. Scapular dyskinesia is also seen in throwers and overhead athletes who have a tight posterior GH joint capsule.[226] During the follow-through of throwing or serving, the tight capsule essentially pulls the scapula along with the humerus, creating excessive scapular protraction during follow-through.[112,225,227] Similarly, excessive protraction that occurs with increased structural or functional kyphosis also produces scapular dyskinesia.

Weakness of the scapular stabilizers can cause decreased elevation, retraction, and/or posterior tilt of the acromion. Lack of proximal stability can also prevent scapulohumeral muscles from generating sufficient force to control superior humeral head translation during active shoulder elevation. Both of these conditions can result in subacromial impingement.[228] Muscular weakness may be due to disuse, abnormally lengthened scapular muscles due to poor postural alignment, or neuropathy.[229] Long thoracic nerve injury, which may occur after a traction injury to the nerve, can cause scapular winging and isolated weakness or paralysis of the serratus anterior muscle. Spinal accessory or dorsal scapular neuropathy[230] can also cause weakness and limitations in active scapular rotation.[229] Likewise, decreased scapular muscle endurance may lead to poor scapular positioning with repetitive overhead movements. This may occur in freestyle swimmers in which full scapular retraction is required during the recovery phase.

Lastly, poor neuromuscular control can lead to inappropriately timed scapular motion, leading to periodic and repeated suboptimal positioning of the humeral head. Because scapular motion is not something individuals can normally observe on themselves, correcting neuromuscular control deficits can be challenging.

History Because scapular dyskinesia may be caused by, or result from, several different pathologies, patients with scapular dyskinesia are quite diverse. The chief complaint of patients with scapular dyskinesia is painful shoulder elevation. Scapular dyskinesia, in itself, is rarely painful. However, scapular dyskinesia may cause impingement, rotator cuff pathology, or muscle spasm or trigger points in the upper trapezius or levator scapulae due to compensatory scapular elevation. Overhead athletes may initially report a feeling of posterior shoulder tightness with cocking and inability to "loosen up" after warming up.[226] Patients with isolated traumatic neuropathies may report the inability to raise their arms overhead.

Key Examination Findings Scapular dyskinesia and scapular malpositioning can be the result of shoulder pain, the cause of shoulder pain, exacerbate existing shoulder pain, or be unrelated to shoulder pain.[231] Therefore, the clinician must first determine whether a relationship exists between altered scapular kinematics and the patient's shoulder pain or functional deficit and, if so, what factors are driving the movement deviations. The clinician should observe the thoracic spine and the resting scapular position both during the history and more formally during structural observation inspecting the medial and inferior scapular borders for symmetry and flushness to the thorax.[228] Next, the clinician stand behind the patient and observe scapular movement during active shoulder flexion and abduction, looking for an abnormal scapulohumeral rhythm as well as winging or tipping of the scapula during the concentric and/or eccentric phases of the movements.[227]

If abnormal scapular motions are noted, the clinician must rule in or rule out concomitant pathology that may result in compensatory scapular dyskinesia, including adhesive capsulitis and rotator cuff tears. If either pathology is found to be present, then the scapular mechanics are clearly the result, rather than the cause of the deviation. If the motion is painful and dyskinesia is present, the motion should be repeated while correcting scapular mechanics using verbal cues or physical assistance, as with the scapular retraction or assistance tests.[226] Pain relief with scapular repositioning suggests scapular dyskinesia is at least partially responsible for the patient's pain complaint. Sometimes, abnormal scapular movement is not noted unless an external load is applied or until fatigue develops. Therefore, clinicians may choose to have the patient perform several repetitions of active range of motion or provide resistance using handheld weights or elastic tubing to detect more subtle scapular dyskinesias.

Shoulder passive range of motion should be examined, and any GIRD or total arc of motion deficits documented. GH joint mobility, particularly posterior humeral glide, should be assessed for restrictions. The pectoralis minor should be assessed for tightness and tenderness at the coracoid attachment. The levator scapulae should be assessed for tenderness, particularly at the superior scapular border attachment, because this muscle may be pathologically lengthened by a protracted scapula, causing undue stress at the attachment point.[226] A corner stretch (Fig. 14-70) may be useful for opening up the anterior chest, stretching the anterior musculature and the GH joint capsule while encouraging shoulder external rotation and thoracic extension. The exercise can be advanced to an isometric exercise to reinforce optimal scapular positioning by having the patient shift slightly back away from the corner, while maintaining scapular retraction and shoulder external rotation actively. Note that the corner stretch exercise should be used with extreme caution in the presence of anterior instability.

Muscle performance testing should include the ST muscles via manual muscle testing and functional testing. For a quick screen of serratus anterior weakness, the clinician may have the patient hold a plank position (Fig. 14-71), either standard or inclined with the hands against a wall just below shoulder height. This

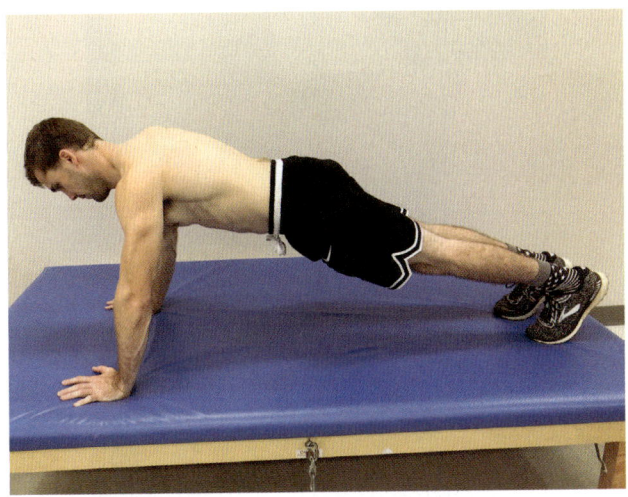

FIGURE 14-71 Plank.

upper extremity weight bearing is frequently enough to reveal scapular winging. For athletes with more subtle problems or impaired neuromuscular control, the clinician may observe the patient's shoulder girdle during overhead movements, such as throwing or serving, or the pain provoking task reported by the patient. Because scapular dyskinesia can lead to impingement of the structures within the subacromial space, the clinician should consider performing special tests for impingement, such as the Neer impingement test, Hawkins-Kennedy impingement test, and the horizontal adduction test.

Differential Diagnoses Differential diagnoses include rotator cuff tear, adhesive capsulitis, and nerve injuries, including the long thoracic nerve, the dorsal scapular nerve, or the spinal accessory nerve (cranial nerve XI).

Rehabilitation Focus and Key Points Interventions must address the specific impairments found in the examination. Posture correction and improving static scapular position, particularly before the patient attempts to raise the arm, are important first steps. Pathologically shortened muscles, such as the pectoralis minor, should be stretched (Fig. 14-72).[112,232] Joint mobilizations, particularly posterior humeral glides, may be required. Patients with increased kyphosis may benefit from thoracic mobilizations and stretching into thoracic extension.[227] Weak scapular stabilizing muscles, such as the serratus anterior, rhomboids, and middle and lower trapezius, should be strengthened. Specifically, the serratus anterior and lower trapezius assist with posterior scapular tilting, the rhomboids and middle trap assist with scapular retraction, and the serratus anterior and upper and lower trapezius assist with upward scapular

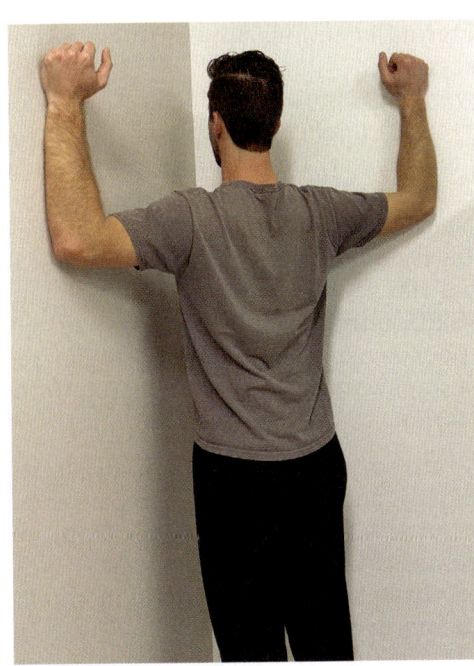

FIGURE 14-70 Corner stretch.

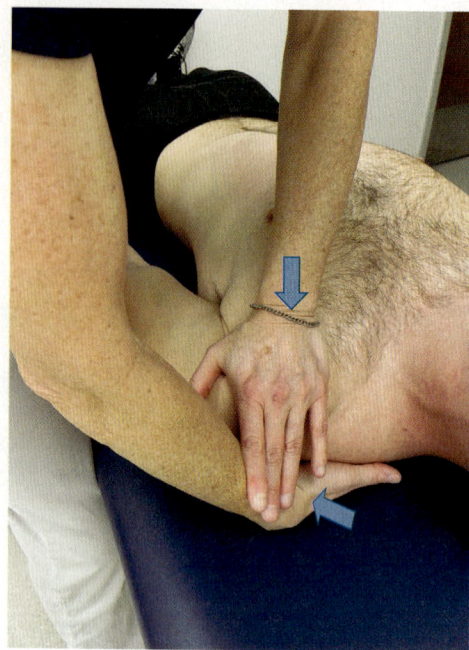

FIGURE 14-72 Manual stretching of the pectoralis minor.

rotation.[233] If the rhomboid or trapezius is ineffective at fully retracting the scapula, the ability to contract in this maximally shortened position should be stressed. If endurance is more problematic than strength, then endurance parameters should be chosen. Biofeedback and video feedback may be beneficial to increase muscle activation and awareness of scapular dyskinesia.[234] Scapular taping may decrease impingement during shoulder elevation[235,236] by improving the resting position, assisting with upward scapular rotation, or providing improved kinesthetic awareness.

Expected Outcomes Because scapular dyskinesia is a functional rather than an anatomic pathology,[231] most patients will have complete resolution of symptoms with a short course of rehabilitation.

Subacromial Impingement Syndrome

Pathology SIS, sometimes referred to as *subacromial pain syndrome*,[237] is shoulder pain due to narrowing of the subacromial space with encroachment of subacromial tissue,[238] such as the rotator cuff, bursa, and long head of the biceps. As such, SIS is the most common cause of shoulder pain[239] and includes pathoanatomic diagnoses such as rotator cuff tendinopathy, partial-thickness rotator cuff tears, bicipital tendinopathy, and subacromial bursitis. Primary impingement occurs when there is a pathologic structural decrease in the subacromial space and may be due to subacromial or AC joint osteophytes, hypertrophy of the coracoacromial ligament, or clavicle fracture malunion.[45]

Secondary impingement occurs when there is a dynamic or functional decrease in the subacromial space.

There are many possible contributing factors to secondary impingement including:

- Rotator cuff dysfunction
- Scapular dyskinesia
- Neuromuscular control
- GH instability
- Hypomobility

The key role the rotator cuff plays in preventing superior humeral head migration has already been discussed.[137] Rotator cuff dysfunction (fatigue, weakness, tensile overload, or pain inhibition) can produce or exacerbate impingement. Scapular dyskinesia, when the scapula fails to attain or maintain an appropriate relationship with the humeral head,[240] can lead to secondary impingement[198] by failing to successfully elevate or posteriorly tilt the acromion during shoulder elevation. Subacromial space and active shoulder elevation progressively decrease from a retracted position to a protracted position.[241,242] Therefore, patients with excessive or inappropriate static and dynamic scapular positioning are at increased risk for impingement due to a functional decrease in the subacromial space. Similarly, excessive anterior humeral glide, as seen in patients with anterior GH instability, can also produce secondary impingement.[45] A downward spiral of tendon degeneration occurs because excessive anterior humeral glide requires greater dynamic control by the rotator cuff while simultaneously compromising cuff integrity by causing impingement. The role of inflammation in SIS continues to be unclear, as corticosteroid injections appear to have some positive effects.[198]

In overhead throwing athletes, posterior (also called internal) impingement[111] can occur. With posterior impingement, the supraspinatus and infraspinatus tendon are compressed against the posterior glenoid during the cocking phase, when the arm is horizontally abducted behind the plane of the body. Additional risk factors for this type of impingement include GIRD, retroversion, poor neuromuscular control, or poor sport-specific form. Chronic (repeated) posterior impingement can lead to a rotator cuff tear or SLAP lesion.

History Patients with SIS report a nontraumatic onset of subacromial and/or deltoid region pain that may be exacerbated with overhead activities, lifting, or reaching. Patients with primary impingement tend to be older and may also note a decrease in shoulder motion. Patients with posterior impingement complain of deep, poorly localized, posterior shoulder achiness or pain. Individuals most at risk for impingement are laborers in jobs requiring repeated overhead activities and athletes, particularly those who participate in overhead sports such as baseball, softball, swimming, and racquet sports.[45] Clinicians should ask patients if they have had a recent change to these types of activities, recent increase in training, or change to a new sport or new position with greater overhead demands (such as a second base person transitioning into the role of catcher or a volleyball setter transitioning into an outside hitter position).

Key Examination Findings Patients with SIS may have a painful arc and will have one or more positive impingement tests,[243] including Neer impingement test,[207] Hawkins-Kennedy impingement test, and the horizontal adduction test. Manual muscle testing of the rotator cuff may be painful, but significant weakness will not be present. There may be decreased serratus anterior or lower trapezius weakness or the inability to maintain a fully retracted position for at least 15 seconds.[122] Those with scapular dyskinesia will have a reduction in pain with the scapular assistance or scapular retraction test.[243] Patients may have positive tests for anterior instability or anterior humeral laxity. Restriction in posterior capsule mobility or GIRD may be present. Individuals with SIS have greater kyphosis and decreased thoracic extension than those without SIS.[244] Patients with posterior impingement are likely to be tender below the posterior acromion and may have a positive relocation test, in that posterior pressure on the humeral head reduces posterior shoulder pain by reducing anterior humeral head translation.[122] Central sensitization may be present.[198]

Differential Diagnoses Differential diagnosis for SIS includes rotator cuff tear and labral pathology.

Rehabilitation Focus and Key Points Interventions for SIS must address the root cause of impingement. Patient education should include optimizing posture and scapular positioning and activity modification. For patients with central sensitization, education must include information about the multifactorial nature of pain and the complex relationship between pain and anatomic pathology. Likewise, the patients should be educated as to what are acceptable pain levels. Pain-reducing methods, including ice, heat, or electrical stimulation can be included as part of, but not in lieu of, therapeutic exercise. Patients with high irritability or high pain levels may benefit from isometric rotator cuff exercises beginning at 50% maximum voluntary isometric contraction intensity, holding up to 30 seconds for several repetitions to assist with pain modulation.[221]

GH and thoracic joint mobilizations can help improve joint mobility.[245] Stretching should address areas of hypomobility. Posterior capsule stretches such as the modified sleeper stretch and horizontal adduction with scapular stabilization can be highly beneficial.[238,246] Thoracic spine extension,[247] such as extending over a low chair back, and pectoral muscle stretching can assist with improving scapular resting position. As always, stretching should be followed by exercises to use or reinforce newly gained ranges. There is conflicting evidence as to the effect of cervical and thoracic manipulation and dry needling on SIS.[243,248]

Shoulder strengthening exercises,[249] with a focus on the rotator cuff and scapular stabilizers, should begin in less challenging positions,[221] such as external rotation with the arm by the side and low rows, before progressing to external rotation in 90° of abduction and high rows. Endurance parameters may be more appropriate than maximal strengthening for some patients, such as a swimmer or drywall installer. Scapular-focused exercises are beneficial for those with poor scapular control.[238] For example, scapular setting, where the patient attempts to isometrically hold a contraction when the shoulder is placed in a position (e.g., 60° of scaption with the scapula manually positioned into retraction, upward rotation, and posterior tilt), may improve muscle activation of the serratus anterior, middle and lower trapezius activation, and increase the subacromial space.[250] Rhythmic stabilization exercises may be useful for improving neuromuscular control, particularly for individuals with instability or scapular dyskinesia. Exercises should begin at lower angles and progress to more challenging positions,[251] such as increased angles of abduction and external rotation required for throwing. Training the entire kinetic chain, including the core and lower extremities,[125] is beneficial for athletes with SIS.

Expected Outcomes Rehabilitation can be expected to lead to consistent improvements in pain,[207] range of motion,[207] strength,[207] and function[252] in about 8 weeks. Individuals with high pain levels or high irritability may benefit from corticosteroid injection.[252] Although, in the past, subacromial decompression (SAD) was a common intervention for patients with SIS, there is now strong evidence against this for individuals with atraumatic SIS,[249,253] because it does not address the functional or dynamic causes of symptoms. However, there is strong evidence that SAD may be beneficial for those failing conservative management.[249] Because type III acromion does encroach upon the subacromial space, SAD may be more likely to be successful in this population.[207]

Glenohumeral Instability

Pathology **Laxity** is an increase in joint mobility that can be assessed by special tests, such as the sulcus sign and load-and-shift tests. Congenital laxity is seen in patients with systemic hypermobility, such as Ehlers-Danlos syndrome or Marfan syndrome. Acquired laxity is the result of activity- or sport-specific demands, such as the increased posterior humeral translation seen in the dominant (trailing) shoulder of golfers due to the repetitive high tensile stress occurring during swing follow-through. Laxity, in itself, need not be a pathologic process. For many activities or sports, a certain amount of laxity is required to be successful. The presence of laxity (generalized laxity with a Beighton score >4[254] or local laxity from sport-specific adaptions or frank dislocation), theoretically predisposes a patient to instability. This loss of passive restraint requires greater strength and neuromuscular control to provide dynamic joint support. Therefore, if an imbalance exists between the static joint constraints (joint capsule, ligaments, labrum, and bony structure) and the dynamic stabilizers (muscle strength, endurance, and dynamic control), instability may result. GH **instability** is a subjective complaint of discomfort or decrease in shoulder function resulting from excessive, symptomatic humeral translation that can occur with or without ligamentous laxity.[255,256] Shoulder pathology may be described along a continuum of instability and impingement (Fig. 14-73).[113] Instability and impingement can both occur in isolation. However, the excessive humeral head translation of GH instability can also lead to secondary impingement, as described previously with posterior impingement. Nearly 70% of patients with instability have positive impingement tests.[257]

Shoulder instability is further categorized by degree, etiology, frequency, and direction (Table 14-17). The GH joint is the most frequently dislocated joint in the body.[258] The incidence of traumatic instability is 1.7% and is greatest in sport participation, particularly collision sports (e.g., American football and wrestling).[259] A one-time traumatic event was responsible for 86% of the cases of shoulder instabilities found in children.[260] Anterior instability is the most frequently seen direction of instability, accounting for about three-quarters of all instabilities.[260] Traumatic anterior instability may result from a fall with the arm abducted and externally rotated. Anterior dislocation is common in wrestling, football, and ice hockey.[143] Anterior humeral subluxation or dislocation can produce a **Bankart lesion**, detachment of the anteroinferior portion of the glenoid labrum, and significant elongation of the IGHLC and anterior capsule. Anterior dislocation can also create a **Hill-Sachs lesion**, which is an osseous deformity of the posterosuperior humeral head from impacting the anterior glenoid.[143] Because of these bony and soft-tissue changes, a substantial number individuals with traumatic anterior instability or dislocation will have a recurrent episode, particularly those younger than 30 years.[143]

Posterior instability accounts for only 2 to 10% of all shoulder instabilities.[261,262] Traumatic posterior instability may be due to a posterior axial load with the shoulder in mid-range flexion, as in a lineman blocking in American football. Likewise, repeated microtrauma can occur from throwing leading to progressive posterior capsular insufficiency.[263] Atraumatic posterior shoulder instability can occur due to seizure, electrocution, or excessive humeral retroversion. Posterior instability is linked to lesions of the posterior labrum, posterior capsule, IGHL, and rotator cuff muscles.[262]

Multidirectional shoulder instability (MDI) is shoulder instability in at least two directions: anterior, posterior, and/or inferior.[264] MDI is generally atraumatic. Individuals with MDI generally have a large, redundant inferior GH joint capsule, causing shoulder laxity[265] or congenital laxity or GH dysplasia. They may participate in an activity requiring global shoulder hypermobility,[266] such as swimming or gymnastics. Those with MDI appear to have reduced joint proprioception, decreased rotator cuff strength, altered neuromuscular control, and scapular dyskinesia.[264] For these reasons, it is not uncommon for MDI to be bilateral. MDI is less

TABLE 14-17
CLASSIFYING SHOULDER INSTABILITY

Etiology	• Traumatic • Atraumatic (voluntary, involuntary) • Overuse • Congenital dysplasia
Degree	• Dislocation • Subluxation • Microinstability
Direction	• Anterior • Posterior • Inferior • Multidirectional
Frequency	• Acute • Recurrent • Chronic

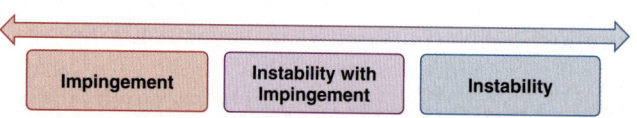

FIGURE 14-73 Continuum of impingement and instability.

common with aging due to natural stiffening of tissues over time.[267]

History Some patients may relate the onset of symptoms to a particular traumatic event, such as a fall, a tackle, or a throw. Individuals with instability generally complain of a feeling of looseness, slippage, or giving way; catching or clicking may also be present. They may report vague shoulder pain, fatigue, or weakness. These individuals commonly report apprehension or symptoms when the arm is in a particular position.[264,266] Patients with anterior instability are likely to experience symptoms when in abduction, external rotation, or horizontal abduction, such as when donning a coat or the cocking phase of throwing. Those with posterior instability may have symptoms while in flexion or internal rotation, or horizontal adduction, such as pushing open a door or a backhand in tennis or push-up variations with a narrow base of support. These patients may complain of tightness in the posterior shoulder[262] due to the increased muscular effort to compensate for lack of static posterior support. Patients with inferior instability may report that carrying heavy items, such as a suitcase, produces symptoms. Patients with Ehlers-Danlos syndrome typically have generalized ligamentous laxity and may present with multidirectional instability. Transient paresthesias due to traction on the brachial plexus are not uncommon in throwers.[113] Some patients may report a "dead arm" in which they lose control of the arm, dropping objects they are holding or the inability to attain the cocking position while attempting to throw due to sudden, transient weakness or pain.[268]

Patients with instability are generally younger than 30 years and may have a previous history of instability or dislocation.[267] The dominant arm more likely to be involved for atraumatic instability,[267] likely as a result of the effect of unilateral sports. Some patients may report or demonstrate the ability to volitionally dislocate the shoulder. Patients with recurrent anterior instability may have a family history of instability.[113]

Key Examination Findings Shoulder range of motion is likely to be excessive in one or more directions, but if painful or apprehensive, motion will appear limited. For example, patients with MDI are likely to have greater than 105° of GH abduction when the scapula stabilized.[149] Patients with instability are likely to have increased GH joint mobility and positive tests for one or more directions of instability.[264,267] However, patients who are painful or apprehensive may guard with testing, making it difficult to detect laxity. The clinician should assess for signs of systemic hypermobility, including checking the patient's Beighton score. Patients with instability may have strength deficits for a variety of reasons. Acutely, there may be weakness due to pain, concomitant impingement, or rotator cuff pathology. The patient may have pre-morbid weakness that exacerbated or led to the instability. EMG studies performed on patients with instability have revealed decreased infraspinatus recruitment, resulting in decreased joint stability and increased anterior humeral translation.[258] Fatigue strength testing may be helpful in assessing impairments in muscle performance. Patients with anterior instability may be tender over the anterior shoulder and greater tuberosity, whereas those with multidirectional instability may have more diffuse joint tenderness anteriorly or posteriorly.[269] Trigger points may be present in the trapezius, levator scapulae, or rhomboids.[269] Impingement tests should be performed to determine the presence of concomitant SIS.

Although not commonly seen in outpatient rehabilitation, direct access practitioners and on-the-field medical providers must be able to identify an acute dislocation. These patients will present with pain and a visible deformity due to humeral head malalignment. Patients with an anterior dislocation will have a significant loss of abduction and internal rotation, whereas those with a posterior dislocation will have a significant loss of adduction and external rotation due to abnormal contact of the humeral head with the glenoid.[270,271] Medical consultation should be sought in such cases. In rare cases, patients may present with chronic shoulder dislocations with atrophy of the deltoid due to axillary nerve palsy, atrophy of the spinati, and/or median or ulnar neuropathy.[272]

Imaging tests will demonstrate an acute dislocation but may be negative with shoulder subluxation or instability. Most patients with repeat anterior dislocations will have radiographic evidence of a Hill-Sachs lesion.[143] Magnetic resonance imaging may reveal concomitant pathology, such as a labral tear or rotator cuff degeneration or tear.[256] The incidence of rotator cuff tears after anterior dislocation is age related: 30% of those over the age of 40 and 80% of those over the age of 60 have concomitant rotator cuff tears.[273]

Differential Diagnoses Differential diagnosis includes subacromial impingement, labral pathology, rotator cuff tear, and fracture.

Rehabilitation Focus and Key Points Conservative rehabilitation for instability should include pain modulation and early controlled motion to prevent disuse atrophy, retard neuromuscular control loss, and improve articular nutrition. There is considerable debate regarding the role of immobilization for

TABLE 14-18	
SHOULDER INSTABILITY PRECAUTIONS	
Direction of Instability	Precautions
Anterior	• Limit abduction • Limit external rotation—particularly in abduction • Limit horizontal abduction • Safe zone: hands should remain anterior to the plane of the scapula
Posterior	• Limit horizontal adduction • Limit internal rotation • Limit weight bearing in 90° flexion • Safe zone: hands should remain posterior to the plane of the scapula
Inferior	• Limit traction forces • Consider elastic resistance tubing rather than free weights for upright exercises • Safe zone: avoid end-range elevation

patients after dislocation. The consensus seems to be in favor of brief immobilization in a sling for comfort as needed.[143] Clinicians must consider the direction(s) of patient instability when designing and progressing rehabilitation programs by prescribing exercises within the safe zones of motion based on the direction of instability (Table 14-18). Aggressive stretching in the direction of dislocation or instability should be avoided until 6 to 10 weeks postinjury, and then only if significant limitations are present.

For acutely unstable patients, rehabilitation should begin with pain modulation, activity modification, and postural correction. For example, a patient with inferior instability who sits with increased kyphosis, protraction, and downwardly rotated scapulae will have little bony stability for the GH joint to prevent inferior humeral head translation. Therefore, for this patient, posture correction and postural exercises should be emphasized early in the rehabilitation process. Active or active-assisted exercise should begin within the safe zone based on the patient's direction of instability. Closed-chain exercises[267] and rhythmic stabilization exercises, initially within safe zones, should be performed, as they assist with muscular co-contraction while providing joint compressive forces to improve joint stability. Scapular stabilizer strengthening progressions can also begin early on.[143,262] Neuromuscular training and/or biofeedback may be useful.[262] Strengthening and endurance training of the rotator cuff and scapular muscles are critical to successful rehabilitation.[262,264,267] Progression from resistance bands to free weights can be particularly beneficial for patients with inferior instability. Exercises are progressed from within the safe zones to more functional or sport-specific positions. For example, a javelin thrower with anterior instability would be progressed from resisted external rotation with the arm by the side, to 45° scaption, and then to 90° scaption. For athletes, progression must also include the entire kinetic chain.[267] For example, a baseball pitcher who does not have adequate lower extremity range, strength, and balance will continue to overstress the anterior GH capsule in an attempt to improve pitch velocity. For some activities, more permanent changes in technique might be recommended. For example, a basketball player with posterior instability should modify bench press and push-ups to a wider hand position so as to provide more bony support during those activities. The use of a brace or shoulder harness can be considered based on the individual's sport-specific demands, timing of competitive season, and symptom response.[143]

Expected Outcomes Compliance with the rehabilitation program appears to be positively correlated with successful conservative management of instability, and patients can expect to have a decrease in pain, increase in strength, and return to function in about 3 months.[262,264] Surgical consult is recommended if recurrent instability is noted after 3 to 6 months of conservative care.[264,274] Because a substantial number young individuals (under 40 years of age) with traumatic anterior dislocation will have recurrent episodes of instability, these patients should be evaluated by an orthopaedist before, or concomitantly with, conservative interventions. Younger patients with atraumatic and repeated instability may also benefit from referral to an orthopaedist.

Rehabilitation after Surgical Stabilization Surgical stabilization followed by rehabilitation is the intervention of choice in younger patients and athletes due to the high recurrence rate of anterior instability and dislocation. Table 14-19 provides details of the multiple types of surgical procedures for patients with recurrent instability, large Bankart lesions, large osseous defects, or the inability to perform sport-specific skills.[143,259,274] Thermal capsular shrinkage is no longer recommended owing to high failure rate.[267,275] Clinicians must know the operative diagnosis, surgical procedure(s) performed, and any surgeon- or patient-specific precautions.

Rehabilitation after instability surgery varies based on procedure(s) but typically includes 2 to 6 weeks of sling immobilization.[267,275] Rehabilitation then includes progressive range of motion and strengthening following the same general procedures outlined for conservative management. All of the listed procedures reliably reduce recurrent instability and improve pain. Open

TABLE 14-19		
SURGICAL PROCEDURES FOR SHOULDER INSTABILITY		
Procedure	Type of Instability	Method
Bankart repair	Anterior	Reattachment of the labrum and repair of the anterior capsule
Remplissage	Anterior	In-setting the posterior capsule and infraspinatus tendon within a large Hill-Sachs defect
Latarjet procedure	Anterior	Transfer of the coracoid process to the anterior glenoid as a bone block to stabilize the joint
Capsular shift	All	The subscapularis is detached, the glenohumeral capsule is split, the bottom part of the capsule is pulled (shifted) up and the top part down decreasing capsular volume
Capsular plication	All	Specific areas of the glenohumeral capsule are sewn upon itself to selectively tighten a portion of the capsule

procedures, such as the capsular shift, are more likely to cause postoperative loss of motion, particularly a loss of external rotation.[274] More than 80% of patients return to same level of sport participation within 6 to 8 months.[259,267,275,276]

However, time to return to sport is at least partially dependent on athlete season, sport, and the procedure(s) performed. Based on a recent systematic review, it appears that athletes undergoing a Latarjet procedure may return to sports in about 6 months, but those participating in collision sports may have a lower level of play.[276]

Labral Pathology

Pathology Some labral pathologies, such as Bankart lesions, have already been discussed within the context of shoulder instability. The next most common labral pathology is the **SLAP lesion**, in which the biceps-labral complex undergoes pathologic changes because of tensile, torsional, or compressive loads. There are four common ways in which a SLAP lesion may occur. First, SLAP lesions may be caused by repetitive tensile overload of the LHBT.[277,278] This is commonly seen in throwing athletes in which the biceps must decelerate the arm during follow-through. Second, repeated torsional forces applied to the biceps anchor during the late cocking phase of throwing (abduction and external rotation) can result in a "peel-back" of the biceps anchor, detaching it from the labrum.[277-279] This may be exacerbated by a tight posterior GH joint capsule due to the resulting anterosuperior shift of the humeral head when the arm is abducted and externally rotated.[280] Third, a SLAP lesion may occur from a one-time trauma.[277-279] A sudden traction force on the arm, as may occur from grabbing a railing during a fall or from the sudden pull of the rope tow while skiing, can pull the biceps away from its attachment. Alternately, compression from a fall on an outstretched hand may also produce a SLAP lesion. Fourth, subtle instability can cause repeated abnormal labral compression, creating a SLAP lesion.[279] As noted previously, the reverse can also occur, in that a SLAP lesion can be the cause, not just the result, of instability.

There are four common types of SLAP lesions (Fig. 14-74), with type II lesions being the most common[278]:

- Type I: fraying
- Type II: detachment of biceps anchor
- Type III: bucket-handle tear of the superior labrum with a normal biceps
- Type IV: bucket-handle tear of the superior labrum that extends into the biceps

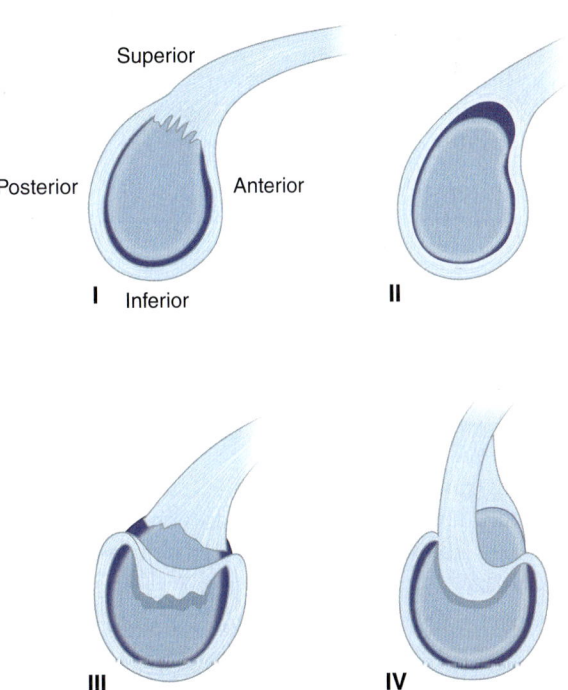

FIGURE 14-74 Common types of labral tears. (Dodson CC, Altchek DW. SLAP lesions: An update on recognition and treatment. *J Orthop Sports Phys Ther*. 2009;39(2):71-80; Figure 1.)

History SLAP lesions are most commonly seen in overhead athletes or workers with significant amounts of over-shoulder height job demands; however, a one-time trauma, as noted previously, is also possible. Individuals with SLAP lesions commonly report poorly localized, deep shoulder pain,[277] although, in throwers, pain is generally posterior. Pain is exacerbated by overhead activity, particularly during the late cocking phase of throwing.[279] Patients may report painful or painless popping, clicking, or catching with overhead movements.[281] Interestingly, individuals who have femoroacetabular impingement are significantly more likely to have SLAP lesions.[282]

Key Examination Findings Patients with labral tears may have positive special tests for labral pathology, including crank test, O'Brien active compression test, and biceps load tests.[279,281] Bicipital pain and positive Speed or Yergason tests may occur due to the stress placed on the biceps anchor.[279] Patients may have scapular dyskinesia, a tight posterior GH capsule, and/or a loss of internal rotation or horizontal adduction, as these appear to be risk factors for SLAP lesions.[279] Special tests for instability, impingement, or contractile lesions may also be positive due to concomitant pathology.[283] Magnetic resonance imaging is the gold standard for identifying SLAP lesions. However, because SLAP lesions can be asymptomatic and most patients can be managed conservatively, imaging is not recommended, except to plan for surgical interventions.

Differential Diagnoses Differential diagnoses include isolated or concomitant GH instability, impingement, or rotator cuff pathology.

Rehabilitation Focus and Key Points Traditionally, individuals with SLAP lesions were referred for surgical interventions.[283] However, it is now believed that most can be successfully managed conservatively.[277,281,284] Initial activity modifications should include limiting activities that stress the biceps and overhead activities, including throwing. Interventions should focus on[281]:

- Activity modification
- Restoring range of motion
- Improving rotator cuff strength and endurance
- Improving scapular muscle strengthen, endurance, and control

During the acute phase, pain and inflammation control along with activity modifications should include limiting activities that stress the biceps and overhead activities, including throwing. Shoulder isometrics, resisted shoulder rotation, and scapular strengthening below 90° of elevation can begin early on using manual resistance, elastic resistance, or dumbbells. Exercise in the plane of the scapula may be better tolerated initially.[285] Posterior humeral glides can improve humeral head positioning and restore internal rotation and horizontal adduction. Exercises can progress into self-stretching of the posterior capsule using horizontal adduction or modified sleeper stretch with the scapula stabilized, this is particularly important if there is a large deficit in internal rotation. Strengthening should be progressed into higher ranges of elevation once lower ranges are tolerated, moving toward sport- or work-specific positions, intensities, and volumes. As noted previously, attention to the entire kinetic chain should be emphasized particularly for overhead athletes. An interval throwing program, particularly for pitchers, can help gradually and methodically increase biceps-labral loading.

Expected Outcomes Conservative management is successful for the vast majority of patients within 3 to 6 months.[277,278,281,284] Patients with high levels of pain or who are progressing more slowly may benefit from one or two corticosteroid injections.[281]

Surgical Interventions for Superior Labrum Anterior and Posterior Lesions Patients who continue to have symptoms after 3 to 6 months of conservative treatment should be referred for a surgical consult.[286] Historically, the intervention of choice for type II SLAP lesions was direct repair to restore the normal anatomic of the biceps-labral connection. However, a SLAP repair tends to result in a decrease in shoulder external rotation,[277] which may be responsible for the fairly poor outcomes for overhead throwing athletes. For example, only 69% of overhead athletes returned to sport[287]; of these, only about half of pitchers returned to their prior level of performance.[287,288] For these reasons, **biceps tenodesis** (releasing the long head of the biceps and reattaching it along the shaft of the humerus) or **biceps tenotomy** (releasing the superior attachment of the long head of the biceps without reattachment) are currently the preferred surgical interventions.[289] Biceps tenodesis has shown to have good results with high return to play and performance rates,[259,290] including when used on middle-aged individuals,[291] military personnel,[292] younger athletes,[293] and athletes with failed SLAP repairs.[294]

Rehabilitation after biceps tenodesis should prioritize the same interventions as noted in conservative management, with the exception of protecting the biceps by waiting 7 to 8 weeks after surgery before initiating resistive elbow flexion exercises.[290] In contrast with a SLAP repair, both the labrum and the biceps must be protected. Unfortunately, although postoperative SLAP repair protocols exist, there is little in the literature to guide these interventions.[295] Most protocols limit shoulder elevation to 90° and shoulder external rotation to about 30° for the first 6 weeks before allowing a gradual increase in motion over the next 6 weeks.[278] Patients generally are able to return to overhead sports 4 to 6 months after tenodesis,[290] but require significantly longer time before return to sport following a SLAP repair.[278]

Biceps Pathology

The long head of the biceps is a key pain generator in the shoulder.[296] The long head of the biceps may be involved due to the close anatomic relationship with the rotator cuff and labrum, the function as a humeral head depressor, and the synovial sheath. There is significant controversy regarding how to manage biceps pathology. Conservative treatment of isolated bicipital tendinopathy generally includes ice and nonsteroidal anti-inflammatory medication, and activity modification to decrease inflammation.[296] Once irritability is reduced, progressive elbow flexion exercises are initiated.

Because the long head of the biceps is a frequent cause of shoulder pain, any abnormality noted in the tendon during a shoulder surgery is typically addressed. Mild fraying of the tendon will be debrided. However, in cases of partial-thickness tearing or significant tissue irritation, the surgeon will typically choose to perform a tenotomy or tenodesis as described earlier in the management of SLAP lesions. Table 14-20 reviews the details of each when used for the management of isolated long head of biceps pathology.[296,297] Traumatic ruptures of the long head of the biceps can occur when attempting to lift or lower a heavy object quickly. This typically results in a so-called "Popeye deformity." While one might be concerned that a tenotomy would result in a loss of elbow flexion and supination power, this has not been consistently seen in the literature.[297]

Suprascapular Neuropathy

The suprascapular nerve is vulnerable to compression or traction at the suprascapular notch or the spinoglenoid notch.[298] For example, the nerve can be compression from a heavy back pack[299] or local ganglion cyst. Nerve traction injuries can occur from repetitive overhead activity in scapular protraction.[300]

Although rare (about 4% of patients),[301] suprascapular neuropathy is more often seen in overhead athletes, causing posterolateral shoulder pain and burning sensation, given the nerve's sensory innervation to the superior and posterior shoulder.[301] If the injury occurs at the suprascapular notch, there will be weakness of shoulder elevation and external rotation,[302] whereas injury at the spinoglenoid notch will result solely in weakness of the infraspinatus.[298] If nerve compression is long-standing, atrophy of the supraspinatus and/or the infraspinatus will be present.[302] Because symptoms are similar to a rotator cuff tear or SIS, sometimes, problems go on for months or years before being properly diagnosed via nerve conduction studies.[303]

Unless a space-occupying lesion such as a large ganglion cyst is present, initial treatment includes range of motion exercises, progressive strengthening, and nonsteroidal anti-inflammatory medication and/or gabapentin to assist with symptom modulation.[298] Corticosteroid injection can assist with diagnosis and may even provide lasting relief.[298] If nerve injury is caused by traction, scapular stabilization and sport-specific training to improve scapular positioning can be highly beneficial.

Patients who fail to respond to conservative care can be successfully treated with arthroscopic nerve decompression. Rehabilitation includes immediate active and passive motion without restriction with progression to strengthening as tolerated.[298] Results are consistently positive for improving pain, restoring strength, and return to functional activities.[298]

DIFFERENTIAL DIAGNOSIS

Pain related to the shoulder region can seem overwhelming to the novice clinician. However, clinicians can begin to narrow down differential diagnoses by symptom location (Fig. 14-75), patient symptoms (Table 14-21), and onset (Fig. 14-76).

TABLE 14-20
TENOTOMY VERSUS TENODESIS FOR LONG HEAD OF BICEPS PATHOLOGY

	Tenotomy	Tenodesis
Surgery and rehabilitation	Simple surgery Consistent pain reduction Cramping sensation common Popeye deformity common	Longer surgery Sling for 4–6 weeks Consistent pain reduction Longer rehabilitation due to the need to protect repair
Most common Patient population	Older individuals	Younger patients, laborers, athletes, individuals conserved about cosmesis

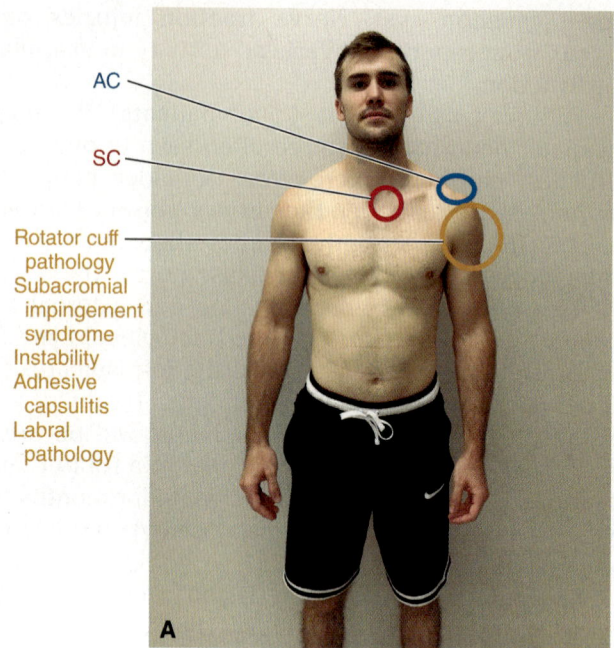 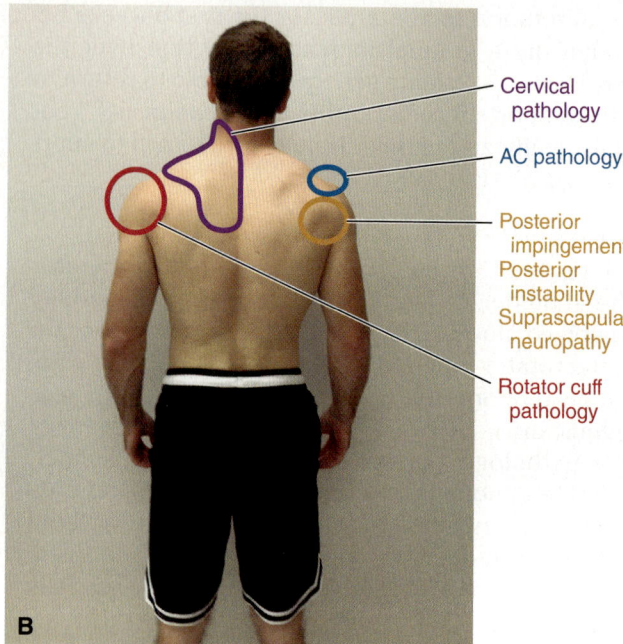

FIGURE 14-75 Shoulder complex pathology based on symptom location. **A.** Anterior shoulder complex. **B.** Posterior shoulder complex. *AC*, acromioclavicular; *SC*, sternoclavicular.

TABLE 14-21	
DIFFERENTIAL DIAGNOSIS OF SHOULDER JOINT COMPLEX PATHOLOGY BY COMPLAINT	
Complaint/Symptom	**Differential Diagnoses**
Stiffness	• Adhesive capsulitis • Glenohumeral osteoarthritis • Scapular dyskinesia • Instability
Weakness	• Rotator cuff tear • Subacromial impingement syndrome • Scapular dyskinesia • Muscle strain • Peripheral nerve injury
Painful arc	• Subacromial impingement syndrome
Instability	• Instability • Labral pathology • Loose body
Mechanical complaints of clicking, locking, catching	• Labral pathology • Osteoarthritis (glenohumeral, acromioclavicular, sternoclavicular) • Acromioclavicular separation • Loose body
Night pain	• Irritable shoulder pathology • Adhesive capsulitis • Rotator cuff pathology • Nonmusculoskeletal condition
Paresthesias	• Cervical dysfunction • Subluxation • Thoracic outlet syndrome • Peripheral nerve injury

ADDITIONAL JOINT MOBILIZATION TECHNIQUES

Clinician- and patient-generated mobilizations can be used to gain range of motion.

Clinician-Generated Joint Mobilizations

The accessory motion procedures described earlier can be used to treat shoulder hypomobility, particularly when using grade III and IV mobilizations and/or performing closer to end-range. However, additional techniques can be valuable for gaining motion in various directions.

Scapular Distraction

Purpose: This is considered a general technique to increase scapular mobility and can also be used as an indirect stretch on the anterior GH capsule to improve shoulder external rotation.

Patient: Sidelying with the elbow resting on the clinician's clavicular region.

Clinician: The clinician's superior hand contacts the patient's acromion. The pads of the clinician's inferior fingers contact the medial border of the scapula.

Mobilization: The scapulae are slowly distracted from the thorax (Fig. 14-77). The mobilization can be modified by adding scapular motion, such as upward rotation.

Inferior Humeral Glide in Flexion

Purpose: To increase joint-play movement necessary for shoulder flexion.

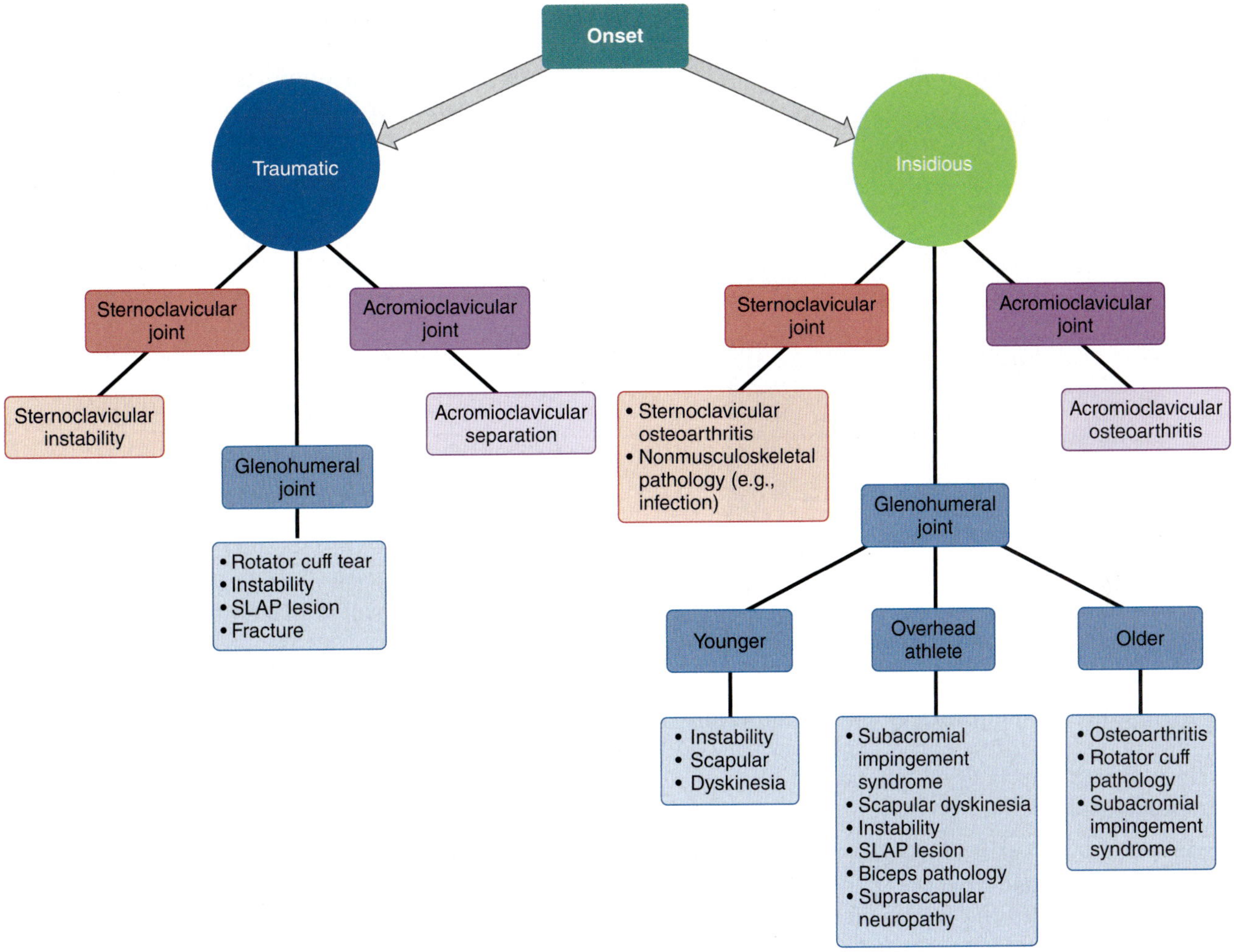

FIGURE 14-76 Shoulder complex pathology based on onset. *SLAP*, superior labrum anterior and posterior.

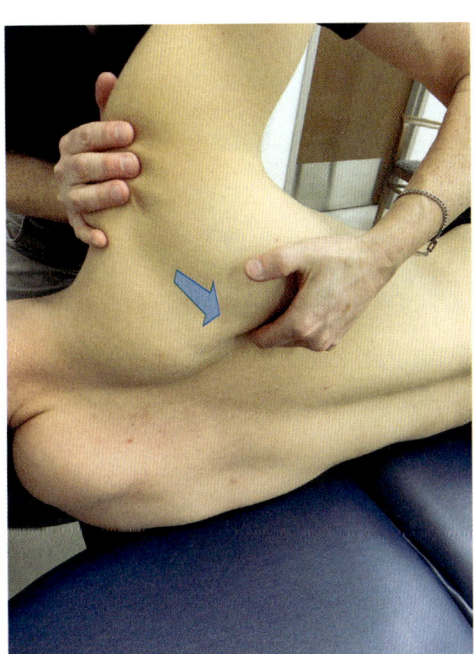

FIGURE 14-77 Scapular distraction.

Patient: Supine with the shoulder in 45 to 100° of flexion with the elbow bent.
Clinician: The clinician grasps the proximal humerus with both hands and fingers interlaced. The clinician's clavicular region supports the patient's distal posterior humerus.
Mobilization: The clinician leans posterior to create an inferior humeral glide. The patient's arm is gradually moved into greater amounts of flexion (Fig. 14-78).

Inferior Humeral Glide in Abduction

Purpose: To increase joint-play movement necessary for shoulder abduction.
Patient: Supine with the shoulder in slight external rotation and varying amounts of abduction or scaption.
Clinician: The clinician supports the patient's arm in with the lateral hand and trunk. The clinician's medial hand contacts the patient's superior proximal humerus (just lateral to the acromion process).

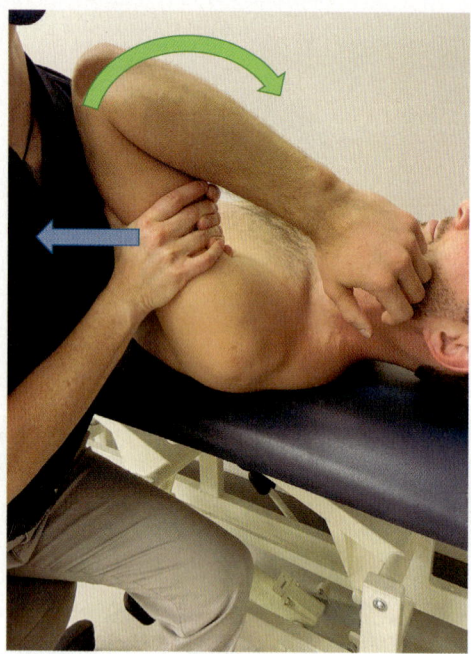

FIGURE 14-78 Inferior humeral glide in flexion.

Mobilization: The clinician shifts weight anteriorly to create an inferior glide of the humerus (Fig. 14-79). The patient's arm is gradually moved into greater amounts of abduction.

Lateral Humeral Distraction With Belt
Purpose: To increase global GH joint-play movement.
Patient: Supine with the arm in 70 to 145° of flexion and the elbow bent 90°.
Clinician: A mobilization belt is looped around the patient's proximal humerus and the clinician's buttocks. The clinician supports the patient's forearm with the superior hand, whereas the inferior hand stabilizes the patient's distal humerus near the elbow.
Mobilization: The clinician creates a distraction force by leaning the hips back into the belt and stabilizing the distal humerus (Fig. 14-80). The patient's arm is gradually moved into greater amounts of flexion. This technique can also be modified to create a mobilization with movement to increase shoulder internal or external rotation by applying the mobilizing force and then performing physiologic rotation.

Prone Humeral Distraction in Flexion
Purpose: To increase joint-play movement necessary for flexion.
Patient: Prone with the arm hanging comfortably into flexion. A towel roll is placed to support the anterior scapula.
Clinician: The clinician grasps the distal humerus with both hands and fingers interlaced.
Mobilization: The clinician's hands apply a distraction force along the long axis of the humerus (Fig. 14-81). This technique can be interspersed with prone pendulum exercises. Alternatively, a lateral distraction force can also be applied.

Patient-Generated Joint Mobilizations
Patients with GIRD would benefit from posterior capsule stretching to improve shoulder internal rotation.

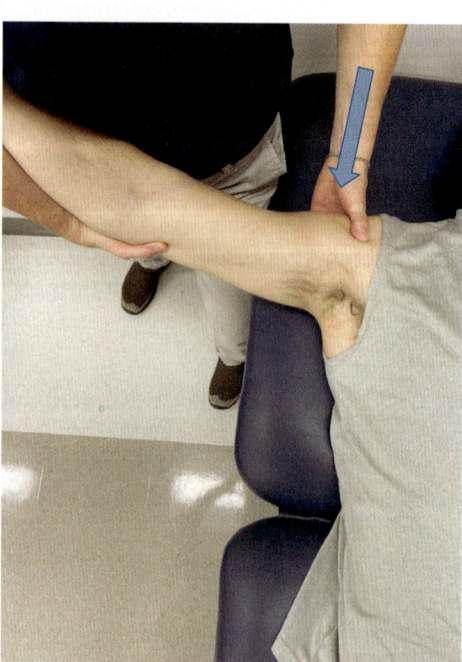

FIGURE 14-79 Inferior humeral glide into abduction.

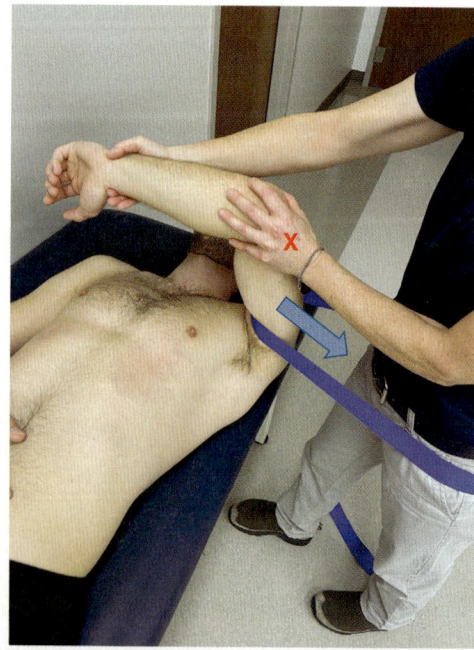

FIGURE 14-80 Lateral humeral distraction with belt.

CHAPTER 14 | SHOULDER COMPLEX

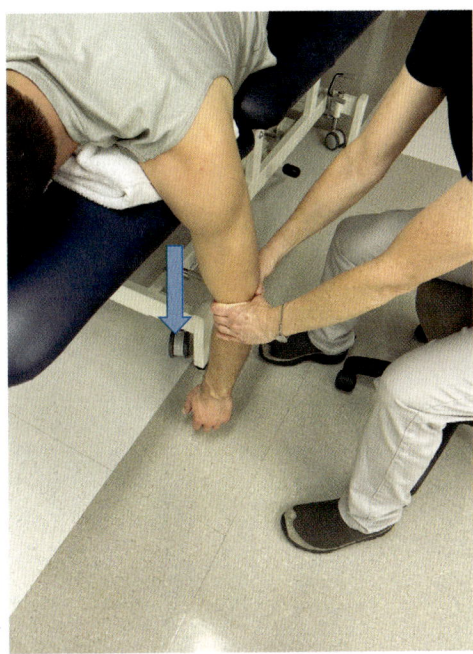

FIGURE 14-81 Prone humeral distraction in flexion.

Sidelying Horizontal Adduction to Stretch the Posterior Capsule

Patient: Three-quarters sidelying on the shoulder to be stretched such that the scapula is stabilized by the patient's body weight. The shoulder should be in 60 to 75° of abduction.

Mobilization: The patient pulls the arm into horizontal adduction (Fig. 14-82).

Modified Sleeper Stretch

Patient: Three-quarters sidelying on the shoulder to be stretched such that the scapula is stabilized by the patient's body weight. The shoulder should be in 60 to 75° of abduction.

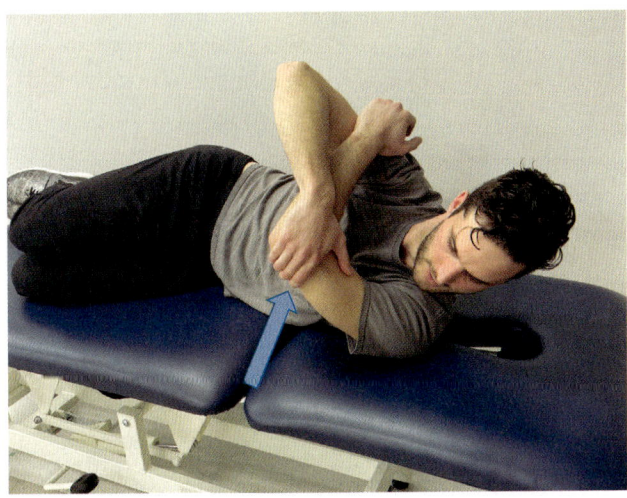

FIGURE 14-82 Sidelying horizontal adduction to stretch the posterior capsule.

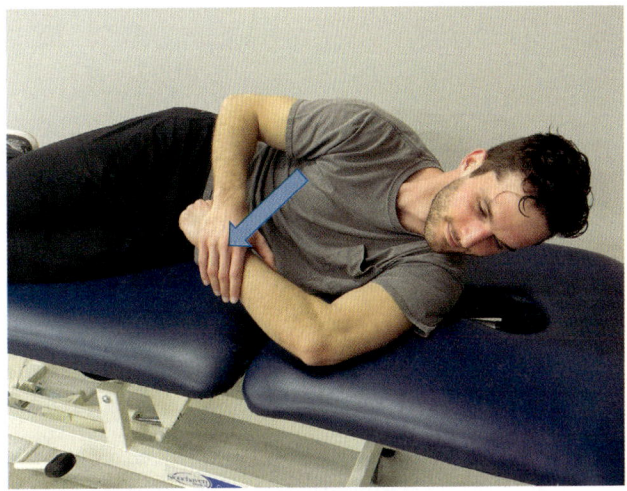

FIGURE 14-83 Modified sleeper stretch to stretch the posterior capsule.

Mobilization: The patient presses the arm into internal rotation (Fig. 14-83).

ADDITIONAL THERAPEUTIC EXERCISES

The exercises discussed throughout this chapter may be beneficial for a wide variety of patients and diagnoses. One of the primary goals of rehabilitation of patients with shoulder pathology is to improve external rotator and scapular muscle strength. This section provides a few examples of common strengthening exercises. There are many excellent resources for exercises for patients with shoulder pathologies.[304,305]

Performing resisted external rotation bilaterally (Fig. 14-84) in lower ranges of elevation is a safe starting

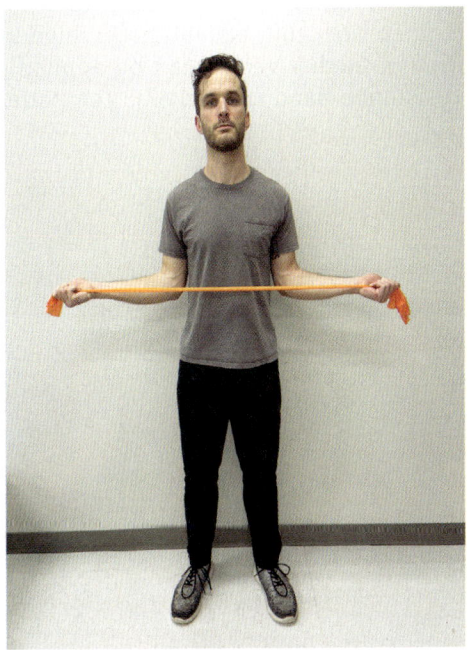

FIGURE 14-84 Resisted external rotation and retraction.

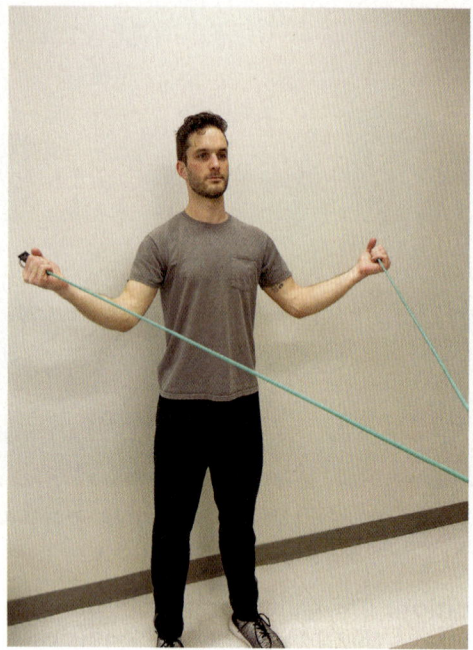

FIGURE 14-85 "W" exercise.

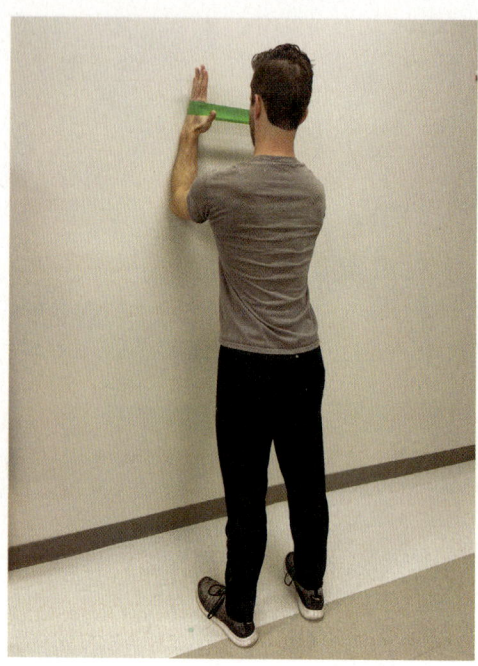

FIGURE 14-87 Bilateral shoulder flexion with a medial vector.

point because the position avoids the common zone of impingement and requires less scapular muscle strength than when performed in higher ranges. The "W" exercise (Fig. 14-85) is a mild progression by having the arms in greater abduction and the angle of resistance requires greater activation of the scapular retractors. Sidelying shoulder flexion from 0 to 90° (Fig. 14-86) is also performed in an impingement-free zone. The weight of the arm, with or without a dumbbell, requires isometric scapular retraction and posterior cuff activation to maintain proper form. To promote posterior cuff activation in higher levels of elevation, a medial vector can be applied using a looped resistance band (Fig. 14-87). The patient then slides the forearms up the wall while maintaining the forearms vertical. Wall angels (Fig. 14-88) require the patient to maintain the forearms against the wall while sliding the arms up into abduction and back down as far possible. This exercise can be extremely challenging as the posterior cuff and scapular muscles must work against normally tight pectoral muscles and internal rotators.

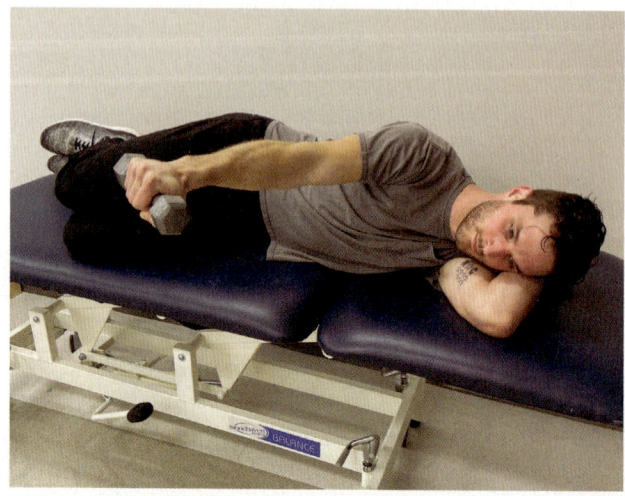

FIGURE 14-86 Sidelying shoulder flexion.

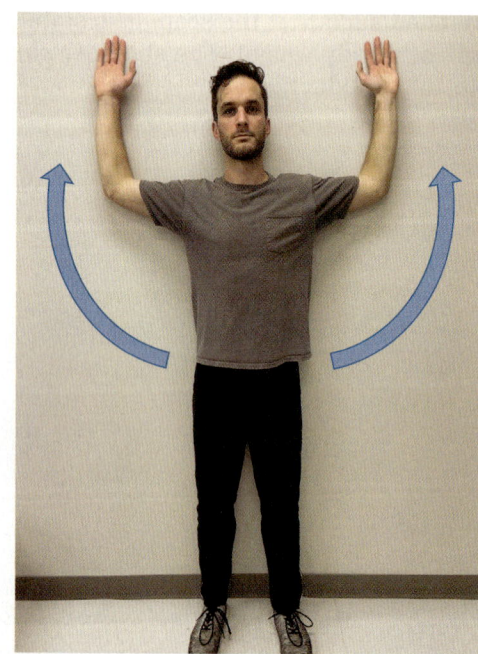

FIGURE 14-88 Wall angels.

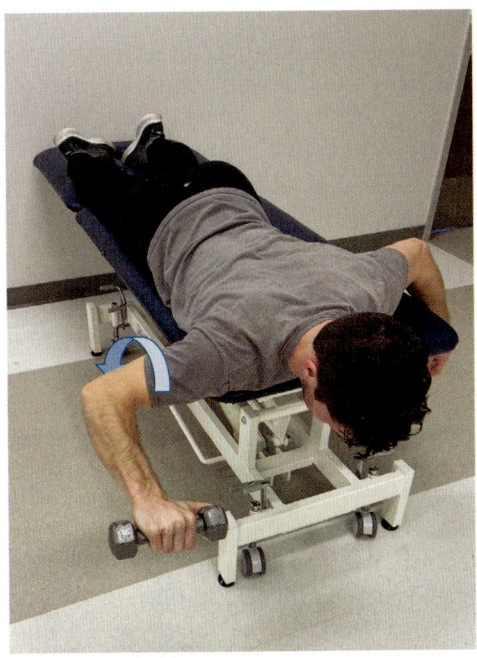

FIGURE 14-89 Prone external rotation.

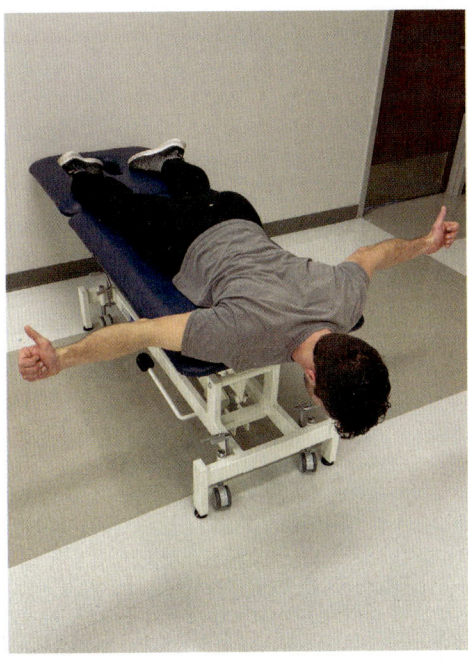

FIGURE 14-91 Prone "T."

Prone exercises can be progressed from active to resisted. Prone-resisted external rotation can be made more challenging by being performed with the humerus off the support surface (Fig. 14-89). Prone ball dribbling can be progressed to a prone ball catch (Fig. 14-90) to improve shoulder external rotator and scapular retractor endurance, which is required for swimming and working overhead. The prone "T" exercise (Fig. 14-91) challenges the middle trapezius muscle, whereas the prone "Y" exercise (Fig. 14-92) targets the lower trapezius. While both exercises also require posterior cuff activation, the prone "Y" exercise is more challenging, given the higher elevation. The "hug-a-tree" exercise (Fig. 14-93) is performed by having the patient attempt to reach around a large imaginary tree against a resistance band emphasizing

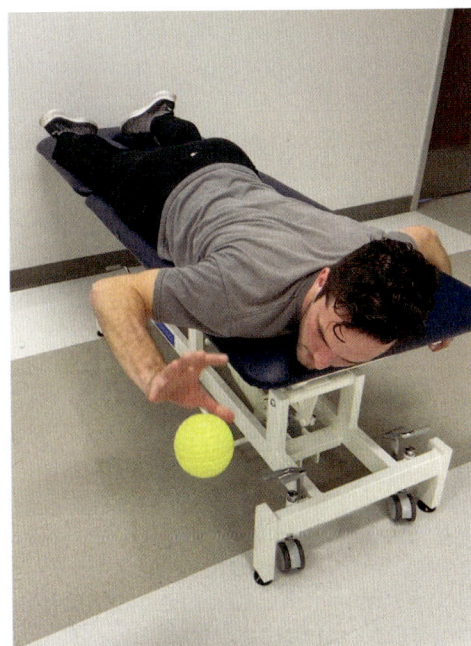

FIGURE 14-90 Prone ball catch.

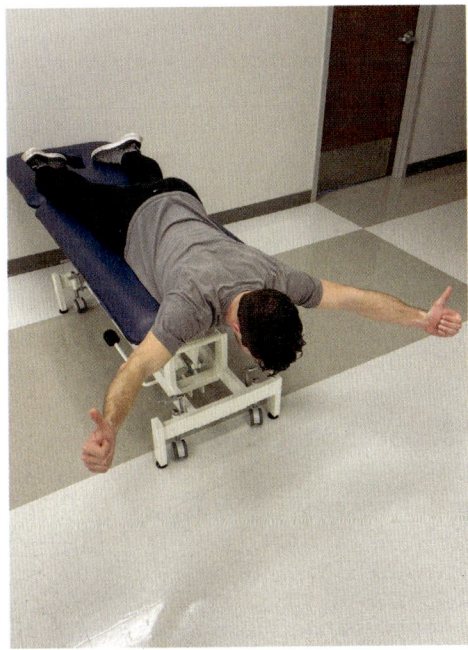

FIGURE 14-92 Prone "Y."

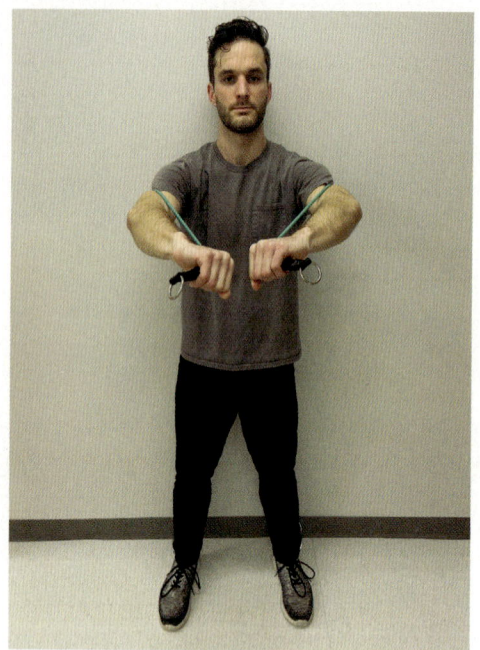

FIGURE 14-93 Hug-a-tree.

serratus anterior activation. The advantages of this exercise are that it is unlikely to create subacromial impingement pain and does not require upper extremity weight bearing like other serratus anterior exercises, such as planks and push-ups. Therefore, the "hug-a-tree" exercise may be easier and also safe for individuals with posterior instability to perform in the early phases of rehabilitation.

The closed kinetic chain upper extremity stability test (CKCUEST) is a challenging, higher level functional performance test for athletes. The test is performed by starting in a tall plank position (Fig. 14-94A) and having the patient reach across the body to touch the tape line with one hand (Fig. 14-94B), followed by the other. The number of line touches the patient can make in 15 seconds is recorded. For the standard test, the tape lines are placed 36 inches apart. A modified version of the test is performed with the tape lines directly under the patient's shoulder and may be more appropriate for smaller patients.[306] Performance can be compared with normative values[307] based on gender and sport.[308] The test can also be used to assess readiness to return to sport.[309]

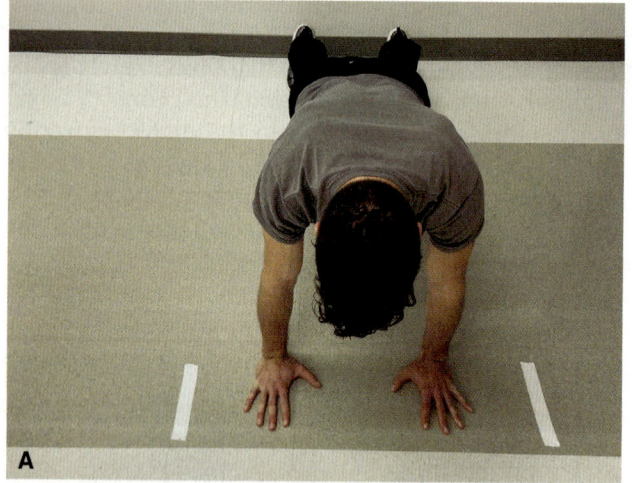
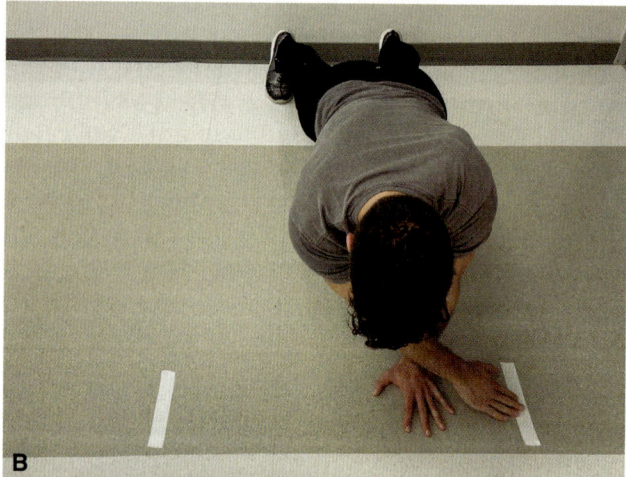

FIGURE 14-94 Closed kinetic chain upper extremity stability test. **A.** Start position. **B.** Cross body tape touch.

CASE STUDY 14-1

Anil: Patient with Intermittent Shoulder Pain

Anil is a 17-year-old baseball player who reports a 3-month history of intermittent pain in his dominant (right) shoulder. He does not recall a particular injury that caused his shoulder pain. The pain occurs during throwing and is beginning to affect his performance. All tests begin with the uninvolved (left) side unless otherwise noted. The physical examination should be organized by position, beginning away and progressing toward the involved area, and providing increasing stress to injured or potentially involved structures. Table 14-22 provides an example of how an experienced clinician might organize the physical examination after performing the history and systems review.

Based on the history, there are no red flags. The patient's history of insidious onset of pain in the throwing arm of a young athlete makes the clinician have an initial hypothesis of instability, scapular dyskinesia. Secondary impingement and rotator cuff pathology should also be considered. The seated examination begins with clearing the cervical spine and elbow of potential involvement. This is followed by a gross appreciation of shoulder active range of motion viewed from both the front and behind to observe quality of motion. The patient reported a painful arc with shoulder flexion, so this motion was immediately followed by the scapular retraction and assistance tests, which revealed resolution of symptoms. The remaining shoulder motions were then assessed, including combined motion. Internal and external rotation range and strength were assessed in sitting for a global understanding of cuff function in a less stressful position before traditional testing in prone. Special tests for systemic hypermobility and GH instability were performed in sitting. Palpation of the region was then performed with emphasis on likely pain generators and areas of potential secondary pathology. Special tests for subacromial impingement were not performed because of their nonspecific nature and the earlier results of scapular dyskinesia testing.

TABLE 14-22
SAMPLE SHOULDER EXAMINATION

Anil, 17-year-old baseball player with reports of intermittent pain in his dominant (right) throwing shoulder

Position	Assessments
Observation	Continues from history
Seated	Cervical flex, ext, lat flex, rot (A, OP) Spurling test Reflexes brachialis, biceps, triceps Dermatomes C4–T1 Finger adduction (A, MMT) Thumb extension (A, MMT) Elbow flex, ext (A, P, MMT) Upper trapezius MMT Shoulder ER arms at side, flex, ext, scaption, abd (A, OP, MMT) Scapular assistance and retraction tests Shoulder combined hand behind neck and behind back reach (A) MMT: ER and IR with arms at sides MMT: shoulder flex, ext, abd Special tests: Beighton, sulcus, load and shift Palpation: including long head of biceps, subacromial region, anterior and posterior shoulder, upper trapezius, levator, and posterior rotator cuff
Supine	PROM: shoulder flex, scap, IR, ER MMT: serratus anterior Glenohumeral accessory motion: anterior, posterior, inferior Special tests: sulcus test in 90° abduction, posterior apprehension, crank, biceps load
Prone	MMT: ER, IR, rhomboid, middle trapezius, lower trapezius Plank hold
Standing	Functional test: mock throwing at slow and then normal speed

A, active; *abd*, abduction; *ER*, external rotation; *ext*, extension; *flex*, flexion; *lat*, lateral; *OP*, overpressure; *MMT*, manual muscle test; *rot*, rotation; *UE*, upper extremity.

Once in supine, the clinician performed passive range testing of the shoulder, noting the presence of GIRD on the involved side. Because no symptoms were created with external rotation, apprehension and relocation testing for anterior instability were not required. GH joint accessory motion was then assessed and perceived to be hypomobile posteriorly. Given the potential for multidirectional instability, the sulcus test was performed in 90° abduction and found to be negative. This was followed by testing for posterior instability and labral pathology. The patient had no complaints of clicking, catching, or locking, making labral pathology unlikely. However, given the patient is an overhead athlete and the potential for a SLAP lesion, the crank and biceps load tests were performed with negative results. The examination continued toward assessing posterior muscle strength, before a plank hold to assess scapular muscle performance and basic core strength. The medial borders of the patient's scapulae failed to remain flush against the thorax after 10 seconds of the plank hold and could not be corrected with cueing. Lastly, mock throwing was performed. In this scenario, the clinician could forgo tests for rotator cuff tears, given the patient's response to active range of motion and manual muscle testing.

The clinician concluded that Anil had right scapular dyskinesia, GIRD, along with weakness and decreased scapular neuromuscular control. Later in the rehabilitation process, the clinician will perform a more thorough evaluation of the patient's throwing mechanics along with core strength and, if needed, lower extremity biomechanics.

CHAPTER SUMMARY

Functional movement of the shoulder involves a complex interaction of the SC, AC, and GH joints and the ST articulation. Shoulder dysfunction may be related to fracture, contractile lesions (impingement, rotator cuff or other muscle/tendon pathology, scapular dyskinesia), and articular pathology (adhesive capsulitis, instability, sprain, dislocation, labral tears, and OA). It is not uncommon for patients to have multiple impairments, such as instability with secondary impingement. Careful examination is required to rule out cervical, elbow, and nonmusculoskeletal pathology. Successful rehabilitation provides a progressive increase in controlled stress to the involved tissues while simultaneously addressing impairments that may have contributed to the patient's symptoms.

REFERENCES

1. Veeger H, van der Helm F. Shoulder function: the perfect compromise between mobility and stability. *J Biomech.* 2007;40(10):2119–2129. doi:10.1016/j.jbiomech.2006.10.016
2. Casier S, Van den Broecke R, Van Houcke J, Audenaert E, De Wilde L, Van Tongel A. Morphologic variations of the scapula in 3-dimensions: a statistical shape model approach. *J Shoulder Elbow Surg.* 2018;27(12):2224–2231. doi:10.1016/j.jse.2018.06.001
3. Bakhsh W, Nicandri G. Anatomy and physical examination of the shoulder. *Sports Med Arthrosc Rev.* 2018;26(3):e10–e22.
4. Ludewig P, Phadke V, Braman J, Hassett D, Cieminski C, LaPrade R. Motion of the shoulder complex during multiplanar humeral elevation. *J Bone Joint Surg Am.* 2009;91(2):378–389. doi:10.2106/jbjs.G.01483
5. Garcia J, Arguello A, Momaya A, Ponce B. Sternoclavicular joint instability: symptoms, diagnosis and management. *Orthop Res Rev.* 2020;12:75–87. doi:10.2147/orr.S170964
6. Bontempo NA, Mazzocca AD, Bontempo NA, Mazzocca AD. Biomechanics and treatment of acromioclavicular and sternoclavicular joint injuries. *Br J Sports Med.* 2010;44(5):361–369. doi:10.1136/bjsm.2009.059295
7. Renfree K, Wright T. Anatomy and biomechanics of the acromioclavicular and sternoclavicular joints. *Clin Sports Med.* 2003;22(2):219–237. doi:10.1016/s0278-5919(02)00104-7
8. Levangie P, Norkin C. *Joint Structure and Function: A Comprehensive Analysis.* 5th ed. F.A. Davis; 2011.
9. Tubbs R, Shah N, Sullivan B, et al. The costoclavicular ligament revisited: a functional and anatomical study. *Rom J Morphol Embryol.* 2009;50(3):475–479.
10. Kihlström C, Möller M, Lönn K, Wolf O. Clavicle fractures: epidemiology, classification and treatment of 2 422 fractures in the Swedish Fracture Register; an observational study. *BMC Musculoskelet Disord.* 2017;18(1):82. doi:10.1186/s12891-017-1444-1
11. Karl J, Olson P, Rosenwasser M. The epidemiology of upper extremity fractures in the United States, 2009. *J Orthop Trauma.* 2015;29(8):e242–e244. doi:10.1097/bot.0000000000000312
12. Postacchini F, Gumina S, De Santis P, Albo F. Epidemiology of clavicle fractures. *J Shoulder Elbow Surg.* 2002;11(5):452–456. doi:10.1067/mse.2002.126613
13. Amer K, Congiusta D, Suri P, Choudhry A, Otero K, Adams M. Clavicle fractures: associated trauma and morbidity. *J Clin Orthop Trauma.* 2021;13:53–56. doi:10.1016/j.jcot.2020.08.020
14. Dempster W. Mechanisms of shoulder movement. *Arch Phys Med Rehabil.* 1965;46:49–70.
15. Barbaix E, Lapierre M, Van Roy P, Clarijs J. The sternoclavicular joint: variants of the discus articularis. *Clin Biomech (Bristol, Avon).* 2000;15(Suppl 1):S3–S7. doi:10.1016/s0268-0033(00)00051-6
16. Moore KL, Dalley AF, Agur AMR. *Clinically Oriented Anatomy.* 8th ed. Wolters Kluwer; 2018.
17. Heers G, Götz J, Schubert T, et al. MR imaging of the intraarticular disk of the acromioclavicular joint: a comparison with anatomical, histological and in-vivo findings. *Skeletal Radiol.* 2007;36(1):23–28. doi:10.1007/s00256-006-0181-6
18. Saccomanno M, de Leso C, Milano G. Acromioclavicular joint instability: anatomy, biomechanics and evaluation. *Joints.* 2014;2(2):87–92. doi:10.11138/jts/2014.2.2.087
19. Salter JG, Nasca R, Shelley B. Anatomical observations on the acromioclavicular joint and supporting ligaments. *Am J Sports Med.* 1987;15(3):199–206. doi:10.1177/036354658701500301
20. Kurata S, Inoue K, Hasegawa H, et al. The role of the acromioclavicular ligament in acromioclavicular joint stability: a cadaveric biomechanical study. *Orthop J Sports Med.* 2021;9(2):2325967120982947. doi:10.1177/2325967120982947
21. Debski R, Parsons I, Woo S, Fu F. Effect of capsular injury on acromioclavicular joint mechanics. *J Bone Joint Surg Am.* 2001;83(9):1344–1351. doi:10.2106/00004623-200109000-00009
22. Lee K, Debski R, Chen C, Woo S, Fu F. Functional evaluation of the ligaments at the acromioclavicular joint during anteroposterior and superoinferior translation. *Am J Sports Med.* 1997;25(6):858–862. doi:10.1177/036354659702500622
23. Fukuda K, Craig E, An K, Cofield R, Chao E. Biomechanical study of the ligamentous system of the acromioclavicular joint. *J Bone Joint Surg Am.* 1986;68(3):434–440.
24. Cullam E, Peat M. Functional anatomy of the shoulder complex. *J Orthop Sports Phys Ther.* 1993;18:342–350.
25. Teece R, Lunden J, Lloyd A, Kaiser A, Cieminski C, Ludewig P. Three-dimensional acromioclavicular joint motions during elevation of the arm. *J Orthop Sports Phys Ther.* 2008;38(4):181–190. doi:10.2519/jospt.2008.2386
26. Conway A. Movements at the sternoclavicular and acromioclavicular joints. *Phys Ther Rev.* 1961;41:421–432.
27. Lawrence R, Braman J, Keefe D, Ludewig P. The coupled kinematics of scapulothoracic upward rotation. *Phys Ther.* 2020;100(2):283–294. doi:10.1093/ptj/pzz165
28. Lugo R, Kung P, Ma C. Shoulder biomechanics. *Eur J Radiol.* 2008;68(1):16–24. doi:10.1016/j.ejrad.2008.02.051
29. Curl L, Warren R. Glenohumeral joint stability. Selective cutting studies on the static capsular restraints. *Clin Orthop Relat Res.* 1996;(330):54–65.
30. Matsen F III, Titelman R, Lippitt S, Rockwood C Jr, Wirth M. Glenohumeral instability. *In:* Rockwood C Jr, Matsen F III, Wirth M, Lippitt S, eds. *The Shoulder.* 3rd ed. Saunders; 2004:655–794.
31. Howell S, Galinat B. The glenoid-labral socket. A constrained articular surface. *Clin Orthop Relat Res.* 1989;(243):122–125.
32. De Filippo M, Schirò S, Sarohia D, et al. Imaging of shoulder instability. *Skeletal Radiol.* 2020;49(10):1505–1523. doi:10.1007/s00256-020-03459-z
33. De Wilde L, Berghs B, Audenaert E, Sys G, Van Maele G, Barbaix E. About the variability of the shape of the glenoid cavity. *Surg Radiol Anat.* 2004;26(1):54–59. doi:10.1007/s00276-003-0167-1
34. Itoi E, Lee S, Berglund L, Berge L, An K. The effect of a glenoid defect on anteroinferior stability of the shoulder after

Bankart repair: a cadaveric study. *J Bone Joint Surg Am.* 2000;82(1):35–46. doi:10.2106/00004623-200001000-00005
35. Burkhart S, De Beer J. Traumatic glenohumeral bone defects and their relationship to failure of arthroscopic Bankart repairs: significance of the inverted-pear glenoid and the humeral engaging Hill-Sachs lesion. *Arthroscopy.* 2000;16(7):677–694. doi:10.1053/jars.2000.17715
36. Harryman D 2nd, Sidles J, Harris S, Matsen F 3rd. The role of the rotator interval capsule in passive motion and stability of the shoulder. *J Bone Joint Surg Am.* 1992;74(1):53–66.
37. Moore S, Musahl V, McMahon P, Debski R. Multidirectional kinematics of the glenohumeral joint during simulated simple translation tests: impact on clinical diagnoses. *J Orthop Res.* 2004;22(4):889–894. doi:10.1016/j.orthres.2003.12.011
38. O'Connell P, Nuber G, Mileski R, Lautenschlager E. The contribution of the glenohumeral ligaments to anterior stability of the shoulder joint. *Am J Sports Med.* 1990;18(6):579–584. doi:10.1177/036354659001800604
39. Jansen J, de Gast A, Snijders C. Glenohumeral elevation-dependent influence of anterior glenohumeral capsular lesions on passive axial humeral rotation. *J Biomech.* 2006;39(9):1702–1707. doi:10.1016/j.jbiomech.2005.04.022
40. Day A, Taylor N, Green R. The stabilizing role of the rotator cuff at the shoulder—responses to external perturbations. *Clin Biomech (Bristol, Avon).* 2012;27(6):551–556. doi:10.1016/j.clinbiomech.2012.02.003
41. Lee S, Kim K, O'Driscoll S, Morrey B, An K. Dynamic glenohumeral stability provided by the rotator cuff muscles in the mid-range and end-range of motion. A study in cadavera. *J Bone Joint Surg Am.* 2000;82(6):849–857. doi:10.2106/00004623-200006000-00012
42. Schenkman M, Rugo de Cartaya V. Kinesiology of the shoulder complex. *J Orthop Sports Phys Ther.* 1987;8(9):438–450. doi:10.2519/jospt.1987.8.9.438
43. An K. Muscle force and its role in joint dynamic stability. *Clin Orthop Relat Res.* 2002;(403 Suppl):S37–S42. doi:10.1097/00003086-200210001-00005
44. Ellenbecker T, Cools A. Rehabilitation of shoulder impingement syndrome and rotator cuff injuries: an evidence-based review. *Br J Sports Med.* 2010;44(5):319–327. doi:10.1136/bjsm.2009.058875
45. Chang W. Shoulder impingement syndrome. *Phys Med Rehabil Clin N Am.* 2004;15(2):493–510.
46. Nadler S, Sherman A, Malanga G. Sport-specific shoulder injuries. *Phys Med Rehabil Clin N Am.* 2004;15(3; vi):607–626.
47. Bigliani L, Kelkar R, Flatow E, Pollock R, Mow V. Glenohumeral stability. Biomechanical properties of passive and active stabilizers. *Clin Orthop Relat Res.* 1996;(330):13–30.
48. Poppen N, Walker P. Forces at the glenohumeral joint in abduction. *Clin Orthop Relat Res.* 1978;(135):165–170.
49. Halder A, Kuhl S, Zobitz M, Larson D, An K. Effects of the glenoid labrum and glenohumeral abduction on stability of the shoulder joint through concavity-compression: an in vitro study. *J Bone Joint Surg Am.* 2001;83(7):1062–1069. doi:10.2106/00004623-200107000-00013
50. Blakely R, Palmer M. Analysis of rotation accompanying shoulder flexion. *Phys Ther.* 1984;64(8):1214–1216. doi:10.1093/ptj/64.8.1214
51. Saha A. The classic. Mechanism of shoulder movements and a plea for the recognition of "zero position" of glenohumeral joint. *Clin Orthop Relat Res.* 1983;(173):3–10.
52. Ludewig P, Cook T. Translations of the humerus in persons with shoulder impingement symptoms. *J Ortho Sports Phys Ther.* 2002;32:248–259.
53. Graichen H, Stammberger T, Bonel H, Englmeier K, Reiser M, Eckstein F. Glenohumeral translation during active and passive elevation of the shoulder—a 3D open-MRI study. *J Biomech.* 2000;33(5):609–613. doi:10.1016/s0021-9290(99)00209-2
54. Poppen N, Walker P. Normal and abnormal motion of the shoulder. *J Bone Joint Surg Am.* 1976;58(2):195–201.
55. Warner J, Bowen M, Deng X, Hannafin J, Arnoczky S, Warren R. Articular contact patterns of the normal glenohumeral joint. *J Shoulder Elbow Surg.* 1998;7(4):381–388. doi:10.1016/s1058-2746(98)90027-1
56. Deutsch A, Altchek D, Schwartz E, Otis J, Warren R. Radiologic measurement of superior displacement of the humeral head in the impingement syndrome. *J Shoulder Elbow Surg.* 1996;5:186–193.
57. Lawrence R, Braman J, Staker J, Laprade R, Ludewig P. Comparison of 3-dimensional shoulder complex kinematics in individuals with and without shoulder pain, part 2: glenohumeral joint. *J Orthop Sports Phys Ther.* 2014;44(9):646–655, b1–b3. doi:10.2519/jospt.2014.5556
58. Chen S, Simonian P, Wickiewicz T, Otis J, Warren R. Radiographic evaluation of glenohumeral kinematics: a muscle fatigue model. *J Shoulder Elbow Surg.* 1999;8(1):49–52. doi:10.1016/s1058-2746(99)90055-1
59. Teyhen D, Miller J, Middag T, Kane E. Rotator cuff fatigue and glenohumeral kinematics in participants without shoulder dysfunction. *J Athl Train.* 2008;43(4):352–358. doi:10.4085/1062-6050-43.4.352
60. Houglum PA, Bertoti DB. *Brunnstrom's Clinical Kinesiology.* 6th ed. F.A. Davis; 2012.
61. Inman V, Saunders J, Abbott L. Observations on the function of the shoulder joint. *J Bone Joint Surg Am.* 1944;26:1–30.
62. McClure P, Michener L, Sennett B, Karduna A. Direct 3-dimensional measurement of scapular kinematics during dynamic movements in vivo. *J Shoulder Elbow Surg.* 2001;10(3):269–277. doi:10.1067/mse.2001.112954
63. Freedman L, Munro R. Abduction of the arm in the scapular plane: scapular and glenohumeral movements. A roentgenographic study. *J Bone Joint Surg Am.* 1966;48:1503–1510.
64. Graichen H, Stammberger T, Bonel H, et al. Magnetic resonance-based motion analysis of the shoulder during elevation. *Clin Orthop Relat Res.* 2000;(370):154–163. doi:10.1097/00003086-200001000-00014
65. Pronk G, van der Helm F, Rozendaal L. Interaction between the joints in the shoulder mechanism: the function of the costoclavicular, conoid and trapezoid ligaments. *Proc Inst Mech Eng H.* 1993;207(4):219–229. doi:10.1243/pime_proc_1993_207_300_02
66. Kibler W, Sciascia A. Current concepts: scapular dyskinesis. *Br J Sports Med.* 2010;44(5):300–305. doi:10.1136/bjsm.2009.058834
67. Guney-Deniz H, Harput G, Toprak U, Duzgun I. Relationship between middle trapezius muscle activation and acromiohumeral distance change during shoulder elevation with scapular retraction. *J Sport Rehabil.* 2019;28(3):266–271. doi:10.1123/jsr.2018-0131
68. Otis J, Jiang C, Wickiewicz T, Peterson M, Warren R, Santner T. Changes in the moment arms of the rotator cuff and deltoid muscles with abduction and rotation. *J Bone Joint Surg Am.* 1994;76(5):667–676. doi:10.2106/00004623-199405000-00007
69. Wickham J, Pizzari T, Stansfeld K, Burnside A, Watson L. Quantifying 'normal' shoulder muscle activity during abduction. *J Electromyogr Kinesiol.* 2010;20(2):212–222. doi:10.1016/j.jelekin.2009.06.004
70. Kronberg M, Németh G, Broström L. Muscle activity and coordination in the normal shoulder. An electromyographic study. *Clin Orthop Relat Res.* 1990;(257):76–85.
71. Payne L, Deng X, Craig E, Torzilli P, Warren R. The combined dynamic and static contributions to subacromial

impingement. A biomechanical analysis. *Am J Sports Med.* 1997;25(6):801–808. doi:10.1177/036354659702500612

72. An Y, Friedman R. Multidirectional instability of the glenohumeral joint. *Orthop Clin North Am.* 2000;31(2):275–285.

73. Huegel J, Williams A, Soslowsky L. Rotator cuff biology and biomechanics: a review of normal and pathological conditions. *Curr Rheumatol Rep.* 2015;17(1):476. doi:10.1007/s11926-014-0476-x

74. Keener J, Wei A, Kim H, Steger-May K, Yamaguchi K. Proximal humeral migration in shoulders with symptomatic and asymptomatic rotator cuff tears. *J Bone Joint Surg Am.* 2009;91(6):1405–1413. doi:10.2106/jbjs.H.00854

75. Oh J, Jun B, McGarry M, Lee T. Does a critical rotator cuff tear stage exist?: a biomechanical study of rotator cuff tear progression in human cadaver shoulders. *J Bone Joint Surg Am.* 2011;93(22):2100–2109. doi:10.2106/jbjs.J.00032

76. Paine R, Voight ML. The role of the scapula. *Int J Sports Phys Ther.* 2013;8(5):617–629.

77. Gooding B, Geoghegan J, Wallace W, Manning P. Scapular winging. *Shoulder Elbow.* 2014;6(1):4–11. doi:10.1111/sae.12033

78. Didesch J, Tang P. Anatomy, etiology, and management of scapular winging. *J Hand Surg Am.* 2019;44(4):321–330. doi:10.1016/j.jhsa.2018.08.008

79. Camargo P, Neumann D. Kinesiologic considerations for targeting activation of scapulothoracic muscles—part 2: trapezius. *Braz J Phys Ther.* 2019;23(6):467–475. doi:10.1016/j.bjpt.2019.01.011

80. Williams P, Warwick R, Myson M, Bannister L, eds. *Gray's Anatomy.* 37th ed. Churchill Livingstone; 1989.

81. Ekstrom R, Donatelli R, Soderberg G. Surface electromyographic analysis of exercises for the trapezius and serratus anterior muscles. *J Orthop Sports Phys Ther.* 2003;33:247–258.

82. Szucs K, Borstad J. Gender differences between muscle activation and onset timing of the four subdivisions of trapezius during humerothoracic elevation. *Hum Mov Sci.* 2013;32(6):1288–1298. doi:10.1016/j.humov.2013.05.003

83. Neumann D. *Kinesiology of the Musculoskeletal System: Foundations for Rehabilitation.* 3rd ed. Elsevier; 2017.

84. Kibler W, Sciascia A, Wilkes T. Scapular dyskinesis and its relation to shoulder injury. *J Am Acad Orthop Surg.* 2012;20(6):364–372. doi:10.5435/jaaos-20-06-364

85. Ludewig P, Braman J. Shoulder impingement: biomechanical considerations in rehabilitation. *Man Ther.* 2011;16(1):33–9. doi:10.1016/j.math.2010.08.004

86. Ludewig P, Cook T, Nawoczenski D. Three-dimensional scapular orientation and muscle activity at selected positions of humeral elevation. *J Orthop Sports Phys Ther.* 1996;24(2):57–65. doi:10.2519/jospt.1996.24.2.57

87. Halder A, Zhao K, Odriscoll S, Morrey B, An K. Dynamic contributions to superior shoulder stability. *J Orthop Res.* 2001;19(2):206–212. doi:10.1016/s0736-0266(00)00028-0

88. McCully S, Suprak D, Kosek P, Karduna A. Suprascapular nerve block results in a compensatory increase in deltoid muscle activity. *J Biomech.* 2007;40(8):1839–1846. doi:10.1016/j.jbiomech.2006.07.010

89. Hoppenfeld S. *Physical Examination of the Spine and Extremities.* Appleton-Century-Crofts; 1976.

90. Reichert B. *Palpation Techniques: Surface Anatomy for Physical Therapists.* Thieme; 2011.

91. van der Windt DA, Koes BW, de Jong BA, Bouter LM. Shoulder disorders in general practice: incidence, patient characteristics, and management. *Ann Rheum Dis.* 1995;54(12):959–964. doi:10.1136/ard.54.12.959

92. McClure P, Michener L. Staged approach for rehabilitation classification: shoulder disorders (STAR-Shoulder). *Phys Ther.* 2015;95(5):791–800.

93. Goodman CC, Fuller KS. *Pathology: Implications for the Physical Therapist.* 5th ed. Elsevier; 2021.

94. Heick J, Peterson S, Jain T. Screening the upper extremity (Independent Study Course 29.3.2). Academy of Orthopaedic Physical Therapy; 2019:1–32.

95. Yocum L. Assessing the shoulder: history, physical examination, differential diagnosis, and special tests used. *Clin Sports Med.* 1983;2(2):281–289.

96. Altchek D, Carson E. Arthroscopic acromioplasty. *Orthop Clin North Am.* 1997;28(2):157–168.

97. Enthoven W, Geuze J, Scheele J, et al. Prevalence and "red flags" regarding specified causes of back pain in older adults presenting in general practice. *Phys Ther.* 2015;96(3):305–312.

98. Boissonnault WG. *Primary Care for the Physical Therapist: Examination and Triage.* St. Elsevier/Saunders; 2011.

99. Finucane LM, Downie A, Mercer C, et al. International framework for red flags for potential serious spinal pathologies. *J Orthop Sports Phys Ther.* 2020;50(7):350–372. doi:10.2519/jospt.2020.9971

100. Lee J. Screening for cancer. In: Goodman CC, Heick J, Lazaro R, eds. *Differential Diagnosis for Physical Therapists: Screening for Referral.* 6th ed. Elsevier; 2018:463–520:chap 13.

101. Thoomes EJ, van Geest S, van der Windt DA, et al. Value of physical tests in diagnosing cervical radiculopathy: a systematic review. *Spine.* 2018;18(1):179–189. doi:10.1016/j.spinee.2017.08.241

102. Hippensteel KJ, Brophy R, Smith MV, Wright RW. A comprehensive review of physical examination tests of the cervical spine, scapula, and rotator cuff. *J Am Acad Orthop Surg.* 2019;27(11):385–394. doi:10.5435/jaaos-d-17-00090

103. Raynor MB, Kuhn JE. Utility of features of the patient's history in the diagnosis of atraumatic shoulder pain: a systematic review. *J Shoulder Elbow Surg.* 2016;25(4):688–694. doi:10.1016/j.jse.2015.09.023

104. Hegedus EJ, Cook C, Lewis J, Wright A, Park JY. Combining orthopedic special tests to improve diagnosis of shoulder pathology. *Phys Ther Sport.* 2015;16(2):87–92. doi:10.1016/j.ptsp.2014.08.001

105. O'Kane JW, Toresdahl BG. The evidenced-based shoulder evaluation. *Curr Sports Med Rep.* 2014;13(5):307–313. doi:10.1249/jsr.0000000000000090

106. McKenzie R, May S. *The Human Extremities: Mechanical Diagnosis and Therapy.* Spinal Publications; 2017.

107. Sandrey MA. Special physical examination tests for superior labrum anterior-posterior shoulder tears: an examination of clinical usefulness. *J Athl Train.* 2013;48(6):856–858. doi:10.4085/1062-6050-48.3.14

108. Kahn A, Cook J. The painful nonruptured tendon: clinical aspects. *Clin Sports Med.* 2003;22(4):711–725.

109. Brooks A, Hammer E. Acute upper extremity injuries in young athletes. *Clin Pediatr Emerg Med.* 2013;14(4):289–303. doi:10.1016/j.cpem.2013.11.001

110. Bonz J, Tinloy B. Emergency department evaluation and treatment of the shoulder and humerus. *Emerg Med Clin North Am.* 2015;33(2):297–310. doi:10.1016/j.emc.2014.12.004

111. Manske RC, Grant-Nierman M, Lucas B. Shoulder posterior internal impingement in the overhead athlete. *Int J Sports Phys Ther.* 2013;8(2):194–204.

112. Kibler WB, Ludewig PM, McClure PW, Michener LA, Bak K, Sciascia AD. Clinical implications of scapular dyskinesis in shoulder injury: the 2013 consensus statement from the

'scapular summit'. *Br J Sports Med.* 2013;47(14):877–885. doi:10.1136/bjsports-2013-092425
113. Greenfield B, Catlin P, Coats P, Green E, McDonald J, North C. Posture in patients with shoulder overuse injuries and healthy individuals. *J Orthop Sports Phys Ther.* 1995;21(5):287–295.
114. Kendall FP, McCreary EK, Provance PG, Rogers MM, Romani WA. *Muscles: Testing and Function with Posture and Pain.* 5th ed. Lippincott Williams & Wilkins; 2005.
115. Sahrmann SA. *Diagnosis and Treatment of Movement Impairment Syndromes.* Mosby; 2002.
116. Levenhagen K, Davies C, Perdomo M, Ryans K, Glichrist L. Diagnosis of upper-quadrant lymphedema secondary to cancer: clinical practice guideline from the oncology section of APTA. *Rehabil Oncol.* 2017;35:E1–E18.
117. Constans J, Salmi LR, Sevestre-Pietri MA, et al. A clinical prediction score for upper extremity deep venous thrombosis. *Thromb Haemost.* 2008;99(1):202–207. doi:10.1160/th07-08-0485
118. American Academy of Orthopedic Surgeons. *America Academy of Orthopedic Surgeons: Joint Motion: Method of Measuring and Recording.* AAOS; 1965.
119. Clarkson HM. *Musculoskeletal Assessment: Joint Range of Motion, Muscle Testing, and Function.* 4th ed. Wolters Kluwer; 2021.
120. Calis M, Akgun K, Birtane M, Karacan I, Clias H, Tuzun F. Diagnostic values of clinical diagnostic tests in subacromial impingement syndrome. *Ann Rheum Dis.* 2000;59:44–47.
121. Redler LH, Dennis ER. Treatment of adhesive capsulitis of the shoulder. *J Am Acad Orthop Surg.* 2019;27(12):e544–e554. doi:10.5435/JAAOS-D-17-00606
122. Wilk KE, Macrina LC, Fleisig GS, et al. Correlation of glenohumeral internal rotation deficit and total rotational motion to shoulder injuries in professional baseball pitchers. *Am J Sports Med.* 2011;39(2):329–335. doi:10.1177/0363546510384223
123. Riley SP, Grimes JK, Apeldoorn AT, Vet R. Agreement and reliability of a symptom modification test cluster for patients with subacromial pain syndrome. *Physiother Res Int.* 2020;25(3):1–7. doi:10.1002/pri.1842
124. Rose MB, Noonan T. Glenohumeral internal rotation deficit in throwing athletes: current perspectives. *Open Access J Sports Med.* 2018;9:69–78. doi:10.2147/OAJSM.S138975
125. Reinold MM, Gill TJ, Wilk KE, Andrews JR. Current concepts in the evaluation and treatment of the shoulder in overhead throwing athletes, part 2: injury prevention and treatment. *Sports Health.* 2010;2(2):101–115.
126. Konin J, Lebscak D, Snyder Valier A. *Special Tests for Orthopaedic Examination.* SLACK Incorporated; 2016.
127. Clarnette RG, Miniaci A. Clinical exam of the shoulder. *Med Sci Sports Exerc.* 1998;30(4 Suppl 1):1–6.
128. Cyriax J. *Textbook of Orthopedic Medicine, Vol. 1: Diagnosis of Soft Tissue Lesions.* 8th ed. Saunders; 1989.
129. Cyriax JH, Cyriax PJ. *Cyriax's Illustrated Manual of Orthopaedic Medicine.* 2nd ed. Butterworth-Heinemann; 1993.
130. Tovin BJ, Greenfield BH. *Evaluation and Treatment of the Shoulder: An Integration of the Guide to Physical Therapist Practice.* F.A. Davis; 2001.
131. Gismervik SO, Drogset JO, Granviken F, Ro M, Leivseth G. Physical examination tests of the shoulder: a systematic review and meta-analysis of diagnostic test performance. *BMC Musculoskelet Disord.* 2017;18(1):41. doi:10.1186/s12891-017-1400-0
132. Holtby R, Razmjou H. Validity of the supraspinatus test as a single clinical test in diagnosing patients with rotator cuff pathology. *J Orthop Sports Phys Ther.* 2004;34:194–200.
133. Itoi E, Kido T, Sano A, Urayama M, Sato K. Which is more useful, the "Full can test" or the "empty can test," in detecting the torn supraspinatus tendon? *Am J Sports Med.* 1999;27(1):65–68.
134. Cotter EJ, Hannon CP, Christian D, Frank RM, Bach BR Jr, Bach BR Jr. Comprehensive examination of the athlete's shoulder. *Sports Health.* 2018;10(4):366–375.
135. Sgroi M, Loitsch T, Reichel H, Kappe T. Diagnostic value of clinical tests for infraspinatus tendon tears. *Arthroscopy.* 2019;35(5):1339–1347. doi:10.1016/j.arthro.2018.12.003
136. Tennent T, Beach W, Meyers J. A review of the special tests associated with shoulder examination: part I: the rotator cuff tests. *Am J Sports Med.* 2003;31(1):154–160.
137. Jancuska J, Matthews J, Miller T, Kluczynski MA, Bisson LJ. A systematic summary of systematic reviews on the topic of the rotator cuff. *Orthop J Sports Med.* 2018;6(9):2325967118797891. doi:10.1177/2325967118797891
138. Biederwolf NE. A proposed evidence-based shoulder special testing examination algorithm: clinical utility based on a systematic review of the literature. *Int J Sports Phys Ther.* 2013;8(4):427–440.
139. Hertel R, Ballmer F, Lombert S, Gerber C. Lag signs in the diagnosis of rotator cuff rupture. *J Shoulder Elbow Surg.* 1996;5(4):307–313.
140. Tokish J, Decker M, Torry M, Hawkins R. The belly-press test for the physical examination of the subscapularis muscle: electromyographical validation and comparison of the lift-off test. *J Shoulder Elbow Surg.* 2003;12(5):427–430.
141. Khazzam M, Gates ST, Tisano BK, Kukowski N. Diagnostic accuracy of the scapular retraction test in assessing the status of the rotator cuff. *Orthop J Sports Med.* 2018;6(10):2325967118799308. doi:10.1177/2325967118799308
142. Mall NA, Foley E, Chalmers PN, Cole BJ, Romeo AA, Bach BR. Degenerative joint disease of the acromioclavicular joint: a review. *Am J Sports Med.* 2013;41(11):2684–2692. doi:10.1177/0363546513485359
143. Donohue MA, Owens BD, Dickens JF. Return to play following anterior shoulder dislocation and stabilization surgery. *Clin Sports Med.* 2016;35(4):545–561. doi:10.1016/j.csm.2016.05.002
144. Tennent T, Beach W, Meyers J. A review of the special tests associated with shoulder examination: part II: laxity, instability, and superior labral anterior and posterior (SLAP) lesions. *Am J Sports Med.* 2003;31(2):301–307.
145. Tzannes A, Paxinos A, Callanan M, Murrell G. An assessment of the interexaminer reliability of tests for shoulder instability. *J Shoulder Elbow Surg.* 2004;13(1):18–23.
146. Speer K, Hannafin J, Altchek D, Warren R. An evaluation of the shoulder relocation test. *Am J Sports Med.* 1994;22(2):177–183.
147. Luime J, Verhagen A, Kuiper J, Burdorf A, Verhaar J, Koes B. Does this patient had an instability of the shoulder or a labrum lesion? *JAMA.* 2004;292(16):1989–1999.
148. Guanche C, Jones D. Clinical testing for tears of the glenoid labrum. *Arthroscopy.* 2003;19(5):517–523.
149. Hegedus EJ, Michener LA, Seitz AL. Three key findings when diagnosing shoulder multidirectional instability: patient report of instability, hypermobility, and specific shoulder tests. *J Orthop Sports Phys Ther.* 2020;50(2):52–54. doi:10.2519/jospt.2020.0602
150. McFarland EG, Campbell G, McDowell J. Posterior shoulder laxity in asymptomatic athletes. *Am J Sports Med.* 1996;24(4):468–471.
151. Stetson W, Templin K. The crank test, the O'Brien test, and routine magnetic resonance imaging scans in the diagnosis of labral tears. *Am J Sports Med.* 2002;30:806–809.

152. Clark RC, Chandler CC, Fuqua AC, Glymph KN, Lambert GC, Rigney KJ. Use of clinical test clusters versus advanced imaging studies in the management of patients with a suspected SLAP tear. *Int J Sports Phys Ther.* 2019;14(3):345–352. doi:10.26603/ijspt20190345
153. Kim S, Ha K, Kim SH, Choi H. Biceps load test II: a clinical test for SLAP lesions of the shoulder. *Arthroscopy.* 2001;17(2):160–164.
154. Kim S, Ha K, Han K. Biceps load test: a clinical test for superior labrum anterior and posterior lesions in shoulders with recurrent dislocations. *Am J Sports Med.* 1999;27:300–303.
155. Dhir J, Willis M, Watson L, Somerville L, Sadi J. Evidence-based review of clinical diagnostic tests and predictive clinical tests that evaluate response to conservative rehabilitation for posterior glenohumeral instability: a systematic review. *Sports Health.* 2018;10(2):141–145. doi:10.1177/1941738117752306
156. Kibler W. Specificity and sensitivity of the anterior slide test in throwing athletes with superior glenoid labral tears. *Arthroscopy.* 1995;11(3):296–300.
157. Holtby R, Razmjou H. Accuracy of the Speed's and Yergason's tests in detecting biceps pathology and SLAP lesions: comparison with arthroscopic findings. *Arthroscopy.* 2004;20(3):231–236.
158. Hulstyn M, Fadale P. Shoulder injuries in the athlete. *Clin Sports Med.* 1997;16(4):663–679.
159. Reid D, Poison K, Johnson L. Acromioclavicular joint separations grades I-III: a review of the literature and development of best practice guidelines. *Sports Med.* 2012;42(8):681–696. doi:10.1007/bf03262288
160. Shamus J, Shamus E. A taping technique for the treatment of acromioclavicular joint sprains: a case study. *J Orthop Sports Phys Ther.* 1997;25(6):390–394.
161. Tibone J, Sellers R, Tonino P. Strength testing after third-degree acromioclavicular dislocations. *Am J Sports Med.* 1992;20(3):328–331. doi:10.1177/036354659202000316
162. Turnbull JR. Acromioclavicular joint disorders. *Med Sci Sports Exerc.* 1998;30(4 Suppl 1):26–32.
163. Meister K. Injuries to the shoulder in the throwing athlete. Part two: evaluation/treatment. *Am J Sports Med.* 2000;28(4):587–601.
164. Martetschläger F, Warth RJ, Millett PJ. Instability and degenerative arthritis of the sternoclavicular joint: a current concepts review. *Am J Sports Med.* 2014;42(4):999–1007. doi:10.1177/0363546513498990
165. Yood R, Goldenberg D. Sternoclavicular joint arthritis. *Arthritis Rheum.* 1980;23(2):232–238.
166. Tasnim S, Shirafkan A, Okereke I. Diagnosis and management of sternoclavicular joint infections: a literature review. *J Thorac Dis.* 2020;12(8):4418–4426. doi:10.21037/jtd-20-761
167. Lacheta L, Dekker TJ, Goldenberg BT, et al. Minimum 5-year clinical outcomes, survivorship, and return to sports after hamstring tendon autograft reconstruction for sternoclavicular joint instability. *Am J Sports Med.* 2020;48(4):939–946. doi:10.1177/0363546519900896
168. Gowd AK, Liu JN, Garcia GH, et al. Figure-of-eight reconstruction of the sternoclavicular joint: outcomes of sport and work. *Orthopedics.* 2019;42(4):205–210. doi:10.3928/01477447-20190523-03
169. Tytherleigh-Strong G, Gill J, Mulligan A, Al-Hadithy N. Arthroscopic excision arthroplasty of the sternoclavicular joint for osteoarthritis: a case series of 50 patients. *Arthroscopy.* 2020;36(5):1223–1229. doi:10.1016/j.arthro.2019.12.005
170. Thomas M, Bidwai A, Rangan A, et al. Glenohumeral osteoarthritis. *Shoulder Elbow.* 2016;8(3):203–214. doi:10.1177/1758573216644183
171. Chillemi C, Franceschini V. Shoulder osteoarthritis. *Arthritis.* 2013;2013:370231. doi:10.1155/2013/370231
172. Macias-Hernandez SI, Morones-Alba JD, Miranda-Duarte A, et al. Glenohumeral osteoarthritis: overview, therapy, and rehabilitation. *Disabil Rehabil.* 2017;39(16):1674–1682. doi:10.1080/09638288.2016.1207206
173. Guo JJ, Wu K, Guan H, et al. Three-year follow-up of conservative treatments of shoulder osteoarthritis in older patients. *Orthopedics.* 2016;39(4):e634–e641. doi:10.3928/01477447-20160606-02
174. Ansok CB, Muh SJ. Optimal management of glenohumeral osteoarthritis. *Orthop Res Rev.* 2018;10:9–18. doi:10.2147/orr.S134732
175. Wolff AL, Rosenzweig L. Anatomical and biomechanical framework for shoulder arthroplasty rehabilitation. *J Hand Ther.* 2017;30(2):167–174. doi:10.1016/j.jht.2017.05.009
176. Bullock GS, Garrigues GE, Ledbetter L, Kennedy J. A systematic review of proposed rehabilitation guidelines following anatomic and reverse shoulder arthroplasty. *J Orthop Sports Phys Ther.* 2019;49(5):337–346. doi:10.2519/jospt.2019.8616
177. Petrillo S, Longo UG, Papalia R, Denaro V. Reverse shoulder arthroplasty for massive irreparable rotator cuff tears and cuff tear arthropathy: a systematic review. *Musculoskelet Surg.* 2017;101(2):105–112. doi:10.1007/s12306-017-0474-z
178. Uschok S, Herrmann S, Pauly S, Perka C, Greiner S. Reverse shoulder arthroplasty: the role of physical therapy on the clinical outcome in the mid-term to long-term follow-up. *Arch Orthop Trauma Surg.* 2018;138(10):1347–1352. doi:10.1007/s00402-018-2977-y
179. Roubal P, Dobritt D, Placzek J. Glenohumeral gliding manipulation following interscalene brachial plexus block in patients with adhesive capsulitis. *J Orthop Sports Phys Ther.* 1996;24(2):66–77.
180. Chan HBY, Pua PY, How CH. Physical therapy in the management of frozen shoulder. *Singapore Med J.* 2017;58(12):685–689. doi:10.11622/smedj.2017107
181. Grubbs N. Frozen shoulder syndrome: a review of literature. *J Orthop Sports Phys Ther.* 1993;18(3):479–487.
182. Hannafin J, Chiaia T. Adhesive capsulitis. *Clin Orthop.* 2000;372:95–109.
183. Vad V, Sakalkale D, Warren R. The role of capsular distention in adhesive capsulitis. *Arch Phys Med Rehabil.* 2003;84:1290–1292.
184. Selley RS, Johnson DJ, Nicolay RW, et al. Risk factors for adhesive capsulitis requiring shoulder arthroscopy: a clinical retrospective case series study. *J Orthop.* 2020;19:14–16. doi:10.1016/j.jor.2019.11.024
185. Kelley M, Shaffer M, Kuhn J, et al. Shoulder pain and mobility deficits: adhesive capsulitis clinical practice guidelines linked to the International Classification of Functioning, Disability, and Health From the Orthopaedic Section of the American Physical Therapy Association. *J Orthop Sports Phys Ther.* 2013;43(5):A1–A31.
186. Lamplot JD, Lillegraven O, Brophy RH. Outcomes from conservative treatment of shoulder idiopathic adhesive capsulitis and factors associated with developing contralateral disease. *Orthop J Sports Med.* 2018;6(7):1–8. doi:10.1177/2325967118785169
187. Cho CH, Lee KL, Cho J, Kim D. The incidence and risk factors of frozen shoulder in patients with breast cancer surgery. *Breast J.* 2020;26(4):825–828. doi:10.1111/tbj.13610
188. Miller M, Wirth M, Rockwood CA. Thawing the frozen shoulder: the "patient" patient. *Orthopedics.* 1996;19(10):849–853.
189. Griggs S, Ahn A, Green A. Idiopathic adhesive capsulitis. A prospective outcome study of nonoperative treatment. *J Bone Joint Surg.* 2000;82:1398–1407.

190. Surendran S, Patinharayil G, Karuppal R, Marthya A, Fazil M, Mohammed Ali S. Arthroscopic capsular release and continuous upper arm brachial block in frozen shoulder—a midterm outcome analysis. *J Orthop.* 2020;21:459–464. doi:10.1016/j.jor.2020.08.033
191. Speed C, Hazleman B. Shoulder pain: 2. *Clin Evid.* 2002(8):1271–1289.
192. Jackins S. Postoperative shoulder rehabilitation. *Phys Med Rehabil Clin N Am.* 2004;15(3, vi):643–682.
193. Rizvi SM, Harisha AJ, Lam PH, Murrell GAC. Factors affecting the outcomes of arthroscopic capsular release for idiopathic adhesive capsulitis. *Orthop J Sports Med.* 2019;7(9):2325967119867621. doi:10.1177/2325967119867621
194. Neviaser R. Tears of the rotator cuff. *Orthop Clin North Am.* 1980;11(2):295–306.
195. Lawrence RL, Moutzouros V, Bey MJ. Asymptomatic rotator cuff tears. *J Bone Joint Surg Rev.* 2019;7(6):e9. doi:10.2106/jbjs.Rvw.18.00149
196. Edwards P, Ebert J, Joss B, Bhabra G, Ackland T, Wang A. Exercise rehabilitation in the non-operative management of rotator cuff tears: a review of the literature. *Int J Sports Phys Ther.* 2016;11(2):279–301.
197. Bedi A, Dines J, Warren R, Dines D. Massive tears of the rotator cuff: current concepts review. *J Bone Joint Surg Am.* 2010;92:194–908.
198. Spargoli G. Supraspinatus tendon pathomechanics: a current concepts review. *Int J Sports Phys Ther.* 2018;13(6):1083–1094.
199. Tempelhof S, Rupp S, Seil R. Age-related prevalence of rotator cuff tears in asymptomatic shoulders. *J Shoulder Elbow Surg.* 1999;8(4):296–299. doi:https://doi.org/10.1016/S1058-2746(99)90148-9
200. Aumiller WD, Kleuser TM. Diagnosis and treatment of cuff tear arthropathy. *JAAPA.* 2015;28(8):33–38. doi:10.1097/01.JAA.0000469435.44701.ce
201. Hio Teng L, Sai Chuen FU, Xin HE, Joo Han OH, Nobuyuki Y, Shu Hang Patrick Y. Risk factors for rotator cuff tendinopathy: a systematic review and meta-analysis. *J Rehabil Med.* 2019;51(9):627–637. doi:10.2340/16501977-2598
202. Orth T, Paré J, Froehlich JE. Current concepts on the genetic factors in rotator cuff pathology and future implications for sports physical therapists. *Int J Sports Phys Ther.* 2017;12(2):273–285.
203. Cordasco F, Bigliani L. Large and massive tears. *Orthop Clin North Am.* 1997;28(2):179–193.
204. Meister K, Seroyer S. Arthroscopic management of the thrower's shoulder: internal impingement. *Orthop Clin North Am.* 2003;34(4):539–547.
205. Breazeak N, Craig E. Partial-thickness rotator cuff tears. *Orthop Clin North Am.* 1997;28(2):145–155.
206. Neer CS II. Anterior acromioplasty for the chronic impingement syndrome in the shoulder: a preliminary report. *J Bone Joint Surg.* 1972;54(1):41–50.
207. Taheriazam A, Sadatsafavi M, Moayyeri A. Outcome predictors in nonoperative management of newly diagnosed subacromial impingement syndrome: a longitudinal study. *MedGenMed.* 2005;7(1):63.
208. Kuhn JE, Dunn WR, Sanders R, et al. Effectiveness of physical therapy in treating atraumatic full-thickness rotator cuff tears: a multicenter prospective cohort study. *J Shoulder Elbow Surg.* 2013;22(10):1371–1379. doi:10.1016/j.jse.2013.01.026
209. Thigpen CA, Shaffer MA, Gaunt BW, Leggin BG, Williams GR, Wilcox RB, 3rd. The American Society of Shoulder and Elbow Therapists' consensus statement on rehabilitation following arthroscopic rotator cuff repair. *J Shoulder Elbow Surg.* 2016;25(4):521–535. doi:10.1016/j.jse.2015.12.018
210. Gerber C, Schneeberger AG, Perren SM, Nyffeler RW. Experimental rotator cuff repair. A preliminary study. *J Bone Joint Surg Am.* 1999;81(9):1281–1290. doi:10.2106/00004623-199909000-00009
211. St Pierre P, Olson EJ, Elliott JJ, O'Hair KC, McKinney LA, Ryan J. Tendon-healing to cortical bone compared with healing to a cancellous trough. A biomechanical and histological evaluation in goats. *J Bone Joint Surg Am.* 1995;77(12):1858–1866.
212. Yi A, Villacis D, Yalamanchili R, Hatch GF 3rd. A comparison of rehabilitation methods after arthroscopic rotator cuff repair: a systematic review. *Sports Health.* 2015;7(4):326–334. doi:10.1177/1941738115576729
213. Shen C, Tang ZH, Hu JZ, Zou GY, Xiao RC, Yan DX. Does immobilization after arthroscopic rotator cuff repair increase tendon healing? A systematic review and meta-analysis. *Arch Orthop Trauma Surg.* 2014;134(9):1279–1285. doi:10.1007/s00402-014-2028-2
214. Hsu JE, Horneff JG, Gee AO. Immobilization after rotator cuff repair: what evidence do we have now? *Orthop Clin North Am.* 2016;47(1):169–177. doi:10.1016/j.ocl.2015.08.017
215. Mazzocca AD, Arciero RA, Shea KP, et al. The effect of early range of motion on quality of life, clinical outcome, and repair integrity after arthroscopic rotator cuff repair. *Arthroscopy.* 2017;33(6):1138–1148. doi:10.1016/j.arthro.2016.10.017
216. Gallagher BP, Bishop ME, Tjoumakaris FP, Freedman KB. Early versus delayed rehabilitation following arthroscopic rotator cuff repair: a systematic review. *Phys Sportsmed.* 2015;43(2):178–187. doi:10.1080/00913847.2015.1025683
217. Karjalainen TV, Jain NB, Heikkinen J, Johnston RV, Page CM, Buchbinder R. Surgery for rotator cuff tears. *Cochrane Database Syst Rev.* 2019;12:Cd013502. doi:10.1002/14651858.Cd013502
218. Olds M, Harman B. Rotator cuff repair protocols: a survey of current New Zealand practice. *N Z J Physiother.* 2017;45:24–30. doi:10.15619/NZJP/45.1.04
219. Kjær BH, Magnusson SP, Henriksen M, et al. Effects of 12 Weeks of progressive early active exercise therapy after surgical rotator cuff repair: 12 weeks and 1-year results from the CUT-N-MOVE randomized controlled trial. *Am J Sports Med.* 2021;49(2):321–331. doi:10.1177/0363546520983823
220. Edwards PK, Ebert JR, Littlewood C, Ackland T, Wang A. A systematic review of electromyography studies in normal shoulders to inform postoperative rehabilitation following rotator cuff repair. *J Orthop Sports Phys Ther.* 2017;47(12):931–944. doi:10.2519/jospt.2017.7271
221. Lewis J. Rotator cuff related shoulder pain: assessment, management and uncertainties. *Man Ther.* 2016;23:57–68.
222. Schmidt CC, Jarrett CD, Brown BT. Management of rotator cuff tears. *J Hand Surg Am.* 2015;40(2):399–408. doi:10.1016/j.jhsa.2014.06.122
223. Klouche S, Lefevre N, Herman S, Gerometta A, Bohu Y. Return to sport after rotator cuff tear repair: a systematic review and meta-analysis. *Am J Sports Med.* 2016;44(7):1877–1887. doi:10.1177/0363546515598995
224. Altintas B, Anderson N, Dornan GJ, Boykin RE, Logan C, Millett PJ. Return to sport after arthroscopic rotator cuff repair: is there a difference between the recreational and the competitive athlete? *Am J Sports Med.* 2020;48(1):252–261.
225. Kibler W. Shoulder rehabilitation: principles and practice. *Med Sci Sports Exerc.* 1998;30(4 Suppl 1):40–50.
226. Burkhart S, Morgan C, Kibler W. The disabled throwing shoulder: spectrum of pathology part III: the SICK scapula, scapular dyskinesis, the kinetic chain, and rehabilitation. *Arthroscopy.* 2003;19(7):722–731.

227. Kibler W. The role of the scapula in athletic shoulder function. *Am J Sports Med.* 1998;26(2):325–337.
228. Kibler W. Rehabilitation of rotator cuff tendinopathy. *Clin Sports Med.* 2003;22(4):837–847.
229. Rubin B, Kibler W. Fundamental principles of shoulder rehabilitation: conservative to postoperative management. *Arthroscopy.* 2002;18(9 Suppl 2):29–39.
230. Muir B. Dorsal scapular nerve neuropathy: a narrative review of the literature. *J Can Chiropr Assoc.* 2017;61(2):128–144.
231. Sciascia A. Evaluating scapular dyskinesis. *Athl Train Sports Health Care.* 2020;12(1):6–10. doi:10.3928/19425864-20191107-01
232. Umehara J, Nakamura M, Nishishita S, Tanaka H, Kusano K, Ichihashi N. Scapular kinematic alterations during arm elevation with decrease in pectoralis minor stiffness after stretching in healthy individuals. *J Shoulder Elbow Surg.* 2018;27(7):1214–1220. doi:10.1016/j.jse.2018.02.037
233. Umehara J, Kusano K, Nakamura M, et al. Scapular kinematic and shoulder muscle activity alterations after serratus anterior muscle fatigue. *J Shoulder Elbow Surg.* 2018;27(7):1205–1213. doi:https://doi.org/10.1016/j.jse.2018.01.009
234. Wan-Yu D, Tsun-Shun H, Yuan-Chun C, et al. Single-session video and electromyography feedback in overhead athletes with scapular dyskinesis and impingement syndrome. *J Athl Train.* 2020;55(3):265–273. doi:10.4085/1062-6050-490-18
235. Ozer ST, Karabay D, Yesilyaprak SS. Taping to improve scapular dyskinesis, scapular upward rotation, and pectoralis minor length in overhead athletes. *J Athl Train.* 2018;53(11):1063–1070. doi:10.4085/1062-6050-342-17
236. Huang T-S, Ou H-L, Lin J-J. Effects of trapezius kinesio taping on scapular kinematics and associated muscular activation in subjects with scapular dyskinesis. *J Hand Ther.* 2019;32(3):345–352. doi:10.1016/j.jht.2017.10.012
237. Veen EJD, Stevens M, Koorevaar CT, Diercks RL. Appropriate care for orthopedic patients: effect of implementation of the Clinical Practice Guideline for Diagnosis and Treatment of Subacromial Pain Syndrome in the Netherlands. *Acta Orthop.* 2019;90(3):191–195. doi:10.1080/17453674.2019.1593641
238. Saito H, Harrold ME, Cavalheri V, McKenna L. Scapular focused interventions to improve shoulder pain and function in adults with subacromial pain: a systematic review and meta-analysis. *Physiother Theory Pract.* 2018;34(9):653–670. doi:10.1080/09593985.2018.1423656
239. Meehan K, Wassinger C, Roy JS, Sole G. Seven key themes in physical therapy advice for patients living with subacromial shoulder pain: a scoping review. *J Orthop Sports Phys Ther.* 2020;50(6):285–293, A1–A12. doi:10.2519/jospt.2020.9152
240. Schmitt L, Snyder-Mackler L. Role of scapular stabilizers in etiology and treatment of impingement syndrome. *J Orthop Sports Phys Ther.* 1999;29(1):31–38.
241. Solem-Bertoft E, Thuomas K, Westerberg C. The influence of scapular retraction and protraction on the width of the subacromial space. *Clin Orthop Rel Res.* 1993;296:99–103.
242. Kebaetse M, McClure P, NPratt N. Thoracic position effect on shoulder range of motion, strength, and three-dimensional scapular kinetics. *Arch Phys Med Rehabil.* 1999;80:945–950.
243. Dunning J, Walsh S, Arias-BurÍA JL, et al. Spinal manipulation and electrical dry needling in patients with subacromial pain syndrome: a multicenter randomized clinical trial. *J Orthop Sports Phys Ther.* 2021;51(2):72–81. doi:10.2519/jospt.2021.9785
244. Hunter DJ, Rivett DA, McKeirnan S, Smith L, Snodgrass SJ. Relationship between shoulder impingement syndrome and thoracic posture. *Phys Ther.* 2020;100(4):677–686. doi:10.1093/ptj/pzz182
245. Land H, Gordon S, Watt K. Effect of manual physiotherapy in homogeneous individuals with subacromial shoulder impingement: a randomized controlled trial. *Physiother Res Int.* 2019;24(2): e1768. doi:10.1002/pri.1768
246. Tahran Ö, Yeşilyaprak SS. Effects of modified posterior shoulder stretching exercises on shoulder mobility, pain, and dysfunction in patients with subacromial impingement syndrome. *Sports Health.* 2020;12(2):139–148. doi:10.1177/1941738119900532
247. Meadows S, Smith G, Vaswani R. Physiotherapist survey: increasing thoracic spine movement within the management of chronic subacromial impingement syndrome. *J Bodyw Mov Ther.* 2020;24(1):93–99. doi:10.1016/j.jbmt.2019.06.013
248. Grimes JK, Puentedura EJ, Cheng MS, Seitz AL. The comparative effects of upper thoracic spine thrust manipulation techniques in individuals with subacromial pain syndrome: a randomized clinical trial. *J Orthop Sports Phys Ther.* 2019;49(10):716–724. doi:10.2519/jospt.2019.8484
249. Nazari G, MacDermid JC, Bobos P. Conservative versus surgical interventions for shoulder impingement: an overview of systematic reviews of randomized controlled trials. *Physiother Can.* 2020;72(3):282–297. doi:10.3138/ptc-2018-0111
250. Kim S-Y, Weon J-H, Jung D-Y, Oh J-S. Effect of the scapula-setting exercise on acromio-humeral distance and scapula muscle activity in patients with subacromial impingement syndrome. *Phys Ther Sport.* 2019;37:99–104. doi:10.1016/j.ptsp.2019.03.006
251. Kara D, Harput G, Duzgun I. Trapezius muscle activation levels and ratios during scapular retraction exercises: a comparative study between patients with subacromial impingement syndrome and healthy controls. *Clin Biomech (Bristol, Avon).* 2019;67:119–126. doi:10.1016/j.clinbiomech.2019.05.020
252. Pasin T, Ataoğlu S, Pasin Ö, Ankarali H. Comparison of the effectiveness of platelet-rich plasma, corticosteroid, and physical therapy in subacromial impingement syndrome. *Arch Rheumatol.* 2019;34(3):308–316. doi:10.5606/ArchRheumatol.2019.7225
253. Hancock MJ. Appraisal of Clinical Practice Guideline: subacromial decompression surgery for adults with shoulder pain: a clinical practice guideline. *J Physiother.* 2019;65(3):177. doi:10.1016/j.jphys.2019.05.002
254. Singh H, McKay M, Baldwin J, et al. Beighton scores and cut-offs across the lifespan: cross-sectional study of an Australian population. *Rheumatology (Oxford).* 2017;56(11):1857–1864.
255. Gibson K, Growse A, Korda L, Wray E, MacDermid J. The effectiveness of rehabilitation for nonoperative management of shoulder instability: a systematic review. *J Hand Ther.* 2004;17(2):229–242.
256. Beasley L, Faryniarz D, Hannafin J. Multidirectional instability of the shoulder in the female athlete. *Clin Sports Med.* 2000;19(2):331–349.
257. Warner J, Micheli L, Arslanian L, Kennedy J, Kennedy R. Patterns of flexibility, laxity, and strength, in normal shoulders and shoulders with instability and impingement. *Am J Sports Med.* 1990;18(4):366–375.
258. McMahon P, Lee T. Muscles may contribute to shoulder dislocation and stability. *Clin Orthop Relat Res.* 2002;1(403):S18–S25.
259. Abdul-Rassoul H, Galvin JW, Curry EJ, Simon J, Li X. Return to sport after surgical treatment for anterior

shoulder instability: a systematic review. *Am J Sports Med.* 2019;47(6):1507–1515. doi:10.1177/0363546518780934

260. Lawton R, Choudhury S, Manst P, Cofield R, Stans A. Pediatric shoulder instability: presentation, findings, treatment, and outcomes. *J Pediatr Orthop.* 2002;22:51–62.

261. Díaz Heredia J, Ruiz Iban MA, Ruiz Diaz R, Moros Marco S, Gutierrez Hernandez JC, Valencia M. The posterior unstable shoulder: natural history, clinical evaluation and imaging. *Open Orthop J.* 2017;11:972–978. doi:10.2174/1874325001711010972

262. McIntyre K, Bélanger A, Dhir J, et al. Evidence-based conservative rehabilitation for posterior glenohumeral instability: a systematic review. *Phys Ther Sport.* 2016;22:94–100. doi:10.1016/j.ptsp.2016.06.002

263. Sekiya JK, Giffin JR, Irrgang JJ, Fu FH, Harner CD. Clinical outcomes after combined meniscal allograft transplantation and anterior cruciate ligament reconstruction. *Am J Sports Med.* 2003;31(6):896–906.

264. Ayekoloye C, Nwangwu O. Multidirectional instability of the shoulder (MDI)—focus on non-operative management. *Eur J Physiother.* 2019;21(4):197–203. doi:10.1080/21679169.2018.1514651

265. Hewitt M, Getelman M, Snyder S. Arthroscopic management of multidirectional instability: pancapsular plication. *Orthop Clin North Am.* 2003;34(4):549–557.

266. Yamaguchi K, Flatow E. Management of multidirectional instability. *Clin Sports Med.* 1995;14(4):885–901.

267. Longo UG, Rizzello G, Loppini M, et al. Multidirectional instability of the shoulder: a systematic review. *Arthroscopy.* 2015;31(12):2431–2443. doi:10.1016/j.arthro.2015.06.006

268. Rowe C, Zarins B. Recurrent transient subluxation of the shoulder. *J Bone Joint Surg Am.* 1981;63(6):863–872.

269. Silliman J, Hawkins R. Classification and physical diagnosis of instability of the shoulder. *Clin Orthop Relat Res.* 1993;291:7–19.

270. Haley CA, Haley CCA. History and physical examination for shoulder instability. *Sports Med Arthrosc Rev.* 2017;25(3):150–155.

271. Allen A, Warner J. Shoulder instability in the athlete. *Orthop Clin North Am.* 1995;26(3):487–504.

272. Moseley H, Overgaard B. The anterior capsular mechanism in recurrent anterior dislocation of the shoulder. *J Bone Joint Surg.* 1962;44B(4):913–927.

273. McCarty E, Ritchie P, Gill H, McFarland EG. Shoulder instability: return to play. *Clin Sports Med.* 2004;23(3):335–352.

274. Chen D, Goldberg J, Herald J, Critchley I, Barmare A. Effects of surgical management on multidirectional instability of the shoulder: a meta-analysis. *Knee Surg Sports Traumatol Arthrosc.* 2016;24(2):630–639. doi:10.1007/s00167-015-3901-4

275. Rolfes K. Arthroscopic treatment of shoulder instability: a systematic review of capsular plication versus thermal capsulorrhaphy. *J Athl Train.* 2015;50(1):105–109. doi:10.4085/1062-6050-49.3.63

276. Hurley ET, Montgomery C, Jamal MS, et al. Return to play after the Latarjet procedure for anterior shoulder instability: a systematic review. *Am J Sports Med.* 2019;47(12):3002–3008. doi:10.1177/0363546519831005

277. Michener LA, Abrams JS, Bliven KCH, et al. National Athletic Trainers' Association Position Statement: evaluation, management, and outcomes of and return-to-play criteria for overhead athletes with superior labral anterior-posterior injuries. *J Athl Train.* 2018;53(3):209–229. doi:10.4085/1062-6050-59-16

278. Christopherson ZR, Kennedy J, Roskin D, Moorman CT. Rehabilitation and return to play following superior labral anterior to posterior repair. *Oper Tech Sports Med.* 2017;25(3):132–144. doi:10.1053/j.otsm.2017.07.002

279. Dodson CC, Altchek DW. SLAP lesions: an update on recognition and treatment. *J Orthop Sports Phys Ther.* 2009;39(2):71–80. doi:10.2519/jospt.2009.2850

280. Ruotolo C, Penna J, Namkoong S, Meinhard B. Shoulder pain and the overhead athlete. *Am J Orthop.* 2003;32(5):248–258.

281. Shin S-J, Lee J, Jeon Y-S, Ko Y-W, Kim R-G. Clinical outcomes of non-operative treatment for patients presenting SLAP lesions in diagnostic provocative tests and MR arthrography. *Knee Surg Sports Traumatol Arthrosc.* 2017;25(10):3296–3302. doi:10.1007/s00167-016-4226-7

282. Vahedi H, Fleischman AN, Salvo JP, Parvizi J, Salvo JP Jr. Higher prevalence of concomitant shoulder labral tears in patients with femoroacetabular impingement. *Arthroscopy.* 2019;35(4):1074–1079. doi:10.1016/j.arthro.2018.10.128

283. Jazrawi L, McCluskey G III, Andrews J. Superior labral anterior and posterior lesions and internal impingement in the overhead athlete. *Instr Course Lect.* 2003;52:43–63.

284. Cvetanovich GL, Gowd AK, Frantz TL, Erickson BJ, Romeo AA. Superior labral anterior posterior repair and biceps tenodesis surgery: trends of the American Board of Orthopaedic Surgery database. *Am J Sports Med.* 2020;48(7):1583–1589. doi:10.1177/0363546520913538

285. Wilk K, Meister K, Andrews J. Current concepts in the rehabilitation of the overhead throwing athlete. *Am J Sports Med.* 2002;30(1):136–151.

286. Gilliam BD, Douglas L, Fleisig GS, et al. Return to play and outcomes in baseball players after superior labral anterior-posterior repairs. *Am J Sports Med.* 2018;46(1):109–115. doi:10.1177/0363546517728256

287. Thayaparan A, Yu J, Horner NS, Leroux T, Alolabi B, Khan M. Return to sport after arthroscopic superior labral anterior-posterior repair: a systematic review. *Sports Health.* 2019;11(6):520–527. doi:10.1177/1941738119873892

288. Douglas L, Whitaker J, Nyland J, et al. Return to play and performance perceptions of baseball players after isolated SLAP tear repair. *Orthop J Sports Med.* 2019;7(3):1–7. doi:10.1177/2325967119829486

289. Dougherty MC, Kulenkamp JE, Boyajian H, Koh JL, Lee MJ, Shi LL. National trends in the diagnosis and repair of SLAP lesions in the United States. *J Orthop Surg.* 2020;28(1):1–5. doi:10.1177/2309499019888552

290. Dunne KF, Knesek M, Tjong VK, et al. Arthroscopic treatment of type II superior labral anterior to posterior (SLAP) lesions in a younger population: minimum 2-year outcomes are similar between SLAP repair and biceps tenodesis. *Knee Surg Sports Traumatol Arthrosc.* 2021;29(1):257–265. doi:10.1007/s00167-020-05971-0

291. Paoli AR, Gold HT, Mahure SA, et al. Treatment for symptomatic SLAP tears in middle-aged patients comparing repair, biceps tenodesis, and nonoperative approaches: a cost-effectiveness analysis. *Arthroscopy.* 2018;34(7):2019–2029. doi:10.1016/j.arthro.2018.01.029

292. Provencher MT, McCormick F, Peebles LA, et al. Outcomes of primary biceps subpectoral tenodesis in an active population: a prospective evaluation of 101 patients. *Arthroscopy.* 2019;35(12):3205–3210. doi:10.1016/j.arthro.2019.06.035

293. Griffin JW, Cvetanovich GL, Kim J, et al. Biceps tenodesis is a viable option for management of proximal biceps injuries in patients less than 25 years of age. *Arthroscopy.* 2019;35(4):1036–1041. doi:10.1016/j.arthro.2018.10.151

294. Frantz TL, Shacklett AG, Martin AS, et al. Biceps tenodesis for superior labrum anterior-posterior tear in the overhead athlete: a systematic review. *Am J Sports Med.* 2021;49(2):522–528. doi:10.1177/0363546520921177

295. Freijomil N, Peters S, Millay A, Sinda T, Sunset J, Reiman MP. The success of return to sport after superior labrum anterior to posterior (SLAP) tears: a systematic review and meta-analysis. *Int J Sports Phys Ther.* 2020;15(5):659–670. doi:10.26603/ijspt20200659
296. Abraham VT, Tan BH, Kumar VP. Systematic review of biceps tenodesis: arthroscopic versus open. *Arthroscopy.* 2016;32(2):365–371. doi:10.1016/j.arthro.2015.07.028
297. MacDonald P, Verhulst F, McRae S, et al. Biceps tenodesis versus tenotomy in the treatment of lesions of the long head of the biceps tendon in patients undergoing arthroscopic shoulder surgery: a prospective double-blinded randomized controlled trial. *Am J Sports Med.* 2020;48(6):1439–1449. doi:10.1177/0363546520912212
298. Nolte PC, Woolson TE, Elrick BP, et al. Clinical outcomes of arthroscopic suprascapular nerve decompression for suprascapular neuropathy. *Arthroscopy.* 2021;37(2):499–507. doi:10.1016/j.arthro.2020.10.020
299. Walsworth M. Diagnosing suprascapular neuropathy in patients with shoulder dysfunction: a report of 5 cases. *Phys Ther.* 2004;84(4):359–372.
300. Memon M, Kay J, Ginsberg L, et al. Arthroscopic management of suprascapular neuropathy of the shoulder improves pain and functional outcomes with minimal complication rates. *Knee Surg Sports Traumatol Arthrosc.* 2018;26(1):240–266. doi:10.1007/s00167-017-4694-4
301. Boykin RE, Friedman DJ, Zimmer ZR, Oaklander AL, Higgins LD, Warner JJP. Suprascapular neuropathy in a shoulder referral practice. *J Shoulder Elbow Surg.* 2011;20(6):983–988. doi:10.1016/j.jse.2010.10.039
302. Millstein E, Snyder S. Arthroscopic evaluation and management of rotator cuff tears. *Orthop Clin North Am.* 2003;34:507–520.
303. Bruce J, Dorizas J. Suprascapular nerve entrapment due to a stenotic foramen: a variant of the suprascapular notch. *Sports Health.* 2013;5(4):363–366. doi:10.1177/1941738113476656
304. Kisner C, Colby LA. *Therapeutic Exercise: Foundations and Techniques.* 7th ed. F.A. Davis; 2018.
305. Haff C, Triplett N. *Essentials of Strength Training and Conditioning.* 4th ed. Human Kinetics; 2015.
306. Hollstadt K, Boland M, Mulligan I. Test-retest reliability of the closed kinetic chain upper extremity stability test (CKCUEST) in a modified test position in Division I collegiate basketball players. *Int J Sports Phys Ther.* 2020;15(2):203–209. doi:10.26603/ijspt20200203
307. Borms D, Cools A. Upper-extremity functional performance tests: reference values for overhead athletes. *Int J Sports Med.* 2018;39(6):433–441. doi:10.1055/a-0573-1388
308. Taylor JB, Wright AA, Smoliga JM, DePew JT, Hegedus EJ. Upper-extremity physical-performance tests in college athletes. *J Sport Rehabil.* 2016;25(2):146–154. doi:10.1123/jsr.2014-0296
309. Pontillo M, Sennett BJ, Bellm E. Use of an upper extremity functional testing algorithm to determine return to play readiness in collegiate football players: a case series. *Int J Sports Phys Ther.* 2020;15(6):1141–1150. doi:10.26603/ijspt20201141

15 | Elbow Complex

Betsy Myers and June Hanks

CHAPTER OBJECTIVES
After reading this chapter, you will be able to:
1. Describe the anatomy of the joints forming the elbow complex to include osteologic ligamentous, capsular, and muscular features.
2. Describe the biomechanics of the articulations of the elbow.
3. Tailor the basic history to a patient with elbow pathology.
4. Describe the components of the physical examination for a patient with elbow pathology.
5. Describe the pathology, history, key examination findings, rehabilitation focus, and expected outcomes of common elbow pathologies.
6. Hypothesize differential diagnoses of elbow symptoms based on location, patient complaint, and onset.
7. Organize the physical examination of a patient with elbow pathology to maximize efficiency.

FUNCTIONAL ANATOMY

The elbow (cubital) complex includes the articulations among the humerus, radius, and ulna forming the humeroulnar, humeroradial, and proximal radioulnar articulations surrounded by one joint capsule.[1] The articulations of the humerus with the ulna and radius are most typically thought of as the elbow joint, with the two articulations acting as one joint to allow the primary motion of flexion and extension. The proximal radioulnar joint movement is pronation and supination of the forearm.[2] The cubital fossa is triangular in shape, bounded proximally by the elbow flexors, laterally by the brachioradialis, and medially by the pronator teres (PT). The combined motions of flexion/extension and pronation/supination at the elbow allow for varied hand positions and functional movements.

Osteology

Landmarks on bones forming the joints of the elbow complex are depicted in Figures 15-1 and 15-2. The distal shaft of the humerus widens to form the medial and lateral supracondylar ridges and epicondyles. The lateral epicondyle provides attachment of the common extensor muscle mass and the lateral collateral ligament complex (LCLC), whereas the more prominent medial epicondyle serves as attachment for the flexor-pronator muscle groups and the medial collateral ligamentous complex.[3] The distal end of the humerus bears two distinctive bony features: the trochlea located medially and the capitulum (capitellum) located laterally. Anteriorly, the coronoid and radial fossae lie immediately proximal to the trochlea and capitulum, respectively. Posteriorly, the deep olecranon fossa lies just above the trochlea and accepts the olecranon process of the ulna during full elbow extension (Fig. 15-3A). The sellar-shaped trochlea looks like a spool. From a mediolateral view, the trochlea is directed anteriorly approximately 45° to the humeral shaft. The trochlear articular surface extends posteriorly, with the medial half extending farther distally than the lateral half. The groove in the trochlea runs obliquely, distally, and laterally, dictating the path for olecranon of the ulna and causing the ulna to angulate laterally on the humerus during elbow extension, which, along with the slight valgus angulation of the trochlear notch of the ulna, creates the "carrying angle" of the elbow, discussed more fully later in this chapter. The capitulum faces anteriorly, forming most of a sphere mediolaterally and half of a sphere anteroposteriorly. During elbow flexion, the coronoid fossa receives the distinct, sharp, superomedial coronoid process of the ulna, and the radial fossa receives the head of the radius (Fig. 15-3B).

The proximal ulna is the larger, medial, and longer bone of the forearm, providing a stabilizing function. Prominent projections are the olecranon and coronoid processes that form the concave trochlear (sigmoid) notch. Posteriorly, the olecranon surface is smooth and subcutaneous, located in a horizontal line with the humeral epicondyles in elbow extension, and descending to form a triangle with humeral epicondyles. The trochlear notch articular surface is divided by the trochlear ridge that articulates with the trochlear groove of the humerus during elbow flexion and extension. The coronoid process fits snugly into the coronoid fossa of the humerus during elbow flexion. Distal to the coronoid process is the tuberosity of the ulna to which the brachialis tendon attaches. The

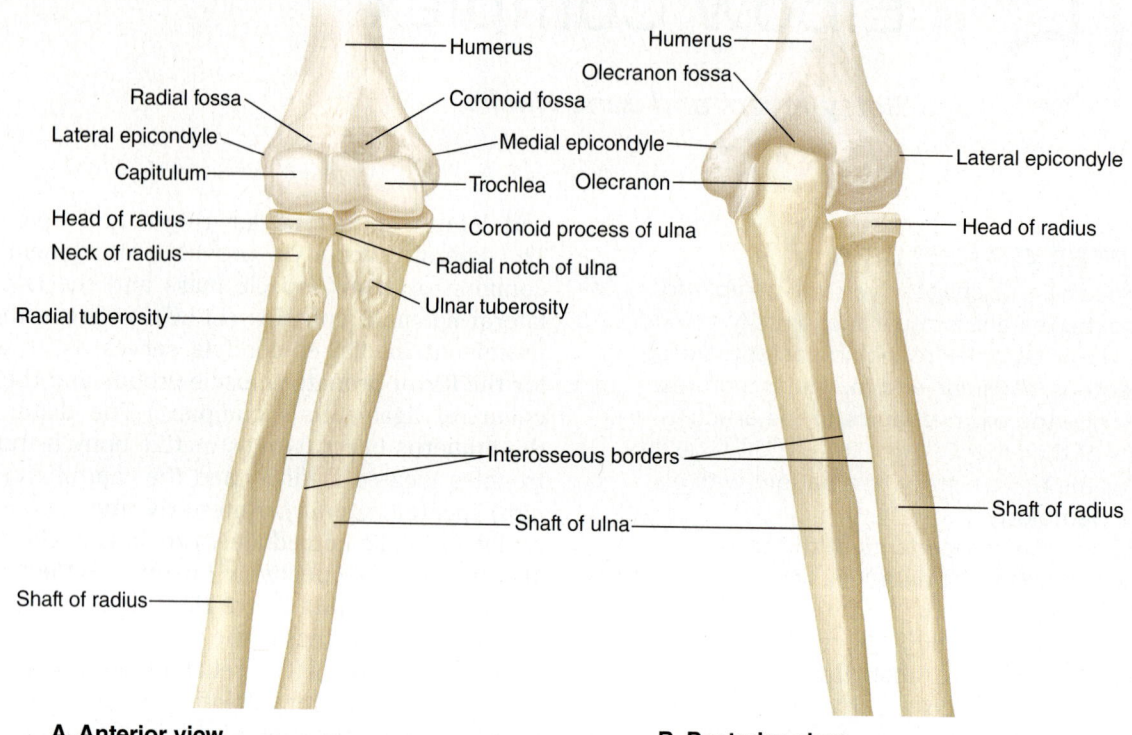

FIGURE 15-1 Bony landmarks of the elbow complex. **A.** Anterior view. **B.** Posterior view. (Gest TR. *Lippincott Atlas of Anatomy*. 2nd ed. Wolters Kluwer; 2020: Plate 2-04.)

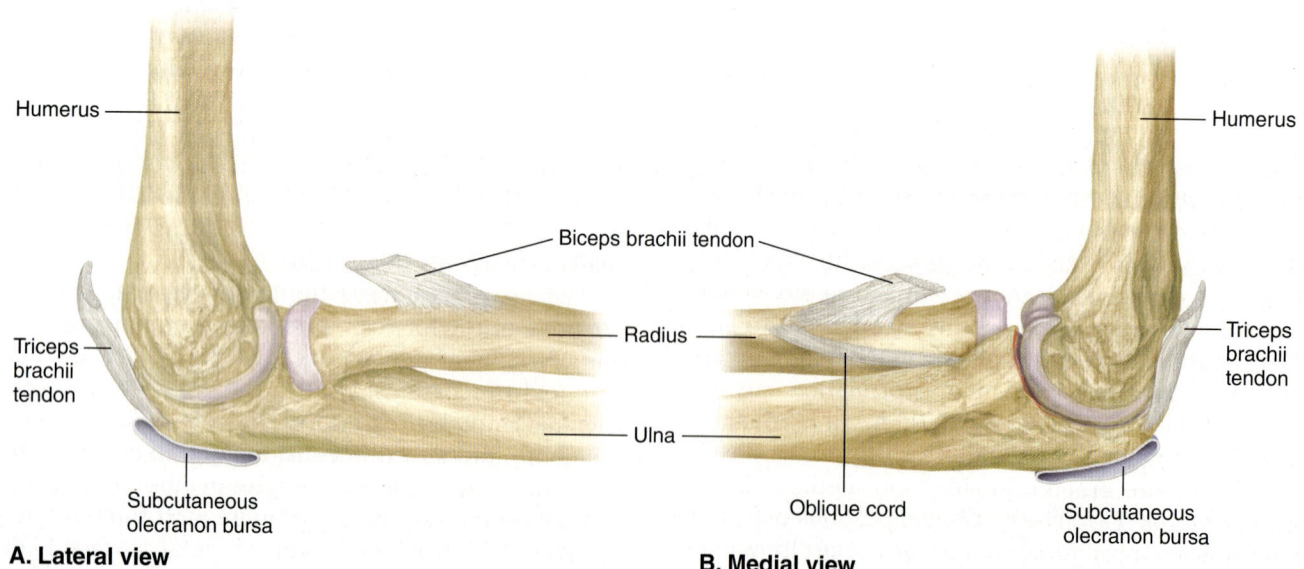

FIGURE 15-2 Elbow complex. **A.** Lateral view. **B.** Medial view. (Gest TR. *Lippincott Atlas of Anatomy*. 2nd ed. Wolters Kluwer; 2020: Plate 2-43B & C.)

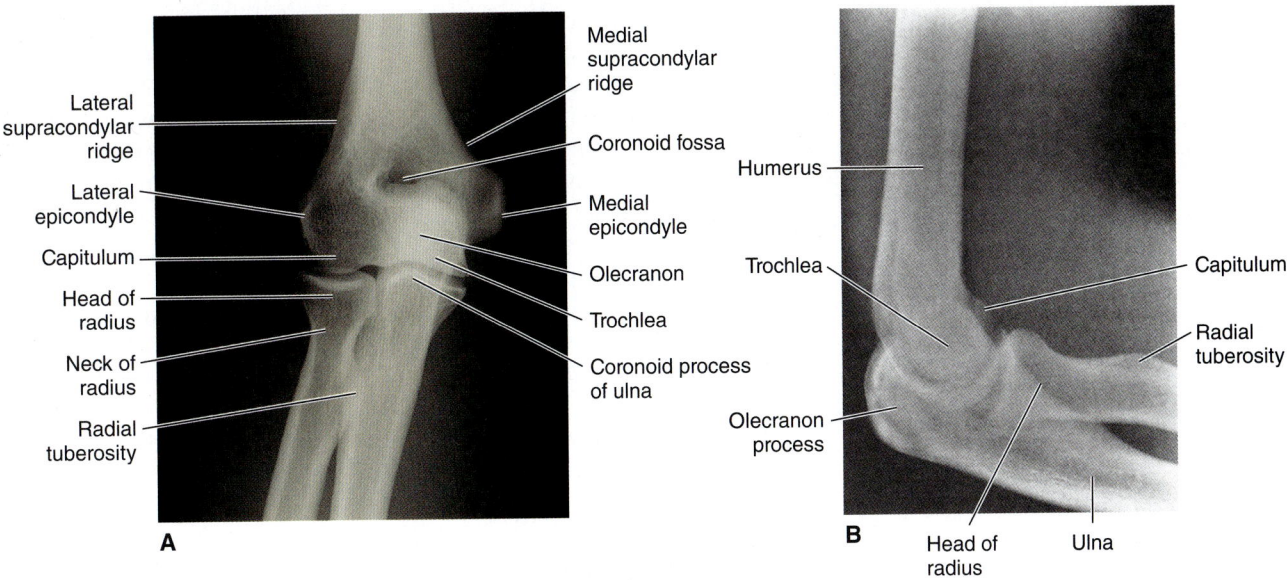

FIGURE 15-3 Radiograph of normal right elbow. **A.** Anterior-posterior view with elbow in extension. The olecranon of the ulna enters the olecranon fossa of the humerus in extension. (Gest TR. *Lippincott Atlas of Anatomy*. 2nd ed. Wolters Kluwer; 2020: Plate 2-05B.) **B.** Lateral view with elbow in partial flexion. Bony limitation to full elbow flexion occurs as the radial head enters the humeral radial fossa, and the tip of the ulnar coronoid process enters the humeral coronoid fossa. (Dudek RW, Louis TM. *High-Yield Gross Anatomy*. 5th ed. Lippincott Williams & Wilkins; 2015: Figure 20.11.)

head of the radius articulates with the radial notch located on the lateral side of the coronoid process, inferior to the trochlear notch. Just distal to the radial notch is the supinator fossa and a prominent ridge, the supinator crest, that serves as attachment for the supinator (Fig. 15-4).[4]

The proximal radius bears a short head, neck, and medially facing radial (biceps) tuberosity. The radial tuberosity, just distal to the medial portion of the radial neck, provides attachment for the biceps brachii. The radial head has an irregular oblong shape owing to the varying thickness of the articular cartilage covering the majority of the peripheral rim.[5] The radial head is concave in the most superior aspect for articulation with the convex capitulum. In a small depression on the lateral posterior aspect of the extended elbow, the posterior surface of the radial head can be palpated.[4]

Joints

The joints of the elbow complex are shown in Figure 15-5. The humeroulnar joint is formed by articulation of the trochlea of the distal humerus and the trochlear notch of the ulna.[1,4] The trochlea extends farther distally on the medial side of the humeroulnar joint, creating the obliquely oriented axis of motion for flexion and extension. The humeroradial joint (also called the *radiocapitular or radiocapitellar joint*) is formed by the articulation of the capitulum of the distal humerus and the head of the radius. The radius and ulna articulate both proximally and distally. The proximal radioulnar joint is formed as the radial head articulates with the radial notch of the ulna, and the distal radioulnar joint is formed by the connection of the head of the ulna and the ulnar notch of the radius. The distal radioulnar joint will be discussed in Chapter 16, Wrist and Hand Complex.

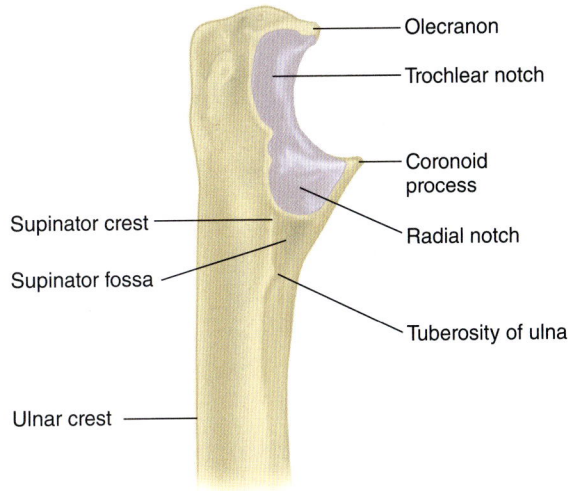

FIGURE 15-4 Proximal ulna. (Modified from Wiesel SW, Albert TJ. *Operative Techniques in Orthopaedic Surgery* (Vol. 3). 3rd ed. Wolters Kluwer; 2022: Figure Pt.7-1.11B.)

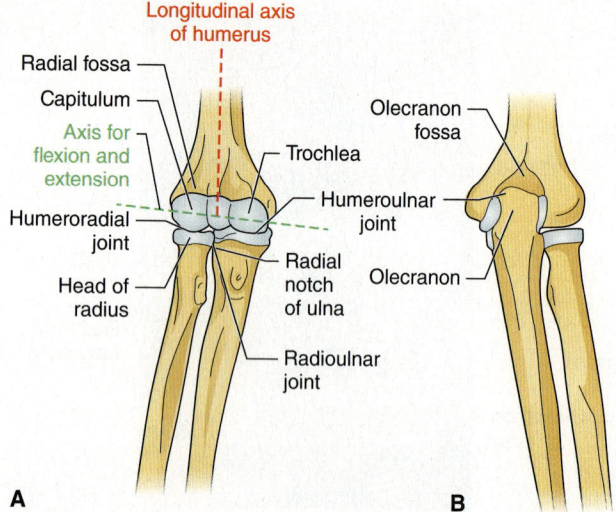

FIGURE 15-5 Joints of the elbow. The axis of motion for flexion and extension (*green dashed line*) is centered in the middle of the trochlea on a line that intersects the longitudinal axis of the humerus (*red dashed line*). (Adapted from Gest TR. *Lippincott Atlas of Anatomy*. 2nd ed. Wolters Kluwer; 2020: Plate 2-04.)

Carrying Angle

The carrying angle is the clinical measurement of the outward angulation (valgus) of the supinated forearm on the extended elbow, generally defined as the angle formed by the intersection of the line along the midshaft of the humerus and the midline of the forearm, though methodologies vary.[6] Reported normal mean values range from 5 to 25°,[6,7] with a greater angle in females and on the dominant side.[6,8,9] Large variations in reported values indicate that comparisons should be made with the contralateral side in the same individual rather than against a normal standard. A normal, excessive valgus and varus angle is shown in Figure 15-6. The carrying angle is more evident when a load is carried in one hand, such as when carrying a bucket. When carrying a load on one side, individuals will typically laterally rotate the arm and supinate the forearm to maximize the space between the carried load and the lower extremity on that side.[6]

Ligaments of Elbow Complex

The primary ligaments of the elbow complex are described in Table 15-1 and depicted in Figures 15-7 and 15-8. The collateral ligaments are thickenings of the joint capsule and provide stabilization for the joint. The medial collateral ligament (MCL), also called the *ulnar collateral ligament*, is triangularly shaped[4] and consists of three bundles: anterior, posterior, and transverse.[10,11] The anterior bundle (AMCL or anterior medial collateral ligament) attaches to the anteroinferior medial

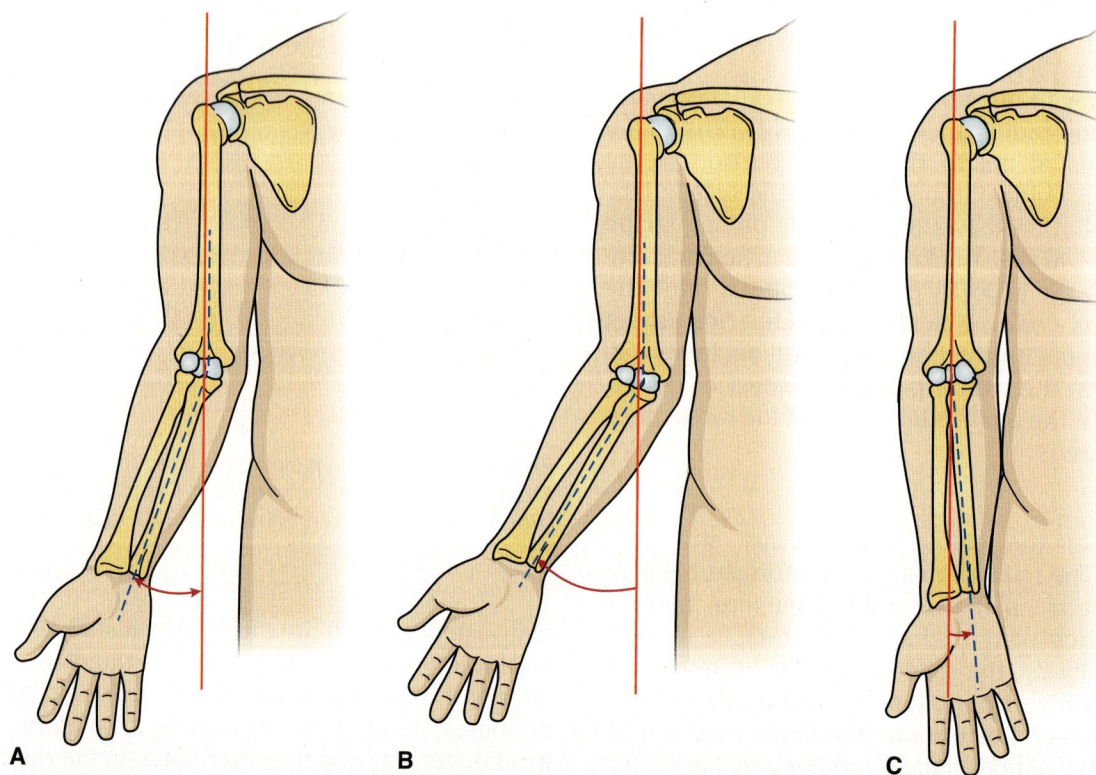

FIGURE 15-6 Carrying angle of elbow, formed by interception of lines along midshaft of humerus and midline of forearm with elbow fully extended and forearm supinated. **A.** Normal carrying angle. **B.** Excessive valgus. **C.** Varus. (Adapted from Nordin M, Frankel VH. *Basic Biomechanics of the Musculoskeletal System*. 5th ed. Wolters Kluwer; 2022: Figure 14-3.)

TABLE 15-1
LIGAMENTS OF THE ELBOW

Ligament/Complex	Characteristics	Attachments	Role/Function
Medial collateral ligament (MCL)	Composed of three bundles: • Anterior (AMCL) • Posterior (PMCL) • Transverse (oblique)	AMCL: medial epicondyle to coronoid process PMCL: medial epicondyle to olecranon medial margin Transverse: olecranon process to coronoid process	AMCL and PMCL: stabilizer for valgus stress and posteromedial instability Transverse: none known
Lateral collateral ligament complex (LCLC)	Composed of: • Radial collateral ligament (RCL) • Lateral ulnar collateral ligament (LUCL) • Annular ligament (AL) • Accessory lateral collateral ligament (ALCL)	RCL: lateral epicondyle to annular ligament LUCL: lateral epicondyle to annular ligament and supinator crest of ulna AL: encircles head of radius ALCL: accessory ligaments to AL (described as anterior/posterior or superior/inferior oblique ligamentous bands)	Stabilizer for varus stress and posterolateral instability AL secures radial head in radial notch of ulna

Modified from Alcid J, Ahmad C, Lee T. Elbow anatomy and structural biomechanics. *Clin Sports Med.* 2004;23(4):503-517; Williams P, Warwick R, Myson M, Bannister L, eds. *Gray's Anatomy.* 37th ed. Churchill Livingstone; 1989.

epicondyle and has an extensive distal attachment to the anteromedial portion of the coronoid process.[4,10,12] The fan-shaped posterior band (PMCL) attaches to the posteroinferior medial epicondyle and the medial margin of the olecranon. Although the AMCL and PMCL may serve as restraints to valgus stress and posteromedial instability,[13] the AMCL is considered the main restrainer and stabilizer,[14-16] particularly to valgus stress.[16,17] The transverse (oblique) bundle passes between the processes of the olecranon and coronoid, does not cross a joint, and does not contribute to stability.[11,14,16]

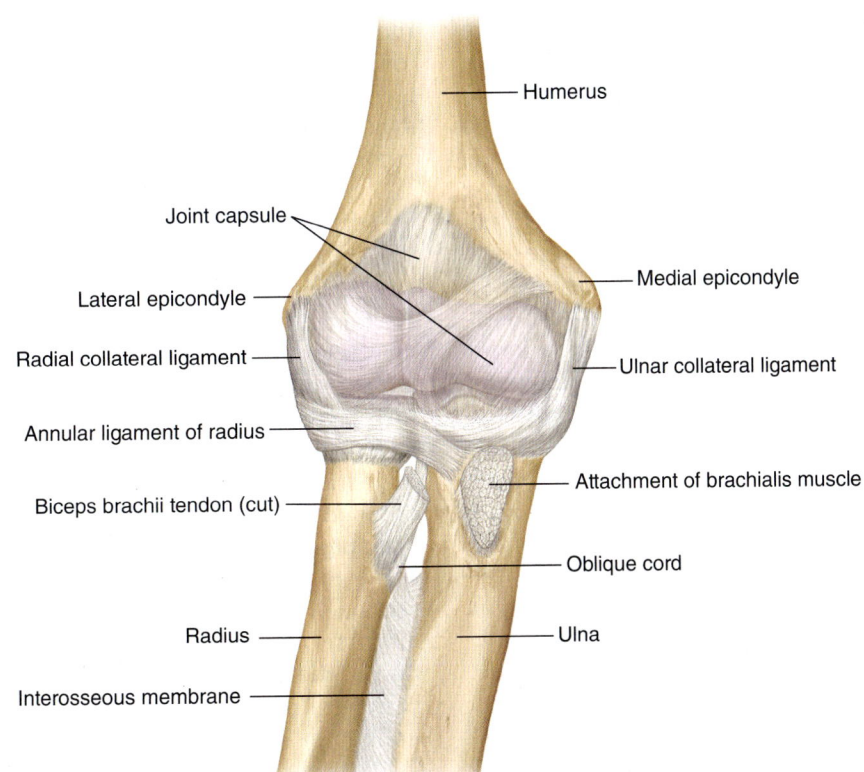

FIGURE 15-7 Anterior elbow, ligaments, and joint capsule. (Gest TR. *Lippincott Atlas of Anatomy.* 2nd ed. Wolters Kluwer; 2020: Plate 2-43A.)

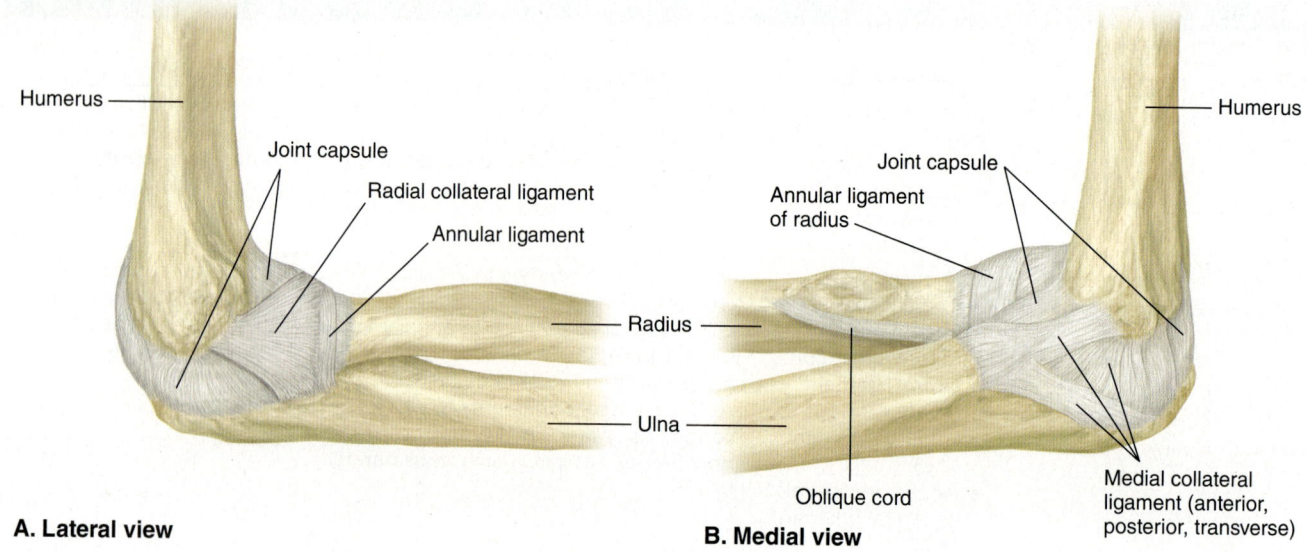

FIGURE 15-8 Ligaments of the elbow joint. **A.** Lateral view. Accessory lateral collateral ligament not shown. **B.** Medial view. Note the anterior, posterior, and transverse bundles of the medial collateral ligament and the association of the joint capsule with the ligaments. (Gest TR. *Lippincott Atlas of Anatomy*. 2nd ed. Wolters Kluwer; 2020: Plate 2-43B & C.)

The LCLC is described with variable nomenclature,[18] but generally is considered a multilayered structure consisting of the radial collateral ligament (RCL), lateral ulnar collateral ligament, (LUCL), annular ligament (AL), and accessory lateral collateral ligaments (ALCLs).[3,19–21] Attachments are described in Table 15-1. The RCL attaches to the inferior portion of the lateral epicondyle and blends distally with the AL, with some fibers attaching to the supinator crest, as well as the supinator.[4] The LUCL passes from the lateral epicondyle superficial to and blending with the AL and attaching to the supinator crest of the ulna. The AL encircles the head of the radius, securing it against the radial notch of the ulna where the proximal radioulnar joint is formed. The AL stabilizes the proximal radioulnar joint along with the associated ALCLs, described by Martin[22] as anterior and posterior ligaments and by others as superior and inferior oblique ligamentous bands.[18,23] A quadrate ligament has been described as a thickening of the joint capsule, attaching just distal to the radial notch of the ulna to the medial surface of the radial neck in line with the bicipital tuberosity, helping to stabilize the proximal radioulnar joint.[24,25] The LCLC is the primary stabilizer for varus stress and posterolateral instability, with some considering the LUCL component to be most critical[1,26] whereas others view the LCLC to function as a stabilizing unit.[12,27,28]

Joint Capsule

A single joint capsule encapsulates all joints of the elbow complex (see Figs. 15-6 and 15-7). The superior portion of the radioulnar joint capsule, deep to the AL, is continuous with this common capsule. The anterior portion of the elbow joint capsule attaches to the anterior distal humerus proximal to the radial and coronoid fossae and passes distally to attach to the rim of the coronoid process and AL. The posterior aspect of the capsule attaches proximally to the distal humerus just above the olecranon fossa area and distally to the olecranon process of the ulna and just below the AL and the lower margins of the radial neck.[1,29] Anterior and posterior fat pads are located between the capsule and the synovium.[30] Medially and laterally, the joint capsule is continuous with the collateral ligaments.[29]

Neurovascular Anatomy

The musculocutaneous, radial, median, and ulnar nerves or branches pass the elbow joint, accompanied by the brachial artery and branches of the deep brachial artery (Figs. 15-9 to 15-11). Branches from the radial, median, and ulnar nerves supply to the elbow joint as they pass distally to the forearm and hand. Traumatic injury or compression to these nerves may result in full or partial paralysis, impaired sensation, pain, and loss of function distal to the injured or compressed nerve. The anatomic course of the major nerves and branches and common sites of entrapment are discussed in this section. The clinical presentation and examination are discussed later in this chapter. (For a complete description of the brachial plexus that includes roots, cords, peripheral nerves, and muscles innervated, see Table 7-7 in Chapter 7, The Physical Examination.)

The musculocutaneous nerve, the continuation of the lateral cord of the brachial plexus, supplies and pierces the coracobrachialis in its course distally to

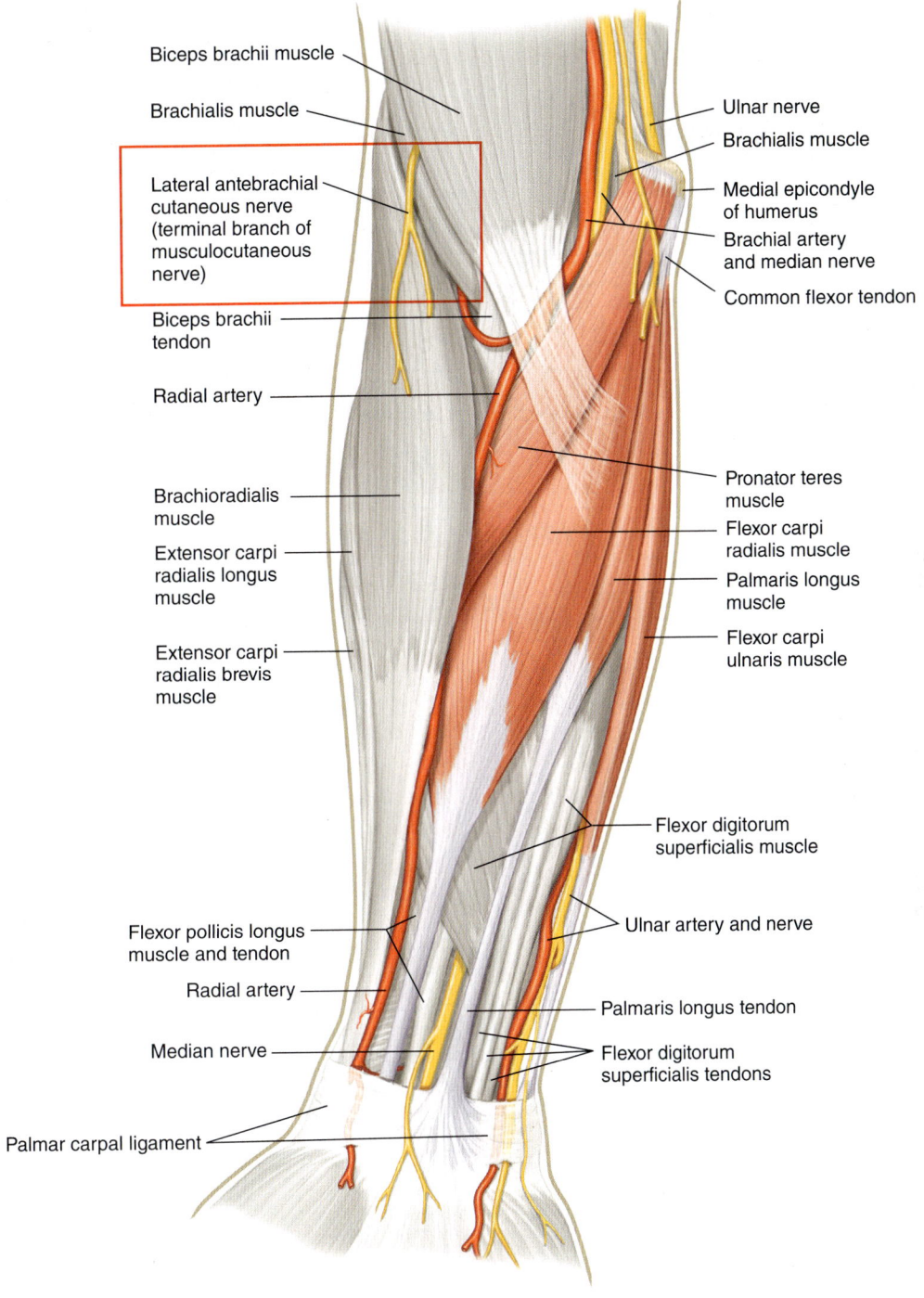

FIGURE 15-9 Anterior arm and forearm, superficial dissection. Box highlights common area of compression of lateral antebrachial cutaneous nerve. (Gest TR. *Lippincott Atlas of Anatomy*. 2nd ed. Wolters Kluwer; 2020: Plate 2-23.)

supply the biceps brachii and brachialis. The musculocutaneous nerve terminates as the lateral antebrachial cutaneous nerve after piercing the deep fascia near the cubital fossa (see Fig. 15-10). A sensory syndrome can be created with injury or compression of the lateral antebrachial cutaneous nerve at the cubital fossa or forearm.[31,32]

The posterior cord yields the axillary nerve that terminates in the arm and the radial nerve that travels down the arm from medial to lateral along the radial (spiral) groove of the humerus, supplying the triceps brachii. The radial nerve pierces the lateral intermuscular septum and enters the anterior compartment of the arm while descending between the

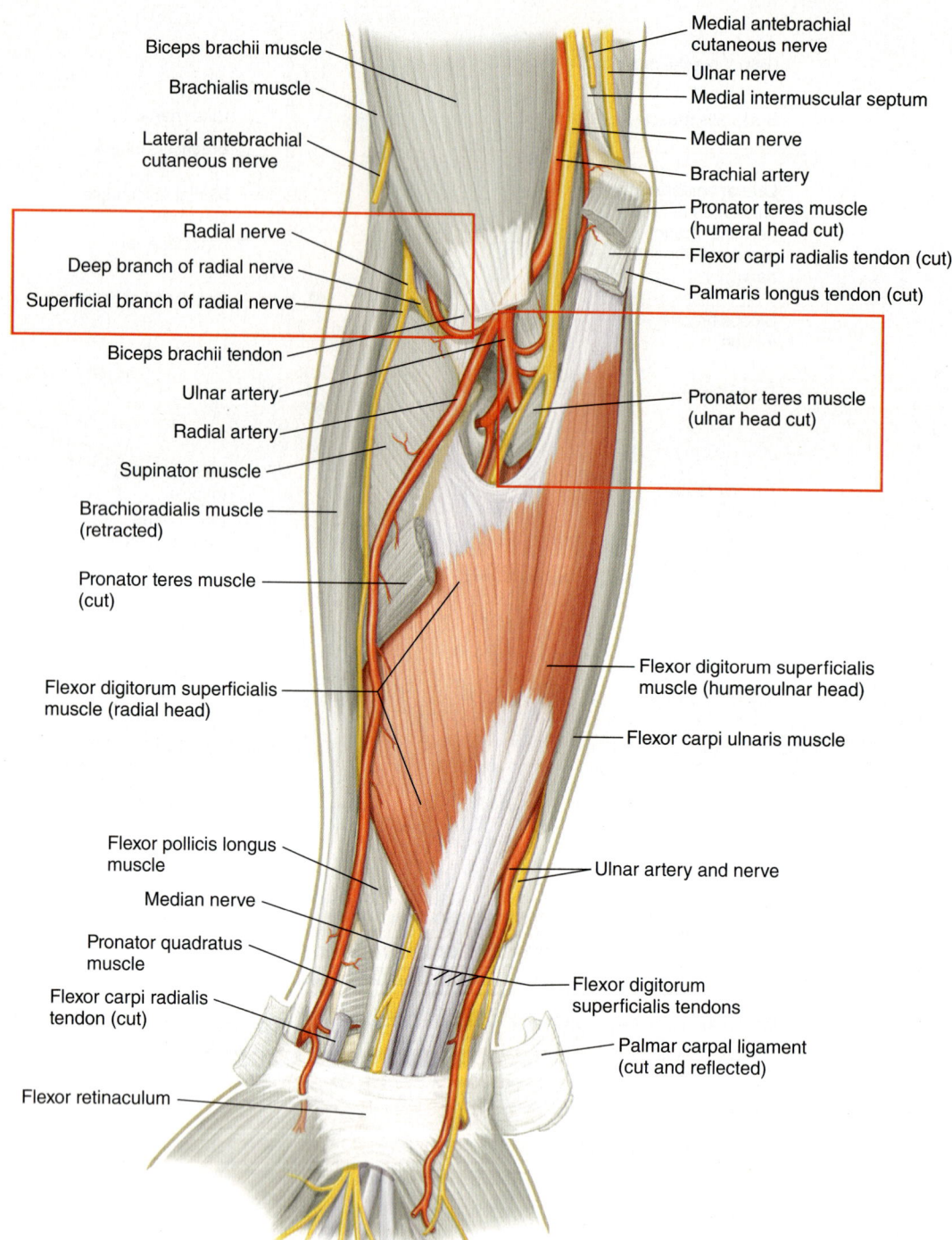

FIGURE 15-10 Anterior arm and forearm, intermediate dissection. Boxes highlight common areas of compression of radial nerve (and branches) and median nerve. (Gest TR. *Lippincott Atlas of Anatomy.* 2nd ed. Wolters Kluwer; 2020: Plate 2-24.)

brachialis and the brachioradialis. The radial nerve then passes anterior to the lateral epicondyle where it divides into two branches: the superficial branch of the radial nerve, supplying the sensation to the dorsal hand and fingers, and the deep branch of the radial nerve (deep radial or posterior interosseous nerve) that pierces the supinator, innervating this muscle and muscles that extend the wrist, fingers, and thumb,[6,33] leading to impaired ability to hold the wrist in extension, due to overpowering by the wrist flexor muscles.[34] Compression of the radial nerve or one of the branches due to trauma or sustained pressure

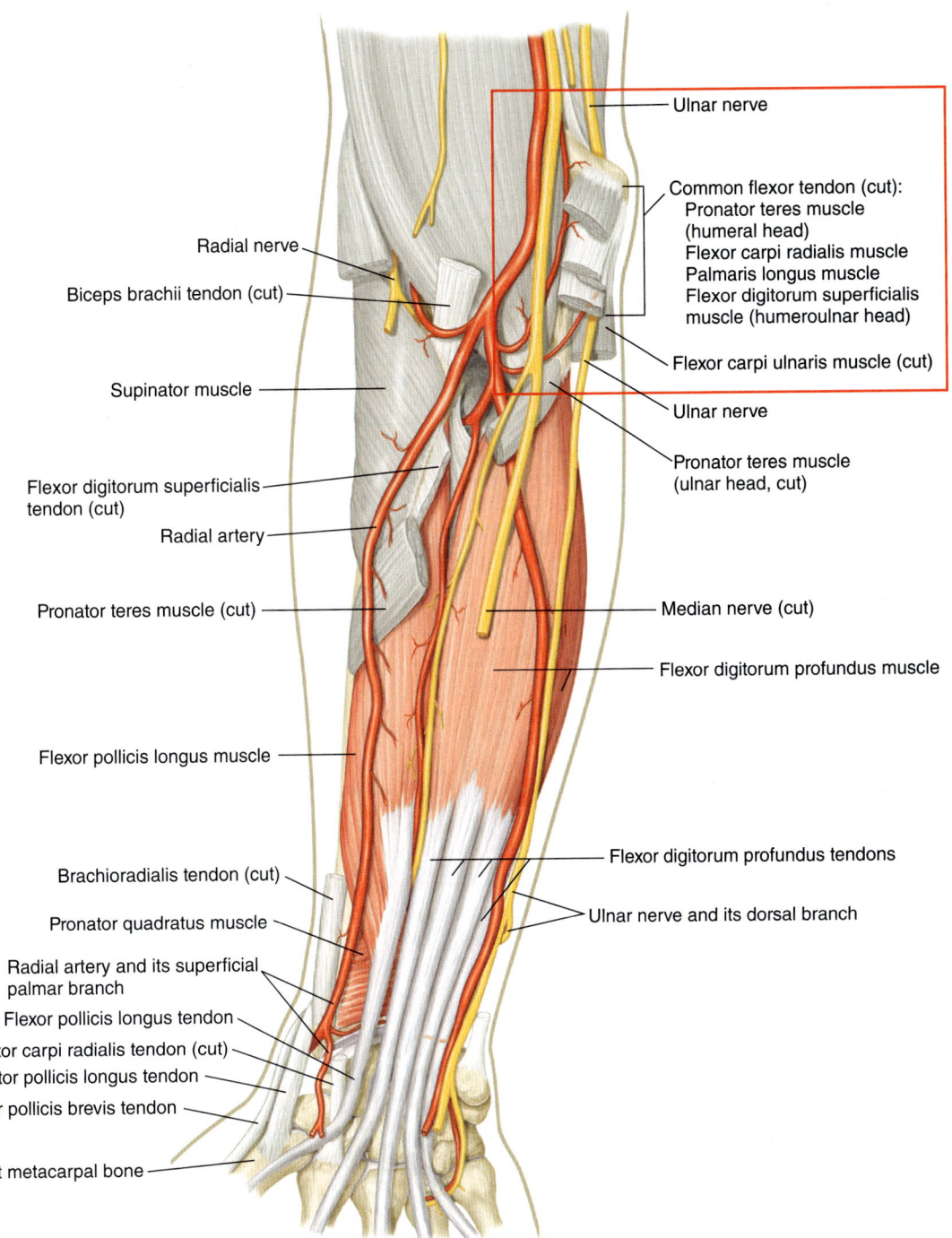

FIGURE 15-11 Anterior arm and forearm, deep dissection. Box highlights common area of compression of ulnar nerve at medial epicondyle and cubital tunnel. (Gest TR. *Lippincott Atlas of Anatomy*. 2nd ed. Wolters Kluwer; 2020: Plate 2-25.)

is not uncommon,[3] particularly as the nerve passes through the triceps,[35,36] at the radial groove of the humerus,[37,38] or as the deep radial nerve passes under a fibrous arch, the arcade of Frohse, along the superficial part of the supinator muscle (see Fig. 15-9).[36,39] Compression of the radial nerve above the elbow may lead to wrist drop.

The median nerve, formed by contributions from the lateral and medial cords of the brachial plexus, descends through the arm with the brachial artery, crossing anterior and lying medial to the brachial artery and biceps tendon and deep to the biceps aponeurosis in the antecubital fossa. The median nerve passes between the humeral (superficial) and ulnar (deep) heads of the PT and between the humeroulnar and the radial heads of the flexor digitorum superficialis (FDS) on its course to supply muscles of the anterior forearm, except for the flexor carpi ulnaris (FCU) and the medial half of the flexor digitorum profundus (FDP), five intrinsic hand muscles, and the thenar side of the palmar skin.[33] While several structures in the elbow region can compress the median nerve at the elbow,[40–43] the PT and associated fibrotic bands are a common cause of compression (see Fig. 15-9).[40,44,45] The biceps brachii aponeurosis, sometimes called the *lacertus fibrosus*, may compress the median nerve.

The ulnar nerve, a continuation of the medial cord of the brachial plexus, descends the arm piercing the medial intermuscular septum and passing anterior to the medial head of the triceps beneath a fascial band, the arcade of Struthers, that connects the triceps medial head to the intermuscular septum of the arm.[46,47] The ulnar nerve passes posterior to the medial epicondyle in the ulnar sulcus (groove), where it is quite superficial and vulnerable. The ulnar nerve continues distally, passing through the cubital tunnel, defined as a passageway whose floor consists of the posterior and transverse bundles of the MCL, the joint capsule, and olecranon. The roof is formed by the cubital tunnel retinaculum (also called *Osborne ligament*), which is a thick, arching, fascial band between the humeral and ulnar heads of the FCU.[48,49] After exiting the cubital tunnel, the ulnar nerve travels distally (see Fig. 15-10) between the FCU heads in the forearm to the wrist and hand. Though the ulnar nerve can be compressed at multiple sites along its course near the elbow, the most common site is in the cubital tunnel.[49,50] The cross-sectional area within the cubital tunnel decreases and ulnar nerve becomes more taut with elbow flexion, potentially contributing to compression.[51,52]

Elbow Complex Movement

The primary movement at the humeroulnar and humeroradial joints is flexion/extension with concurrent conjunct rotation, given that the ulna moves into slight pronation in extension and supination in flexion. Extension is limited by approximation of the olecranon in the olecranon fossa as well as tension in the anterior capsule and muscles. Full flexion is limited by soft-tissue approximation and entry of the radial head and tip of the ulnar coronoid processes into their respective fossae on the humerus (see Fig. 15-3). Normal extension is 0° to slight hyperextension, and flexion range is 140°[53] to approximately 150°.[1,54] The humeroradial and radioulnar joints allow approximately 80° of pronation and supination. Individuals with elbow movement limitations may still have functional use of the upper extremity, because only 30° to 130° of flexion/extension and 50° of rotation are required to perform most daily tasks.[53,55]

Pronation and supination movement of the forearm occurs at the radioulnar joints. Proximally, the radial head rotates (spins) on the capitulum within the AL and radial notch of the ulna. The distal radioulnar joint is formed by articulation between the convex ulnar head and the concave ulnar notch of the radius. In the supinated position, the radius is lateral and parallel to the ulna. With pronation, the radius moves anteromedially across the ulna, with the proximal radius remaining lateral and the distal radius, carrying the hand and moving to a medial position relative to the ulna (Fig. 15-12).[4]

Muscles

Attachments of muscles surrounding the elbow joint are listed in Table 15-2. The prime mover for elbow extension is the three-headed triceps brachii that inserts distally by a broad tendon to the olecranon. The anconeus crosses the elbow, and, along with the extensor carpi radialis longus (ECRL) and extensor carpi radialis brevis (ECRB), extensor digitorum (ED), extensor

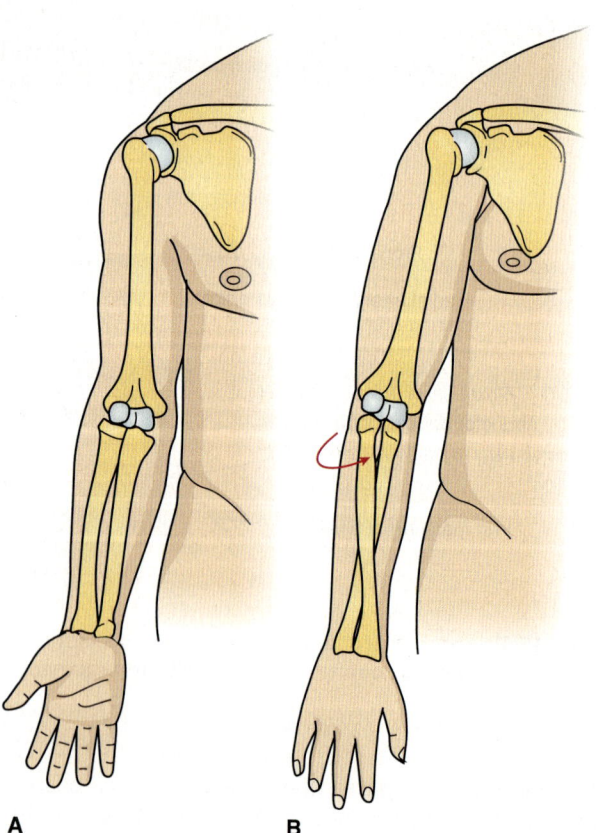

FIGURE 15-12 Supinated (**A**) and pronated (**B**) position of the forearm. Movement occurs at the proximal and distal radioulnar joints. (Adapted from Hamill J, Knutzen KM, Derrick TR. *Biomechanical Basis of Human Movement.* 5th ed. Wolters Kluwer; 2022: Figure 5-21.)

TABLE 15-2
PRIME MOVERS OF ELBOW

Group	Muscle (Innervation)	Attachments	Feature
Elbow extensors	Triceps brachii (radial nerve)	• Long head: infraglenoid tubercle of scapula to proximal end of olecranon • Medial head: posterior surface of humerus, inferior to radial groove to proximal end of olecranon • Lateral head: posterior surface of humerus superior to radial groove to proximal end of olecranon	Primary elbow extensor The long head resists dislocation of the glenohumeral joint; medial head is workhorse; lateral head is strongest, but recruited mostly against resistance
	Anconeus (radial nerve)	Lateral epicondyle of humerus to lateral surface of olecranon	Triangularly shaped; partially blends with medial head of triceps muscle; assists extension of elbow and tenses joint capsule to prevent pinching during extension
Elbow flexors	Brachialis (musculocutaneous nerve; lateral part by branch of radial nerve)	Distal half of anterior surface of humerus to coronoid process and tuberosity of ulna	Primary elbow flexor, working in all elbow positions; not affected by pronation or supination position of forearm
	Biceps brachii (musculocutaneous nerve)	• Short head: coracoid process to tuberosity of radius and fascia of forearm via bicipital aponeurosis • Long head: supraglenoid tubercle of scapula to tuberosity of radius and fascia of forearm via bicipital aponeurosis and indirect attachment to ulna via fascia	Elbow flexor; forearm supinator; long head resists dislocation of shoulder Action affected by position of forearm (strongest in supination)
	Brachioradialis (radial nerve)	Proximal two-thirds of supraepicondylar ridge of distal humerus to lateral surface of distal radius just proximal to styloid process	Weak elbow flexor; strongest when forearm is in midposition
Forearm pronators	Pronator teres (median nerve)	• Humeral head: medical epicondyle of humerus (part of common flexor origin) to middle convexity of lateral surface of radius • Ulnar head: coronoid process to middle convexity of lateral surface of radius	Forearm pronator
	Pronator quadratus (anterior interosseous nerve from median nerve)	Distal quarter of anterior ulna surface to distal quarter of anterior radius surface	Forearm pronator; quadrangular shape; helps bind the radius and ulna together
Forearm supinators	Supinator (deep branch of radial nerve)	Lateral epicondyle of humerus; radial collateral and annular ligaments; supinator fossa; crest of ulna to lateral, posterior and anterior surfaces of proximal third of radius	Forearm supinator; rotates radius to turn palm anteriorly, if elbow is extended; rotates radius to turn palm superiorly, if elbow is flexed

Adapted from Moore KL, Dalley AF, Agur AMR. *Clinically Oriented Anatomy*. 8th ed. Wolters Kluwer; 2018; Levangie P, Norkin C. *Joint Structure and Function: A Comprehensive Analysis*. 5th ed. F.A. Davis; 2011.

digiti minimi (EDM), and extensor carpi ulnaris (ECU) have proximal attachment to the lateral humeral condyle via the common extensor tendon and help stabilize the elbow joint during functional movement. The elbow and wrist extensor muscles are depicted in Figure 15-13.

Only three (biceps brachii, brachialis, and brachioradialis) of the nine muscles crossing the anterior aspect elbow joint contribute significantly to elbow joint movement. The brachialis is the main elbow flexor, participating in elbow flexion in all positions of the forearm. The contribution of the biceps brachii to elbow flexion is greatest when the elbow is flexed approximately 90° and the forearm is supinated. The brachioradialis is a weak flexor of the elbow, with greatest contribution occurring with the forearm in a neutral position. The supinator, PT, flexor carpi radialis (FCR), FCU, FDS, humeroulnar

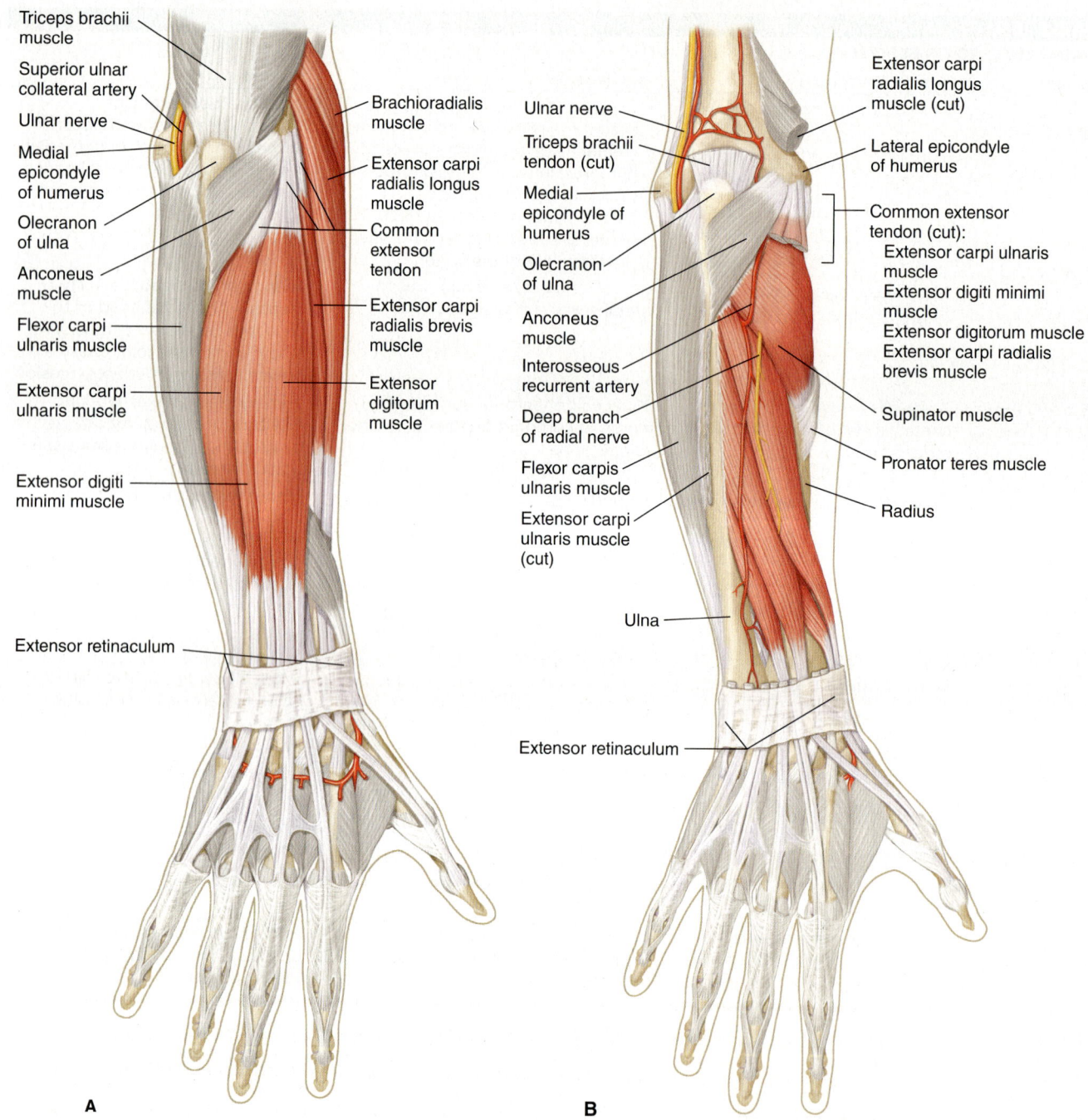

FIGURE 15-13 Elbow and wrist extensors. **A.** Superficial dissection. **B.** Deep dissection. (Gest TR. *Lippincott Atlas of Anatomy*. 2nd ed. Wolters Kluwer; 2020: Plates 2-29 and 2-30.)

head, and palmaris longus (PL) have a common origin from the medial epicondyle of the humerus and may weakly flex the elbow. These muscles are depicted in Figures 15-8 to 15-10.

The PT and the distally located pronator quadratus act to pronate the forearm. The supinator is a forearm supinator, along with the biceps brachii, particularly when the forearm is pronated. The common extensor and common flexor origins attach to their respective epicondyles outside the articular capsule.

Although the primary actions of the ECRL, ECRB, ED, EDM, ECU, FCR, FCU, FDS, and PL are at the wrist, hand, and fingers, these muscles have proximal attachment to the distal humerus common extensor or flexor sites. One of the main functions of the elbow is to position the wrist and hand for functional movements. Pathology of these muscles at the elbow can lead to significant functional deficits. For example, the repetitive use of the muscles attaching to the lateral humeral condyle, such as could occur with hammering, sawing, or gripping, may lead to cellular and tissue changes that thin and disrupt collagen fibers, changing the vascularity and cellular content and leading to chronic inflammation.

Stability of Elbow Joint

The stability of the elbow complex is provided by the interdependence of bony and ligamentous structures along with the forearm musculature.[20,56]

Passive stabilizers include the articulations, joint capsule, and ligaments. Muscles about the elbow provide dynamic stabilization.[3,57] Primary stabilizers include the humeroulnar bony congruency, AMCL, and LCLC, whereas the anterior capsule, forearm musculature, and radial head are secondary.[12,56,58]

Although at maximal degrees of elbow extension, small amounts of frontal plane laxity occur,[59] the elbow is inherently stable in this position. The valgus carrying angle of the humeroulnar joint predisposes the joint to valgus stress. The primary bony stability is provided at the humeroulnar joint, with contributions from both the olecranon and coronoid processes.[60] Stability is enhanced in extension as the olecranon locks into the olecranon fossa. In flexion, stability is increased as the coronoid process engages into the coronoid fossa[12,17] and the radial head meets the radial fossa.[12]

The interdependence of bony and ligamentous structures is demonstrated in cadaver studies in which stability is tested during serial resection of the olecranon or coronoid process, with and without intact ligamentous structures. The importance of the coronoid process to stability is highlighted by studies of serial olecranon resection indicating that upward of 70% of olecranon resection can occur before gross instability is observed as long as stabilizing ligaments remain intact.[59–62] The studies of the coronoid process underscore its contribution to resist posterior ulnar subluxation and posteromedial and posterolateral rotatory forces, with and without ligamentous deficiency.[59,63–65] Valgus laxity is greater with resection of the MCL than with resection of the radial head. Removal of both the MCL and the radial head results in gross instability.[56] These findings support the role of the MCL as a primary stabilizer, whereas the bony support of the radial head provides secondary stabilization.[2]

The individual elbow complex ligaments provide both frontal plane and rotary stabilities. The MCL, particularly the anterior portion, the AMCL, is crucial for stabilization against the valgus and pronation rotatory stresses throughout the range of motion.[20,66] During overhead motions such as throwing, the MCL may take up as much as 50% of the valgus stress.[67] With repetitive overhand throwing, laxity of the MCL leads to a valgus extension overload, resulting in posteromedial osteophytes from the repetitive wedging of the olecranon in the olecranon fossa.[3,68] The posterior bundle of the MCL provides greater restraint to valgus forces as elbow flexion range increases.[1]

The anterior joint capsule contributes resistance to varus and valgus stress and distraction, primarily when the elbow is in extension.[14,15,17] By virtue of anatomic connections, the anterior capsule likely limits posterior dislocation.[15,20] As the elbow moves toward flexion, the ligaments contribute more whereas the joint capsule contributes less to stability.

The muscles crossing the elbow joint contribute to compression of the joint surfaces and thereby help to stabilize the joint.[2] The wrist extensors and anconeus are dynamic stabilizers against varus stress,[69–71] whereas the pronator-flexor muscle group stabilizes against valgus stress,[1] such as occurs in overhand throwing.[72] For example, loading of the PT relieves the valgus stress to the elbow,[72] and in the presence of MCL deficiency, the FCU and FDS act as primary and secondary stabilizers, respectively.[72,73] In high-level baseball pitchers, the forces generated across the elbow exceed the tensile strength of the AMCL, indicating muscular forces are important as stabilizers of the elbow.[3]

Although technically not part of the elbow joint complex, the interosseous membrane (IOM), a ligamentous complex that binds together the radius and the ulna in the forearm, contributes to stability by transmitting compression forces proximally from the radius to the ulna and subsequently through the elbow, as well as distally through the wrist.[74] This transfer of compressive force distributes the load between the humeroulnar and humeroradial joints, such that the shared compressive force reduces the load to either joint individually.[75] The majority of fibers of the IOM form the central band, whose fibers are obliquely oriented distally and medially from the radius to the ulna (see Fig. 15-6).[74,76] Less substantial ligamentous bands of the IOM have been observed, including a proximal oblique cord, accessory band, and dorsal oblique cord, whose functions are not clearly defined.[75,76] Contraction of elbow flexors, pronators, and supinators, which have distal attachment to the radius, results in a pulling of the radius proximally against the capitulum, particularly when the elbow is near extension. The IOM central band helps to shift some of the compression force of weight bearing through the hand from the radius to the ulna, thereby protecting the humeroulnar joint.[77,78] The fiber orientation of the central band does not favor resistance of distally applied forces to the radius, such as when holding a heavy bucket or suitcase. The distraction force slackens the IOM, requiring other tissues such as the AL or brachioradialis to resist the load by holding the radius against the capitulum.[69,79] Chronic application of large distractive loads could result in tears to the IOM and reduced elbow stability.[77]

ARTHROKINEMATICS

The three joints of the elbow complex allow for the independent osteokinematic movements of flexion/extension (through the humeroulnar and humeroradial joints) and pronation/supination (through the radioulnar joints). The tight fit of the articular surfaces guides and restricts movement at the elbow.

Arthrokinematics of the Humeroulnar Joint

The concave sagittal plane and convex frontal plane orientation of the sellar-shaped trochlear notch of the ulna fits snugly to the trochlea of the ulna, although the articulation is not equally congruent throughout the range of motion (Fig. 15-14). Extension is limited by the bony articulation of the olecranon in the olecranon fossa along with the extensibility of the anterior soft tissues (elbow flexors, anterior joint capsule, anterior fibers of the AMCL). In flexion, the concave surface of the trochlear notch rolls and slides on the convex trochlea with full flexion requiring elongation of the posterior soft tissues, including the posterior joint capsule, elbow extensors, portions of the collateral ligaments, and the ulnar nerve.[80] Repetitive flexion activities can lead to irritation of the ulnar nerve, resulting in neuropathy, which is sometimes treated with decompression or transposition of the nerve to a location anterior to the medial epicondyle.[80,81]

Arthrokinematics of Humeroradial Joint

The cuplike concave depression (fovea) of the proximal radial head articulates with the convex capitulum, compressed against the capitulum by contracting muscles during flexion and extension. The mediolateral axis of rotation is the center of the capitulum. The radial fovea rolls and slides on the capitulum, as depicted in Figure 15-15. The humeroradial joint is a significant secondary stabilizer resisting valgus stress.[66] Refer to the previous section in this chapter on elbow stability for a discussion of impact of the IOM on resistance of compression and distraction forces on the humeroradial joint.

Arthrokinematics of the Proximal Radioulnar Joint

The articulation of the radius and ulna proximally and distally allows forearm rotation (pronation and supination) to occur about the axis of rotation that extends from the radial head through the ulnar head and passing through both joints.[82] The transfer of forces through the IOM reduces stress to the proximal radioulnar joint, providing some protection.[77]

Rotation of the hand can occur without concurrent rotation of the ulna or the humerus. Supination and pronation at the proximal radioulnar joint occurs as the radial head spins within the fibro-osseous ring formed by the radial notch and AL. Owing to the intimate fit

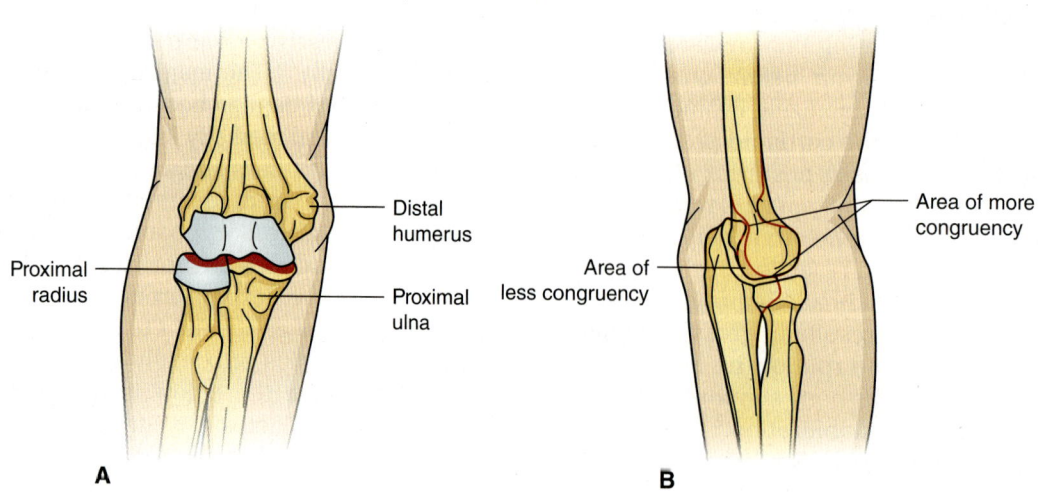

FIGURE 15-14 Articulation of trochlear notch of ulna with distal humerus. **A.** Anterior view demonstrating relative congruency. **B.** Lateral view demonstrating areas of congruency and noncongruency. (Adapted from Oatis, CA. *Kinesiology: The Mechanics and Pathomechanics of Human Movement*. 3rd ed. Wolters Kluwer; 2017: Figures 11.13 and 11.14.)

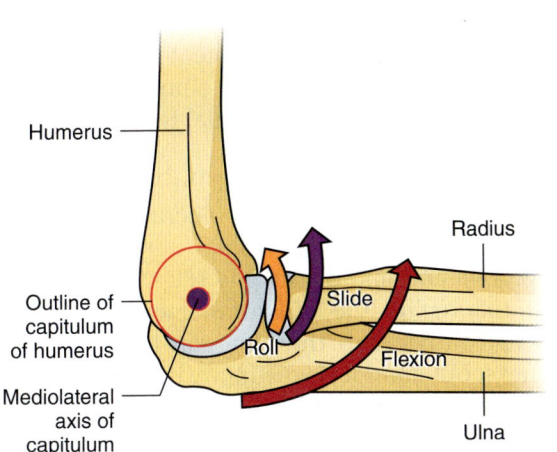

FIGURE 15-15 Sagittal section of elbow at 90° flexion. Mediolateral axis of rotation is the center of capitulum. (Adapted from Gest TR. *Lippincott Atlas of Anatomy*. 2nd ed. Wolters Kluwer; 2020: Plate 2-43B.)

of the radial head within the space, expected roll-and-slide arthrokinematic movement is not observed.[83] The ulna connects firmly to the humerus at the humeroulnar joint and remains relatively stationary during rotational movement of the forearm, although a slight counterrotation of the ulna relative to the radius at the humeroulnar joint has been described.[84] The lack of direct connection between the distal ulna and the wrist-hand complex allows the carpal bones and radius to rotate freely around the ulna. With the humerus free to rotate at the glenohumeral joint, the ulna can rotate during pronation and supination.[79]

In upper extremity weight bearing with the radius and hand fixed, pronation and supination occurs at the proximal radioulnar joint by rotation of the AL and radial notch of the ulna around the fixed radial head. For example, consider a gymnast with hands placed on the parallel bars, such that the elbows are straight, wrists extended, and hands firmly fixed (Fig. 15-16). In this situation, the movement of forearm pronation and supination involves internal and external rotation of the humerus at the glenohumeral joint owing to the tight bony articulations at the humeroulnar joint. With a starting point of the forearm in full supination (i.e., radius and ulna are parallel), the muscular force couple creating pronation is that of the infraspinatus externally rotating the humerus on the fixed scapula and the pronator quadratus rotating the ulna on the fixed radius. The AL and radial notch of the ulna rotate around the fixed radial head, and the capitulum spins relative to the fovea of the fixed radius.[79]

PALPATION

Palpation of the elbow involves locating bony prominences (medially, laterally, and posteriorly) and identifying the cubital fossa (anterior), surrounding musculature, and nerves.

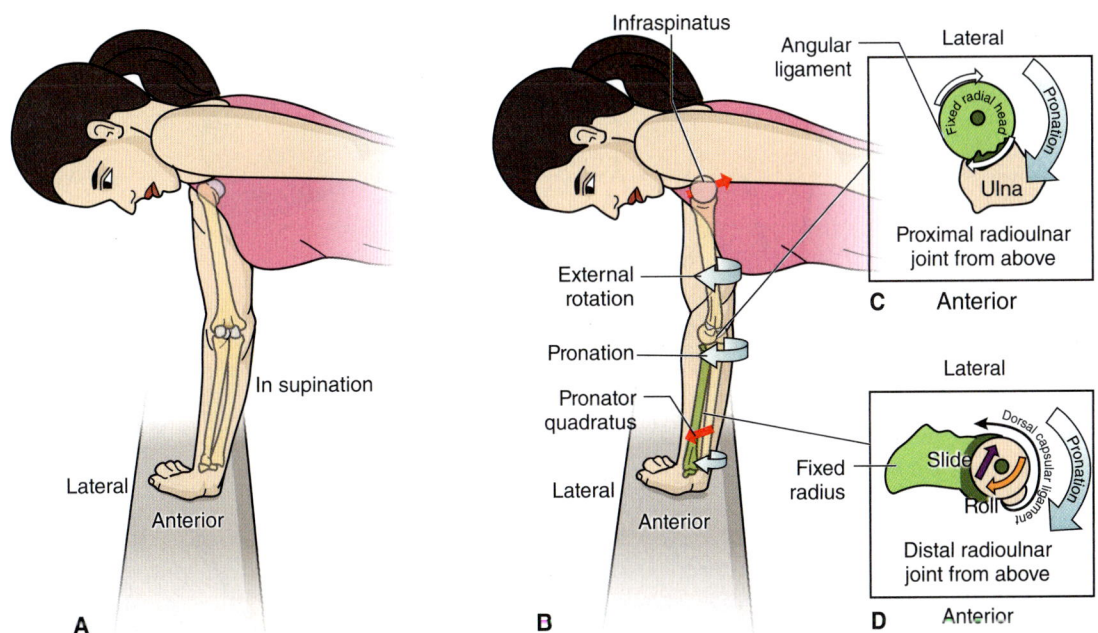

FIGURE 15-16 Gymnast shown supporting her upper body weight through the right forearm, which is in full supination (i.e., the bones of the forearm are parallel). **A.** The radius is fixed, but the humerus and ulna are free to rotate. **B.** The humerus and ulna have rotated externally from the initial position (**A**), showing pronation of the forearm as the ulna rotates around the fixed radius. The force couple between the infraspinatus and pronator quadratus muscles is demonstrated. The two insets show a superior view of the arthrokinematics at the proximal (**C**) and distal (**D**) radioulnar joints.

With the patient's elbow straight, the clinician can easily palpate the medial and lateral epicondyles of the distal humerus as large, subcutaneous bony prominences located on the distal medial and lateral end of the humerus, respectively. Just proximal to the epicondyles, the supracondylar ridges can be felt. On the posterior elbow between and in line with the epicondyles, the olecranon can be felt. With the elbow bent 90°, a triangle is formed between the epicondyles and the olecranon (Fig. 15-17). An appreciable deviation in the relative orientation of these bony prominences suggests an anatomic disruption, such as fracture or dislocation, and warrants further investigation.

After palpating the proximal posterior border of the olecranon, the elbow can be partially extended as the palpating fingers move superiorly, allowing palpation of the olecranon fossa. Moving the fingers laterally, the lateral epicondyle and lateral supracondylar ridge can be felt. With the patient's elbow at 90° and forearm in neutral (neither pronated nor supinated), the muscle mass of the brachioradialis, ECRL, and ECRB can be palpated between the lateral epicondyle and the midpoint of the anterior cubital fossa. The brachioradialis muscle becomes particularly prominent with resisted elbow flexion with the forearm in this neutral position. With movement of the fingers laterally to the lateral epicondyle, inferolaterally, and just below the lateral epicondyle, the radial head can be palpated in the depression just medial and posterior to the wrist extensor group muscular attachment. Supination and pronation of the forearm with the elbow partially bent facilitates identification of the radial head as it rotates within the AL.

On the posteromedial side of the elbow between the medial epicondyle and the olecranon, the ulnar groove can be palpated. The ulnar nerve can be felt in the groove and just proximally (Fig. 15-18). Just inferior to this region, the MCL attachment between the medial epicondyle and the ulna can be checked for tenderness, but cannot be distinctly palpated because of the thickness of overlying tissues. Moving the palpating fingers to the anterior medial epicondyle, the common wrist flexor attachments can be felt. To identify the location of the superficial pronator-flexor muscles and tendons, the clinician can place the palm and extended fingers of the opposite hand on the anterior forearm, as shown in Figure 15-19.

INTRODUCTION TO THE EXAMINATION OF THE ELBOW

Most elbow conditions are either traumatic, from falls or athletics, or due to degenerative conditions, from overhead throwing or repetitive use in occupations requiring manual labor. Peripheral nerve injuries are more common in the elbow/forearm region than in the shoulder or lower extremity and must be considered

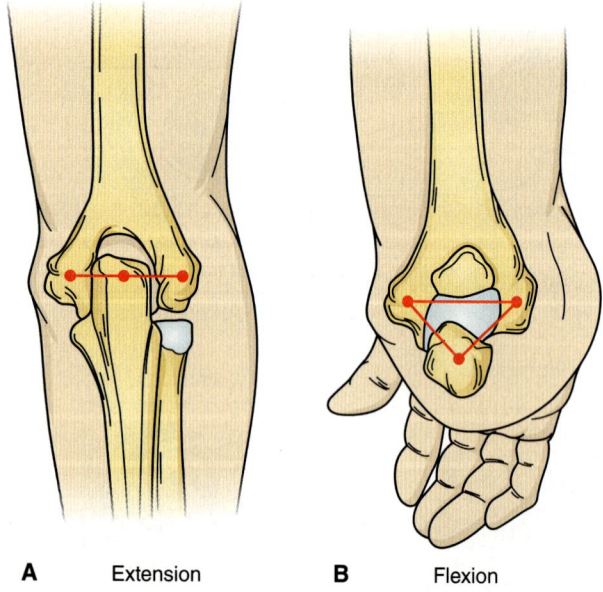

A Extension **B** Flexion

FIGURE 15-17 Bony prominences of the elbow shown in posterior view with elbow extended. The epicondyles and olecranon are in a straight line when the elbow is extended (**A**) and form a triangle when the elbow is flexed 90° (**B**). (Adapted from Oatis, CA. *Kinesiology: The Mechanics and Pathomechanics of Human Movement*. 3rd ed. Wolters Kluwer; 2017: Figure 11.9.)

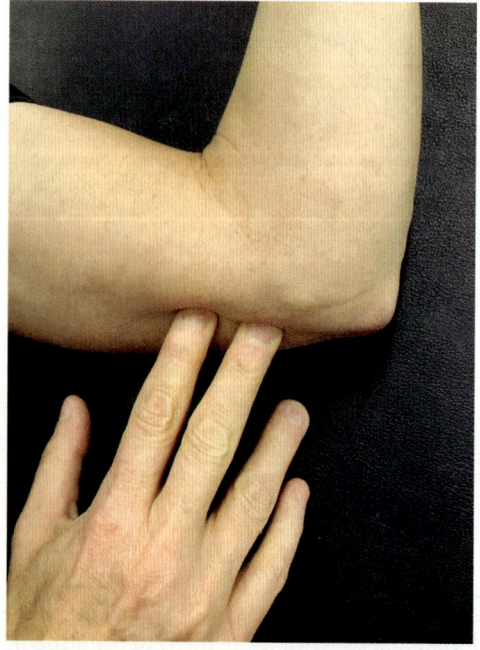

FIGURE 15-18 Palpation of ulnar nerve just proximal to medial epicondyle.

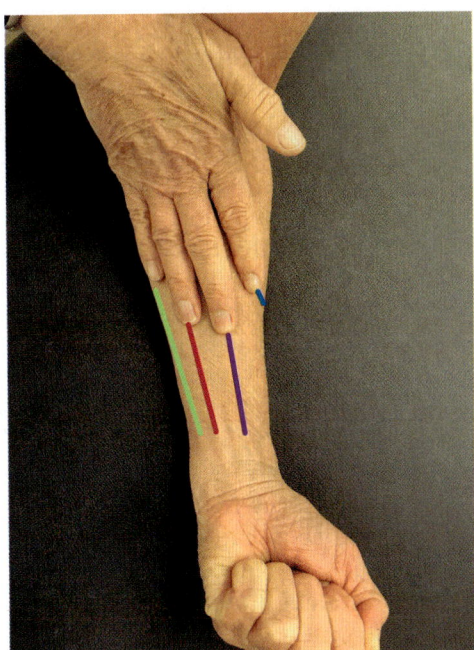

FIGURE 15-19 Orientation of pronator-flexor muscles in the anterior forearm. With the hand placed as shown, the path of muscle-tendons toward their attachments can be identified: index finger to PT, middle finger to FCR, ring finger to palmaris longus and fifth to FCU. *FCR* flexor carpi radialis; *FCU*, flexor carpi ulnaris; *PT*, pronator teres.

in cases of paresthesias, weakness, or atrophy. The elbow is largely derived from C6 and C7 nerve roots and may, therefore, be the site of referred pain from other structures of the same derivation.

PATIENT HISTORY: ELBOW COMPLEX

As noted with other body regions, the history is critical to guiding an efficient and effective physical examination for patients with elbow/forearm symptoms. Unlike the lower extremity, the elbow functions more often in the open kinetic chain, making it less affected by conditions of the contralateral extremity.

Review of Systems

It is important to know about prior elbow and forearm injuries, even if remote. For example, degenerative changes of the radiohumeral or humeroulnar joint may result from a childhood fracture. Likewise, the clinicians must be aware of any prior surgeries in the region because MCL reconstruction can injure the medial antebrachial cutaneous nerve, whereas a distal biceps repair may affect the lateral antebrachial cutaneous nerve.[85] The clinician must ask about any systemic diseases, such as rheumatoid arthritis or gout, as these often involve the elbow.

Onset

Understanding the mechanism of onset of elbow symptoms can help with developing diagnostic hypotheses. The possibility of fracture must be considered in cases of traumatic onset of elbow pain, whereas overuse injuries, such as tendinopathy, should be considered in individuals who participate in throwing or swinging sports. An insidious onset of elbow symptoms in an older individual would be suggestive of osteoarthritis (OA).

Location of Symptoms

Localization of symptoms can be useful in creating diagnostic hypotheses because many elbow conditions create local symptoms that are amenable to palpation. For example, medial elbow symptoms in a tennis player are suggestive of pronator-flexor pathology, whereas lateral symptoms are suggestive of lateral epicondylalgia. Vague or poorly localized symptoms may be referred due to nerve compression.[86]

Chief Complaint

Clinicians should determine the quality, severity, and irritability of symptoms. Mechanical symptoms, such as catching, clicking, or locking, suggest intra-articular pathology.[87] Numbness, tingling, or shooting symptoms suggest involvement of one of several peripheral nerves that cross this region. Muscle atrophy and motor weakness also suggest nerve compression. For example, anterior interosseous syndrome involves only the motor branch and leaves the patient with an inability to position the fingers, such that the thumb and index finger form a circle whereas the other fingers are straight. Instability suggests ligamentous pathology.

Clinicians should determine exacerbating and relieving activities, asking specifically about symptoms with lifting, carrying, gripping, swinging, and throwing. For example, most individuals with ulnar collateral ligament injuries have medial elbow symptoms during the late cocking phase of throwing.[88]

Personal Factors

Knowing patient hand dominance and sport or vocation is critical to understanding tissue loading and assists with preliminary differential diagnoses. Has the patient started a new job, changed to a new racquet with a wider grip, attempted a new pitch, or altered exercise habits recently that may have contributed to the chief complaint?

Outcome Measures

The Disabilities of Arm, Shoulder, and Hand Questionnaire (see Chapter 14, Shoulder Complex) and the Patient-Specific Functional Scale (see Chapter 6, Patient History) can be useful outcome tools for patients with elbow symptoms. Elbow-specific outcome measures include the Patient-Rated Elbow Evaluation, American Shoulder and Elbow Surgeons Elbow Form, the Elbow Self-Assessment Score, and the Oxford Elbow Score (Table 15-3).

PHYSICAL EXAMINATION: ELBOW COMPLEX

As noted in Chapter 13, Upper Quarter Screen, the physical examination is composed of the systems review, the quarter screen, the clearing examination, and the joint-specific examination. However, the clinician must first be alert to any potential red flags. For the elbow complex, the most common red flags to consider are fracture and dislocation.

Elbow fracture should be considered in individuals with a traumatic onset of elbow pain, particularly those who are older or have a history of osteoporosis. Clinical tests to identify elbow fracture include[89,90]:

- The elbow extension test
- The elbow flexion test

To perform the tests, the patient flexes both shoulders to 90° and then attempts to fully straighten or bend both elbows. The inability to fully actively straighten or bend the elbow is considered a positive test. Negative tests have been shown to adequately rule out elbow fractures in children and adults.[90,91] Unfortunately, while isolated bony tenderness helps rule in fracture in other regions, the same is not true for the elbow.[89]

In the pediatric population, nursemaid's elbow or distal subluxation of the radial head must be considered. A history of a sudden onset of elbow pain, typically after a traction type injury, such as a parent grabbing a child by the hand to prevent the child from falling, warrants further investigation.[92] The typical presentation of a patient with a radial head subluxation would be a child between the ages of 1 and 4 years who is in mild distress without excessive effusion or deformity, refuses to use the arm, and holds the arm in elbow flexion and forearm pronation.[93] Although radiographs are generally not helpful in diagnosis, a closed reduction may relieve symptoms and allow return to function.[94]

Once the patient has been cleared of any red flags and the history and systems review have been performed, the clinician should perform an upper quarter

TABLE 15-3
COMMON OUTCOME TOOLS FOR PATIENTS WITH SHOULDER PATHOLOGIES

Tool	Tool Basics
Patient-Rated Elbow Evaluation (PREE)*,†	• 20 items divided into two sections: pain (5) and function (15) • Scoring: 0-100, with higher scores indicating greater limitation • Minimum clinically important difference 7 points • Common diagnoses: elbow osteoarthritis, after elbow surgery, epicondylalgia
American Shoulder and Elbow Surgeons Elbow Form (pASES-e)*,‡	• 18 items divided into three sections: pain (0-10), function (0-3), and satisfaction (0-10) • Scoring: overall percentage with lower scores indicating greater limitation • Minimal detectable change: 16 points • Common diagnoses: elbow osteoarthritis, after elbow surgery, various elbow pathologies
Elbow Self-Assessment Score (ESAS)‡	• Scoring: converted to a percentage, with lower scores indicating greater limitation • 22 items rated 0-10 • Domains: pain, elbow function, and quality of life • Common diagnoses: elbow osteoarthritis, fracture or dislocation in the elbow region, epicondylalgia
Oxford Elbow Score	• 12 items rated 1-5, with lower scores indicating higher function • Domains: pain, elbow function, social/psychological • Scoring: 0-48 • Common diagnoses: elbow osteoarthritis

*Vincent JI, MacDermid JC, King GJW, Grewal R, Lalone E. Establishing the psychometric properties of 2 self-reported outcome measures of elbow pain and function: a systematic review. *J Hand Ther.* 2019;32(2):222-232; Vincent JI, MacDermid JC, King GJW, Grewal R. Linking of the Patient Rated Elbow Evaluation (PREE) and the American Shoulder and Surgeons e Elbow questionnaire (pASES-e) to the International Classification of Functioning Disability and Health (ICF) and hand core sets. *J Hand Ther.* 2015;28(1):61-68.
†Macdermid JC, Silbernagel KG. Outcome evaluation in tendinopathy: foundations of assessment and a summary of selected measures. *J Orthop Sports Phys Ther.* 2015;45(11):950-964.
‡Beirer M, Friese H, Lenich A, et al. The Elbow Self-Assessment Score (ESAS): development and validation of a new patient-reported outcome measurement tool for elbow disorders. *Knee Surg Sports Traumatol Arthrosc.* 2017;25(7):2230-2236.

screen (UQS) and a clearing examination (in this case, active and passive shoulder and wrist range of motion) to ensure that the area of pathology has been narrowed down to the elbow/forearm region and any proximal potential contributing factors have been identified. All components of the joint-specific examination need not be performed on every patient. Like the UQS, the experienced clinician will titrate the joint-specific examination based on the patient history, presentation, and goals. In practice, the joint-specific examination is organized by position and should proceed from uninvolved (or less involved) to involved side but is presented here by category to aide conceptualization.

Structure

Observe the patient's general appearance and body structure. The elbow should be observed for symmetry in elbow's carrying angle, atrophy, and edema. An increased carrying angle (cubital valgus) (see Fig. 15-6) has been seen in professional baseball players, possibly due to repetitive valgus stress.[86] An elbow with effusion is often held in about 70° of flexion (the open-packed position) as this is the position with the greatest capsular volume.[95] Because abnormal findings at the shoulder or the scapula may affect elbow kinematics,[95] the patient's posture should be observed in both sitting and standing.

Skin

Clinicians should inspect the skin for scars, effusion, or localized areas of edema, such as olecranon bursitis. Redness, drainage, or more generalized edema is suggestive of infection.

Range of Motion

Active physiologic elbow, forearm, and wrist range of motion and passive overpressure should be assessed and compared with normative values (Table 15-4).[54] It is common for individuals to have elbow hyperextension, but this should be symmetrical side to side.[87] Recall, full motion is not necessary for most daily activities. Baseball players, particularly pitchers, typically have about a 5°[96] loss of elbow extension.[97] Forearm motion should be assessed with the elbow in 90° of flexion and adducted to the body to prevent glenohumeral joint compensation.[87] Wrist flexion and extension range of motion is key to include as part of the standard examination not only as part of a clearing examination as the joint distal to the elbow, but because the wrist flexors and extensors are commonly involved in elbow pathologies, such as epicondylalgia.

The clinician should note any changes in symptoms with motion. Mechanical symptoms such as clicking and locking are more suggestive of loose bodies within the joint,[87,95] whereas crepitus may indicate OA. Elbow effusion frequently results in a capsular pattern of restriction in which flexion is more limited than extension. Pain with extension may be the result of posterior impingement and is often seen in throwers and gymnasts.[85]

The normal endfeel for flexion is soft-tissue opposition, but may be bony in extremely slender individuals. The normal endfeel for extension is firm or bony. Endfeels for pronation and supination are typically firm due to capsular or ligamentous restriction, but may muscular as well. A premature hard endfeel may represent bony impingement due to osteophyte formation or abnormal fracture healing.[86] A premature soft endfeel is common with effusion or soft-tissue swelling.

TABLE 15-4

PASSIVE RANGE OF MOTION NORMATIVE VALUES

Motion	Normative Value (degrees)
Elbow flexion	0–150
Elbow extension	0
Supination	0–80–90
Pronation	0–80–90
Wrist flexion	0–80
Wrist extension	0–70
Wrist radial deviation	0–20
Wrist ulnar deviation	0–30

Muscle Length

When working with patients with elbow pathology, the clinician must be mindful of the effect of two-joint muscles (Table 15-5), such as the long head of the biceps brachii. Normal long head of biceps length is 60° of shoulder extension with the elbow straight. If shoulder extension measured in the standard position (with the elbow flexed) is greater than when measured with the elbow extended, a restriction in the long head of the biceps is confirmed. Targeting the supinator for stretching may be beneficial for radial tunnel syndrome[98] or supinator strains. To minimize the impact of the biceps on range of motion, the elbow should not be extended. To provide a consistent position for tracking changes in muscle length over time, the standard measurement position of 90° of elbow flexion is recommended. The ECRL proximal attachment is high enough on the supracondylar region to impact elbow extension range of motion, whereas the remaining wrist muscles is inconsequential. Because several wrist flexors and extensors cross both the elbow and the wrist, it may be wise to perform stretches with the elbow in 90° flexion as well as fully extended. Additional two-joint muscles of the forearm and hand are discussed in Chapter 16, Wrist and Hand Complex.

TABLE 15-5
TARGETED STRETCHING OF MUSCLES ABOUT THE ELBOW

Muscle	Method*
Biceps brachii	Shoulder extension, forearm pronation, followed by elbow extension
Supinator	Elbow flexed 90° followed by forearm pronation
Pronator teres	Forearm supination, followed by elbow extension
Extensor carpi radialis longus	Elbow extension, wrist ulnar deviation, followed by wrist flexion
Extensor carpi radialis brevis	Elbow flexed 90°, wrist ulnar deviation, followed by wrist flexion
Flexor carpi radialis†	Wrist ulnar deviation, followed by wrist extension
Flexor carpi ulnaris†	Wrist radial deviation, followed by wrist extension

*Performing stretches in the order indicated is recommended because the last motion provides a large arc of motion that can be measured to track changes over time.
†These muscles are extremely weak elbow flexors and, therefore, may be slightly affected by elbow position. It may be beneficial to stretch them with the elbow extended and flexed 90°.

TABLE 15-6
TARGETING SPECIFIC MUSCLES VIA MANUAL MUSCLE TESTING

Muscle	Method
Biceps brachii	Resist elbow flexion at 90° with the forearm supinated
Brachioradialis	Resist elbow flexion at 90° with the forearm in neutral
Brachialis	Resist elbow flexion at 90° with the forearm pronated
Pronator teres	Resist forearm pronation with the elbow in midrange
Pronator quadratus	Resist forearm pronation with the elbow at end-range flexion
Supinator	Resist forearm supination with • elbow 90° flexed, arm by side • elbow extended, shoulder extended • elbow flexed, shoulder 90° flexed Resistance with elbow fully flexed significantly reduces biceps assistance

Muscle Performance

Manual muscle testing is the most common method of assessing muscle performance of elbow flexor and extensors and forearm pronators and supinators. Kendall[99] recommends precise positioning when attempting to target one muscle over another (Table 15-6). This is particularly useful for identifying muscle strains, tendinopathies, and nerve entrapments. Measuring grip strength using a handheld dynamometer (Fig. 15-20) is particularly useful for objectifying strength deficits, and pain-free grip strength can be used for tracking changes in patients with epicondylaglia[100] or peripheral nerve pathologies.

Sensory Tests

As noted previously in this chapter, the musculocutaneous, radial, median, and ulnar nerves and branches may be compressed or irritated in multiple locations in the distal arm and elbow region. Therefore, the clinician must be keenly aware of the normal sensory nerve distribution of the upper extremity (see Fig. 7-5). Individuals with paresthesias, atrophy, or profound

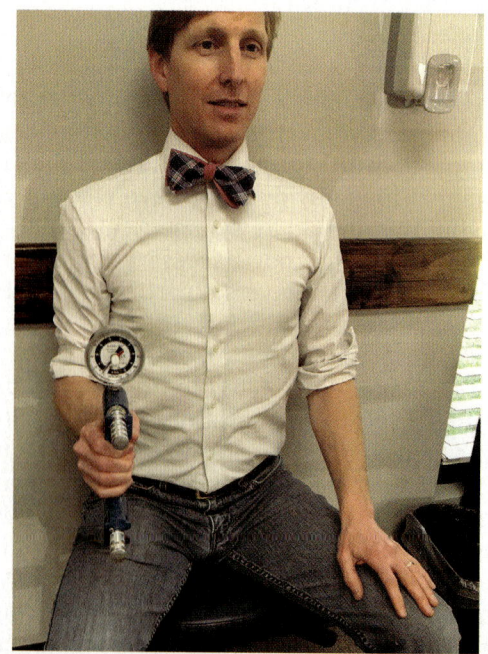

FIGURE 15-20 Grip testing using a handheld dynamometer.

weakness and a negative upper quarter neurologic screen should be carefully assessed for peripheral nerve injuries. For example, compression of the ulnar nerve at the cubital tunnel (cubital tunnel syndrome) can lead to altered sensation along the ulnar side of the hand and fourth and fifth digits along with difficulties performing normal daily activities such writing due to weakness of hand muscles that are innervated by the ulnar nerve.[101]

Reflexes

If a patient reports paresthesias, the clinician should assess the biceps, brachioradialis, and triceps reflexes to assess possible upper or lower motor neuron involvement. The Hoffman test (described in Chapter 13, Upper Quarter Screen) may be used to help identify an upper motor neuron lesion.[102]

Neurodynamic Testing

Neurodynamic testing, including the upper limb tension test (ULTT) (described in Chapter 17, Cervical and Thoracic Spine), should be performed on patients with suspected cervical or upper thoracic pathology with symptoms into the upper extremity. Positive findings mandate a closer examination of spinal structures.

Accessory Motion

Joints should be assessed for hypermobility or hypomobility and the presence or absence of pain.

Humeroulnar Lateral Tilt

Purpose: To assess joint-play movement necessary for terminal elbow extension.
Patient: Supine with arm by the side, elbow near end-range extension. A small towel roll can be placed under the distal humerus.
Clinician: Supports the patient's arm just proximal to the elbow with the superior hand. Grasps the forearm with the inferior hand. For improved support and control, the clinician can hold the forearm against the trunk.
Mobilization: While stabilizing the arm, the clinician creates a medial glide (tilt) with the inferior hand (Fig. 15-21). The mobilization can also be performed in reverse, with the forearm being stabilized and the mobilization being performed by having the superior hand glide the humerus medially.

Humeroulnar Medial Tilt

Purpose: To assess joint-play movement necessary for terminal elbow extension.
Patient: Supine with arm by the side, elbow near end-range extension. A small towel roll can be placed under the distal humerus.
Clinician: Supports the patient's arm just proximal to the elbow with the superior hand. Grasps the forearm with the inferior hand. For improved support and control, the clinician can hold the forearm against the trunk.
Mobilization: While stabilizing the arm, the clinician creates a medial glide (tilt) with the inferior hand (Fig. 15-22). The mobilization can also be performed in reverse, with the forearm being stabilized and the mobilization being performed by having the superior hand glide the humerus laterally.

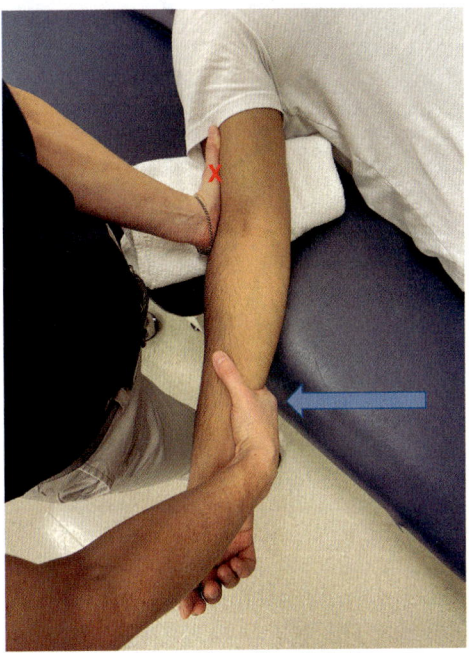

FIGURE 15-21 Humeroulnar lateral tilt.

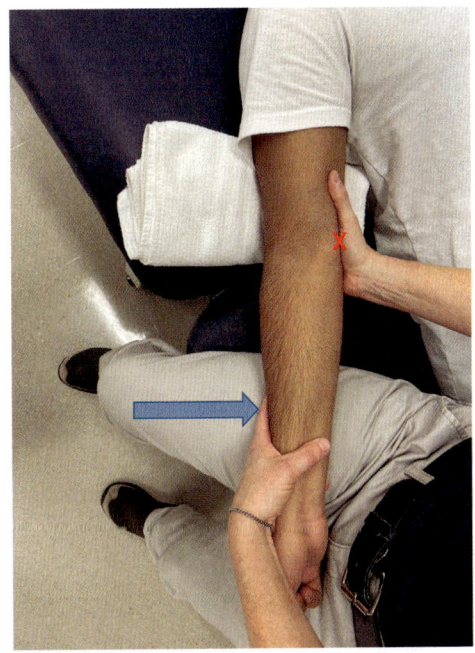

FIGURE 15-22 Humeroulnar medial tilt.

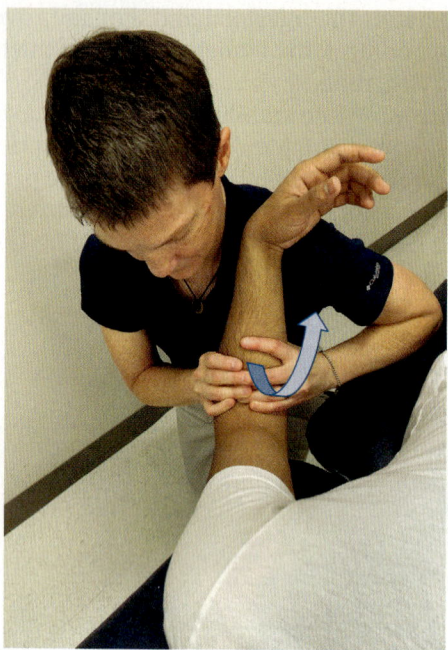

FIGURE 15-23 Humeroulnar distraction.

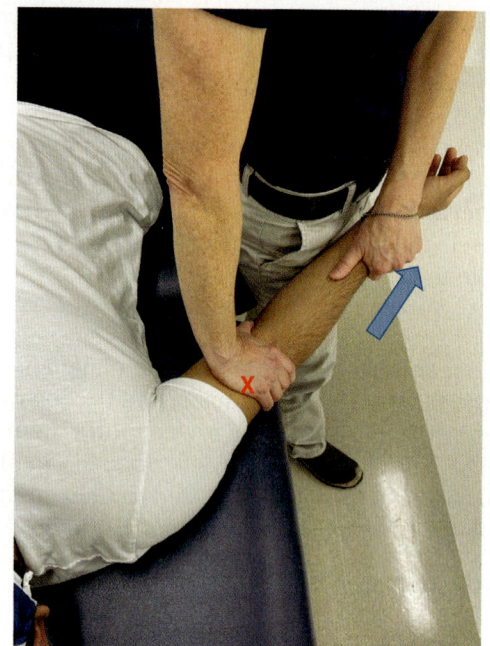

FIGURE 15-24 Humeroradial distraction.

Humeroulnar Distraction

Purpose: To assess global joint mobility.
Patient: Supine with arm by the side.
Clinician: The clinician supports the forearm on the clavicular region so that the elbow is in approximately 70° of flexion. The clinician grasps the proximal ulnar with both hands, interlacing the fingers if desired.
Mobilization: The clinician creates a distraction force by leaning backward (Fig. 15-23). When used to gain motion, the patient is positioned near end-range flexion and the clinician leans backward and uses the hands to create a scooping motion toward elbow flexion.

Humeroradial Distraction

Purpose: To assess global joint mobility.
Patient: Supine with arm by the side and elbow extended and forearm supinated.
Clinician: While stabilizing the distal humerus against the table with the superior hand, the clinician grasps lateral forearm with thenar eminence and the distal radius with the fingers wrapping around posteriorly.
Mobilization: The clinician creates a longitudinal distraction force by rotating the trunk to the left (Fig. 15-24).

Proximal Radioulnar Dorsal Glide (and Dorsal Radiohumeral Glide)

Purpose: To assess joint-play movement necessary for pronation and extension.
Patient: Supine with arm by the side and elbow extended and forearm supinated.
Clinician: The clinician stabilizes the proximal ulna with the medial hand. The clinician moves the flexor-pronator mass laterally to contact the radial head with the thumb of the lateral hand. The fingers then wrap around the posterior radius.
Mobilization: The mobilizing hand glides the radius posteriorly (Fig. 15-25). This mobilization also creates a dorsal glide of the radius on the humerus, which can be used to increase elbow extension. The mobilization to gain more elbow extension can be made more aggressive by positioning the elbow near end-range extension.

Proximal Radioulnar Ventral Glide (and Ventral Radiohumeral Glide)

Purpose: To assess joint-play movement necessary for supination and flexion.
Patient: Supine with arm by the side and elbow comfortably flexed.
Clinician: The inferior hand stabilizes the ulna. The superior hand displaces the extensor muscles dorsally to allow the thenar eminence to more directly contact the radial head.
Mobilization: A ventral glide is created by the thenar eminence (Fig. 15-26). Note that a dorsal glide can be performed by pulling dorsally with the fingers of the superior hand. The mobilization to gain more elbow flexion can be made more aggressive by positioning the elbow near end-range flexion.

CHAPTER 15 | ELBOW COMPLEX

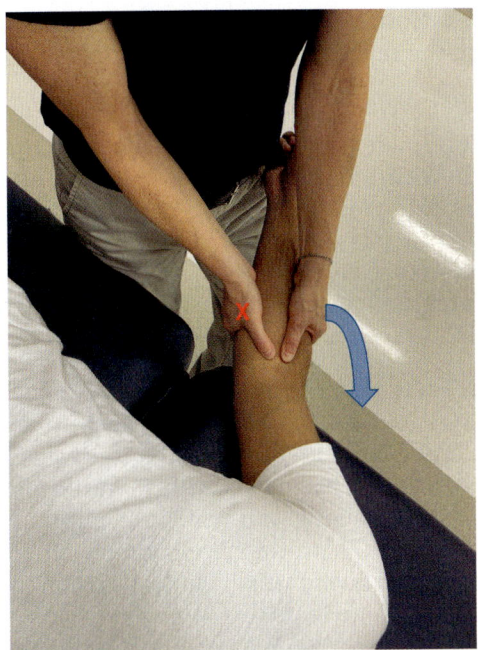

FIGURE 15-25 Proximal radioulnar dorsal glide (and dorsal radiohumeral glide).

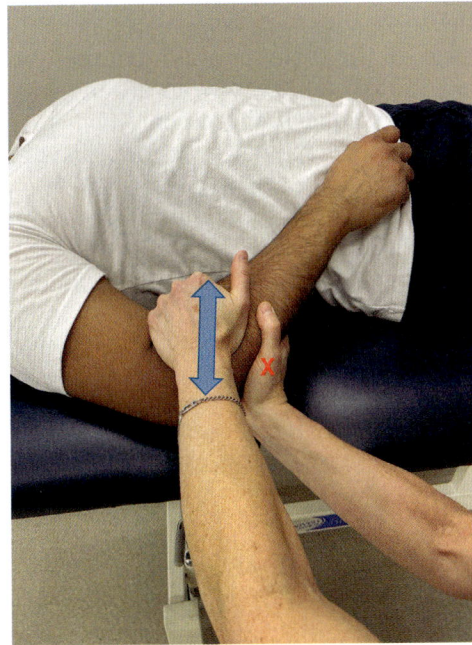

FIGURE 15-26 Proximal radioulnar ventral glide (and ventral radiohumeral glide).

Distal Radioulnar Dorsal Glide

Purpose: To assess joint-play movement necessary for supination.
Patient: Seated with the forearm resting on the table, forearm in about 10° of supination.
Clinician: The clinician stabilizes the distal ulna with the lateral hand. The thenar eminence of the mobilizing hand contacts the distal radius and the fingers wrap around to contact the dorsal radius. The mobilization can be made more aggressive for gaining supination by placing the patient near end-range supination.
Mobilization: A dorsal glide is created by the thenar eminence (Fig. 15-27).

Distal Radioulnar Ventral (or Palmar) Glide

Purpose: To assess joint-play movement necessary for pronation.
Patient: Seated with the forearm resting on the table, forearm in about 10° of supination.
Clinician: The clinician stabilizes the distal ulna with the lateral hand. The thenar eminence of the mobilizing hand contacts the distal radius and the fingers wrap around to contact the ventral radius.
Mobilization: A ventral glide is created by the thenar eminence (Fig. 15-28). The mobilization can be made more aggressive for gaining pronation by placing the patient near end-range pronation.

Special Tests/Provocative Testing

Clinicians should choose which special/provocative tests to perform based on the patient history and physical examination to this point in order to help rule in and rule out competing differential diagnoses. For elbow/forearm pathology, these tests may be grossly grouped into three main categories: epicondylalgia, instability, and peripheral nerve pathology (Fig. 15-29).

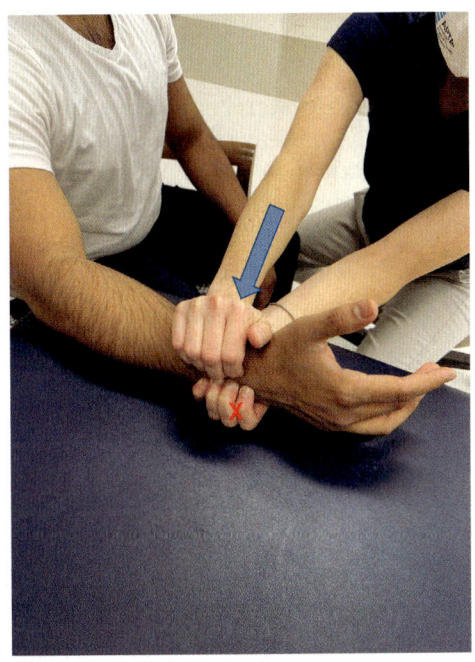

FIGURE 15-27 Distal radioulnar dorsal glide.

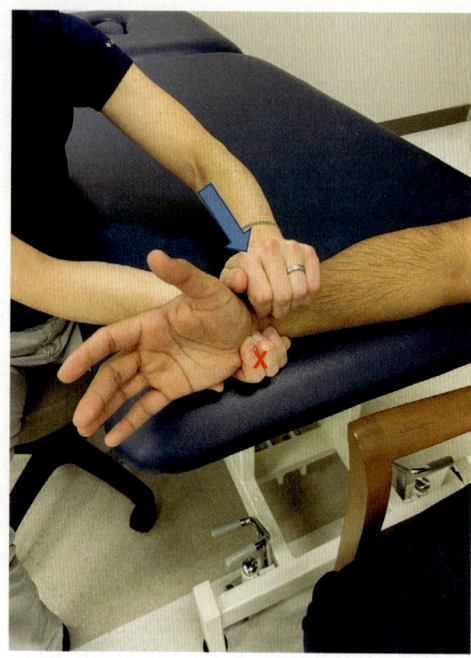

FIGURE 15-28 Distal radioulnar ventral (or palmar) glide.

Special Tests for Epicondylalgia

Resisted Wrist Extension and Radial Deviation Test (aka Cozen Test)

Purpose: To identify lateral epicondylalgia.
Method: With the patient seated, forearm pronated and supported on the table, the clinician resists wrist extension and radial deviation[87] by applying pressure against the dorsal 2nd metacarpal (Fig. 15-30).
Interpretation: A positive test is reproduction of pain in the region of the lateral epicondyle.

Resisted Third Finger Extension Test (aka Maudsley Test)

Purpose: To identify lateral epicondylalgia.
Method: With the patient seated, forearm pronated, hand supported on a table, the clinician resists third finger extension (Fig. 15-31).[87]
Interpretation: A positive test is reproduction of pain in the region of the lateral epicondyle.

Passive Lateral Epicondylalgia Test (Mill Test)

Purpose: To identify lateral epicondylalgia.
Method: With the patient seated or standing, the elbow is extended with the forearm pronated, then the wrist is passively moved into flexion and ulnar deviation (see Fig. 15-42B).[103]
Interpretation: A positive test is reproduction of pain in the region of the lateral epicondyle.

Special Tests for Elbow Instability

Valgus elbow instability is a common pathology seen in throwing athletes and can be identified using the valgus stress test or the moving valgus stress test. Varus instability is seen less frequently and can be identified via the varus stress test. Posterolateral rotatory elbow instability (PLRI) can be identified clinically using the chair push-up or push-up tests.

Valgus Stress Test

Purpose: To identify injury to the MCL, particularly the anterior bundle.[98,104,105]
Method: With the patient seated or standing and elbow flexed 20 to 30°, the clinician places the superior hand on the distal lateral humerus to create a medial force. The fingers wrap around the arm to palpate the medial humeroulnar joint space. The clinician supports the patient's forearm with the inferior hand and trunk. The clinician then creates a valgus stress on the elbow by rotating the trunk to the right (Fig. 15-32).
Interpretation: A positive test is reproduction of the patient's medial elbow pain, palpable joint gapping, or lack of a firm endfeel.

Moving Valgus Stress Test

Purpose: To identify injury to the AMCL by performing a dynamic stress to the MCL that simulates the throwing motion.[98,104,106]

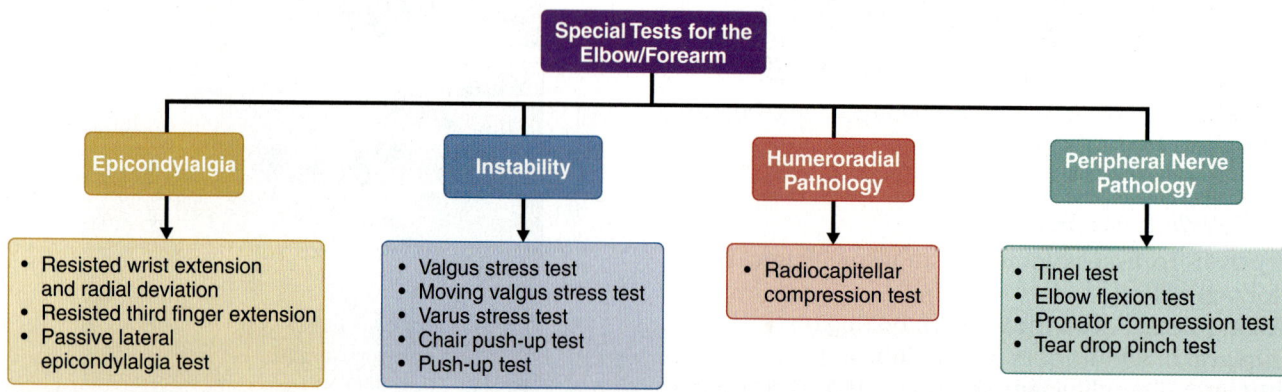

FIGURE 15-29 Special tests for elbow and forearm pathology.

CHAPTER 15 | ELBOW COMPLEX 537

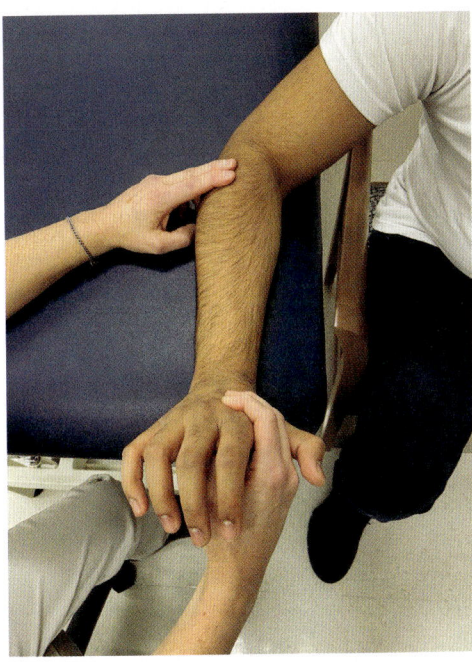

FIGURE 15-30 Resisted wrist extension and radial deviation test (aka Cozen test).

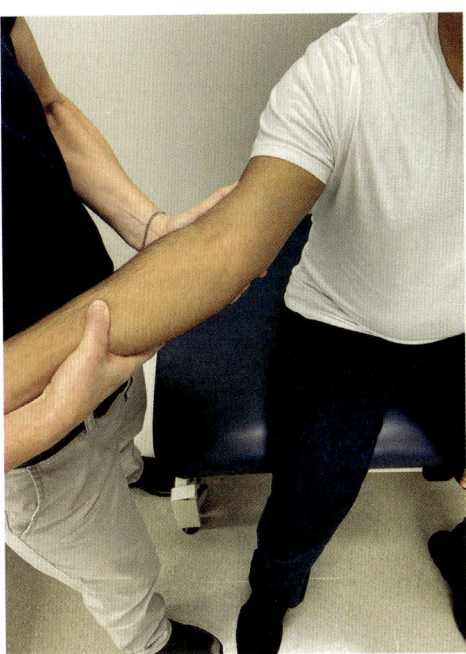

FIGURE 15-32 Valgus stress test.

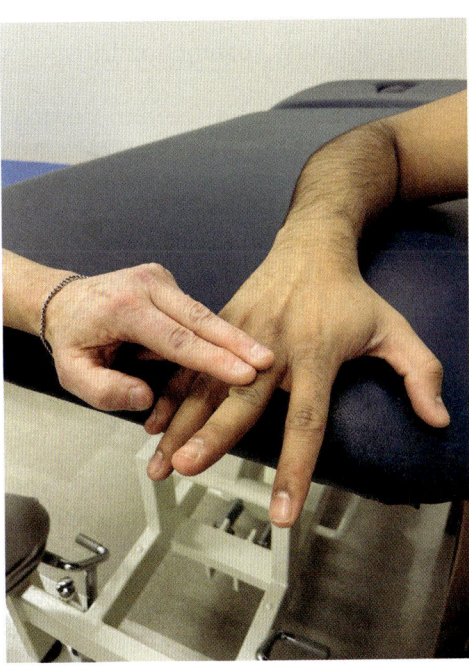

FIGURE 15-31 Resisted third finger extension test (aka Maudsley test).

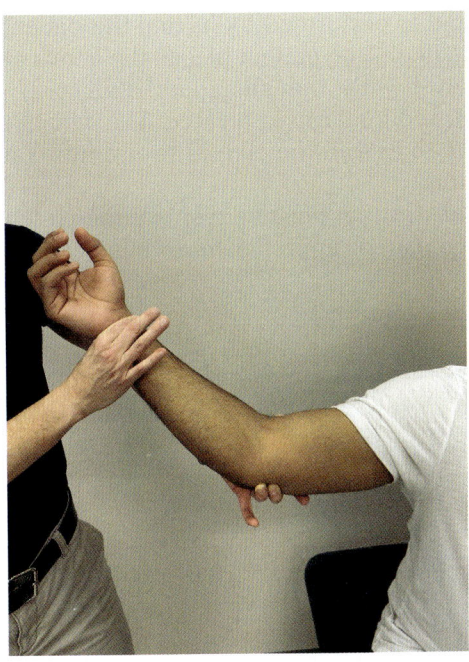

FIGURE 15-33 Moving valgus stress test.

Method: With the patient seated or standing and shoulder abducted to 90°, and the elbow maximally flexed, the clinician applies a valgus force to the elbow. While maintaining the valgus stress, the elbow is extended (Fig. 15-33).

Interpretation: A positive test is reproduction of the patient's medial elbow pain between 70 and 120° of elbow flexion.

Varus Stress Test

Purpose: To identify injury to the RCL.[105]

Method: With the patient seated or standing and elbow flexed 20 to 30°, the clinician places the medial hand on the distal medial humerus to create a medial force. The fingers can be wrapped around the arm to palpate the lateral humeroulnar joint space. The clinician supports the patient's forearm with the lateral hand and trunk. The clinician then creates a varus stress on the elbow by rotating the trunk to the left (Fig. 15-34).

Interpretation: A positive test is reproduction of the patient's lateral elbow pain or increased varus laxity compared to the contralateral side.

Chair Push-Up Test

Purpose: To identify PLRI.[98,107]
Method: The seated patient places the hands on the armrest of the chair with shoulders abducted, elbows flexed, and forearms supinated. The patient then extends the elbows to rise off the chair (Fig. 15-35).
Interpretation: A positive test is if the patient experiences pain or apprehension while performing the test.

Push-Up Test

Purpose: To identify PLRI.[98,107]
Method: The push-up test is a more stressful alternative and is performed by having the patient prone on the floor. The patient places the hands at shoulder level with the shoulders abducted, elbows flexed, and forearms supinated. The patient then attempts to extend the elbows to rise into a push-up position.
Interpretation: A positive test is if the patient experiences pain or apprehension while performing the test.

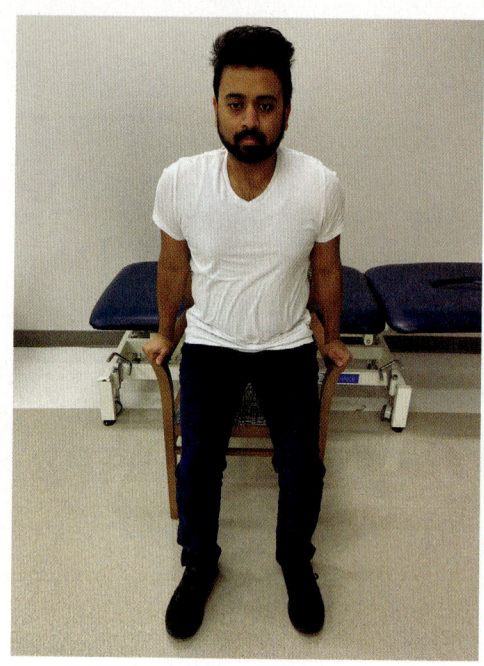

FIGURE 15-35 Chair push-up test.

Special Test for Humeroradial Pathology

Radiocapitellar Compression Test

Purpose: To identify osteochondritis dissecans (OCD).
Method: With the patient's forearm resting on the table, the clinician stabilizes the patient's humerus with the lateral hand and grasps the patient's hand in a "handshake" position with the medial hand. The clinician applies an axial load to the radius with the medial hand and then rotates the patient's forearm into pronation and supination (Fig. 15-36).
Interpretation: A positive test is recreation or exacerbation of pain in the humeroradial joint region with testing. The test may also be positive with humeroradial arthritis or radial head fracture.

Special Tests for Peripheral Nerve Pathology
A Tinel test, tapping over an affected superficial nerve, is likely to provoke the patient's paresthesias within the sensory distribution of the nerve. For example, to help identify cubital tunnel syndrome, the clinician would tap posterior to the medial epicondyle of the humerus in the region of the ulnar nerve (see Fig. 15-49) and a positive test would be the production or exacerbation of paresthesias in the ulnar wrist, ulnar hand, the fifth finger, and half of the fourth finger.[86,104]

Elbow Flexion Test

Purpose: To identify ulnar nerve pathology at the cubital tunnel.[50,86,98]
Method: The patient sits with the elbows flexed and wrists extended for 1 to 3 minutes (Fig. 15-37).

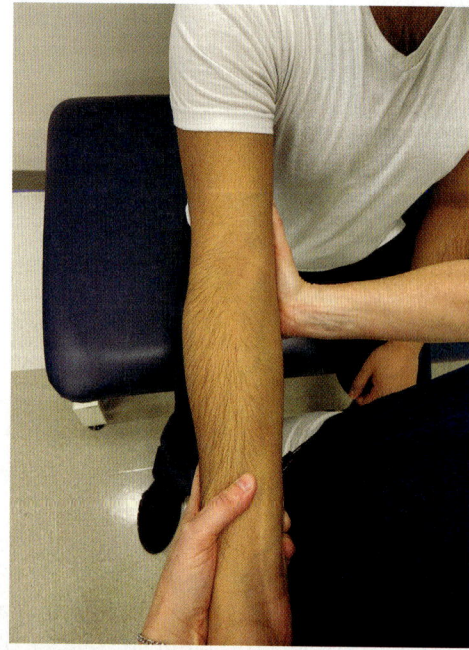

FIGURE 15-34 Varus stress test.

the proximal volar forearm just proximal and lateral to the PT muscle belly for 30 to 60 seconds (Fig. 15-38).

Interpretation: A positive test is production or exacerbation of paresthesias in the thenar eminence, index, middle, and radial half of the fourth fingers.

Tear Drop Pinch Test

Purpose: To identify an anterior interosseous nerve lesion.

Method: The patient attempts to make a circle by touching the tips of the index finger and thumb.

Interpretation: If a teardrop shape (Fig. 15-39) is made rather than a circle due weakness of the anterior interosseous innervated flexor pollicis longus

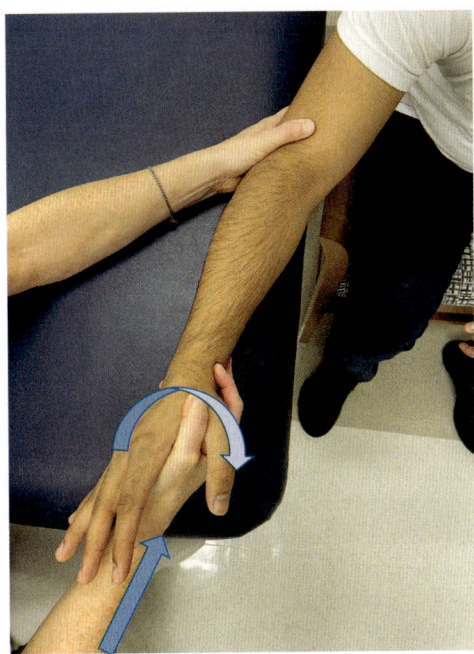

FIGURE 15-36 Radiocapitellar compression test.

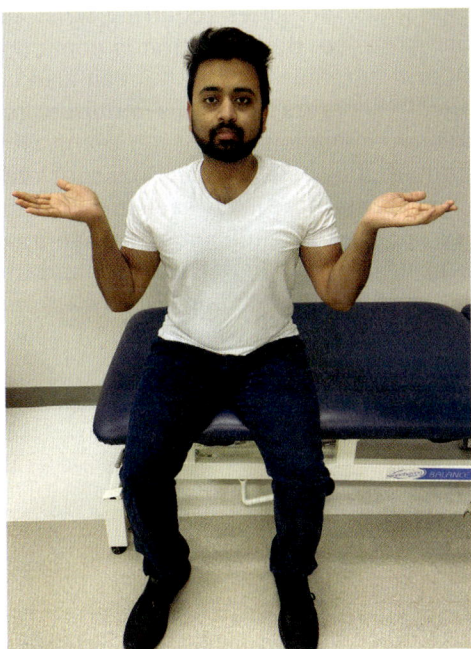

FIGURE 15-37 Elbow flexion test.

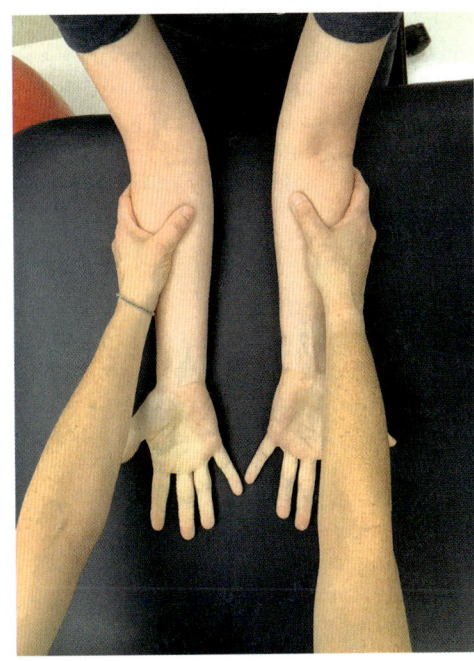

FIGURE 15-38 Pronator compression test.

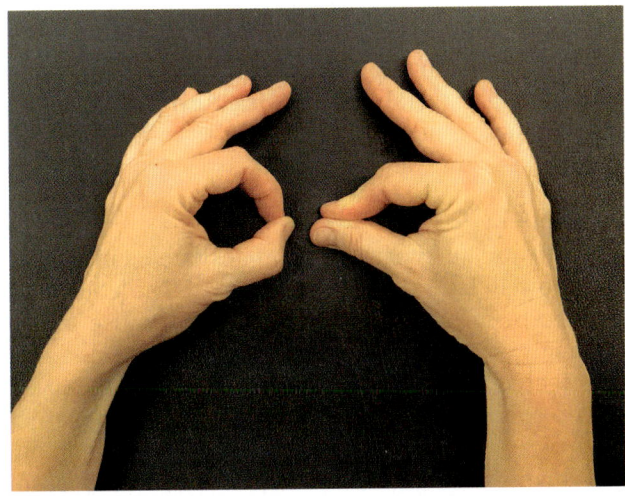

FIGURE 15-39 Teardrop pinch test. Normal on left, positive on right.

Interpretation: A positive test is production or exacerbation of paresthesias in the ulnar wrist/hand or the fifth and ulnar half of the fourth digit.

Pronator Compression Test

Purpose: To identify pronator syndrome.[108,109]

Method: With the patient seated and forearms resting on the table in supination, the clinician compresses

(FPL) and FDP being unable to flex the interphalangeal (IP) joint of the thumb and distal interphalangeal (DIP) of index finger.[108,110]

Palpation

Clinicians should palpate structures for tenderness as noted in the palpation section. Many important elbow structures are superficial, honest tissues, simplifying identification of many pathologies. For example, warmth and edema of the posterior olecranon can indicate olecranon bursitis,[87] gout,[87] or infection,[87] where tenderness in an adolescent male thrower may indicate an olecranon stress fracture.[111] Tenderness of the epicondyle in a skeletally immature patient may indicate an epiphyseal plate injury.[86] The ulnar nerve is superficial posterior to the medial epicondyle, and palpation or percussion, which reproduces a patient's symptoms, is consistent with ulnar neuritis or cubital tunnel syndrome. An MCL injury is a common source of elbow instability. When acutely injured, there may be tenderness when palpating the sulcus just distal to the medial epicondyle.[86]

Functional Testing

Functional testing for the elbow complex can include a wide variety of tasks. Lower level function can be assessed by observing the patient perform fine motor tasks, such as tip-to-tip pinch or manipulating objects of daily living, such as writing with a pen. Higher level functional tasks may include weight-bearing tasks such as using an arm rest to rise from sitting or performing a push-up. Video analysis of faster activities, such as swinging a racquet or throwing a ball, can provide insights into biomechanical faults that may be the source of or contributing to the patient's chief complaint.

COMMON ELBOW PATHOLOGIES

This section contains details on the most common or most problematic elbow pathologies, including epicondylalgia, instability, OA, fracture, compression neuropathies, tendon ruptures, bursitis, apophysitis, OCD, and internal derangement.

Lateral Epicondylalgia

Pathology The most common lesion occurring at the elbow is lateral epicondylalgia.[112] The condition has also been coined "tennis elbow," because of the frequency with which recreational tennis players are affected. Although historically referred to as *lateral epicondylitis*, researchers have failed to detect signs of an inflammatory process.[87] Lateral epicondylalgia most frequently affects the extensor carpi radialis brevis (ECRB), just distal to its attachment on the epicondyle. It is thought that this tendon is more susceptible to progressive overload because of the common functional activities and the unique location of the ECRB (Fig. 15-40). Functionally, tasks like a backhand in tennis and using hedge clippers are performed with the forearm in pronation and the elbow at, or near, full extension as an external load is applied. In pronation, the oval-shaped radial head is positioned with its taller diameter more vertical, acting as a fulcrum over which the ECRB tendon is stretched. This fulcrum creates a compressive force to the ECRB tendon, which, when coupled with the tensile load from functional activities, creates the combined loading that is characteristic of tendinopathy. The ECRL is not at risk for compression by the radial head, regardless of forearm position, owing to its more proximal attachment on the lateral supracondylar ridge. Occasionally, the extensor carpi digitorum or the ECU is involved.[112] Recall that tenocyte proliferation, collagen abnormalities, tendon disrepair, neovascularization, and central sensitization are common features of tendinopathy.[113]

History Patients with lateral epicondylalgia report a gradual onset of lateral elbow pain that is exacerbated with gripping and activities requiring wrist extensor activation. As noted, the condition is common in the dominant arm of tennis players but can also occur in middle-aged[100] laborers with jobs requiring repeated wrist extensor activation, such as gripping. Occasionally, individuals may have an acute onset of lateral epicondylalgia. This is more likely seen in individuals new to a job or sport or a significant acute overload, such as a patient who rents a hedge trimmer and performs several hours of hedge trimming in a day. Alternatively, a middle-aged individual who begins a new fitness

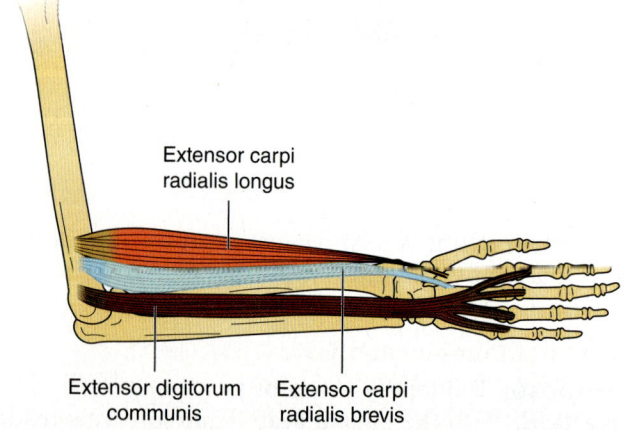

FIGURE 15-40 Biomechanics of lateral epicondylalgia.

class with repeated bouts of battle rope exercises may experience an acute onset of symptoms the day after exercise. However, these individuals rarely seek treatment resulting from the obvious acute tissue overload and isolated nature of these types of occurrences.

Key Examination Findings Individuals with lateral epicondylalgia have pain with grip testing,[86] and at least a 5 to 10% decrease in grip strength[103] can be expected. In addition, an 8% reduction in grip strength when tested with the elbow extended compared to the standard test position of 90° of elbow flexion is highly suggestive of lateral epicondylalgia.[114] Key positive examination findings include:

- Painful weakness with gripping
- Positive resisted wrist extension and radial deviation test
- Positive resisted third finger extension test
- Pain with passive wrist flexion and ulnar deviation with the elbow extended

The proximal extensor forearm, particularly the ECRB, may be to tender to palpation and trigger points may be present. With isolated exceptions, individuals with lateral epicondylalgia do not present with a loss of elbow joint range.

Differential Diagnoses Differential diagnoses include cervical referred pain or radiculopathy, radial tunnel syndrome,[115] posterior interosseous nerve entrapment, and humeroradial arthritis.[98,116] In younger individuals, clinicians must consider **OCD** and **Panner disease**.

Rehabilitation Focus and Key Points Rehabilitation involves activity modification, symptom modulation, and progressive loading of the affected tissues (Fig. 15-41). Short-term activity modification reduces tendon overload.[117] For example, a tennis player with moderate irritability may be allowed to practice forehands and forehand volleys, but avoid backhands and serves. Modifying racquet and tool grip size can significantly decrease the load on the wrist extensors, as increased wrist extensor force is needed to counterbalance the increased gripping force required for a handle that is either too large or too small.[117] A counterforce elbow brace can provide immediate reduction of activity-related symptoms by reducing load proximal to the brace.[100,117,118] Form correction is particularly important in sports to help resolve symptoms and reduce recurrence. For tennis, key technique errors to identify and correct are leading with the elbow during a backhand swing, excessive pronation to create top spin on a forehand, and excessive wrist flexion snap during serves.[112]

Educating patients about central sensitization can be particularly beneficial for those with work-related symptoms. Such education would include discussing the difference between hurt and harm as well as the natural recovery process (i.e., that the vast majority of individuals with lateral epicondylalgia fully recover within a year).[118] Ice can assist with pain modulation[117] owing to its analgesic qualities.

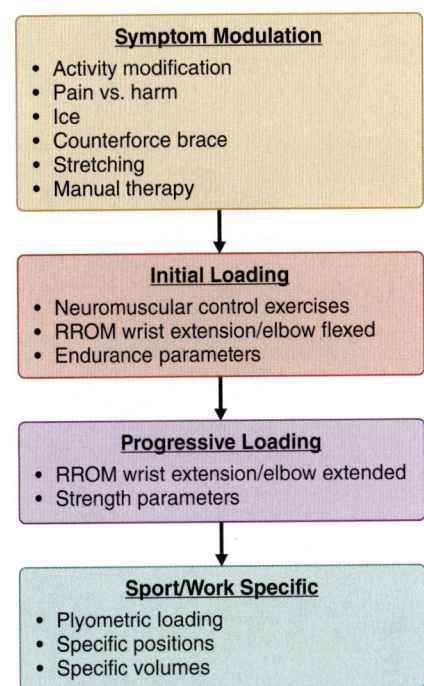

FIGURE 15-41 Treatment progression for lateral epicondylalgia. *RROM*, resisted range of motion.

Wrist extensor stretching can help with improving tissue extensibility, with a common exercise prescription being three repetitions of 30-second holds one or more times per day (Fig. 15-42).[117,119] The stretch can be individually titrated by altering the amount of radial or ulnar deviation. Neuromuscular control exercises, such as the palm-slide exercise (Fig. 15-43), can help with reducing accessory muscle activation. For this exercise, the patient slowly extends the wrist with a focus on raising the knuckles while keeping the fingers in relaxed contact with the support surface. Although an active warm-up may be beneficial for patients with lateral epicondylalgia, an upper body ergometer (UBE) should not be initiated until after tissue irritability has been reduced.[117] Instrument-assisted soft-tissue mobilization and deep friction massage[100] may also be beneficial.[117]

There is conflicting information regarding exercise prescription, particularly in regard to allowable pain with exercise.[119] As a general guideline, pain should not exceed 5/10 on a visual analog scale. Isometric wrist extension with the elbow flexed 90° held for 30 to 60 seconds at an intensity that does not increase

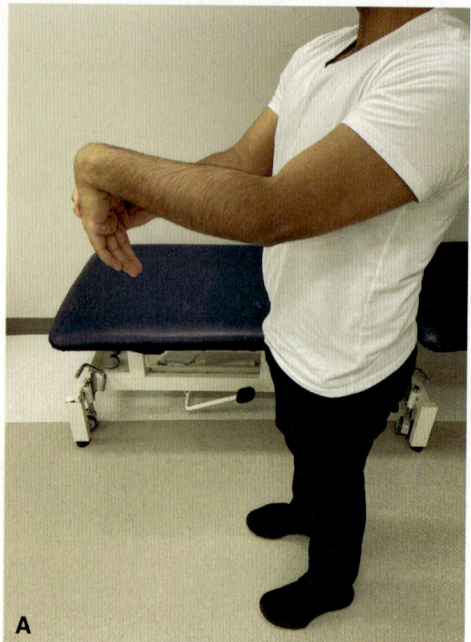 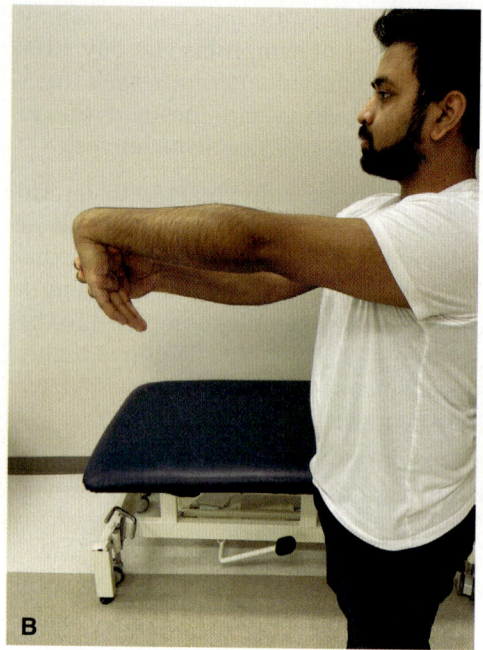

FIGURE 15-42 Wrist extensor stretching. **A.** Elbow flexed. **B.** Elbow extended.

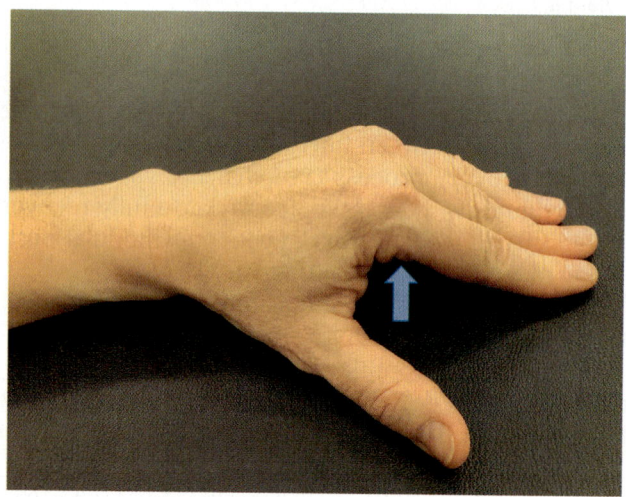

FIGURE 15-43 Palm-slide exercise.

pain greater than 5/10 can have a pain-modulating effect[116] and, therefore, should be initiated early in the rehabilitation to provide a well-tolerated, low load to the tendon. This should be progressed in intensity as symptoms allow, followed by resistive wrist extension including both concentric and eccentric contractions. Initially, resisted wrist extension with a looped resistance band or cuff weight may be better tolerated than the gripping required to use a dumbbell. Tendon load is gradually progressed in intensity. Once tolerating heavy resistance, combined tendon loading can be initiated by lowering the resistance, but placing the elbow in a more functional (typically extended) position.[117] As with other tendinopathies, a return to plyometric loading, such as that required to perform a backhand in tennis, is initiated followed by and a gradual progression to sport-specific positions and volumes.

Mobilization with Movement

Purpose: A lateral elbow mobilization with movement[100,116,117] can help improve pain-free gripping (Fig. 15-44).

Patient: Supine with elbow extended and forearm pronated.

Clinician: Standing with knees slightly bent and a mobilization belt looped over the patient's proximal forearm and inferior shoulder. Proximal hand stabilizes the patient's distal arm, where the distal hand stabilizes the distal forearm against the support surface.

Mobilization: The clinician applies a lateral mobilization via the belt by straightening the knees. Once the glide is applied, the patient performs a gripping activity, such as making a fist or squeezing a ball, and holds this position for 6 to 10 seconds. The grip is released, then the mobilization is released. The procedure is repeated for 6 to 10 repetitions.

Varus and valgus tilts can also assist with symptom modification.[117] Exercises to address any deficits in the kinetic chain that may have contributed to lateral epicondylalgia can be initiated at any phase in the rehabilitation process. Improvements in pain-free grip strength is a reliable measure to detect progress over the course of treatment.[100]

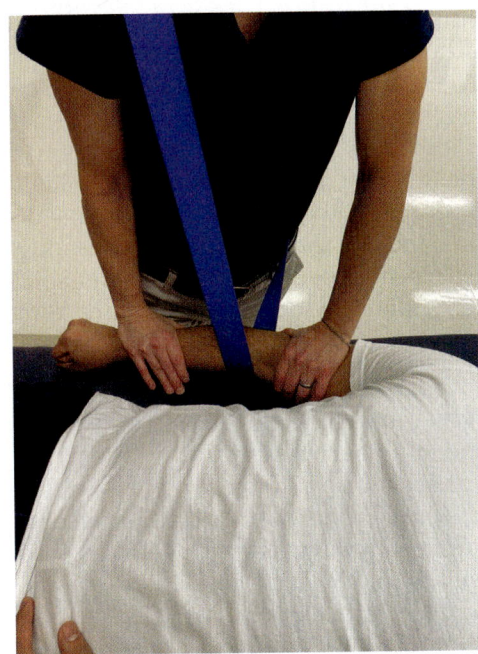

FIGURE 15-44 Lateral elbow mobilization with movement.

Expected Outcomes Nearly all patients with lateral epicondylalgia will have complete and lasting symptom resolution within a year.[120] Patients who fail to improve despite 6 to 12 months of conservative management may benefit from referral.[116,118,121] Corticosteroid injections, although potentially reducing symptoms in the short term, appear to be potentially harmful in the long term.[112] Platelet-rich plasma (PRP) injections[122,123] and arthroscopic debridement of the ECRB appear to lead to consistently positive outcomes.[112] However, it is possible that the benefits of surgery are more in the forced activity reduction required postoperatively.[120]

Medial Epicondylalgia

Pathology Medial epicondylalgia is far less common than its counterpart, lateral epicondylalgia.[124] Both are degenerative, overuse conditions that require the same general treatment strategies. Medial epicondylalgia involves the pronator-flexor group near the medial epicondyle. In the older population, the condition is often called "golfer's elbow" as it is a common overuse injury from exacerbated by poor form of repeated excessive wrist flexion and pronation.[87] The condition is common in throwers, with pain most often occurring during late cocking and early acceleration[87] due to the increased valgus stress the muscles must counteract[125] or at ball release[126] as the extremity moves into forearm pronation and wrist flexion. Other sports, such as bowling, javelin, and weightlifting, are also prone to medial epicondylalgia. Individuals with occupations that require repetitive wrist flexion and forearm pronation, such as some factory jobs, are also more at risk.

Acute strains of the common flexor tendons can occur in high-level athletes,[125] but the majority of cases are chronic, overuse injuries.

History Patients with medial epicondylalgia report a gradual onset of medial elbow pain that is exacerbated by wrist flexion, pronation, or pulling activities. For example, tennis players may report pain with forehand, but not backhand strokes. Pain may radiate into the medial forearm. In addition to the sports noted previously, workers who require repeated or forceful gripping are more at risk for medial epicondylalgia.[124] They may note a recent change in equipment or job duties. A bowler may have changed to a new ball weight, changed the finger positions, started attempting a new spin technique, or increased practice time. Throwers are likely to report an increase in activity, change in position, or attempts at a new technique.

Key Examination Findings Patients with medial epicondylalgia are typically tender to palpation just distal to the medial epicondyle over the PT or, occasionally, the FCR.[86] Skeletally immature individuals may have tenderness along the medial epicondyle.[86] Although a mild elbow flexion contracture is not uncommon for throwers,[125] range of motion is generally unrestricted. Patients may have pain with resisted forearm pronation and/or wrist flexion, particularly if biased toward the FCR. Acutely, stretching these tissues may create mild symptoms.

To rule out an MCL injury in throwers, clinicians should perform the valgus stress test and the moving valgus stress test (described later in this chapter).[125] Because many laborers with medial epicondylalgia also have concomitant musculoskeletal pathologies, such as lateral epicondylalgia or rotator cuff pathology,[124] a thorough examination of the kinetic chain, workplace, and tools is recommended.

Differential Diagnoses Differential diagnosis includes MCL injury,[125] acute rupture of the common flexor tendon,[125] and ulnar nerve pathology.[124,125] The clinician must consider the possibility of an avulsion fracture in adolescents with an acute onset of severe medial elbow pain, accompanied by swelling or ecchymosis from a throw.[127]

Rehabilitation Focus and Key Points As with lateral epicondylalgia, treatment involves activity modification, symptom modulation, and progressive loading of the affected tissues. For athletes, a 2- to 6-week period of limited throwing is recommended.[125] Stretching and soft-tissue mobilization of the pronator-flexors can begin immediately.[124] Wrist flexors can be stretched in the open kinetic chain similar to the wrist extensor stretching noted previously or can be performed in a weight-bearing position (Fig. 15-45). Care should be taken to avoid including the fingers because the resulting passive insufficiency of the FDS and profundus will preclude stretching of the wrist flexors and progressive strengthening of the wrist flexors and forearm pronators, followed by a progressive return to sport-specific activities and loading.[125]

Expected Outcomes The majority of patients have full symptom resolution without residual deficits with conservative interventions.[125] Rarely, surgery is required without overt tendon rupture. As with lateral epicondylalgia, there seems to be a potential role for PRP injection in the treatment of medial epicondylalgia.[128]

Elbow Dislocation and Instability

The common types of elbow instability are dislocation, MCL sprain and valgus instability, and PLRI. Elbow instability may occur due to trauma, overuse,[12] bony dysplasia, Ehlers-Danlos syndrome, rheumatoid arthritis, or may develop iatrogenically after a surgery.[129] Isolated RCL sprains are far less common than ulnar side injuries[130] and are generally the result of landing on an outstretched hand.[85]

Elbow Dislocation The elbow is the second most commonly dislocated joint (behind the shoulder).[131] Elbow dislocation is more common in collegiate wrestlers, gymnasts, and football players, primarily the result of trauma.[132] Management consists of reduction and assessment for concomitant injuries, such as fracture, ligament rupture, and neurovascular damage. If no postreduction instability is noted, rehabilitation can begin within the first week of injury with early active assisted range of motion (AAROM) in a hinged elbow brace. The most common complication with conservative management is postdislocation stiffness. Individuals with less than 30° of extension after 4 to 8 weeks should be fitted for a static progressive splint.[133] Surgical intervention is the norm if the orthopaedist notes residual instability with postreduction testing or with fracture dislocations.[133] Postoperative rehabilitation is dependent upon the location of fracture, direction of instability, and stabilization methods performed.

Medial Collateral Ligament Sprain and Valgus Instability Valgus instability arises as a result of damage to the MCL, particularly the anterior bundle.[12] As noted previously, from 20 to 120° of elbow flexion, the MCL is the primary restraint to valgus stresses,[97] which can be extremely high during overhand throwing. A recent survey noted of professional baseball players noted a significant increase in MCL reconstruction, with 20% of pitchers reporting having undergone the procedure.[134] Although the literature largely focuses on baseball, athletes participating in softball, javelin, water polo, tennis, golf, wrestling, and football quarterbacks may also sustain an MCL injury.[135] An MCL rupture increases the demand on the flexor-pronators to provide dynamic control of valgus stresses during throwing. In addition, chronically increased valgus increases traction on the ulnar nerve, putting athletes at risk for ulnar neuropathy; produces lateral compression that can lead to OCD of the capitulum[85,95]; and creates posterior shearing forces that can lead to posterior elbow pain and osteophyte formation.[98,126] Risk factors for MCL injuries include playing baseball year-round, longer seasons, pitching, and pitch volume.[136,137]

Injuries to the MCL are sometimes divided into levels of severity:

- Sprain—pain without MCL laxity with valgus testing
- Partial-thickness tear—pain with minimal laxity with valgus testing
- Complete rupture—obvious laxity with valgus testing

Unfortunately, laxity can be difficult to identify in clinical testing, even for complete MCL ruptures.[137] However, this does not mean that imaging, such as magnetic resonance imaging, should occur before a trial of conservative interventions.

Individuals with an MCL injury may report an acute onset of medial elbow pain during an overhead throw, with or without a "popping" sensation. They are unable to continue throwing due to medial elbow pain that occurs during late cocking or early acceleration phase of throwing.[136] Conversely, many athletes report a gradual increase in medial elbow pain along with decrease in accuracy, throwing endurance, and ball

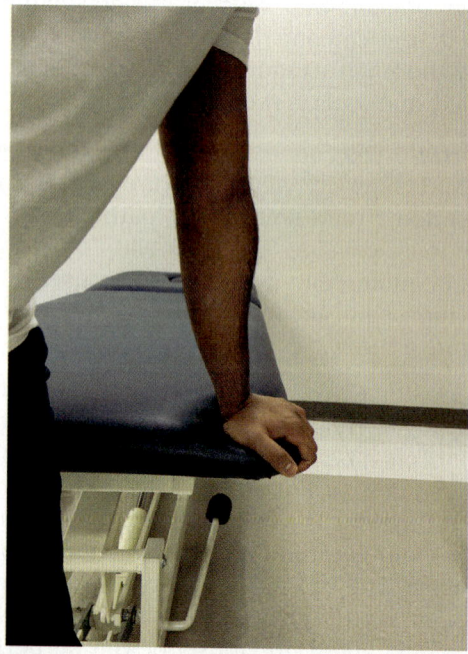

FIGURE 15-45 Weight-bearing wrist flexor stretching.

velocity.[98] Some may complain of elbow tightness.[126] Symptoms are generally only noticed during throwing or similar motions and not with activities of daily living.[126]

Key physical examination findings for MCL sprain include a positive valgus stress test and moving valgus stress test.[12,136] Tenderness over the MCL is common.[88,104,126] Ecchymosis, if present, is a sign of MCL rupture,[98] but is not universally observed.[126] A thorough examination of the overhead athlete must look beyond identification of an MCL injury and examine relative components of the cervical/thoracic spine and shoulder girdle in addition to the elbow, forearm, and wrist.[126] Many athletes with MCL injury have been noted to have elbow flexion contractures and significant glenohumeral internal rotation deficits (GIRD),[98] which may contribute to increased valgus stress. Likewise, pronator-flexor weakness or endurance deficit may contribute to valgus stress by causing microinstability or be the result of increased valgus stress.[126] Grip strength should be evaluated to help assess ulnar nerve integrity, although weakness is generally only present with advanced pathology.[126] Upper extremity sensation should also be assessed.

Multiple structures must be considered in the differential diagnosis of medial elbow symptoms, including MCL injury, medial epicondylalgia, pronator syndrome, and ulnar nerve pathology.[126] These pathologies are discussed elsewhere in this chapter.

There is ongoing debate regarding the management of MCL injuries. Although the number of MCL surgeries has increased significantly, this has not led to consistent improvement in outcomes, including return to play. The current consensus is to avoid surgery unless an athlete fails 3 to 6 months of conservative interventions.[137] PRP injections may be a beneficial adjunct to conservative management.[136] In younger athletes, partial-thickness tears are more common, so the potential for full recovery is likely better with conservative management.[138] In addition, amateur athletes may not require surgery[137] because medial elbow instability is not disabling for activities of daily living and most sporting activities.

Rehabilitation for MCL injuries should be progressive (Fig. 15-46) and include abstinence from overhead throwing or similar activities for at least 6 weeks for partial-thickness tears[137] and 8 to 12 weeks for full-thickness[136] MCL injuries. During this time, the athlete should focus on fitness of the remaining kinetic chain, including lower extremity conditioning as well as strengthening of the core, scapular, and rotator cuff[137] muscles. In addition, elbow flexion contractures and GIRD should be addressed with stretching, joint mobilizations, and manual therapy.[121] Elbow, forearm, and wrist strengthening[137] should begin with low-load, high repetition exercises that avoid valgus stress before progressing to heavy strength training. The "Throwers Ten Program" contains a series of throwing-specific exercises for strengthening the forearm, elbow, shoulder, scapular muscles, and trunk and is recommended for injury prevention and elbow rehabilitation.[121] Muscular endurance and dynamic stability training, including rhythmic stabilization exercises, should be incorporated into a holistic rehabilitation program.[121] Upper extremity plyometrics are then added to the program. Once the athlete tolerates all strength training and symptoms have resolved, a sport-specific movement analysis should be performed and an interval throwing program initiated that addresses any biomechanical errors noted. Such training is critical to resolution of symptoms and successful return to sport.

Operative management via direct repair appears to have limited success, and therefore, MCL reconstruction, typically using a PL graft, is the most common surgical intervention. There are currently multiple variations in operative technique,[137] so rehabilitation guidelines are difficult to generalize, particularly in the early postsurgical period. The elbow is typically immobilized for about a week in 90° of flexion. Isometric exercise and ice may be initiated immediately postoperatively. Elbow range of motion puts only a mild stress on the graft and need not be restricted,[121] allowing for progression of elbow range as tolerated with a goal of full motion by 6 weeks postsurgery. Therefore, elbow range is progressively increased as tolerated with a goal of full motion by postoperative week 6. After this point, progressive resistance exercises, such as the "Throwers Ten Program," can begin for the shoulder, elbow, and wrist.[121] Exercises are progressed to more sport-specific angles with increase in elbow valgus stress at about 3 months. An interval throwing program is generally started at 4 to 5 months postsurgery.[136] Throwing gradually progresses in distance, volume, and intensity based on the athlete's position. Outcomes for baseball players after MCL surgery appear to be highly variable, with 67 to 100% of athletes[136,139] returning to sport in 17 to 20 months.[139] Pitchers appear to fare far worse in terms of percentage returning to play and sport performance,[139] and as many as 50% return to the disabled list.[136]

Because of the prolonged loss of playing time and limited success for long-term return to competitive sport, prevention of MCL injuries has gained attention. Limiting pitch counts,[137] discouraging pitching (if not playing) on multiple leagues,[137] and an emphasis on proper throwing mechanics[137] in addition to encouraging youth athletes to participate in a variety of sports are imperative. As athletes mature and progress from youth sports, an arm-care program may be beneficial. In one study, a series of nine stretches for the forearm,

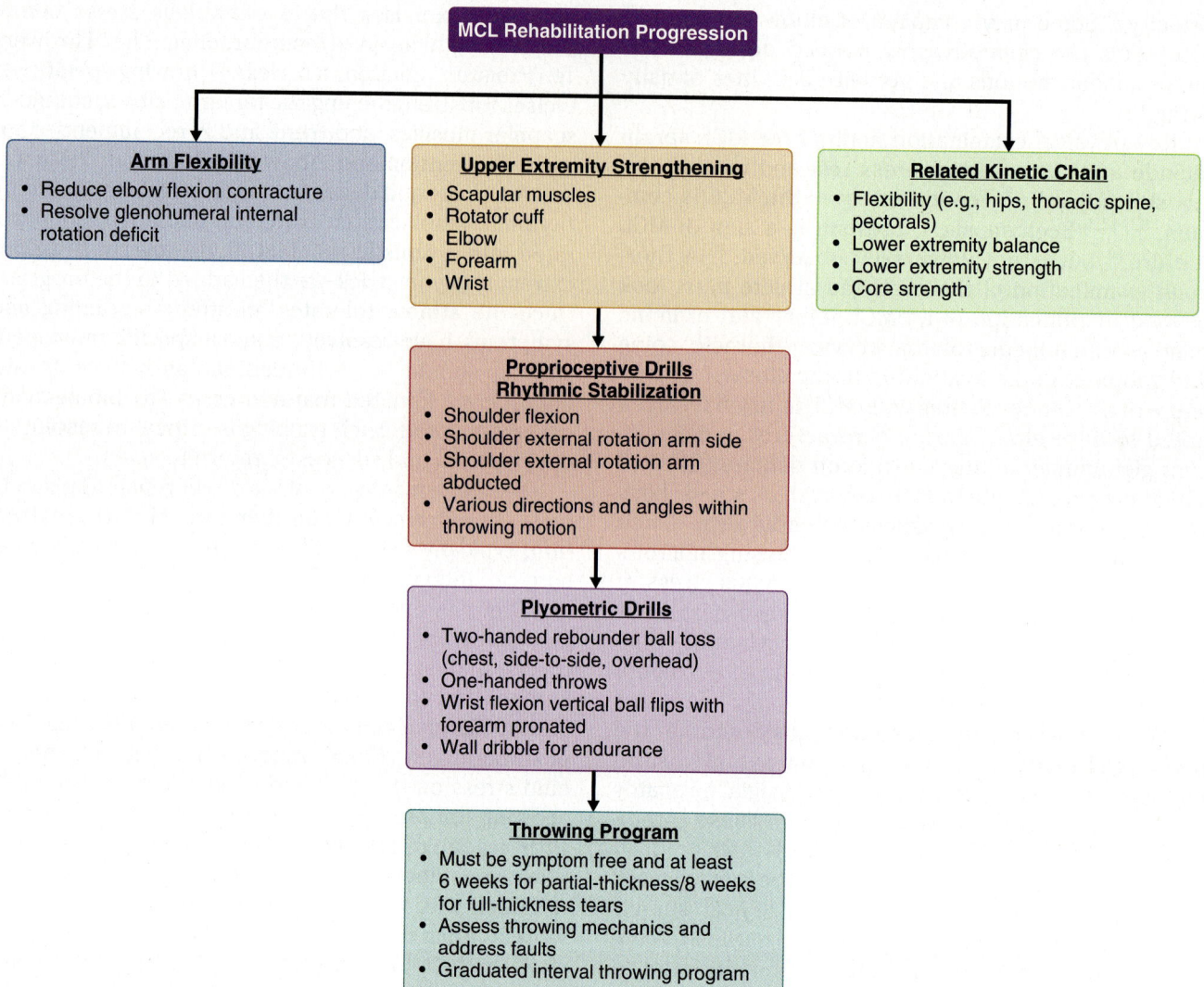

FIGURE 15-46 Medial collateral ligament (MCL) rehabilitation. *ER,* external rotation; *GIRD,* glenohumeral internal rotation deficit; *LE,* lower extremity; *UE,* upper extremity.

elbow, shoulder, trunk, and hips resulted in a significant decrease in medial elbow injuries,[140] while a separate study with a modification of the exercise regime that included single leg balance and a simulated pitching motion reduced both shoulder and elbow injuries.[141] The "Throwers Ten Program" is a holistic strengthening program that may assist with injury prevention. Lastly, attention should be paid to identifying and resolving any lower extremity range, strength, and balance deficits, as these have been found to be independently correlated with elbow injuries in baseball players.[142]

Posterolateral Rotatory Instability PLRI is the most common type of chronic elbow instability[129,143,144] and is a result of RCL rupture and radial head posterolateral subluxation,[12] with or without capsular damage. The typical mechanism of onset is a fall on an outstretched hand.[143] Patients with PLRI report mechanical symptoms, such as clunking, clicking, or a feeling of instability in the elbow. Lateral elbow pain may be present.[144] Patients with PLRI generally do not have a loss of motion or grip strength, but may be tender along the RCL and lateral elbow.[145] Several tests for PLRI have been described. However, many are not useful when used in a nonsedated patient. The reproduction of symptoms or apprehension with the chair push-up and push-up tests is consistent with PLRI.[98,107,144] Alternatively, the tabletop relocation test[146] has been described in which the patient places the supinated hand with the elbow extended on a tabletop. The patient then places weight through the hand and slowly flexes the elbow.[144] A positive test is determined by the report of posterolateral elbow pain or apprehension with the test and symptom improvement if the test is repeated with the clinician applying pressure with the thumb to prevent posterior subluxation of the radial head. Although frequently mentioned in the literature, there is minimal data to support the tabletop relocation test.[12] Patients with suspected PLRI should referred for further evaluation as conservative management is seldom effective.[144] Surgical options include repair and reconstruction of affected tissues.[145]

Rehabilitation after surgery generally includes progressive range of motion with splinting used to protect the involved tissues.[145] Varus and valgus stresses should be avoided. Full extension is generally achieved by 8 weeks, and elbow strengthening is initiated at around 12 weeks after surgery.[145] High-level activities, particularly those involving varus stress, may be limited for up to 6 months.[145] Unfortunately, recurrent instability after surgery may be as high as 25%.[144]

Elbow Osteoarthritis

Pathology Elbow OA affects nearly 4% of men over the age of 40.[147] Unlike the weight-bearing joints of the knee and hip, primarily age-related elbow OA is rare.[148] Secondary elbow OA occurs in athletes, such as those in throwing and swinging sports or weight lifting; manual laborers, including those working with hammers and pneumatic or vibrating tool[149]; or after prior trauma, including fracture or dislocation.[150] Elbow OA may also result from diseases, such as rheumatoid arthritis and gout.[148]

History Patients with elbow OA report loss of motion with end-range pain that limits functional activities.[149] Complaints such as catching and locking are common.[151] Patients may have concomitant ulnar nerve symptoms[149] due to osteophytes encroaching on the cubital tunnel.[151]

Key Examination Findings Bony enlargement, intermittent effusion, and joint warmth are common. Loss of motion in a capsular pattern in which flexion is more limited than extension (typically 15 to 115°)[151] and with equal limitations of flexion and extension. Crepitus is common, and end-range pain will be present if the tissues are irritable. Joint mobility will be globally restricted. Strength deficits may be present due to disuse.

Differential Diagnoses Differential diagnosis includes rheumatoid arthritis and gout.

Rehabilitation Focus and Key Points Ice, heat, and nonsteroidal anti-inflammatory medications commonly help alleviate pain.[151,152] Injections with corticosteroid or hyaluronic acid may be useful adjuncts for symptom modulation.[149,152] Early motion exercises including frequent elbow flexion/extension and pronation/supination can assist with joint nutrition and the perception of stiffness. Manual therapy, including soft-tissue mobilization, joint mobilization combined with stretching, and active range of motion exercises, is recommended. Patients can be taught self-distraction mobilization (Fig. 15-47) to supplement clinician mobilizations. Ultrasound to the anterior capsule may be beneficial in combination with stretching to improve elbow extension range of motion. Low-load, long-duration stretching is particularly useful and may be better tolerated than aggressive static stretching. Stretching into a bony endfeel is counterproductive and should be avoided as it is likely a bony block due to osteophyte formation and will only exacerbate symptoms. Pronator-flexor strengthening has been recommended owing to the potential to unload the elbow from valgus stresses. General strengthening may be beneficial in cases of deconditioning. Occupation-specific strengthening and worksite assessment may be beneficial for laborers.

Expected Outcomes Little is reported in the literature regarding outcomes for conservative management of elbow OA. Anecdotally, significant gains in range of motion, decreases in pain, and improvements in function are seen after 4 to 6 weeks of rehabilitation. However, range of motion gains will not be as substantial as those obtained through surgical interventions.

Surgical Options Surgical options for patients with elbow OA who fail conservative interventions include debridement and partial or total joint arthroplasty. Surgery is most commonly performed when the involved upper extremity is the dominant one.[149] Arthroscopic debridement is appropriate for younger patients and often includes anterior capsulotomy, removal of loose bodies, and resection of osteophytes.[149] Occasionally, ulnar nerve transposition is needed.[149]

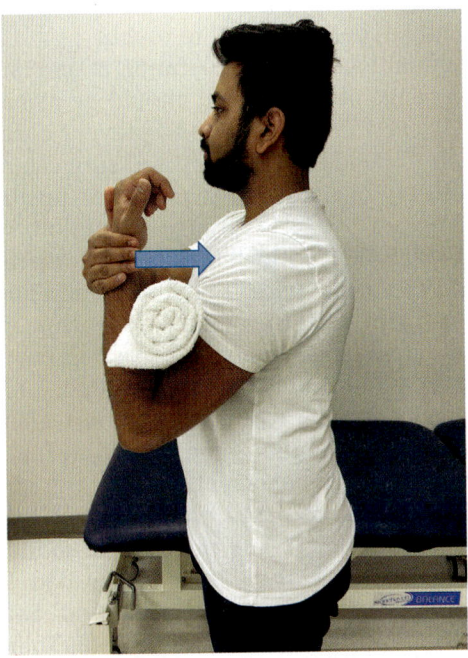

FIGURE 15-47 Self-distraction mobilization.

After debridement, immediate passive range of motion, AAROM, and active range of motion are encouraged. Resisted exercises are generally begun 4 to 6 weeks after surgery,[151] once range of motion has been improved and is less of a priority. Debridement yields a consistent increase in elbow range of motion, although younger patients typically have larger gains than older patients,[149] and most are able to return to throwing as early as 2 months after surgery.[151] Postoperative range of motion can be expected to improve to 4 to 130°[151] with postsurgical therapy. In contrast, elbow arthroplasty is more commonly performed on older individuals, patients with rheumatoid arthritis, or after prior surgical procedures.[152] Arthroplasty results in improvements in pain, total arc of elbow flexion/extension motion, and function.[153]

Fractures in the Region of the Elbow

Fractures in the elbow region are typically the result of a fall on an outstretched arm. Isolated single-bone fracture is possible, but injury to multiple structures is common. Table 15-7 provides details of common fractures within the elbow region. Distal radius fractures, such as a Colles fracture, are discussed in Chapter 16, Wrist and Hand Complex. Decisions are based on the bone fractured; concomitant injuries to bones, joints, and soft tissue; and patient age.

Key examination findings after fracture include a loss of motion in the elbow and forearm in a capsular pattern. Ecchymosis will be present if seen shortly after fracture. Distal arm, elbow, and hand edema are to be expected due to both the injury and postinjury immobilization. Clinicians should observe for signs of complex regional pain syndrome, such as generalized edema, trophic changes of the skin and nails, dysesthesias, and hypersensitivity to touch.

The initial focus of rehabilitation is on restoration of elbow range of motion and should be managed aggressively early in the process to prevent contracture formation.[154] Pending the injury and surgical intervention, this may begin as early as 1 week postinjury. A home program of passive range of motion, AAROM, and active range of motion of the elbow, forearm, wrist, and hand can assist with edema reduction and range recovery. To prevent secondary adhesive capsulitis, shoulder active range of motion exercises, particularly external rotation, should also be included.

After consultation with the surgeon to determine fracture stability, gentle grade I/II mobilizations can assist with pain management, whereas grades III/IV should be utilized to assist with range of motion. In addition to frequent bouts of range of motion exercises, contract-relax stretching and low-load, long-duration stretching are frequently required. Soft-tissue mobilization may assist with tone reduction, allowing an increase in motion. Dynamic splinting should be considered as an early option if motion is difficult to achieve. However, it is imperative the clinician be aware of fracture alignment, as range of motion limited by poor fracture alignment will not be resolve with rehabilitation.

If fracture fixation is adequate, gentle strengthening may also begin early in the rehabilitation process.[154] Beginning with endurance strengthening for the elbow/forearm, a home program should also incorporate total arm strength because an elbow rehabilitation program is not complete without the inclusion of the shoulder complex and hand rehabilitation. Nerve gliding exercises, if needed, should not be initiated until 6 to 8 weeks after surgery to allow adequate time for healing and inflammation resolution.[154] Common postfracture problems include post-traumatic OA, heterotopic ossification, and osteochondrosis of the capitulum.

Stress Fractures in the Elbow Region

Stress fractures within the elbow region are overuse injuries more commonly seen in athletes who participate in throwing sports, but may also occur in gymnasts, tennis players, and golfers.[155] Olecranon stress fractures are the most common type of stress fracture about the elbow and typically result from repetitive hyperextension with or without valgus overload. Radial head stress fractures may be seen in skeletally immature female gymnasts.[155] Magnetic resonance imaging is the diagnostic imaging of choice for stress fractures and can assist with early identification.

Presentation varies based on involved bone, sport, and severity. The prototypical case would be a 12- to 16-year-old, male baseball pitcher or catcher playing year-round baseball.[111] Patients typically report vague posterior elbow pain, decreased throwing velocity, and decreased ball control. Clinically, the patient will have pain to palpation of the olecranon and pain with resisted elbow extension. There may be a slight loss of passive elbow extension due to pain.[111]

Conservative management is the mainstay of treatment for elbow stress fractures. Treatment includes activity modification, ice, and nonsteroidal anti-inflammatory medications. Maintaining or attaining full body fitness including lower extremity, core, rotator cuff strength should be emphasized early in the rehabilitation process. Optimization of sport-specific mechanics and volume moderation as described previously are critical components for returning to sport. Prevention is the ideal strategy and should include encouraging children to participate in a variety of sports, monitoring training loads including participation in multiple leagues or year-round play. Conservative treatment for olecranon stress fractures is likely to require about 3 months, compared to 7 months for those

TABLE 15-7
COMMON FRACTURES WITHIN THE ELBOW REGION

Fracture	Fracture Features

Distal humerus	• Onset
	  • Older individuals falls
	  • Young men: high energy trauma
	• Operative treatment decreases risk of postoperative stiffness by allowing early mobilization
	• Complications common including heterotopic bone formation, ulnar neuritis, hardware-related problems

Medial epicondyle	• Isolated avulsion fractures in adolescent boys during throwing activities • Nonoperative management unless largely displaced, but may result in future instability
Olecranon	• Various presentations from simple to comminuted • Fall landing directly on the point of the elbow • Avulsion fracture due to forceful triceps contraction • More common in individuals over the age of 50 • Surgical management is the norm and may involve plating or k-wires • Overall outcome is good
Coronoid	• Frequent concurrent injuries including posterior dislocation, radial head fracture, and/or ligament rupture • Isolated fracture may be managed nonoperatively • Complex fractures managed via ORIF to restore buttress function of coronoid and retain elbow stability
Radial head	• Most common elbow fracture • Primarily due fall on outstretched arm • May have MCL injury if onset result of valgus trauma or concomitant elbow dislocation • ORIF likely, radial head replacement option for older patients • Complications more common after ORIF
Combined Fractures	**Fracture Features**
Monteggia fractures	• Fracture of the proximal third of the ulna with radial head dislocation, may have additional associated injuries • More commonly seen in osteoporotic individuals who fall • Given difficulty of diagnosis in pediatric patients, delayed presentation possible • Surgical management required • Early (after the first week) AROM • Complications common: malunion, nonunion, ulnar neuritis
Galeazzi fracture	• Radial fracture with disruption of DRUJ dorsally or ventrally • Result of axial load to the forearm, typically during a fall • Children typically treated with closed reduction and immobilization • Adults treated with ORIF and repair of additional structures as needed
Essex-Lopresti injury	• Radial head fracture with proximal migration damaging intraosseous membrane and distal radioulnar joint • Humeroradial injury may occur at time of injury or chronically • Radial shortening can lead to future wrist and distal ulnar pain • Result of axial load to the wrist, commonly due to a fall

AROM, active range of motion; DRUJ, distal radioulnar joint; MCL, medial collateral ligament; ORIF, open reduction internal fixation.
Adapted from Midtgaard KS, Ruzbarsky JJ, Hackett TR, Viola RW. Elbow fractures. *Clin Sports Med.* 2020;39(3):623–636; Avasthi A, Peach C. Fractures of the proximal radius and ulna. *Orthop Trauma.* 2019;33(5):322–329; Desai A, Amer M, Tourret L, Phadnis J. Forearm fracture dislocations. *Orthop Trauma.* 2019;33(5):330–340.

undergoing surgical intervention.[111] However, many individuals will fail to be able to return to sport without surgical interventions. Those failing to improve with 3 to 6 months of conservative care[156] would benefit from a surgical consult.

Nerve Compression In the Elbow Region

Pathology Most compression neuropathies, also referred to as *peripheral nerve entrapments*, occur in the upper extremity, particularly the elbow/forearm region. Figure 15-48 summarizes areas about the elbow where the ulnar, median, and radial nerves are most vulnerable to compression. As described previously in this chapter, a nerve crossing the elbow may be compressed during passage through a narrow space, generally bordered by bone or thickened, dense connective tissue. Narrowing of the space due to positioning, inflammation, or a space-occupying lesion can lead to alterations in neuronal blood flow, fibrosis, and nerve conduction changes.[39] If compression continues, axonal degeneration can occur.[39] Nerve damage can result from a low level of compression over a long period of time, a higher degree of compression over a shorter period of time (such as inflammation after a humerus fracture), or intermittent compression with traction (such as during the cocking phase of throwing).[157] In addition, nerve conduction can be damaged by a **double-crush injury**, when a nerve is compressed at more than one point. In such as case, less compression is needed to adversely affect nerve function.[158] A double-crush injury is best explained using a simple water hose analogy. Consider using a hose to wash a car. The water is turned on, and a full stream of water flows through the hose. As one progresses around the car, the hose may get kinked under one of the tires, decreasing the flow of water from the hose. If the person continues to walk around the car and the hose becomes kinked under a second tire, the water from the hose maybe decreased to a trickle or blocked entirely. A similar type of compression can occur to a nerve coursing through the upper extremity. For example, consider a middle-aged patient who decides to train for a long bicycle century (100 miles). If the patient has a small osteophyte in the cervical spine reducing the space available for the C8 nerve root and then rides for 2 hours, the patient may report tingling and numbness anywhere in the distribution of the ulnar nerve, such as in the fifth and ulnar half of the fourth digit. These symptoms are consistent with ulnar nerve compression in the hand (at the tunnel of Guyon), but may also be associated with compression in the neck or anywhere about the elbow, such as the cubital tunnel, as vibration through the handlebars may irritate the ulnar nerve. The example demonstrates the importance of conducting a thorough cervical examination on any patient suspected of having an upper extremity compression neuropathy. The patient's symptoms may improve with treatment directed solely toward the elbow or hand (use of cycling gloves and/or reducing vibration through a more shock-absorbing fork or tires) or solely toward the cervical spine (cervical manipulation). However, the patient may require interventions directed toward both areas of nerve compression for full symptom resolution. Predisposing factors for compression neuropathies include diabetes, hypothyroidism, and smoking.[158]

Compression Neuropathies of the Ulnar Nerve

The ulnar nerve is prone to compression in multiple places.[50,101] Compression of the ulnar nerve at the tunnel of Guyon is discussed in Chapter 16, Wrist and Hand Complex. Cubital tunnel syndrome, compression of the ulnar nerve at the cubital tunnel, is the second most common nerve-entrapment syndrome, after carpal tunnel syndrome.[159] Risk factors for cubital tunnel syndrome include male sex, occupations requiring repetitive elbow flexion or direct pressure over the elbow, and increased cubital valgus.[160] In throwers, cubital tunnel syndrome may be the result of combination of compression and traction to the nerve.[108] Nerve compression may also result from compression or tension after elbow fracture or dislocation.

Individuals with cubital tunnel syndrome report medial elbow aching and pain, fatigue with repetitive tasks,[108] clumsiness or loss of fine motor coordination, and/or difficulty crossing the fingers[39] and decreased pinch/grip strength[160] due to interossei weakness. Symptoms may be worsened with activities requiring prolonged or repeated elbow flexion.[86,104]

Individuals with cubital tunnel syndrome will have weakness of ulnar innervated muscles, resulting in decreases in grip and pinch strength.[86] Individuals commonly present with weakness of wrist flexion with ulnar deviation (FCU), index finger abduction (first dorsal interossei), and thumb adduction (adductor pollicis). Fine motor dexterity may also be reduced.[85] Advanced cubital tunnel syndrome will present with atrophy of the first dorsal interossei or hypothenar eminence.[50,85,160] There may be slight clawing of the fourth and fifth digits, though less than what is seen with more distal compression. Semmes-Weinstein monofilament testing will reveal abnormal sensation of the ulnar wrist and hand as well as the fifth and half of the fourth finger.[86] The elbow flexion test and the Tinel sign at the

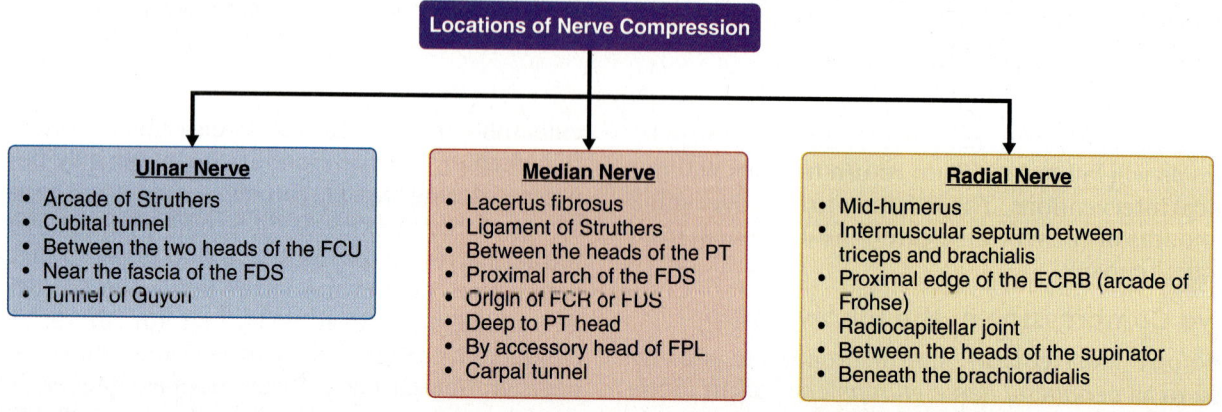

FIGURE 15-48 Common locations of upper extremity nerve compression. *ECRB*, extensor carpi radialis brevis; *FCR* flexor carpi radialis; *FCU*, flexor carpi ulnaris; *FDS*, flexor digitorum superficialis; *FPL*, flexor pollicis longus; *PT*, pronator teres.

cubital tunnel (Fig. 15-49) may be positive. The ULTT with ulnar nerve bias may be positive (refer to Chapter 17, Cervical and Thoracic Spine). In some individuals, ulnar nerve hypermobility may be present, which may produce ulnar neuritis. To assess for ulnar nerve mobility, the clinician should flex and extend the elbow while palpating the ulnar nerve at the cubital tunnel gently to observe for nerve subluxation or dislocation.[157] Differential diagnoses include C8/T1 radiculopathy, thoracic outlet syndrome, ulnar nerve compression at the tunnel of Guyon, and medial epicondylalgia.[50,101]

Interventions for cubital tunnel include relative rest and nonsteroidal anti-inflammatory medication.[157,161] For throwing athletes, up to 6 weeks of limited throwing frequency is recommended. Elbow pads during occupations requiring weight bearing through the elbows and night splinting[50] with the elbow in about 45°[121] (the position of maximal cubital tunnel space and limited nerve tension)[101] can be beneficial. Progressive strengthening exercises can be initiated immediately. Manual therapy to improve soft-tissue restrictions in the FCU and FDS may be beneficial. Addressing any sport-specific biomechanical errors[157] is critical to reducing symptoms and preventing recurrence.

Compression Neuropathies of the Median Nerve

Median nerve entrapment can create pronator syndrome, anterior interosseous nerve syndrome, and carpal tunnel syndrome, pending the site of compression (Table 15-8).[86,87,108,109] Carpal tunnel syndrome (discussed in detail in Chapter 16, Wrist and Hand Complex) and pronator syndrome commonly coexist with overlapping symptoms.[162] Pronator syndrome is commonly seen in pitchers, tennis players, weight lifters, and in occupations requiring repeated gripping, such as carpentry, cooking, and some assembly line work.[108,109]

Individuals with pronator syndrome report an aching pain in the volar forearm and paresthesias in the thenar eminence, index, middle, and radial half of the fourth fingers.[108] Patients report loss of pinch strength and fine motor skills and overall hand clumsiness.[86] This is in contrast to carpal tunnel syndrome, where the palmar cutaneous nerve branches off before the carpal tunnel and thenar eminence sensation is not affected.[108] Weakness may be found on physical examination of the PT, FPL, FDP of the index and ring finger, and FCR.[86] The patient may have a positive Tinel sign and positive pronator compression test.[108,109] The ULTT with median nerve bias may be positive (refer to Chapter 17, Cervical and Thoracic Spine). Differential diagnosis for median nerve compression neuropathies includes cervical and brachial plexus pathology. Because pronator syndrome can coexist with medial epicondylalgia and ulnar collateral ligament injuries, the clinician should specifically assess for these pathologies.

Interventions for pronator syndrome parallel those for cubital tunnel syndrome and include relative rest and nonsteroidal anti-inflammatory medication. Short-term use of a posterior elbow splint to keep the forearm in neutral rotation with the elbow in midrange[110] or an extended position can be beneficial.[157] Soft-tissue mobilization to the PT may decrease muscle tension and improve mobility of tissue around the nerve.[109] Symptom-free median nerve glides have been suggested.[109,110] The patient is progressed to light resistance, high-volume pronation and supination exercises as able.[109]

Anterior interosseous nerve syndrome occurs when there is compression of the anterior interosseous nerve, which is a purely motor portion of the medial nerve that branches off distal to the site of compression for PT syndrome. As such, anterior interosseous nerve syndrome results in only motor deficits to the PT, FPL, and FDP of the index and ring finger, with sparing of more distal median nerve innervated muscles and normal sensory function. The patient may be unable to form a circle with the thumb and index finger. When asked to do so, the IP joint of the thumb is collapses into extension as a result of recruitment of the ulnarly innervated adductor pollicis and weakness of the FPL (see Fig. 15-39).[108,110]

Compression Neuropathies of the Radial Nerve

The radial nerve can be compressed at various points along its path.[86] Radial tunnel syndrome and posterior interosseous entrapment are pathologies of the radial nerve with some degree of controversy because of their infrequency and somewhat varying presentations.[161] Radial tunnel syndrome presents as vague pain in the region of the lateral elbow, dorsal forearm,

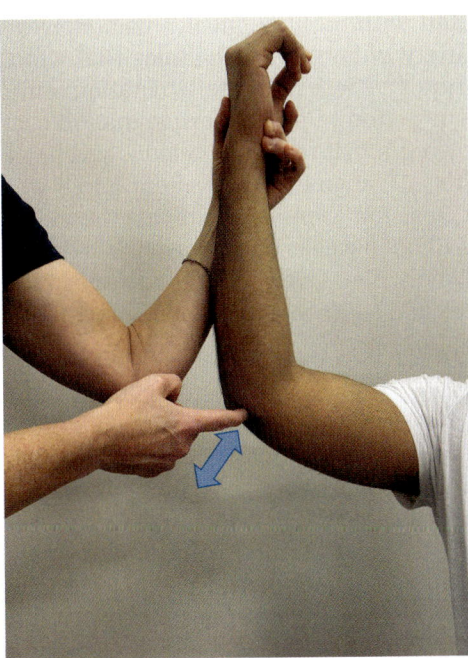

FIGURE 15-49 Tinel test at the cubital tunnel.

TABLE 15-8
COMPRESSION NEUROPATHIES OF THE MEDIAN NERVE

	Pronator Syndrome	Anterior Interosseous Nerve Syndrome	Carpal Tunnel Syndrome
Site of nerve compression	Lacertus fibrosus Ligament of Struthers Between the heads of the PT* Proximal arch of the FDS	Origin of FCR Origin of FDS Deep to PT head By accessory head of FPL	Carpal tunnel
Area of paresthesia	Volar forearm and paresthesias in the thenar eminence, index, middle, and radial half of the fourth fingers	None	Middle finger and radial half of the fourth finger
Night pain	Uncommon	Not present	Consistently present

FCR, flexor carpi radialis; *FDS*, flexor digitorum superficialis; *FPL*, flexor pollicis longus; *PT*, pronator teres.
*Most common site of pathology.

and radial wrist[86] and is thought to be due to compression at the arcade of Frohse.[161] Repeated forearm rotation, such as occurs in swimmers and tennis players,[108] may contribute to the compression. There is typically tenderness to palpation or pressure applied in this region about 3 to 5 cm distal to the lateral epicondyle.[85,108] Pain with resisted supination is suggestive of radial nerve compression at the arcade of Frohse.[85] The posterior interosseous nerve, a deep branch of the radial nerve after it pierces the supinator, may become compressed at the edge of the supinator distal to the muscular branches to the ECRL.[115] Weakness of the ECRB and extensor digitorum communis (EDC) with intact sensation is suggestive of posterior interosseous nerve entrapment[85] and has been seen in weight lifters, tennis players, and gymnasts.[157] The ULTT with radial nerve bias may be positive (refer to Chapter 17, Cervical and Thoracic Spine). Differential diagnoses includes lateral epicondylalgia and PLRI.[85] Treatment for radial nerve entrapments parallel those mentioned previously and include nonsteroidal anti-inflammatory medications, activity modification, soft-tissue mobilization, biomechanics assessment, and progressive strengthening. A counterforce elbow brace, as may be used for "tennis elbow," should be avoided[161] as this increases nerve compression.

Biceps and Triceps Injuries at the Elbow

Strains of the biceps brachii and triceps brachii are common and generally result from an acute bout of exercise or activity that overloads the muscle, particularly those requiring eccentric activity. Strains can be identified by local muscle pain that is exacerbated by active and resisted muscle contraction of the affected muscle and, if severe, by lengthening of the affected muscle. While athletes may receive treatment for such injuries, formal rehabilitation is seldom required. Treatment would involve ice, activity modification, and symptom-modulated AAROM or active range of motion exercise. Once symptoms resolve, progressive strengthening, beginning with endurance parameters, should be initiated. If onset was the result of a training error, care should be taken to modify training progression to prevent recurrence. Biceps and triceps tendinopathies at the elbow are extremely rare.

Distal Biceps Rupture Distal biceps rupture is a relatively rare clinical entity and occurs as a result of forceful eccentric contraction of the biceps. Rupture more commonly affects males between the ages of 40 and 60.[163] Risk factors include being male, tobacco or steroid use, and obesity.[163] Acute ruptures are seldom seen in the outpatient rehabilitation setting but can be readily identified by the "Popeye" deformity (a ball-shaped deformity in the anterior arm formed as the torn biceps retracts), anterior arm ecchymosis, and weakness in elbow flexion and supination. Elderly patients and those with low upper extremity demands may be treated nonoperatively with overall excellent function other than a loss of supination strength. Younger, active individuals are treated with early surgical repair. However, there are a variety of surgical techniques that will affect rehabilitation.[163] Generally, rehabilitation progression includes a period of postoperative immobilization, followed by a gradual return of flexion, and finally extension, with full range expected about 6 to 8 weeks after surgery. Resisted exercises involving the biceps can be initiated about 8 weeks after surgery and gradually progressed thereafter. Overall, biceps repair has excellent outcomes and a low rate of complications.[163]

Distal Triceps Rupture Triceps ruptures are more common in patients with systemic diseases, such as rheumatoid arthritis and diabetes.[164] In athletes, acute triceps ruptures are most common in weight lifting and American football during forceful eccentric contraction and are often associated with a history of steroid use.[164,165] Complete ruptures are rarely seen within the outpatient setting but are readily identifiable by history of acute onset of pain and loss of function coupled with ecchymosis and the inability to actively straighten the elbow.[164] A palpable defect is generally present[165] but may be missed clinically.

Complete ruptures are typically managed surgically with repair within the first 3 weeks for best results.[165] Postoperatively, the elbow is immobilized in 30 to 45° of flexion for 2 weeks, after which range is gradually increased to full by 6 to 8 weeks postoperatively. Active elbow extension is typically initiated about 4 weeks after surgery with resisted exercise as soon as 6 to 8 weeks with gradual progression following.[165]

Partial-thickness triceps tears are generally managed conservatively with 3 to 4 weeks of immobilization in 30° of elbow flexion followed by a gradual, progressive increase in stress to the triceps.[165] A full recovery can be expected.

Olecranon Bursitis

Olecranon bursitis presents local edema and warmth over the posterior elbow.[95] Onset is usually due to a one-time trauma of bumping the olecranon on an object, but can occur due to repeated compression and friction of weight bearing on the elbow. Because the bursa is extracapsular, elbow and forearm range of motion are preserved, and strength testing is normal. However, local tenderness is common. Olecranon bursitis is generally self-limiting, and treatment includes avoiding weight bearing over the affected bursa. Elbow pads may be beneficial either short term, whereas the bursa is inflamed, or long term for occupations requiring repeated or prolonged forearm/elbow weight bearing. Differential diagnosis includes gout, rheumatoid arthritis, or infection. Patients presenting with constitutional signs and symptoms, drainage, erythema, or a history of gout or rheumatoid arthritis should be referred to a primary care provider for further evaluation.

Medial Apophysitis

Medial apophysitis, also known as *Little Leaguer elbow*, is commonly seen in skeletally immature adolescents where the physis is weaker than the MCL.[130] The condition is characterized by insidious onset of progressive medial elbow pain that occurs with throwing activities. The cause of injury includes repetitive valgus stress with tension forces on the medial epicondyle via the MCL and the flexor-pronator muscle mass. These valgus stresses result in repetitive microtrauma to the medial epicondylar apophysis. Individuals present with vague medial elbow pain with throwing and decreased throwing abilities (decreased velocity and accuracy). These signs in combination with tenderness of the medial epicondyle in a skeletally immature patient are suggestive of medial apophysis injury.[86] In the absence of an avulsion fracture, treatment involves limiting valgus stress, ice, and symptom-modulated range of motion exercise. Elbow, forearm, and wrist isometrics are progressed to strengthening once pain free.[121] A gradual return to throwing with attention to ensuring proper mechanics is imperative. As with other throwing-related pathologies, clinicians should be sure to address the entire kinetic chain for optimal outcomes.

Osteochondritis Dissecans and Panner Disease

OCD is caused by repetitive valgus stress[121] or axial loading.[130] In the elbow, OCD is most commonly seen at the humeroradial joint.[127] Athletes with OCD generally have a gradual onset of vague lateral elbow pain. Management of OCD continues to evolve. Currently, conservative management is the rule with 3 to 6 weeks of immobilization with the elbow in 90° of flexion.[121] Once symptoms resolve, isometric and resistive exercises are gradually progressed. Surgery, including microfracture, osteochondral autograft, or osteochondral implantation, is reserved for unstable lesions in adolescents over the age of 14.[127] Panner disease is similar to OCD but involves the entire capitellum and generally affects younger individuals.[127] Panner disease appears to be self-limiting with restrictions in provocative activities, such as throwing.[127]

Internal Derangement

Internal derangement can occur when loose bodies are present within the joint, leading to a noncapsular loss of motion with limitation of flexion or extension. Forearm rotation is generally unaffected or minimally affected. Patients report the joint periodically locks, with full extension or flexion being limited with a hard endfeel. Range of motion returns gradually over several days. Frequent occurrences can lead to a reactive OA, even in adolescents.

Three different clinical pictures can be considered depending on the age group in which they appear: adolescents, adults, or the elderly.

- In adolescence: the condition does not occur before the age of 14 and usually results from OCD. Arthroscopic removal of the loose bodies is the normal course of treatment.
- In a normal joint in adulthood: the cause is usually traumatic, the injury having chipped off one or more pieces of cartilage. A very clear noncapsular pattern is found with limitation on either flexion or extension, depending on the position of the fragment. The loose bodies can shift position, allowing full motion to occur. If pain or functional limitations persist, arthroscopic removal is recommended.
- In an arthritic joint in middle aged or older: the symptoms are of repeated bouts of pain and a noncapsular pattern of restriction lasting for about a week. Between bouts, a capsular pattern of elbow range of motion restriction persists. The loose bodies may be visible on radiograph. Given the intermittent nature of the problem and spontaneous reduction, surgery is rarely required.

Differential diagnosis includes gout, rheumatoid arthritis, or infection.

DIFFERENTIAL DIAGNOSIS

Differential diagnosis of elbow pathology can be simplified by considering the patient's chief complaint (Table 15-9), symptom location (Fig. 15-50), and onset (Fig. 15-51). Because fracture and dislocation have their own unique presentations, these have not been considered in the differential diagnoses. OA of the elbow generally causes a more global, aching sensation, but posterior pain with extension can be noted with posterior osteophytes. Medial elbow pain can be difficult to differentiate. Table 15-10 highlights the typical findings for the most common medial elbow pathologies.

ADDITIONAL JOINT MOBILIZATION TREATMENT TECHNIQUES

The accessory motion procedures described earlier can be used to treat elbow and forearm hypomobility, particularly when using grade III and IV mobilizations and/or performing closer to end range. This section provides additional manual techniques to improve range of motion.

Humeroulnar Distraction Mobilization

Purpose: To improve humeroulnar joint mobility and elbow flexion.
Patient: Supine with arm by the side, elbow bent, forearm supinated.
Clinician: The clinician stabilizes the wrist with the inferior hand and grasps the proximal forearm close to the joint line with the superior hand pronated.
Mobilization: The clinician glides the proximal ulna inferiorly by weight shifting from the right to the left, creating joint distraction (Fig. 15-52). The mobilization can be performed near end-range flexion to more specifically improve elbow flexion range of motion.

Posterior Radiohumeral Mobilization

Purpose: To improve elbow extension.
Patient: Supine with arm by the side, elbow near end-range extension, forearm supinated.
Clinician: The clinician supports the wrist with the inferior hand and grasps the proximal radius close to the joint line with the superior hand pronated.
Mobilization: The clinician glides the proximal radius posteriorly (Fig. 15-53).

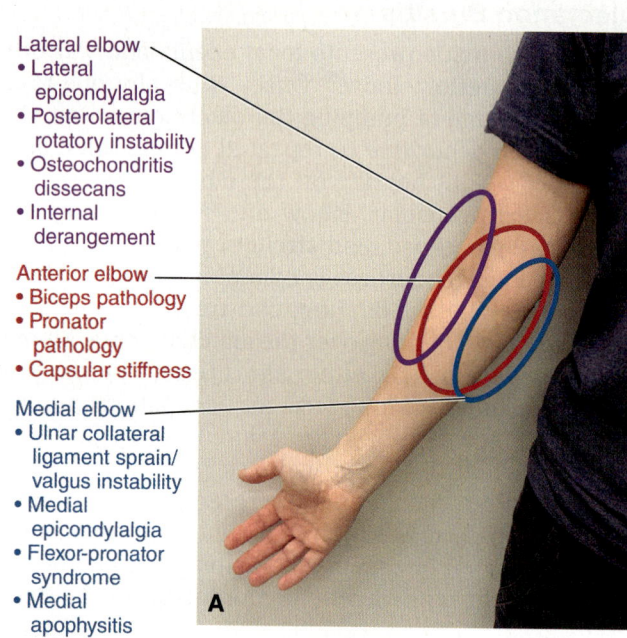

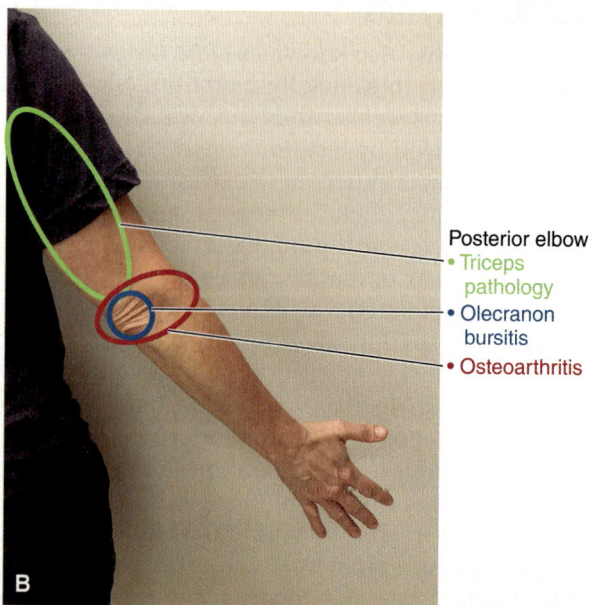

FIGURE 15-50 Elbow pathology by symptom location. **A.** Anterior view. **B.** Posterior view.

TABLE 15-9
DIFFERENTIAL DIAGNOSIS OF ELBOW PATHOLOGY BY COMPLAINT

Complaint/Symptom	Differential Diagnoses
Stiffness	• Osteoarthritis • Postimmobilization
Weakness	• Strain • Tendon rupture • Epicondylalgia • Peripheral nerve compression neuropathy
Instability	• Instability/ligament sprain
Mechanical complaints of clicking, locking, catching	• Osteoarthritis • Internal derangement • Instability
Paresthesias	• Cervical dysfunction • Thoracic outlet syndrome • Peripheral nerve compression neuropathy

CHAPTER 15 | ELBOW COMPLEX

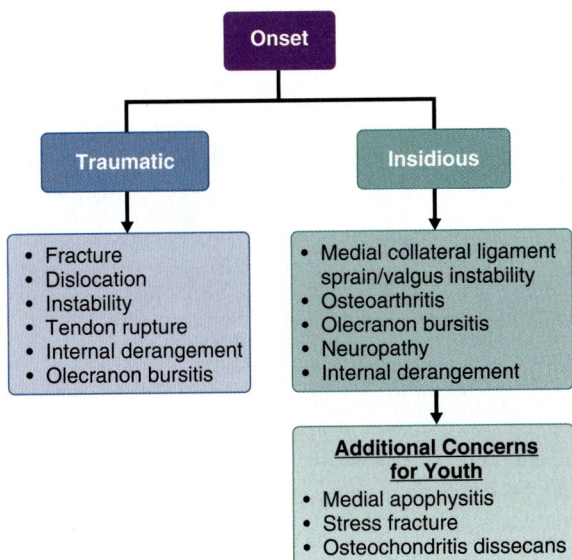

FIGURE 15-51 Elbow pathology based on typical onset.

TABLE 15-10
DIFFERENTIAL DIAGNOSIS OF MEDIAL ELBOW SYMPTOMS

Pathology	Examination Findings
MCL sprain/valgus instability	Positive valgus stress test or moving valgus stress test Tenderness along the MCL Pain during late cocking/early acceleration phase of throwing Activities of daily living relatively unaffected
Medial epicondylalgia	Pain with MMT of wrist flexors or pronators Mild pain with stretching of the flexor carpi radialis or pronator teres Tenderness of the flexor/pronators More painful during acceleration and/or release phases of throwing Pain with activities requiring repeated or resisted wrist flexion or forearm pronation
Pronator syndrome	Paresthesias into the volar forearm, thenar eminence, and radial digits Weakness of median nerve innervated FPL, index and ring finger FDP, and FCR Positive tinel of the median nerve in the forearm; pronator compression test
Ulnar nerve pathology	Positive tinel at the cubital tunnel Paresthesias or decreased sensation of the fourth and fifth digits Painless decrease in grip strength Symptoms with repeated elbow flexion/extension Report of clumsiness or first dorsal interossei atrophy in advanced pathology
Medial apophysitis	Skeletally immature Tenderness of the medial epicondyle

FCR, flexor carpi radialis; *FDP*, flexor digitorum profundus; *FPL*, flexor pollicis longus; *MCL*, median collateral ligament, *MMT*, manual muscle test.

Radioulnar Spreading

Purpose: To improve forearm supination.
Patient: Supine with arm by the side, elbow near end-range extension, forearm near end-range supination.
Clinician: The clinician grasps the ulna with the lateral hand and the radius with the medial hand.
Mobilization: The clinician moves the radius into supination stretching the IOM and pronators (Fig. 15-54). The clinician's hands can be move further superior or inferior along the patient's forearm to better target the stretch.

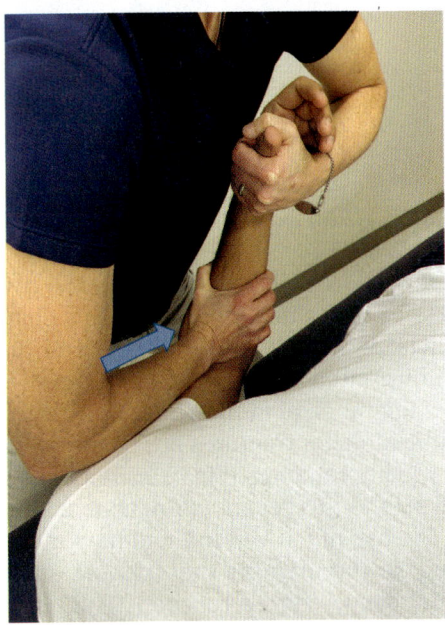

FIGURE 15-52 Humeroulnar distraction mobilization.

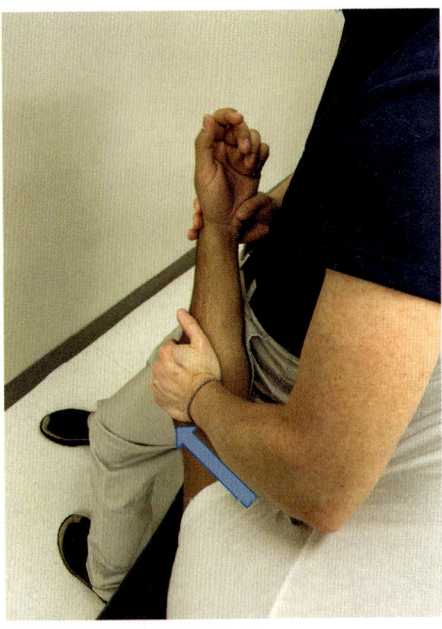

FIGURE 15-53 Posterior radial mobilization.

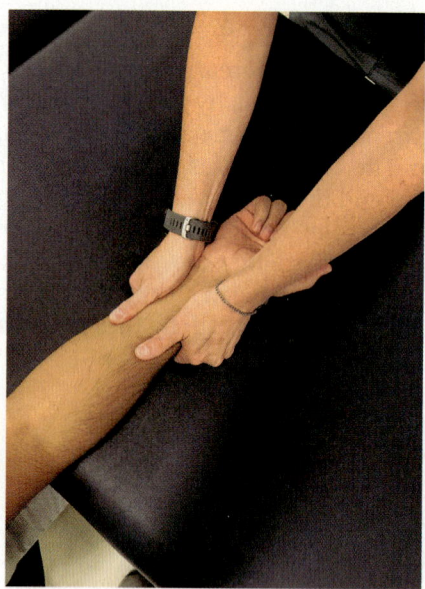

FIGURE 15-54 Radioulnar spreading.

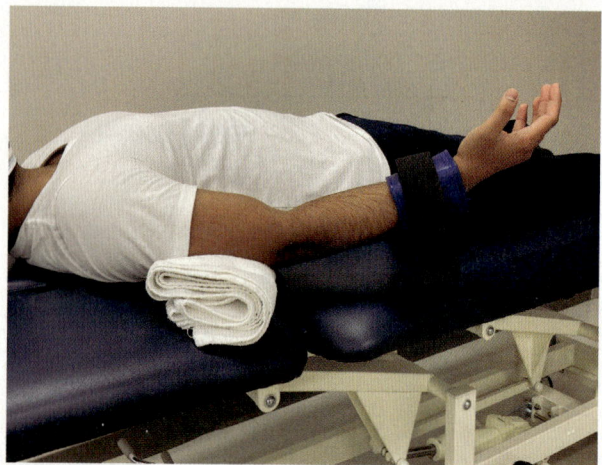

FIGURE 15-55 Low-load, long-duration stretch for elbow extension range of motion.

ADDITIONAL THERAPEUTIC EXERCISES

The exercises described throughout this chapter may be beneficial for a variety of patients and diagnoses. This section contains additional examples of exercises for improving range of motion, strength, and function.

Elbow flexion contractures are common. Low-load, long-duration stretching (Fig. 15-55) can be a well-tolerated method to regain elbow extension range of motion. The use of a towel roll and having the motion performed at the edge of the support surface help ensure end range can be reached. The use of a cuff weight allows the patient to relax, rather than contract muscles to grip a free weight or other weighted object.

Pronation (Fig. 15-56A) and supination (Fig. 15-56B) can be assisted or resisted with the use of an object with an offset weight, such as a hammer. By holding further away from the weighted end, the intensity of the stretch is increased. If performed as a continuous motion, this same setup becomes a strengthening exercise for the pronators and supinators.

A flexible resistance bar can be used for pronation strengthening by grabbing the horizontal bar with both hands palms up (supinated). The patient moves both hands into pronation against the resistance of the bar (Fig. 15-57A). For supination strengthening, the horizontal bar is grasped with palms down (pronated). The patient moves both hands into supination (Fig. 15-57B).

Wrist extensor strengthening can be performed with a flexible resistance bar or free weight. In the early phases of rehabilitation for lateral epicondylalgia, the forearm should be in a more neutral position (Fig. 15-58A) or the elbow in about 90° of flexion (Fig. 15-58B). In later phases,

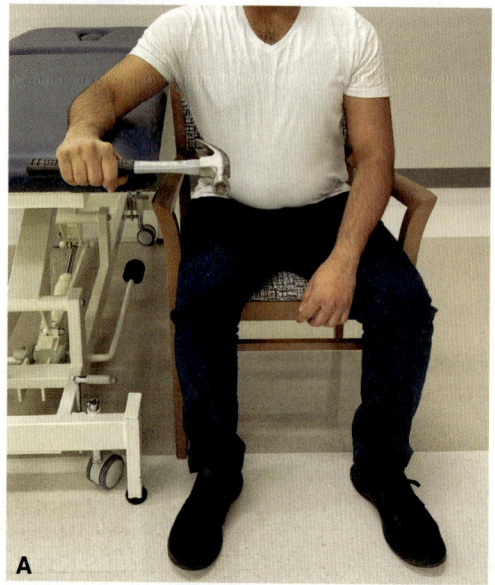
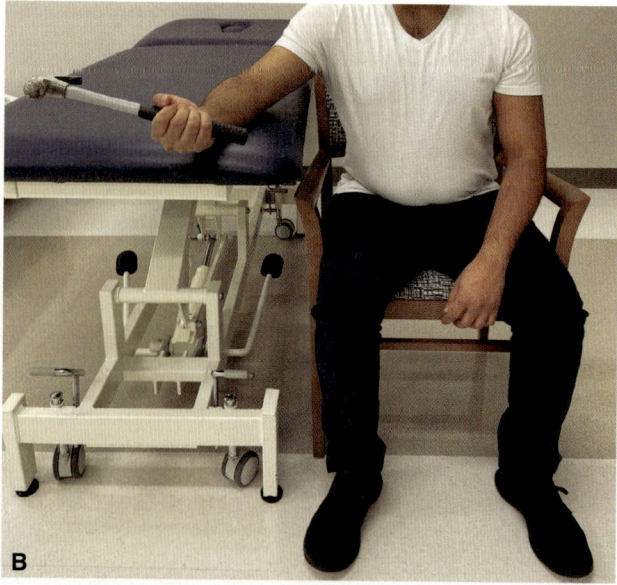

FIGURE 15-56 Static stretch to increase pronation (**A**) and supination (**B**).

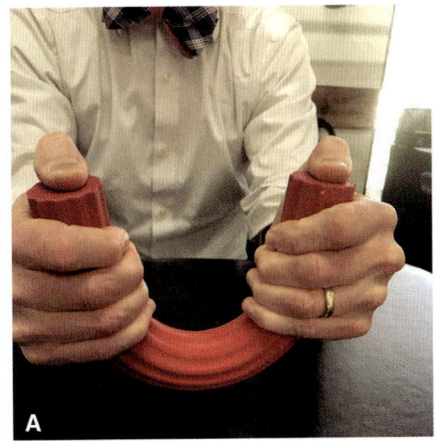
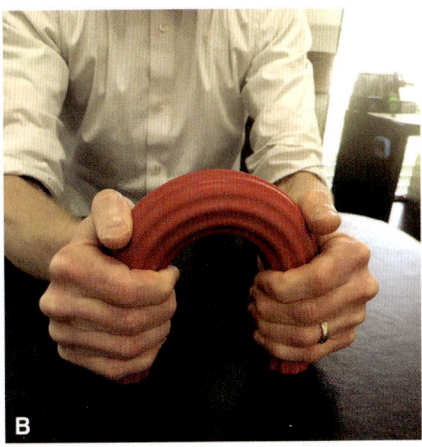

FIGURE 15-57 Flexible resistance bar for pronation (**A**) and supination (**B**) strengthening.

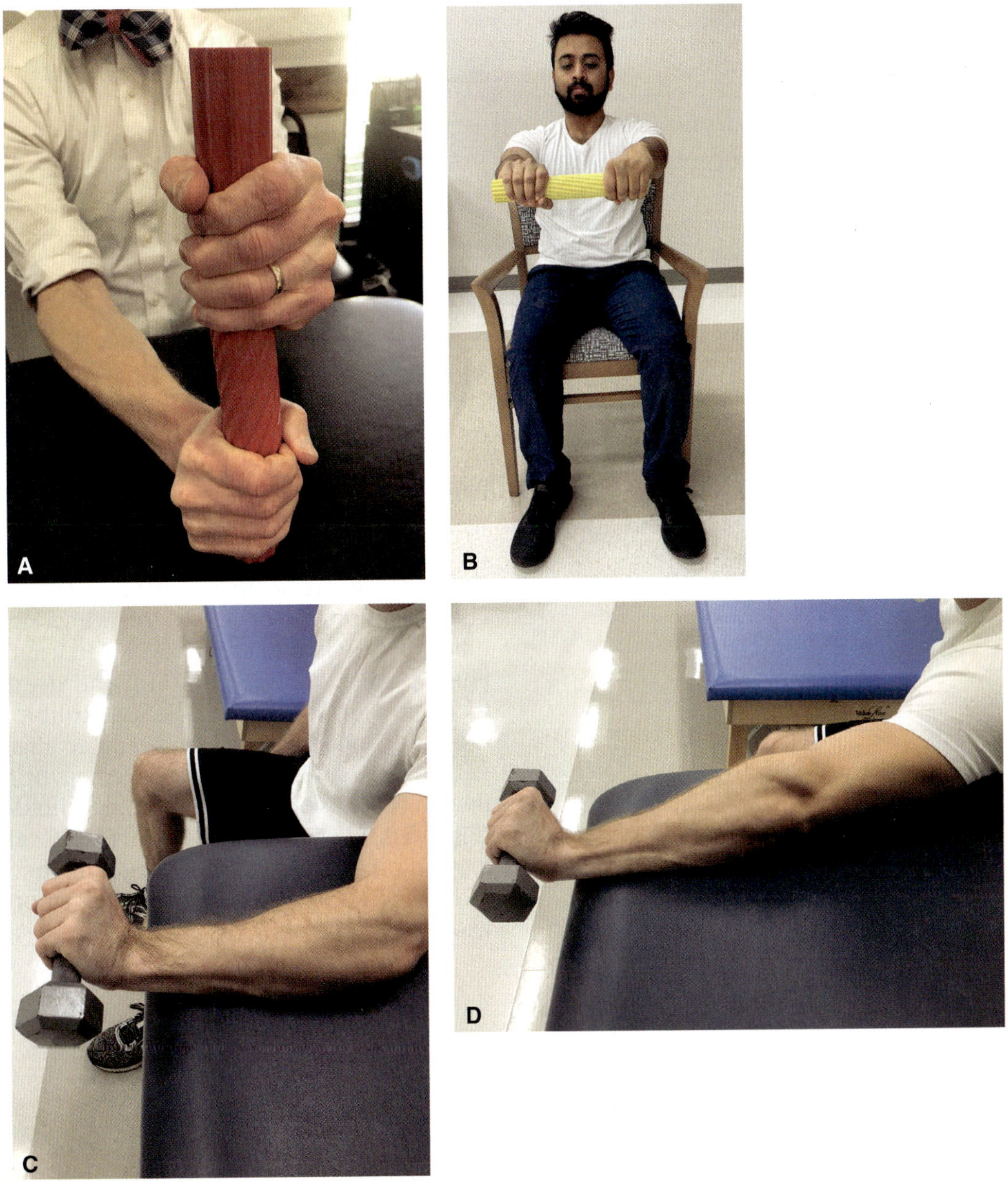

FIGURE 15-58 Wrist extensor strengthening can be progressed from early-phase exercises using a flexible resistance bar with elbow flexed and neutral forearm (**A**) and forearm pronated (**B**) to late phase using a dumbbell with forearm pronated (**C**) and elbow extended (**D**).

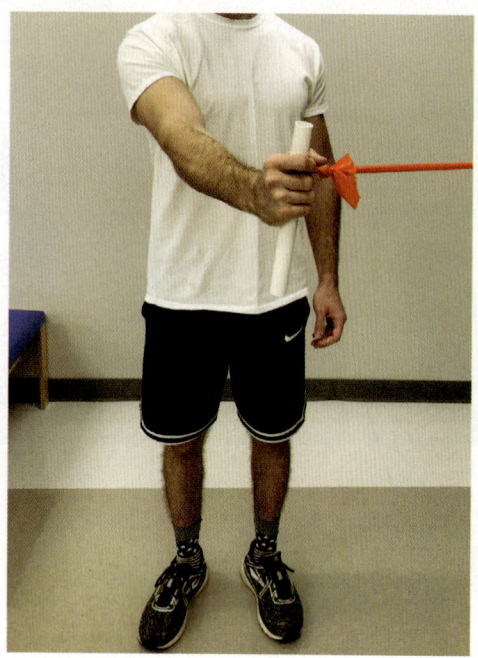

FIGURE 15-59 Simulated backhand with posterior vector.

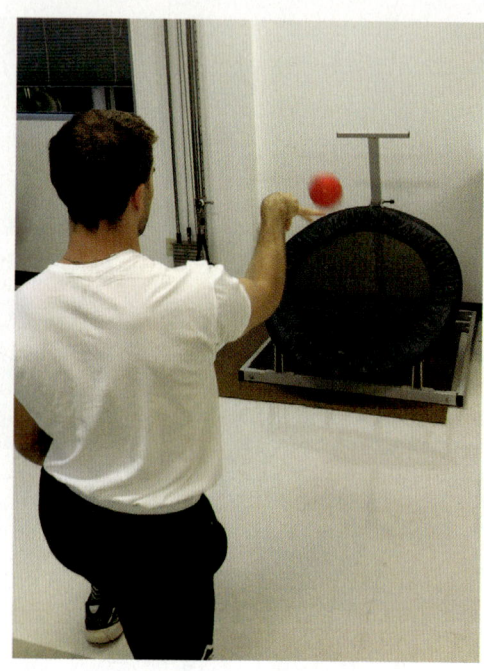

FIGURE 15-61 Rebounder ball toss.

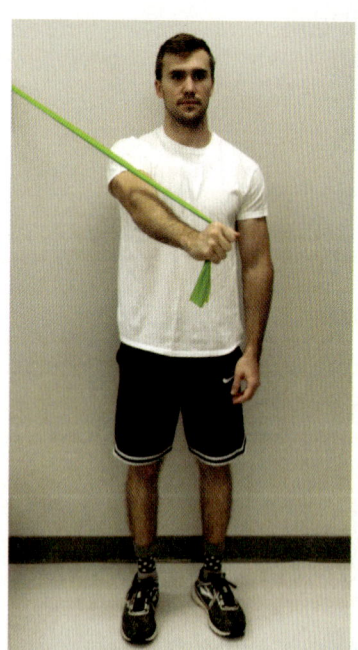

FIGURE 15-60 D2 extension with resistance band.

the forearm can be pronated and the elbow extended (Fig. 15-58C, D).

For athletes in racquet sports, a posterior vector can be added to a simulated backhand to require increased isometric wrist extensor activity (Fig. 15-59). A racquet can also be used for this activity.

There are several progressions for throwing athletes. A "D2 extension pattern of the upper extremity" (the motion of grabbing and buckling a seatbelt) using a resistance band or cable column is an early functional exercise to incorporate the entire kinetic chain required for overhead throwing (Fig. 15-60). Plyometric exercises can be progressed from two-handed chest passes, sideways passes, and overhead passes to single arm (Fig. 15-61). The wall dribble requires the athlete to maintain proper scapular alignment while performing small arc throws, using primarily wrist flexion, or larger arcs, by adding shoulder rotation (Fig. 15-62). Using the support of the table, the ball flip is a plyometric exercise targeting the wrist flexors (Fig. 15-63). For athletes in racquet sports, a similar exercise can be performed while holding a racquet.

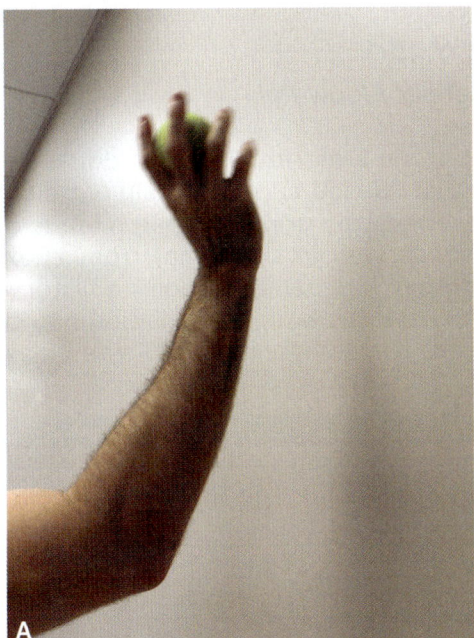
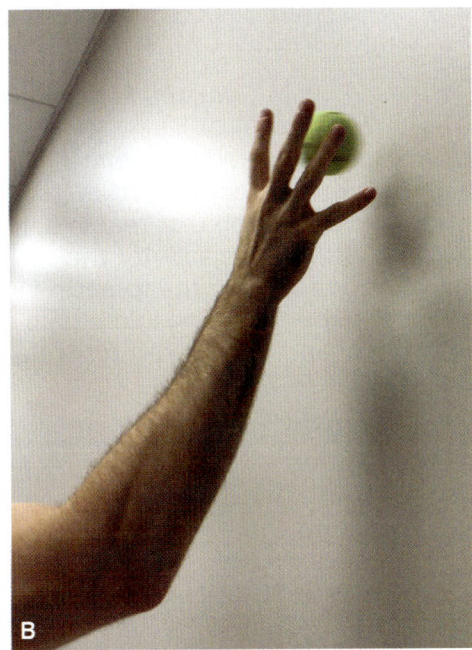

FIGURE 15-62 Wall dribble exercise. **A.** Eccentric catch phase. **B.** Concentric throw phase.

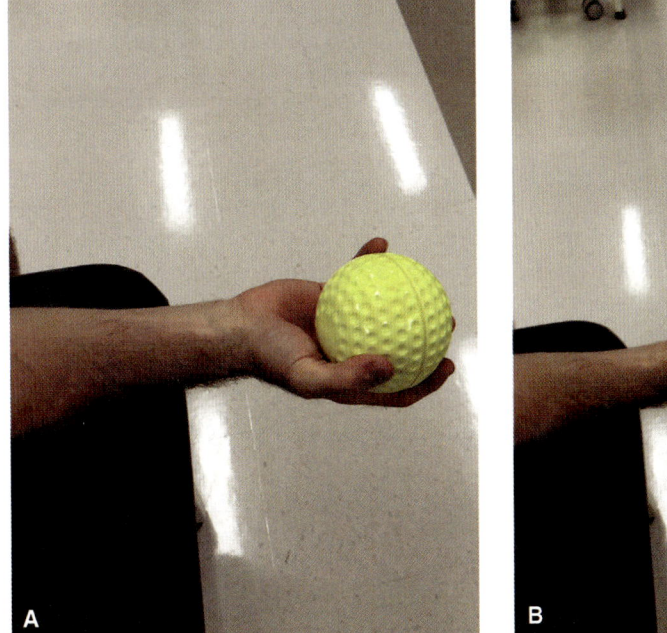
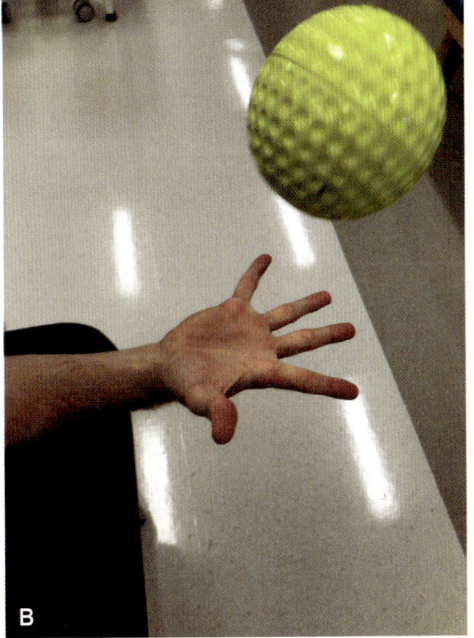

FIGURE 15-63 Ball flip exercise. **A.** Eccentric catch phase. **B.** Concentric throw phase.

CASE STUDY 15-1
Hiroshi: Patient with Lateral Elbow Pain

Hiroshi is a 47-year-old assembly line worker who reports a 2-month history of dominant (right) lateral elbow pain. He does not recall a particular injury that caused his elbow pain but did note that he was just transferred to a new job that requires him to repeatedly grip and stretch fabric over a frame. When asked to demonstrate this activity, the clinician observes Hiroshi moving from a flexed elbow to an extended elbow position with the forearm in pronation. The patient reports a history of diabetes and a distant history of participating in multiple sports while growing up, including playing American football in high school and college. All tests begin with the uninvolved (left) side unless otherwise noted (see Table 15-11).

TABLE 15-11

SAMPLE ELBOW EXAMINATION

Hiroshi, a 47-year-old assembly line worker with a 2-month history of dominant (right) lateral elbow pain

Position	Assessments
Observation	Observe motion noted to be problematic by patient
Seated	Shoulder flex, ext, abd (A, OP, MMT)
	Shoulder behind neck and behind back combined plan motion (A)
	MMT shoulder IR, ER with arm at side
	Elbow flex, ext (A, P, MMT)
	Forearm pro, sup (A, OP, MMT)
	Wrist flex, ext, RD, UD (A, P, MMT)
	Handheld dynamometer: maximal grip, maximal pain-free grip strength
	Special tests: humeroradial compression test, resisted wrist extension and radial deviation, passive wrist flexion with the elbow extended
	Palpation: including the lateral epicondyle, supracondylar ridge, radial head, and muscles of the extensor forearm

A, active; *abd*, abduction; *ext*, extension; *ER*, external rotation; *flex*, flexion; *IR*, internal rotation; *MMT*, manual muscle test; *OP*, overpressure; *P*, passive; *pro*, pronation; *RD*, radial deviation; *sup*, supination; *UD*, ulnar deviation.

Based on the history, there are no red flags. The patient's history of insidious onset of elbow pain that coincided with a change in job tasks makes the clinician have an initial hypothesis of lateral epicondylalgia. The patient's age and prior sporting history make OA a potential competing diagnosis. The seated examination began by observing the motion the patient notes to be most problematic. This was believed to be safe, given the lack of red flags and the patient is currently working without restriction. By learning more about the exact functional activity aggravating the patient's symptoms, the clinician is able to target the physical examination more precisely. The clinician then obtained an overall sense of shoulder function in the seated position. The clinician decided there was no need for more specific assessments of rotator cuff strength and precise manual muscle testing in the prone position was deferred.

Sensory testing and other neurologic assessments were deferred because the patient did not report any neurologic symptoms. Goniometric measurement using standardized test positions and accessory motion testing were not performed because range of motion was normal and instability was not part of the initial working hypotheses for differential diagnosis. Maximal grip testing was performed to compare dominant and nondominant sides. Because pain-free grip strength is a valid measure of change over time, a grip strength test was performed to allow comparison later in the rehabilitation process. The radiocapitellar compression test was chosen because the clinician wanted to clearly rule out the potential for articular surface changes, given Hiroshi's prior sporting history. This could have been deferred, given there was no range deficit noted. However, because increased stress to the lateral joint surface did not change Hiroshi's symptoms, the clinician was satisfied that OA was no longer a potential cause of symptoms. Special tests for lateral epicondylalgia (resisted wrist extension and radial deviation; and passive wrist flexion with the elbow extended) were positive for reproducing the patient's symptoms. Therefore, the resisted third finger extension test was not considered necessary. The clinician concluded that Hiroshi had right lateral epicondylalgia.

CHAPTER SUMMARY

Understanding normal anatomy and biomechanics of the elbow complex is a critical precursor to identifying pathologies in the region. Differential diagnosis of patients with elbow or forearm symptoms begins with a thorough history. An upper quarter neurologic screen and assessment of peripheral nerve status for patients presenting with paresthesias, atrophy, or reports of clumsiness/decreased coordination are essential to diagnosis and intervention planning. Severity, delay in diagnosis, or improper management of fractures or dislocations in the elbow region is likely to lead to future motion loss, instability, or functional impairment. Elbow overuse injuries are common and may benefit from examination and intervention strategies that consider the entire kinetic chain. Dysfunction of the shoulder or wrist and hand may lead to altered movement patterns that affect the elbow, particularly in repetitive activities that involve overhead movements or forearm pronation and supination.

REFERENCES

1. Martin S, Sanchez E. Anatomy and biomechanics of the elbow joint. *Semin Musculoskelet Radiol.* 2013;17(5):429–436. doi:10.1055/s-0033-1361587
2. Dipaola M, Geissler W, Osterman A. Complex elbow instability. *Hand Clin.* 2008;24(1):39–52. doi:10.1016/j.hcl.2007.11.010
3. Alcid J, Ahmad C, Lee T. Elbow anatomy and structural biomechanics. *Clin Sports Med.* 2004;23(4):503–517, vii. doi:10.1016/j.csm.2004.06.008
4. Williams P, Warwick R, Myson M, Bannister L, eds. *Gray's Anatomy.* 37th ed. Churchill Livingstone; 1989.
5. Giannicola G, Sedati P, Polimanti D, Cinotti G, Bullitta G. Contribution of cartilage to size and shape of radial head circumference: magnetic resonance imaging analysis of 78 elbows. *J Shoulder Elbow Surg.* 2016;25(1):120–126. doi:10.1016/j.jse.2015.07.003
6. Van Roy P, Baeyens J, Fauvart D, Lanssiers R, Clarijs J. Arthro-kinematics of the elbow: study of the carrying angle. *Ergonomics.* 2005;48(11–14):1645–1656. doi:10.1080/00140130500101361
7. Hoppenfeld S. *Physical Examination of the Spine and Extremities.* Appleton-Centruy-Crofts; 1976.
8. Yilmaz E, Karakurt L, Belhan O, Bulut M, Serin E, Avci M. Variation of carrying angle with age, sex, and special reference to side. *Orthopedics.* 2005;28(11):1360–1363.
9. Paraskevas G, Papadopoulos A, Papaziogas B, Spanidou S, Argiriadou H, Gigis J. Study of the carrying angle of the human elbow joint in full extension: a morphometric analysis. *Surg Radiol Anat.* 2004;26(1):19–23. doi:10.1007/s00276-003-0185-z
10. Farrow L, Mahoney A, Stefancin J, Taljanovic M, Sheppard J, Schickendantz M. Quantitative analysis of the medial ulnar collateral ligament ulnar footprint and its relationship to the ulnar sublime tubercle. *Am J Sports Med.* 2011;39(9):1936–1941. doi:10.1177/0363546511406220
11. Floris S, Olsen B, Dalstra M, Søjbjerg J, Sneppen O. The medial collateral ligament of the elbow joint: anatomy and kinematics. *J Shoulder Elbow Surg.* 1998;7(4):345–351. doi:10.1016/s1058-2746(98)90021-0
12. Karbach LE, Elfar J. Elbow instability: anatomy, biomechanics, diagnostic maneuvers, and testing. *J Hand Surg Am.* 2017;42(2):118–126. doi:10.1016/j.jhsa.2016.11.025
13. Pollock J, Brownhill J, Ferreira L, McDonald C, Johnson J, King G. Effect of the posterior bundle of the medial collateral ligament on elbow stability. *J Hand Surg Am.* 2009;34(1):116–123. doi:10.1016/j.jhsa.2008.09.016
14. Morrey B, An K. Articular and ligamentous contributions to the stability of the elbow joint. *Am J Sports Med.* 1983;11(5):315–319. doi:10.1177/036354658301100506
15. Safran M, Baillargeon D. Soft-tissue stabilizers of the elbow. *J Shoulder Elbow Surg.* 2005;14 (1 Suppl S):179s–185s. doi:10.1016/j.jse.2004.09.032
16. Callaway G, Field L, Deng X, et al. Biomechanical evaluation of the medial collateral ligament of the elbow. *J Bone Joint Surg Am.* 1997;79(8):1223–1231. doi:10.2106/00004623-199708000-00015
17. Bryce C, Armstrong A. Anatomy and biomechanics of the elbow. *Orthop Clin North Am.* 2008;39(2):141–154, v. doi:10.1016/j.ocl.2007.12.001
18. Barnes J, Chouhan V, Egekeze N, Rinaldi C, Cil A. The annular ligament-revisited. *J Shoulder Elbow Surg.* 2018;27(1):e16–e19. doi:10.1016/j.jse.2017.07.031
19. Mesgarzadeh M, Revesz G, Bonakdarpour A. Femoral neck torsion angle measurement by computed tomography. *J Comput Assist Tomogr.* 1987;11(5):799–803. doi:10.1097/00004728-198709000-00011
20. Tarassoli P, McCann P, Amirfeyz R. Complex instability of the elbow. *Injury.* 2017;48(3):568–577. doi:10.1016/j.injury.2013.09.032
21. Mehta J, Bain G. Posterolateral rotatory instability of the elbow. *J Am Acad Orthop Surg.* 2004;12(6):405–415. doi:10.5435/00124635-200411000-00005
22. Martin B. The annular ligament of the superior radio-ulnar joint. *J Anat.* 1958;92(3):473–482.
23. Bozkurt M, Acar H, Apaydin N, et al. The annular ligament: an anatomical study. *Am J Sports Med.* 2005;33(1):114–118. doi:10.1177/0363546504266070
24. Tubbs R, Shoja M, Khaki A, et al. The morphology and function of the quadrate ligament. *Folia Morphol (Warsz).* 2006;65(3):225–227.
25. Spinner M, Kaplan E. The quadrate ligament of the elbow—its relationship to the stability of the proximal radio-ulnar joint. *Acta Orthop Scand.* 1970;41(6):632–647. doi:10.3109/17453677008991554
26. O'Driscoll S. Elbow instability. *Acta Orthop Belg.* 1999;65(4):404–415.
27. Dunning C, Zarzour Z, Patterson S, Johnson J, King G. Ligamentous stabilizers against posterolateral rotatory instability of the elbow. *J Bone Joint Surg Am.* 2001;83(12):1823–1828. doi:10.2106/00004623-200112000-00009
28. Cohen M, Hastings H 2nd. Rotatory instability of the elbow. The anatomy and role of the lateral stabilizers. *J Bone Joint Surg Am.* 1997;79(2):225–233.
29. Williams P. *Gray's Anatomy: The Anatomical Basis of Medicine and Surgery.* 38th ed. Churchill Livingstone; 1995.
30. Daniels D, Mallisee T, Erickson S, Boynton M, Carrera G. The elbow joint: osseous and ligamentous structures. *Radiographics.* 1998;18(1):229–236. doi:10.1148/radiographics.18.1.9460127
31. Floranda E, Jacobs B. Evaluation and treatment of upper extremity nerve entrapment syndromes. *Prim Care.* 2013;40(4):925–943, ix. doi:10.1016/j.pop.2013.08.009
32. Dailiana Z, Roulot E, Le Viet D. Surgical treatment of compression of the lateral antebrachial cutaneous nerve.

J Bone Joint Surg Br. 2000;82(3):420–423. doi:10.1302/0301-620x.82b3.10098
33. Moore KL, Dalley AF, Agur AMR. *Clinically Oriented Anatomy.* 8th ed. Wolters Kluwer; 2018.
34. Ljungquist K, Martineau P, Allan C. Radial nerve injuries. *J Hand Surg Am.* 2015;40(1):166–172. doi:10.1016/j.jhsa.2014.05.010
35. Latef T, Bilal M, Vetter M, Iwanaga J, Oskouian R, Tubbs R. Injury of the radial nerve in the arm: a review. *Cureus.* 2018;10(2):e2199. doi:10.7759/cureus.2199
36. Bumbasirevic M, Palibrk T, Lesic A, Atkinson H. Radial nerve palsy. *EFORT Open Rev.* 2016;1(8):286–294. doi:10.1302/2058-5241.1.000028
37. Chang G, Ilyas A. Radial nerve palsy after humeral shaft fractures: the case for early exploration and a new classification to guide treatment and prognosis. *Hand Clin.* 2018;34(1):105–112. doi:10.1016/j.hcl.2017.09.011
38. Shao Y, Harwood P, Grotz M, Limb D, Giannoudis P. Radial nerve palsy associated with fractures of the shaft of the humerus: a systematic review. *J Bone Joint Surg Br.* 2005;87(12):1647–1652. doi:10.1302/0301-620x.87b12.16132
39. Doughty CT, Bowley MP. Entrapment neuropathies of the upper extremity. *Med Clin North Am.* 2019;103(2):357–370. doi:10.1016/j.mcna.2018.10.012
40. Caetano E, Vieira L, Sprovieri F, Petta G, Nakasone M, Serafim B. Anatomical variations of pronator teres muscle: predispositional role for nerve entrapment. *Rev Bras Ortop.* 2017;52(2):169–175. doi:10.1016/j.rboe.2017.02.003
41. Soubeyrand M, Melhem R, Protais M, Artuso M, Crézé M. Anatomy of the median nerve and its clinical applications. *Hand Surg Rehabil.* 2020;39(1):2–18. doi:10.1016/j.hansur.2019.10.197
42. Tubbs R, Marshall T, Loukas M, Shoja M, Cohen-Gadol A. The sublime bridge: anatomy and implications in median nerve entrapment. *J Neurosurg.* 2010;113(1):110–112. doi:10.3171/2009.10.Jns091251
43. Seitz W Jr, Matsuoka H, McAdoo J, Sherman G, Stickney D. Acute compression of the median nerve at the elbow by the lacertus fibrosus. *J Shoulder Elbow Surg.* 2007;16(1):91–94. doi:10.1016/j.jse.2006.04.005
44. Hartz C, Linscheid R, Gramse R, Daube J. The pronator teres syndrome: compressive neuropathy of the median nerve. *J Bone Joint Surg Am.* 1981;63(6):885–890.
45. Jacobson J, Fessell D, Lobo Lda G, Yang L. Entrapment neuropathies I: upper limb (carpal tunnel excluded). *Semin Musculoskelet Radiol.* 2010;14(5):473–486. doi:10.1055/s-0030-1268068
46. Siqueira M, Martins R. The controversial arcade of Struthers. *Surg Neurol.* 2005;64(Suppl 1):17–20; discussion S1:20–21. doi:10.1016/j.surneu.2005.04.017
47. Caetano E, Sabongi Neto J, Vieira L, Caetano M. The arcade of Struthers: an anatomical study and clinical implications. *Rev Bras Ortop.* 2017;52(3):331–336. doi:10.1016/j.rboe.2016.07.006
48. Palmer B, Hughes T. Cubital tunnel syndrome. *J Hand Surg Am.* 2010;35(1):153–163. doi:10.1016/j.jhsa.2009.11.004
49. Granger A, Sardi J, Iwanaga J, et al. Osborne's ligament: a review of its history, anatomy, and surgical importance. *Cureus.* 2017;9(3):e1080. doi:10.7759/cureus.1080
50. Staples JR, Calfee R. Cubital tunnel syndrome: current concepts. *J Am Acad Orthop Surg.* 2017;25(10):e215–e224. doi:10.5435/JAAOS-D-15-00261
51. James J, Sutton L, Werner F, Basu N, Allison M, Palmer A. Morphology of the cubital tunnel: an anatomical and biomechanical study with implications for treatment of ulnar nerve compression. *J Hand Surg Am.* 2011;36(12):1988–1995. doi:10.1016/j.jhsa.2011.09.014
52. Iba K, Wada T, Aoki M, Oda T, Ozasa Y, Yamashita T. The relationship between the pressure adjacent to the ulnar nerve and the disease causing cubital tunnel syndrome. *J Shoulder Elbow Surg.* 2008;17(4):585–588. doi:10.1016/j.jse.2007.12.003
53. Nordin M, Frankel VH. *Basic Biomechanics of the Musculoskeletal System.* 4th ed. Lippincott Williams & Wilkins; 2012.
54. American Academy of Orthopedics Surgeons. *America Academy of Orthopedic Surgeons: Joint Motion: Method of Measuring and Recording.* American Academy of Orthopedic Surgeons; 1965.
55. Morrey BF, Askew LJ, Chao EY. A biomechanical study of normal functional elbow motion. *J Bone Joint Surg Am.* 1981;63(6):872–877.
56. Morrey B, An K. Stability of the elbow: osseous constraints. *J Shoulder Elbow Surg.* 2005;14(1 Suppl S):174s–178s. doi:10.1016/j.jse.2004.09.031
57. O'Driscoll S, Jupiter J, King G, Hotchkiss R, Morrey B. The unstable elbow. *Instr Course Lect.* 2001;50:89–102.
58. McKee M, Schemitsch E, Sala M, SW OD. The pathoanatomy of lateral ligamentous disruption in complex elbow instability. *J Shoulder Elbow Surg.* 2003;12(4):391–396. doi:10.1016/s1058-2746(03)00027-2
59. Wilps T, Kaufmann R, Yamakawa S, Fowler J. Elbow biomechanics: bony and dynamic stabilizers. *J Hand Surg Am.* 2020;45(6):528–535. doi:10.1016/j.jhsa.2020.01.016
60. An K, Morrey B, Chao E. The effect of partial removal of proximal ulna on elbow constraint. *Clin Orthop Relat Res.* 1986;(209):270–279.
61. Kamineni S, Hirahara H, Pomianowski S, et al. Partial posteromedial olecranon resection: a kinematic study. *J Bone Joint Surg Am.* 2003;85(6):1005–1011. doi:10.2106/00004623-200306000-00004
62. Bell T, Ferreira L, McDonald C, Johnson J, King G. Contribution of the olecranon to elbow stability: an in vitro biomechanical study. *J Bone Joint Surg Am.* 2010;92(4):949–957. doi:10.2106/jbjs.H.01873
63. Closkey R, Goode J, Kirschenbaum D, Cody R. The role of the coronoid process in elbow stability. A biomechanical analysis of axial loading. *J Bone Joint Surg Am.* 2000;82(12):1749–1753. doi:10.2106/00004623-200012000-00009
64. Schneeberger A, Sadowski M, Jacob H. Coronoid process and radial head as posterolateral rotatory stabilizers of the elbow. *J Bone Joint Surg Am.* 2004;86(5):975–982. doi:10.2106/00004623-200405000-00013
65. Beingessner D, Dunning C, Stacpoole R, Johnson J, King G. The effect of coronoid fractures on elbow kinematics and stability. *Clin Biomech (Bristol, Avon).* 2007;22(2):183–190. doi:10.1016/j.clinbiomech.2006.09.007
66. Morrey B, Tanaka S, An K. Valgus stability of the elbow. A definition of primary and secondary constraints. *Clin Orthop Relat Res.* 1991;(265):187–195.
67. Fleisig G, Andrews J, Dillman C, Escamilla R. Kinetics of baseball pitching with implications about injury mechanisms. *Am J Sports Med.* 1995;23(2):233–239. doi:10.1177/036354659502300218
68. Wilson F, Andrews J, Blackburn T, McCluskey G. Valgus extension overload in the pitching elbow. *Am J Sports Med.* 1983;11(2):83–88. doi:10.1177/036354658301100206
69. Kincaid B, An K. Elbow joint biomechanics for preclinical evaluation of total elbow prostheses. *J Biomech.* 2013;46(14):2331–2341. doi:10.1016/j.jbiomech.2013.07.027
70. Funk D, An K, Morrey B, Daube J. Electromyographic analysis of muscles across the elbow joint. *J Orthop Res.* 1987;5(4):529–538. doi:10.1002/jor.1100050408

71. Buchanan T, Rovai G, Rymer W. Strategies for muscle activation during isometric torque generation at the human elbow. *J Neurophysiol.* 1989;62(6):1201–1212. doi:10.1152/jn.1989.62.6.1201
72. Lin F, Kohli N, Perlmutter S, Lim D, Nuber G, Makhsous M. Muscle contribution to elbow joint valgus stability. *J Shoulder Elbow Surg.* 2007;16(6):795–802. doi:10.1016/j.jse.2007.03.024
73. Park M, Ahmad C. Dynamic contributions of the flexor-pronator mass to elbow valgus stability. *J Bone Joint Surg Am.* 2004;86(10):2268–2274. doi:10.2106/00004623-200410000-00020
74. Poitevin L. Anatomy and biomechanics of the interosseous membrane: its importance in the longitudinal stability of the forearm. *Hand Clin.* 2001;17(1):97–110, vii.
75. Morrey B, An K, Stormont T. Force transmission through the radial head. *J Bone Joint Surg Am.* 1988;70(2):250–256.
76. Noda K, Goto A, Murase T, Sugamoto K, Yoshikawa H, Moritomo H. Interosseous membrane of the forearm: an anatomical study of ligament attachment locations. *J Hand Surg Am.* 2009;34(3):415–422. doi:10.1016/j.jhsa.2008.10.025
77. McGinley J, Kozin S. Interosseous membrane anatomy and functional mechanics. *Clin Orthop Relat Res.* 2001;(383):108–122. doi:10.1097/00003086-200102000-00013
78. Ofuchi S, Takahashi K, Yamagata M, Rokkaku T, Moriya H, Hara T. Pressure distribution in the humeroradial joint and force transmission to the capitellum during rotation of the forearm: effects of the Sauvé-Kapandji procedure and incision of the interosseous membrane. *J Orthop Sci.* 2001;6(1):33–38. doi:10.1007/s007760170022
79. Neumann D. *Kinesiology of the Musculoskeletal System: Foundations for Rehabilitation.* 3rd ed. Elsevier; 2017.
80. Topp K, Boyd B. Structure and biomechanics of peripheral nerves: nerve responses to physical stresses and implications for physical therapist practice. *Phys Ther.* 2006;86(1):92–109. doi:10.1093/ptj/86.1.92
81. Caliandro P, La Torre G, Padua R, Giannini F, Padua L. Treatment for ulnar neuropathy at the elbow. *Cochrane Database Syst Rev.* 2016;11(11):CD006839. doi:10.1002/14651858.CD006839.pub4
82. Chin A, Lloyd D, Alderson J, Elliott B, Mills P. A marker-based mean finite helical axis model to determine elbow rotation axes and kinematics in vivo. *J Appl Biomech.* 2010;26(3):305–315. doi:10.1123/jab.26.3.305
83. Baeyens J, Van Glabbeek F, Goossens M, Gielen J, Van Roy P, Clarys J. In vivo 3D arthrokinematics of the proximal and distal radioulnar joints during active pronation and supination. *Clin Biomech (Bristol, Avon).* 2006;21(Suppl 1):S9–S12. doi:10.1016/j.clinbiomech.2005.09.008
84. Kleinman W, Graham T. The distal radioulnar joint capsule: clinical anatomy and role in posttraumatic limitation of forearm rotation. *J Hand Surg Am.* 1998;23(4):588–599. doi:10.1016/s0363-5023(98)80043-9
85. Hsu SH, Moen TC, Levine WN, Ahmad CS. Physical examination of the athlete's elbow. *Am J Sports Med.* 2012;40(3):699–708. doi:10.1177/0363546511428869
86. Smith MV, Lamplot JD, Wright RW, Brophy RH. Comprehensive review of the elbow physical examination. *J Am Acad Orthop Surg.* 2018;26(19):678–687. doi:10.5435/JAAOS-D-16-00622
87. Laratta J, Caldwell JM, Lombardi J, Levine W, Ahmad C. Evaluation of common elbow pathologies: a focus on physical examination. *Phys Sportsmed.* 2017;45(2):184–190. doi:10.1080/00913847.2017.1292831
88. Zouzias IC, Byram IR, Shillingford JN, Levine WN. A primer for physical examination of the elbow. *Phys Sportsmed.* 2012;40(1):51–61. doi:10.3810/psm.2012.02.1951
89. Joshi N, Lira A, Mehta N, Paladino L, Sinert R. Diagnostic accuracy of history, physical examination, and bedside ultrasound for diagnosis of extremity fractures in the emergency department: a systematic review. *Acad Emerg Med.* 2013;20(1):1–15. doi:10.1111/acem.12058
90. Appelboam A, Reuben AD, Benger JR, et al. Elbow extension test to rule out elbow fracture: multicentre, prospective validation and observational study of diagnostic accuracy in adults and children. *Br Med J.* 2008;337:a2428. doi:10.1136/bmj.a2428
91. Darracq MA, Vinson DR, Panacek EA. Preservation of active range of motion after acute elbow trauma predicts absence of elbow fracture. *Am J Emerg Med.* 2008;26(7):779–782. doi:10.1016/j.ajem.2007.11.005
92. Johnson MK. Nursemaid's elbow reduction. *Adv Emerg Nurs J.* 2019;41(4):330–335. doi:10.1097/TME.0000000000000270
93. Campo TM. A case of subluxation of the radial head: Nursemaids' elbow. *Adv Emerg Nurs J.* 2011;33(1):8–14. doi:10.1097/tme.0b013e318208ca79
94. Genadry KC, Monuteaux MC, Neuman MI, Lipsett SC. Management and outcomes of children with nursemaid's elbow. *Ann Emerg Med.* 2021;77(2):154–162. doi:10.1016/j.annemergmed.2020.09.002
95. Redler LH, Watling JP, Ahmad CS. Physical examination of the throwing athlete's elbow. *Am J Orthop.* 2015;44(1):13–18.
96. Wright RW, Steger-May K, Wasserlauf BL, et al. Elbow range of motion in professional baseball pitchers. *Am J Sports Med.* 2006;34(2):190–193.
97. Cain EL, Dugas JR, Wolf RS, Andrews JR. Elbow injuries in throwing athletes: a current concepts review. *Am J Sports Med.* 2003;31(4):621–635. doi:10.1177/03635465030310042601
98. Hausman MR, Lang P. Examination of the elbow: current concepts. *J Hand Surg Am.* 2014;39(12):2534–2541. doi:10.1016/j.jhsa.2014.04.028
99. Kendall F, McCreary E, Provance P, Rogers M, Romani W. *Muscles: Testing and Function with Posture and Pain.* 5th ed. Lippincott, Williams, and Wilkins; 2005.
100. Bisset LM, Vicenzino B. Physiotherapy management of lateral epicondylalgia. *J Physiother.* 2015;61(4):174–181. doi:10.1016/j.jphys.2015.07.015
101. Andrews K, Rowland A, Pranjal A, Ebraheim N. Cubital tunnel syndrome: anatomy, clinical presentation, and management. *J Orthop.* 2018;15(3):832–836. doi:10.1016/j.jor.2018.08.010
102. Grijalva R, Hsu F, Wycliffe N, et al. Hoffman sign. *Spine (Phila Pa 1976).* 2015;40(7):475–479.
103. Zwerus EL, Somford MP, Maissan F, Heisen J, Eygendaal D, van den Bekerom MP. Physical examination of the elbow, what is the evidence? A systematic literature review. *Br J Sports Med.* 2018;52(19):1253–1260. doi:10.1136/bjsports-2016-096712
104. Smith AM, Driscoll SW. Diagnosing medial elbow pain in throwers: the use of provocative testing has improved clinical evaluation. *J Musculoskel Med.* 2005;22:305–316.
105. Konin J, Lebscak D, Snyder VA. *Special Tests for Orthopaedic Examination.* SLACK Incorporated; 2016.
106. O'Driscoll SWM, Lawton RL, Smith AM. The "moving valgus stress test" for medial collateral ligament tears of the elbow. *Am J Sports Med.* 2005;33(2):231–239. doi:10.1177/0363546504267804
107. Regan W, Lapner PC. Prospective evaluation of two diagnostic apprehension signs for posterolateral instability of the elbow. *J Shoulder Elbow Surg.* 2006;15(3):344–346. doi:10.1016/j.jse.2005.03.009

108. Cass S. Upper extremity nerve entrapment syndromes in sports: an update. *Curr Sports Med Rep.* 2014;13(1):16–21. doi:10.1249/JSR.0000000000000025
109. Bair MR, Gross MT, Cooke JR, Hill CH. Differential diagnosis and intervention of proximal median nerve entrapment: a resident's case problem. *J Orthop Sports Phys Ther.* 2016;46(9):800–808. doi:10.2519/jospt.2016.6723
110. Lee MJ, LaStayo PC. Pronator syndrome and other nerve compressions that mimic carpal tunnel syndrome. *J Orthop Sports Phys Ther.* 2004;34(10):601–609. doi:10.2519/jospt.2004.34.10.601
111. Greif DN, Emerson CP, Allegra P, Shallop BJ, Kaplan LD. Olecranon stress fracture. *Clin Sports Med.* 2020;39(3):575–588. doi:10.1016/j.csm.2020.02.005
112. Keijsers R, de Vos RJ, Kuijer PPF, van den Bekerom MP, van der Woude HJ, Eygendaal D. Tennis elbow. *Shoulder Elbow.* 2019;11(5):384–392. doi:10.1177/1758573218797973
113. Scott A, Backman L, Speed C. Tendinopathy: update on pathophysiology. *J Orthop Sports Phys Ther.* 2015;45(11):833–841.
114. Dorf ER, Chhabra AB, Golish SR, McGinty JL, Pannunzio ME. Effect of elbow position on grip strength in the evaluation of lateral epicondylitis. *J Hand Surg.* 2007;32(6):882–886. doi:https://doi.org/10.1016/j.jhsa.2007.04.010
115. Cutts S, Gangoo S, Modi N, Pasapula C. Tennis elbow: a clinical review article. *J Orthop.* 2020;17:203–207. doi:10.1016/j.jor.2019.08.005
116. Coombes BK, Bisset L, Vicenzino B. Management of lateral elbow tendinopathy: one size does not fit all. *J Orthop Sports Phys Ther.* 2015;45(11):938–949. doi:10.2519/jospt.2015.5841
117. Day JM, Lucado AM, Uhl TL. A comprehensive rehabilitation program for treating lateral elbow tendinopathy. *Int J Sports Phys Ther.* 2019;14(5):818–829.
118. Lai WC, Erickson BJ, Mlynarek RA, Wang D. Chronic lateral epicondylitis: challenges and solutions. *Open Access J Sports Med.* 2018;9:243–251. doi:10.2147/OAJSM.S160974
119. Keating C, Bodnar R, Joseph J, Knapp S, Legpage M, Solger G. Effectiveness of painful loading in lateral elbow tendinopathy on pain outcomes: a systematic literature review. *Orthop Pract.* 2020;22(4):208–214.
120. Meunier M. Lateral epicondylitis/extensor tendon injury. *Clin Sports Med.* 2020;39(3):657–660. doi:10.1016/j.csm.2020.03.001
121. Wilk KE, Arrigo CA. Rehabilitation of elbow injuries: nonoperative and operative. *Clin Sports Med.* 2020;39(3):687–715. doi:10.1016/j.csm.2020.02.010
122. Hastie G, Soufi M, Wilson J, Roy B. Platelet rich plasma injections for lateral epicondylitis of the elbow reduce the need for surgical intervention. *J Orthop.* 2018;15(1):239–241. doi:10.1016/j.jor.2018.01.046
123. Stafford Ii CD, Colberg RE, Garrett H. Orthobiologics in elbow injuries. *Clin Sports Med.* 2020;39(3):717–732. doi:10.1016/j.csm.2020.02.008
124. Amin NH, Kumar NS, Schickendantz MS. Medial epicondylitis: evaluation and management. *J Am Acad Orthop Surg.* 2015;23(6):348–355. doi:10.5435/JAAOS-D-14-00145
125. Alrabaa RG, Dantzker N, Ahmad CS. Injuries and conditions affecting the elbow flexor/pronator tendons. *Clin Sports Med.* 2020;39(3):549–563. doi:10.1016/j.csm.2020.02.001
126. Ciccotti MC, Ciccotti MG. Ulnar collateral ligament evaluation and diagnostics. *Clin Sports Med.* 2020;39(3):503–522. doi:10.1016/j.csm.2020.02.002
127. Leahy I, Schorpion M, Ganley T. Common medial elbow injuries in the adolescent athlete. *J Hand Ther.* 2015;28(2):201–211. doi:10.1016/j.jht.2015.01.003
128. Tarpada SP, Morris MT, Lian J, Rashidi S. Current advances in the treatment of medial and lateral epicondylitis. *J Orthop.* 2018;15(1):107–110. doi:10.1016/j.jor.2018.01.040
129. Marinelli A, Guerra E, Rotini R. Elbow instability: are we able to classify it? Review of the literature and proposal of an all-inclusive classification system. *Musculoskelet Surg.* 2016;100(Suppl 1):61–71. doi:10.1007/s12306-016-0424-1
130. Kheterpal AB, Bredella MA. Overuse injuries of the elbow. *Radiol Clin North Am.* 2019;57(5):931–942. doi:10.1016/j.rcl.2019.03.005
131. de Haan J, Schep NWL, Tuinebreijer WE, Patka P, den Hartog D. Simple elbow dislocations: a systematic review of the literature. *Arch Orthop Trauma Surg.* 2010;130(2):241–249. doi:10.1007/s00402-009-0866-0
132. Goodman AD, Lemme N, DeFroda SF, Gil JA, Owens BD. Elbow dislocation and subluxation injuries in the National Collegiate Athletic Association, 2009–2010 through 2013–2014. *Orthop J Sports Med.* 2018;6(1):2325967117750105. doi:10.1177/2325967117750105
133. Rezaie N, Gupta S, Service BC, Osbahr DC. Elbow dislocation. *Clin Sports Med.* 2020;39(3):637–655. doi:10.1016/j.csm.2020.02.009
134. Leland DP, Conte S, Flynn N, et al. Prevalence of medial ulnar collateral ligament surgery in 6135 current professional baseball players: a 2018 update. *Orthop J Sports Med.* 2019;7(9):2325967119871442. doi:10.1177/2325967119871442
135. Zaremski JL, Vincent KR, Vincent HK. Elbow ulnar collateral ligament: injury, treatment options, and recovery in overhead throwing athletes. *Curr Sports Med Rep.* 2019;18(9):338–345. doi:10.1249/JSR.0000000000000629
136. Cain EL, Ochsner MG III. Ulnar collateral ligament reconstruction. *Clin Sports Med.* 2020;39(3):523–536. doi:10.1016/j.csm.2020.02.003
137. Daruwalla JH, Daly CA, Seiler JG III. Medial elbow injuries in the throwing athlete. *Hand Clin.* 2017;33(1):47–62. doi:10.1016/j.hcl.2016.08.013
138. Savoie FH III, O'Brien M. Sprains, strains, and partial tears of the medial ulnar collateral ligament of the elbow. *Clin Sports Med.* 2020;39(3):565–574. doi:10.1016/j.csm.2020.02.007
139. Coughlin RP, Gohal C, Horner NS, et al. Return to play and in-game performance statistics among pitchers after ulnar collateral ligament reconstruction of the elbow: a systematic review. *Am J Sports Med.* 2019;47(8):2003–2010. doi:10.1177/0363546518798768
140. Sakata J, Nakamura E, Suzuki T, et al. Efficacy of a prevention program for medial elbow injuries in youth baseball players. *Am J Sports Med.* 2018;46(2):460–469. doi:10.1177/0363546517738003
141. Sakata J, Nakamura E, Suzuki T, et al. Throwing injuries in youth baseball players: can a prevention program help? A randomized controlled trial. *Am J Sports Med.* 2019;47(11):2709–2716. doi:10.1177/0363546519861378
142. Deal MJ, Richey BP, Pumilia CA, et al. Regional interdependence and the role of the lower body in elbow injury in baseball players: a systematic review. *Am J Sports Med.* 2020;48(15):3652–3660. doi:10.1177/0363546520910138
143. Camp CL, Smith J, O'Driscoll SW. Posterolateral rotatory instability of the elbow: part I. Mechanism of injury and the posterolateral rotatory drawer test. *Arthrosc Tech.* 2017;6(2):e401–e405. doi:10.1016/j.eats.2016.10.016
144. Conti Mica M, Caekebeke P, van Riet R. Lateral collateral ligament injuries of the elbow—chronic posterolateral rotatory instability (PLRI). *EFORT Open Rev.* 2016;1(12):461–468. doi:10.1302/2058-5241.160033

145. Streubel PN, Cohen MS. Diagnosis and treatment of posterolateral rotatory instability. *Oper Tech Sports Med.* 2017;25(4):319–326. doi:10.1053/j.otsm.2017.08.013
146. Arvind CHV, Hargreaves DG. Tabletop relocation test: a new clinical test for posterolateral rotatory instability of the elbow. *J Shoulder Elbow Surg.* 2006;15(6):707–708. doi:10.1016/j.jse.2006.01.005
147. Stanley D. Prevalence and etiology of symptomatic elbow osteoarthritis. *J Shoulder Elbow Surg.* 1994;3(6):386–389. doi:10.1016/S1058-2746(09)80024-4
148. Spahn G, Lipfert J, Maurer C, et al. Risk factors for cartilage damage and osteoarthritis of the elbow joint: case-control study and systematic literature review. *Arch Orthop Trauma Surg.* 2017;137(4):557–566. doi:10.1007/s00402-017-2654-6
149. Sochacki KR, Jack RA, Hirase T, et al. Arthroscopic debridement for primary degenerative osteoarthritis of the elbow leads to significant improvement in range of motion and clinical outcomes: a systematic review. *Arthroscopy.* 2017;33(12):2255–2262. doi:10.1016/j.arthro.2017.08.247
150. Heijink A, Vanhees M, Ende K, et al. Biomechanical considerations in the pathogenesis of osteoarthritis of the elbow. *Knee Surg Sports Traumatol Arthrosc.* 2016;24(7):2313–2318. doi:10.1007/s00167-015-3518-7
151. Jhan S-W, Chou W-Y, Wu K-T, Wang C-J, Yang Y-J, Ko J-Y. Outcomes and factors of elbow arthroscopy upon returning to sports for throwing athletes with osteoarthritis. *J Orthop Surg Res.* 2018;13(1):280. doi:10.1186/s13018-018-0992-x
152. Kotzamitelos D, Bhalaik V, Kent M, et al. Management of elbow (ulnohumeral) arthritis in the young active patient. *Orthop Trauma.* 2020;34(4):219–227. doi:https://doi.org/10.1016/j.mporth.2020.05.005
153. Kim DM, Han M, Jeon I-H, Shin MJ, Koh K-H. Range-of-motion improvement and complication rate in open and arthroscopic osteocapsular arthroplasty for primary osteoarthritis of the elbow: a systematic review. *Int Orthop.* 2020;44(2):329–339. doi:10.1007/s00264-019-04458-z
154. Midtgaard KS, Ruzbarsky JJ, Hackett TR, Viola RW. Elbow fractures. *Clin Sports Med.* 2020;39(3):623–636. doi:10.1016/j.csm.2020.03.002
155. McBride AP, Brais G, Wood T, Ek ET, Hoy G. Stress reactions and fractures around the elbow in athletes. *J Sci Med Sport.* 2021;24(5):425–429. doi:10.1016/j.jsams.2020.10.010
156. Smith SR, Patel NK, White AE, Hadley CJ, Dodson CC. Stress fractures of the elbow in the throwing athlete: a systematic review. *Orthop J Sports Med.* 2018;6(10):2325967118799262. doi:10.1177/2325967118799262
157. Schickendantz MS, Yalcin S. Conditions and injuries affecting the nerves around the elbow. *Clin Sports Med.* 2020;39(3):597–621. doi:10.1016/j.csm.2020.02.006
158. Kumar SD, Bourke G. Nerve compression syndromes at the elbow. *Orthop Trauma.* 2016;30(4):355–362. doi:10.1016/j.mporth.2016.05.012
159. An TW, Evanoff BA, Boyer MI, Osei DA. The prevalence of cubital tunnel syndrome: a cross-sectional study in a U.S. metropolitan cohort. *J Bone Joint Surg Am.* 2017;99(5):408–416. doi:10.2106/JBJS.15.01162
160. Lauretti L, D'Alessandris QG, De Simone C, et al. Ulnar nerve entrapment at the elbow. A surgical series and a systematic review of the literature. *J Clin Neurosci.* 2017;46:99–108. doi:10.1016/j.jocn.2017.08.012
161. Strohl AB, Zelouf DS. Ulnar tunnel syndrome, radial tunnel syndrome, anterior interosseous nerve syndrome, and pronator syndrome. *Instr Course Lect.* 2017;66:153–162.
162. Asheghan M, Hollisaz M, Aghdam A, Khatibiaghda A. The prevalence of pronator teres among patients with carpal tunnel syndrome: cross-sectional study. *Int J Biomed Sci.* 2016;12(3):89–94.
163. Tjoumakaris FP, Bradley JP. Distal biceps injuries. *Clin Sports Med.* 2020;39(3):661–672. doi:10.1016/j.csm.2020.02.004
164. Shuttlewood K, Beazley J, Smith CD. Distal triceps injuries (including snapping triceps): a systematic review of the literature. *World J Orthop.* 2017;8(6):507–513. doi:10.5312/wjo.v8.i6.507
165. Walker CM, Noonan TJ. Distal triceps tendon injuries. *Clin Sports Med.* 2020;39(3):673–685. doi:10.1016/j.csm.2020.03.003

16 | Wrist and Hand Complex

Betsy Myers, June Hanks, and Zachary Sutton

CHAPTER OBJECTIVES
After reading this chapter, you will be able to:
1. Describe the anatomy of the joints forming the wrist and hand complex to include osteologic ligamentous, capsular and muscular features.
2. Describe the biomechanics of the articulations of the wrist and hand.
3. Tailor the basic history to a patient with wrist and hand pathology.
4. Describe the components of the physical examination for a patient with wrist or hand pathology.
5. Describe the pathology, history, key examination findings, rehabilitation focus, and expected outcomes of common wrist and hand pathologies.
6. Hypothesize differential diagnoses of wrist and hand symptoms based on location, patient complaint, and onset.
7. Organize the physical examination of a patient with wrist or hand pathology to maximize efficiency.

FUNCTIONAL ANATOMY

The complex anatomic arrangement among the multiple structures of the upper extremity allows for remarkable precision and dexterity in use of the hand during functional activity. The bone and soft tissues (joint capsules, ligaments, muscles, and tendons) of wrist and hand work in a coordinated manner to allow individuals to interact with the environment for activities such as reaching and grasping. Dysfunction of single or multiple components risks compromise to function, with each part influencing other components.

OSTEOLOGY

The wrist and hand complex includes the distal radius and ulna, with the remaining bones organized into three groups based on structure and function: 8 carpal bones, arranged in proximal distal rows; 5 metacarpal bones; and 14 phalanges (Fig. 16-1). The bony curvatures provide for a range of congruency in articulations, and bony projections provide attachments for tendons and ligaments that direct movement.

Distal End of Radius and Ulna

The distal radius is larger, wider, and extends farther distally than the ulna. The distal articular end of the radius is concave in shape, with the articular surface angulated toward the medial direction in the frontal plane approximately 25° (ulnar tilt) (Fig. 16-2A) and about 10° anteriorly in the sagittal plane (palmar tilt) (Fig. 16-2B).[1] The distal end of the radius bears two adjacent fossae for articulation with the scaphoid and lunate carpal bones (Fig. 16-3). The lateral distal radius forms the distal radial styloid that extends farther distally than the scaphoid and lunate. The dorsal surface of the distal radius is irregularly shaped, with a prominent tubercle (Lister tubercle) and a smooth groove just medial to the tubercle for passage of the tendon of the extensor pollicis longus (EPL).[2]

The distal ulna consists of a rounded head facing laterally toward the radius and a medial end that forms the ulnar styloid process. The ulnar head fits into the ulnar notch of the radius and the distal end is separated from the carpal bones by an articular disc, the triangular fibrocartilage (TFC) (Fig. 16-3). The TFC is a component of the triangular fibrocartilage complex (TFCC).[3] The TFC attaches to the sigmoid notch and lunate fossa of the distal radius and becomes wedge shaped along the ulnar border. On radiograph (Fig. 16-4), the space for the TFCC is clearly seen between the ulnar styloid process and the lunate.

Carpals

The eight carpal bones are arranged in two transverse rows. Described from lateral to medial, the proximal row contains the scaphoid (navicular), lunate, triquetrum, and pisiform, and the distal row consists of the trapezium, trapezoid, capitate, and hamate (see Figs. 16-1 and 16-4). Each carpal bone has unique features, impacting the congruency among the articulations. No tendons insert to the proximal row of carpal bones, making motion of these bones dependent on

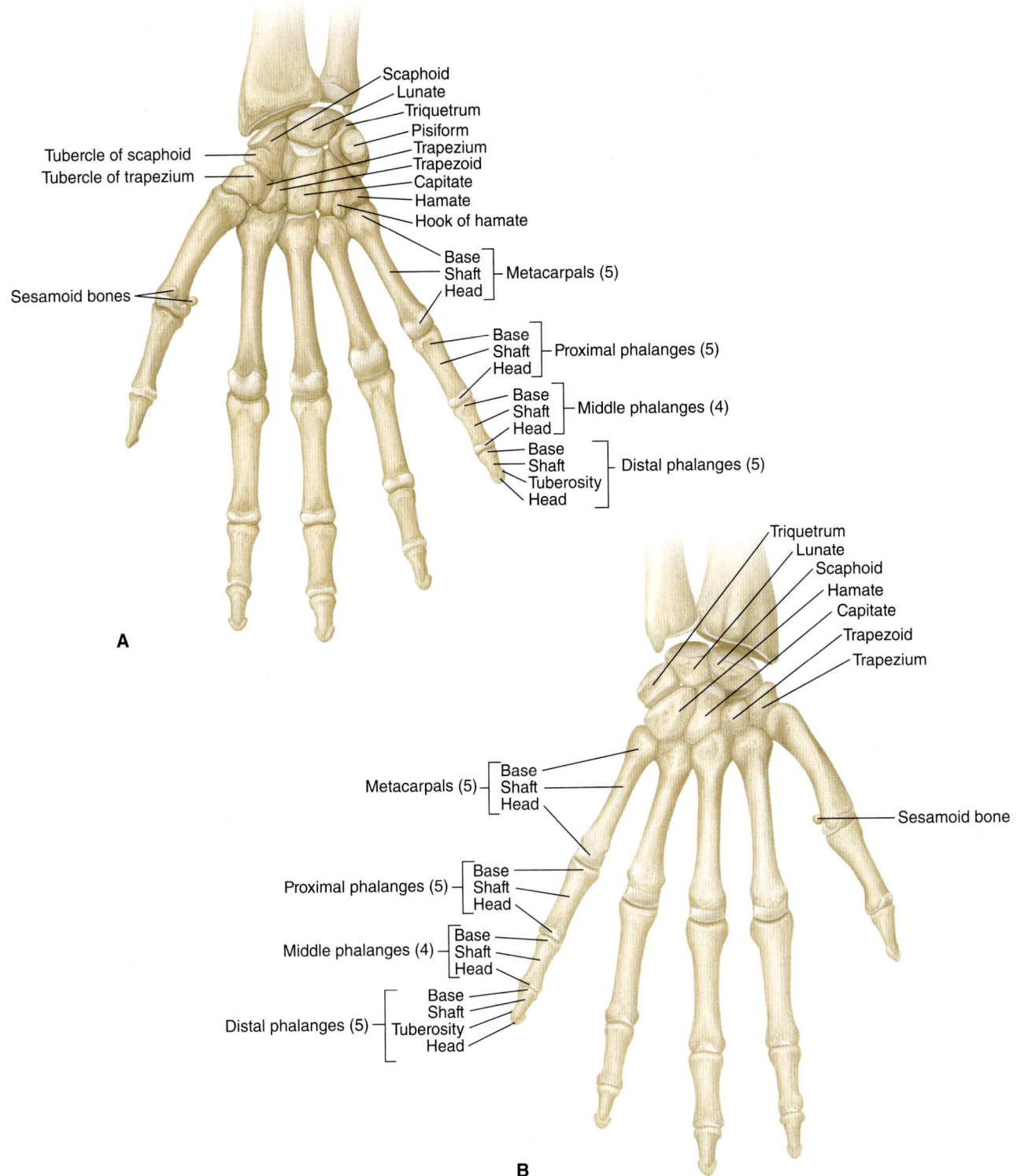

FIGURE 16-1 Distal radius, ulna, carpals, metacarpals, and phalanges. **A.** Anterior view. **B.** Posterior view. (Gest TR. *Lippincott Atlas of Anatomy*. 2nd ed. Wolters Kluwer; 2020: Plates 2-31 and 2-32.)

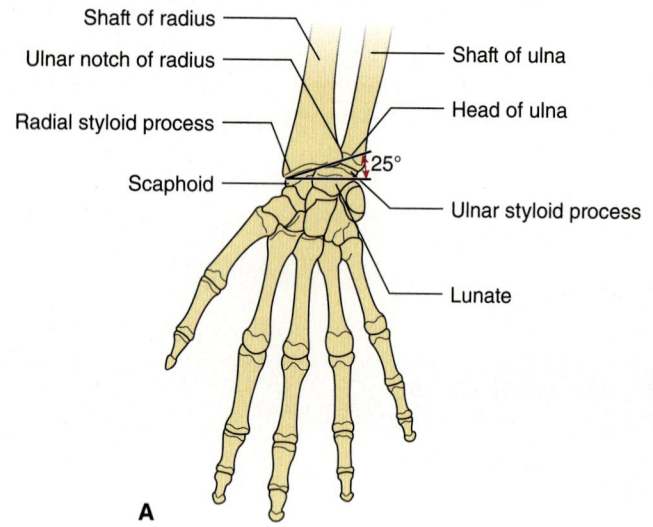
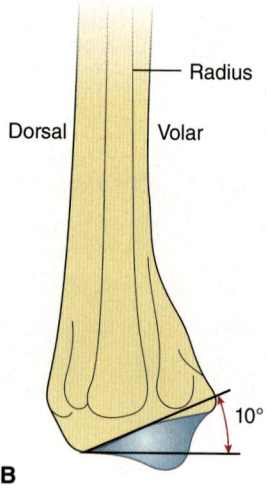

FIGURE 16-2 Tilt of distal radius. **A.** Anterior view of radius (with ulna and carpal bones) showing ulnar tilt of about 25°. **B.** Lateral view of radius showing palmar tilt of about 10°. (Adapted from Oatis CA. *Kinesiology: The Mechanics and Pathomechanics of Human Movement.* 3rd ed. Wolters Kluwer; 2017: Figure 14.4A.)

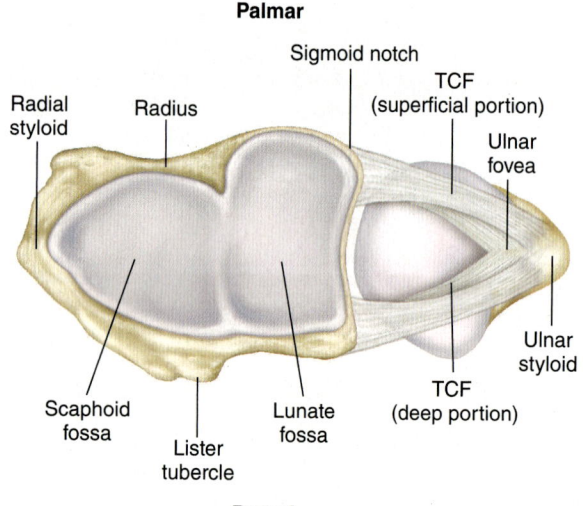

FIGURE 16-3 Distal radius and ulna with triangular fibrocartilage (TFC). Axial view. (Modified from Chung KC. *Grabb and Smith's Plastic Surgery.* 8th ed. Wolters Kluwer; 2020: Figure 75.1.)

movement of neighboring joints and tension in connecting ligaments. The distal row of carpals is strongly bound together by ligaments, causing the bones to move together as a functional unit.[4] The relationship of the carpal bones to the joints of the wrist and hand is shown in Figure 16-5.

Scaphoid The proximal pole of the scaphoid articulates with the scaphoid fossa of the radius, and the distal pole articulates with the trapezium and trapezoid. The distal pole of the scaphoid, which can be palpated as a blunt tubercle (scaphoid tubercle) at the distal wrist crease on the palmar side, serves as an attachment for the flexor retinaculum. The central portion is narrow. The concave distal-medial portion articulates with the capitate, whereas a small medially directed facet articulates with the lunate, forming the scapholunate joint (SLJ). The scaphoid is the most commonly fractured carpal bone, followed by the lunate and triquetrum.[1]

Lunate The lunate is positioned centrally in the proximal row between the scaphoid and the triquetrum. The lunate is crescent shaped on a lateral view and square shaped from an anteroposterior view (see Fig. 16-4). On an anteroposterior radiograph, a change to a triangular shape suggests instability, avascular necrosis, or some other pathology.[5] The proximal convex portion articulates with the lunate fossa of the radius, and the distal concave portion articulates with the capitate and part of the hamate. The bony shape, absence of muscular attachments, and deficiency of strong ligamentous attachment to the firmly held capitate lead to the potential for instability of the lunate.

Triquetrum The triquetrum articulates with the lunate and can be palpated just distal to the ulnar styloid process. The medial side of the long, flat triquetrum articulates with the hamate. On the palmar surface, a facet accepts the pea-shaped pisiform to which attaches the flexor carpi ulnaris (FCU) tendon, abductor digiti minimi muscle, the transverse carpal ligament, and multiple additional ligaments.[5]

CHAPTER 16 | WRIST AND HAND COMPLEX   569

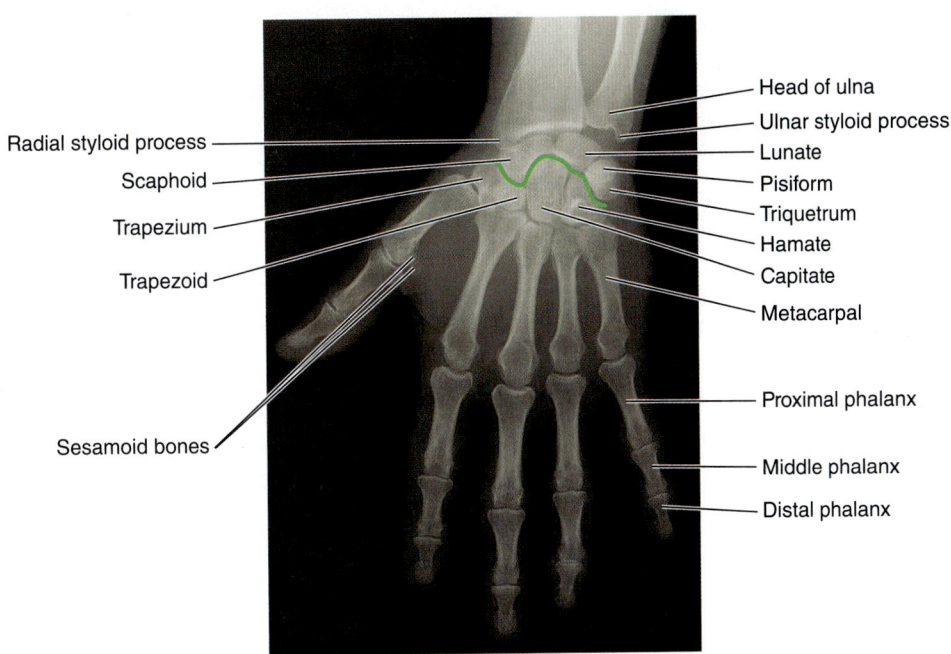

FIGURE 16-4 Radiograph of right wrist and hand, anterior view. Note space between head of ulna and carpal bones of wrist, indicating the location of the triangular fibrocartilaginous cartilage and associated structures (forming the triangular fibrocartilaginous complex). The green line shows the S-shaped midcarpal joint. (Gest TR. *Lippincott Atlas of Anatomy*. 2nd ed. Wolters Kluwer; 2020: Plate 2-05.)

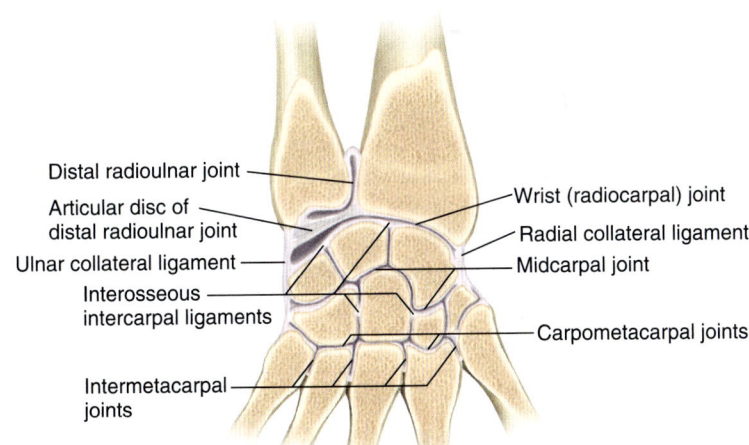

FIGURE 16-5 Joints of the wrist and hand (excluding digits). (Gest TR. *Lippincott Atlas of Anatomy*. 2nd ed. Wolters Kluwer; 2020: Plate 2-44.)

Hamate The hamate, the most medial of the distal row of carpals, is wedged between the triquetrum and the capitate. Distally, the hamate articulates with the bases of 4th and 5th metacarpal bones. The proximal portion articulates with the lunate. A large bony projection from the palmar surface, the hook of the hamate, provides attachment for the transverse carpal ligament.

Capitate The largest of the carpal bones is the centrally located capitate, called the "keystone" of the distal row of carpal bones because of its stability between the hamate and trapezoid and the attachment of short, strong ligaments passing among these bones. The large proximal end articulates with the deep cavities of the scaphoid and lunate. Distally, the capitate articulates directly with 3rd metacarpal base and, to some extent, the bases of 2nd and 4th metacarpal bases. The strong attachment of the capitate to 3rd metacarpal provides significant stability to the entire wrist and hand complex.[1,5]

Trapezoid The trapezoid is wedged between the capitate and the trapezium. The trapezoid has a concave-shaped proximal articulation with the scaphoid and a convex-shaped distal articulation with 2nd metacarpal base.[6,7]

Trapezium The most lateral of the distal row of carpals is the trapezium, an asymmetrically shaped bone that articulates with the scaphoid proximally. The distal portion of the bone bears a small facet for articulation with 2nd metacarpal base and a large distolateral surface for articulation with 1st metacarpal base, forming 1st carpometacarpal (CMC) joint.[7] A tubercle extending from the palmar side of the trapezium provides, along with the scaphoid tubercle, attachment for the lateral side of the transverse carpal ligament (aka the flexor retinaculum). Immediately medial to the palmar tubercle is a deep groove for the flexor carpi radialis (FCR).[1,7]

Metacarpals

Each of the five metacarpals has a base (proximal), shaft, and head (distal). The metacarpal bones vary in length, with 1st being the shortest, 2nd the longest, and 3rd through 5th gradually decreasing in length. The metacarpal bases articulate with one or more of the carpal bones. The sellar shape of the 1st metacarpal base is oriented such that the concave surface articulates with the trapezium during thumb flexion and extension and the convex surface articulates with the trapezium during thumb abduction and adduction. The remaining metacarpal bases are somewhat planar shaped with small facets to articulate with adjacent metacarpal bases. The dorsal side of the metacarpal heads is prominent, particularly with the fist clenched. Just proximal to the metacarpal head is the narrow neck, which is a common fracture site.

The heads of metacarpals 2 through 5 are biconvex, articulating with the proximal phalanx of the associated digit. With the hand in a resting, relaxed position, metacarpals 2 through 5 align beside one another and 1st metacarpal rotates toward the midline of the hand, facilitating movement of the thumb across the palm of the hand for activities such as grasping and pinching.

Phalanges

There are 14 phalangeal bones: three for digits 1 to 4 and two for the thumb. As with the metacarpals, each phalangeal bone consists of a base, shaft, and head. The shaft is convexly shaped dorsally and flat with a gentle concave curvature on the palmar side. The base of each phalanx is concave in shape, whereas the head is convex. The heads of the proximal and middle phalangeal bones bear a bicondylar facet that allows a snug fit within the concavity of the articulating base of the adjacent joint surface. The articular contour of the bicondylar hinge provides stability between the phalanges, limiting motion to flexion and extension. The articulations among the phalanges are proximal or distal, referred to as the *proximal interphalangeal* (PIP) and *distal interphalangeal* (DIP) joints, respectively.

Arches

The relaxed hand demonstrates a natural concavity of the palmar surface as the bones form arches: two transverse and one longitudinal (Fig. 16-6). The proximal transverse arch is more stable than the distal and is located at the level of the distal carpal bones, with the capitate serving as the keystone. The distal transverse arch passes through all of the metacarpal heads, with 3rd metacarpal head as the keystone. The longitudinal arch is composed of metacarpals 2 through 5 along with the associated carpal bones and

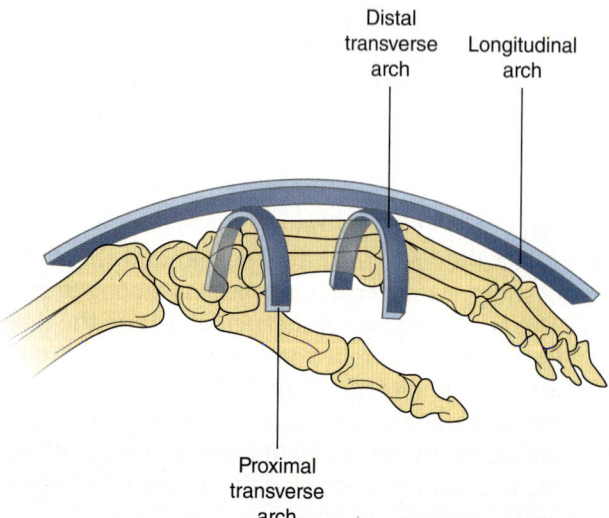

FIGURE 16-6 Arches of hand. Mediolateral view. (Strickland JW. Anatomy and kinesiology of the hand. In Fess EE, Philips CA, eds. *Hand Splinting: Principles and Methods*. 2nd ed. Mosby; 1987:3–41. Copyright © 1987 Elsevier. With permission.)

phalanges. The relatively rigid CMC joints forming the proximal portion of the longitudinal arch contribute significantly to hand stability. The 2nd and 3rd metacarpal bones are considered the keystone to the longitudinal arch, with the thumb and fourth and fifth digits moving about 2nd and 3rd. The hand arches are interlinked, providing the functional stability necessary to grasp and manipulate objects of varying size and shape.

JOINTS OF THE WRIST AND HAND COMPLEX

The joints proximal to the wrist complex allow placement of the hand in space, with the shoulder serving as a base of support and the elbow allowing the hand to move toward or away from the body. The forearm adjusts the position of the hand as an object is approached. The object is grasped by coordinated activation of forearm and hand muscles acting from these stable bases. The following joints are discussed in this chapter: distal radioulnar joint (DRUJ); wrist complex, composed of the radiocarpal and midcarpal joints; and hand complex, composed of intercarpal, CMC, metacarpophalangeal (MCP), PIP, and DIP joints. Ligaments are discussed briefly in this section and in more detail later in this chapter.

Distal Radioulnar Joint

The DRUJ, briefly discussed in Chapter 15, Elbow Complex, is described in more detail in this section. The DRUJ consists of articulation of the ulnar side of the distal radius along the distal interosseous border, forming the concave, semi-cylindrical sigmoid (ulnar) notch,[8] the head of the ulna,[2,3,9] and the articular disc. The convex-shaped ulnar head is covered with articular cartilage and bears an articular surface for union with the ulnar notch. The TFC attaches along the rim of the ulnar notch with the apex attaching at the base of the ulnar styloid process and the anterior and posterior edges continuous with the deep layers of ligaments about the wrist (see Fig. 16-3). The TFC separates the joint cavities of the DRUJ and wrist joint (see Fig. 16-5) and is part of a collective group of connective tissues known as the TFCC (Fig. 16-7).[3,10] The TFCC is a primary stabilizer of the DRUJ.[11] During pronation and supination of the DRUJ, various portions of the surrounding deep and superficial dorsal and palmar radioulnar ligaments tighten, contributing to stability.[12,13]

Movement of the DRUJ is linked with that of the proximal radioulnar joint (PRUJ) such that movements in the joints accompany each other. During pronation with the hand free to move, the radius crosses over the ulna at the PRUJ as the radial head spins on the capitulum of the humerus and within the radial notch

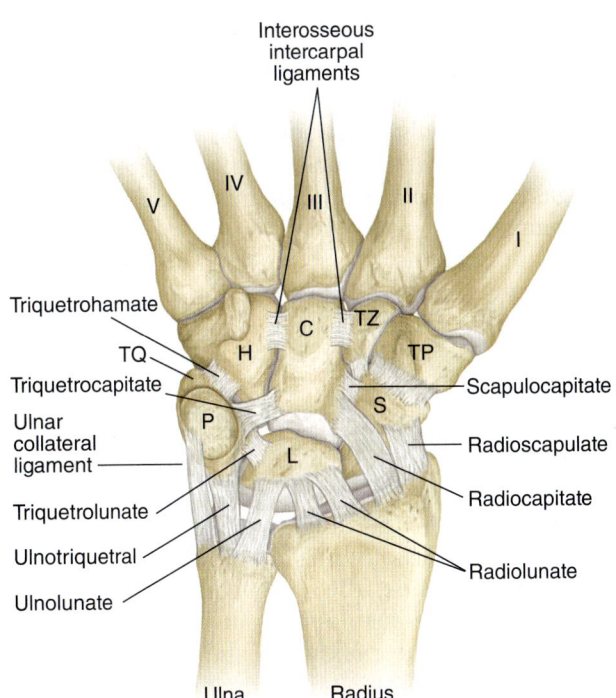

FIGURE 16-7 Right wrist and hand, palmar side. Components of the triangular fibrocartilage complex can be seen between the distal ulna and the lunate and triquetrum. *C*, capitate; *H*, hamate; *L*, lunate; *P*, prestyloid recess; *S*, scaphoid; *TP*, trapezium; *TQ*, triquetrum (the pisiform is not shown); *TZ*, trapezoid.

and annular ligament. The ulna moves posterolaterally and distally, serving as a pivot point around which the radius and connected hand move during pronation and supination[9,14] with the TFC moving beneath the ulnar head.[13] Joint congruency is maximal at the midposition between pronation and supination.[13] As explained in Chapter 15, Elbow Complex, compressive loads, as occurs during a push-up, are transmitted to the radius and ulna through the DRUJ.

Radiocarpal Joint

The radiocarpal joint is formed by articulation between the radius and the scaphoid (laterally), the lunate (medially), and the TFCC. With the wrist in a neutral position, the TFCC articulates primarily with the lunate and triquetrum. As noted previously, the TFCC is part of the DRUJ, helping to stabilize the joint. The TFCC separates the distal ulna from direct articulation with carpal bones and provides shock absorption between the ulna and carpal bones[15] and is part of both the DRUJ and the radiocarpal joint. The TFCC consists of the TFC and multiple fibrous attachments that support the radioulnar joint. The specific components of the

TFCC are variably described,[16–19] but are typically designated as follows:
- Palmar components:
  - Palmar radioulnar ligament
  - Ulnocarpal ligamentous complex (ulnotriquetral ligament, ulnocapitate ligament, and ulnolunate ligament)
- Ulnar components:
  - Triangular ligament
  - Ulnar collateral ligament (UCL)
  - Meniscal homolog (thickened portion forming ulnocarpal meniscus)[16]
- Dorsal components:
  - Dorsal radioulnar ligament
  - Extensor carpi ulnaris (ECU) tendon sheath

Figures 16-7, 16-8, and 16-9 show the components of the TFCC along with other ligaments of the hand.

On the ulnar side, the TFC apex firmly attaches to the fovea at the base of the ulnar styloid, sharing attachment with the radioulnar and ulnocarpal ligaments. On the radial side of the ulnar surface, the TFC more loosely attaches to hyaline cartilage of the ulna and to the radius (see Figs. 16-3 and 16-5). The components for the TFCC fill the space between the distal

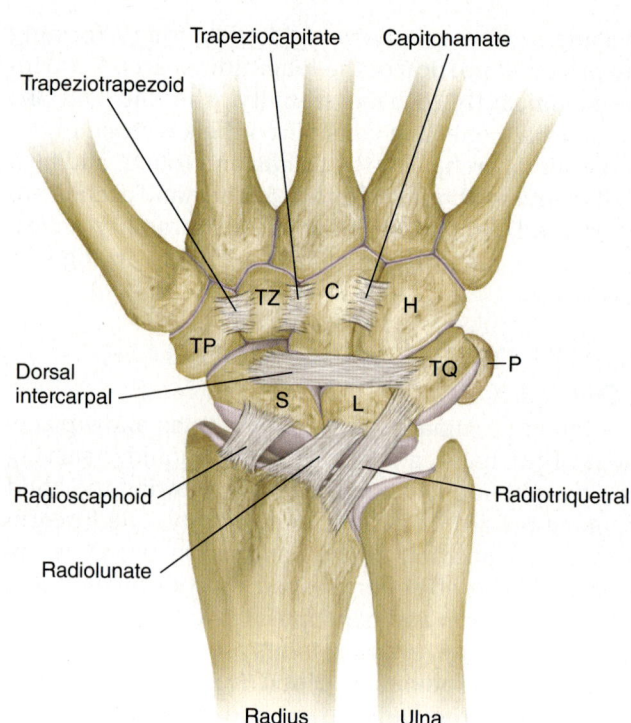

FIGURE 16-9 Ligaments of wrist. Dorsal view of right hand. C, capitate; H, hamate; L, lunate; P, pisiform; S, scaphoid; TP, trapezium; TQ, triquetrum; TZ, trapezoid.

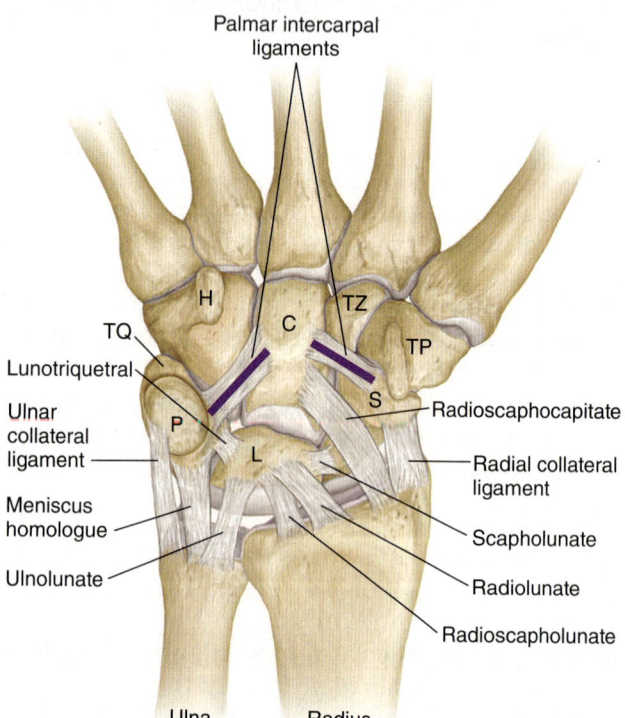

FIGURE 16-8 Ligaments of the right wrist, palmar view. The palmar intercarpal ligaments form a distal inverted "V" (purple) converging toward the capitate. The short palmar intrinsic ligaments are not shown. C, capitate; H, hamate; L, lunate; P, pisiform; S, scaphoid; TP, trapezium; TQ, triquetrum; TZ, trapezoid.

ulna and the triquetrum.[17,20,21] Blood supply to the TFCC is minimal, with central and radial portions being avascular.

Variations in articular surface of the geometry of the radius are common and even subtle differences influence the synergy of wrist joint movement with movement of the other joints in the hand.[22] The frontal plane (ulnar tilt) and sagittal plane (palmar tilt) angulations of the distal radius (see Fig. 16-2) impact range of motion (ROM) at the wrist. The ulnar tilt allows greater ulnar than radial deviation, due to the bony impingement of the lateral (radial side) carpal bones with the radius styloid process at end-range radial deviation. In addition, the ulnar tilt of the radius promotes sliding of the carpal bones in the ulnar direction.[23] Compression forces must be resisted by passive tension in the ligaments crossing the radiocarpal joint. Weakening of these ligaments in inflammatory disease, such as rheumatoid arthritis (RA), may lead to excessive ulnar translation, altering the mechanics of the wrist (Fig. 16-10). The palmar tilt allows greater flexion than extension at the wrist joint and is used to assess angular deformities with distal radius fractures.[24] Distal radius fractures, such as the very common Colles fracture or the less common Smith fracture, impact the normal tilt, as fragments displace dorsally or ventrally,

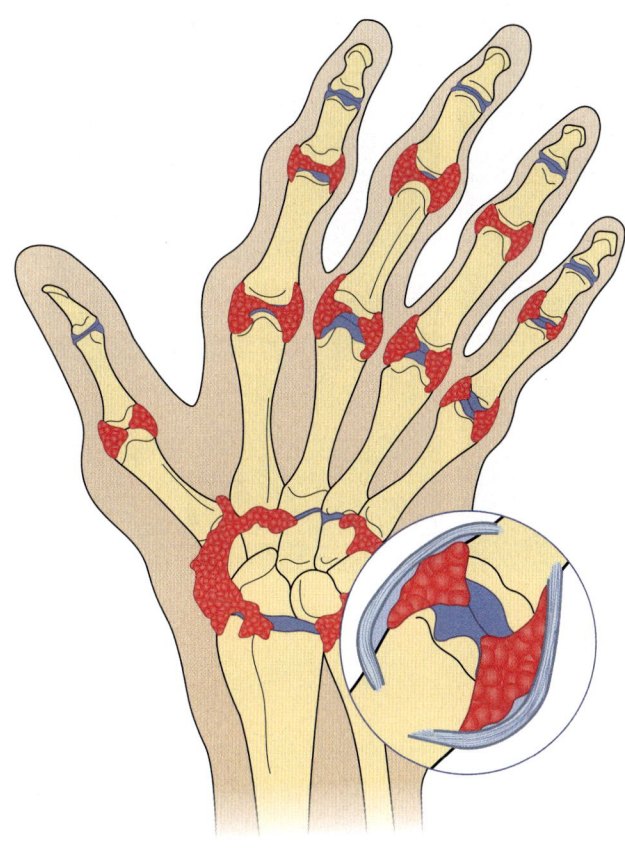

FIGURE 16-10 Rheumatoid arthritis affecting joints of the wrist and hand. (Adapted from Anatomical Chart Company. *Understanding Arthritis.* Wolters Kluwer/Anatomical Chart Company; 2004.)

respectively (Fig. 16-11). A change in the distal radial tilt can lead to significant motion loss and instability at the wrist if the bony alignment cannot be properly restored.

Midcarpal and Intercarpal Joints

The articulations between the proximal and distal row of carpal bones form the midcarpal joint, which is S shaped (see Fig. 16-4). With the exception of attachments to the pisiform, no extrinsic muscles attach to the carpal bones. Movement between the carpal bones (intercarpal joints) is small, especially compared to movement at the midcarpal and radiocarpal joints,[25,26] but is essential for proper wrist positioning. The shape of the intercarpal articulations varies greatly, allowing varying gliding and rotary motions. The intercarpal ligaments are stretched with intercarpal motion, contributing to the dissipation of forces across the wrist.

The radiocarpal and midcarpal joints move simultaneously to permit large motions and varied positions. The distal row of carpal bones is firmly held together by ligaments and primarily moves together as a unit with little individual bone motion. The proximal carpal bones are less stable and are more likely to dislocate. During wrist flexion and extension, the proximal and distal carpal bones move together on the radius (Fig. 16-12), following the convex-on-concave principle (Chapter 3, Arthrology). With wrist extension, the convex lunate rolls dorsally while sliding palmarly on the radius. Simultaneously, at the midcarpal joint, the head of the capitate follows the same pattern, rolling dorsally and sliding palmarly on the lunate. The combination of arthrokinematic movement over both the radiocarpal and midcarpal joints allows for greater total ROM, while requiring only moderate motion at any individual joint, thus providing greater stability. During wrist extension, the palmar ligaments further add to wrist stability. This stability is helpful particularly with activities of weight bearing through the upper limb on an extended wrist, such as crawling on the hands and knees or performing a push-up. The arthrokinematics occurring during wrist flexion are similar, but in opposite directions, with stabilizing ligamentous contributions from the dorsally located ligaments. Figure 16-12 depicts the sliding and rolling movements at the lunate and capitate, but does not include movement of all carpal bones. As an example, the scaphoid moves similarly to the lunate during wrist flexion and extension, except that the size and shape of the scaphoid allows the bone to move at a faster speed than the lunate. This means that, in a normal wrist at the end of full wrist flexion or extension, the scaphoid is slightly displaced from the lunate, the degree of which is determined by the specific scaphoid shape of an individual and the restraint provided by the scapholunate ligament.

With wrist ulnar and radial deviation, the convex-on-concave principles apply with movement at the radiocarpal and midcarpal joints, as shown in Figure 16-13. The scaphoid and lunate are bound tightly together by the scapholunate ligament. With ulnar deviation, the proximal carpal bones (scaphoid, lunate, and triquetrum) roll in an ulnar direction and slide radially on the radius.[1,5] At the midcarpal joint, the capitate rolls ulnarly and slides radially. With radial deviation, similar arthrokinematic movement occurs, but in the opposite direction and, to a lesser extent, due to limitations at the radiocarpal joint imposed by the radial styloid process. With both ulnar and radial deviations, the majority of motion occurs at the midcarpal joint, with one study demonstrating midcarpal joint motion accounting for approximately 85% or ulnar deviation and 60% of radial deviation.[25]

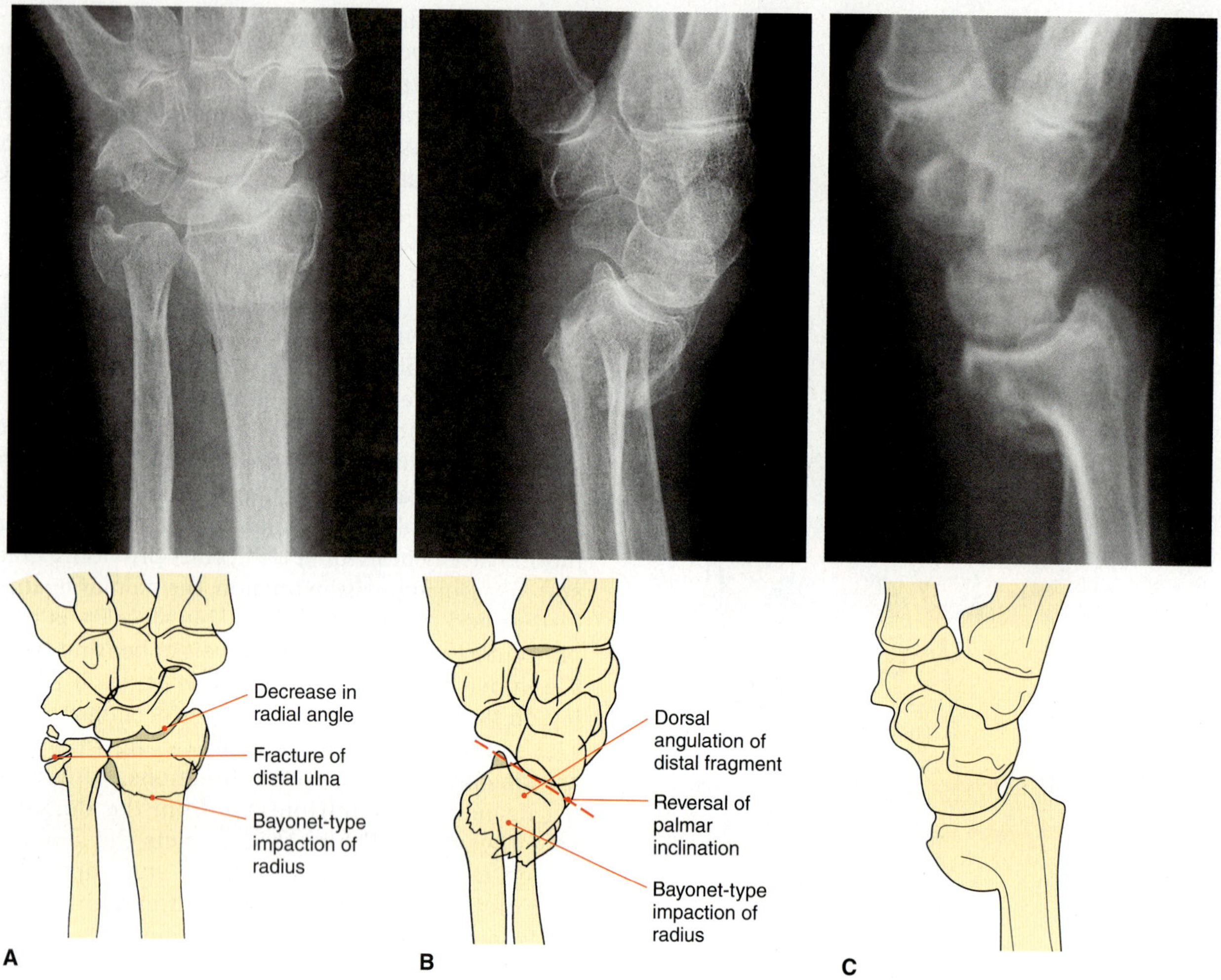

FIGURE 16-11 **A.** Colles fracture. (Greenspan A, Beltran J. *Orthopaedic Imaging: A Practical Approach*. 7th ed. Wolters Kluwer; 2021: Figure 7.11.) **B.** Smith fracture with dorsal angulation. (Brant WE, Helms CA. *Fundamentals of Diagnostic Radiology*. 4th ed. Lippincott Williams & Wilkins; 2012: Figure 42.33.) **C.** Smith fracture with ventral angulation.

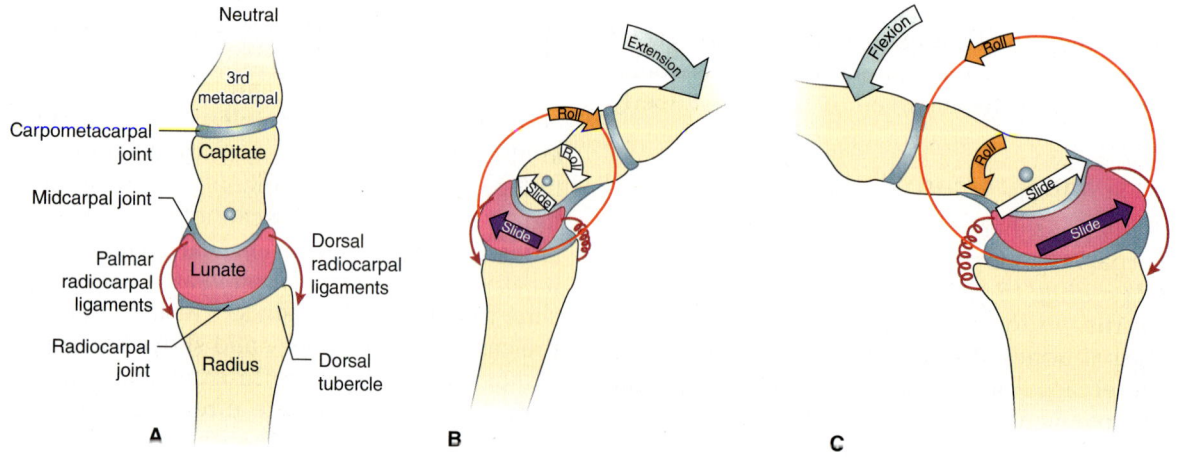

FIGURE 16-12 Simplified model showing arthrokinematic movement at the radiocarpal and midcarpal joint during wrist sagittal plane movement of extension and flexion. Lateral view. **A.** Neutral position. **B.** Wrist extension. **C.** Wrist flexion. (Modified from Neumann D. *Kinesiology of the Musculoskeletal System: Foundations for Rehabilitation*. 3rd ed. Elsevier; 2017: Figure 7-15.)

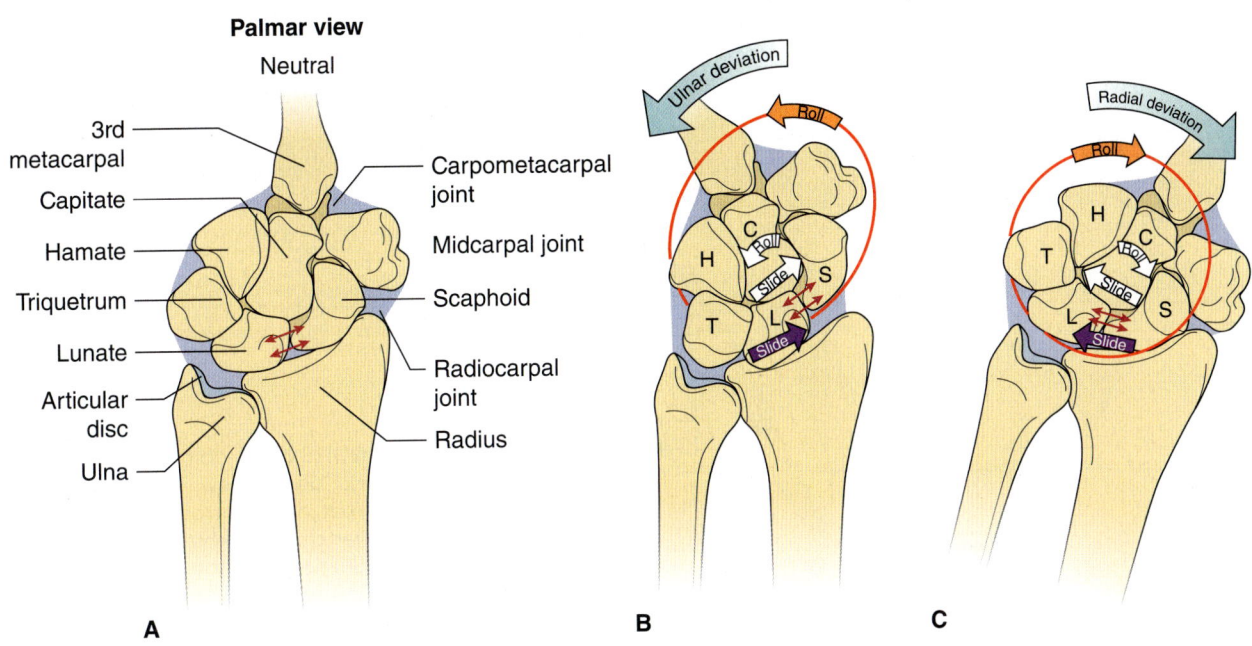

FIGURE 16-13 Simplified model showing arthrokinematic movement at the radiocarpal and midcarpal joints during radioulnar deviation. **A.** Neutral position. **B.** Ulnar deviation. **C.** Radial deviation. (Roentgenogram courtesy of Alex Norman, M. D.; drawings adapted with permission from Taleisnik J. *The Wrist*. Churchill Livingstone; 1985.)

In addition, this study[25] and others[26–29] demonstrate combined out-of-plane motions with wrist radioulnar deviation. With radial deviation, the scaphoid and lunate flex and twist on the radius and the capitate extends on the scaphoid/lunate (with the converse motions occurring in ulnar deviation) to produce the frontal plane radioulnar deviation.[26] The sagittal plane motion of flexion and extension with radioulnar deviation is greater at the scaphoid than at the lunate, stressing the scapholunate ligament. In a normal wrist, such stress to the scapholunate ligament is well tolerated. However, injury to the scapholunate ligament impacts arthrokinematics of the entire proximal row of carpals.

Carpometacarpal Joints

The distal row of carpal bones articulates with the bases of the long metacarpal bones, forming the CMC joints. The sellar shape of 1st CMC allows extensive movement and opposition, such that the thumb can easily touch the tips of the other digits. The mobility and complexity of 1st CMC subjects the joint to degenerative changes with overuse. Compared to 1st CMC joint, 2nd and 3rd CMC joints are flatter with interlocking joint surfaces, with the shape and strong surrounding ligaments forming the central stabilizing pillar of the hand (Fig. 16-14). The 4th and 5th CMC joints are flatter still, with the metacarpal bases matching the slightly convex hamate. The 4th and 5th CMC joints contribute to hand mobility by flexing and rotating toward 3rd metacarpal, allowing a cupping motion as the ulnar border of the hand folds toward the center. The mobility of 4th and 5th CMC joints is easily visualized as one moves from a relaxed to clenched fist position, thereby enhancing grasping capability.

Metacarpophalangeal Joints

The articulation of the metacarpal heads and proximal phalanx forms the MCP joints. The connective tissues surrounding the joints provide stability. The joint capsule of each MCP contains collateral ligaments on the radial and ulnar sides, with an embedded palmar (volar) plate (Fig. 16-15). The collateral ligaments attach just proximal to the metacarpal head and then separate into a thick dorsal part that attaches to the palmar aspect of the proximal phalanx, and a thinner accessory part that fans out, attaching to the edge of the palmar plate (Fig. 16-16). The palmar plate is composed of thick fibrocartilage that is thinner and more elastic proximally where it attaches to the metacarpal just proximal to the head. The palmar plate is thick and stiff distally where it attaches to the proximal phalangeal base.[30] Attaching to the anterior (palmar) surface of the palmar plate is the fibrous digital sheath of the extrinsic finger flexors. The composition

576 SECTION IV | UPPER QUARTER

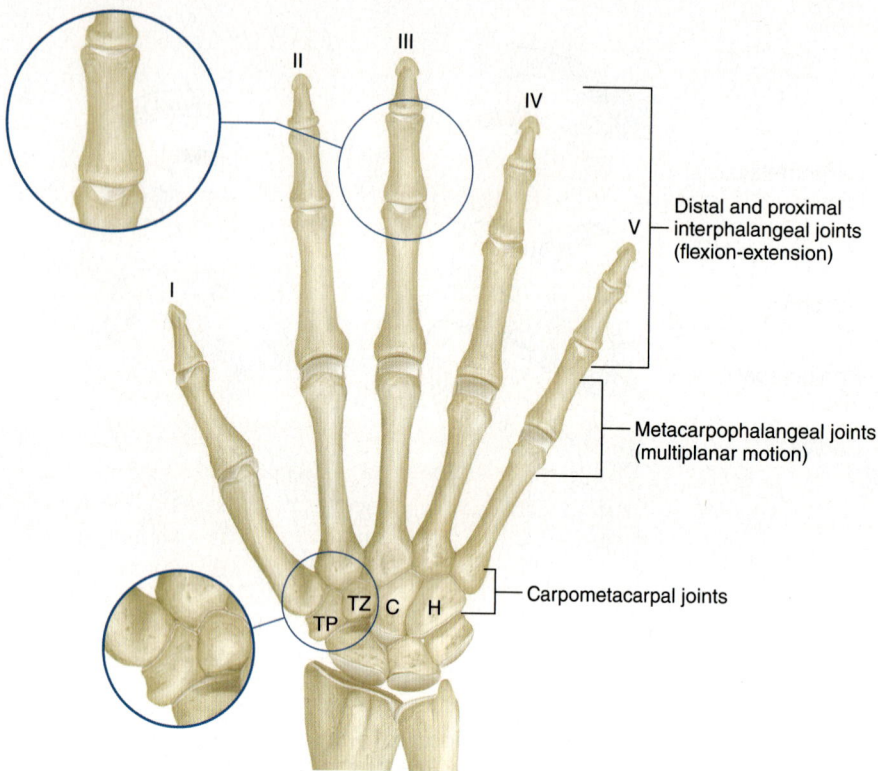

FIGURE 16-14 Joints of the wrist and hand, dorsal view. The 1st carpometacarpal joint (bottom inset) shows the sellar shape of the articulating surfaces between the trapezium and 1st metacarpal, with the convexity of one fitting into the concavity of the other. The top inset shows the articular contour of a typical interphalangeal joint. (Gest TR. *Lippincott Atlas of Anatomy*. 2nd ed. Wolters Kluwer; 2020: Plate 2-04.)

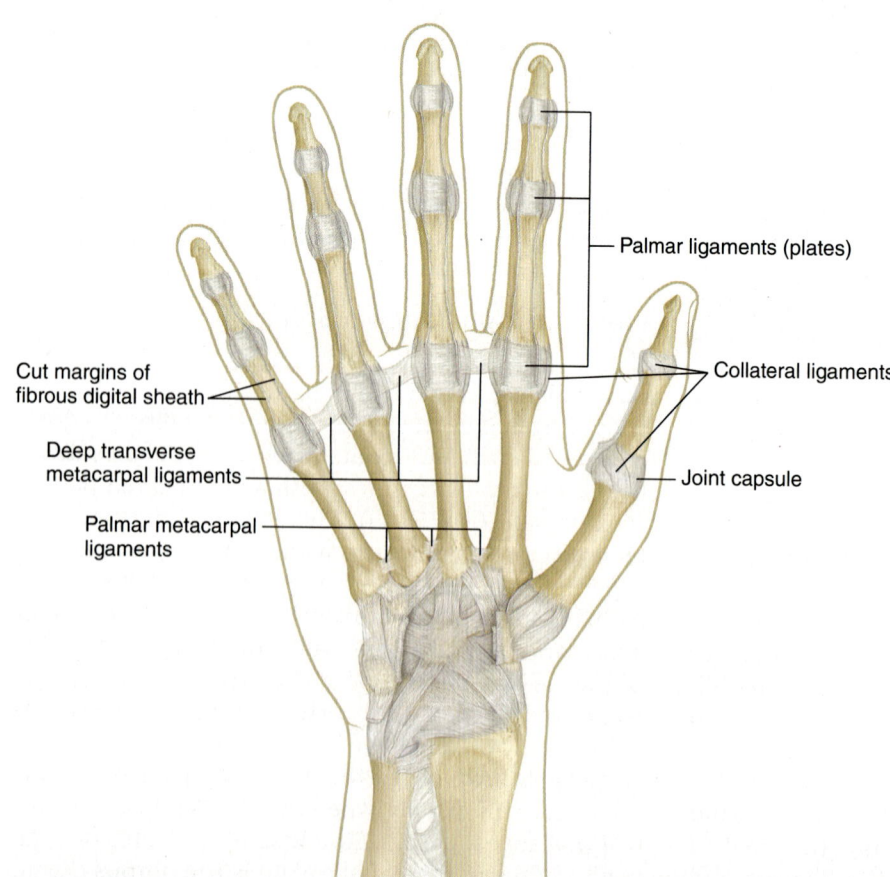

FIGURE 16-15 Ligaments of the hand with palmar plate identified. (Gest TR. *Lippincott Atlas of Anatomy*. 2nd ed. Wolters Kluwer; 2020: Plate 2-45A.)

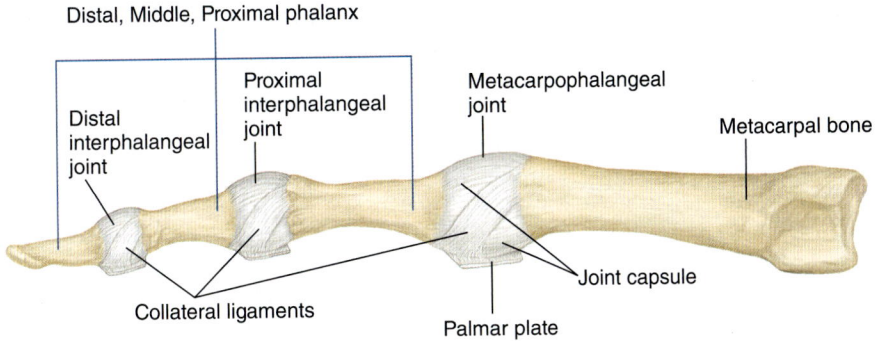

FIGURE 16-16 Ligaments of the metacarpal and interphalangeal joints. (Gest TR. *Lippincott Atlas of Anatomy*. 2nd ed. Wolters Kluwer; 2020: Plate 2-45B.)

and location of the palmar plate strengthens the MCP joint overall and helps to limit extension.[31] The deep transverse metacarpal ligaments form wide interconnecting bands that bind together the metacarpals 2 through 5 to maintain the transverse arch and further increase stability.[32] The proximal phalanx can be passively moved on the metacarpal head into distraction-compression, axial rotation, and translation side to side and anterior to posterior. The motion of the thumb MCP limits extension to 0° and flexion to 50°, whereas the MCPs 2 through 5 permit 25° extension, 20° abduction and adduction, and 90 to 115° flexion, with greatest flexion demonstrating 4th and 5th MCPs. The increased ROM of 4th and 5th MCPs allows for a tighter grasp in a pistol-grip shape. Handles that incorporate this shape are typically more comfortable and allow a stronger grip.

With the digits free to move, the concave-shaped proximal phalanx moves on the convex metacarpal head, with expected roll-and-slide arthrokinematic movement during flexion/extension and abduction/adduction. Although the thumb MCP osteokinematic movement is more limited than the other digits, the arthrokinematic movement is similar. The thumb collateral ligaments are particularly vulnerable to rupture when subjected to large abduction forces.

Interphalangeal Joints

The interphalangeal (IP) joints, the PIP and DIP joints, are formed by articulation of the respective proximal with middle and middle with DIP heads and bases (Fig. 16-16). A tongue-in-groove articulation is formed as the convexly shaped bicondylar phalangeal head with intervening groove fits snugly with the reciprocally concave facets and ridge of the adjoining phalangeal base. Like the MCP, the IP joints have a palmar plate that adds to joint stability, particularly in limiting extension.[33] Unlike the MCP joint, the collateral ligament of the IP joints maintains tension throughout the ROM, likely because of the nearly spherical bicondylar phalangeal heads. A fibrous tissue called the *check-rein ligament* blends with the periosteum to reinforce the proximal attachment of the palmar plate. Check-rein ligaments are not present at the palmar plate of the DIP.

Active movement at the IP joints is limited to flexion and extension. The tongue-in-groove IP joint shape restricts axial rotation. The roll-slide convex-on-concave arthrokinematic movement of the MCP joints occurs at the IP joints.

LIGAMENTS OF THE WRIST AND HAND COMPLEX

The small size and seemingly inconspicuous nature make ligaments of the wrist and hand complex difficult to isolate from surrounding connective tissues. The ligaments of the wrist maintain the intercarpal alignment and transfer forces across the carpus. The hand ligaments are extremely intricate with the bones, surrounding joint capsules, and tendinous sheaths. All ligaments of the wrist and hand assist with stabilization of the associated joints to allow surrounding muscles and tendons to provide efficient functional movement.

Ligaments of the Wrist

Ligaments about the wrist are classified as extrinsic or intrinsic. The extrinsic ligaments have proximal attachment to a bone of the forearm, attaching distally to the wrist close to the joint capsule and providing structural support to the wrist. The intrinsic ligaments have both attachments within the wrist and bind the carpal bones together, allowing them to move in collective patterns.[34] While ligaments are generally named by the bones to which they attach, there is some inconsistency in naming of ligaments, in part due to variations in dimensions and structure. Refer to Table 16-1 for a listing of wrist ligaments. See Figures 16-7, 16-8, and 16-9 for ligaments of the wrist.

Small ligaments of the wrist and hand play a critical role in alignment of bones and the transfer of forces across the bony segments. Forces produced by muscles are stored in the stretched ligaments, helping to control the complex accessory movements.[1]

TABLE 16-1
EXTRINSIC AND INTRINSIC LIGAMENTS OF THE WRIST

Location		Subcomponents
Extrinsic ligaments	Dorsal radiocarpal	
	Radial collateral*	
	Palmar radiocarpal	• Radioscaphocapitate • Radiolunate long (aka radiolunotriquetral) • Radiolunate short (aka radioscapholunate)
	TFCC	• Articular disc (TFC) • DRUJ capsular ligaments (dorsal and palmar) • Palmar ulnocarpal ligament (ulnotriquetral, ulnolunate) • Ulnar collateral ligament† • Fascial sheath enclosing tendon of ECU
Intrinsic ligaments	Short (distal row)	• Dorsal • Palmar • Interosseous
	Intermediate	• Lunotriquetral • Scapholunate
	Long	• Palmar intercarpal ("distal inverted V") with lateral leg (capitate to scaphoid), medial leg (capitate to triquetrum) • Dorsal intercarpal (trapezium-scaphoid-lunate-triquetrum)

DRUJ, distal radioulnar joint; *ECU*, extensor carpi ulnaris; *TFC*, triangular fibrocartilage; *TFCC*, triangular fibrocartilage complex.
*Excluded from some lists as a distinct entity.
†Thickening of ulnar side joint capsule; often blends with ulnotriquetral to reinforce the ulnar side of the wrist.

The mechanoreceptors embedded within the wrist ligaments, particularly the dorsal ligaments,[35,36] are activated by stretching or loading and contribute to proprioception (joint position and kinesthetic sense).[36,37] The proprioceptive information from the ligaments and joint capsules influences muscle activation, contributing dynamic joint stability to compliment the static ligamentous stability.[35,36] Sensory signals from richly innervated ligaments provide information regarding joint angle, movement velocity, and intra-articular pressure,[38] leading to a protective dynamic stability from specific muscles, thus enhancing the stability provided by the ligaments.[39] For example, the dorsal radiocarpal ligament attaches to the radius, scaphoid, and lunate and provides some support to the SLJ. Although this dorsally located ligament is not a primary stabilizer of the SLJ,[4] the relatively large number of mechanoreceptors within the ligament[35,36] plays a prominent large role in wrist joint proprioception.

The movement of the wrist joint is driven by muscle, but the ligaments guide the movements. Major ligaments of the wrist are commonly referred to as an "inverted double V system," with variations noted among anatomists regarding the actual ligaments forming distal and proximal V. In general, the distal V is formed by the medial and lateral portions of the palmar intercarpal ligament as it converges on the capitate, and the more proximal V is composed of attachments of the palmar ligaments converging on the lunate (Fig. 16-17).[1,5] Even when in a wrist neutral position, there is some tension within the ligaments. With radioulnar deviation, passive tension is placed on the ligaments opposite the side of deviation, providing stability to the carpal bones.

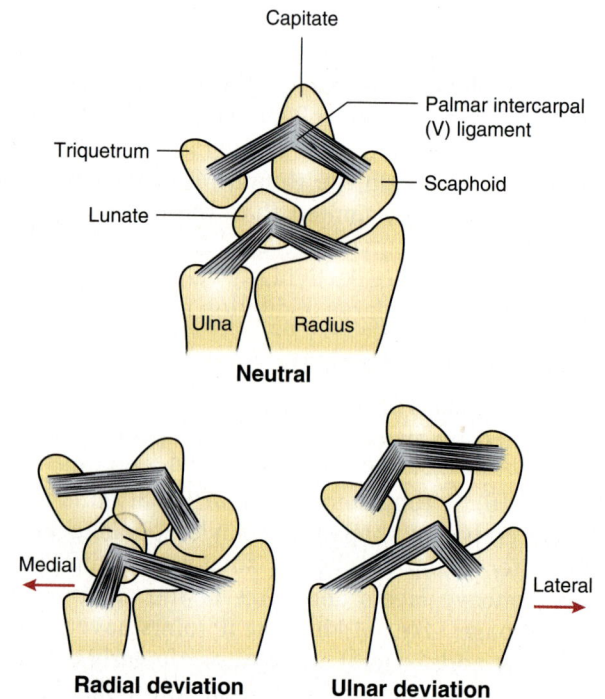

FIGURE 16-17 Inverted double V system of palmar ligaments. (Taleisnik J. *The Wrist*. Churchill Livingstone; 1985.)

Ligaments of the Hand

Table 16-2 provides a summary of primary ligaments associated with joints of the hand. With the exception of the thumb, the major ligaments associated with the CMC, MCP, and IP joints have been described in the previous section on the joints. Refer to Figures 16-15 and 16-16 for details.

Stabilization of the thumb CMC joint is provided largely by ligaments surrounding the joint and by extrinsic thumb muscles rather than by bony congruency. The CMC ligaments of the thumb are not consistently described in the literature, and the functional importance of each is debated.[40] Neumann[1] describes five thumb CMC joint ligaments: anterior (palmar) oblique, posterior oblique, ulnar collateral, radial collateral, and intercarpal ligaments. The strongest and thickest of these are radial collateral and posterior oblique ligaments,[41,42] which are both primary stabilizers when the thumb is in an opposed position. Instability due to ligamentous laxity may lead to degenerative changes in the joint.[43]

MUSCLES OF THE WRIST AND HAND COMPLEX

The muscles of the wrist and hand complex can be divided into extrinsic and intrinsic muscles. Both the proximal and distal attachments of the intrinsic muscles are within the hand. In contrast, the extrinsic muscle bellies are located proximal to the wrist, with proximal attachments about the elbow and forearm and distal attachments in the hand. The extrinsic flexors lie in the anterior compartment of the forearm and flex the wrist and digits, whereas the extrinsic extensors lie in the posterior compartment of the forearm and extend the wrist and digits. The muscles acting on the wrist and hand are numerous without excessive bulkiness due to the design of the intrinsic and extrinsic muscles, in combination with the fascial and ligamentous structures. The intrinsic muscles work together to balance the opposing forces of the extrinsic muscles. This section provides an overview of the muscles of the wrist and hand complex.

The extrinsic muscles in the anterior compartment of the arm can be subdivided into superficial, intermediate, and deep groups. The forearm pronators, the pronator teres, and pronator quadratus were discussed in Chapter 15, Elbow Complex, and are listed with other forearm anterior compartment muscles, though these pronators do not cross the wrist. The intrinsic muscles of the hand can be grouped by relationship to the first digit (thenar muscles), fifth digit (hypothenar muscles), and short muscles (lumbricals and interossei). Table 16-3 outlines the attachments

TABLE 16-2
LIGAMENTS ASSOCIATED WITH JOINTS OF THE HAND

Digit(s)	Joint	Ligaments
Thumb	CMC	• Anterior (palmar) oblique • Posterior oblique • Ulnar collateral • Radial collateral • Posterior oblique
	MCP and IP	• Radial collateral* • Ulnar collateral*
Digits 2-5	CMC	• Dorsal CMC • Palmar CMC • Intermetacarpal
	MCP and PIP	• Radial collateral* • Ulnar collateral* • Palmar plate • Check-rein
	DIP	• Radial collateral • Ulnar collateral

The joint capsule of each joint contributes additional support.
*Includes cord and accessory parts.
CMC, carpometacarpal; DIP, distal interphalangeal; IP, interphalangeal; MCP, metacarpophalangeal; PIP, proximal interphalangeal

TABLE 16-3
EXTRINSIC MUSCLES OF THE WRIST (ANTERIOR AND POSTERIOR COMPARTMENTS)

Location	Muscle	Proximal Attachment	Distal Attachment
Posterior forearm compartment (superficial layer)	Brachioradialis	Proximal 2/3 of supracondylar ridge of humerus	Proximal to radius styloid process on lateral surface of distal end
	ECRL	Lateral supracondylar ridge of humerus	Dorsal aspect of base of 2nd metacarpal
	ECRB	Common extensor origin (lateral epicondyle of humerus)	Dorsal aspect of base of 3rd metacarpal
	Extensor digitorum		Extensor expansion of medial four digits
	ECU	Lateral epicondyle of humerus and posterior border of ulna	Dorsal aspect of 5th metacarpal

(continued)

TABLE 16-3 (continued)
EXTRINSIC MUSCLES OF THE WRIST (ANTERIOR AND POSTERIOR COMPARTMENTS)

Location	Muscle	Proximal Attachment	Distal Attachment
Posterior forearm compartment (deep layer)	Supinator	Lateral epicondyle of humerus, radial collateral and annular ligaments, ulnar crest	Lateral, posterior, and anterior surfaces of proximal radius
	Extensor indicis	Posterior surface of distal 1/3 of ulna and interosseous membrane	Extensor expansion of second digit
Posterior forearm (emerging muscles of thumb)	APL	Posterior surface of proximal 1/2 of ulna, radius, and interosseous membrane	Base of 1st metacarpal
	EPB	Posterior surface of middle 1/3 of ulna and interosseous membrane	Dorsal aspect of base of distal phalanx of thumb
	EPL	Posterior surface of distal 1/3 of radius and interosseous membrane	Dorsal aspect of base of proximal phalanx of thumb
Anterior forearm compartment (superficial layer)	Pronator teres		
	Ulnar head	Coronoid process	Midportion of lateral radius
	Humeral head	Common flexor origin (medial epicondyle of humerus)	
	FCR		Base of 2nd metacarpal
	PL		Distal half of flexor retinaculum and apex of palmar aponeurosis
	FCU		
	Humeral head		Pisiform, hook of hamate, 5th metacarpal
	Ulnar head	Olecranon and posterior ulna border	
Anterior forearm compartment (intermediate layer)	FDS		
	Humeroulnar head	Common flexor origin (medial epicondyle of humerus) and coronoid process	Shafts of middle phalanges of digits 2-5
	Radial head	Superior 1/2 of anterior border of radius	
Anterior forearm compartment (deep layer)	FDP	Proximal 3/4 of medial and anterior surfaces of ulna and interosseous membrane	Bases of distal phalanges digits 2-5
	FPL	Anterior surface of radius and adjacent interosseous membrane	Base of distal phalanx of thumb
	Pronator quadratus	Distal quarter of anterior surface of ulna	Distal quarter of anterior surface of radius

APL, abductor pollicis longus; *ECRB*, extensor carpi radialis brevis; *ECRL*, extensor carpi radialis longus; *ECU*, extensor carpi ulnaris; *EDI*, extensor digiti minimi; *EPB*, extensor pollicis brevis; *EPL*, extensor pollicis longus; *FCR*, flexor carpi radialis; *FCU*, flexor carpi ulnaris; *FDP*, flexor digitorum profundus; *FDS*, flexor digitorum superficialis; *FPL*, flexor pollicis longus.
Adapted from Moore KL, Dalley AF, Agur AMR. *Clinically Oriented Anatomy*. 8th ed. Wolters Kluwer; 2018.

of the extrinsic muscles. The superficial and deep extensors of the wrist are shown in Figures 16-18 and 16-19, respectively. Note the extensor retinaculum at the posterior wrist. The superficial, intermediate, and deep muscles of the anterior forearm are shown in Figures 16-20, 16-21, and 16-22, respectively. Note that the flexor retinaculum in Figure 16-20 has been removed in Figures 16-21 and 16-22.

Table 16-4 outlines the attachments of intrinsic muscles of the hand. The muscles are shown in superficial, intermediate, and deep dissection schematics in Figures 16-23, 16-24, 16-25, and 16-26, respectively.

The extrinsic and intrinsic muscles work together to produce the many motions of the wrist and hand. Table 16-5 groups the muscles by action and includes the nerve supply to each.

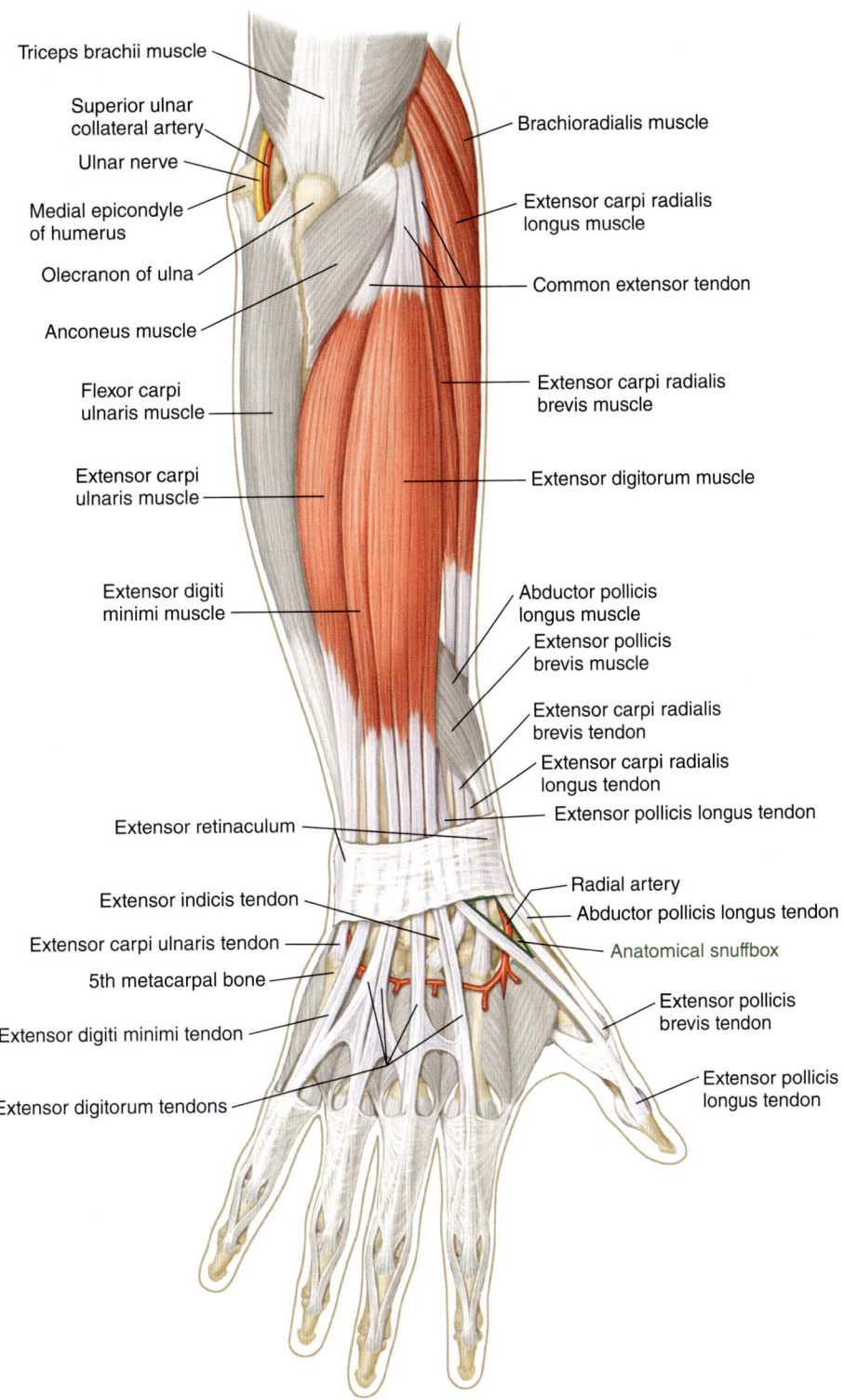

FIGURE 16-18 Superficial extensors of wrist. (Gest TR. *Lippincott Atlas of Anatomy*. 2nd ed. Wolters Kluwer; 2020: Plate 2-29.)

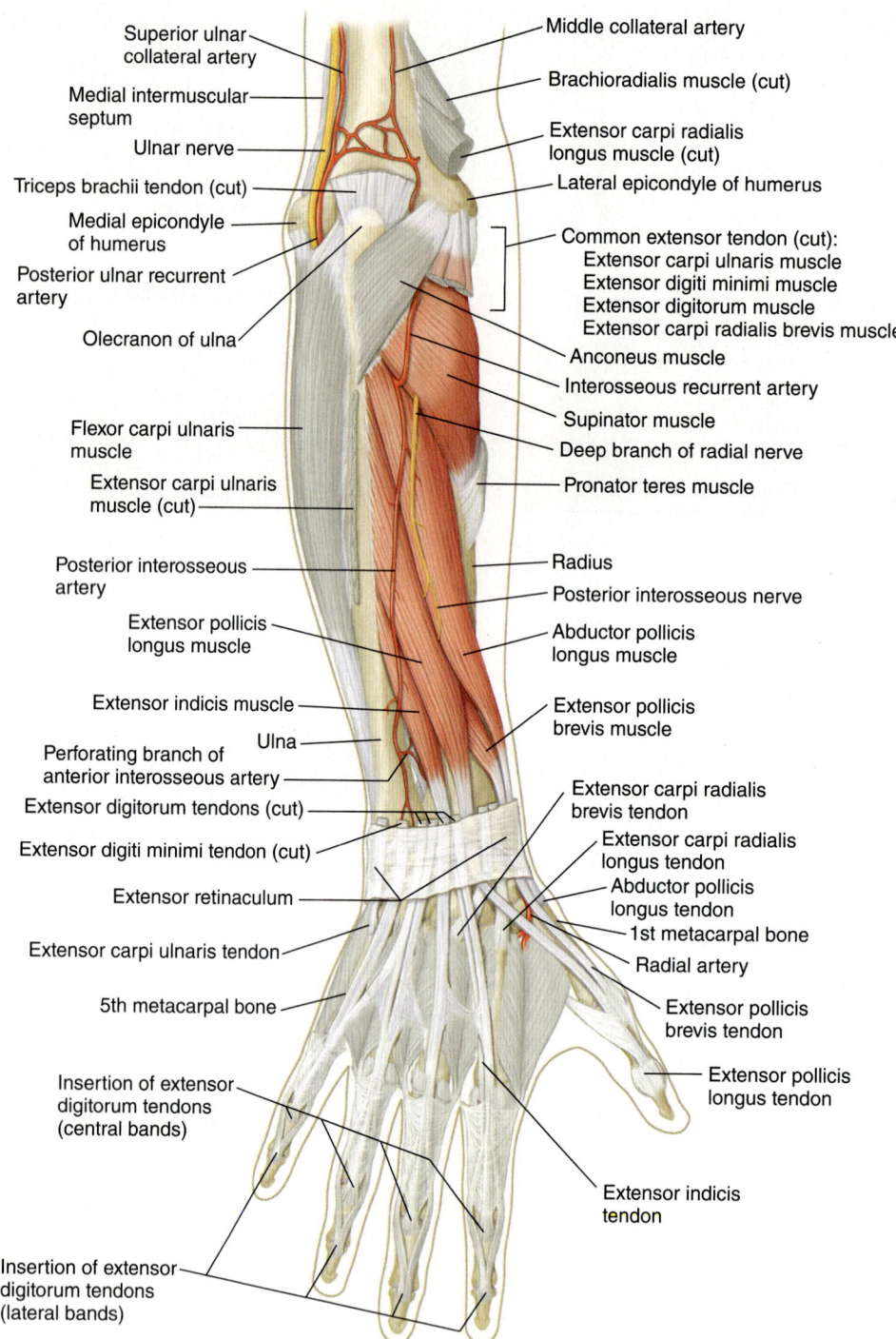

FIGURE 16-19 Deep extensors of wrist. (Gest TR. *Lippincott Atlas of Anatomy*. 2nd ed. Wolters Kluwer; 2020: Plate 2-30.)

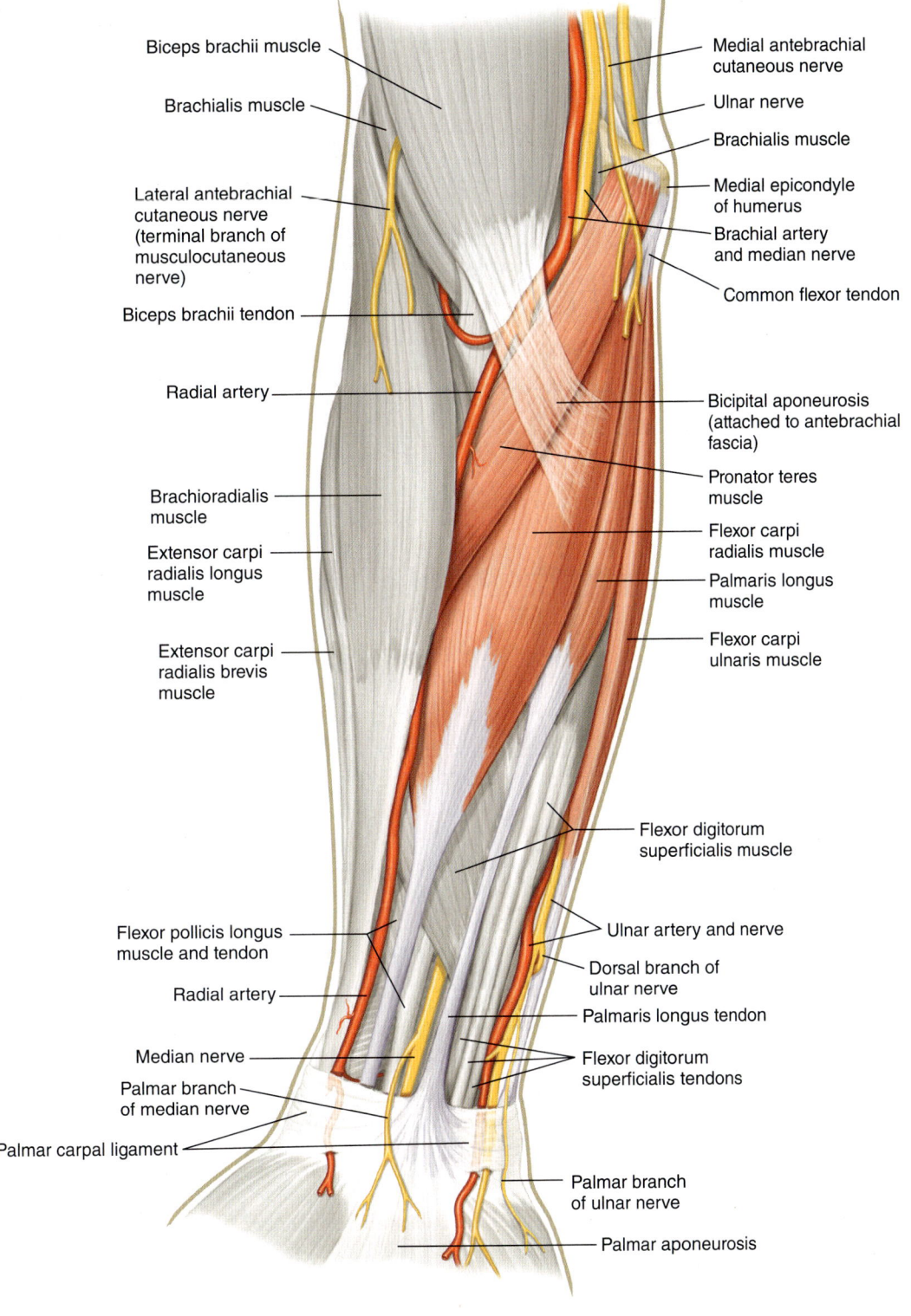

FIGURE 16-20 Superficial flexors of wrist. (Gest TR. *Lippincott Atlas of Anatomy*. 2nd ed. Wolters Kluwer; 2020: Plate 2-23.)

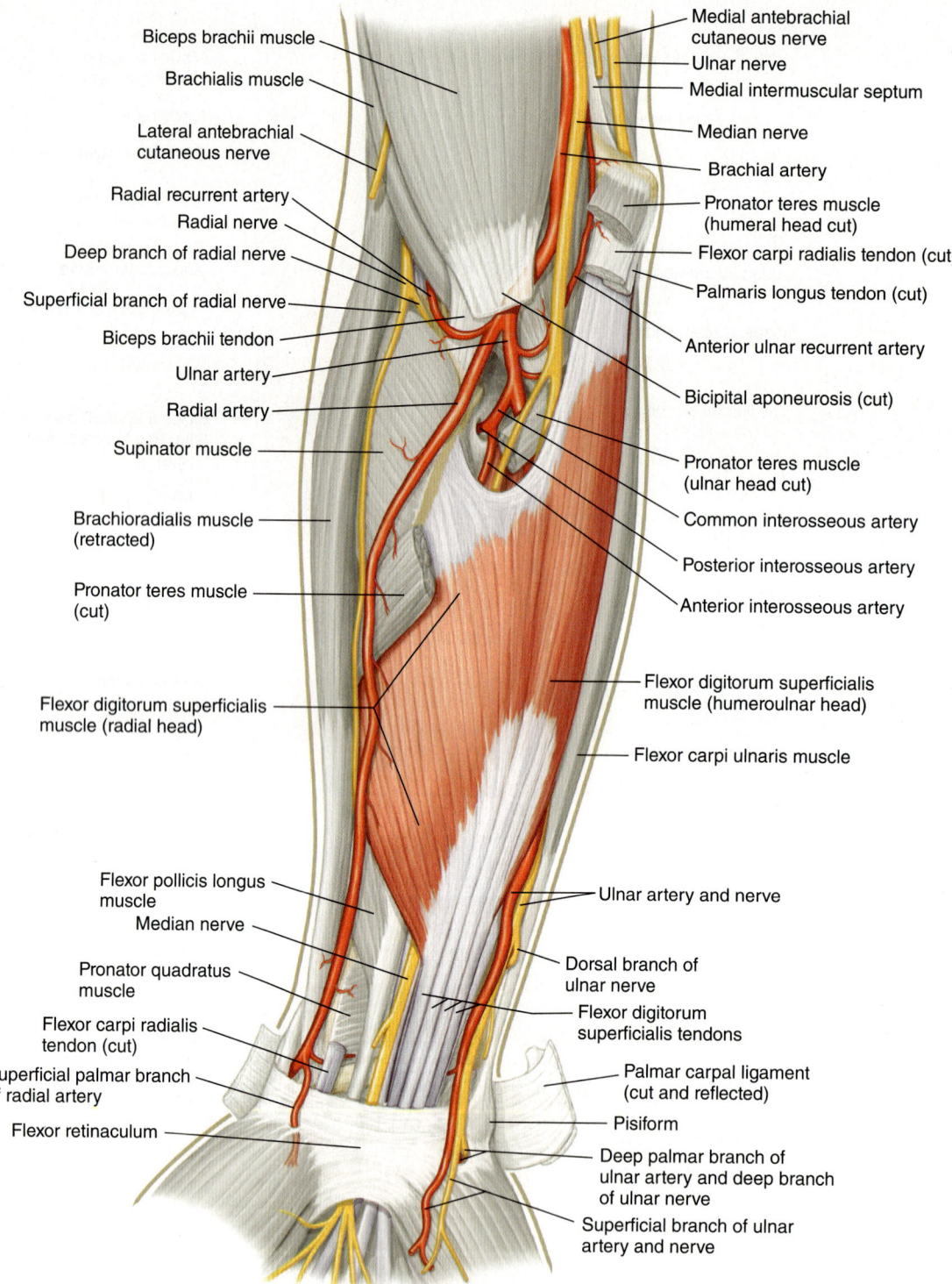

FIGURE 16-21 Intermediate flexors of wrist. (Gest TR. *Lippincott Atlas of Anatomy*. 2nd ed. Wolters Kluwer; 2020: Plate 2-24.)

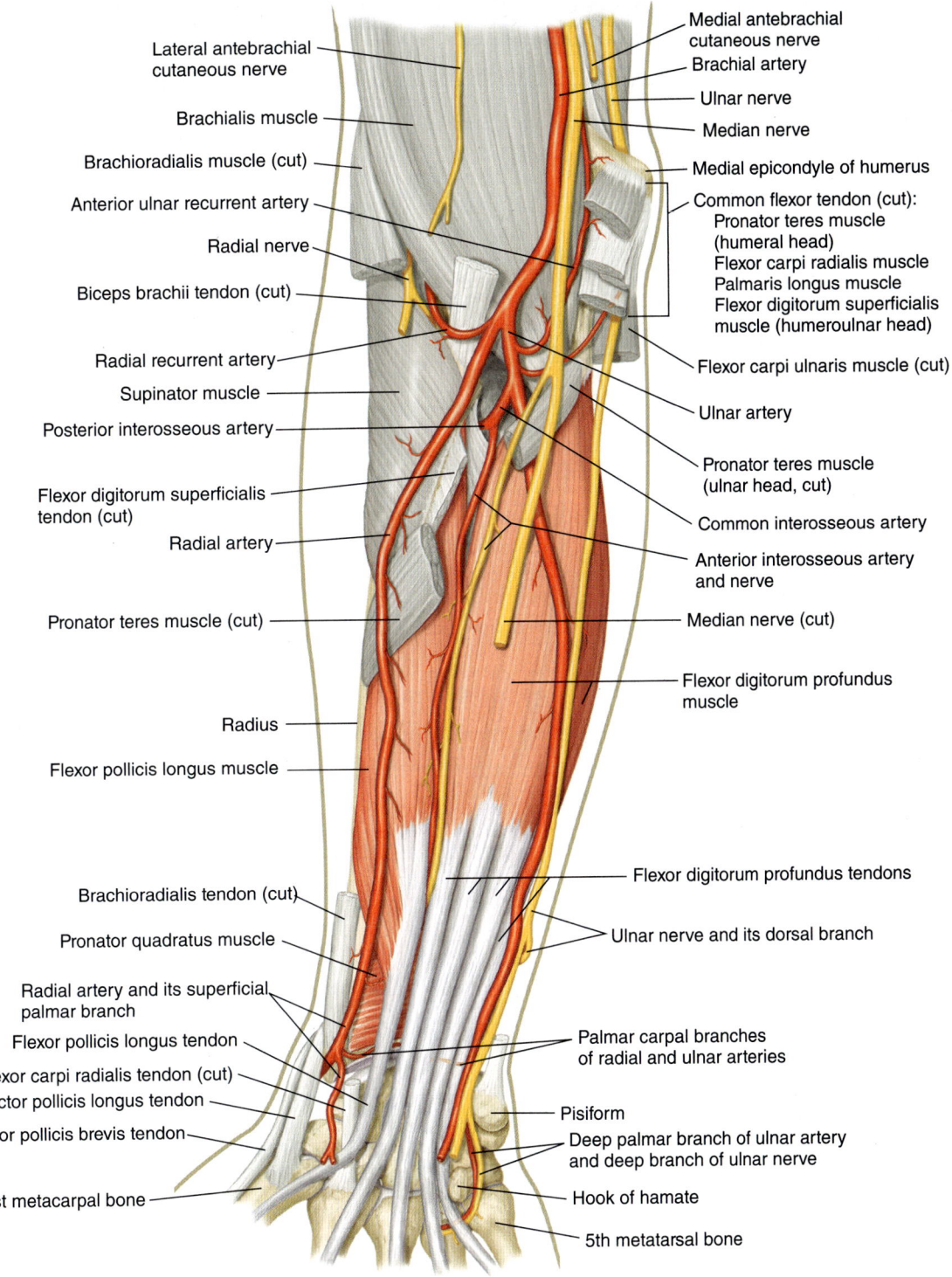

FIGURE 16-22 Deep flexors of wrist. (Gest TR. *Lippincott Atlas of Anatomy*. 2nd ed. Wolters Kluwer; 2020: Plate 2-25.)

TABLE 16-4
INTRINSIC HAND MUSCLES (GROUPED BY LOCATION)

Location	Muscle	Proximal Attachment	Distal Attachment
Thenar	Opponens pollicis	Flexor retinaculum, tubercles of scaphoid and trapezium	Lateral side of 1st metacarpal
	ABD-PB		Base of proximal phalanx of thumb, lateral side
	FPB		
	Superficial head		
	Deep head		
	ADDP		
	Oblique head	Bases of 2nd and 3rd metacarpals, capitate, and adjacent carpals	Base of proximal phalanx of thumb, medial side
	Transverse head	Anterior surface of shaft of 3rd metacarpal	
Hypothenar	ABD-DM	Pisiform	Base of proximal phalanx of fifth digit, medial side
	FDMB	Hook of hamate and flexor retinaculum	
	Opponens digiti minimi		Medial border of 5th metacarpal
Short muscles	Lumbricals		
	1st and 2nd	Lateral two tendons of FDP	Lateral sides of extensor expansions digits 2–5
	3rd and 4th	Medial three tendons of FDP	
	Dorsal interossei (1st–4th)	Adjacent sides of two metacarpals	Bases of proximal phalanges; extensor expansions of digits 2–4
	Palmar interossei (1st–3rd)	Palmar surfaces metacarpals 2, 4, 5	Bases of proximal phalanges; extensor expansions digits 2, 4, 5

ABD-DM, abductor digiti minimi; *ABD-PB*, abductor pollicis brevis; *ADDP*, adductor pollicis; *FDMB*, flexor digiti minimi brevis; *FPB*, flexor pollicis brevis.
Adapted from Moore KL, Dalley AF, Agur AMR. *Clinically Oriented Anatomy.* 8th ed. Wolters Kluwer; 2018.

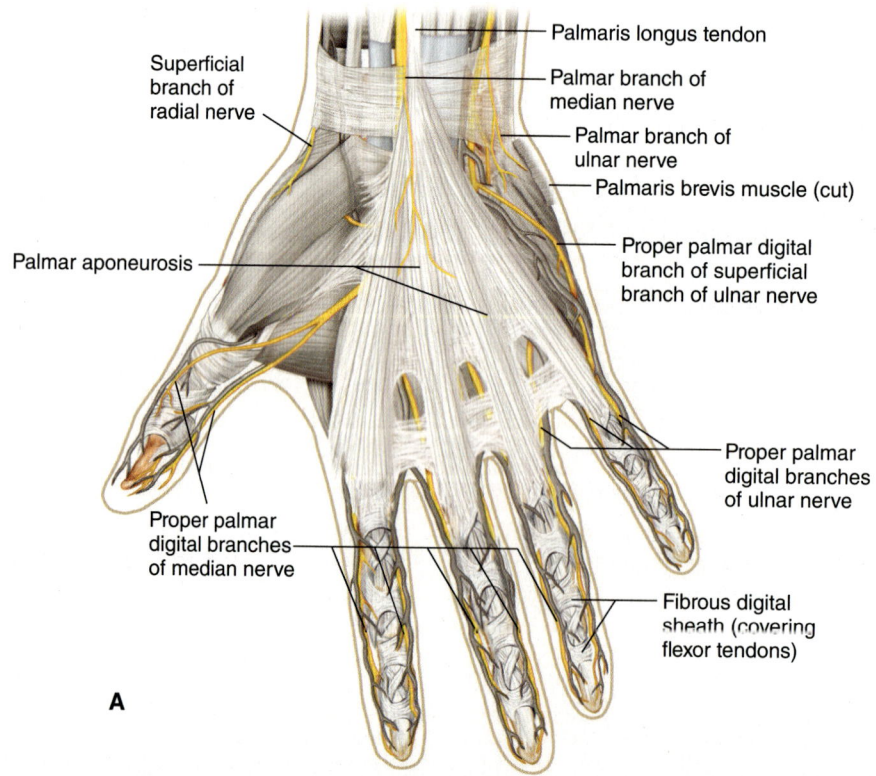

FIGURE 16-23 Schematic of hand dissection, superficial. Palmar view. **A.** Palmar aponeurosis and flexor tendon sheaths.

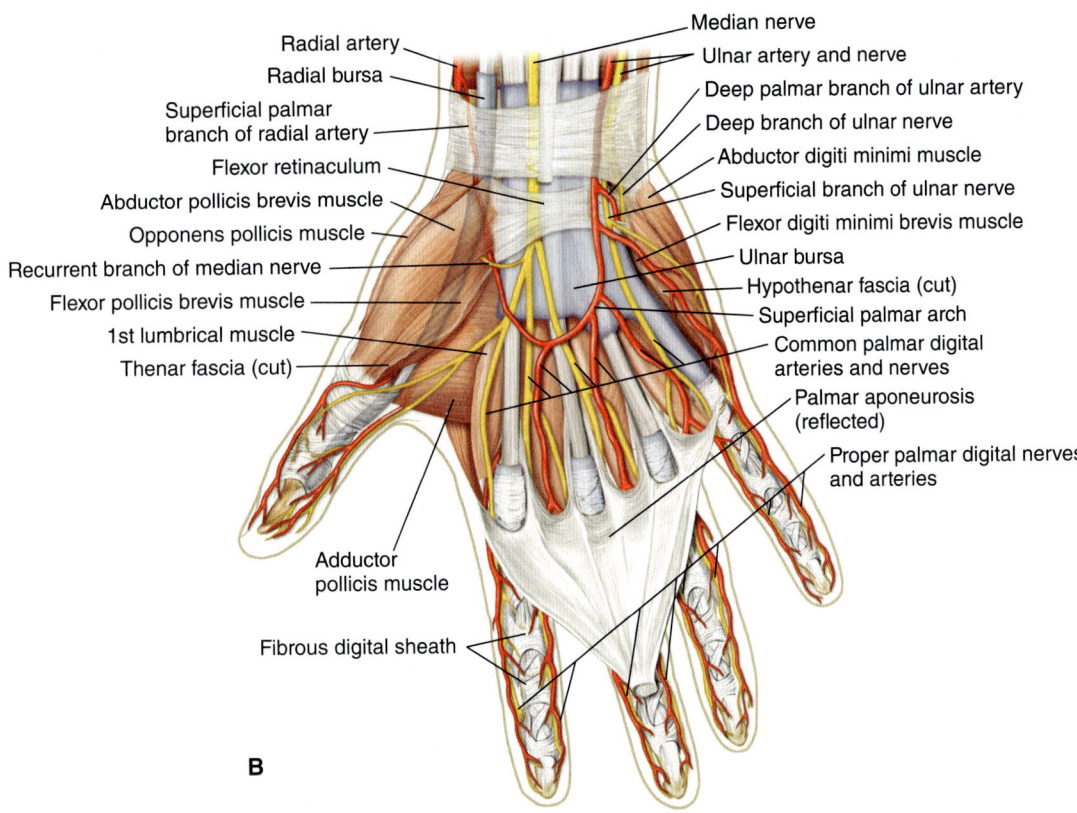

FIGURE 16-23 (continued) **B.** Palmar aponeurosis reflected. (Gest TR. *Lippincott Atlas of Anatomy*. 2nd ed. Wolters Kluwer; 2020: Plates 2-33A and 2.34A.)

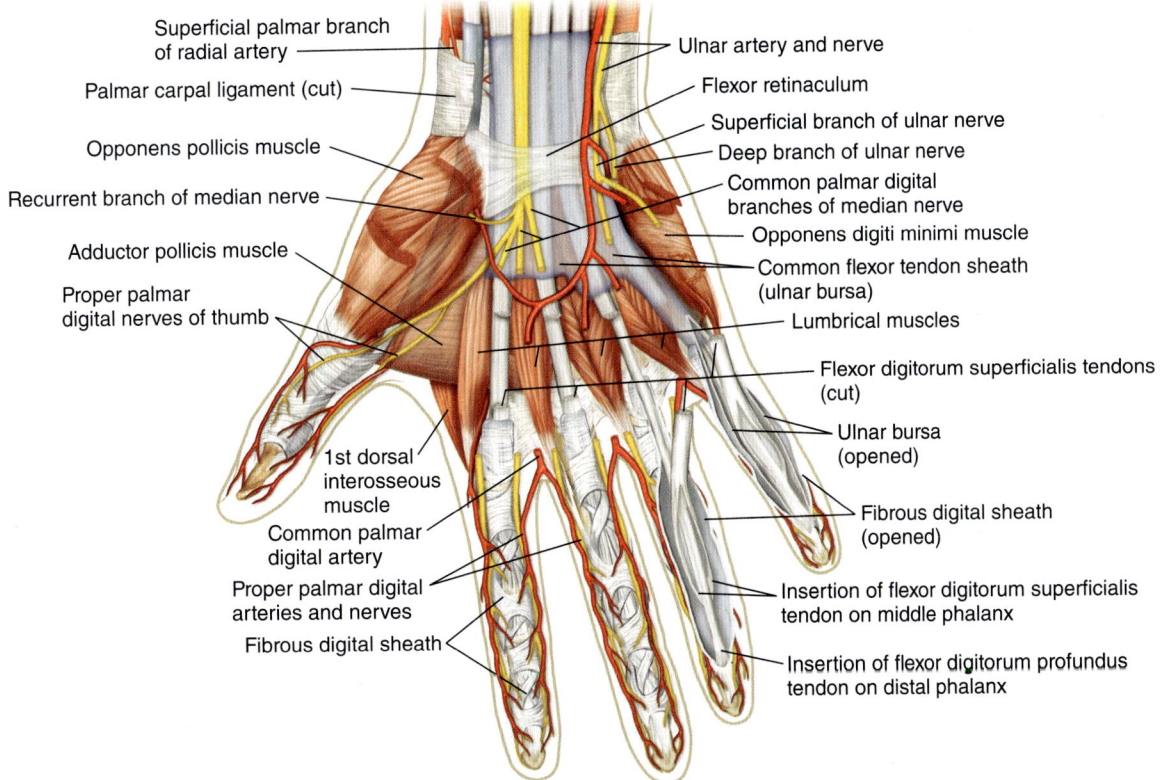

FIGURE 16-24 Schematic of hand dissection, intermediate. Palmar view. (Gest TR. *Lippincott Atlas of Anatomy*. 2nd ed. Wolters Kluwer; 2020: Plate 2-34B.)

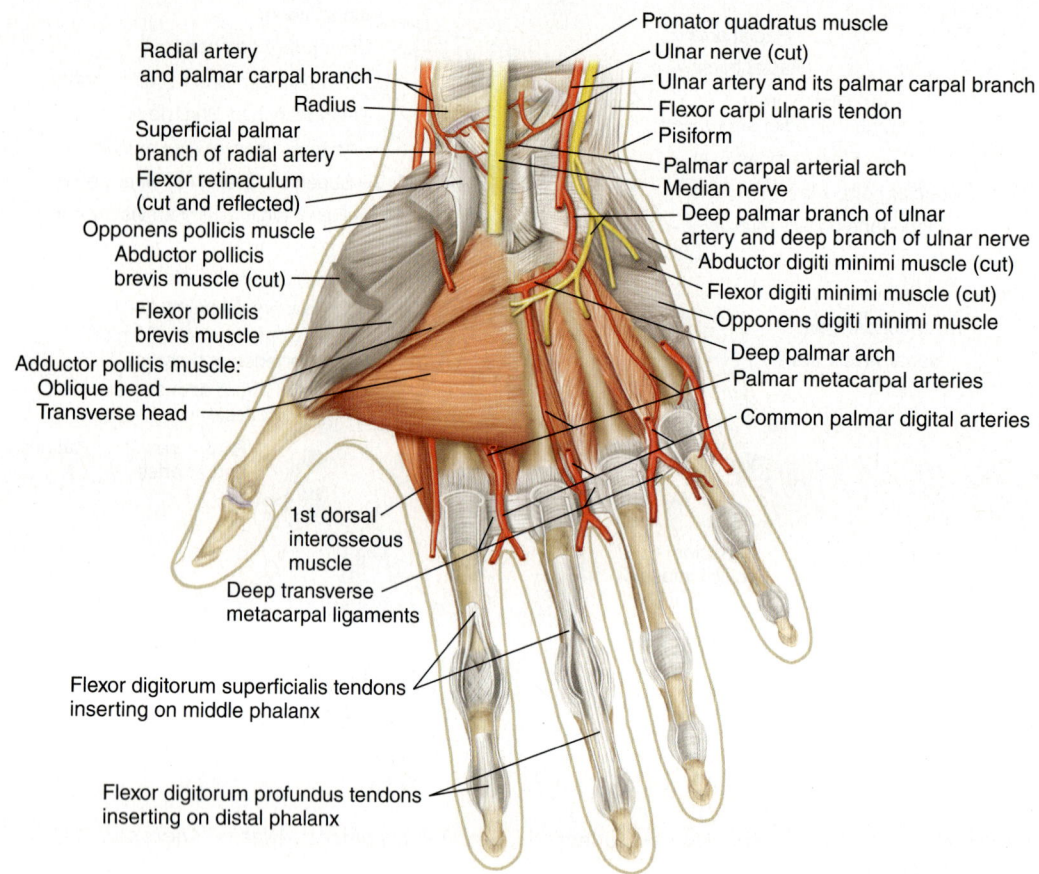

FIGURE 16-25 Schematic of hand dissection, deep. Palmar view. (Gest TR. *Lippincott Atlas of Anatomy*. 2nd ed. Wolters Kluwer; 2020: Plate 2-35A.)

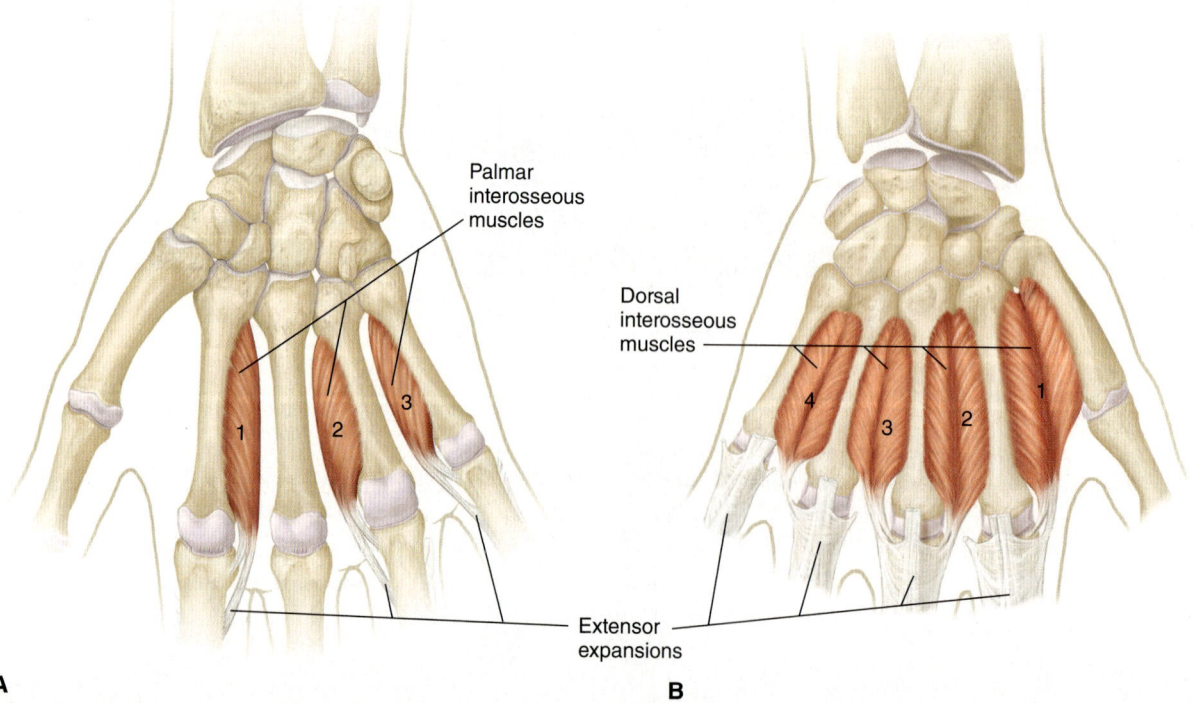

FIGURE 16-26 Schematic of hand interossei dissection, deep. Palmar view. **A.** Palmar interossei. **B.** Dorsal interossei. (Gest TR. *Lippincott Atlas of Anatomy*. 2nd ed. Wolters Kluwer; 2020: Plate 2-35B & C.)

TABLE 16-5
MUSCLES OF WRIST AND HAND (GROUPED BY ACTION)

Action	Muscles	Nerve Supply
Wrist extension	ECRL	Radial
	ECRB	Posterior interosseous
	ECU	
Wrist flexion	FCR	Median
	FCU	Ulnar
Wrist ulnar deviation	FCU	Ulnar
	ECU	Posterior interosseous
Wrist radial deviation	FCR	Median
	ECRL	Radial
	APL	Posterior interosseous
	EPB	
Finger extension	Extensor digitorum	Posterior interosseous
	Extensor indicis	
	EDM	
Finger flexion	FDP	Anterior interosseous: lateral two digits
		Ulnar: medial two digits
	FDS	Median
	Lumbricals	1st and 2nd: median
		3rd and 4th: ulnar
	Interossei	Ulnar
	FDMB	
Abduction of fingers	Dorsal (posterior) interossei	Ulnar
	ABD-DM	
Adduction of fingers	Palmar (anterior) interossei	Ulnar
Extension of thumb	EPL	Posterior interosseous
	EPB	
	ABD-PL	
Flexion of thumb	FPB	Superficial head: median
		Deep head: ulnar
	FPL	Anterior interosseous
	Opponens pollicis	Median
Abduction of thumb	ABPL	Posterior interosseous
	ABD-PB	Median
Adduction of thumb	ADDP	Ulnar
Opposition of thumb and fifth digit	Opponens pollicis	Median
	FPB	Superficial head: median
	ABD-PB	Median
	Opponens digiti minimi	Ulnar

The posterior interosseous nerve is a branch of the deep radial nerve, supplying muscles in the posterior forearm.

ABD-DM, abductor digiti minimi; *ABD-PB*, abductor pollicis brevis; *ABD-PL*, abductor pollicis longus; *ADDP*, adductor pollicis; *ECRB*, extensor carpi radialis brevis; *ECRL*, extensor carpi radialis longus; *ECU*, extensor carpi ulnaris; *EDI*, extensor digiti minimi; *EPB*, extensor pollicis brevis; *EPL*, extensor pollicis longus; *FCR*, flexor carpi radialis; *FCU*, flexor carpi ulnaris; *FDMB*, flexor digiti minimi brevis; *FDP*, flexor digitorum profundus; *FDS*, flexor digitorum superficialis; *FPB*, flexor pollicis brevis; *FPL*, flexor pollicis longus.

Adapted from Dutton M. *Dutton's Orthopedic Examination, Evaluation and Intervention.* 4th ed. McGraw Hill; 2016.

SPECIFIC ANATOMIC REGIONS OF THE WRIST AND HAND COMPLEX

The complexity of wrist and hand movement requires unique configurations of bones and connective tissues to perform tasks, such as holding and picking up a cup, gripping a hammer, or holding a broom handle while sweeping. The anatomic relationships among connective tissues are described in this section.

Extensor Retinaculum and Expansion

At the dorsal and lateral wrist, the tendons of the extensor muscles of the forearm pass under the extensor retinaculum, a thickened portion of the fascia on the posterior distal forearm that attaches to the radius and ulna (see Figs. 16-18 and 16-19). The extensor retinaculum forms osseofibrous tunnels for the tendons, holding the tendons close to the wrist to prevent bowstringing (protrusion beyond the contour of the bent limb). The extensor tendons enter synovial tendon sheaths as they pass, reducing friction. The tendons of the extensor muscles of the forearm pass beneath the extensor retinaculum in six synovial tendon sheaths, to form compartments, as shown in Figure 16-27.

While passing toward the distal attachments, the finger extensor tendons spread out and form intertendinous connections near the MCP joints. These connections limit independent extension of digits 2 through 5, particularly digit 4. Extending farther distally, the four tendons flatten and spread into a triangularly shaped aponeurosis named the *extensor expansion* (aka extensor digital expansion or extensor hood) (Fig. 16-28). Passing over the dorsal MCP joint, the extensor expansion is anchored to the dorsal MCP joint by palmar ligaments, a portion of the MCP joint capsule. The extensor expansion continues distally,

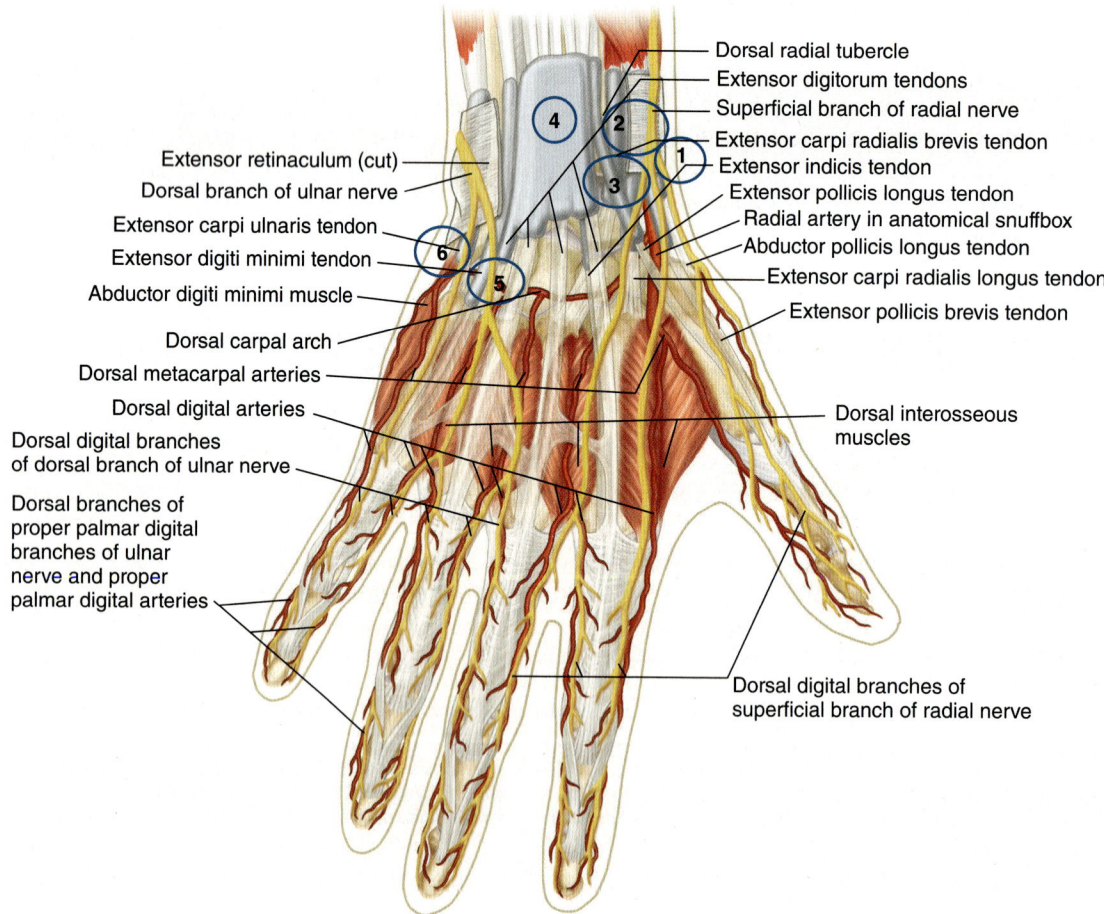

FIGURE 16-27 Extensor retinaculum and extensor tendon. The tendons within the numbered compartments are (1) extensor pollicis brevis, abductor pollicis longus; (2) extensor carpi radialis brevis, extensor carpi radialis longus; (3) extensor pollicis longus; (4) extensor digitorum, extensor indicis; (5) extensor digiti minimi; and (6) extensor carpi ulnaris. (Gest TR. *Lippincott Atlas of Anatomy*. 2nd ed. Wolters Kluwer; 2020: Plate 2-41.)

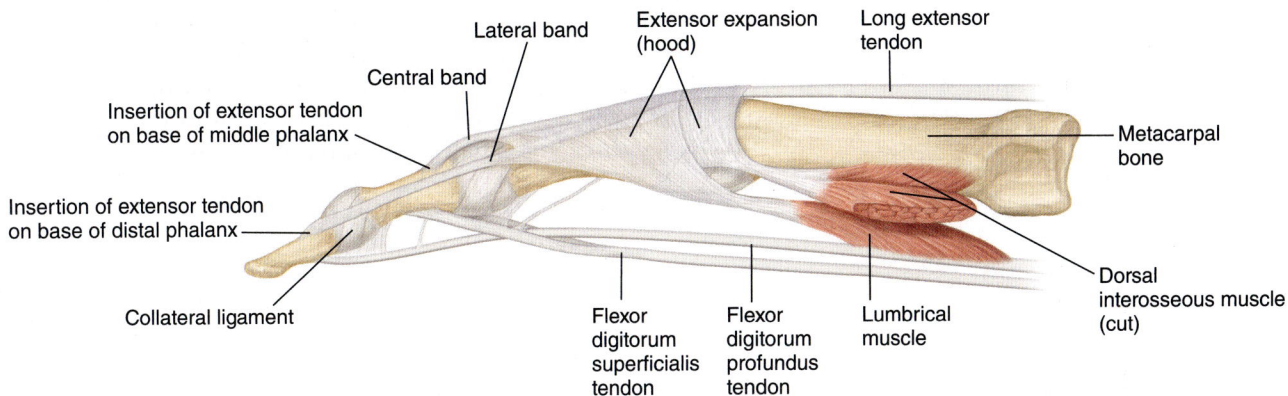

FIGURE 16-28 Extensor expansion and smaller ligaments of the digits. (Gest TR. *Lippincott Atlas of Anatomy*. 2nd ed. Wolters Kluwer; 2020: Plate 2-45C.)

dividing into a median band that attaches to the middle phalangeal base and two lateral bands that flank the median band to attach to the DIP base. The retinacular ligament passes from the flexor digital sheaths on the proximal phalanx to join the extensor expansion attachment to the distal phalanx. Tension in the retinacular ligament during DIP joint flexion pulls the PIP into flexion. Likewise, with extension of the PIP, the DIP is pulled into near-complete extension. The extensor digitorum acts primarily to extend the proximal phalanx, and through the extensor expansion, is able to extend the middle and distal phalanges. The lumbricals and interossei have distal attachment into the extensor expansion.

Palmar Aponeurosis and Flexor Tendon Sheaths

The fascia covering the palm and hand is a continuation of the fascia of the forearm and dorsal hand. Thin over the thenar and hypothenar eminences, the palmar fascia is thick centrally, forming the palmar aponeurosis. Refer to Figure 16-23, which shows the palmar aponeurosis intact (A) and reflected distally (B). As the palmar aponeurosis extends distally, four bands extend and attach to the proximal phalanges, converging with the flexor tendon sheaths. The synovial sheaths of the flexor digitorum superficialis (FDS) and flexor digitorum profundus (FDP) tendons are formed at the wrist deep to the flexor retinaculum and spread out distally toward their respective digits, providing a tube-like structure for passage of the synovial membranes and tendons in route to distal attachments. The synovial sheaths continue to the bases of the proximal phalanges and merge with the extensions of the palmar aponeurosis to form fibrous digital sheaths. The fibrous tendon sheaths and palmar surface of the phalanges combine to form an osseofibrous tunnel that is reinforced by thickenings of the fibrous digital sheath. The thickenings form five annular (A1, A2, A3, A4, and A5) and three cruciform (C1, C2, and C3) bands that act as pulleys as the tendons pass traverse through the tunnel (Fig. 16-29). The bands prevent bowstringing of the tendons and help transfer forces during flexion of the digits.[44,45] Injury or inflammation to the flexor tendon sheath risks compromise to the glide of the tendons housed within the sheath.

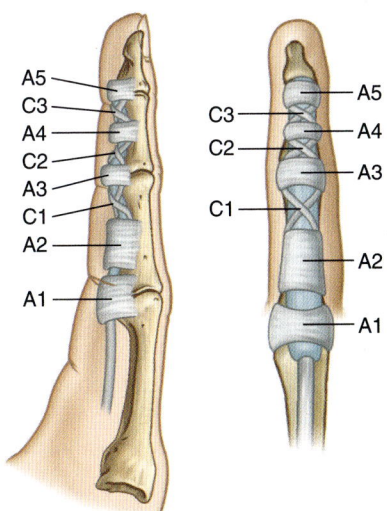

FIGURE 16-29 The annular and cruciate bands of the flexor tendon sheath-pulley system. **A.** Lateral view, **B.** Palmar view. *A*, annular; *C*, cruciate. (Anderson MK, Barnum M. *Foundations of Athletic Training: Prevention, Assessment, and Management*. 6th ed. Wolters Kluwer; 2017: Figure 19.4.)

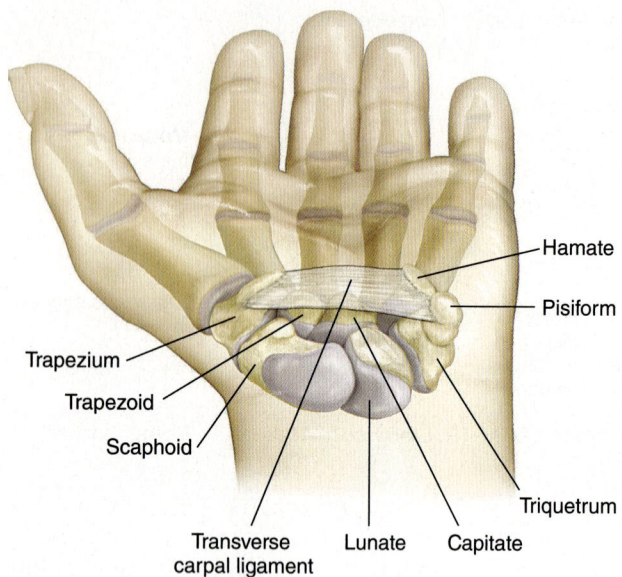

FIGURE 16-30 Carpal tunnel.

Carpal Tunnel

The palmar side of the carpal bones are shaped such that articulation among them forms a concavity. The wide, strong transverse carpal ligament has an attachment to the hook of the hamate and pisiform on the ulnar side and the trapezium and scaphoid on the radial side, covering the concavity and creating a passageway named the *carpal tunnel* (Fig. 16-30). The transverse carpal ligament serves as an attachment for intrinsic and extrinsic muscles. Along with the median nerve, nine extrinsic muscle tendons pass through the tunnel: FDS (four), FDP (four), and flexor pollicis longus (FPL) (one).

Anatomical Snuffbox

The triangular depression on the lateral dorsum of the hand, most clearly seen when the thumb is actively extended, is the anatomical snuffbox (see Fig. 16-18). The borders listed in the following are described from the anatomic position:

- Ulnar (medial) border—the tendon of the EPL
- Radial (lateral) border—the tendons of extensor pollicis brevis (EPB) and abductor pollicis longus (APL)
- Proximal border—styloid process of the radius
- Floor—scaphoid and trapezium
- Roof—skin

The contents of the anatomical snuffbox include the radial artery, which crosses the floor and turns medially passing between the heads of the adductor pollicis (ADDP) muscle. The blood supply to the scaphoid bone travels from distal to proximal, significantly impacting blood flow to the bone if the artery is injured in a scaphoid fracture, as commonly occurs with horizontal fractures of the bone. The superficial branch of the radial nerve is located in the skin and subcutaneous tissue supplying the skin of the lateral three and a half digits and back of the hand.

NERVES SUPPLYING THE WRIST AND HAND

The three peripheral nerves supplying the skin and muscle of the wrist and hand (Table 16-5) are the median, ulnar, and radial nerves formed by the C5-T11 nerve roots. The course of the nerves in the arm and forearm is described in Chapter 15, Elbow Complex. Compression of one of the nerves at any point in its course can lead to motor and sensory deficits that are most commonly manifested in the forearm or hand.

Median Nerve

The median nerve is formed by contributions of the lateral and medial cords of the brachial plexus and has no branches in the axilla or arm. The median nerve supplies all of the muscles in the anterior forearm (except for the FCU and ulnar half of the FDP) and five intrinsic muscles of the hand. The median nerve enters the hand through the carpal tunnel and supplies the first two lumbricals and thenar muscles and skin of the hand, as shown in Figure 16-31. A palmar cutaneous branch of the median nerve, supplying the central palm, does not pass through the carpal tunnel.

Ulnar Nerve

The ulnar nerve is the terminal branch of the medial cord of the brachial plexus. The ulnar nerve supplies the FCU and ulnar half of the FDP before continuing distally at the wrist through the ulnar canal (aka Guyon canal) and then dividing into a superficial cutaneous branch (supplying skin on the anterior ulnar palmar surface) and a deep branch that supplies all muscles of the hand, except those supplied by the median nerve (Fig. 16-32). Just proximal to the wrist, the ulnar nerve gives off a palmar cutaneous branch that traverses distally to supply the skin on the medial side of the palm. A dorsal cutaneous branch supplies a portion of the ulnar dorsum of the hand and the fifth and the medial half of the fourth finger.

Radial Nerve

The radial nerve is a terminal branch of the posterior cord of the brachial plexus and supplies the muscles on the posterior arm and forearm. The radial nerve supplies skin on the dorsum of the hand, but does not supply any muscles in the hand (Fig. 16-33). A summary of sensory supply to the distal wrist and hand is shown in Figure 16-34.

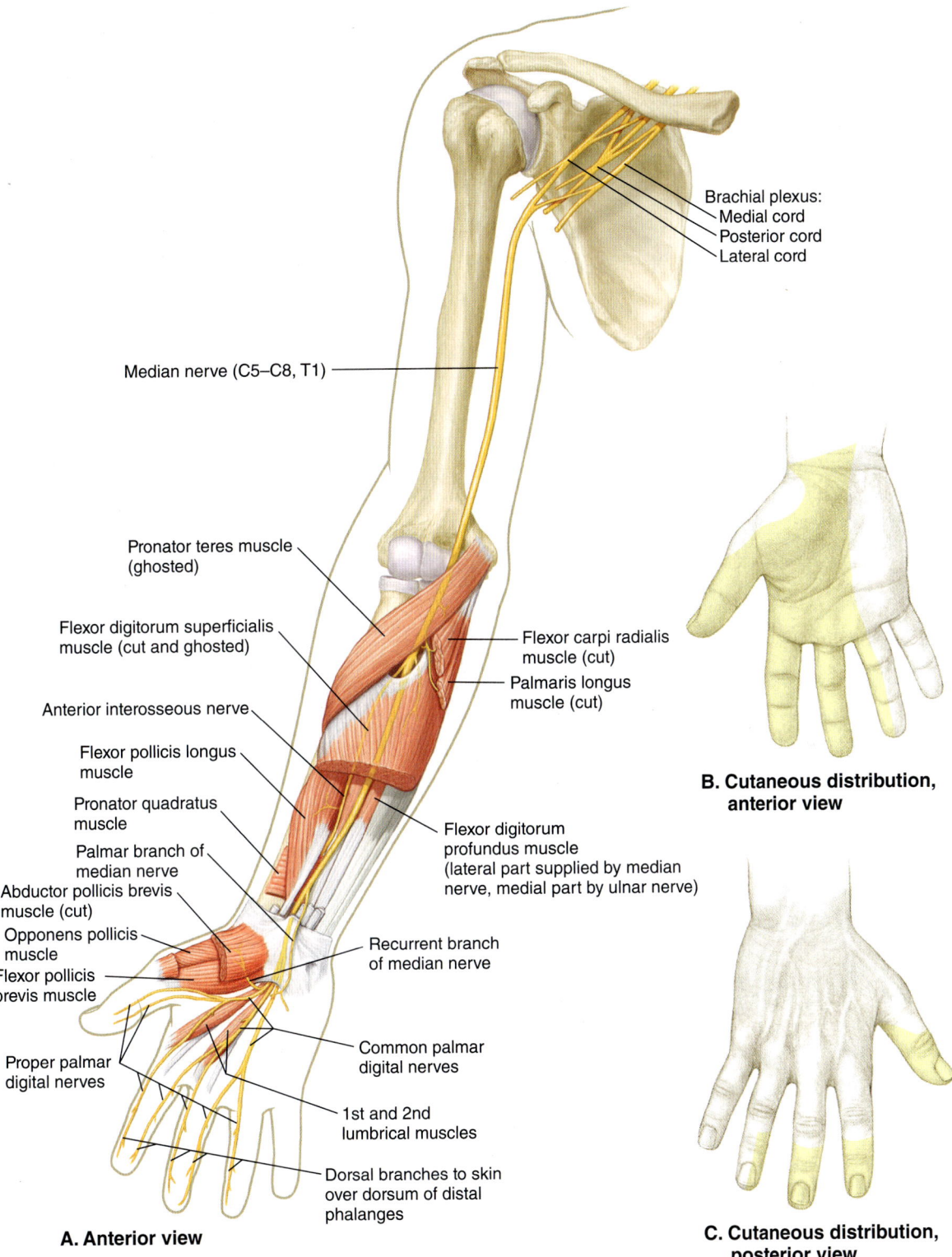

FIGURE 16-31 Median nerve. **A.** Course of the median nerve including motor and sensory supply. Cutaneous distribution: **B.** Anterior view. **C.** Posterior view. (Gest TR. *Lippincott Atlas of Anatomy*. 2nd ed. Wolters Kluwer; 2020: Plate 2-50A-C.)

594 SECTION IV | UPPER QUARTER

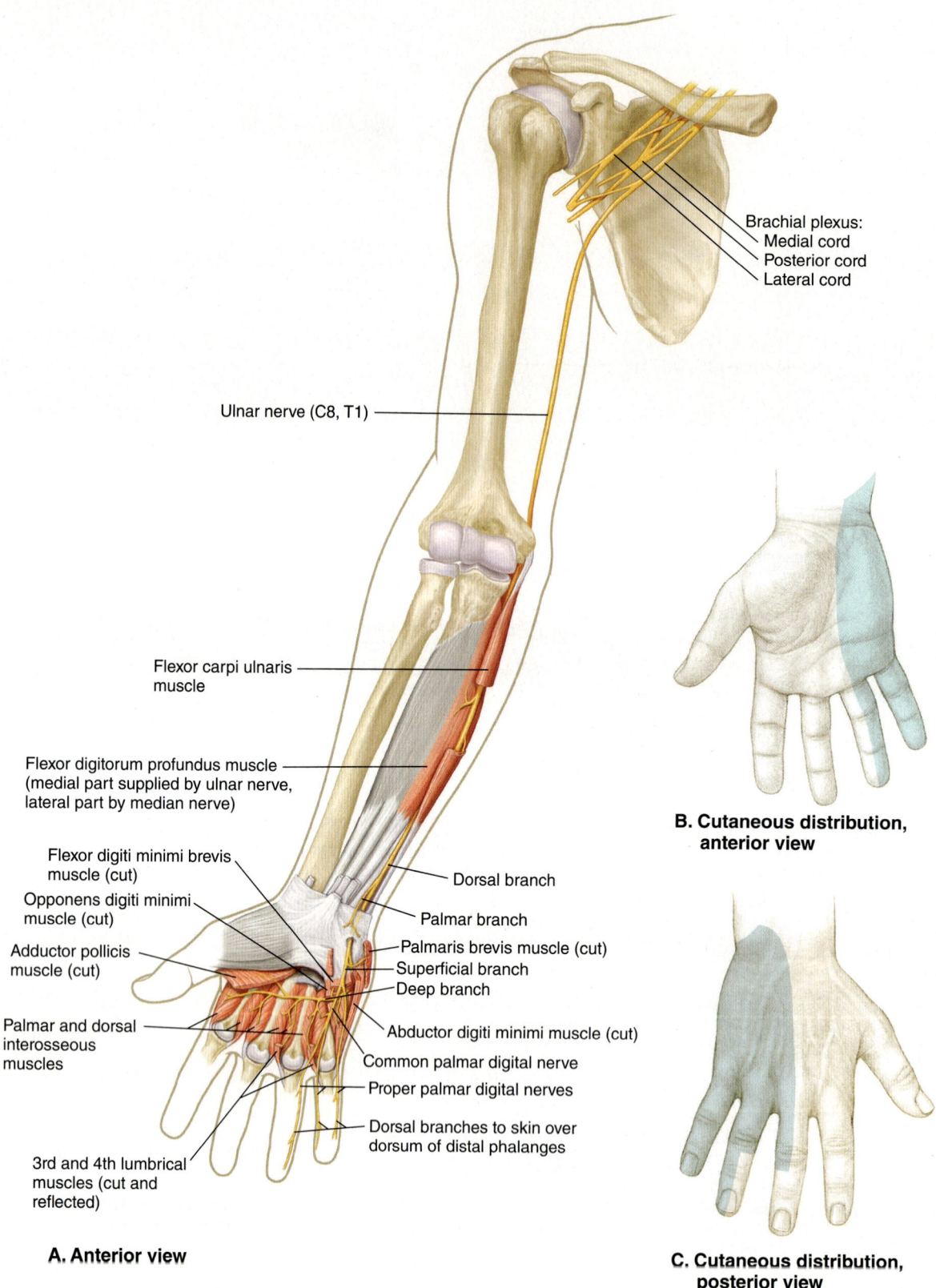

FIGURE 16-32 Ulnar nerve. **A.** Course of the ulnar nerve including motor and sensory supply. Cutaneous distribution: **B.** Anterior view. **C.** Posterior view. (Gest TR. *Lippincott Atlas of Anatomy*. 2nd ed. Wolters Kluwer; 2020: Plate 2-51A-C.)

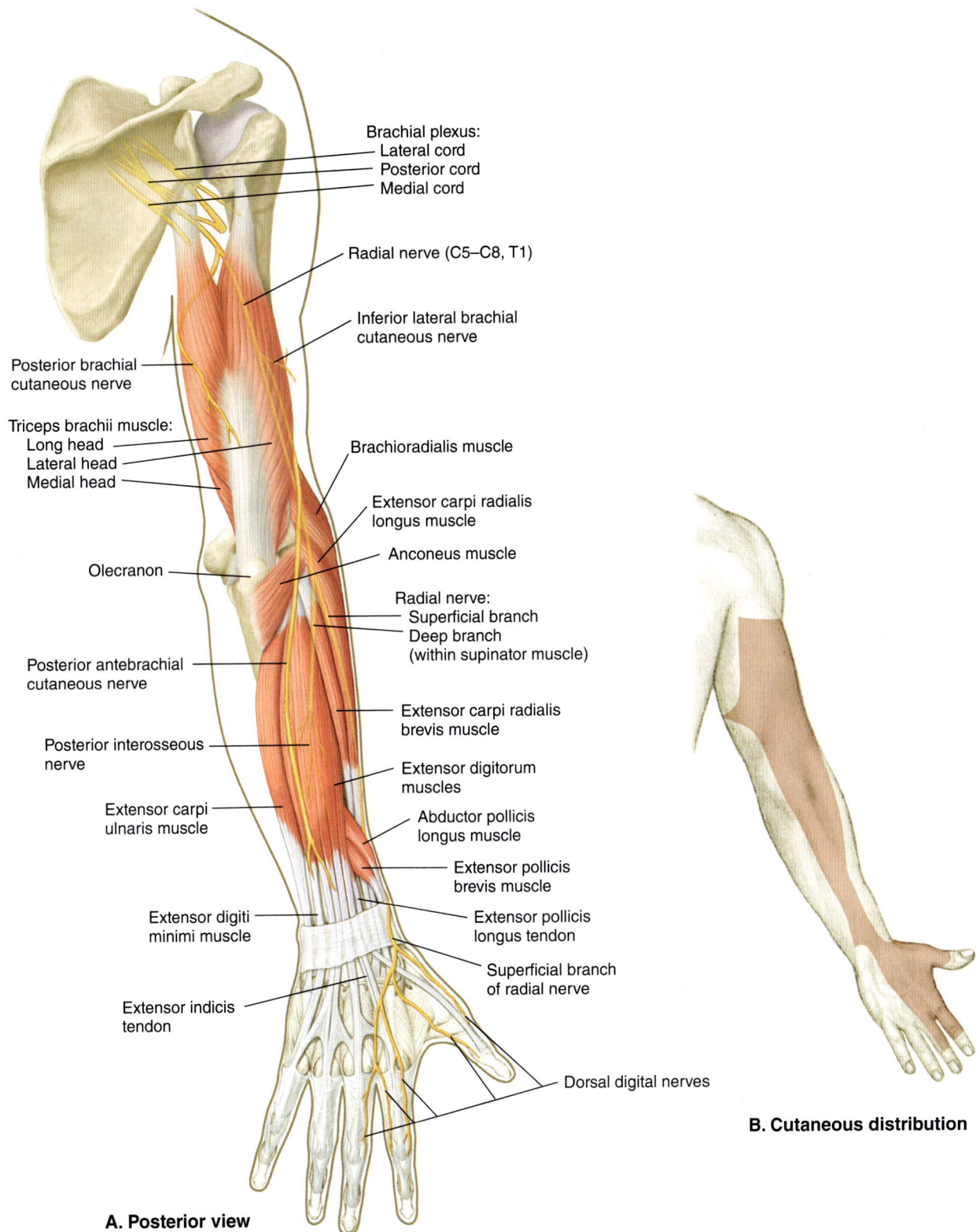

FIGURE 16-33 Radial nerve. **A.** Course of the radial nerve including motor and sensory supply. **B.** Cutaneous distribution. *C,* cervical; *T,* thoracic. (Gest TR. *Lippincott Atlas of Anatomy.* 2nd ed. Wolters Kluwer; 2020: Plate 2-52A & B.)

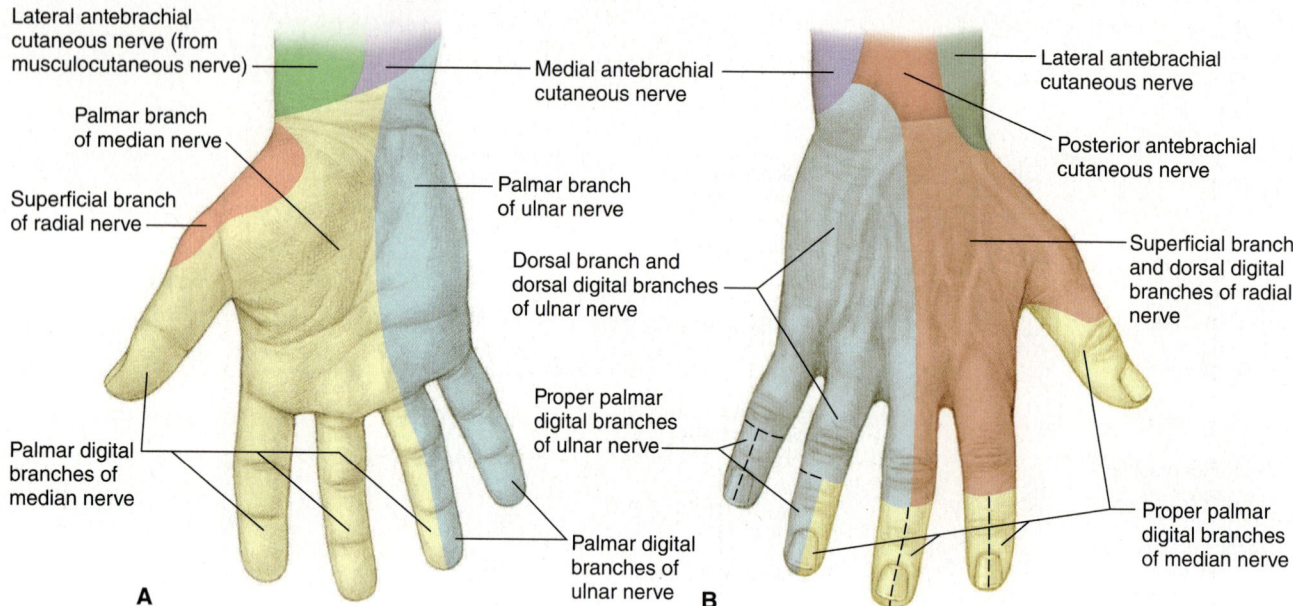

FIGURE 16-34 Summary of sensory supply to the distal wrist and hand. **A.** Palmar view. **B.** Dorsal view. (Gest TR. *Lippincott Atlas of Anatomy.* 2nd ed. Wolters Kluwer; 2020: Plates 2-33B and 2-39B.)

PALPATION OF THE WRIST AND HAND

Palpation of the wrist and hand should begin with the patient in a relaxed position with the hand resting on a surface.

Bony Palpation

The radial and ulnar styloid processes should be identified to provide a starting point for palpation. In the description here, the patient has the forearm pronated with the palm facing downward toward the surface. The clinician places a cupped hand with the thumb and index finger palpating either side of the patient's wrist joint. The clinician's other hand can be used to gently move the patient's wrist into radial and ulnar deviation. The radial styloid is palpated on the radial side just proximal to the wrist as the patient's wrist is moved into ulnar deviation. Likewise, the ulnar styloid is identified as the distinctive distal end of the ulna when the patient's wrist is moved into radial deviation. From this point, the clinician should identify the radial styloid and palpate proximally until the bony prominence is obscured by soft tissue; then return to the wrist to confirm the location of the radial styloid. The ulnar styloid location can be confirmed in a similar manner on the ulnar side.

Moving from the radial styloid approximately one-third of the way across the dorsal wrist, a small bony prominence, Lister tubercle, can be felt. Moving toward the distal ulna, the ulnar styloid process can be grasped between the clinician's thumb and index finger. Returning to Lister tubercle and moving distally toward 3rd metacarpal, the clinician can palpate the lunate, capitate, and 3rd metacarpal bone in a straight line. Just proximal to the base of 3rd metacarpal, the largest carpal bone, the capitate, can be felt. With the wrist in a neutral position, the small depression of the capitate's dorsal surface can be felt. When the wrist is flexed, the capitate moves and this depression is no longer felt. Proceeding proximally, the lunate can be palpated, in line with Lister tubercle.

Returning to the radial styloid process and moving slightly distal, the anatomical snuffbox can be seen and palpated and made easier when the patient extends the thumb away from the fingers. The scaphoid forms the floor, and tendons form the borders of the anatomical snuffbox.

Moving the patient into supination, the triquetrum can be palpated at the palmar and ulnar side of the wrist, just distal to the midportion of the distal ulna. Moving slightly distally and toward the ulnar side of the hand, the pea-shaped pisiform bone can be easily palpated on top of the triquetrum. The hamate is located slightly distal and radial to the pisiform bone, in line with the midportion of the patient's web space formed by the thumb and index finger. The hook of the hamate is deep under layers of soft tissue; therefore, pressure must be firm to feel the bone. The pisiform and hook of the hamate form the borders of the ulnar tunnel (tunnel of Guyon) through which the ulnar nerve and artery pass. Deep palpation of the ulnar nerve may produce neurologic symptoms, even in nonpathologic hand.

The long bones of the hand can be palpated from the proximal bases to the more distal heads. The MCP joints are easily identified as the knuckles. The PIP and DIP joints of digits 2 through 5 can be felt on all sides.

Soft-Tissue Palpation

Palpation of the wrist extensor tendons is typically done with reference to the extensor tendon compartments (see Fig. 16-27). Palpation should begin with location of the radial styloid process and anatomical snuffbox, then moving across the dorsal wrist toward the ulnar side. Having the patient gently contract the muscle whose tendon is being palpated aids the palpation process. For example, palpation of the ECU tendon is facilitated by having the patient gently extend and ulnarly deviate the wrist. The tendon should be palpated along its course to the distal attachment. Refer to Table 16-3 for distal attachments and to Figures 16-18 and 16-19 for the location of the extensor tendons.

The tendons of the wrist flexors can be identified most easily by starting with palpation of the distal attachment while the patient gently contracts the muscle. Combining wrist flexion with radioulnar deviation may help differentiate the FCU and FCR from the other wrist flexors. The deep wrist flexor tendons cannot be palpated at the wrist. Refer to Figure 16-20 for a review of superficial tendons on the flexor side of the wrist.

The thenar eminence is located on the palmar and radial sides at the base of the thumb and is composed of three intrinsic muscles contributing to thumb motion. The hypothenar eminence is located on the palmar and ulnar sides at the base of the fifth digit and is composed of three intrinsic muscles that move the small digit. The muscle bellies can be palpated as a group in both the thenar and hypothenar eminences, but it is difficult to delineate specific muscles.

INTRODUCTION TO THE EXAMINATION OF THE WRIST AND HAND COMPLEX

The hand is perhaps the most vital functional unit of the upper extremity. Wrist and hand conditions may begin with trauma, such as a fracture from falling on an outstretched hand, or have an insidious onset, such as carpal tunnel syndrome (CTS). If trauma was involved, the clinician should attempt to discern the mechanism of injury. When there is no apparent reason for symptoms, the clinician must be prepared to direct the line of questioning to elicit information concerning more proximal regions. The wrist and hand are innervated by C6 through T1 nerve roots. Because pain is more commonly referred in a proximal-to-distal direction, a more proximal cause should be considered.

PATIENT HISTORY: WRIST AND HAND COMPLEX

The patient history provides key insights to direct an efficient physical examination. The patient interview should elicit specific information related to the patient's health history and demographics and review of systems (refer to Chapter 6, Patient History). The clinician must understand the patient's symptoms and determine the acuity, severity, irritability, and stability of the condition as well as the functional implications of the patient's condition. In addition, the following specific information should be obtained when interviewing patients with possible wrist and hand disorders.

Hand Dominance

The clinician should ask if the symptoms involved the patient's dominant or nondominant hand. While some wrist/hand tasks, such as keyboarding, require bilateral hand use, others, such as handwriting, do not. In addition, most tools are designed with a dominant right upper extremity in mind.

Occupation and Recreational Activities

In addition to determining hand dominance, the clinician must understand the patient's occupation and recreational demands. Jobs that expose workers to vibration, such as the use of power tools, or external pressure on the wrist are risk factors for CTS. Many wrist and hand injuries are the result of overuse from repetitive microtrauma. This can occur with factory line work, jobs that require repeated grasping or tool use, or recreational activities, such as kayaking and rock climbing.

Mechanism of Onset

Common lesions at, or about, the wrist vary in onset, from insidious (CTS, osteoarthritis [OA], RA, and trigger finger) to those in which a trauma is definitely recalled (fracture, lunate dislocation, capsuloligamentous sprains, and tendon rupture). If a traumatic event is cited, the examiner should attempt to determine the exact mechanism of injury. A fall on an outstretched hand (sometimes referred to as a *FOOSH injury*) can damage various structures based on the direction of the fall and the position of the wrist and hand. If a fall did occur, the clinician should understand the circumstances surrounding the incident. For example, does the patient require additional balance screening, such as the Berg Balance test (Chapter 11, Hip), or was the fall due to random bad luck. Clinicians should also query the patient if there was a break in skin integrity from the incident because bacteria can enter the hand and create an infection that can rapidly spread proximally within a synovial tendon sheath.

Chief Complaint

The clinician should understand the patient's chief complaint. Does the hand hurt with certain activities, such as gripping or weight bearing? Is the main patient complaint related to stiffness, as can occur with OA, or to weakness or lack of dexterity, as with a distal peripheral nerve injury? Is the patient experiencing clicking or catching as might occur with a TFCC injury[46] or trigger finger?[47] The clinician must ask questions to elicit information about more proximal regions so as not to confound distal symptoms with a more proximal pathology, particularly if the onset is insidious.

Reports of tingling, numbness, or paresthesias require a thorough examination of proximal structures, including an upper quarter neurologic screen. This is essential with the wrist and hand because of the potential for double-crush syndrome (Chapter 15, Elbow Complex). A clinical example in the wrist and hand would be when the C7 nerve root is compressed at the cervical spine and the median nerve (to which C7 contributes) is compressed at the carpal tunnel. Although improvement in symptoms may occur with treatment of one region, optimal results are more likely if both areas of compression are addressed.[48] The clinician must also consider that (diagnosed or previously undiagnosed) diabetes can cause peripheral neuropathy, including bilateral paresthesias, loss of protective sensation, and weakness.

Prior History

The clinician should learn of past injuries to the upper extremity. A radial fracture as a child may arrest the radial growth plates, causing the radius to be shorter than the ulna (positive ulnar variance). This results in increased compressive forces on the TFCC during upper extremity weight bearing.[49] Risk factors for complex regional pain syndrome (CRPS) include recent carpal tunnel surgery,[50] distal radius fractures,[50] and individuals with a history of depression.[51] In addition to a history of diabetes, clinicians should consider that patients with a history of OA in other joints may be experiencing a similar degeneration to joints of the wrist and/or hand.[52] Lastly, clinicians should consider that patients with pain in the wrist, PIP, and/or MCP joints may be experiencing symptoms of an autoimmune disease, such as RA. Symptoms of RA tend to be bilateral and progressive and include swelling, motion loss, and eventual joint deformity.

Outcome Measures

The Patient-Specific Outcome Tool, Disabilities of the Arm, Shoulder, and Hand (DASH), and Quick-DASH (introduced in Chapter 6, Patient History, and Chapter 14, Shoulder Complex) might be applicable to any patient with an upper extremity disorder. The shorter version of the DASH, the Quick-DASH, is a frequently used outcome measure for patients with hand dysfunction. Additional region-specific outcome tools are listed in Table 16-6.[53]

PHYSICAL EXAMINATION: WRIST AND HAND

As noted earlier in the text, the physical examination is composed of the systems review, the quarter screen, the clearing examination, and the joint-specific examination. However, the clinician must first be alert to any potential red flags, such as a fracture or tendon rupture. A fracture should be considered

TABLE 16-6
COMMON OUTCOME TOOLS FOR PATIENTS WITH WRIST/HAND PATHOLOGIES

Tool	Tool Basics
Patient-Rated Wrist and Hand Evaluation	• Designed for use with wrist and hand pathologies • Two subscales pain (5 items) and function (10 items) rated on a 0-10 scale with lower scores indicating greater function • Total scores range 0-100 • MCID: 11-14 points
Functional Index for Hand Osteoarthritis	• Specific to hand osteoarthritis • 10 items rated on a 0-4 scale with lower scores indicating greater function • Validated but limited information on MDC
Australian Canadian Osteoarthritis Hand Index	• Designed for hand osteoarthritis but also used for other hand conditions • 15 items related to pain, stiffness, and function rated 0-4 with lower scores indicating fewer symptoms and greater function • MCID: 2.0
Boston Carpal Tunnel Syndrome Questionnaire	• Specific to carpal tunnel syndrome • Two subcomponents: severity of symptoms (11 items) and functional abilities (8 items) rated on a 0-5 scale with lower scores indicating fewer symptoms and greater function • MCID: 0.75

MCID, minimal clinically important difference; *MDC*, minimal detectable change.

a differential diagnosis if the patient had an acute trauma, such as landing on an outstretched hand. The potential for a fracture after a fall is particularly important to consider for older patients, those with a history of (or likelihood for) osteoporosis/osteopenia, and those under the influence of a substance affecting balance, such as alcohol or sleep medications. In these cases, the clinician should immediately assess for fracture.

In addition to information gained from the patient history, fracture should be suspected if there is visible acute deformity, ecchymosis, protective spasm, and report of a deep constant ache.[54] Because scaphoid fractures are common,[55] its presence should be suspected in a patient with a traumatic onset of radial-sided wrist or thumb pain. The clinician should assess the following key areas in an attempt to determine whether imaging is warranted[54–57]:

- Tenderness in the snuffbox
- Pain with the scaphoid compression test (Fig. 16-35)[58]
- Tenderness of the scaphoid tubercle

If these tests are positive, the examination should be halted, and the patient should be referred for radiographs.[59] If the patient also has pain with active thumb ROM, the specificity for fracture is improved.[55] Unfortunately, negative initial imaging does not rule out the possibility of scaphoid fracture.[60] Patients may benefit from immobilization with reassessment after 2 weeks. If minimal or no improvement is noted after 2 weeks, the patient should be referred for repeat radiographs.

Clinical suspicion for non–scaphoid carpal and radial fractures should be raised in cases of isolated bony tenderness.[61] For children with pain in the region of the wrist and a history of trauma, radiographs should be requested if there is bony tenderness to the distal radius or anatomical snuffbox and more than a 20% decrease in grip strength compared to the contralateral side.[62]

Acute tendon rupture may be the result of a laceration, a sudden increase in tendon tension, or trauma, such as when the distal phalanx is hit by an object. The most common tendon injuries that rehabilitation professionals must be able to quickly identify are jersey finger and mallet finger. Jersey finger is a rupture of the FDP, so named because of the occurrence in sports when a player grips the shirt of an opposing player who is trying to get away. A patient with jersey finger presents with an acute inability to flex the DIP joint. In order to regain function, early surgical management is required. Mallet finger is the acute rupture of the terminal tendon and results in the inability to extend the DIP joint. Mallet finger can occur with or without an avulsion fracture (Fig. 16-36). The DIP joint will remain in a flexed position owing to the unopposed

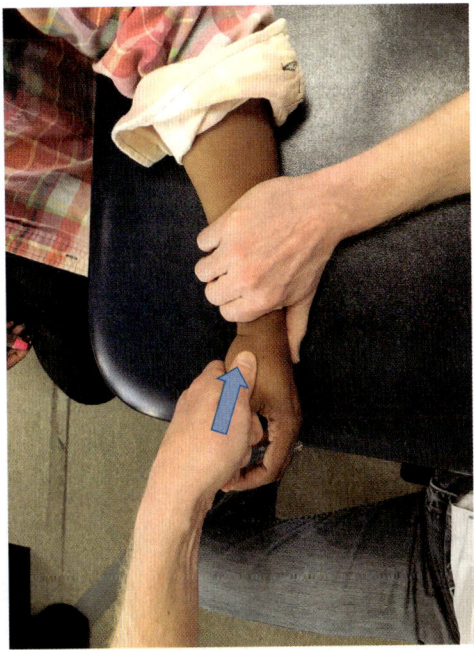

FIGURE 16-35 Scaphoid compression test. While supporting the patient's forearm, the clinician applies an axial load to the scaphoid through 1st metacarpal.

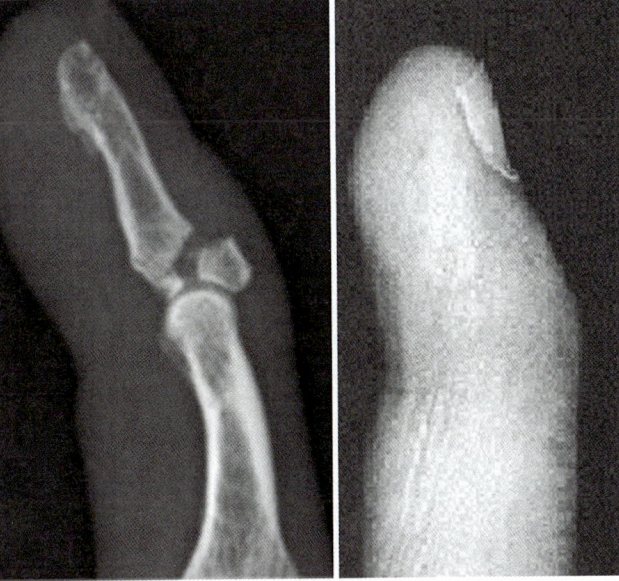

FIGURE 16-36 Lateral radiograph of a patient with an avulsion fracture and mallet finger. (Yoon JO, Baek H, Kim JK. The outcomes of extension block pinning and nonsurgical management for mallet fracture. *J Hand Surg Am.* 2017;42:387.e1–387.e7; Kalainov DM, Hoepfner PE, Hartigan BJ, Carroll C, Genuario J. Nonsurgical treatment of closed mallet finger fractures. *J Hand Surg Am.* 2005;30:580–586.)

action of the FDP. Mallet finger requires prolonged immobilization of the DIP in an extended position to prevent a DIP flexion contracture (a so-called *mallet finger deformity*).

Once the patient has been cleared of any red flags and the history and systems review have been performed, the clinician should perform an upper quarter screen. Next, the clinician should perform a clearing examination (in this case, elbow flexion/extension and forearm pronation supination) before moving to the joint-specific wrist and hand examination.

Structure and Posture

Observe the general appearance of the patient's arm and hand including the patient's overall posture and use of the arm, bony alignment, soft tissue, and skin and nails. Having the patient place both hands on the treatment table allows for easy side-to-side comparisons.

Limb Posture and Use Observe the patient's resting hand posture. Normally, the fingers are relaxed in slight flexion. Note how the patient uses the hand to complete paperwork or perform fine motor skills, such as removing a pen cap or handling the papers. Do all fingers move in synchrony or is use of one digit avoided? Note the use of the arms during transitional movements, such pushing through the upper extremities to rise from a chair.

Bony Structure and Alignment Observe the shape of the digits. In addition to mallet finger previously described, there are numerous structural changes that can occur in the hand (Fig. 16-37). Bony enlargements, such as Heberden nodes or Bouchard nodes affecting the DIP and PIP, respectively, are indicative of degenerative joint disease. A swan-neck deformity (PIP extension with DIP flexion), Boutonniere deformity (PIP flexion with DIP extension), or ulnar drift (MCP joint angulation) may occur with RA. A Colles fracture may lead to characteristic "dinner-fork" deformity.[63]

Peripheral nerve lesions can also lead to hand and wrist abnormalities in structure and alignment, due to full or partial paralysis with subsequent force imbalances among muscle groups. Damage to the radial nerve can lead to wrist drop. Damage to the ulnar nerve affecting the interossei muscles can lead to clawing of the fourth and fifth digits (Fig. 16-38).

Soft Tissue Observe for edema and muscle atrophy. Finger and dorsal hand edema are common with acute injuries or after immobilization of the upper extremity. However, redness along with swelling is suggestive

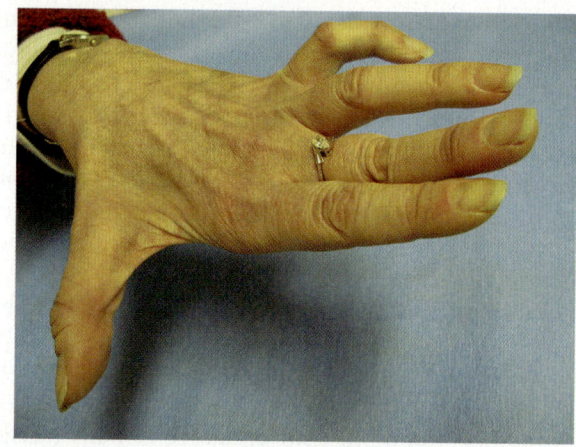

FIGURE 16-38 Ulnar nerve paralysis leading to clawing of digits 4 and 5. Note the muscle atrophy in the interossei. (Maschke SD, Graham TJ, Evans PJ. *Master Techniques in Orthopaedic Surgery: The Hand.* 3rd ed. Wolters Kluwer; 2016: Figure 17-9.)

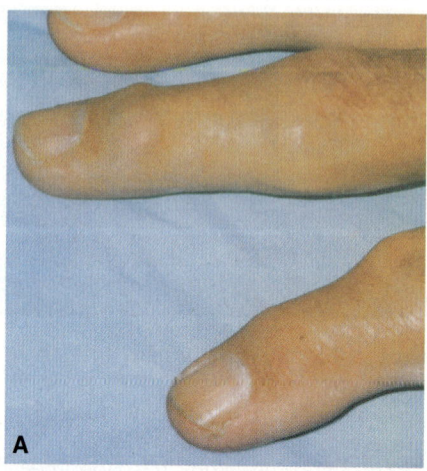
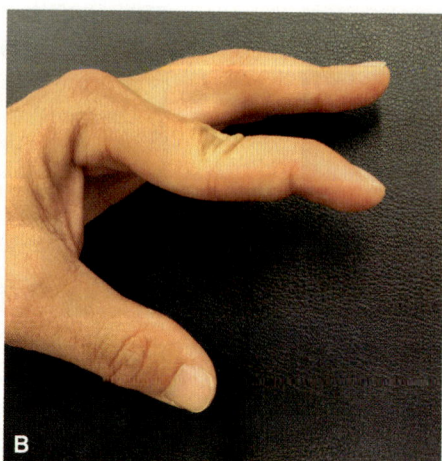
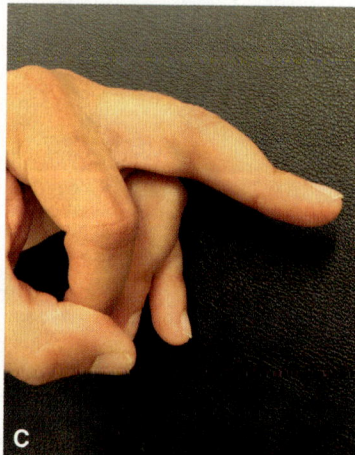

FIGURE 16-37 Structural changes of the hand. **A.** Heberden nodes. (From Berg D. *Atlas of Adult Physical Diagnosis.* Wolters Kluwer; 2005. ISBN: 9780781741903, published 9/5/2005.) **B.** Swan-neck deformity of the index finger. **C.** Boutonniere deformity of the third finger.

of cellulitis or infection.[64] Volumetric or circumferential measurements can be used to track changes over time.[63,65] A ganglion cyst, a fluid-filled cyst primarily found on the dorsal wrist, is usually asymptomatic.[64] Local swelling can occur with tenosynovitis or joint effusion. Atrophy may be seen with peripheral nerve lesions. For example, prolonged compression of the median nerve at the carpal tunnel can lead to atrophy of the muscles of the thenar eminence.

Skin and Nails

The skin and nails should be observed. Chronic smokers frequently have yellow tinged nails. Clubbing of the nails is a potential indicator of pulmonary pathology.[66] Color changes in the skin may indicate vasomotor changes, such as those occurring with CRPS.[66] Scarring can limit joint motion. A palmar nodular-like thickening proximal to the A1 pulley suggests trigger finger that can lead to snapping or locking of the digit.[47] Dupuytren contracture, discussed later in this chapter, is a thickening and shortening of the palmar fascia that can cause an MCP flexion deformity.[67]

Range of Motion

Active and passive movement should be performed to assess the quantity and quality of movement and compared to normative values (Table 16-7).[68,69] At times, it may be useful to utilize composite motion

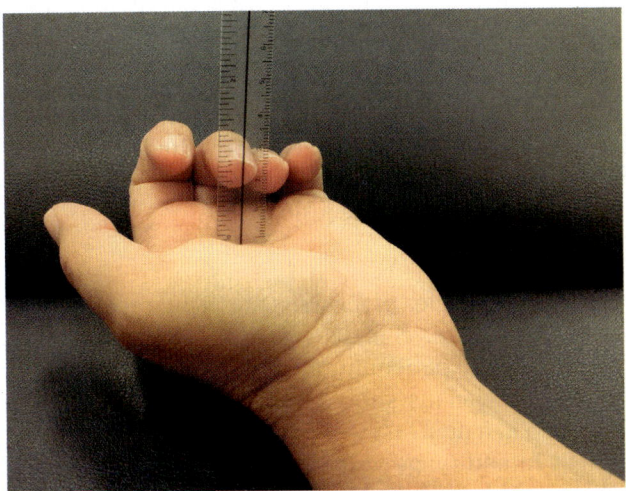

FIGURE 16-39 Composite finger flexion.

measurements. Composite finger flexion provides a quick look at functional digit flexion and is particularly useful if multiple digits are limited by measuring the distance from the fingertip to a fixed point in the palm (Fig. 16-39). However, it is less reliable than goniometric measurements.[70] Opposition, a combination of CMC, MCP, and IP joint motion, should allow the thumb to touch the base of the fifth digit. Any deficit in motion can be measured as the distance between the tip of the thumb and the base of the fifth digit.

A normal endfeel of a healthy wrist should be firm ligamentous or capsular endfeel. A springy endfeel may indicate soft-tissue obstruction or carpal malalignment, whereas a hard endfeel may indicate severe OA.[63] For the fingers, a normal endfeel should be a firm ligamentous or capsular endfeel. However, soft-tissue approximation may also occur with finger PIP flexion and 1st CMC flexion. Capsular patterns of restriction for the wrist and hand are listed in Table 16-8.[71–74]

Strains and sprains of the wrist are quite common and can frequently be identified based on the tissue's response to active and passive motion. If there is a noncontractile lesion, active and passive motion in the same direction is likely to be painful or restricted, as both will put tension on the injured tissue. In contrast, if there is a contractile lesion, active muscle

TABLE 16-7
PASSIVE RANGE OF MOTION NORMATIVE VALUES

Joint	Motion	Normative Value (Degrees)
Wrist	Flexion	0–80
	Extension	0–70
	Radial deviation	0–20
	Ulnar deviation	0–30
Finger MCP	Flexion	0–90
	Extension	0–45
PIP	Flexion	0–100
	Extension	0
DIP	Flexion	0–90
	Extension	0
Thumb CMC	Flexion	0–15
	Extension	0–20
	Palmar abduction	0–70
	Palmar adduction	0
Thumb MCP	Flexion	0–50
	Extension	0
Thumb IP	Flexion	0–80
	Extension	0–30

CMC, carpometacarpal; *DIP*, distal interphalangeal; *IP*, interphalangeal; *MCP*, metacarpophalangeal; *PIP*, proximal interphalangeal.

TABLE 16-8
CAPSULAR PATTERN FOR THE WRIST AND HAND

Joint	Motion Restriction
Wrist	Limitation: flexion = extension
Midcarpal	Limitation: equal all directions
Trapeziometacarpal	Limitation of abduction > extension
Carpometacarpals 2–5	Limitation of flexion > extension
Upper extremity digits	Limitation of flexion > extension

contraction is likely to be painful and may be weak. There may also be pain with active and passive lengthening of the tissue. With a minor contractile lesion, resistance may need to be applied to create sufficient stress on the injured tissue. Refer to Chapter 2, Tissue Behavior, Healing, and Repair, for additional information regarding soft-tissue lesions.

Muscle Length

Most of the muscles of the wrist and hand cross several joints. Therefore, clinicians should be precise when positioning the patient for measuring joint motion. For example, clinicians should be sure to measure finger IP flexion in a neutral wrist position, as positioning the patient in end-range wrist flexion would lengthen the EDC over the wrist, potentially limiting digit flexion.

Muscle Performance

After performing the upper quarter screen, specific muscle performance testing of the wrist and hand should be performed. Strength of individual muscles and muscle groups may be assessed using manual muscle testing (MMT).[75] Grip strength should be assessed using a handheld dynamometer (see Fig. 15-20), and any pain with testing should be noted. It may be useful to obtain both maximal grip and maximal pain-free grip strength. Grip strength should vary based on grip width, with maximal grip generally at midrange. Changing grip width on the dynamometer allows the clinician to bias more toward a particular muscle group. For example, FDP has increased contribution to grip strength when using wider grips. Patients whose grip strength fails to vary with changes in grip width may benefit from a more detailed assessment of psychosocial factors. Grip strength can be compared bilaterally as well as with normative values based on age and gender.

Pinch assessment using a pinch gauge (Fig. 16-40) can also provide objective measures of strength that can be compared bilaterally and with normative values.[76] A three-point pinch, sometimes referred to as a *three-jaw chuck or palmar pinch*, is assessed by placing the palmar surfaces of the second and third digits on one side of the pinch gauge and the pad of the thumb on the other. A two-point pinch, sometimes called *tip-to-tip pinch*, is assessed using the tips of the thumb and index finger. A lateral pinch, sometimes referred to as *key pinch*, is assessed by squeezing the pinch gauge between the thumb pad and the radial aspect of the index finger.

Sensory Tests

The clinician must have a working knowledge of the sensory distribution of upper extremity peripheral nerves (refer to Fig. 13-3 in Chapter 13, Upper Quarter Screen) as peripheral nerve injuries, such as carpal or ulnar tunnel syndrome, are common. Light-touch sensation can be screened using a paper clip.[63] However, more specific assessment should be performed if the clinician suspects a peripheral nerve injury. Patients with intact light-touch sensation should be able to detect the 3.22 Semmes Weinstein monofilaments in the hand (~68 mg of force).[65,76] Static two-point discrimination can be assessed using 4 to 5 mm as the threshold for normal sensation (Fig. 16-41).[76]

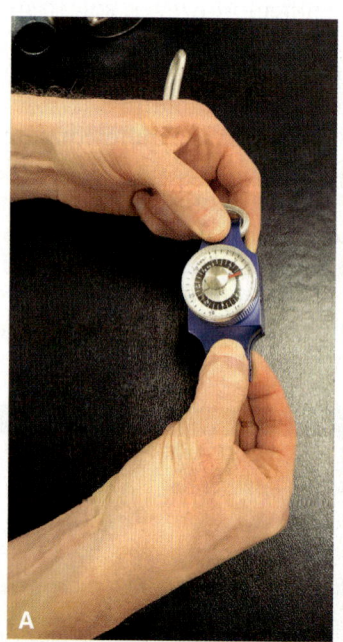
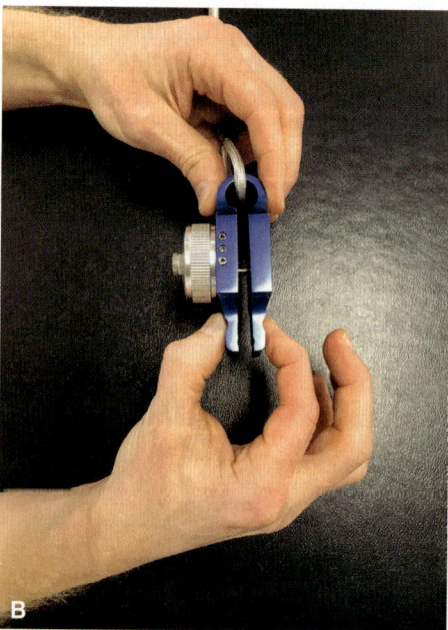
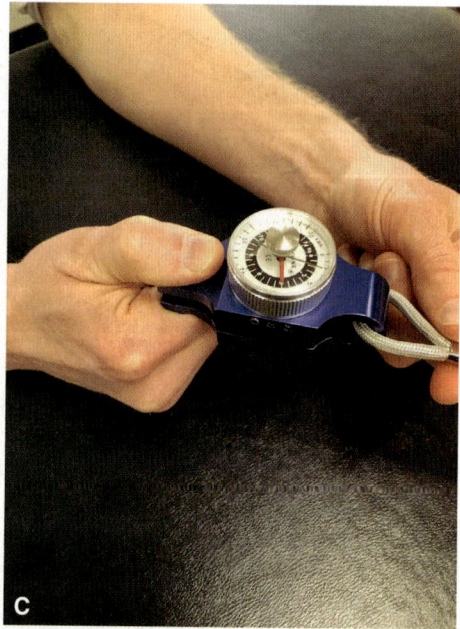

FIGURE 16-40 Pinch testing. **A.** Three-point pinch. **B.** Two-point pinch. **C.** Lateral pinch.

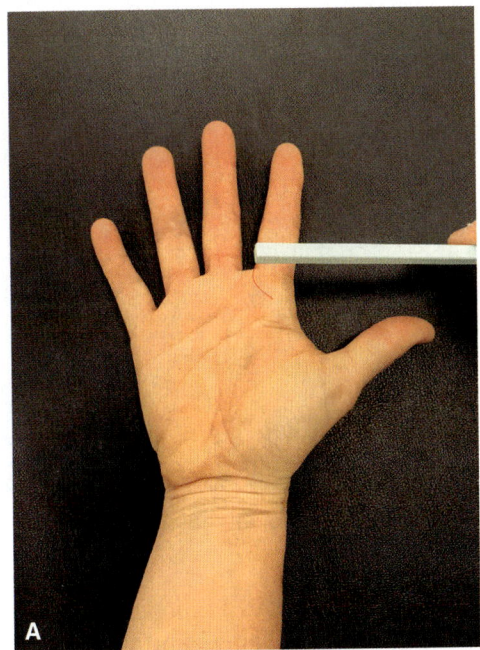
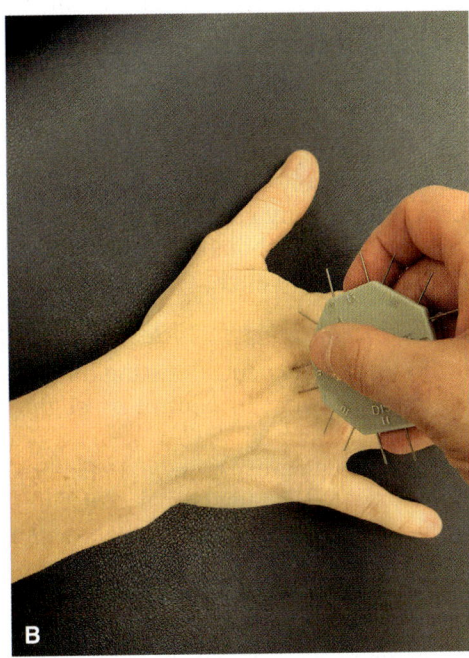

FIGURE 16-41 Sensory testing of the hand. **A.** Semmes Weinstein monofilament. **B.** Two-point discrimination tool.

Reflexes

If a patient reports paresthesias or if nerve involvement is suspected, the clinician should assess upper extremity reflexes, biceps, brachioradialis, triceps, and the Hoffman test, to assess for possible upper or lower motor neuron involvement. Refer to Chapter 13, Upper Quarter Screen, for more information on upper extremity reflex testing.

Vascular Testing

Clinicians should assess the radial and ulnar pulses if vascular pathology is suspected. The assessment should be made using the tips of the index and middle fingers over the respective arteries on the radial or ulnar side of the volar wrist surface.

Neurodynamic Testing

Neurodynamic testing, such as the upper limb tension tests, may be required for patients reporting paresthesias in the hand as part of the upper quarter screen. Although these tests are less accurate than the lower extremity equivalent, the straight leg raise, they can still provide clinical insight into nerve involvement.[77,78] Chapter 17, Cervical and Thoracic Spine, provides details on how to perform and interpret these tests.

Accessory Motion

Joints should be assessed for hypomobility and hypermobility, as well as the presence or absence of pain with accessory motion testing. In the wrist and hand, this can be quite complex, given the numerous joints involved. Joint hypomobility is common after immobilization, fracture, and with acute or chronic swelling. In contrast, isolated joint hypermobility frequently occurs after trauma, such as a wrist sprain, and with RA. Degenerative arthritis of the digits generally leads to hypomobility; however, at 1st CMC joint, hypermobility is more common. Clinicians may need to assess the mobility of the following joint complexes: DRUJ, radiocarpal joint, midcarpal joint, MCP joint, and IP joint. Chapter 15, Elbow Complex, contains details on assessing and treating the radioulnar joints.

Table 16-9 contains specific accessory motions (joint mobility) in the wrist and forearm to be assessed. When performing radiocarpal glides, the clinician

TABLE 16-9
FOREARM AND WRIST ACCESSORY MOTION ASSESSMENT

Joint	Mobilization	Motion Facilitated
Proximal radioulnar joint	Dorsal glide	Pronation
	Ventral glide	Supination
Distal radioulnar joint	Dorsal glide	Supination
	Ventral glide	Pronation
Radiocarpal joint	Dorsal glide	Flexion
	Palmar glide	Extension
	Ulnar glide	Radial deviation
	Radial glide	Ulnar deviation
Midcarpal joint	Dorsal glide	Flexion
	Palmar glide	Extension
	Ulnar glide	Radial deviation
	Radial glide	Ulnar deviation

must consider the palmar tilt of the distal radius (see Fig. 16-2). Therefore, the glide is not purely palmar, but on a slight angle. In addition, in patients with distal radius fractures, it is common that the dorsal distal radius is compressed, decreasing this palmar tilt. Therefore, clinicians must rely closely on the endfeel during assessments. If obtaining a bony endfeel, rather than a capsular endfeel, the clinician should repeat the mobilization using a slightly altered angle.

Palmar Radiocarpal and Midcarpal Glides

Patient: Seated with forearm in neutral resting on the treatment table and the wrist in neutral or slight ulnar deviation.

Clinician: The stabilizing hand grasps the patient's distal forearm just proximal to the radiocarpal joint. The mobilizing hand contacts the proximal carpals with the first web space and supports the patient's hand by wrapping the fingers around toward the palm.

Mobilization: The clinician applies a palmar glide with the mobilizing hand (Fig. 16-42).

Modifications: When used as a treatment technique to improve accessory motion, the wrist can be placed in varying degrees of wrist extension. To direct the mobilization to the midcarpal joint, the stabilizing hand encircles the proximal row of carpals, whereas the mobilizing hand contacts the distal carpal row.

Dorsal Radiocarpal and Midcarpal Glides

Patient: Seated with forearm supinated resting on the treatment table and the wrist in neutral or slight ulnar deviation.

Clinician: The stabilizing hand grasps the patient's distal forearm just proximal to the radiocarpal joint. The mobilizing hand contacts the proximal carpals with the first web space and supports the patient's hand by wrapping the fingers around toward the palm.

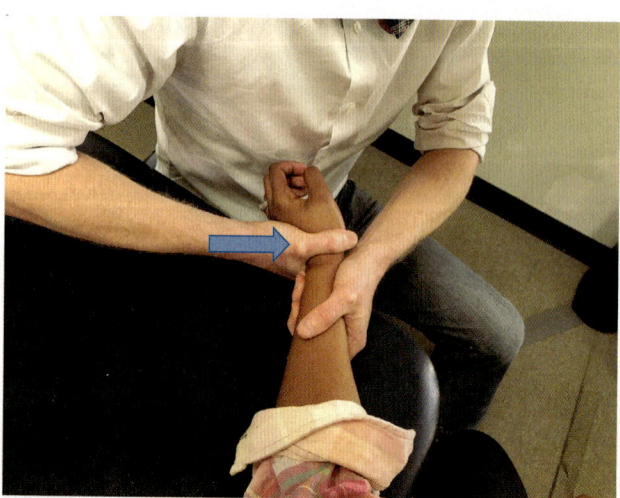

FIGURE 16-42 Palmar radiocarpal glide.

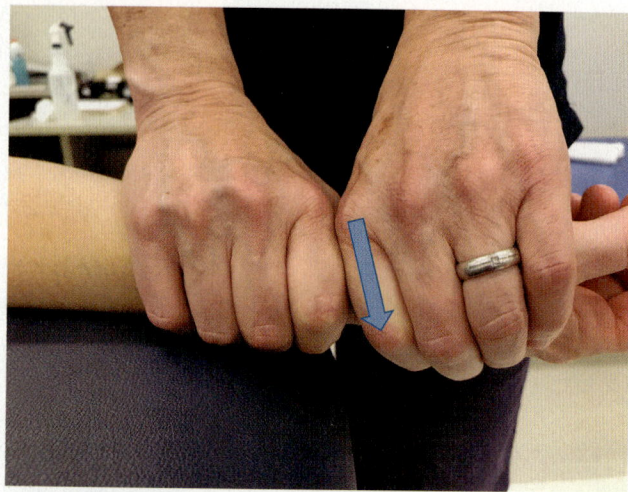

FIGURE 16-43 Dorsal radiocarpal glide.

Mobilization: The clinician applies a palmar glide with the mobilizing hand (Fig. 16-43).

Modifications: The forearm can be neutral, as in Figure 16-43. When used as a treatment technique to improve accessory motion, the wrist can be placed in varying degrees of wrist flexion. To direct the mobilization to the midcarpal joint, the stabilizing hand encircles the proximal row of carpals, whereas the mobilizing hand contacts the distal carpal row.

Radiocarpal and Midcarpal Distraction Radiocarpal or midcarpal distraction can be performed in numerous ways. Most simply, the clinician can use the same hand holds and positioning as used in the dorsal radiocarpal and midcarpal glides but simply apply a distracting force perpendicular to the joint surface with the mobilizing hand.

Ulnar Radiocarpal and Midcarpal Glides

Patient: Seated with forearm in neutral resting on the treatment table and the wrist in neutral or slight ulnar deviation.

Clinician: The stabilizing hand grasps the patient's distal forearm just proximal to the radiocarpal joint. The mobilizing hand contacts the proximal carpals with the first web space and supports the patient's hand by wrapping the fingers around the hand.

Mobilization: The clinician applies an ulnar glide with the mobilizing hand (Fig. 16-44).

Modifications: When used as a treatment technique to improve accessory motion, the wrist can be placed in varying degrees of wrist flexion. To direct the mobilization to the midcarpal joint, the stabilizing hand encircles the proximal row of carpals, whereas the mobilizing hand contacts the distal carpal row.

Radial Radiocarpal and Midcarpal Glides Nearly identical positioning can be used to perform a radial

CHAPTER 16 | WRIST AND HAND COMPLEX

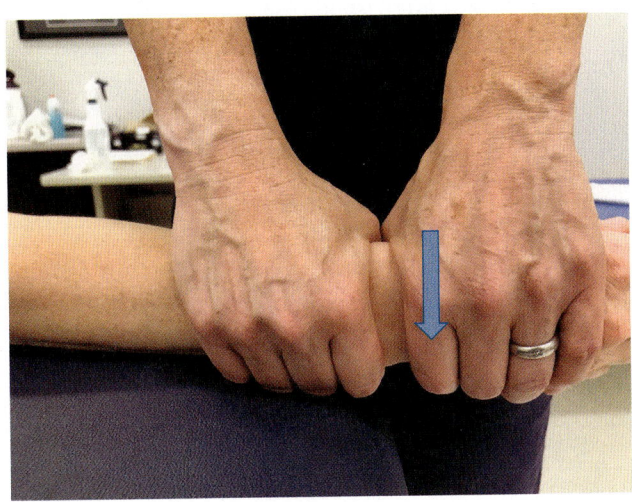

FIGURE 16-44 Ulnar radiocarpal glide.

TABLE 16-10
HAND ACCESSORY MOTION ASSESSMENT

Joint	Mobilization	Motion Facilitated
Metacarpophalangeal joint	Dorsal glide	Extension
	Palmar glide	Flexion
	Radial glide	Abduction of digits 2-3 Adduction digits 4-5
	Ulnar glide	Adduction of digit 2 Abduction of digits 3-5
	Distraction	Global joint play
Intermetacarpal joints	Dorsal glide	Hand opening
	Palmar glide	Opposition
Interphalangeal joints	Dorsal glide	Extension
	Palmar glide	Flexion
	Distraction	Global joint play
Thumb carpometacarpal	Dorsal glide	Abduction
	Palmar glide	Adduction
	Radial glide	Extension
	Ulnar glide	Flexion
	Distraction	Global joint play

glide, but with the index finger of the mobilizing hand wrapping around the patient's wrist to contact the ulnar border of the radiocarpal or midcarpal joints. Alternatively, the patient can be positioned with the forearm pronated so that the thumb is pointing down. This position is generally used for the treatment of limited ulnar deviation as it provides the clinician with improved leverage.

Isolated Carpal Glides Isolated intercarpal joint mobility testing (Fig. 16-45) should be performed if an intercarpal ligament sprain is suspected. Kaltenborn[79] created a system of sequentially assessing individual carpal mobility:

- Stabilize capitate and glide trapezoid, scaphoid, and lunate.
- Stabilize lunar and hamate and glide capitate.
- Stabilize scaphoid and glide the trapezoid and trapezium together.
- Stabilize the radius and glide the scaphoid and lunate.
- Stabilize the ulna and glide the triquetrum.
- Stabilize the triquetrum and glide the hamate and pisiform.

Table 16-10 contains specific hand accessory motions to be assessed.

Intermetacarpal Joint Mobilization

Patient: Hand resting comfortably on the table forearm in pronation.
Clinician: The stabilizing hand stabilizes a metacarpal between the thumb and the index finger. The mobilizing hand grasps the adjacent metacarpal between the thumb and the index finger and applies a dorsal or palmar force (Fig. 16-46).

Metacarpophalangeal Joint Mobilization

Patient: Hand resting comfortably on the table with the joint to be assessed in the loose-packed position.
Clinician: The stabilizing hand supports the patient's hand and stabilizes the proximal bone by grasping dorsally and palmarly with the thumb and index finger. The mobilizing hand grasps the distal bone between the thumb and the index finger and applies a dorsal, palmar, or distracting force (Fig. 16-47). To perform radial and ulnar glides, the clinician's mobilizing hand is shifted to contact the radial and ulnar surfaces of the patient's phalange.

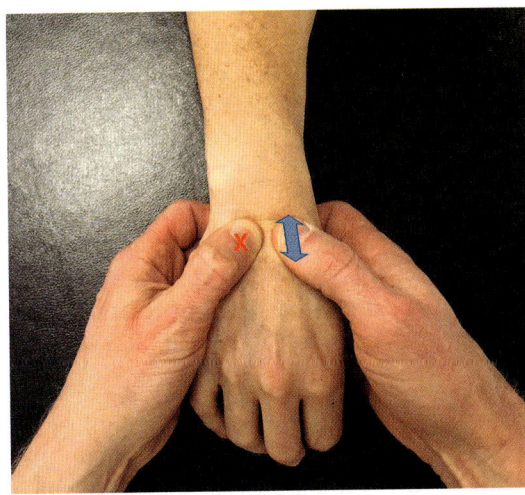

FIGURE 16-45 Dorsal and palmar intercarpal glides.

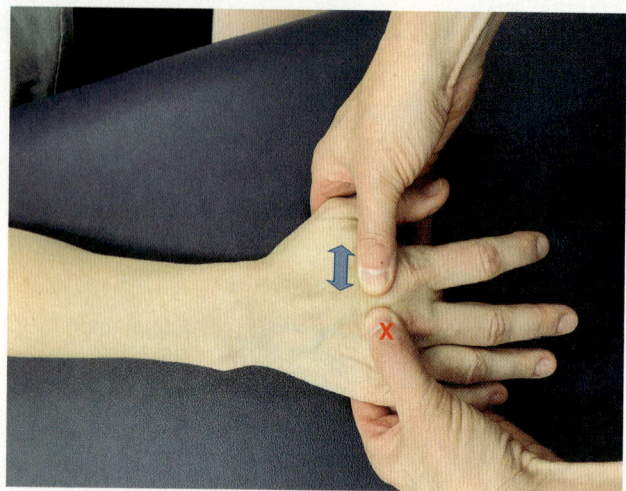

FIGURE 16-46 Dorsal and palmar intermetacarpal glides.

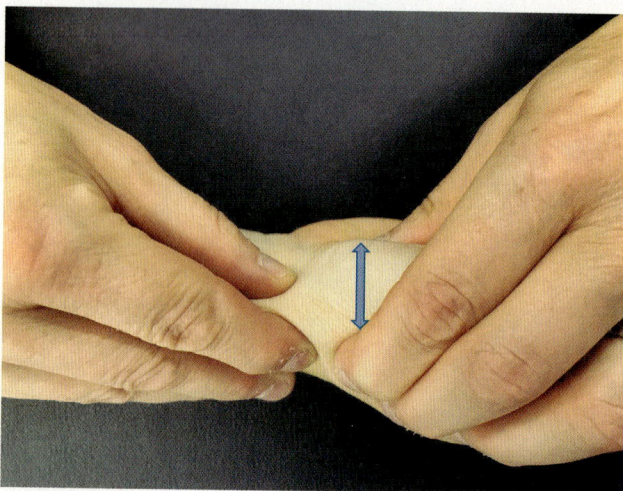

FIGURE 16-48 Dorsal and palmar thumb carpometacarpal glides.

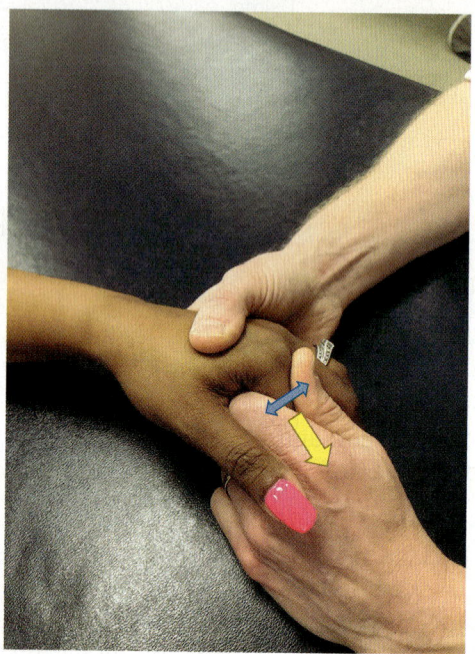

FIGURE 16-47 Metacarpophalangeal joint mobilizations. Dorsal and palmar glides (*blue arrow*) and distraction (*yellow arrow*) of the proximal phalanx on the metacarpal.

Interphalangeal Joint Mobilizations The joint-play movements for the IP joints of the fingers are similar to the MCP; the clinician's hand position simply shifts to the joint to be assessed, stabilizing proximally and mobilizing distally.

Thumb Carpometacarpal Joint Mobilization

Patient: Hand resting comfortably on the table forearm in pronation.
Clinician: The stabilizing hand supports the patient's hand and stabilizes the trapezium dorsally and palmarly with the thumb and index finger. The mobilizing hand grasps 1st metacarpal between the thumb and the index finger and applies a dorsal, palmar, or distracting force. To perform radial and ulnar glides, the clinician's mobilizing hand is shifted to contact the radial and ulnar surfaces of the patient's 1st metacarpal (Fig. 16-48).

Special Tests/Provocative Testing

Clinicians should choose which special/provocative tests to perform based on the patient history and physical examination to this point in order to help rule in and rule out competing differential diagnoses. For wrist and hand pathology, these tests may be grossly grouped into five main categories. Tests are performed to identify OA, instability, tendon pathology, TFCC pathology, and peripheral nerve injury (Fig. 16-49).

Special Tests for Osteoarthritis

Carpometacarpal Grind Test
Purpose: To identify CMC OA.
Method: The clinician grasps the 1st metacarpal, provides an axial load to compress the CMC joint (performing the scaphoid compression test as in Fig. 16-35), then rotates the metacarpal.
Interpretation: The test is positive if there is pain with or without crepitus.[46,80]

Special Tests for Ligament/Instability
The following special tests assist with identifying ligament or wrist instability: scaphoid shift test, the Ballottement test, piano key test, midcarpal shift test, ulnar and radial collateral stress tests, and the digital stress test.

Scaphoid Shift Test (aka the Watson Test)
Purpose: To identify scapholunate instability.[63,80]
Method: With the patient's elbow resting on the table and the wrist in ulnar deviation and slight extension, the clinician places a thumb on the scaphoid

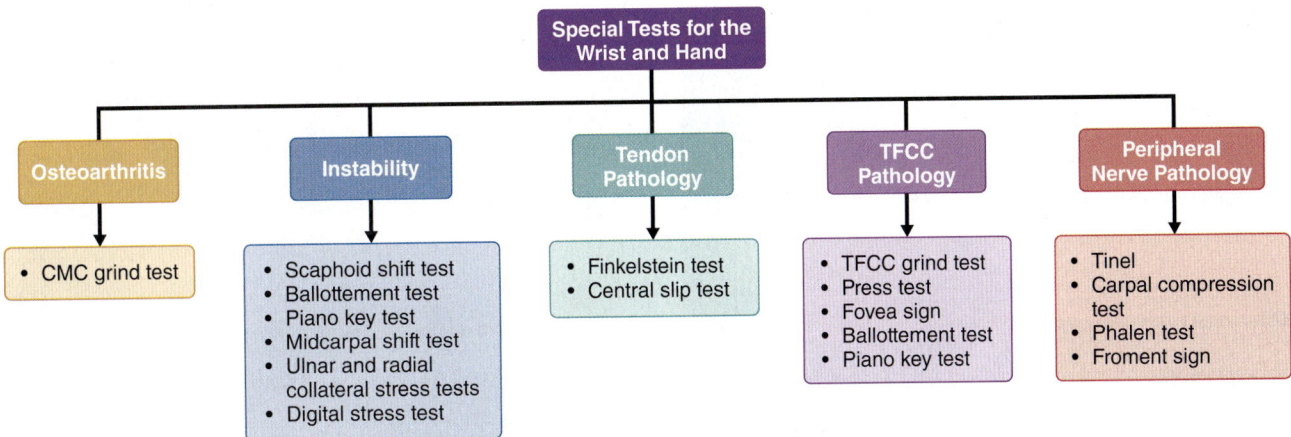

FIGURE 16-49 Special tests for the wrist and hand. *CMC*, carpometacarpal; *TFCC*, triangular fibrocartilage complex.

tubercle, creating dorsal pressure. This pressure is maintained while moving the wrist into radial deviation and slight flexion (Fig. 16-50).

Interpretation: A positive test is when the scaphoid remains extended when the wrist is brought into radial deviation, creating a dorsal subluxation and report of pain. When the clinician releases the pressure, a snapping occurs as the scaphoid self-reduces.

Ballottement Test

Purpose: To test for lunotriquetral instability.[81]

Method: With the patient's forearm pronated and wrist in neutral, the clinician stabilizes the lunate dorsally and palmarly with the radial hand. With the ulnar hand, the clinician contacts the triquetrum with the thumb dorsally and the index finger palmarly. The clinician uses the ulnar hand to glide the pisotriquetral dorsally and palmarly (Fig. 16-51).

Interpretation: A positive test for lunotriquetral instability is pain or laxity with testing.

Piano Key Test

Purpose: To identify a TFCC tear or DRUJ instability.[82]

Method: With the patient's forearm resting on the table in pronation, the clinician stabilizes the radius and wrist with the medial hand by placing the thumb on the dorsal radius and the index finger along the volar aspect of the proximal carpal row. The clinician grasps the ulnar styloid process with the thumb and index finger of the lateral hand and uses the thumb to perform a palmar glide on the distal ulna (Fig. 16-52).

Interpretation: A positive test for a TFCC tear is recreation of the patient's pain. A positive test for radioulnar joint instability is excessive ulnar mobility with the test.

Midcarpal Shift Test

Purpose: To identify midcarpal instability.[81]

Method: With the patient's forearm pronated and radially deviated, the clinician grasps the distal carpal row and then provides a palmar force using the

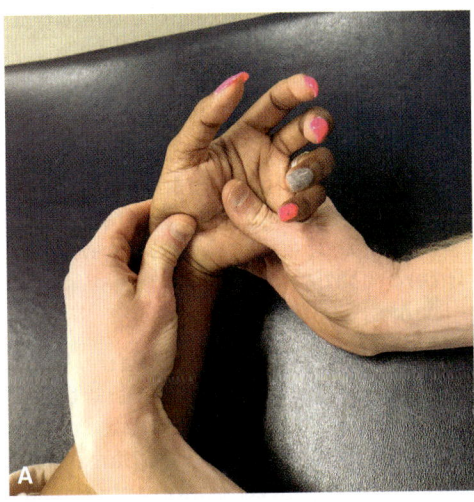
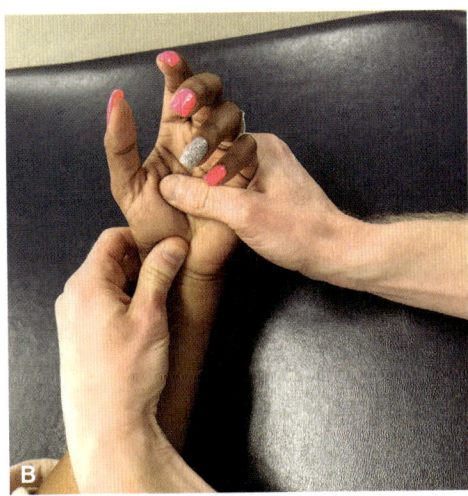

FIGURE 16-50 The scaphoid shift test. **A.** Start position. **B.** End position.

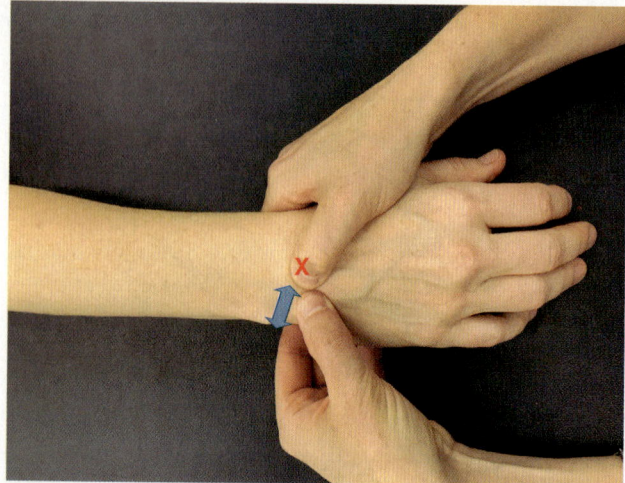

FIGURE 16-51 Ballottement test.

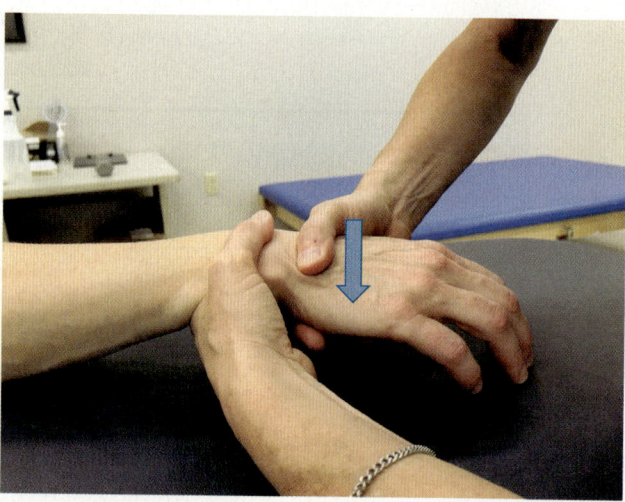

FIGURE 16-53 Midcarpal shift test.

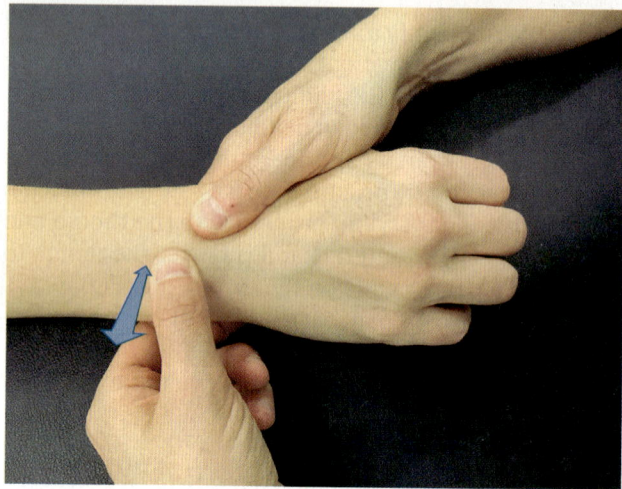

FIGURE 16-52 Piano key test.

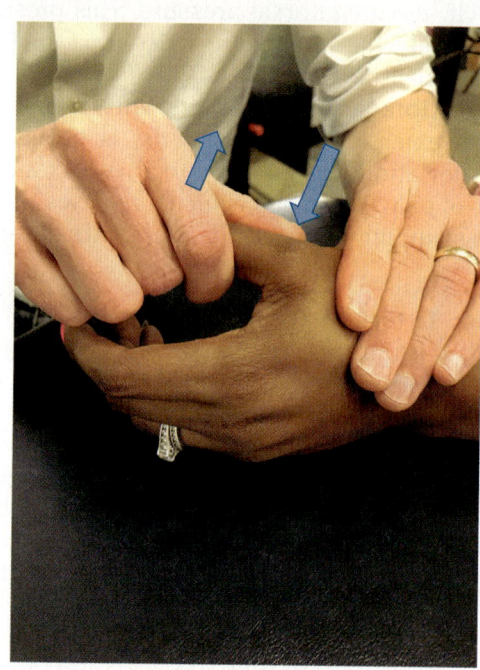

FIGURE 16-54 Ulnar collateral stress test.

thumb. While maintaining this palmar force, the clinician then moves the patient's wrist into ulnar deviation (Fig. 16-53).

Interpretation: A positive test is reproduction of the patient's pain and a clunking sensation as the wrist is moved from radial to ulnar deviation.

Ulnar and Radial Collateral Stress Test

Purpose: To identify injury to the UCL or radial collateral ligament (RCL) of the thumb.[83]

Method: The clinician holds the patient's hand and creates a valgus (UCL) or varus (RCL) stress to the MCP joint of the thumb (Fig. 16-54).

Interpretation: Both tests are graded similarly.
  Grade 1: pain along the involved ligament without laxity
  Grade 2: laxity with a firm endfeel, with or without pain, indicates a partial ligament rupture
  Grade 3: laxity with a soft or empty endfeel implies a complete ligament rupture

Digital Stress Test

Purpose: To identify a collateral ligament injury at the MCP, PIP, or DIP joint.[84]

Method: With the joint in slight flexion, a varus or valgus stress is applied. The tests are performed identically to the thumb collateral stress tests.

Interpretation: A positive test is if the test produces pain or laxity is present.

Special Tests for Tendon Pathology Finkelstein test and the central slip test are used to identify tendon pathology. Recall that the presence of mallet finger or the inability to extend the PIP joint is indicative of a rupture of the terminal tendon, whereas an inability to flex the DIP joint is consistent with a rupture of the FDP.

Finkelstein Test

Purpose: To identify de Quervain tenosynovitis involving the EPB and/or the APL.[46]

Method: The clinician stabilizes the patient's forearm with the wrist in a neutral position, the patient's thumb is flexed into palm and then the patient closes the fingers around the thumb to maintain this position. If no symptoms are present with thumb flexion, the patient's wrist is then passively ulnarly deviated (Fig. 16-55).

Interpretation: A positive test is recreation of the patient's radial wrist pain. It should be noted that this test is normally uncomfortable in unaffected individuals, making it even more important to perform the test on the asymptomatic side first.

Alternate test: Given the pain noted with testing, an alternate test has been proposed.[85] The patient first actively ulnarly deviates the wrist, then the clinician passively moves the wrist to end-range ulnar deviation. Finally, the clinician passively palmarflexes the thumb. The test is stopped as soon as symptoms pare provoked.

Central Slip Test

Purpose: To identify a rupture of the central slip.[33]

Method: Have the patient positioned with the palm down and PIP joint of the finger to be tested at the edge of a table. The clinician applies pressure against the dorsum of the middle phalanx and then asks the patient to extend the finger. The patient should be able to do so while the DIP remains relaxed (Fig. 16-56).

Interpretation: A positive test is if the DIP extends or hyperextends (by way of the lateral bands) in an attempt to extend the finger and the examiner feels little pressure from the middle phalanx.

Special Tests for Triangular Fibrocartilage Complex Pathology There are three special tests to help identify TFCC pathology: the TFCC grind test, the press test, and the fovea sign. The piano key test may also be positive.

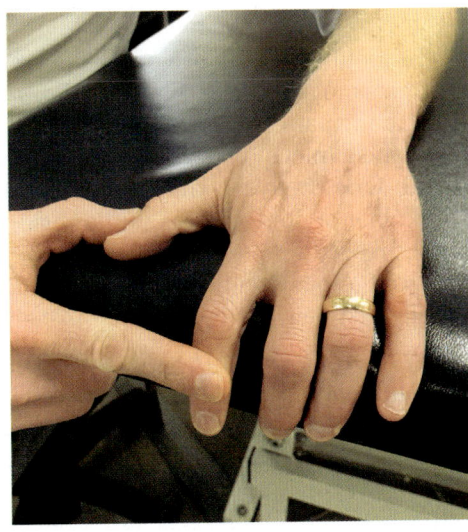

FIGURE 16-56 Central slip test.

Triangular Fibrocartilage Complex Grind Test

Purpose: To identify a TFCC lesion or ulnotriquetral ligament pathology.[86]

Method: With the patient's forearm pronated and wrist in ulnar deviation, the clinician applies an axial load to the wrist while pronating and supinating the patient's forearm (Fig. 16-57).

Interpretation: A positive test is the reproduction of ulnar-sided wrist pain.

Press Test

Purpose: To identify a TFCC lesion.[86–88]

Method: The seated patient places hands on the arm rests of chair or on the support surface and presses down trying to lift the body off the support surface.

Interpretation: A positive test is the reproduction of ulnar-sided wrist pain.

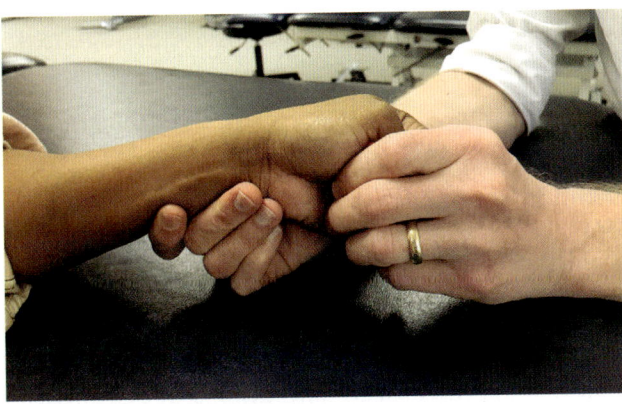

FIGURE 16-55 Finkelstein test.

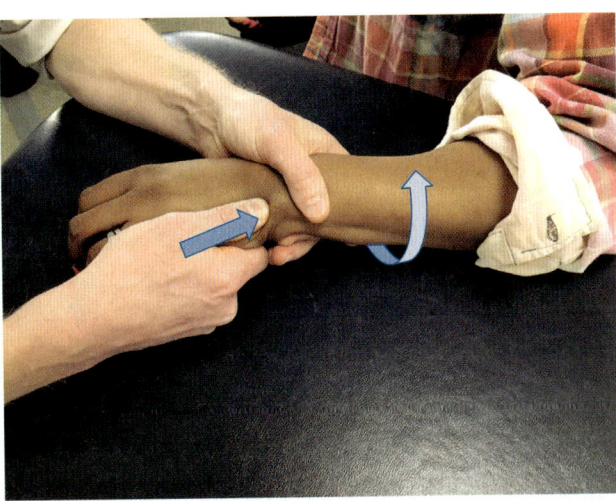

FIGURE 16-57 Triangular fibrocartilage complex grind test.

Fovea Sign

Purpose: To identify a TFCC lesion or ulnotriquetral ligament pathology.[86,89]

Method: With the patient's elbow flexed 90° and wrist in neutral, the clinician presses deeply on the ulnar side of the wrist between the ECU, the FCU, pisiform, and ulnar styloid process in the region of the TFCC (Fig. 16-58).[87]

Interpretation: A positive test is the reproduction of ulnar-sided wrist pain.

Special Tests for Nerve Pathology The Tinel test, as described in Chapter 9, Ankle and Foot, can be used to identify potential nerve irritation or entrapment by tapping over the median nerve at the carpal tunnel or the ulnar nerve at the tunnel of Guyon.[46,80] The carpal compression test and Phalen test attempt to create median nerve symptoms by compressing the median nerve. Froment sign helps identify motor weakness due to ulnar nerve or anterior interosseous nerve pathology. The tear drop sign, presented in Figure 15-39, Chapter 15, Elbow Complex, is when the patient attempts to make a circle by touching the tips of the index finger and thumb as a means of identifying an anterior interosseous nerve lesion.

Carpal Compression Test

Purpose: To identify CTS.[46,80,90]

Method: With the patient in supination and neutral wrist, the clinician compresses the median nerve at the carpal tunnel with both thumbs for up to 30 seconds (Fig. 16-59).

Interpretation: A positive test is pain or paresthesias in the distal distribution of the median nerve.

Phalen Test

Purpose: To identify CTS.[46,76,80]

Method: The patient maintains full wrist flexion for up to 60 seconds. Commonly performed bilaterally simultaneously by having the patient put dorsal wrists together (Fig. 16-60).

Interpretation: A positive test is pain or paresthesias in the distal distribution of the median nerve.

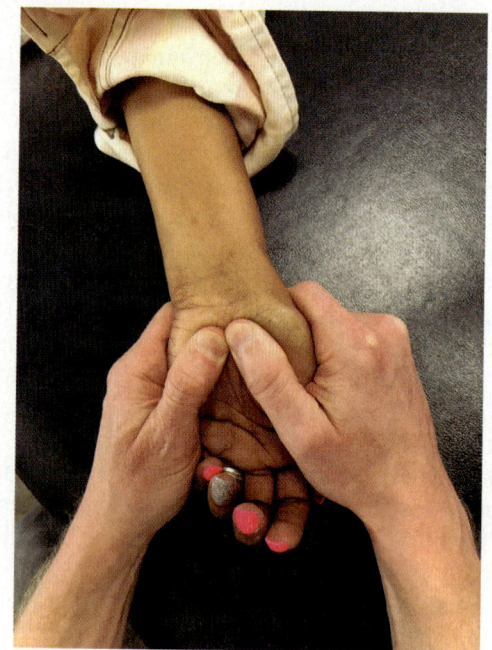

FIGURE 16-59 Carpal compression test.

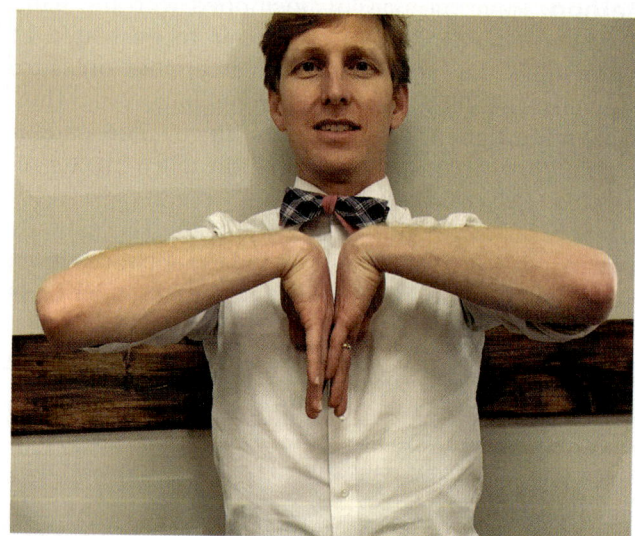

FIGURE 16-60 Phalen test.

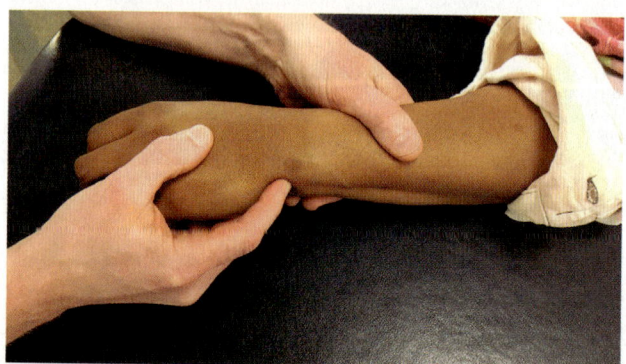

FIGURE 16-58 Fovea sign.

Froment Sign

Purpose: To identify an ulnar nerve lesion.

Method: The patient attempts to hold a lateral/key pinch to prevent the clinician from pulling out a piece of paper between the thumb and the index finger (Fig. 16-61).

Interpretation: A test is positive if the patient flexes the thumb IP joint due to weakness of the ulnar nerve innervated ADDP and deep head of the flexor pollicis brevis (FPB).

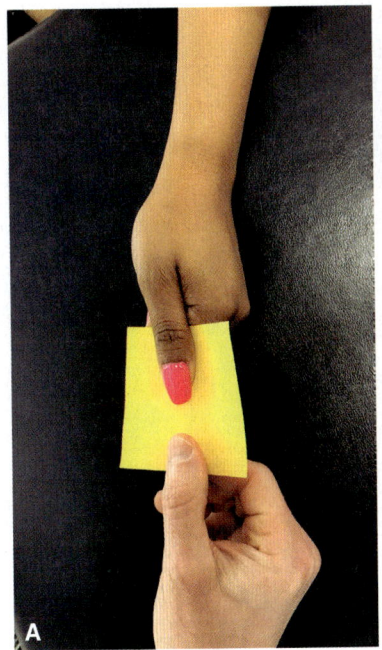 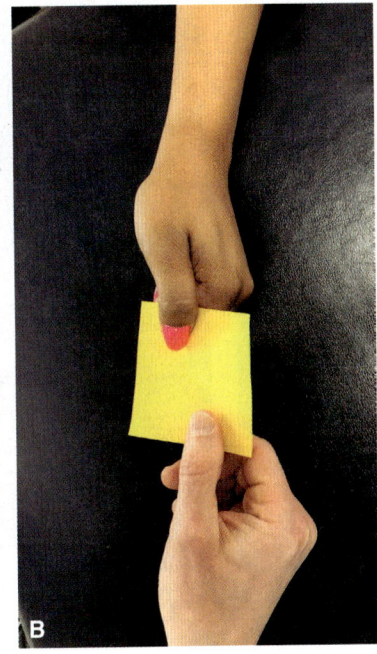

FIGURE 16-61 Froment sign. **A.** Negative test. **B.** Positive test.

Special Considerations with Palpation

Clinicians should palpate structures in the area of symptoms for tenderness, as noted in the section on palpation. The potential to identify factures in the region based on bony tenderness has been already discussed. Because many structures within the wrist and hand are superficial, palpation can be quite useful in identifying additional pathologies as well. For patients without neurologic signs and symptoms, this makes for the rare situations when palpation might be beneficial earlier in the examination, even for patients without potential fracture. Dorsally and radially, clinicians should palpate along the extensor compartments and the extrinsic tendons of the thumb to identify areas of local swelling indicative of tenosynovitis. The palm with its dense fascia rarely swells, but dorsal hand edema is common with hand and upper extremity injuries and may pit to the touch. Palmarly, tenderness along the palmar radiocarpal ligaments would be consistent with a wrist sprain. Tenderness of the ulnar wrist, a positive fovea sign, is suggestive of a TFCC injury or ulnotriquetral ligament pathology.[86,89] Tenderness along the medial or lateral joint lines of the fingers with a history of trauma should make clinicians consider the possibility of a collateral ligament sprain. Thickening of the palmar fascia or the first annular (A1) pulley is an indication of Dupuytren contracture or trigger finger, respectively. Warmth and swelling over the joints may represent an acute flare-up of RA, whereas bony enlargement is more consistent with degenerative joint disease.

Functional Testing

Functional assessment of the hand should include examining how the patient grips, pinches, and performs a variety of specific tasks.

Power Grips A power grip is a forceful act resulting in flexion at all fingers. The thumb, when used, acts as a stabilizer to the object held between the fingers and the palm. This typically involves clamping an object with partially flexed fingers against the palm of the hand, with counterpressure from the adducted thumb. The finger flexors contract isometrically with varying intensity based on the weight, size, and shape of the object. With all power grips, the hand is kept stable and the power movements are produced by either radial or ulnar deviation of the wrist, as in the action of hammering, by supination and pronation of the wrist, and by extension of the elbow. The four phases of a power grip occur in sequence: (1) opening the hand, (2) positioning the fingers, (3) approaching the fingers to the object, and (4) transitioning to a static hold, or grip. The three main types of power grip include cylindrical, spherical, and hook (Fig. 16-62). A hook grip does not involve the thumb and is used functionally for carrying objects, such as a briefcase. The strength of a hook grip is derived primarily from the FDS.

Precision Grip Precision grip (Fig. 16-63) shares the first three steps of the power grip sequence, followed by dynamic movement rather than a static phase. Hence, *precision handling* may be a better term. For precision handling, the object is picked up

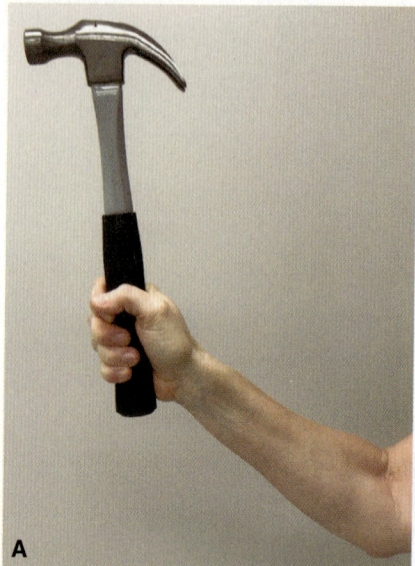
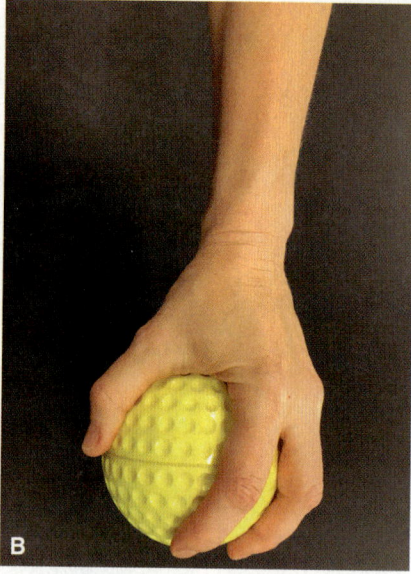
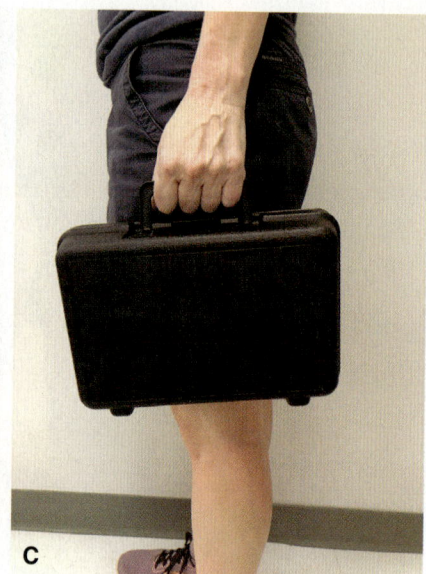

FIGURE 16-62 Power grips. **A.** Cylindrical grip. **B.** Spherical grip. **C.** Hook grip.

and manipulated by the fingers and thumb. The object is not in contact with the palm. Rather, the object is manipulated between the opposing thumb and the fingers—mainly against the next index finger or the index and third finger. The most sensitive surface of the fingers is used to allow delicate adjustments in object manipulation. There are three types of precision grip. Palmar pinch is used when holding a pencil—the pad of the thumb is opposed to the pad of one or more fingers. Lateral pinch or opposition is used when holding a key or a piece of paper—the palmar aspect of the thumb pad presses on the radial surface of the proximal phalanx of the index finger. Tip prehension is used to pick up small objects such as a pin—the tip of the pad is opposed to the tip of the index (or middle) finger. Tip prehension is the finest and most precise grip and is easily upset by any pathology of the hand because it requires a whole range of movements and fine muscle control.

Specific Hand Function The patient should be observed performing a variety of functional tasks involving power grip, precision grip, and various types of object manipulation.

- Picking up a coin
- Turning a key

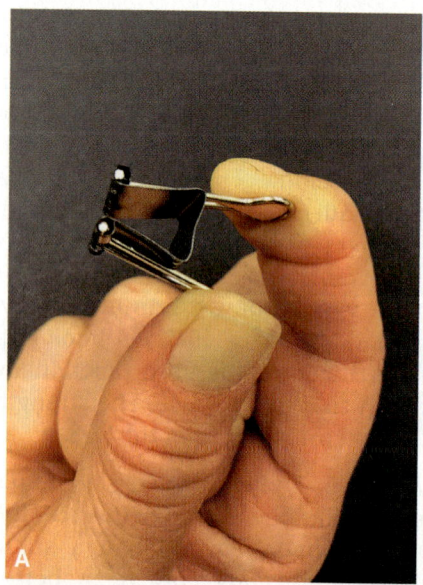
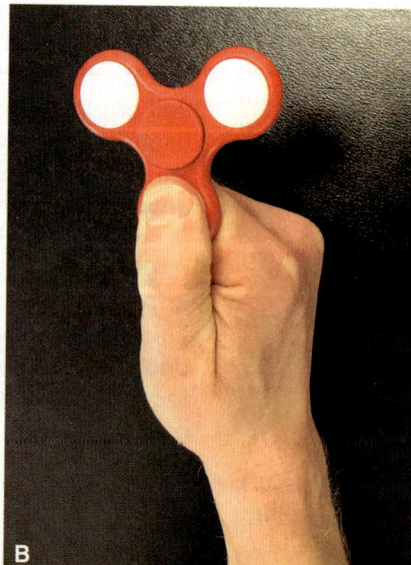
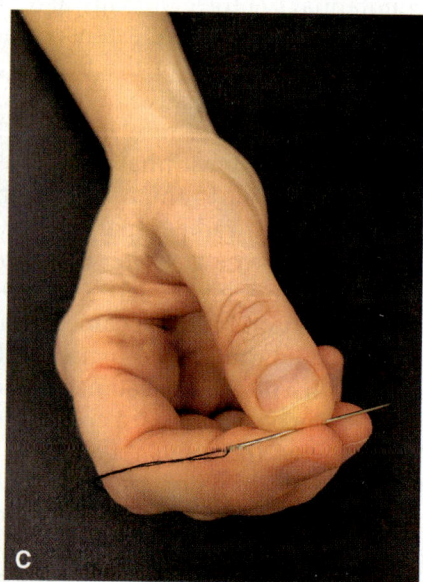

FIGURE 16-63 Precision grip. **A.** Palmar pinch. **B.** Lateral pinch. **C.** Tip prehension.

- Fastening a button
- Tying a shoelace
- Writing
- Keyboarding
- Opening a jar

Patients should also be observed performing the tasks most related to their occupation or activities of daily living that are problematic. There are several standardized hand function tests to provide a systematic and holistic understanding of a patient's abilities (Table 16-11).

COMMON WRIST AND HAND PATHOLOGIES

Common pathologies include ligament sprain and resulting instability, tendon pathology, arthritis, fracture, peripheral nerve injuries, and TFCC pathology. This section begins with pathologies related to the thumb, followed by the digits, palm, and wrist. Lastly, fracture and peripheral nerve injuries are presented.

Ulnar Collateral Ligament Injuries

Pathology UCL dysfunction is the most common cause of ulnar-sided thumb pain. The IP joint of the thumb is very stable; varus and valgus forces are well controlled during functional gripping demands. However, the ulnar side of the MCP joint is vulnerable to instability owing to its location between the stable IP joint and sellar-shaped CMC joint. The ulnar side of the MCP joint is stabilized by the UCL. Damage to the UCL may be the result of acute trauma, repetitive stress, or

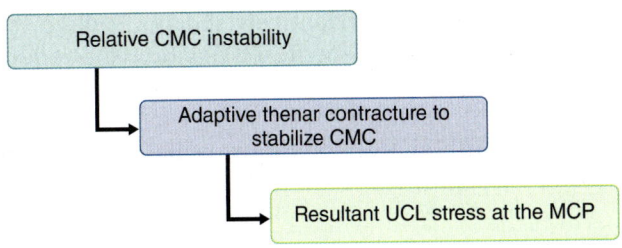

FIGURE 16-64 Cascade causing ulnar collateral ligament (UCL) pathology. *CMC,* carpometacarpal joint; *MCP,* metacarpophalangeal joint.

secondary instability from chronic OA changes. Acute trauma is often associated with falling or with direct valgus force to the distal thumb. Repetitive stresses, such as unusual manipulation of objects during a routine household task or prolonged one-time projects, can overload the UCL. This overuse injury is commonly referred to as "skier's thumb" or "gamekeeper's thumb" because of the repeated valgus stress of using ski poles or a gaming joystick. OA at the CMC can lead to a cascade of changes, ultimately stressing the UCL (Fig. 16-64).

The following are the details of the three-part cascade:

1. OA of the CMC joint reduces joint space, causing capsular and ligamentous laxity such that joint alignment is not maintained. The CMC joint gradually subluxes, and the CMC joint complex demonstrates a zigzag pattern.

TABLE 16-11

STANDARDIZED HAND FUNCTION TESTS

Assessment	Description
Jebsen hand function test	• This test has seven different timed tests performed with each hand: writing, card turning, picking up objects, stacking, using eating utensils, and moving light and heavy objects. • Times can be compared with normative data based on age and gender. • Population: wide range of nonspecific hand conditions including osteoarthritis, rheumatoid arthritis, post-hand surgery, and patients with upper motor neuron lesions.
Minnesota rate of manipulation test	• This test assesses hand eye coordination as well as hand dexterity. • The patient must move wooden or plastic cylinders from one board to another as fast as possible using first one hand, then the other, then using both hands. • Specific tests include placing, turning, and displacing. • The test may be useful for occupations that require rapid gross motor function of the hands and for rating of hand impairment. • Normative data based on age are available.
Hand tool dexterity test	• This timed test assesses hand dexterity for using tools, such as bolts and wrenches. • The test may be appropriate for individuals with factory jobs or for vocational assessment.
Perdue pegboard test	• This test has four components that assess hand dexterity and bimanual skill. • The patient places as many pegs into a series of holes as possible in 30 seconds with one hand, then the other. The test is repeated with both hands simultaneously. Lastly, the patient has 1 minute for both hands to place a pin followed by stacking three objects on the pin. • The test is scored by the number of pins placed in the time allotted. • Normative data were obtained on factory workers.

2. The thenar muscles adaptively shorten, pulling 1st metacarpal into a palmarflexed position and reducing grip width.
3. In order to open the hand wide, for example, to grasp a cup, 1st MCP joint must radially deviate to compensate for lost CMC motion. Thus, with each grip, microstresses are applied to the UCL.

History Patients with UCL injuries will report ulnar-sided MCP pain. Pain and/or difficulty with gripping can be expected. Those with acute trauma or repetitive motion injuries will link these to the root cause of their symptoms. In contrast, individuals with CMC OA will report a more subtle progression of symptoms. When asked, they will note a gradual decrease in gripping ability.

Key Examination Findings Although the intensity of symptom varies, patients with all mechanisms of onset will exhibit UCL tenderness. UCL stress testing will be painful, and the presence of laxity suggests a grade 2 or 3 injury. Patients with CMC OA may also have thumb CMC and MCP deformities or Heberden (DIP) or Bouchard (PIP) nodes. In addition, for patients with thumb CMC OA, the long-standing palmarflexed thumb position often leads to first dorsal interosseous atrophy and weakness.

Differential Diagnosis Patients with a history of trauma who present with first dorsal interosseous swelling should be referred for imaging to rule out fracture.

Rehabilitation Focus and Key Points The plan of care is guided by acuity and sprain grade.[91] Grade 3 UCL injuries should be referred for a surgical consultation. Initially, grade 1 and 2 UCL injuries should be protected via taping or a hand-based CMC orthosis.[92]

Grade 1 and 2 acute traumatic or repetitive stress injuries should be braced for 2 to 6 weeks with gentle active range of motion (AROM) exercises beginning after 3 weeks. Activities that stress the UCL, such as biking, bench press, and some tool use, should be gradual progressed once motion is full and pain free and stress testing is negative.

For patients with CMC OA, rehabilitation must work toward restoring thumb alignment at the CMC and MCP joints, else UCL microtrauma will continue. A hand-based CMC orthosis may be required for longer periods of time, pending the degree of joint dysfunction. Strengthening of the first dorsal interossei is crucial to achieving a safer functional thumb position and thus less need for compensation at the MCP joint.

Expected Outcomes The greater the laxity and instability, the greater the challenge to perform everyday activities without pain. Patients who receive proper education regarding activity modification and are adherent with joint protection strategies will have higher functional gains and outcome scores. Full recovery can be expected in about 3 weeks for grade 1 injuries, whereas grade 2 injuries may take up to 2 months.

Rehabilitation after Ulnar Collateral Ligament Reconstruction Patients with grade 3 UCL sprains are typically managed with UCL reconstruction. Ongoing communication between the clinician and surgeon is needed to understand the surgical procedure and patient-specific precautions for progressive loading of the MCP joint. Often, active thumb ROM is initiated early in the postoperative period before passive range of motion (PROM) to avoid overstressing the reconstruction. Full MCP joint ROM should be expected by about 6 weeks after surgery, at which point gentle strengthening of the thumb and hand can begin. However, the clinician valgus stresses should be avoid for at least 8 weeks and progressed gradually so as not to stress the reconstruction.[93]

Flexor Pollicis Longus Tenosynovitis

Pathology The tendinous sheath of the FPL is often called the *radial bursa* and extends from radial and superficial carpal tunnel before angling around the scaphoid and trapezium to the thumb. This location as well as the two annular pulleys are areas of potential compression and irritation of the tendon and tendon sheath.

History Patients with FPL tenosynovitis complain of palmar thumb pain. This pain is associated with movement, and patients often report the onset was after an activity that required repeated thumb use, such as gripping, rock climbing, or texting.[94] Symptoms can also arise after internal fixation of a distal radius fracture.[95]

Key Examination Findings The classic presentation of FPL tenosynovitis is pain with active motion but pain-free MMT. Active and resisted thumb IP flexion ROM will increase pain along the palmar side of the thumb due to the tendon sliding within the inflamed sheath. Resisted isometrics do not exacerbate symptoms, given the lack of relative motion between the tendon and the tendon sheath. If an annular pulley is involved, a click may be present with active thumb flexion and extension. Local palmar thumb pain may be less related to tendon pathology and more related to pulley pathology.

Differential Diagnosis Differential diagnosis includes a sprain or rupture of the annular pulley. Rock climbing utilizes a number of grips that often require sustained forces for long periods of time. The efficiency of these holds relies on the integrity of the pulley system. Although the FPL is less likely to be involved than the long finger flexors, if bowstringing of the FPL is found on examination, referral to a hand physician is warranted. If bowstring of the FPL is not observed, but concomitant involvement of the annular is suspected, "H" or cruciate taping can help protect from further injury, particularly if the climber is unwilling to undergo short-term activity modification.

Rehabilitation Focus and Key Points Reducing tissue irritability is the first treatment priority. The source of the overuse injury must be identified, and this activity should be modified, if possible. For example, splinting or supportive taping may allow continued activity while protecting the tissue from undue irritation. Nonsteroidal anti-inflammatory medications may be beneficial.[94] Soft-tissue mobilization and myofascial release to the proximal portion of the FPL can be beneficial. However, cross-friction (aka deep friction) massage over the inflamed tendon should be avoided. Likewise, active exercises or exercises that increase tendon excursion are contraindicated for patients with high levels of irritability, particularly if high repetitions are prescribed. Once irritability is reduced to low levels, the clinician can initiate an isometric progression. Isometric thumb exercises can be initiated when pain free, beginning in midrange to minimize tendon compression against the pulleys in flexed position and against phalanx in the extended position. Isometrics are progressed in time and intensity. A good guideline for when a patient is ready to advance to AROM exercise is when the patient is able to perform 10 repetitions of 60-second isometric holds without symptoms.

Expected Outcomes Outcomes are extremely variable owing to difficulty with adherence to recommended activity modifications. Patients with FPL tenosynovitis often check their ability to resume normal activities, thus re-irritating the condition. Thus, patient education regarding FPL tenosynovitis pathology is critical. Those who are adherent should expect to be able to resume modified activity in 10 to 21 days. Patients with high irritability may benefit from a corticosteroid injection.[94]

First Carpometacarpal Joint Osteoarthritis

Pathology First CMC joint OA is common in older adults.[96] The degenerative process causes pain and relative instability. Given the importance of the thumb in most functional activities, thumb CMC OA can be quite disabling. As noted previously, CMC OA is the initial event in the cascade leading to chronic microtrauma of the UCL.

History Patients with CMC OA will report pain in the region of the snuffbox with thumb movement.[96] Pain is usually worse in the morning but improves with movement or with the use of heat (e.g., heating pad or hot water). Activities that increase joint compressive forces, such as forceful gripping, pinching, or radial deviation, will be painful. This may lead patients to avoiding even basic activities of daily living. In the elderly, this can negatively impact nutrition.[97]

Key Examination Findings While a patient may come for treatment specific to the CMC joint, most patients will also have OA of other joints in both hands, including motion loss and bony enlargements (Fig. 16-65). Common impairments specific to CMC OA found on evaluation include:

- Thenar contracture with limited thumb abduction
- Decreased CMC joint ROM
- Weakness of the intrinsic muscles of the hand, which may progress to atrophy of the first dorsal interosseous muscle
- MCP joint ulnar laxity

The CMC grind test is often positive. Accessory motion may be decreased in multiple joints. Grip and pinch strength are decreased and may be painful if irritability is high.

Differential Diagnosis CMC OA is a pathology of chronicity. Scaphoid fracture or instability should be considered in patients reporting a traumatic onset of symptoms.

Rehabilitation Focus and Key Points Rehabilitation addresses patient-specific impairments found in the examination (Fig. 16-66).[92,96,98]

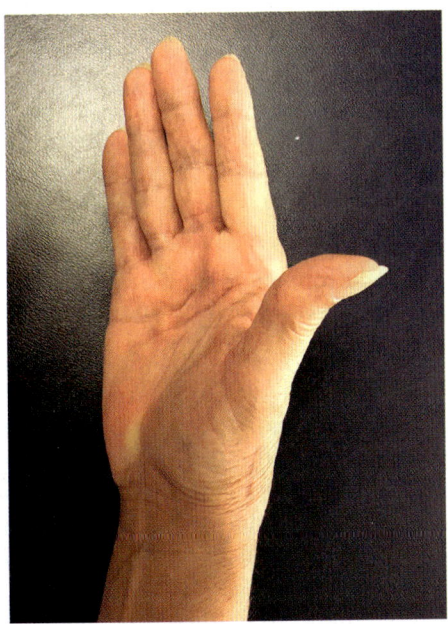

FIGURE 16-65 Patient with carpometacarpal joint osteoarthritis.

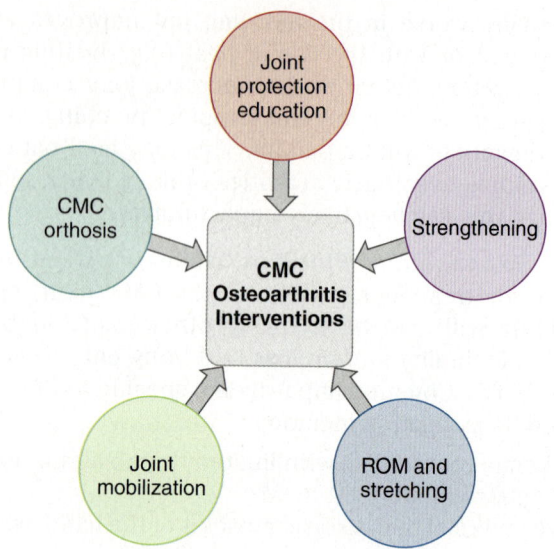

FIGURE 16-66 Carpometacarpal (CMC) joint osteoarthritis interventions. *ROM*, range of motion.

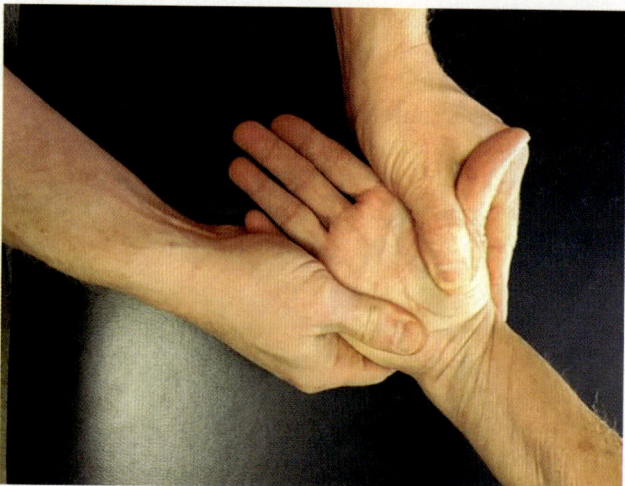

FIGURE 16-68 Manual stretching to improve carpometacarpal joint motion.

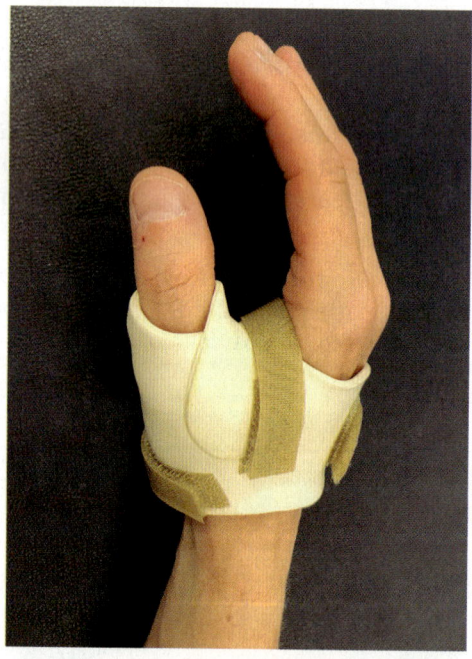

FIGURE 16-67 Custom-made hand-based carpometacarpal orthosis. (Orthosis courtesy of Cindy Poole, OTD.)

Prefabricated CMC joint orthoses are available, or they can be custom made (Fig. 16-67).[92,96,99]

The materials vary, but the most common in order of stability are neoprene, soft rubber, and thermo-moldable plastic. Orthoses that provide greater stability are more likely to limit functional activities. Therefore, clinicians must carefully assess each patient's desired activities and opinions regarding bracing before deciding upon the ideal orthotic. Joint protection is more than a short-term restriction of movement with an orthosis. In the truest sense, it is activity modification, and these modifications often need to be permanent to successfully manage symptoms and slow disease progression. Clinicians should identify the activities each patient needs to perform that stresses the CMC joint and create successful adaptations as well as behavior cues for the patient to make joint protection strategies habitual.[100]

CMC joint mobilization is an effective intervention for patients with CMC OA and must consider the sellar-shaped joint when trying to gain motion.[99] Joint distraction can be a very useful technique, particularly to decrease pain in patients with high irritability. Manual therapy is best followed by stretching to improve CMC range, particularly thumb abduction (Fig. 16-68).[52] A simple ball rolling exercise with the thumb can help train improved dynamic thumb alignment to improve web space (Fig. 16-69).[52] Strengthening of the first dorsal interosseous muscle may be best added once adequate ROM has been restored.

Most hand OA management guidelines recommend exercise, both short and long term, including ROM and local muscle strengthening.[98] However, there is limited evidence to help direct exercise prescription. Most exercise programs consist of two to four sets of up to 10 repetitions. ROM exercises are generally prescribed two or more times per day, whereas strengthening exercises are prescribed anywhere from 3 to 7 days per week, pending intensity level and phase of rehabilitation.[52] Clinicians should train patients to pinch without hyperextending at the MCP joint or adducting at the CMC joint.[101] Incorporating functional, task-specific exercises, such as knitting, computer gaming, or musical instrument playing, appears to both increase adherence and improve function.[52] Given that most patients have multijoint involvement, general aerobic

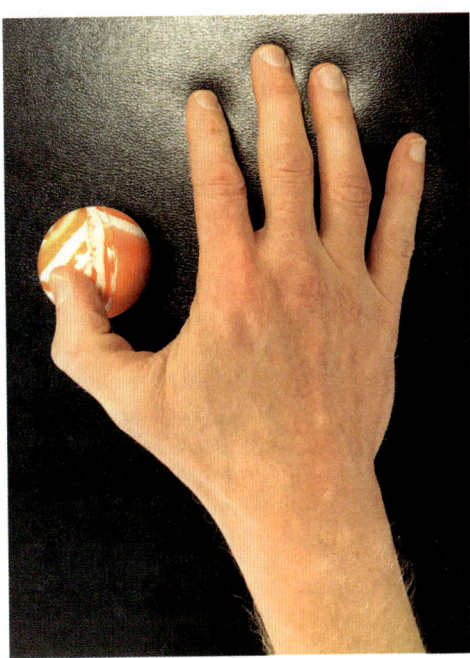

FIGURE 16-69 Thumb ball rolling exercise.

exercise[98] and basic arthritis principles discussed within the lower extremity chapters, such as weight management and the use of ergonomic aides, should be incorporated into the plan of care. Nonsteroidal anti-inflammatory medications may be beneficial.[100,101]

Expected Outcomes Joint mobility exercises, stretching, and strengthening lead to improvements in pain[98] and hand function[98] in 4 to 12 weeks.[52,102,103] Optimal results appear to require a multimodal approach that includes exercise and bracing.[103,104] Clinicians must alert patients that it may take time before improvements in impairments and function are noticed because of the chronicity and degenerative nature of CMC OA.[105] By providing patients with an outline of the plan of care, including expected time frames for milestones, adherence may be improved. For example, thenar flexibility often takes 3 to 6 weeks of regular stretching to improve. Also, patients must understand that due to the bony changes, it may not be possible to restore full motion and normal function. Restoration of first dorsal interosseous muscle strength, particularly with severe atrophy, can take months. Once joint mobility and thenar flexibility have been maximized, patients should be provided with a home exercise program that includes intrinsic hand strengthening to continue independently. Patients who fail to show improvement after 6 weeks of rehabilitation should be referred for further evaluation because the likelihood for successful conservative management after this point is low.[101]

First Carpometacarpal Arthroplasty

There are a number of surgical options for patients with CMC OA who have continued pain and functional limitations. Ligament reconstruction and tendon interposition (LRTI) with trapeziectomy is a commonly performed procedure.[100] The FCR is commonly interposed, or placed within, the vacant space of the trapezium.[106] It has been stated that "hand therapy is essential after arthroplasty around the wrist."[107] Clinicians should obtain a copy of the operative report and communicate with the surgeon to clarify postoperative restrictions and treatment progressions.

Patients are typically placed in a protective splint after surgery. However, early active motion is encouraged to promote mobility and function.[108] Edema control should be encouraged via manual lymph drainage, elevation, and gentle ROM exercise. It is not unusual for patients to continue to have ADDP contracture and generalized joint laxity at the MCP that clinicians should try to address. Progression to hand intrinsic strengthening is important for creating lasting functional improvements. As with conservative care, patients should be educated on joint protection strategies. Ergonomic modifications may be needed for occupational demands. For example, changing from a spherical grip to a hook grip in which the thumb is not involved.

Finger Osteoarthritis

Pathology The two main types of digit arthritis are RA and OA. In the hand, these are often easily distinguishable because they typically affect different joints. RA is most often found in the MCPs, whereas OA is most often found in the PIP joints (Bouchard nodes) and DIP joints (Heberden nodes). While isolated joints can be affected with RA or OA, patients tend to have the majority of the joints in the same level (MCP, PIP, or DIP) affected.

History Patients typically present to the clinic after chronic changes have settled insidiously over a number of years and their perspective on quality is associated with the number of joints affected.[109] Patients typically start to seek treatment when the condition has begun to limit their ability to perform activities of daily living.

Key Examination Findings Bony deformity at multiple joints at a specific level (MCP, PIP, or DIP) is a classic observation. ROM of the affected joints is typically reduce but may still be functional. Patients with finger OA typically have hypomobile joints. In contrast, the MCP joints of patients with chronic RA are typically hypermobile, unstable, and present with a characteristic drift of the digits in the ulnar direction (Fig. 16-70). The ulnar drift is due to swelling of

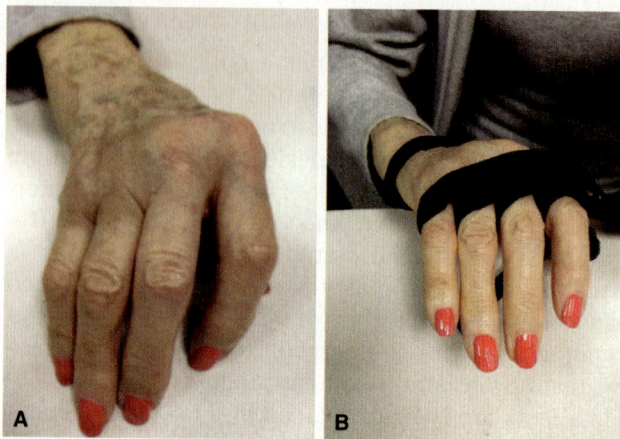

FIGURE 16-70 **A.** Ulnar drift of the metacarpals. **B.** Orthosis to help correct ulnar drift. (Jacobs MA, Austin NM. *Orthotic Intervention for the Hand and Upper Extremity: Splinting Principles and Process.* 3rd ed. Wolters Kluwer; 2022: Figure 11-20.)

the MCP joints and damage to the joint capsule and surrounding structures from chronic inflammation as well as the relative dominance of the ulnar side forces within the hand. While occurring most commonly with inflammatory arthritic conditions, ulnar drift sometimes occurs with OA due to damage to the joint cartilage. Grip and pinch strength are typically reduced and may be painful during flare-ups.

Differential Diagnosis Differential diagnosis should include gout, particularly if the patient's presentation has an acute onset that is limited to a single joint or the patient has a history of gout in the lower extremity.

Rehabilitation Focus and Key Points Because of the relative instability of joints with RA, joint protection and activity modification are the primary interventions.[110] Commonly, grip strengthening exercises emphasize the extrinsic flexors (FDS and FDP), but extrinsic flexor strengthening is contraindicated because they contribute to ulnar drift. For example, with increasing grip intensity, the patient will move into wrist radial deviation and MCP joint ulnar deviation, resulting in increased tissue stress. Properly crafted therapeutic exercise can help improve MCP joint alignment by focusing on the intrinsic hand muscles, particularly the lumbricals, which have a radial bias.[52,110,111] An example is "radial finger walking": the patient maintains the palm flat on the table and slides the fingers in a radial direction. Clinicians should ensure patients do not substitute by recruiting the extensor digitorum. Radial finger walking can help maintain joint alignment and reduce the malalignment that occurs with forceful gripping and pinching. As with CMC OA, static orthoses may help improve joint alignment,[92] but at the cost of restricting some function. Gloves that encourage radial deviation are sometimes a useful compromise between function and protection (Fig. 16-70B).

Similar to patients with CMC OA, patients with finger OA often report that heating pads and/or paraffin help reduce joint stiffness. Reductions in ROM, particularly flexion, can impact function. However, patients are often concerned by the appearance of limited finger extension.

Joint mobilizations and stretching may need to be supplemented with a static progressive orthosis. Although these devices can be fabricated, there are a number of affordable prefabricated devices to improve both flexion and extension that are easy for patients to do independently. For patients in whom ROM remains limited, ergonomic aides, such as large handled utensils, or using foam to increase utensil girth can be extremely helpful to maintain function (Fig. 16-71).[112]

Expected Outcomes Prevention of joint deformities is key for patients with RA, as once irreparable joint damage occurs, it is difficult to manage symptoms or improve function without orthosis or adaptive equipment. In addition, because patients often do not seek medical care until a deformity has already occurred, abnormal motor patterns and adaptive disuse atrophy are often quite profound, requiring more extensive rehabilitation and reducing the potential to achieve optimal results.

Because patients with finger OA do not have instability, they have a much lower risk of deformity and do not present with as much hand weakness. Grip and pinch strength are often regained in a relatively short

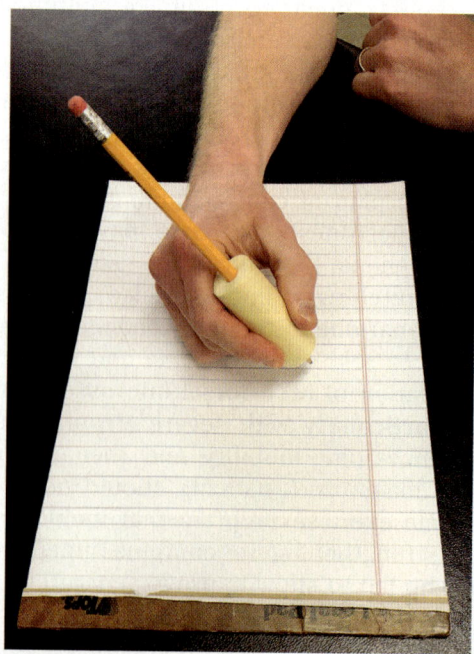

FIGURE 16-71 Foam tubing to widen pencil/pen grip.

period of time, and there are no problems associated with abnormal motor patterns. Although the prognosis for patients with finger OA is good, patients and clinicians must remember that OA is still a degenerative process that patients will need to manage long term.

Surgical management for finger arthritis is seldom required. However, patients may benefit from pharmacologic interventions, such as nonsteroidal anti-inflammatories. In some cases, arthrodesis (fusing) or arthroplasty (replacement) of the involved joint(s) may be warranted.[100]

Extensor Tendon Disruption

Pathology Pathologies along the dorsal finger are related to disruption of the extensor tendon. Each joint has a specific pathology that occurs when a portion of the extensor tendon mechanism is disrupted at that joint (Table 16-12). Prompt identification of central slip and terminal tendon disruption is required because permanent deformity and functional loss is likely without early intervention.

History Laceration and acute trauma are the most common causes of these dorsal finger injuries, although sagittal band rupture can occur insidiously in the elderly due to chronic microtrauma. Patients with lacerations are generally managed surgically and are beyond the scope of this textbook.

Key Examination Findings With acute injury, the clinician will be able to manipulate the finger into full flexion and full extension of the MCP, PIP, and DIP joints (Fig. 16-72). Normally, the intact sagittal band will maintain the extensor tendon centered on top of the MCP throughout flexion and extension. Patients with sagittal band rupture will demonstrate ulnar or radial deviation of the tendon when the patient actively moves into flexion.

A central slip rupture results in a Boutonniere deformity: MCP extension, PIP flexion, and DIP hyperextension. This position occurs because the central slip no longer applies a counterforce to the flexors at

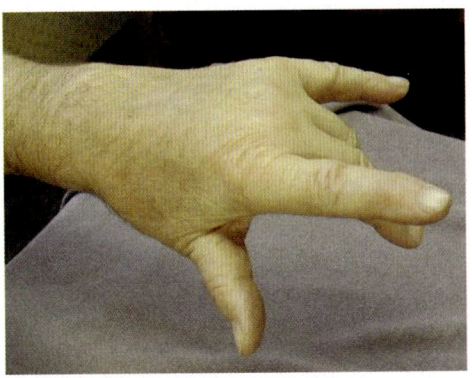

FIGURE 16-72 Rupture of the extensor digitorum communis tendons to the long and ring fingers. (Lubahn JD, Wolfe TL. Surgical treatment and rehabilitation and tendon ruptures in the rheumatoid hand. In: Mackin EJ, Callahan AD, Skirven TM, et al, eds. *Rehabilitation of the Hand and Upper Extremity*. 5th ed. Mosby; 2002:1598–1607.)

the PIP joint. However, the influence of the extensor tendon on the finger is not completely lost. Rather, its force is now fully directed on the terminal tendon, creating DIP hyperextension. It is not uncommon for a patient with a central slip rupture to forego medical intervention until a contracture of the extensor tendon and PIP capsule occurs; with these patients, the clinician will not be able to correct the deformity with passive manipulation.

Patients with a ruptured terminal tendon will be unable to actively extend the DIP. With a terminal tendon rupture, patients tend to seek medical attention more immediately. Early intervention may prevent contracture of the DIP capsule.

Differential Diagnosis Clinicians must consider the potential for concomitant avulsion fracture, which requires imaging to rule out.

Rehabilitation Focus Patients rarely seek care for an acute sagittal band rupture. In fact, it is most often found by clinicians while examining a separate patient complaint. Given the lack of functional limitation from the rupture, the patient may not be interested in addressing any type of intervention. However, the clinician should explain the pathology and recommend the patient limit full finger flexion by increasing the girth of objects the patient commonly uses, such as knives, pens, and toothbrushes, to prevent tendon irritation due to repeated subluxation during finger flexion.

For patients with extensor tendon irritation, in addition to the activity modifications noted earlier, kinesiology tape can be applied to the dorsal MCP to reduce flexor capacity and provide proprioceptive awareness of tendon and joint position.

A relative motion orthosis can be prescribed. The device is inexpensive, simple to make from thermoplastic materials, easily donned and doffed, and places

TABLE 16-12
EXTENSOR TENDON RUPTURE

Joint	Location of Rupture	Deformity
Metacarpophalangeal	Sagittal band	Ulnar or radial deviated extensor tendon subluxation (aka "boxer's knuckle")
Proximal interphalangeal	Central slip	Boutonniere deformity
Distal interphalangeal	Terminal tendon	Mallet finger

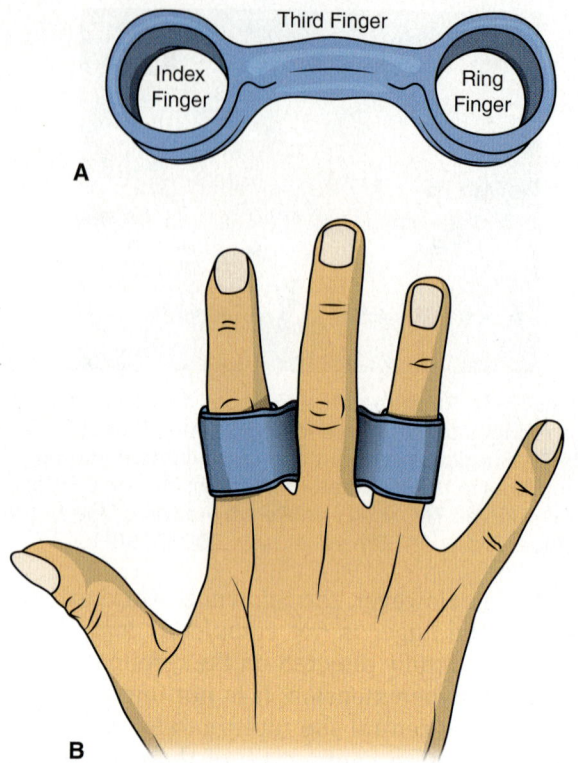

FIGURE 16-73. Relative motion orthosis (A) to reduce left third metacarpophalangeal joint flexion (B).

the pathologic finger in relative MCP extension compared to the other fingers, thus reducing the chance of subluxation and irritation (Fig. 16-73). To better imagine how the orthosis works to prevent third finger MCP flexion, place a pen over the dorsal aspect of the index and ring finger, but under the palmar aspect of the third finger. It is now easy to understand how 3rd MCP is prevented from fully flexing and maintained in a more extended position.

For acute injuries or patients with high irritability, a custom-made hand-based orthosis should be fabricated to hold the pathologic MCP joint in extension for 6 weeks.[113] For this orthosis, the palm will be the base, and the orthosis will extend along the palmar aspect of proximal phalanx of the affected finger. Because the subluxation of the extensor tendon occurs solely with MCP flexion, the other joints are free to move.

With dorsal finger injuries at the PIP and DIP, there is often a conservative period of immobilization before surgical intervention is considered. Patients with an acute central slip injury should be placed in a long finger orthosis (maintaining the MCP and PIP extended) for 6 weeks to allow scar tissue formation. They should be educated that any movement into flexion will result in complete disruption of any healing that has already occurred, and a new 6-week period of immobilization must be restarted. The orthosis should permit DIP motion to preserve ROM and tendon gliding. If immobilization is successful in restoring the integrity of the central slip, gentle AROM can begin while continuing to wear the orthosis for an additional 2 weeks during activities of daily living. After 8 weeks of immobilization, PIP PROM can begin to resolve any residual joint tightness.[114] To encourage PIP motion at this point, a relative motion orthosis can be crafted that reduces affected MCP flexion, thus requiring increased PIP flexion during functional activities.

For patients with a chronic Boutonniere deformity, the goal is to improve passive PIP extension. This is generally done via low-load, prolonged stretching with serial splinting for profound contractures or a static progressive orthosis for milder cases (Fig. 16-74). While these can be custom-made, prefabricated, spring-based splints for finger extension can be used. Ultimately, even if ROM is restored for the patient with a Boutonniere deformity, the integrity of the central slip will not be fully restored and an imbalance at the PIP joint will remain. These patients would benefit from long-term joint protection after ROM is normalized. A number of inexpensive, fashionable joint protection orthoses are available.

Patients with a ruptured terminal tendon should be immediately placed in an orthosis with slight hyperextension of the DIP (the PIP and MCP can be unrestricted). Although prefabricated orthoses appear to have a higher risk of skin complications compared to custom-made orthoses, there are no differences in treatment outcomes.[115] The orthosis must be worn for 6 weeks. When removed for handwashing or other

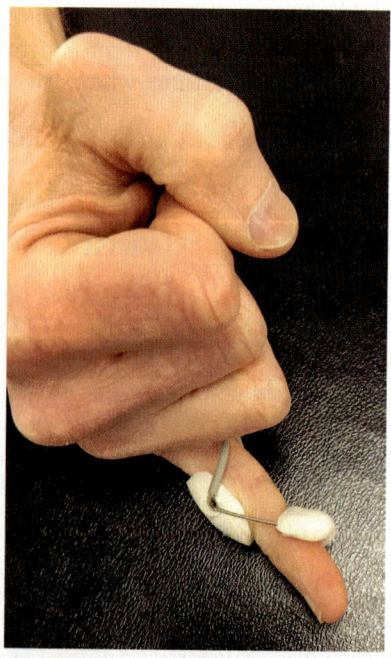

FIGURE 16-74 Splint for proximal interphalangeal extension.

purposes, the DIP must be manually held in extension. If the DIP ever moves out of the extended position, the timeline for orthotic immobilization starts a new. After 6 weeks, the orthosis is removed and the joint examined. If the DIP joint cannot be maintained in a fully extended position without support (i.e., an extension lag is present), an additional week of immobilization is added along with bracing and reassessment until the goal of no extension lag is reached.

Expected Outcome Outcomes for dorsal finger injuries are quite varied. For patients with sagittal band ruptures who adhere to activity modification, tendon irritation and symptoms resolve within 2 to 3 weeks. However, patients should be made aware that repeated periods of protection may be required in the future. Patients with central slip injuries and a Boutonniere deformity can be challenging to treat conservatively. If conservative immobilization is unsuccessful, surgical intervention may be needed for synovectomy, terminal tenotomy, extensor reconstruction, or salvage surgery.[114] In contrast, patients with terminal tendon ruptures tend to have an excellent prognosis with conservative interventions if patients are adherent with maintaining the DIP extended at all times during the 6-week immobilization period. Patients who fail conservative interventions should be referred for a surgical consult.

Dupuytren Contracture

Dupuytren contracture is a benign, insidious overproduction of fibrous tissue within the palmar fascia. The condition primarily affects older men of European descent.[116] Patients typically do not seek medical interventions until limited ROM starts to interfere with functional activities. For examples, patients initially will have difficulty fully extending the involved finger, making keyboarding, performing push-ups, or even placing the hand in a pocket or gloves difficult. Because the condition is progressive, the affected finger will gradually curl into the palm, interfering with grip. Dupuytren contracture can be recognized by a palpable thickening near the distal palmar crease that limits MCP extension of the affected finger(s), most commonly the long and ring fingers.[116] Multiple fingers can be involved, and, in severe cases, PIP extension can also be limited.[116]

Differential diagnosis includes trigger finger (discussed in the following section), which occurs just distal to Dupuytren contracture, or an MCP capsular restriction. Examining MCP motion in varying positions of PIP and DIP motion provides accurate diagnosis. First, place the hand in the starting position of DIP and PIP joint extension and MCP joint flexion. Next, while maintaining IP extension, the MCP joint is extended and the amount of MCP joint ROM is noted. Lastly, the DIP and PIP joints are flexed, and the clinician attempts to extend the MCP joint. If there is an increase in MCP extension with the DIP and PIP joints flexed, the long finger flexors are limiting ROM and Dupuytren contracture is confirmed. If there is no change in MCP extension with DIP and PIP flexion, an MCP capsular restriction is present and the patient may benefit from joint mobilizations.

Deep tissue mobilization, therapeutic ultrasound, and manual stretching have limited effectiveness, so interventions should focus on sustained stretching to the affected area. Low-load, long-duration stretching with a static progressive orthosis is an effective conservative intervention, but patient adherence tends to be limited. Given the progressive nature of Dupuytren contracture even if an improvement in MCP extension occurs, the patient will need to continue to utilize the orthosis long term to maintain the ROM gained. Therefore, patients wanting a long-term solution are typically managed surgically.[67] Surgical interventions include fasciectomy, fasciotomy, or injection of a solution that reduces the contracture strength, followed by a forceful manipulation to break the scar tissue.[116,117] Surgical interventions require aggressive postoperative ROM and the use of an orthotic to maintain gained extension.[67] Regrettably, even if full motion is restored, the 5-year recurrence rate is nearly 50%.[116] Therefore, many patients forego surgery.[67] In extreme cases of functional limitation due to a chronically flexed digit, finger amputation can result in improved function.

Trigger Finger

Trigger finger (aka stenosing tenosynovitis) is caused by friction and inflammation of the FDS with development of an inflammatory nodule near the distal palmar crease. Although other pulleys may be involved, the A1 pulley is most common. When the finger is flexed, the nodule moves proximally through the A1 pulley. As the patient attempts to extend the finger, the nodule must be pulled distally through the A1 pulley, creating a palpable (and sometimes audible) click. Often, the finger will become nearly locked in a flexed position and require the finger to be passively pulled back to extension.

Patients with trigger finger report an insidious onset of finger clicking and occasional locking. There may be a recent history of an activity that required increased grip frequency or force. Relative rest by avoiding gripping improves the condition, but the clicking and/or locking return when the patient resumes the repetitive activity. Examination reveals tenderness proximal to the A1 pulley, and a small palpable thickness may be present. When palpating this area during finger flexion and extension, a click, catch, or even locking of the finger is observable. This is in contrast to the painless, consistent stiffness, and deformity of Dupuytren contracture.

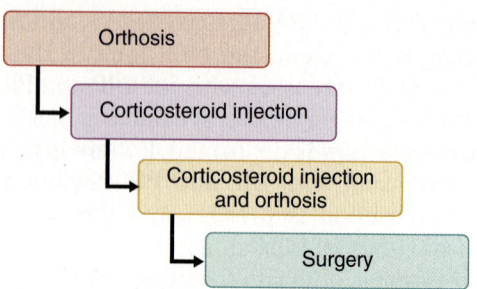

FIGURE 16-75 Trigger finger treatment progression.

Successful management of trigger finger requires identification and modification of the offending activity/activities. Once inflammation and friction have been controlled, normal tendon gliding will be restored. The short-term use of an orthotic (or kinesiology tape) to keep the MCP joint extended can be extremely beneficial, particularly for individuals with high irritability or who are unable or unwilling to avoid the provocative activities. Figure 16-75 demonstrates a proposed multidisciplinary trigger finger treatment progression schema.[67] The vast majority of cases resolve with conservative interventions. However, patients with long-standing symptoms before seeking medical care tend to have worse results.

Patients who fail conservative management for trigger finger generally report good results with surgical interventions.[67] Surgery involves decompression (partial or complete release) of the A1 pulley. Postoperative rehabilitation focuses on preserving the gliding ability of the flexor tendons. Because scar tissue formation can occur quickly after surgery, PROM (tendon gliding) should begin on the day of surgery. Although the tendon itself is not damaged during surgery, AROM should be limited to that required for activities of daily living for the first 2 weeks to help control local inflammation. Finger flexor strengthening exercises can be initiated as early as 3 weeks postoperatively if AROM is full and symptom free.

Complete release of the A1 pulley typically results in bowstringing of the flexor tendons at the MCP. However, most patients will still result improved function after surgery because of the significant disability created by the trigger finger before surgery.

Swan-Neck Deformity

Pathology A swan-neck deformity is caused by damage to the PIP volar plate.[118] This can occur in two ways. First, hyperextension of the PIP joint ruptures the palmar plate. Without an intact palmar plate, the extensor hood goes unchecked and pulls the PIP into hypertension. Hyperextension of the PIP joint alters the moment arm of the extensor mechanism, changing it into a DIP flexor. Alternatively, a swan-neck deformity can result from an untreated mallet finger.[118] Rupture of the terminal tendon means the extensor mechanism force is solely placed at the central slip insertion. This force and resultant adaptive shortening cause microtrauma to the volar plate. Volar plate instability results in PIP joint hyperextension. Patients with RA or cerebral palsy[115] often develop swan-neck deformities. For patients with a recent PIP hyperextension, treatment consists of immobilization of the PIP joint for 3 to 6 weeks. An orthosis that limits PIP hyperextension is the treatment of choice for patients with chronic swan-neck deformities[118]; however, adherence is limited. Swan-neck deformities can be functionally limiting. Surgical correction generally results in functional benefit. Surgery for swan-neck deformity is typically more successful than for Boutonniere deformity.[119]

Rehabilitation after Finger Flexor Repair

Finger flexor lacerations can result from falling with a breakable object in hand or accidently slicing the hand with a knife or piece of machinery. Complete tendon lacerations need prompt evaluation by a hand surgeon as the tendons will retract and may become difficult to fully mobilize back to their normal anatomic attachment site. Finger flexor tendon injuries are often identified by zone (Fig. 16-76).

Zone 1 includes the FDP. Zone 2 includes FDP and FDS and is often referred to as "No Man's Land" because it is the most complex region to address surgically. Prognosis for Zone 2 is reduced compared with other zones because of the increased likelihood of scar tissue formation within the extensive pulley system.

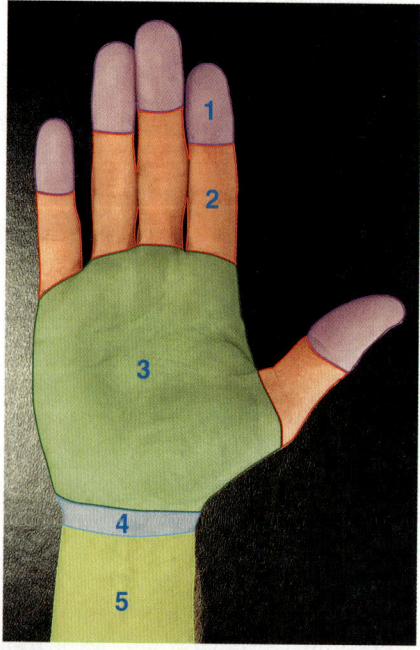

FIGURE 16-76 Flexor zones. Zone 1 (purple), zone 2 (tan), zone 3 (green), zone 4 (blue), zone 5 (light green).

Zone 3 includes the tendons of the FDP and FDS, and the lumbricals and interosseous muscles and may include damage to the median and/or ulnar nerve as well as the ulnar artery and the superficial palmar artery. Zone 4 includes all the contents of the carpal tunnel. Zone 5 includes all of the anatomic structures of zone 4, as well as the FCU, pronator quadratus, and brachioradialis muscles. Lacerations may involve one or all structures within the zone. Some patients may have multiple hand lacerations, affecting different zones and/or different digits.

Owing to the complexity of surgery and the potential complications of tendon rupture and contracture formation, rehabilitation after flexor tendon repair is dominated by protocols. Protocols provide consistency of treatment and help assure that the interventions are performed consistently at a particular time. However, patients vary in surgical procedure, presentation, and healing capacity. From a surgical standpoint, beyond the zone of repair, type of fixation affects the integrity of the repair. For example, an eight-strand repair is nearly twice as strong as a four-strand repair.[120] In addition, tendon quality may affect repair strength. Patient factors, such as being a smoker or having diabetes or peripheral vascular disease, are known to adversely affect healing rates.

During the first 2 weeks after flexor tendon repair, the risk of rupture with active contraction or passive overstretching is high. However, because scar tissue begins to form within the first 3 days after repair, strict immobilization also poses some degree of risk. Thus, surgeons and clinicians need to critically appraise each patient's situation to assure the best outcome. This section includes some basic information regarding the three main types of flexor tendon repair protocols: PROM, early AROM, or a hybrid often referred to as the *Pyramid of Progressive Force*.

Passive Range of Motion Protocol The Modified Duran protocol is a commonly used PROM protocol that is considered traditional and "safe." PROM helps lubricate the affected tendon, and it is thought to be beneficial to perform PROM before AROM.[121] The Modified Duran protocol generally uses a dorsal blocking orthosis that allows 20° of wrist flexion with MCP joints in a loose-packed position. Adherence to the orthosis can be a challenge; thus, patient education is crucial. Exercises during the first 4 weeks of rehabilitation include passive flexion of DIP, PIP, and MCP joints; passive protected extension; and up to 30° of wrist extension with the digits flexed.

Early Active Motion Protocol The early active motion protocol gained popularity as means of reducing scarring and the challenges of restoring finger ROM when following the more conservative PROM protocol. The early active motion protocol significantly reduces finger contractures without increasing the risk of tendon rupture.[122] An orthosis (the Manchester short splint) is used and allows for wrist mobility, but protects against full extension of all of the finger joints.[123] With the early active motion protocol, the patient is allowed to actively flex up to one-third of normal motion during postoperative weeks 1 to 4. Full active flexion ROM is permitted after the fourth week.

Pyramid of Progressive Force Unlike the previous protocols, the pyramid of progressive force is based on a gradual increase in tissue stress and the patient's response. The pyramid of progressive force application[124] begins with low levels of tendon stress. Patients failing to gain motion are progressed to the next level of force. Specifically, at each visit, the clinician will categorize the patient's postoperative ROM improvement as responsive or unresponsive. If the patient's ROM is unresponsive, the clinician progresses to the next level of the pyramid. If the patient's ROM is responsive, the clinician maintains the current level of exercise until the patient's ROM is no longer responsive with that level of exercise. This method provides the least amount of force necessary to improve motion.

Regardless of the protocol followed, clinicians must make efforts to control edema. Edema increases friction between the tendon and the surrounding tissue and makes it difficult to gain motion. Edema can be minimized via manual lymphatic drainage,[125] compression wrapping, elevation, and active motion of the elbow and shoulder.

Subacute Rehabilitation of the Postoperative Hand When a patient exhibits a limitation of ROM, the clinician needs to determine whether this limitation is related to the joint capsule or tendon contracture by examining the effect of isolated and combined joint motion as discussed earlier. Capsular restrictions should be treated with joint mobilization and isolated joint stretching in a position that does not increase tension on the extrinsic tendons. For example, a patient with limited MCP flexion may be treated with grade 3 to 4 palmar glides of the proximal phalanx, followed by passive stretching into MCP flexion with the involved digit (or wrist) to avoid excessive stretch of the extensors.

After the first 3 weeks of flexor tendon repair, the traditional, bulky postoperative orthosis can be replaced with a relative motion orthosis.[126] Patient adherence is improved with this smaller device, and the patient may be able to return to regular activities of daily living sooner while still providing adequate protection of the repaired tendon.

Tendon gliding is very common exercise routine that follows the pyramid of progressive force concepts. Figure 16-77 provides examples of common

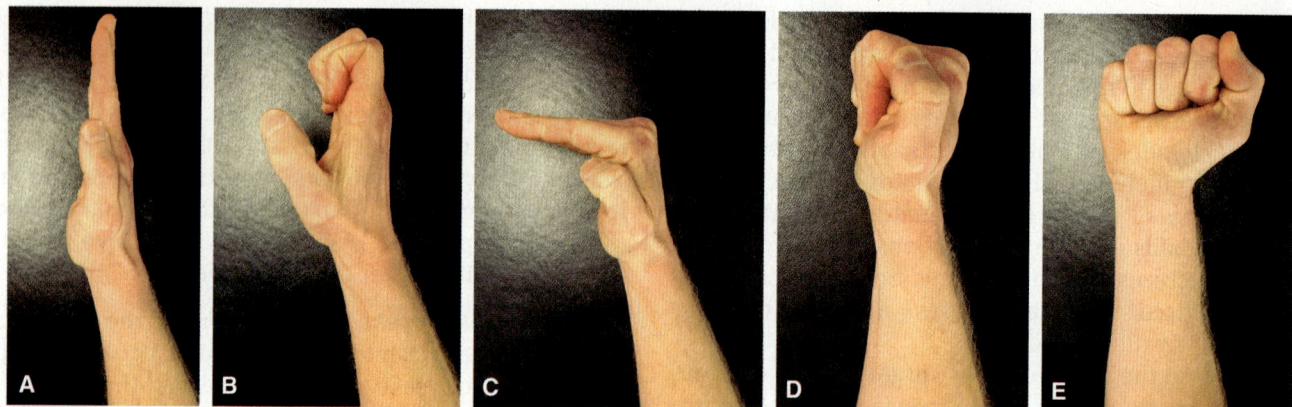

FIGURE 16-77 Tendon gliding positions. **A.** Straight hand. **B.** Hook fist. **C.** Metacarpophalangeal flexion (tabletop). **D.** Straight fist. **E.** Full composite fist.

tendon gliding positions. The straight hand places both the FDS and the FDP on stretch, particularly when combined with wrist extension. The hook fist partially shortens both the FDS and the FDP. MCP flexion (aka tabletop position) shortens the lumbricals and interosseous muscles. A straight fist maximally shortens the FDS, but not the FDP. The full composite fist maximally shortens the FDP and places all joints at end-range flexion.

Radial Wrist Pain

After scaphoid fracture, the three most common causes of radial wrist/forearm symptoms are de Quervain tenosynovitis, intersection syndrome, and Wartenberg syndrome. Table 16-13 provides a summary of the key features of each pathology. All three conditions are often chronic in nature and related to overuse, particularly activities requiring repeated wrist ulnar deviation. De Quervain and intersection syndrome are identical, except that the symptoms are either distal (de Quervain) or proximal (intersection syndrome) to the extensor retinaculum. Wartenberg syndrome is the only condition to involve a nerve, and therefore, the presence of tingling or paresthesias, rather than pain, is a key distinguishing feature.

Although these three pathologies have separate anatomic causes, interventions are similar.[127] Clinicians must first identify the source of the overuse activity and provide appropriate activity modifications. A patient may temporarily change to using the contralateral hand or use a power screwdriver rather than a manual one. Assembly line workers may be temporarily reassigned to an alternate job. Kayakers and paddlers may utilize alternately designed paddles or may need to modify their stroke to correct excessive ulnar deviation, particularly if combined with wrist flexion.

An orthotic that prevents ulnar deviation will reduce tendon friction. Orthotics appear to be more effective when combined with a corticosteroid injection.[128] Patients with Wartenberg syndrome should use caution with wrist jewelry and watches because they may cause external compression of the superficial radial nerve. Wrist deviation range and wrist joint mobility should be assessed, as a loss of motion typically leads to increased muscular recruitment to attain end-range positions that may increase tendon stress. Resisted testing of the EPB and APL is typically painful, and strength may be inhibited due to pain. If strengthening is required, it should begin with symptom-free isometrics before progressive to resisted ROM exercise. Strengthening exercises should be used with caution, gradually increasing in repetition based on work/recreational demands, and using precise positioning, given the potential to increase tendon friction.

TABLE 16-13
COMMON OVERUSE INJURIES CAUSING RADIAL WRIST/FOREARM SYMPTOMS

	De Quervain	*Intersection Syndrome*	*Wartenberg Syndrome*
Pathology	Friction between the APL and EPB in the first dorsal compartment of the wrist	Friction between the APL and EPB as they move over the ECRL/ECRB in the forearm	Compression of the superficial radial nerve between the ECLR and BR in the forearm
Finkelstein test	Positive for pain	Positive for pain	Produces tingling sensation
Tinel test	Negative	Negative	Positive

APL, abductor pollicis longus; *ECRB*, extensor carpi radialis brevis; *ECRL*, extensor carpi radialis longus; *EPB*, extensor pollicis brevis.

Assuming patients are able to perform the necessary activity modifications to decrease tissue irritability, most symptoms are fully resolved within 3 to 6 weeks of conservative care.[127]

Triangular Fibrocartilage Complex Injury

TFCC injuries are one of the most common causes of ulnar wrist pain.[129] Most TFCC injuries are traumatic in onset, such as a FOOSH on an extended wrist or a rotational injury, such as when the wrist and hand are twisted into hypersupination.[86] However, degenerative lesions and repetitive motion lesions from repetitive ulnar deviation may also damage the TFCC. Patients will report ulnar-sided wrist pain that is exacerbated with weight-bearing pain through the hand or carrying heavy objects.[86] Patients may also note difficulty with activities requiring end-range pronation, wrist extension, or ulnar deviation. Patients may report the wrist feels unstable.[129]

Key Examination Findings Key indicators of a TFCC injury include a positive fovea sign, a positive TFCC grind test, and/or a positive press test.[130] Patients typically also have pain with end-range pronation and ulnar deviation. Edema is rare unless there are concomitant injuries, such as a fracture.

Differential Diagnosis Differential diagnoses include FCU or ECU tendinopathy, ulnar impaction syndrome, and distal radioulnar sprains.[130]

Rehabilitation Focus and Key Points Minor injuries to the TFCC can be managed conservatively with a period of immobilization followed by active and active-assisted wrist motions. Forearm rotation and strengthening should be resumed gradually as symptoms allow. Some patients may find relief with taping procedures that limit DRUJ motion.[89] Anti-inflammatory medications or corticosteroid injections can be beneficial,[89] particularly for athletes and workers who are unable to avoid provoking activities.

Expected Outcomes The prognosis for conservative management of TFCC injuries is unclear. Some literature suggests that conservative treatment should be limited to isolated ulnar styloid fracture without TFCC tear, while any involvement of the TFCC proper should be surgically repaired.[131] More recent literature suggests that early diagnosis and management of TFCC injuries lead to improved outcomes.[89] However, patients with DRUJ instability respond less favorably to immobilization and should be referred for further evaluation if symptoms persist.[129]

Rehabilitation after Triangular Fibrocartilage Complex Repair Surgery Various surgical interventions can address TFCC pathology, including debridement, suture, fixation of TFCC to the fovea or styloid notch, tendon graft reconstruction, and arthroplasty. Clinicians involved in the postoperative rehabilitation process must acquire the operative report and discuss postoperative rehabilitation protocol directly with the surgeon. Patients undergoing an open TFCC repair are typically placed in a long arm splint with the elbow at 90° of flexion and forearm in neutral position for 4 to 6 weeks,[132] after which the goal is to restore functional wrist motion followed by forearm rotation. Strengthening should be delayed and begin cautiously to avoid premature loading of the TFCC.[49,107] Athletes and patients with occupations requiring aggressive forearm rotation activity are typically able to return to activity within 3 to 6 months.[85,107]

Wrist Instability

There are multiple pathologies that can lead to wrist instability. If the instability is within one carpal row, such as a scaphoid-lunate tear, it is considered intercalated or dissociative. However, if the instability is in both the proximal and distal row of carpals, then it is considered nondissociative and is more commonly referred to as *midcarpal instability*. Midcarpal instability is often associated with distal radius fractures.[82]

The lunate is the key to understanding many aspects of wrist instability and nomenclature. Recall that the scaphoid, lunate, and triquetrum are all part of the proximal row of carpals. These carpal bones do not merely rest in place; the scaphoid and triquetrum each have a bias that is mediated by their relationship with the lunate. The scaphoid has a bias to move toward a flexed position, whereas the triquetrum has a bias toward extension. The lunate provides the balance between these two opposing biases and helps maintain the carpals in a neutral position. The lunate is inherently unstable because of its lack of muscular attachments. Therefore, when there is a disruption between the lunate and either of its adjacent carpals, the scaphoid or the triquetrum, the lunate will be pulled into the biased position of the carpal to which it still has a ligamentous attachment (Table 16-14).[82]

The mechanism of injury that is most characteristic and stress tests for each type of instability are listed in Table 16-14. After an acute injury, patients will report pain and have diffuse dorsal wrist swelling with limited ROM.[133] Typical chronic presentation of wrist instability is the report of central wrist pain and may describe clicking with wrist motion or a clunk with weight bearing through the hand in addition to reporting the wrist feels as if it will "give way."[82]

Treatment for wrist instability involves 4 to 12 weeks of immobilization in an orthosis that stabilizes the wrist but allows hand mobility. The dart thrower's motion orthosis is increasingly being used in the treatment of proximal row wrist sprains and postoperative

TABLE 16-14
SCAPHOID-LUNATE-TRIQUETRUM COMPLEX PATHOLOGY

Schematic	Ligament Status	Lunate	Pathology	Onset	Stress Test
S-L-T	Intact	Stable	None	NA	Negative
S**x**L-T	Scapholunate ligament rupture	Extends with triquetrum	Dorsal* intercalated segmental instability (DISI)	FOOSH in ulnar deviation	Positive scaphoid shift test
S-L**x**T	Lunotriquetral ligament rupture	Flexes with scaphoid	Volar* intercalated segmental instability (VISI)	FOOSH in radial deviation	Positive Ballottement test
SLT **XXX** TzCH	One or more ligaments between carpal rows	NA	Midcarpal instability	Generalized ligamentous laxity†	Positive midcarpal shift test

C, capitate; H, hamate; L, lunate; S, scaphoid; T, triquetrum; Tr, trapezium; **X**, ruptured.
*Nomenclature is based on lunate malposition.
†May also occur due to a fall.

rehabilitation. A dart thrower's motion orthosis is a hinged device that allows a small diagonal arc of motion akin to dart throwing: moving from radial deviation and some extension into ulnar deviation and slight flexion. Because the radiocarpal ligaments are not stressed during this motion, the orthosis protects ligament integrity while reducing the effects of prolonged, static immobilization.[134,135] Immobilization is followed by early motion exercises to help resolve wrist stiffness.

Strengthening exercises for patients with subacute and chronic injuries may benefit consideration for the ligament involved. For example, for scapholunate ligament injuries, strengthening should begin with muscles that help compress the scaphoid to the lunate to help improve wrist stability. This would include muscles such as the extensor carpi radialis brevis (ECRB), extensor carpi radialis longus (ECRL), APL, and FCU. In contrast, patients with lunotriquetral ligament injuries should initially focus on strengthening of the pronators and ECU. Once strengthening is tolerated, clinicians should focus on restoring the proprioceptive control to optimize wrist function.[136–138]

Patients who have a sedentary physical demand occupation can often resume unrestricted work for 4 weeks, whereas athletes and heavy physical demand occupations may need 3 to 6 months of modified duty. Unfortunately, up to 24% of patients may develop chronic instability.[77] Patients who fail conservative interventions should be referred to a hand specialist.

Scapholunate advanced collapse (aka an SLAC wrist) can result from a chronic, untreated scapholunate ligament injury. In an SLAC wrist, the scapholunate interval widens and the capitate drifts into the interval.[133] These misaligned carpals cause instability and abnormal forces across the radiocarpal and midcarpal joints, ultimately leading to progressive arthritis, pain, and loss of wrist function. Patients typically report morning and overuse stiffness. Examination will reveal positive instability tests, generalized wrist weakness, as well as decreased grip strength, decreased wrist motion, and tenderness along the scaphoid, capitate, and lunate. Conservative management for an SLAC wrist includes following basic arthritis and joint protection principles. Mid-ROM mobility exercises and manual distraction help reduce symptoms. Patients may benefit from generalized wrist strengthening, including diagonal motions, such as a dart thrower's motion. Carpal excision and fusion is a potential surgical solution that tends to result in significant pain relief, but with nearly 50% loss of wrist flexion and extension range.[139]

Fracture

Distal Radius Fractures In Colles fracture, the most common distal radius fracture, the distal radius fracture segment is displaced dorsally. Colles fractures typically occur from a FOOSH with the wrist extended. In contrast, a Smith fracture is when the fracture segment rests in a volar position and is the result of a FOOSH with the wrist flexed (Fig. 16-78). Distal radius fractures may be managed conservatively or with open reduction and internal fixation (ORIF). The main benefit of ORIF is that patients are safely able to begin mobility exercises just after surgery[140] whereas conservative casting and immobilization typically requires 4 to 6 weeks for appropriate callus formation. Clinicians should communicate with the managing health care provider to understand fracture alignment and any additional injuries sustained.

Regardless of the management approach, typical examination findings include hand edema, limited ROM, limited joint mobility, and weakness.[141] Motion loss typically includes the hand, wrist, and forearm, with the most substantial deficits at the wrist and into supination. Clinicians should assess shoulder ROM, both due to the habitually holding of the extremity close to the body as if in a sling and because limited

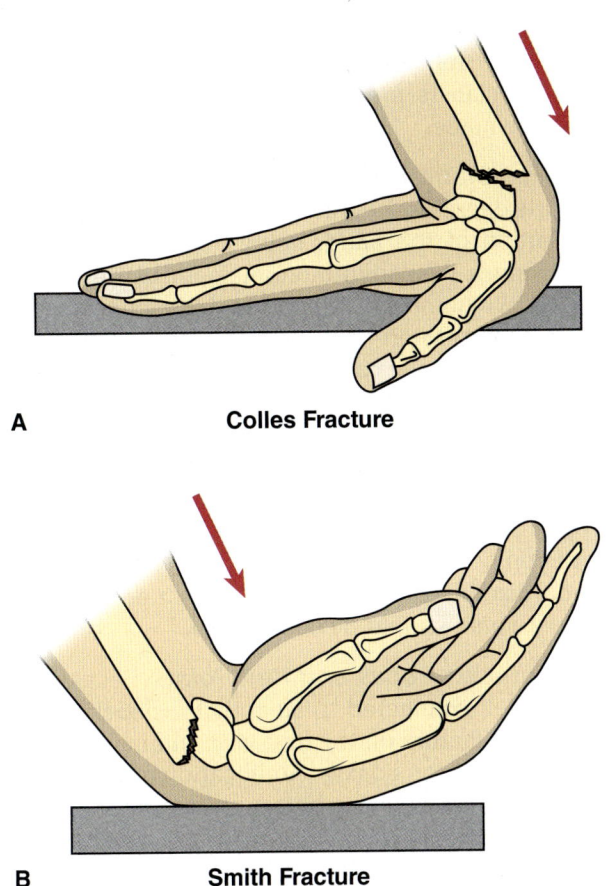

FIGURE 16-78 Mechanism of injury for Colles fracture (**A**) and Smith fracture (**B**). (Adapted from Anatomical Chart Company. *Hand and Wrist*. Wolters Kluwer/Anatomical Chart Company; 2004.)

hand use precludes the need to reach in various directions. Sensory deficits are uncommon, but clinicians should screen sensation. Muscle performance assessment of the upper extremity should minimally include pinch, grip, wrist, and forearm strength testing. Because the majority of distal radius fractures are the result of falls, clinicians must be sure to learn the details of the injury and determine whether balance or vestibular assessment is indicated.

Edema management, if present, must be an initial treatment priority because edema can reduce and complicate finger gliding, capsular mobility, and hand intrinsic strength. Self and clinician manual lymphatic drainage as well as specialized compression wrapping can be implemented by those with appropriate training. Therapeutic exercise after distal radius fracture is highly beneficial.[142] Passive motion of the long finger tendons and intrinsics promotes tendon health, lubricates the synovium, and helps avoid adhesions. Tendon gliding exercises should be encouraged. Joint mobilizations and stretching are key to restoring motion. However, clinicians must make note of motion

endfeels. Early in the rehabilitation process, stiffness is likely due to immobilization and endfeels are likely to be capsular. However, later on, a bony endfeel is an indication of bony malalignment, and further efforts to gain range in that direction will be unsuccessful (Fig. 16-78). Strengthening should include hand intrinsic and extrinsic strengthening as well as the wrist musculature. Clinicians should also consider the overall strength and endurance of the now deconditioned upper extremity. Clinicians can often begin to improve proximal strength impairments, even when the distal restrictions limit AROM and strengthening.

Once initial immobilization and edema-related stiffness resolves, sometimes symptoms of wrist instability, such as clicking or popping, will develop; this is likely the result of ligamentous damage at the time of fracture. Midcarpal instability is often following a distal radius fracture.[82] The clinician should perform instability testing and consider incorporating treatment for scapholunate instability, lunotriquetral instability, or midcarpal instability. In addition to strengthening the wrist muscles including the FCR, FCU, ECR, and ECU, the clinician should utilize the diagonal "dart thrower's motion" pattern and incorporate proprioceptive exercises.

Average duration of rehabilitation ranges from 4 to 12 weeks.[142] Patients typically require 4 to 6 weeks to achieve maximal ROM, while grip and intrinsic strengthening takes somewhat longer. Compliant patients can often progress to an independent home exercise program after functional ROM has been achieved and manual mobilization is not required for goal achievement.

Scaphoid Fracture The scaphoid is susceptible to fracture from a FOOSH, particularly if the wrist is in extension. A horizontal fracture across the scaphoid can disrupt blood flow and lead to avascular necrosis. If left untreated, this necrosis can cause an SLAC wrist. With the loss of the bony foundation of the proximal scaphoid, the capitate can migrate proximally, creating instability in both the proximal and distal carpal rows. To prevent this severely damaging and debilitating condition, early identification and proper treatment of scaphoid fractures are crucial.

Conservative treatment of scaphoid fractures includes casting or rigid orthosis, such as a thumb spica, to protect movement of 1st metacarpal and wrist. Nondisplaced or minimally displaced scaphoid waist fractures are generally well healed within 6 weeks.[143] Although wrist stiffness can be expected upon cast/orthosis removal, this generally resolves without the need for formal rehabilitation.

Surgical fixation using a percutaneous screw or k-wire (aka Kirschner wire) may be required for displaced fractures,[143,144] proximal pole fractures,[143] or those fractures that fail to demonstrate timely callus formation. Postoperative rehabilitation is typically not required, but some patients may benefit from a short course of treatment to address residual stiffness if function is limited.

Hand Fractures Hand fractures occur with various types of trauma, such as falls, crush injury, tendon avulsion, and direct trauma. Swelling may be present but is not universal. Pain often limits patient attempts at active motion and is a key indicator of fracture in athletes. Immobilization of stable, extra-articular phalanx fracture helps reduce pain and maintain fracture congruence.[145,146] Immobilization typically lasts 3 to 6 weeks pending bone, fracture size, and patient-specific factors such as osteoporosis.[147] Most patients with simple, closed hand fractures do not require rehabilitation unless there is residual joint stiffness.

Unstable or displaced hand fractures are treated with ORIF with a k-wire, screws, pins, or plates. Surgery may be performed on stable fractures to allow quicker return to competitive sports for athletes.[146] Because of the structure of the palmar plate, the IP joints are typically immobilized in extension to decrease the risk of developing a flexion contracture. If needed, postoperative rehabilitation begins once the fracture is deemed stable and the initial focus is controlling swelling and improving ROM. Frequent bouts of PROM, active-assisted ROM, and AROM exercises should be prescribed as part of a home exercise program. Joint mobilizations may be beneficial. Patients can progress to strengthening exercises once range is no longer a priority.

Carpal Tunnel Syndrome

Pathology CTS is compression of the median nerve in the space under the transverse carpal ligament. Increased pressure within the carpal tunnel, nerve fibrosis, nerve ischemia, and compression from adjacent structures all appear to contribute to patient symptoms.[76] Compression or irritation of the median nerve can occur from static positioning, such as holding a mobile phone for prolonged periods of time with wrist flexion or extension bias, or from repetitive digital flexor activity, such as keyboarding. CTS can also occur with fluid overload, such as during pregnancy. Patients who are female, over 45 years of age,[148] or have diabetes or thyroid disease are also at increased risk of CTS.[76]

History Patients with CTS will report paresthesias in the volar aspect of the thumb, index, and middle finger. They will often report nocturnal symptoms that require shaking of the hand to abolish.[76] Clinicians should ask about activities or occupational tasks that place the patient at risk for CTS. Patients with diabetes should be asked about the blood sugar control, and appropriate follow-ups (patient education or referral to specialists in endocrinology and/or nutrition) should be made.

Key Examination Findings Patients with CTS present with decreased light touch in the median nerve distribution of the hand, being unable to sense the 3.22 Semmes Weinstein monofilament and having decreased two-point discrimination.[76] Phalen test, carpal tunnel compression test, and/or Tinel testing of the median nerve at the carpal tunnel may be positive. Clinicians must carefully screen the cervical spine to rule out or address the potential for a double-crush injury. Grip and pinch strength should be assessed and compared bilaterally and with normative values.[76] Thenar atrophy is noted with severe or prolonged median nerve compression.[76] ROM testing is typically normal. Standardized hand function tests, such as the Perdue pegboard test, should be considered.[76]

Rehabilitation Focus and Key Points Because CTS is often well connected to an activity, clinicians must identify the factors on the first visit and make activity, environmental, or dosing modifications. Ergonomics, posture, and setup of machinery or computers all need to be considered. The CTS clinical practice guideline reports limited evidence to support neurodynamic mobilizations.[76] However, a trial of nerve glides, using a test-treat-retest paradigm, may be warranted.

Mobilization to the pisiform theoretically loads and lengthens the transverse carpal ligament, allowing more space for the median nerve. Patient self-mobilization, as noted in Figure 16-79, may be helpful.[149] Soft-tissue mobilization and myofascial release of the FDS and FDP may be indicated if the CTS is more likely related to fingering friction rather than postural disposition. Nocturnal splints with the wrist in a neutral position are commonly provided for patients who are experiencing night pain due to improper positioning. To patients who are experiencing night pain, these splints may be more effective when used in combination with other interventions,[150] such as limited daytime repetitive wrist activities. Patients should be treated holistically by addressing known risk factors, such as obesity, deconditioning, smoking, and diet.[76]

Outcomes Outcomes for patients with CTS are quite varied. Conservative management should be considered for patients with mild symptoms.[151] The addition of nonsteroidal anti-inflammatory medication or corticosteroid injections may be beneficial.[151] Without modification of exacerbating activities, the prognosis for symptom resolution is limited. Patients with severe symptoms or who fail to improve with conservative management should be referred for further evaluation.

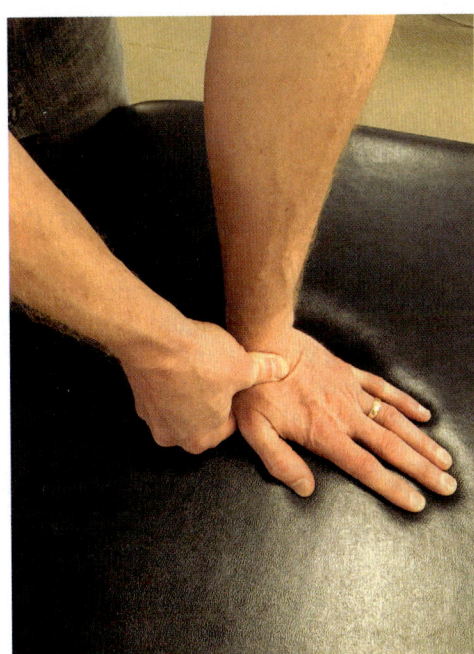

FIGURE 16-79 Self-mobilization for carpal tunnel syndrome.

Surgical release of the carpal tunnel may provide lasting symptom relief for these individuals.[151]

Ulnar Nerve Compression at the Tunnel of Guyon

Although much less common in CTS or cubital tunnel syndrome, the ulnar nerve is at risk for compression in the tunnel of Guyon, leading to sensory and potentially motor deficits pending the exact zone of injury.[152] Compression can occur from space-occupying ganglion cysts, swelling and displacement associated with hook of the hamate fractures, and positional compression, such as prolonged cycling.

Patients with ulnar neuropathy at the tunnel of Guyon report numbness and tingling in the ulnar nerve distribution of the hand. This can be transient and noted only during activity, as in the case of a recreational cyclist. In cases of insidious onset, clinicians should thoroughly evaluate the cervical spine and the more proximal segments of the ulnar nerve for possible involvement. Patients with mild or intermittent symptoms are likely to have full symptom resolution with conservative care. Patient education, activity modification, and ergonomic changes, such as the use of cycling gloves, are the mainstay of treatment.

Patients with prolonged or high nerve compression, such as from a large ganglion cyst, will have more constant symptoms, which may progress to causing weakness of the ulnar innervated hand intrinsics, intrinsic atrophy, and a positive Froment sign. Patients with atrophy or whose onset of symptoms began after hamate fracture should be referred for further evaluation. Surgical treatment may involve excision of space-occupying cysts, release of fibrous bands, or removal of bony protrusions. Patients undergoing surgical management rarely require postoperative treatment.

Complex Regional Pain Syndrome

CRPS is a debilitating pain condition that can occur after surgery or minimal trauma. The pathophysiology of CRPS is not completely understood. It is a complex condition involving peripheral and central nervous system sensitization, autonomic dysfunction, and psychological distress.[153,154] Although CRPS can occur in the lower extremity, most commonly after an ankle sprain, it is more prevalent in the upper extremity, particularly after distal radius facture,[155] shoulder surgery,[156] and stroke. CRPS affects women more than men.[157] Patients with CRPS present with two or more of the characteristics noted in Table 16-15.[157–159] Patients may also have coexisting psychological or emotional conditions. Most cases of CRPS affect only one limb.[158]

Individuals with CRPS typically have sustained a minor injury, fracture, or recent surgery and have pain disproportionate to the degree of injury. The involved extremity is typically swollen and discolored (Fig. 16-80). Often, patients will demonstrate kinesiophobia and catastrophizing.[157] If the upper extremity is involved, the patient will typically hold the limb in a sling-type position and refrain from using it. Light touch, even from clothing, is perceived to be incredibly painful.

Recovery is optimized by early recognition, intensive rehabilitation, and a multidisciplinary approach that includes pain management and psychological treatment if warranted.[158] Therefore, it is critical that clinicians identify the classic signs and symptoms of CRPS and consult with additional health care providers. Early motion and avoidance of immobilization

TABLE 16-15	
CHARACTERISTICS OF COMPLEX REGIONAL PAIN SYNDROME	
Characteristics	*Example*
Sensory changes	Hyperalgesia
Vasomotor changes	Changes in skin color (local areas of white, red, blue) Changes in skin temperature (local areas of cold or hot)
Sweating or edema	Edema Changes in sweating or asymmetries of sweating
Motor or trophic changes	Nail, hair changes (thin, brittle) Changes in skin texture Weakness, tremor Decreased range of motion Bone changes (osteopenia)

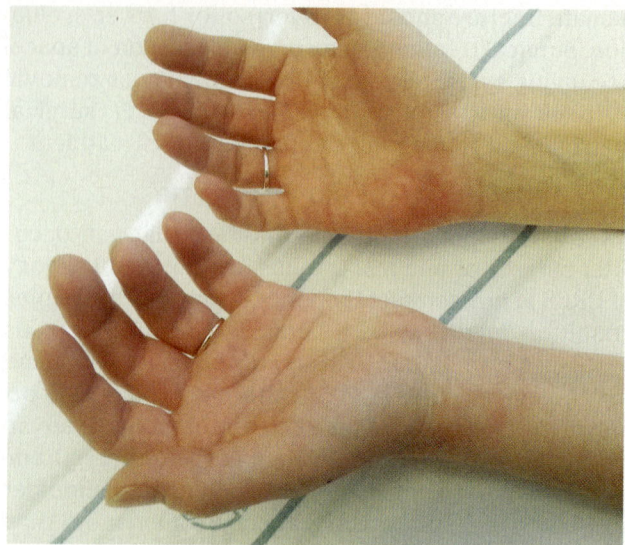

FIGURE 16-80 Physical changes of a patient with complex regional pain syndrome: the left hand has color changes and appears glossy. (Hoppenfeld JD. *Fundamentals of Pain Medicine: How to Diagnose and Treat Your Patients.* Wolters Kluwer Health; 2014: Figure 7-2.)

are considered a critical first step in the management of CPRS.[158] Intermittent elevation and hourly gentle AROM, such as gripping, can assist with edema management. Manual lymph drainage can also help reduce edema.[153] Progressive desensitization can be used to help decrease hypersensitivity.[153] For example, a patient may slide a piece of silky fabric over the affected area and the contralateral side. This smooth, soft material provides a mild stress to the local sensory fibers. As the patient becomes less sensitive to this (the silk feels like silk rather than needles or a threat), rougher material, such as cotton, are introduced. This is progressed to more abrasive materials, such as blue jeans. Graded motor imagery and mirror therapy may be beneficial in reducing pain and improving function.[160] It is postulated that these aide in cortical reorganization.[157] In addition, clinicians should encourage a graded return to activity.[153] Medications, such as analgesics,[158] gabapentin, and amitriptyline, can provide significant pain reduction.[161] Psychological treatment, including cognitive–behavioral therapy, should be considered.[157] Additional intervention options, if more conservative methods fail, include sympathetic nerve blocks, spinal cord stimulation, and dorsal root ganglion neurostimulation.[154,162]

The majority of patients will recover within 6 to 12 months.[158] However, up to 20% of patient will have persistent symptoms.[158] Chapter 19, Pain Management: A Mechanisms Centered Approach, provides additional details on the holistic management of patients with chronic pain.

DIFFERENTIAL DIAGNOSIS

Clinicians should consider the patient's chief complaint (Table 16-16), symptom location (Fig. 16-81), and onset (Fig. 16-82) to begin narrowing down differential diagnoses for patients with wrist and hand pathology.

ADDITIONAL JOINT MOBILIZATION TREATMENT TECHNIQUES

The accessory motion procedures described earlier can be used to treat wrist and hand hypomobility, particularly when using grade 3 and 4 mobilizations and/or performing closer to end-range. This section provides additional manual techniques to improve ROM.

TABLE 16-16

DIFFERENTIAL DIAGNOSIS OF WRIST AND HAND PATHOLOGY BY COMPLAINT

Complaint/Symptom	Differential Diagnoses
Weak	Tendon rupture Osteoarthritis Peripheral nerve injury
Paresthesias	Cervical dysfunction Carpal tunnel syndrome Wartenberg syndrome Ulnar nerve compression
Unstable, catching	TFCC pathology Scapholunate ligament sprain Lunotriquetral ligament sprain Midcarpal instability Ulnar collateral ligament sprain
Stiffness	Osteoarthritis Post-immobilization
Difficulty opening fingers or hand	Dupuytren contracture Trigger finger Carpometacarpal joint osteoarthritis Finger osteoarthritis
Deformity	Osteoarthritis Rheumatoid arthritis Extensor tendon disruption Peripheral nerve injury
Pain with gripping	Flexor pollicis longus tenosynovitis Carpometacarpal joint osteoarthritis
Pain with ulnar deviation	de Quervain tenosynovitis Intersection syndrome Wartenberg syndrome TFCC pathology
Pain with weight bearing	TFCC pathology Scapholunate ligament sprain Lunotriquetral ligament sprain Midcarpal instability

TFCC, triangular fibrocartilage complex.

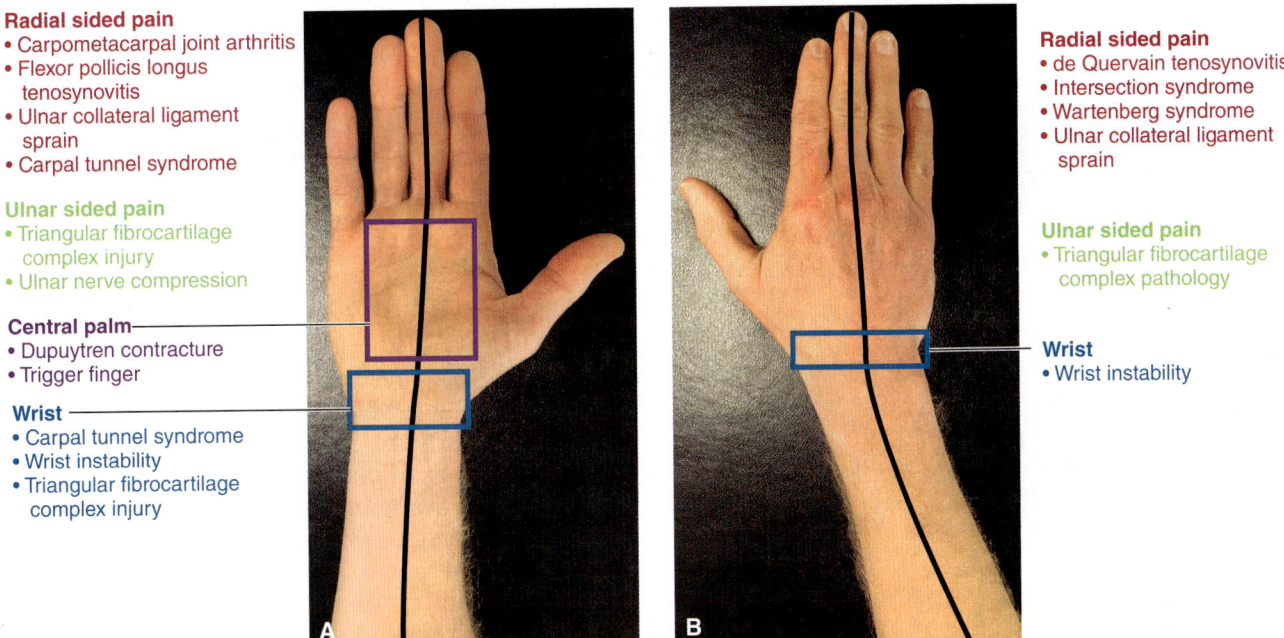

FIGURE 16-81 Wrist and hand pathology by symptom location. **A.** Palmar view. **B.** Dorsal view.

Palmar Radiocarpal Glide with Movement

Purpose: To improve wrist extension ROM.
Patient: Forearm pronated resting at the edge of the treatment table.
Clinician: The clinician places the fourth or fifth finger on the dorsal aspect of the proximal row of carpals and wraps the thumbs around the patient's palm to support the hand. The table is used to stabilize the forearm.

Mobilization: The clinician applies a palmar force to the proximal row of carpals while moving the wrist into further extension (Fig. 16-83). The mobilization can be performed targeting the midcarpal joint by having the clinician contact the dorsal aspect of the distal row of carpals.

Palmar Glide of Scaphoid

Purpose: To improve wrist extension.

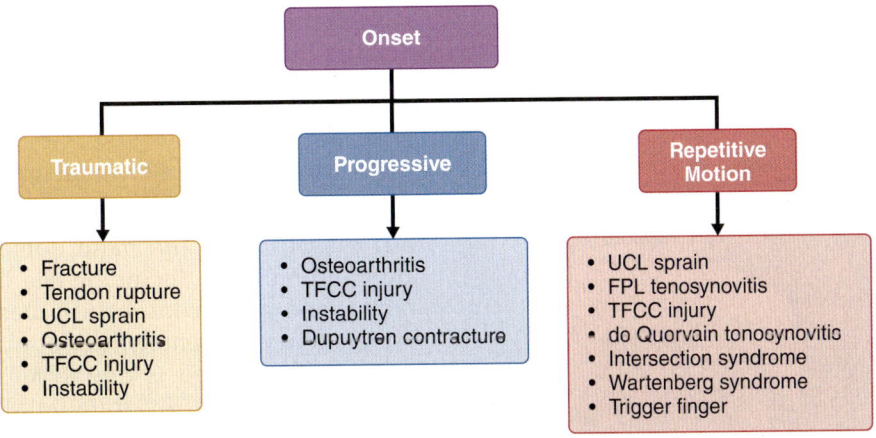

FIGURE 16-82 Wrist and hand pathology based on typical onset. *FPL*, flexor pollicis longus; *TFCC*, triangular fibrocartilage complex; *UCL*, ulnar collateral ligament.

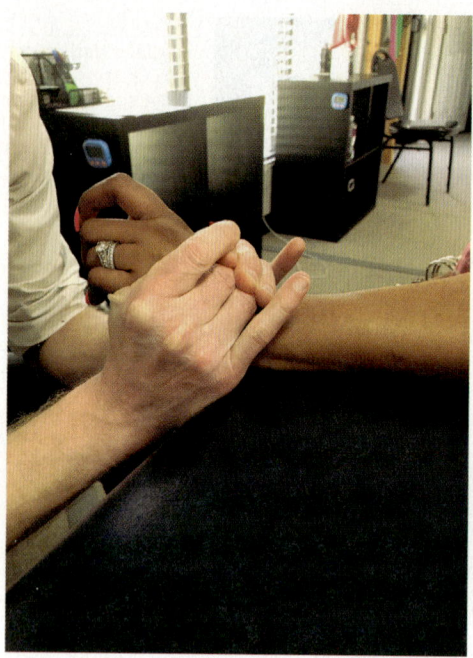

FIGURE 16-83 Palmar radiocarpal glide with movement.

Patient: Forearm pronated resting at the edge of the treatment table.

Clinician: The clinician contacts the dorsal scaphoid with the thumbs and supports the patient's hand by wrapping the fingers around the patient's palm.

Mobilization: The clinician applies a palmar force to the scaphoid (Fig. 16-84). The mobilization can be performed with movement similar to the previous treatment technique.

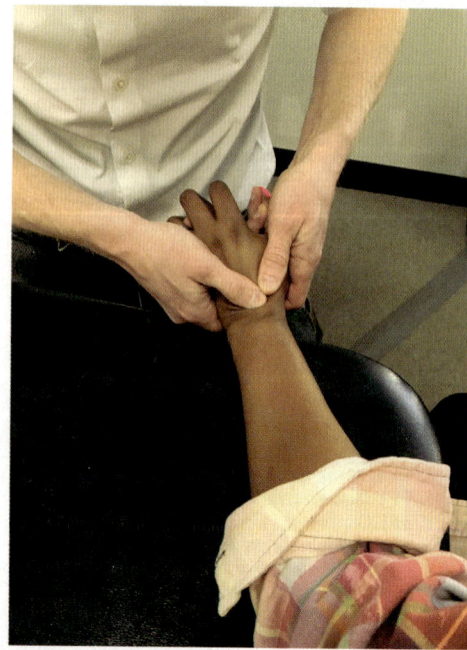

FIGURE 16-84 Palmar glide of scaphoid.

ADDITIONAL THERAPEUTIC INTERVENTIONS

The interventions described throughout this chapter may be beneficial for a variety of patients and diagnoses. This section contains additional examples of exercises for improving ROM and strength, as well as joint protection strategies that can lead to improved function.

Interventions for Range of Motion

The complexity of the joints and multijoint muscles of the fingers requires careful evaluation and management. Finger joints should be stretched individually, not solely grossly, to ensure each joint is moved to end-range. ROM and muscle elongation may be easier after an active warm-up. Performing AROM within a fluidotherapy unit may help gain motion. Likewise, clinicians may use paraffin to assist with skin mobility, joint motion, and pain modulation. Either painting or dipping the hand into paraffin to create multiple layers, then covering the area in plastic wrap or a plastic bag and toweling for 10 to 20 minutes before stretching may be useful. For a more aggressive stretch, a joint can be place on stretch and taped into that position and then dipped into the paraffin or placed under a hot pack.

When stretching the wrist joint, simultaneous elongation over the joints of the hand should be avoided, as this creates passive insufficiency of the finger flexors and extensors, thereby prematurely limiting wrist motion. To stretch the FDS and FDP, the standing patient can place the hand on a table, then actively (or use the other hand to) extend the joints distal to proximal until the hand is flat on the table. Once the fingers are fully extended, the patient can use the other hand to maintain finger extension while the trunk is moved to extend the wrist until a comfortable stretch is felt. Stretching can also be performed from distal to proximal. For example, to stretch the EDC, the patient can actively or passively flex the DIP, PIP, and MCP in succession. Then, maintaining full finger flexion, being to flex the wrist until a stretch is felt.

Interventions for Strengthening

Fine motor control occurs via the long finger flexors, but the power of the hand comes from the intrinsic hand muscles, including the lumbricals and the dorsal and palmar interossei. Despite their varying attachments, ultimately, the power the intrinsic finger muscles deliver is due to MCP flexion with DIP and PIP extension. By training MCP flexion with IP extension, grip strength can reliably be improved. The addition of finger abduction (emphasis on the

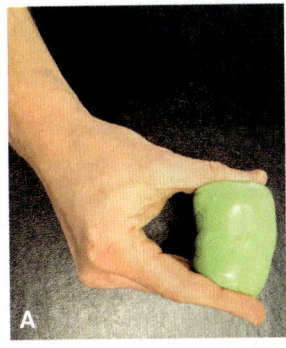 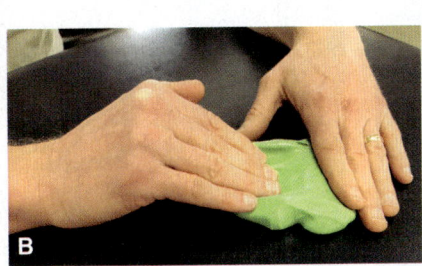 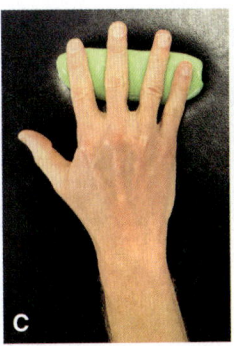 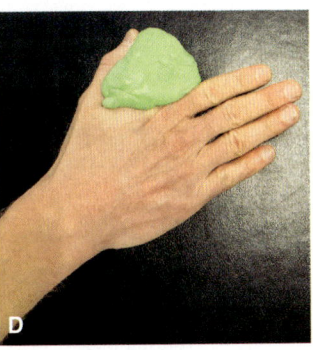

FIGURE 16-85 Putty for intrinsic strengthening. **A.** MCP flexion with IP joints extended. **B.** MCP flexion with wrist extension. **C.** MCP flexion and adduction. **D.** Thumb adduction. *IP*, interphalangeal; *MCP*, metacarpophalangeal.

dorsal interossei) and finger adduction (emphasis on the palmar interossei) may prove beneficial as well. Squeezing large objects, such as a tennis ball, should not be encouraged unless functionally relevant, as this recruits the FDS and FDP, rather than the hand intrinsics. It is important to incorporate wrist strengthening as a stable wrist is required to balance out the influence of the long flexors. There are multiple ways in which putty can be used to strength the intrinsics without over-recruiting the FDS and FDP (Fig. 16-85).

Joint Protection Strategies

Joint protection is a form of activity modification that may require frequent cues and repetitive practice to change a patient's typical movement patterns. Some joint protection strategies are listed as follows:

- Pour with two hands, not one.
- Use cups with larger handles and support with contralateral hand as needed.
- Plates and papers: support in supination (palms up) rather than grasping in pronation (palms down).
- When cooking, stir with a neutral forearm (thumbs up), rather than pronated (thumbs down).
- Writing utensils: using foam to widen utensil size can reduce the force required to hold and joint compressive forces.
- Opening jars: use pads to help increase transfer of force and do not allow fingers to deviate away from neutral.
- Pots: lift with two hands on handle or one hand on handle and on under the opposite side.

Although research is lacking for joint protection in arthritic hands,[163] clinicians may choose to apply these joint protection strategies to improve patient function in a safe manner.

Short-term use of a prefabricated wrist orthosis (Fig. 16-86) can be useful for individuals with severe wrist sprains or for nighttime use for individuals with CTS.

Athletic taping during activities can allow individuals to safely participate in sporting activities. Thumb spica taping, and variations thereof, can be used to protect individuals with thumb CMC pathology or collateral ligament sprains (Fig. 16-87).

H-taping can be used for rock climbers or other types of pulley injuries (Fig. 16-88). The taping helps offload the pulleys during gripping activities, such as the crimp grip used in rock climbing.

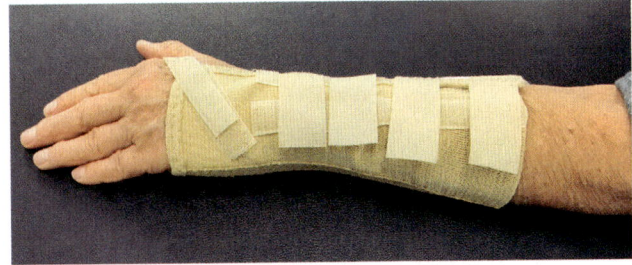

FIGURE 16-86 Prefabricated wrist orthosis.

634 SECTION IV | UPPER QUARTER

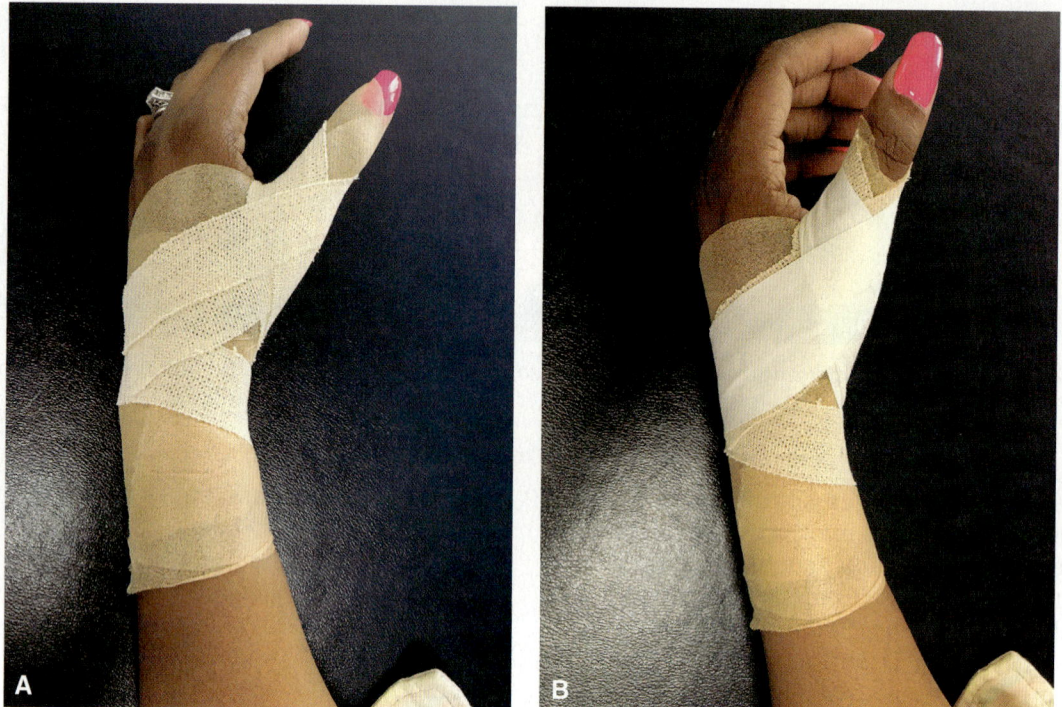

FIGURE 16-87 Wrist and hand pathology by symptom location. **A.** Palmar view. **B.** Dorsal view.

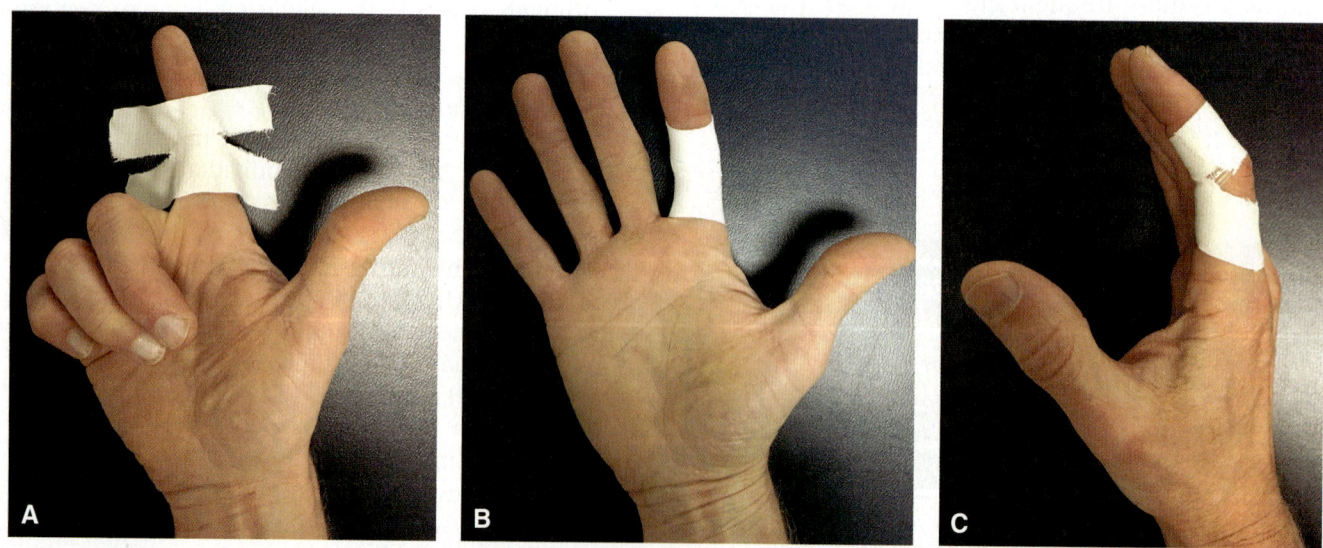

FIGURE 16-88 H-taping. **A.** Initial tape placement. Completed taping volar (**B**) and radial (**C**) views.

CASE STUDY 16-1
Ruth: Patient with Wrist Pain

Ruth is a 64-year-old female who reports falling 3 days ago landing on her outstretched dominant hand. She does not recall what made her fall and is unsure of how her hand/wrist were positioned at the time of the fall. She reports her wrist was immediately sore and assumed it would resolve with ice and time. Because her wrist felt only somewhat better, she decided to have the injury assessed by a clinician. When describing the location of her pain, Ruth points to her radial and palmar right wrist. All tests begin with the uninvolved (left) side unless otherwise noted. The examination should begin away and progress toward the involved area and provide increasing stress to injured or potentially involved structures. Table 16-17 provides an example of how an experienced clinician might organize the physical examination after performing the history and systems review.

TABLE 16-17

SAMPLE WRIST EXAMINATION

Ruth: 64-year-old female with right wrist pain after a fall

Position	Assessments
Observation	Continues from history
Seated	Palpation: bony palpation of the scaphoid, radius, ulna as well as the remaining carpals, and palmar wrist. Scaphoid compression test Thumb flex, ext, abd, add, opposition (A, P, MMT) Elbow flex, ext (A, P, MMT) Forearm pronation, supination (A, P, MMT) Finger composite flexion (A) Wrist resisted isometric testing: flex, ext, ulnar deviation, radial deviation Wrist ulnar deviation, radial deviation, flex, ext (A, P, MMT) Grip Pinch: lateral, 3-point Wrist accessory motion: palmar, dorsal, radial, ulnar Special tests: midcarpal shift test, scaphoid shift test
Standing	Gait Balance assessment: Berg balance test

A, active; *abd*, abduction; *add*, adduction; *ext*, extension; *flex*, flexion; *MMT*, manual muscle test; *P*, passive range of motion.

Based on the history, the clinician's initial hypotheses were fracture and wrist sprain. The examination begins with bony palpation, scaphoid compression test, and assessment of thumb active motion to determine the need for radiographs. As the results were negative, the clinician continued in the same region to assess for tenderness of the wrist ligaments, radial wrist, and proximal thumb. After noting full and symptom-free thumb motion, MMT was performed. The clinician then moved more proximally to clear involvement of the elbow and forearm. Moving back distally, the clinician cleared the fingers via assessing composite flexion, knowing the grip and pinch strength would be assessed shortly. Having cleared proximal and distal joints, the examination continued with wrist-specific assessments. Given the patient's noted pain with movement, testing began with resisted isometric testing in a neutral position to obtain a cursory understanding as to if a contractile lesion may be present. This was followed by a comparison of active and passive wrist motion while noting symptom provocation. Resisted MMT was performed as AROM was full. To complete the muscle performance assessment, grip and pinch testing were performed. The wrist-specific examination concluded with assessment of joint mobility and instability to thoroughly investigate the clinician's hypothesis of wrist sprain. Once the wrist-specific examination was complete, the clinician chose to assess the patient's gait and perform a balance assessment to determine whether the patient may benefit from balance training to decrease the risk of future falls.

CHAPTER SUMMARY

Traumatic, degenerative, and repetitive motion injuries are common in the wrist and hand. Patient symptoms may also be referred from more proximal regions. Examination and treatment of patients with wrist or hand symptoms begins with a thorough history to determine whether the symptoms are from local tissues or referred from other areas. An upper quarter screen and clearing joints proximal and distal joints, including consideration for multijoint structures, help further elucidate the source of the patient complaint. The wrist and hand joint-specific examination is further fine-tuned based on the history and basic examination findings to include selected accessory motion testing, special tests, and palpation. Rehabilitation strategies for the wrist and hand must consider the intricate biomechanics of the region and be individualized for each patient for best outcomes.

REFERENCES

1. Neumann D. *Kinesiology of the Musculoskeletal System: Foundations for Rehabilitation.* 3rd ed. Elsevier; 2017.
2. Obert L, Loisel F, Gasse N, Lepage D. Distal radius anatomy applied to the treatment of wrist fractures by plate: a review of recent literature. *SICOT J.* 2015;1:14. doi:10.1051/sicotj/2015012
3. af Ekenstam F, Hagert C. Anatomical studies on the geometry and stability of the distal radio ulnar joint. *Scand J Plast Reconstr Surg.* 1985;19(1):17–25. doi:10.3109/02844318509052861
4. Kitay A, Wolfe S. Scapholunate instability: current concepts in diagnosis and management. *J Hand Surg Am.* 2012;37(10):2175–2196. doi:10.1016/j.jhsa.2012.07.035
5. Wadsworth C. The wrist and hand. In: *Current Concepts of Orthopaedic Physical Therapy.* (Independent Study Course 16.2.6): 1–60.
6. Moore KL, Dalley AF, Agur AMR. *Clinically Oriented Anatomy.* 8th ed. Wolters Kluwer; 2018.
7. Williams P, Warwick R, Myson M, Bannister L, eds. *Gray's Anatomy.* 37th ed. Churchill Livingstone; 1989.
8. Tolat A, Stanley J, Trail I. A cadaveric study of the anatomy and stability of the distal radioulnar joint in the coronal and transverse planes. *J Hand Surg Br.* 1996;21(5):587–594. doi:10.1016/s0266-7681(96)80136-7
9. Mauck B, Swigler C. Evidence-based review of distal radius fractures. *Orthop Clin North Am.* 2018;49(2):211–222. doi:10.1016/j.ocl.2017.12.001
10. Zancolli E. *Anatomy of the Hand: Anatomy of the TFCC. Hand Clin.* 2013;17(1):146–147.
11. Ahn A, Chang D, Plate A. Triangular fibrocartilage complex tears: a review. *Bull NYU Hosp Jt Dis.* 2006;64(3–4):114–118.
12. Schuind F, An K, Berglund L, et al. The distal radioulnar ligaments: a biomechanical study. *J Hand Surg Am.* 1991;16(6):1106–1114. doi:10.1016/s0363-5023(10)80075-9
13. af Ekenstam F. Anatomy of the distal radioulnar joint. *Clin Orthop Relat Res.* 1992;(275):14–18.
14. Haugstvedt J, Langer M, Berger R. Distal radioulnar joint: functional anatomy, including pathomechanics. *J Hand Surg Eur Vol.* 2017;42(4):338–345. doi:10.1177/1753193417693170
15. Jawed A, Ansari M, Gupta V. TFCC injuries: how we treat? *J Clin Orthop Trauma.* 2020;11(4):570–579. doi:10.1016/j.jcot.2020.06.001
16. Palmer A, Werner F. The triangular fibrocartilage complex of the wrist—anatomy and function. *J Hand Surg Am.* 1981;6(2):153–162. doi:10.1016/s0363-5023(81)80170-0
17. Moradi A, Binava R, Vahedi E, Ebrahimzadeh M, Jupiter J. Distal radioulnar joint prosthesis. *Arch Bone Joint Surg.* 2021;9(1):22–32. doi:10.22038/abjs.2020.53537.2659
18. Palmer A. Triangular fibrocartilage complex lesions: a classification. *J Hand Surg Am.* 1989;14(4):594–606. doi:10.1016/0363-5023(89)90174-3
19. Skalski M, White E, Patel D, Schein A, RiveraMelo H, Matcuk G Jr. The traumatized TFCC: an illustrated review of the anatomy and injury patterns of the triangular fibrocartilage complex. *Curr Probl Diagn Radiol.* 2016;45(1):39–50. doi:10.1067/j.cpradiol.2015.05.004
20. Palmer A, Glisson R, Werner F. Relationship between ulnar variance and triangular fibrocartilage complex thickness. *J Hand Surg Am.* 1984;9(5):681–682. doi:10.1016/s0363-5023(84)80013-1
21. Chidgey L, Dell P, Bittar E, Spanier S. Histologic anatomy of the triangular fibrocartilage. *J Hand Surg Am.* 1991;16(6):1084–1100. doi:10.1016/s0363-5023(10)80073-5
22. Su F, Chou Y, Yang C, Lin G, An K. Movement of finger joints induced by synergistic wrist motion. *Clin Biomech (Bristol, Avon).* 2005;20(5):491–497. doi:10.1016/j.clinbiomech.2005.01.002
23. Arimitsu S, Murase T, Hashimoto J, et al. A three-dimensional quantitative analysis of carpal deformity in rheumatoid wrists. *J Bone Joint Surg Br.* 2007;89(4):490–494. doi:10.1302/0301-620x.89b4.18476
24. Arik A, Tanrikulu S, Demiray T, Leblebicioglu G. Radial reference points for measuring palmar tilt and ulnar variance on lateral wrist radiographs. *J Hand Surg Asian Pac Vol.* 2020;25(1):95–103. doi:10.1142/s2424835520500137
25. Kaufmann R, Pfaeffle J, Blankenhorn B, Stabile K, Robertson D, Goitz R. Kinematics of the midcarpal and radiocarpal joints in radioulnar deviation: an in vitro study. *J Hand Surg Am.* 2005;30(5):937–942. doi:10.1016/j.jhsa.2005.05.016
26. Kobayashi M, Berger R, Nagy L, et al. Normal kinematics of carpal bones: a three-dimensional analysis of carpal bone motion relative to the radius. *J Biomech.* 1997;30(8):787–793. doi:10.1016/s0021-9290(97)00026-2
27. Short W, Werner F, Fortino M, Mann K. Analysis of the kinematics of the scaphoid and lunate in the intact wrist joint. *Hand Clin.* 1997;13(1):93–108.
28. Ruby L, Cooney WP III, An K, Linscheid R, Chao E. Relative motion of selected carpal bones: a kinematic analysis of the normal wrist. *J Hand Surg Am.* 1988;13(1):1–10. doi:10.1016/0363-5023(88)90189-x
29. Moritomo H, Murase T, Goto A, Oka K, Sugamoto K, Yoshikawa H. Capitate-based kinematics of the midcarpal joint during wrist radioulnar deviation: an in vivo three-dimensional motion analysis. *J Hand Surg Am.* 2004;29(4):668–675. doi:10.1016/j.jhsa.2004.04.010
30. Pang E, Yao J. Anatomy and biomechanics of the finger proximal interphalangeal joint. *Hand Clin.* 2018;34(2):121–126. doi:10.1016/j.hcl.2017.12.002
31. Lee S, Ng Z, Fogg Q. Three-dimensional analysis of the palmar plate and collateral ligaments at the proximal interphalangeal joint. *J Hand Surg Eur Vol.* 2014;39(4):391–397. doi:10.1177/1753193413492288
32. al-Qattan M, Robertson G. An anatomical study of the deep transverse metacarpal ligament. *J Anat.* 1993;182(Pt 3)(Pt 3):443–446.
33. Carruthers K, Skie M, Jain M. Jam injuries of the finger: diagnosis and management of injuries to the interphalangeal joints across multiple sports and levels of experience. *Sports Health.* 2016;8(5):469–478.
34. Berger R. The anatomy of the ligaments of the wrist and distal radioulnar joints. *Clin Orthop Relat Res.* 2001;(383):32–40. doi:10.1097/00003086-200102000-00006

35. Hagert E. Proprioception of the wrist joint: a review of current concepts and possible implications on the rehabilitation of the wrist. *J Hand Ther*. 2010;23(1):2–17. doi:10.1016/j.jht.2009.09.008
36. Hagert E, Garcia-Elias M, Forsgren S, Ljung B. Immunohistochemical analysis of wrist ligament innervation in relation to their structural composition. *J Hand Surg Am*. 2007;32(1):30–36. doi:10.1016/j.jhsa.2006.10.005
37. Vekris M, Mataliotakis G, Beris A. The scapholunate interosseous ligament afferent proprioceptive pathway: a human in vivo experimental study. *J Hand Surg Am*. 2011;36(1):37–46. doi:10.1016/j.jhsa.2010.10.002
38. Mataliotakis G, Doukas M, Kostas I, Lykissas M, Batistatou A, Beris A. Sensory innervation of the subregions of the scapholunate interosseous ligament in relation to their structural composition. *J Hand Surg Am*. 2009;34(8):1413–1421. doi:10.1016/j.jhsa.2009.05.007
39. Sjölander P, Johansson H, Djupsjöbacka M. Spinal and supraspinal effects of activity in ligament afferents. *J Electromyogr Kinesiol*. 2002;12(3):167–176. doi:10.1016/s1050-6411(02)00017-2
40. Lin J, Karl J, Strauch R. Trapeziometacarpal joint stability: the evolving importance of the dorsal ligaments. *Clin Orthop Relat Res*. 2014;472(4):1138–1145. doi:10.1007/s11999-013-2879-9
41. Ladd A, Weiss A, Crisco J, et al. The thumb carpometacarpal joint: anatomy, hormones, and biomechanics. *Instr Course Lect*. 2013;62:165–179.
42. Ladd A, Lee J, Hagert E. Macroscopic and microscopic analysis of the thumb carpometacarpal ligaments: a cadaveric study of ligament anatomy and histology. *J Bone Joint Surg Am*. 2012;94(16):1468–1477. doi:10.2106/jbjs.K.00329
43. Pellegrini V Jr. Osteoarthritis of the trapeziometacarpal joint: the pathophysiology of articular cartilage degeneration. I. Anatomy and pathology of the aging joint. *J Hand Surg Am*. 1991;16(6):967–974. doi:10.1016/s0363-5023(10)80054-1
44. Zafonte B, Rendulic D, Szabo R. Flexor pulley system: anatomy, injury, and management. *J Hand Surg Am*. 2014;39(12):2525–2532; quiz 2533. doi:10.1016/j.jhsa.2014.06.005
45. Lin G, Cooney W, Amadio P, An K. Mechanical properties of human pulleys. *J Hand Surg Br*. 1990;15(4):429–434. doi:10.1016/0266-7681(90)90085-i
46. Day CS, Wu WK, Smith CC. Examination of the hand and wrist. *N Eng J Med*. 2019;380(12):e15. doi:10.1056/NEJMvcm1407111
47. Huisstede BM, Hoogvliet P, Coert JH, Friden J. Multidisciplinary consensus guideline for managing trigger finger: results from the European HANDGUIDE Study. *Phys Ther*. 2014;94(10):1421–1433.
48. Kane PM, Daniels AH, Akelman E. Double crush syndrome. *J Am Acad Orthop Surg*. 2015;23(9):558–562. doi:10.5435/JAAOS-D-14-00176
49. Altman E. The ulnar side of the wrist: clinically relevant anatomy and biomechanics. *J Hand Ther*. 2016;29(2):111–122. doi:10.1016/j.jht.2016.03.012
50. Petersen PB, Mikkelsen KL, Lauritzen JB, Krogsgaard MR. Risk factors for post-treatment complex regional pain syndrome (CRPS): an analysis of 647 cases of CRPS from the Danish Patient Compensation Association. *Pain Pract*. 2018;18(3):341–349. doi:10.1111/papr.12610
51. Elsharydah A, Loo NH, Minhajuddin A, Kandil ES. Complex regional pain syndrome type 1 predictors—epidemiological perspective from a national database analysis. *J Clin Anesth*. 2017;39:34–37. doi:10.1016/j.jclinane.2017.03.027
52. Brosseau L, Thevenot O, MacKiddie O, et al. The Ottawa Panel guidelines on programmes involving therapeutic exercise for the management of hand osteoarthritis. *Clin Rehabil*. 2018;32(11):1449–1471. doi:10.1177/0269215518780973
53. Naughton N, Algar L. Linking commonly used hand therapy outcome measures to individual areas of the International Classification of Functioning: a systematic review. *J Hand Ther*. 2019;32(2):243–261.
54. Streppa J, Schneidman V, Biron A. Requesting wrist radiographs in emergency department triage: developing a training program and diagnostic algorithm. *Adv Emerg Nurs J*. 2014;36(1):62–77. doi:10.1097/TME.0000000000000005
55. Tsyrulnik A. Emergency department evaluation and treatment of wrist injuries. *Emerg Med Clin North Am*. 2015;33(2):283–296. doi:10.1016/j.emc.2014.12.003
56. Urch EY, Lee SK. Carpal fractures other than scaphoid. *Clin Sports Med*. 2015;34(1):51–67. doi:10.1016/j.csm.2014.09.006
57. Burrows B, Moreira P, Murphy C, Sadi J, Walton DM. Scaphoid fractures: a higher order analysis of clinical tests and application of clinical reasoning strategies. *Man Ther*. 2014;19(5):372–378. doi:10.1016/j.math.2014.05.007
58. Chen SC. The scaphoid compression test. *J Hand Surg*. 1989;14B:323–325.
59. Avery DM III, Rodner CM, Edgar CM. Sports-related wrist and hand injuries: a review. *J Orthop Surg Res*. 2016;11(1):99. doi:10.1186/s13018-016-0432-8
60. Shymko M. Fractures of the scaphoid. *Radiol Technol*. 2017;89(2):177–181.
61. Mahmood B, Lee S. Carpal fractures other than scaphoid in the athlete. *Clin Sports Med*. 2020;39(2):353–371.
62. Pershad J, Monroe K, King W, Bartle S, Hardin E, Zinkan L. Can clinical parameters predict fractures in acute pediatric wrist injuries? *Acad Emerg Med*. 2000;7(10):1152–1155. doi:10.1111/j.1553-2712.2000.tb01267.x
63. Porretto-Loehrke A, Schuh C, Szekeres M. Clinical manual assessment of the wrist. *J Hand Ther*. 2016;29(2):123–135. doi:10.1016/j.jht.2016.02.008
64. Saccomano SJ, Ferrara LR. Assessment and management of wrist pain. *Nurse Pract*. 2017;42(8):15–19. doi:10.1097/01.NPR.0000520834.99158.4e
65. Llanos C, Gan EY, Chen J, Lee M-J, Kilbreath SL, Dylke ES. Reliability and validity of physical tools and measurement methods to quantify hand swelling: a systematic review. *Phys Ther*. 2021;101(2):pzaa206. doi:10.1093/ptj/pzaa206
66. Goodman CC, Heick J, Lazaro RT. *Differential Diagnosis for Physical Therapists: Screening for Referral*. 6th ed. Elsevier; 2018.
67. Huisstede BM, Hoogvliet P, Coert JH, Fridén J. Dupuytren disease: European hand surgeons, hand therapists, and physical medicine and rehabilitation physicians agree on a multidisciplinary treatment guideline: results from the HANDGUIDE study. *Plast Reconstr Surg*. 2013;132(6):964e–976e. doi:10.1097/01.prs.0000434410.40217.23
68. Clarkson HM. *Musculoskeletal Assessment: Joint Range of Motion, Muscle Testing, and Function*. 4th ed. Wolters Kluwer; 2021.
69. American Academy of Orthopedic Surgeons. *American Academy of Orthopedic Surgeons: Joint Motion: Method of Measuring and Recording*. AAOS; 1965.
70. Ellis B, Bruton A. A study to compare the reliability of composite finger flexion with goniometry for measurement of range of motion in the hand. *Clin Rehabil*. 2002;16(5):562–570. doi:10.1191/0269215502cr513oa
71. Kaltenborn F. *Manual Mobilization of the Joints: The Extremities*. 5th ed. Olaf Norlis Bokhandel; 1999.
72. Kaltenborn F, Evjenth O, Kaltenborn T, Vollowitz E. *The Spine: Basic Evaluation and Mobilization Techniques*. 2nd ed. Olaf Norlis Bokhandel Universitetsgaten; 1993.

73. Cyriax J. *Textbook of Orthopedic Medicine: Diagnosis of Soft Tissue Lesions.* Vol 1. 8th ed. Saunders; 1989.
74. Edmond S. *Manipulations and Mobilizations: Extremity and Spinal Techniques.* Mosby; 1993.
75. Kendall FP, McCreary EK, Provance PG, Rogers MM, Romani WA. *Muscles: Testing and Function with Posture and Pain.* 5th ed. Lippincott Williams & Wilkins; 2005.
76. Erickson M, Lawrence M, Stegink Jansen C, Coker D, Amadio P, Cleary C. Hand pain and sensory deficits: carpal tunnel syndrome. *J Orthop Sports Phys Ther.* 2019;49(5):CPG1–CPG85. doi:10.2519/jospt.2019.0301
77. Thoomes EJ, van Geest S, van der Windt DA, et al. Value of physical tests in diagnosing cervical radiculopathy: a systematic review. *Spine.* 2018;18(1):179–189. doi:10.1016/j.spinee.2017.08.241
78. Lemeunier N, Silva-Oolup S, Chow N, et al. Reliability and validity of clinical tests to assess the anatomical integrity of the cervical spine in adults with neck pain and its associated disorders: part 1—a systematic review from the Cervical Assessment and Diagnosis Research Evaluation (CADRE) Collaboration. *Eur Spine J.* 2017;26(9):2225–2241. doi:10.1007/s00586-017-5153-0
79. Kaltenborn F. *Manual Mobilization of the Joints: The Extremities.* Vol 1. 7th ed. Norli; 2011.
80. Valdez K, LaStayo P. The value of provocative tests for the wrist and elbow: a literature review. *J Hand Ther.* 2013;26(1):32–42.
81. O'Brien L, Robinson L, Lim E, O'Sullivan H, Kavnoudias H. Cumulative incidence of carpal instability 12–24 months after fall onto outstretched hand. *J Hand Ther.* 2018;31(3):282–286.
82. Newton AW, Hawkes DH, Bhalaik V. Clinical examination of the wrist. *Orthop Trauma.* 2017;31(4):237–247. doi:10.1016/j.mporth.2017.05.009
83. Daley D, Geary M, Gaston R. Thumb metacarpophalangeal ulnar and radial collateral ligament injuries. *Clin Sports Med.* 2020;39:443–455.
84. Konin J, Lebscak D, Snyder Valier A. *Special Tests for Orthopaedic Examination.* SLACK Incorporated; 2016.
85. Dawson C, Mudgal CS. Staged description of the Finkelstein test. *J Hand Surg.* 2010;35(9):1513–1515. doi:https://doi.org/10.1016/j.jhsa.2010.05.022
86. Kirchberger MC, Unglaub F, Mühldorfer-Fodor M, et al. Update TFCC: histology and pathology, classification, examination and diagnostics. *Arch Orthop Trauma Surg.* 2015;135(3):427–437. doi:10.1007/s00402-015-2153-6
87. Spies CK, Langer M, Müller LP, Oppermann J, Unglaub F. Distal radioulnar joint instability: current concepts of treatment. *Arch Orthop Trauma Surg.* 2020;140(5):639–650.
88. Lester B, Hallbrecht J, Levy I, Gaudinez R. "Press test" for office diagnosis of triangular fibrocartilage complex tears of the wrist. *Ann Plast Surg.* 1995;35(1):41–45.
89. Dineen H, Greenberg J. Ulnar-sided wrist pain in the athlete. *Clin Sports Med.* 2020;39(2):373–400.
90. MacDermid JC, Doherty T. Clinical and electrodiagnostic testing of carpal tunnel syndrome: a narrative review. *J Orthop Sports Phys Ther.* 2004;34(10):565–588.
91. Ritting AW, Baldwin PC, Rodner CM. Ulnar collateral ligament injury of the thumb metacarpophalangeal joint. *Clin J Sport Med.* 2010;20(2):106–112. doi:10.1097/JSM.0b013e3181d23710
92. Kolasinski SL, Neogi T, Hochberg MC, et al. 2019 American College of Rheumatology/Arthritis Foundation Guideline for the management of osteoarthritis of the hand, hip, and knee. *Arthritis Rheumatol.* 2020;72(2):220–233. doi:10.1002/art.41142
93. Başar H, Özden E, Başar B. The effects of rehabilitation on the outcomes of surgically treated acute and chronic thumb metacarpophalangeal ulnar collateral ligament ruptures. *Hand Surg Rehabil.* 2020;39(4):291–295. doi:10.1016/j.hansur.2020.03.002
94. Johnson JD, Gaspar MP, Shin EK. Stenosing tenosynovitis due to excessive texting in an adolescent girl: a case report. *J Hand Microsurg.* 2016;8(1):45–48. doi:10.1055/s-0035-1571263
95. Azzi AJ, Aldekhayel S, Boehm KS, Zadeh T. Tendon rupture and tenosynovitis following internal fixation of distal radius fractures: a systematic review. *Plast Reconstr Surg.* 2017;139(3):717e–724e. doi:10.1097/prs.0000000000003076
96. Villafañe JH, Valdes K, Pedersini P, Berjano P. Thumb carpometacarpal osteoarthritis: a musculoskeletal physiotherapy perspective. *J Bodyw Mov Ther.* 2019;23(4):908–912.
97. Hickson M. Malnutrition and ageing. *Postgrad Med J.* 2006;82(963):2–8. doi:10.1136/pgmj.2005.037564
98. Sankah BEA, Stokes M, Adams J. Exercises for hand osteoarthritis: a systematic review of clinical practice guidelines and consensus recommendations. *Phys Ther Rev.* 2019;24(3/4):66–81.
99. Bertozzi L, Valdes K, Vanti C, Negrini S, Pillastrini P, Villafañe JH. Investigation of the effect of conservative interventions in thumb carpometacarpal osteoarthritis: systematic review and meta-analysis. *Disabil Rehabil.* 2015;37(22):2025–2043.
100. Kloppenburg M, Kroon FP, Blanco FJ, et al. 2018 update of the EULAR recommendations for the management of hand osteoarthritis. *Ann Rheum Dis.* 2019;78(1):16–24. doi:10.1136/annrheumdis-2018-213826
101. Tsehaie J, Spekreijse KR, Wouters RM, et al. Predicting outcome after hand orthosis and hand therapy for thumb carpometacarpal osteoarthritis: a prospective study. *Arch Phys Med Rehabil.* 2019;100(5):844–850. doi:10.1016/j.apmr.2018.08.192
102. Cantero-Téllez R, Villafañe JH, Valdes K, Berjano P. Effect of immobilization of metacarpophalangeal joint in thumb carpometacarpal osteoarthritis on pain and function. A quasi-experimental trial. *J Hand Ther.* 2018;31(1):68–73. doi:10.1016/j.jht.2016.11.005
103. Shankland B, Beaton D, Ahmed S, Nedelec B. Effects of client-centered multimodal treatment on impairment, function, and satisfaction of people with thumb carpometacarpal osteoarthritis. *J Hand Ther.* 2017;30(3):307–313. doi:10.1016/j.jht.2017.03.004
104. Wouters RM, Tsehaie J, Slijper HP, Hovius SER, Feitz R, Selles RW. Exercise therapy in addition to an orthosis reduces pain more than an orthosis alone in patients with thumb base osteoarthritis: a propensity score matching study. *Arch Phys Med Rehabil.* 2019;100(6):1050–1060. doi:10.1016/j.apmr.2018.11.010
105. Buhler M, Chapple CM, Stebbings S, Sangelaji B, Baxter GD. Effectiveness of splinting for pain and function in people with thumb carpometacarpal osteoarthritis: a systematic review with meta-analysis. *Osteoarthritis Cartilage.* 2019;27(4):547–559. doi:10.1016/j.joca.2018.09.012
106. Vermeulen GM, Slijper H, Feitz R, Hovius SE, Moojen TM, Selles RW. Surgical management of primary thumb carpometacarpal osteoarthritis: a systematic review. *J Hand Surg Am.* 2011;36(1):157–169. doi:10.1016/j.jhsa.2010.10.028
107. Crosby CA, Reitz JL, Mester EA, Grenier ML. Rehabilitation following thumb CMC, radiocarpal, and DRUJ arthroplasty. *Hand Clin.* 2013;29(1):123–142. doi:10.1016/j.hcl.2012.08.025
108. Wouters RM, Tsehaie J, Hovius SER, Dilek B, Selles RW. Postoperative rehabilitation following thumb base surgery: a

systematic review of the literature. *Arch Phys Med Rehabil.* 2018;99(6):1177–1212.e2. doi:10.1016/j.apmr.2017.09.114
109. López López CO, Alvarez-Hernández E, Medrano Ramirez G, et al. Hand function in rheumatic diseases: patient and physician evaluations. *Int J Rheum Dis.* 2014;17(8):856–862. doi:10.1111/1756-185x.12466
110. Kroon FPB, Carmona L, Schoones JW, Kloppenburg M. Efficacy and safety of non-pharmacological, pharmacological and surgical treatment for hand osteoarthritis: a systematic literature review informing the 2018 update of the EULAR recommendations for the management of hand osteoarthritis. *RMD Open.* 2018;4(2):e000734. doi:10.1136/rmdopen-2018-000734
111. Lamb SE, Williamson EM, Heine PJ, et al. Exercises to improve function of the rheumatoid hand (SARAH): a randomised controlled trial. *Lancet.* 2015;385(9966):421–429. doi:10.1016/s0140-6736(14)60998-3
112. Valdes K, Marik T. A systematic review of conservative interventions for osteoarthritis of the hand. *J Hand Ther.* 2010;23(4):334–350; quiz 351. doi:10.1016/j.jht.2010.05.001
113. Bellemère P. Treatment of chronic extensor tendons lesions of the fingers. *Chir Main.* 2015;34(4):155–181. doi:10.1016/j.main.2015.05.001
114. Williams K, Terrono AL. Treatment of boutonniere finger deformity in rheumatoid arthritis. *J Hand Surg.* 2011;36(8):1388–1393. doi:https://doi.org/10.1016/j.jhsa.2011.05.029
115. Witherow EJ, Peiris CL. Custom-made finger orthoses have fewer skin complications than prefabricated finger orthoses in the management of mallet injury: a systematic review and meta-analysis. *Arch Phys Med Rehabil.* 2015;96(10):1913–1923.e1. doi:10.1016/j.apmr.2015.04.026
116. Mella JR, Guo L, Hung V. Dupuytren's contracture: an evidence based review. *Ann Plast Surg.* 2018;81(6S Suppl 1):S97–S101. doi:10.1097/sap.0000000000001607
117. Soreide E, Murad MH, Denbeigh JM, et al. Treatment of Dupuytren's contracture: a systematic review. *Bone Joint J.* 2018;100-B(9):1138–1145. doi:10.1302/0301-620x.100b9.Bjj-2017-1194.R2
118. Fox PM, Chang J. Treating the proximal interphalangeal joint in swan neck and boutonniere deformities. *Hand Clin.* 2018;34(2):167–176. doi:10.1016/j.hcl.2017.12.006
119. Elzinga K, Chung KC. Managing swan neck and boutonniere deformities. *Clin Plast Surg.* 2019;46(3):329–337. doi:10.1016/j.cps.2019.02.006
120. Nelson GN, Potter R, Ntouvali E, et al. Intrasynovial flexor tendon repair: a biomechanical study of variations in suture application in human cadavera. *J Orthop Res.* 2012;30(10):1652–1659. doi:10.1002/jor.22108
121. Wu YF, Tang JB. Tendon healing, edema, and resistance to flexor tendon gliding: clinical implications. *Hand Clin.* 2013;29(2):167–178. doi:10.1016/j.hcl.2013.02.002
122. Starr HM, Snoddy M, Hammond KE, Seiler JG III. Flexor tendon repair rehabilitation protocols: a systematic review. *J Hand Surg Am.* 2013;38(9):1712–1717.E14. doi:10.1016/j.jhsa.2013.06.025
123. Peck FH, Roe AE, Ng CY, Duff C, McGrouther DA, Lees VC. The Manchester short splint: a change to splinting practice in the rehabilitation of zone II flexor tendon repairs. *Hand Ther.* 2014;19(2):47–53. doi:10.1177/1758998314533306
124. Groth GN. Pyramid of progressive force exercises to the injured flexor tendon. *J Hand Ther.* 2004;17(1):31–42. doi:10.1197/j.jht.2003.10.005
125. Knygsand-Roenhoej K, Maribo T. A randomized clinical controlled study comparing the effect of modified manual edema mobilization treatment with traditional edema technique in patients with a fracture of the distal radius. *J Hand Ther.* 2011;24(3):184–193; quiz 194. doi:10.1016/j.jht.2010.10.009
126. Henry SL, Howell JW. Use of a relative motion flexion orthosis for postoperative management of zone I/II flexor digitorum profundus repair: a retrospective consecutive case series. *J Hand Ther.* 2020;33(3):296–304. doi:10.1016/j.jht.2019.05.002
127. Huisstede BM, Gladdines S, Randsdorp MS, Koes BW. Effectiveness of conservative, surgical, and postsurgical interventions for trigger finger, Dupuytren disease, and de quervain disease: a systematic review. *Arch Phys Med Rehabil.* 2018;99(8):1635–1649.e21. doi:10.1016/j.apmr.2017.07.014
128. Abi-Rafeh J, Kazan R, Safran T, Thibaudeau S. Conservative management of de quervain stenosing tenosynovitis: review and presentation of treatment algorithm. *Plast Reconstr Surg.* 2020;146(1):105–126. doi:10.1097/prs.0000000000006901
129. Crosby NE, Greenberg JA. Ulnar-sided wrist pain in the athlete. *Clin Sports Med.* 2015;34(1):127–141.
130. DaSilva MF, Goodman AD, Gil JA, Akelman E. Evaluation of ulnar-sided wrist pain. *J Am Acad Orthop Surg.* 2017;25(8):e150–e156. doi:10.5435/jaaos-d-16-00407
131. Atzei A, Luchetti R. Foveal TFCC tear classification and treatment. *Hand Clin.* 2011;27(3):263–272. doi:10.1016/j.hcl.2011.05.014
132. Doarn MC, Wysocki RW. Acute TFCC injury. *Oper Tech Sports Med.* 2016;24(2):123–125.
133. Montero Lopez NM, Paksima N. Perilunate injuries and dislocations: etiology, diagnosis, and management. *Bull Hosp Jt Dis.* 2018;76(1):33–37.
134. Bergner JL, Farrar JQ, Coronado RA. Dart thrower's motion and the injured scapholunate interosseous ligament: a scoping review of studies examining motion, orthoses, and rehabilitation. *J Hand Ther.* 2020;33(1):45–59. doi:10.1016/j.jht.2018.09.005
135. Moritomo H, Apergis EP, Garcia-Elias M, Werner FW, Wolfe SW. International Federation of Societies for Surgery of the Hand 2013 Committee's report on wrist dart-throwing motion. *J Hand Surg Am.* 2014;39(7):1433–1439. doi:10.1016/j.jhsa.2014.02.035
136. Hagert E, Forsgren S, Ljung BO. Differences in the presence of mechanoreceptors and nerve structures between wrist ligaments may imply differential roles in wrist stabilization. *J Orthop Res.* 2005;23(4):757–763. doi:10.1016/j.orthres.2005.01.011
137. Salva-Coll G, Garcia-Elias M, Hagert E. Scapholunate instability: proprioception and neuromuscular control. *J Wrist Surg.* 2013;2(2):136–140. doi:10.1055/s-0033-1341960
138. Hincapie OL, Elkins JS, Vasquez-Welsh L. Proprioception retraining for a patient with chronic wrist pain secondary to ligament injury with no structural instability. *J Hand Ther.* 2016;29(2):183–190. doi:10.1016/j.jht.2016.03.008
139. d'Almeida MA, Sturbois-Nachef N, Amouyel T, Chantelot C, Saab M. Four-corner fusion: clinical and radiological outcome after fixation by headless compression screws or dorsal locking plate at minimum 5 years' follow-up. *Orthop Traumatol Surg Res.* 2021;107(5):102886. doi:10.1016/j.otsr.2021.102886
140. Clementsen S, Hammer OL, Šaltytė Benth J, Jakobsen RB, Randsborg PH. Early mobilization and physiotherapy vs. late mobilization and home exercises after ORIF of distal radial fractures: a randomized controlled trial. *JB JS Open Access.* 2019;4(3):e0012.1–e0012.11. doi:10.2106/jbjs.Oa.19.00012
141. Skorupińska A, Tora M, Bojarska-Hurnik S. Classification and elements of distal radius fractures treatment. *Physiotherapy.* 2015;23(1):40–46.

142. Ziebart C, Nazari G, MacDermid JC. Therapeutic exercise for adults post-distal radius fracture: an overview of systematic reviews of randomized controlled trials. *Hand Ther*. 2019;24(3):69–81. doi:10.1177/1758998319865751
143. Clementson M, Björkman A, Thomsen NOB. Acute scaphoid fractures: guidelines for diagnosis and treatment. *EFORT Open Rev*. 2020;5(2):96–103. doi:10.1302/2058-5241.5.190025
144. Borges CS, Ruschel PH, Pignataro MB. Scaphoid reconstruction. *Orthop Clin North Am*. 2020;51(1):65–76. doi:10.1016/j.ocl.2019.08.010
145. Gaston RG, Chadderdon C. Phalangeal fractures: displaced/nondisplaced. *Hand Clin*. 2012;28(3):395–401, x. doi:10.1016/j.hcl.2012.05.032
146. Wahl EP, Richard MJ. Management of metacarpal and phalangeal fractures in the athlete. *Clin Sports Med*. 2020;39(2):401–422. doi:10.1016/j.csm.2019.12.002
147. Weber DM, Seiler M, Subotic U, Kalisch M, Weil R. Buddy taping versus splint immobilization for paediatric finger fractures: a randomized controlled trial. *J Hand Surg Eur Vol*. 2019;44(6):640–647. doi:10.1177/1753193418822692
148. Wainner RS, Fritz JM, Irrgang JJ, Delitto A, Allison S, Boninger ML. Development of a clinical prediction rule for the diagnosis of carpal tunnel syndrome. *Arch Phys Med Rehabil*. 2005;86(4):609–618. doi:10.1016/j.apmr.2004.11.008
149. Shem K, Wong J, Dirlikov B. Effective self-stretching of carpal ligament for the treatment of carpal tunnel syndrome: a double-blinded randomized controlled study. *J Hand Ther*. 2020;33(3):272–280. doi:10.1016/j.jht.2019.12.002
150. Mansiz Kaplan B, Akyuz G, Kokar S, Yagci I. Comparison of the effectiveness of orthotic intervention, kinesiotaping, and paraffin treatments in patients with carpal tunnel syndrome: a single-blind and randomized controlled study. *J Hand Ther*. 2019;32(3):297–304. doi:10.1016/j.jht.2017.12.006
151. Wahab KW, Sanya EO, Adebayo PB, Babalola MO, Ibraheem HG. Carpal tunnel syndrome and other entrapment neuropathies. *Oman Med J*. 2017;32(6):449–454. doi:10.5001/omj.2017.87
152. Maroukis BL, Ogawa T, Rehim SA, Chung KC. Guyon canal: the evolution of clinical anatomy. *J Hand Surg Am*. 2015;40(3):560–565. doi:10.1016/j.jhsa.2014.09.026
153. Packham T, Holly J. Mechanism-specific rehabilitation management of complex regional pain syndrome: proposed recommendations from evidence synthesis. *J Hand Ther*. 2018;31(2):238–249. doi:10.1016/j.jht.2018.01.007
154. Shim H, Rose J, Halle S, Shekane P. Complex regional pain syndrome: a narrative review for the practising clinician. *Br J Anaesth*. 2019;123(2):e424–e433. doi:10.1016/j.bja.2019.03.030
155. Rolls C, McCabe C, Llewellyn A, Jones GT. What is the incidence of complex regional pain syndrome (CRPS) type I within four months of a wrist fracture in the adult population? A systematic review. *Hand Ther*. 2020;25(2):45–55. doi:10.1177/1758998320910179
156. Martel M, Laumonerie P, Pecourneau V, Ancelin D, Mansat P, Bonnevialle N. Type 1 complex regional pain syndrome after subacromial shoulder surgery: incidence and risk factor analysis. *Indian J Orthop*. 2020;54(Suppl 1):210–215. doi:10.1007/s43465-020-00174-8
157. Kessler A, Yoo M, Calisoff R, Zasler N. Complex regional pain syndrome: an updated comprehensive review. *NeuroRehabilitation*. 2020;47(3):253–264. doi:10.3233/NRE-208001
158. Cowell F, Gillespie S, Narayan B, Goebel A. Complex regional pain syndrome (CRPS) in orthopaedics: an overview. *Orthop Trauma*. 2019;33(4):217–223. doi:10.1016/j.mporth.2019.05.003
159. Kortekaas MC, Niehof SP, Stolker RJ, Huygen FJPM. Pathophysiological mechanisms involved in vasomotor disturbances in complex regional pain syndrome and implications for therapy: a review. *Pain Pract*. 2016;16(7):905–914. doi:10.1111/papr.12403
160. Méndez-Rebolledo G, Gatica-Rojas V, Torres-Cueco R, Albornoz-Verdugo M, Guzmán-Muñoz E. Update on the effects of graded motor imagery and mirror therapy on complex regional pain syndrome type 1: a systematic review. *J Back Musculoskelet Rehabil*. 2017;30(3):441–449. doi:10.3233/BMR-150500
161. Javed S, Abdi S. Use of anticonvulsants and antidepressants for treatment of complex regional pain syndrome: a literature review. *Pain Manag*. 2021;11(2):189–199. doi:10.2217/pmt-2020-0060
162. Deer TR, Hunter CW, Mehta P, et al. A systematic literature review of dorsal root ganglion neurostimulation for the treatment of pain. *Pain Med*. 2020;21(8):1581–1589. doi:10.1093/pm/pnaa005
163. Bobos P, Nazari G, Szekeres M, Lalone EA, Ferreira L, MacDermid JC. The effectiveness of joint-protection programs on pain, hand function, and grip strength levels in patients with hand arthritis: a systematic review and meta-analysis. *J Hand Ther*. 2019;32(2):194–211. doi:10.1016/j.jht.2018.09.012

17 | Cervical and Thoracic Spine

Betsy Myers and June Hanks

CHAPTER OBJECTIVES
After reading this chapter, you will be able to:
1. Tailor the basic history to a patient with cervicothoracic pathology.
2. Describe the components of the physical examination for a patient with cervicothoracic pathology.
3. Describe the pathology, history, key examination findings, rehabilitation focus, and expected outcomes of common cervicothoracic pathologies.
4. Describe interventions for patients with nonspecific neck pain and neck pain presumed to be from pathoanatomic causes.
5. Organize the physical examination of a patient with cervicothoracic pathology to maximize efficiency.

INTRODUCTION TO THE EXAMINATION OF CERVICAL AND THORACIC SPINE

Neck pain is extremely common. The 12-month prevalence of neck pain is 30 to 50% in the general population. However, only about 2 to 10% of individuals with neck pain will have limited function.[1] Roughly a quarter of individuals with neck pain will have a recurrence.[2] Neck pain is more common in women and peaks at middle age. Risk factors for neck pain include smoking, a sedentary lifestyle, and poor psychological health.[1] Chapter 4, Spine Osteology and Arthrology, provides detailed anatomy and biomechanics of the cervical and thoracic spine. The spine's complexity, including the intimate relationship with the cervical vasculature and central nervous system, can be daunting. This chapter adapts the history and physical examination to patients with suspected pathology of the cervical or thoracic spine to best guide patient management. The chapter concludes with additional exercise ideas and manual therapy techniques, which may be appropriate for a wide variety of patients with cervicothoracic dysfunction.

PATIENT HISTORY

A detailed history is paramount for patients with complaints within the head, neck, and trunk. The clinician must not only investigate spine-specific questions to help guide the physical examination but also identify red flags and symptoms referred from non-neuromusculoskeletal sources.

Review of Systems
The clinician must review systems that:
- Can refer symptoms to the patient's area of complaint.
- Can cause the symptoms described by the patient.
- Are involved in the patient's past medical history.

When evaluating patients with pain in the region of the head, neck, or trunk, clinicians should review the cardiovascular, pulmonary, gastrointestinal, genitourinary, endocrine, and psychiatric systems as well as the eyes, ears, nose, and throat.

Eyes, Ears, Nose, and Throat Patients with poor vision are likely to adopt poor postural habits when working at a computer, reading, or working on fine motor tasks in order to better see to perform the task. For example, an accountant with an inappropriate eyeglass prescription is likely to sit in excessive thoracic flexion, with a forward head and upper cervical spine extension in order to better see the computer screen. Patients may have an appropriate prescription for distance and reading, but it may not be adequate for working at a computer. Without identifying poor vision as a causative or perpetuating factor in a patient's suboccipital headache, symptom resolution will be more difficult and recurrence highly probable. The presence of diplopia, dysarthria, and/or dysphagia should raise concerns for vertebral artery or internal carotid cervical artery dysfunction.[3] Clinicians should ask about patient difficulty hearing and the presence of tinnitus (ringing in the ears). A patient presenting with complaints of dizziness but also having tinnitus is more likely to be describing symptoms consistent with Meniere disease rather than cervicogenic dizziness.

Cardiovascular and Pulmonary Systems The cardiovascular system generally refers pain to the chest, left arm, and left jaw, whereas an abdominal aortic aneurysm (AAA) can cause abdominal or mid-back pain.[4-6] A cause for immediate referral is the presence of an abdominal aorta pulse width greater than 4.0 cm or a patient report of a pulsing sensation in the back or abdomen.[7] Patients should be asked about the presence of dizziness, fainting, or headaches. Hypertension is a risk factor for cervical arterial disease,[8] myocardial infarction, and cerebrovascular accidents. Therefore, assessment of blood pressure is of prime importance.

A variety of pulmonary diseases can refer pain to the neck and thoracic region, including lung cancer, bronchitis, and pneumonia.[6,7] Smoking increases the risk of cervical **spondylosis**[9] as well as increasing the risk of cancer.[7] Patients should be asked about shortness of breath and the presence of a cough or fever.

Gastrointestinal and Genitourinary Systems
Thoracic pain may be referred from the gallbladder, pancreas, or intestines.[7] Esophagitis or esophageal cancer may cause cervical or thoracic pain. Therefore, the clinician should ask about the presence of nausea, vomiting, or if symptoms change as the result of eating. To better understand the potential for poor bone density, the clinician should ask older patients if they have had a bone density test, the results, and the use of any medications prescribed for osteoporosis. Females should be asked about their last menstrual cycle, surgical history of hysterectomy or oophorectomy, and hormone replacement therapy. Bowel or bladder dysfunction may indicate cervical myelopathy[9] and may be cause for immediate referral.

Psychiatric System Poor psychological health is a risk factor for neck pain.[9] The presence of psychological factors such as a passive coping style, anxiety, depression, kinesiophobia, catastrophizing, and lack of satisfaction at work are associated with worse outcomes[10] and an increased risk for chronic pain.[11] The clinician should screen for these factors. The use of the Pain Catastrophizing Scale (PCS) or the Fear-Avoidance Beliefs Questionnaire (FABQ) may be beneficial. See Chapter 19, Pain Management: A Mechanism-Centered Approach, for additional information.

General Medical Information

Clinicians should thoroughly review the patient's general medical history. Medication reconciliation can provide insights into the patient's current condition (relief of symptoms with the use of muscle relaxers) and undisclosed medical conditions (use of diuretic to manage hypertension or the use of antidepressants), as well as identify potential problems such as polypharmacy and adverse drug reactions. Specifically asking about prior surgeries or problems with the neck or upper extremities may help with differential diagnosis. For example, a patient reporting a history of hand numbness and tingling that was treated with carpal tunnel surgery may have been exhibiting signs of cervical radiculopathy or a double-crush injury (see Chapter 15, Elbow Complex). Likewise, a patient reporting a history of back surgery for stenosis may have global spondylosis or may be experiencing cervical stenosis due to a congenitally narrow spinal canal. A recent tooth procedure or illness increases the suspicion for an abscess or infection.

The clinician should determine the results of recent imaging, if performed, and obtain the imaging and reports. For example, a patient with a prior history of low back pain (LBP) may not have been informed of the presence of a thoracic compression fracture because it was an incidental finding unrelated to the patient's complaint of LBP. However, the presence of an old osteoporotic fracture should raise the suspicion for additional compression fractures and will influence intervention options.

Lifestyle and Occupation

Clinicians should inquire about work, exercise, and leisure activities to best understand the physical demands of patients' daily lives, identify potential predisposing or exacerbating factors, as well as any repetitive stresses that may be related to their chief complaint. Neck and thoracic pain are common among individuals who sit for prolonged periods of time. Clinicians should understand the patient's office and home workstation arrangement, including desk height, chair characteristics, the use of external monitors, phones or headsets, and the use of eyewear. Patients should be asked about smoking history, as smoking increases the risk of lung cancer.

Patients should be asked about leisure activity. A patient who enjoys reading for pleasure but who works at a seated job all day may benefit from the addition of a type of leisure activity that does not involve sitting. Likewise, patients should be asked about nighttime rituals, such as reading or watching television in bed, as prolonged time in suboptimal postures may contribute to the patients' complaints.

History of Neck Pathology

Patients should be asked about prior neck injuries, trauma, or motor vehicle accidents. The clinician should ask about prior interventions and the short- and long-term impact. Patients with a fixed mindset as to what interventions will be beneficial are less likely to be adherent to suggestions that do not match their beliefs. Neck pain recurrence is not uncommon and may indicate lack of identification and correction of causative and contributing factors.

Chief Complaint

The clinician must understand the patient's chief complaint and the impact on patient function. Stiffness suggests spondylosis, whereas bilateral upper extremity paresthesias or weakness is consistent with myelopathy. The clinician should ask about pain, paresthesias, weakness, stiffness, headaches, dizziness, and decreased balance.

Onset

Patients should be asked about the timing and possible causes for their symptoms. An insidious onset of neck or thoracic pain is not uncommon. However, a 72-year-old patient reporting symptoms that began after a fall should be suspected of having a fracture. A headache that occurs daily at the end of a work shift may indicate inadequate ergonomic setup, suboptimal posture, or psychological stress. Symptoms present for less than 3 months have a better overall prognosis than those present for longer.

Location and Intensity of Symptoms

Clinicians should thoroughly investigate the location of current and prior symptoms and whether the current symptoms are central, bilateral, or unilateral. Symptoms in the neck or scapular region may be referred from the facet joints or present due to spondylosis. Symptoms into the upper extremity may indicate radiculopathy. The patient should be asked if symptoms are constant or intermittent. Intermittent symptoms are likely to be mechanical in nature, whereas constant symptoms may represent inflammation or chronic pain. Similar to the lumbar spine, tracking a patient's symptoms helps to identify patterns, such as centralization or peripheralization (Fig. 17-1). (Chapter 12, Lumbar Spine and Sacroiliac Joint, provides details regarding centralizations, peripheralization, and directional preference.)

Symptom Quality

Symptom quality can help shape the clinician's diagnostic hypotheses. A dull aching pain is consistent with facet arthropathy or spondylosis, whereas shooting or burning pain raises suspicion of radiculopathy. Headache quality is extremely important to identify. A severe, intense, "thunder-clap" headache should make the clinician suspect an aneurysm. Dizziness is not uncommon with cervical pathology. However, vertigo (feeling as though the room is spinning) suggests a vestibular pathology.

Symptom Behavior

Patients should be questioned about aggravating and remitting factors. The patient history can help identify if the patient has a directional preference. For example, the vast majority of patients with signs and symptoms of cervical radiculopathy have a directional preference of extension and centralize with repeated extension with retraction.[12] Patients should specifically be asked about bending the head down forward (as in reading a book, phone, or tablet), looking up, turning (as in checking traffic before crossing the street or looking back while driving a car in reverse), sitting, walking, and sleeping. Patients should be asked about sleep positions as well as the use and type of pillows. A patient who regularly sleeps in a chair due to gastroesophageal reflux disease (GERD) may have neck pain from sleeping with the head sagged in an awkward position. Likewise, sleeping supine with two large pillows is likely to perpetuate a forward head position throughout the day, increasing strain on the neck and upper back. Patients should be asked to describe the 24-hour pattern of symptoms. Symptoms that occur

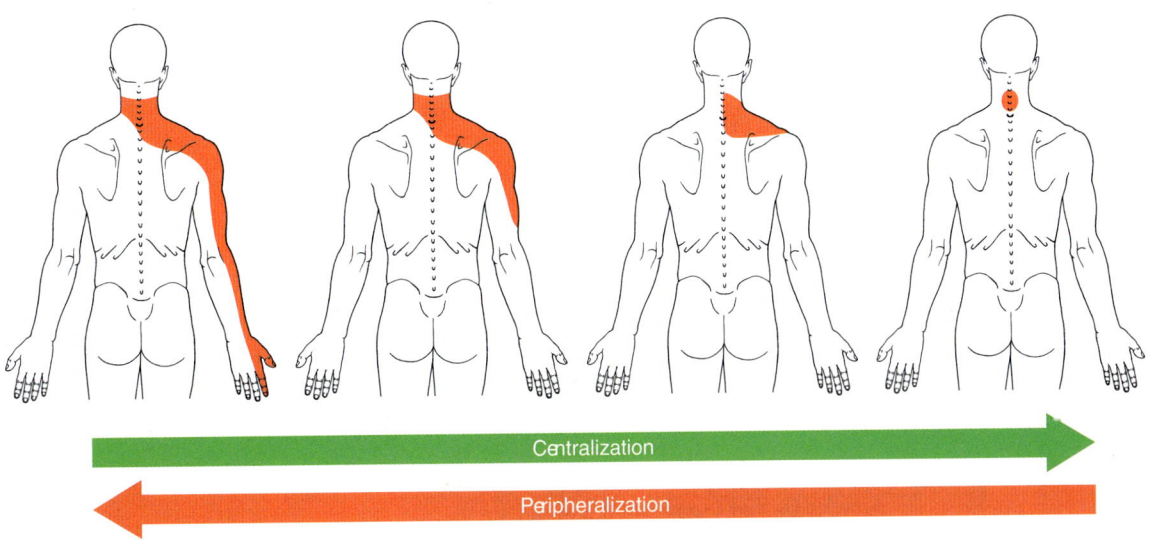

FIGURE 17-1 Centralization and peripheralization of symptoms in the cervical spine.

as the day goes on may have a postural or endurance component, whereas morning stiffness that goes away within 30 minutes is more consistent with spondylosis. However, stiffness lasting longer than 30 minutes or so may indicate a systemic inflammatory disease, such as ankylosing spondylitis.

Red Flag Screening for Cervicothoracic Pathology

Red flag screening for cervicothoracic pathology deserves special attention as several pathologies may be life-threatening, if missed.[11,13,14] Potentially life-threatening conditions include:

- Fracture
- Brain aneurysm or mass lesion
- Vertebrobasilar artery insufficiency or cervical artery dissection
- Cervical myelopathy
- Upper cervical spine instability
- Cancer
- Infection

Clinicians should consider the possibility of inflammatory arthritis for patients with morning stiffness and swelling in multiple joints.[11] Medical consultation is advised as the patient is likely to benefit from additional medical evaluation and pharmacologic interventions.

Fracture Routine imaging is not recommended on any clinical practice guideline.[10] However, clinicians should follow the Canadian C-spine rule for patients reporting a major trauma, such as a motor vehicle accident or a fall from a height, who have not been medically evaluated and cleared of a fracture or other condition requiring further medical testing (Fig. 17-2).[15] If cleared, the examination can proceed. The Canadian C-spine rule appears to be accurate than using the National Emergency X-Radiography Utilization Study (NEXUS) criteria.[16]

Brain Aneurysm or Mass Lesion Patient's reporting a sudden, intense, "thunder-clap" headache may be experiencing intracerebral pathology such as a mass lesion or ruptured cerebral aneurysm and require immediate referral.[10]

Vertebrobasilar Insufficiency or Cervical Artery Dissection The vertebral and internal carotid arteries are closely associated with the cervical spine and may be subject to compromise, particularly in the case of trauma. Patients with sudden, intense neck pain or headache who are exhibiting the "5D's and 3N's" listed in Table 17-1 may be exhibiting signs of **vertebrobasilar insufficiency** (VBI) or cervical artery dissection and should be immediately referred for further medical evaluation.[7,10,13,17]

Cervical Myelopathy One of the first steps of the evaluation of patient with neck pain is to differentiate between central and peripheral nervous system involvement. Cervical spondylitic (degenerative) myelopathy is the most common cause of spinal cord dysfunction.[18,19] Age-related degenerative changes including osteophytes, hypertrophy of the posterior longitudinal ligament (PLL) and ligamentum flavum,

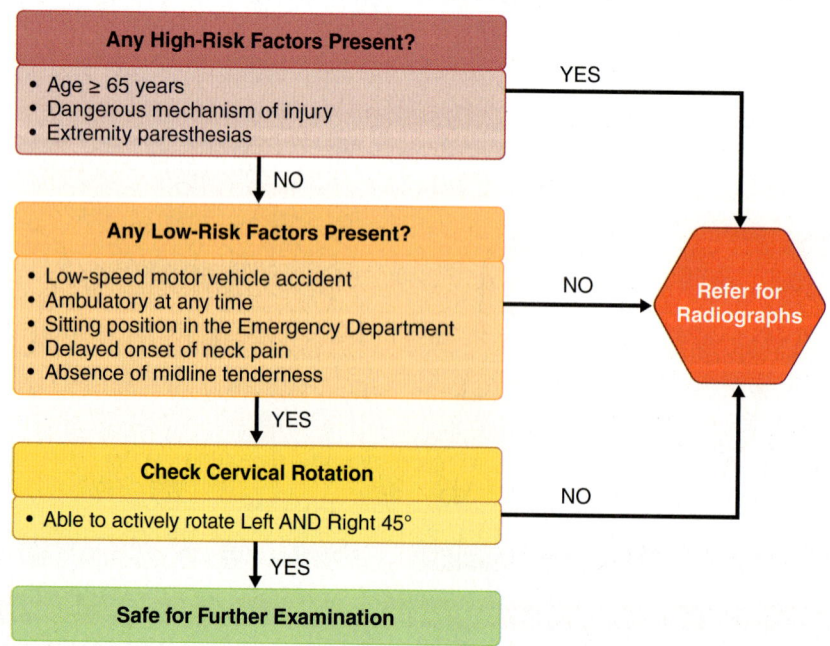

FIGURE 17-2 Canadian C-spine rule.

TABLE 17-1	
5D'S AND 3N'S VERTEBROBASILAR INSUFFICIENCY	
Diplopia	**N**ausea
Dizziness	**N**umbness
Drop attacks	**N**ystagmus
Dysarthria	
Dysphagia	

disc degeneration, and postural and positioning changes can all cause or exacerbate central canal stenosis.[19,20] Congenital spinal canal narrowing may increase the risk of cervical myelopathy.[19,20] Cervical myelopathy leads to compression of the spinal cord, with the most affected regions being the lateral corticospinal tracts and the anterior and posterior spinocerebellar tracts (Fig. 17-3).[21]

Patients with cervical myelopathy may present with complaints of neck pain, stiffness, or upper extremity radicular pain, leading clinicians to incorrectly suspect cervical radiculopathy.[21] Delay in diagnosis may contribute to lasting functional loss. Therefore, clinicians must conduct a thorough history and physical examination with particular consideration for possible red flags. On more careful review, patients with cervical myelopathy will present with one or more of the signs and symptoms noted in Table 17-2.[19-27] Upper extremity weakness that is greater than lower extremity weakness should make clinicians highly suspicious of the presence of cervical myelopathy.[19] If the clinician suspects cervical myelopathy, the patient should be referred for further medical management. Cervical myelopathy is generally managed via surgical decompression, which may include single or multilevel laminectomy and fusion.[20] However, mild cases may be treated conservatively with careful observation.[19]

Upper Cervical Spine Instability Clinicians should consider the integrity of the upper cervical spine ligaments before commencing physical therapy. Patients with cervical spine instability may present with occipital numbness and headaches as well as severely limited cervical range of motion (CROM). They may report a feeling of head instability, the need to support their head, or feeling a lump in their throat.[8] These ligaments may become incompetent after a trauma, such as a fall in an elderly individual or a motor vehicle accident in a younger person. Instability between C1 and C2 may develop in up to 65% of individuals with rheumatoid arthritis[28] and 20% of individuals with Down syndrome.[29] The diagnostic accuracy of all clinical tests for instability is limited.[30] A positive alar ligament test or positive Sharp-Purser test requires referral. However, clinicians cannot be certain of the absence of instability if both tests are negative. Therefore, clinicians should consider the entirety or the patient history and physical examination, observe for signs and symptoms of myelopathy, and refer or consult with other medical providers as needed.

Cancer Clinicians should be suspicious of the potential for cancer in patients over the age of 50 years who report a history of cancer, significant unexplained weight loss, constant pain that is unrelieved by position or movement, or night pain.[13] The most

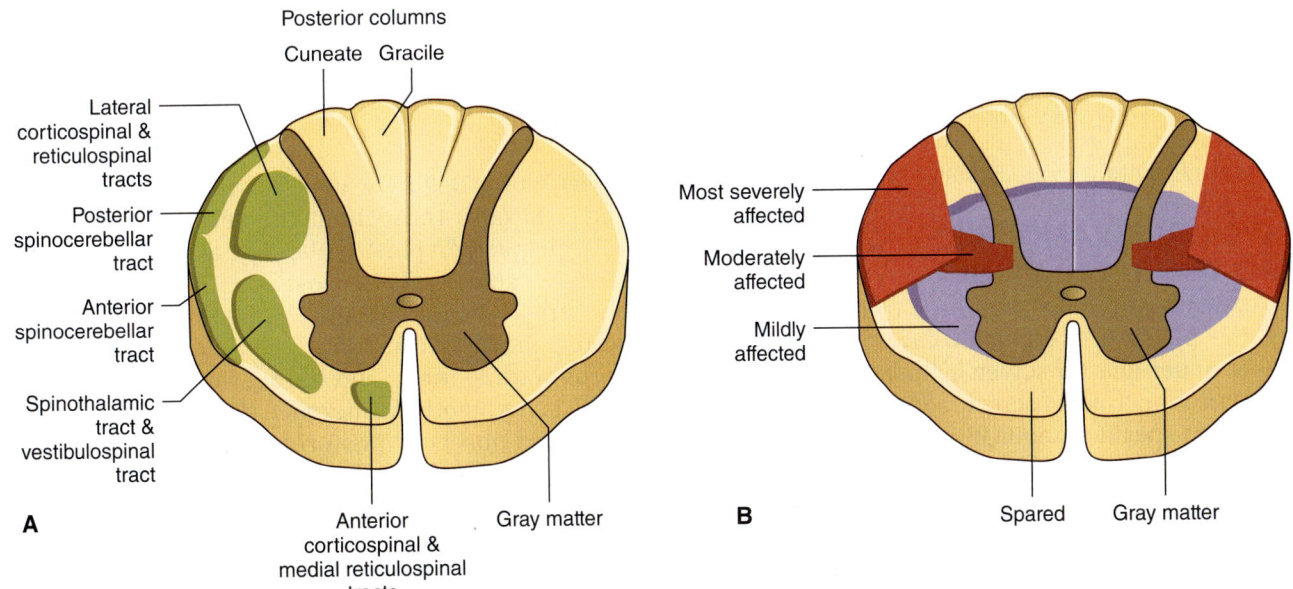

FIGURE 17-3 Cervical myelopathy. **A.** Normal spinal cord anatomy. **B.** Spinal cord regions affected with cervical myelopathy.

TABLE 17-2
SIGNS AND SYMPTOMS OF CERVICAL MYELOPATHY

Patient Symptoms	Clinical Signs
Hand clumsiness, changes in handwriting Paresthesias in one or more extremities Upper extremity weakness Legs feeling as if they will give way, falls Changes in bowel/bladder function*	Hyperreflexia Clonus Positive Babinski reflex Positive Hoffman sign Upper extremity weakness, that is likely bilateral Lower extremity weakness that is bilateral Decreased hand dexterity Gait changes including decreased step length, decreased speed, and ataxia Decreased single limb balance

*Rare as this requires the presence of significant central stenosis.

TABLE 17-3
COMMON OUTCOME TOOLS FOR PATIENTS WITH NECK PAIN

Tool	Tool Basics
Neck Disability Index (NDI)	• 10 items scored 0-5, with higher scores indicating greater disability • Scoring may be reported on a 0-50 scale or changed to a percentage of perceived disability • Assesses frequency and severity of neck pain and headaches as well as the influence of neck pain on broad categories of functional tasks • Minimum detectable change varies between 5 and 10 points based on the type of neck condition
Patient-Specific Functional Scale (PSFS)	• Patients note two to five activities they are having difficulty performing due to neck pain • Activities are rated on a 0-10 scale, with 0 = unable to perform, 10 = able to perform as well as before the condition • Minimum clinically important difference = 1.3 points
Pain Catastrophizing Scale (PCS)	• 13 items rated 0-4, with higher scores indicative of greater tendency to magnify the threat of pain or feel helpless to control pain • Scores of 30 or more represent a clinically relevant level of catastrophizing

significant risk factor is a history of prior cancer.[7] Cancers of the breast, prostate, and lung are most likely to metastasize to bone. The most frequent sites for metastases are the vertebra, pelvis, ribs, sternum, femur, and skull. Patients who are smokers or have a history of smoking are at increased risk of lung cancer. Although the clinician *may* choose to continue with the evaluation, referral is required and treatment should be delayed until medical clearance is obtained.

Infection Patients with a temperature greater than 100°F, a history of recent infection or surgery, or a history of drug use or immunosuppression may be experiencing an infection.[13] Although the clinician *may* choose to continue with the evaluation, consultation or referral is required before treatment.

Outcome Measures Patient-reported outcome measures can provide insights into the patient's functional difficulties and help identify the potential for pain-associated psychological distress and fear-avoidance beliefs. The Neck Disability Index (NDI), the Patient-Specific Functional Scale (PSFS), and the PCS are the most commonly researched and validated outcome tools for patients with neck pain (Table 17-3).[14,31–33]

PHYSICAL EXAMINATION: CERVICAL AND THORACIC SPINE

For patients with suspected neck or thoracic pathology, the physical examination includes the systems review, upper quarter screen including a thorough upper quarter neurologic screen, a clearing examination, and a joint-specific examination. Because of the close relationship between the lumbar and thoracic spine, the motion and muscle performance examinations are closely linked. Likewise, the shoulder has multiple links to the cervical and thoracic spine. Clearing of the shoulder joint may consist of active ROM (AROM) with overpressure for flexion, abduction, hand behind head, and hand behind back. A Cyriax screen using resisted isometric testing with the shoulder in a neutral position for the shoulder flexion/extension, rotation, abduction, and adduction can help screen the muscles of the shoulder. However, more detailed muscle performance assessments may be needed for the axiohumeral and scapulothoracic muscles. Assessment of the temporomandibular joint is rarely required unless symptoms specific to the jaw are noted.

Observation

Observation begins when first meeting the patient and continues throughout the session. For patients with suspected spinal pathology, assessment should include typical resting postures. This is best done unobtrusively, for example, while the patient is completing intake information, when meeting the patient in the waiting room, and during the history, because there is frequently a difference between habitual postures and observed postures. Likewise, the clinician should start to consider if a patient's postures are fixed or chosen, and if any deviations from normal might contribute to the patient's symptoms, might contribute to future problems, or are irrelevant. Note, for example, if the patient holds the head and neck rigidly, turning the entire trunk to address the

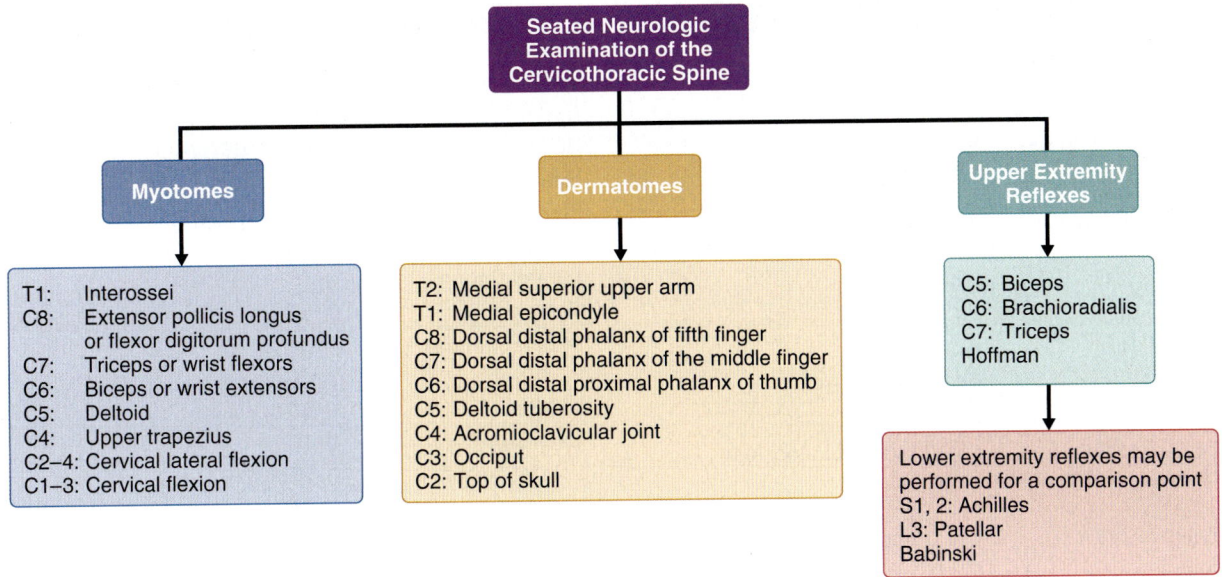

FIGURE 17-4 Seated neurologic examination of the cervicothoracic spine.

clinician or raising paperwork up closer to eye level to prevent the need for cervical flexion. Observe if the patient's shoulders appear level or if one is higher than the other, potentially indicating the presence of a scoliosis. Observe the patient's fine motor control when completing intake forms.

Neurologic Examination of the Cervical and Thoracic Spine

Upper extremity strength and paresthesias from cervical spine pathology can change as a result of changes in neck loading.[34] Therefore, the examination of the neurologic status of the upper quarter is performed in the seated position before assessment of CROM (Fig. 17-4). Because symptoms are in the head and neck, the basic upper quarter neurologic screen should be expanded to include testing of the C2–C4 dermatomes. C2–C4 myotomes (C1–C3: cervical flexion, C2–C4: cervical lateral flexion) have significant overlap and will be considered when assessing muscle performance later in the examination.

To perform the Hoffman reflex, the clinician holds the seated patient's middle phalanx of the third digit and flicks the distal phalanx into flexion (Fig. 17-5). An abnormal response (positive Hoffman sign) is involuntary flexion of the thumb and index finger. The Hoffmann test is a sensitive, but nonspecific test for upper motor neuron lesion, such as cervical myelopathy.[35]

A cranial nerve screening assessment is required for patients with:
- History of trauma
- Headache
- Dizziness

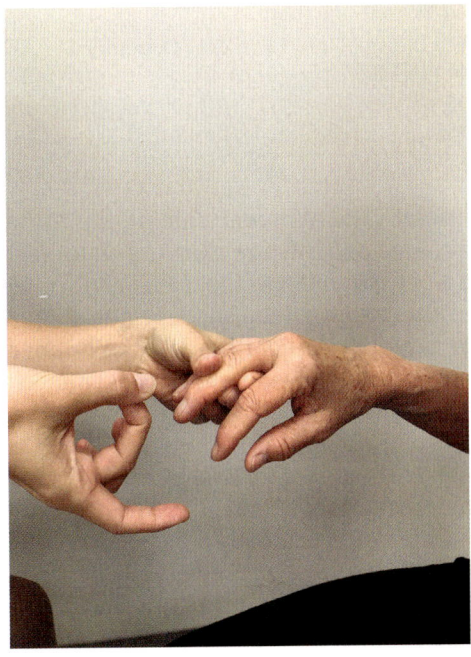

FIGURE 17-5 Hoffman reflex.

There are multiple ways one can assess the cranial nerves. Table 17-4 outlines a possible quick cranial nerve screen that is organized in the order in which the clinician would efficiently perform it rather than in numbered nerve order. Any positive tests require consultation or referral.

Structure and Posture

Observe the patient's overall structure and posture with the patient standing barefoot from a posterior

TABLE 17-4	
QUICK CRANIAL NERVE SCREEN EXAMPLE	
Assessment	Cranial Nerve (CN)
Patient is asked to follow the clinician's finger making an H shape in front of the patient's face	CN IV Trochlear CN VI Abducens CN III Oculomotor
Examine pupil response to light	CN III Oculomotor
Close eyes	CN VII Facial
Raise eyebrows	CN VII Facial
Smile	CN VII Facial
Clench jaw	CN V Trigeminal
Stick-out tongue	CN XII Hypoglossal
Rub fingers together or crinkle paper by patient's ears	CN VIII Vestibulocochlear
Shoulder shrug	CN XI Accessory
Swallow and speak without hoarseness	CN IX Glossopharyngeal CN X Vagus
Read a word or count number of fingers presented in front of patient	CN II Optic
Identify the smell of coffee	CN I Olfactory
Assess balance or walking	CN VIII Vestibulocochlear if desired

TABLE 17-5	
NORMATIVE VALUES FOR RANGE OF MOTION OF THE CERVICAL AND THORACOLUMBAR SPINE	
Cervical Motion	Normative Value (degrees)
Protrusion	Visual observation
Retraction	Visual observation
Flexion	0–80
Extension	0–30
Lateral flexion	0–35
Rotation	0–60 or 80
Thoracolumbar Motion	
Flexion	0–80
Extension	0–30
Lateral flexion	0–35
Rotation	0–45

and lateral view. When examining the thoracic spine, ideally, male patients are shirtless and female patients are in a gown opened to the back or sports bra to maximize visualization of the entire region. Palpate the iliac crests, inferior scapular borders, and upper trapezius regions to obtain a general feel for symmetry between the left and right sides. Observe the course of the patient's spinal curvatures, noticing if the curves are smooth and neither excessive nor reduced. Observe for the presence of scoliosis (see Fig. 4-4 in Chapter 4, Spine Osteology and Arthrology), a lateral spinal curvature that may be accompanied by a posterior rib hump. If scoliosis is suspected, having the patient flex the trunk will make any posterior rib hump more prominent. Note the general muscular contours for atrophy, hypertrophy, or hypertonicity of the paraspinals, upper trapezius, and cervical musculature.

Cervical and Thoracic Range of Motion

Cervical and thoracic AROM should be assessed and should include protrusion, retrusion, flexion, extension, lateral flexion, and rotation. Thoracic AROM can also be assessed with the patient seated straddling the corner of the table to help stabilize the pelvis. Cervical passive range of motion (PROM) should be assessed in supine. The clinician should assess movement quantity, pain provocation, and endfeel using normative values (Table 17-5). Measurement can be made with a goniometer or with the CROM device.[36] A capsular pattern of restriction for the cervical facet joints would be a limitation of ipsilateral lateral flexion and rotation with a mild loss of extension.[37,38] Patients with spondylosis are likely to have limited extension with end-range pain. Patients with whiplash-associated disorder (WAD) may have globally limited motion with guarding.

Many times patients lack retraction range and present with a forward head. In these cases, it may be useful to have the patient stand with the back to the wall and attempt to retract the cervical spine and posteriorly translate the head as far as possible while keeping the chin and eyes level with the horizon. The clinician then measures the horizontal distance from the most posterior portion of the patient's occiput to the wall. The clinician can attempt to target rotation between C1 and C2 by performing the cervical flexion-rotation test (Fig. 17-6).

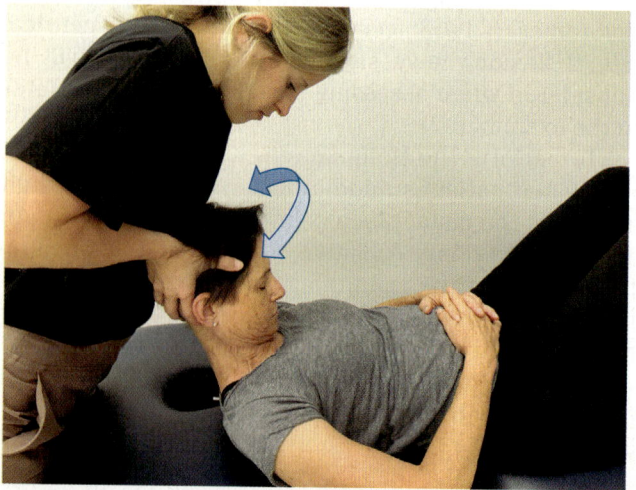

FIGURE 17-6 Cervical flexion-rotation test.

Cervical Flexion-Rotation Test
Purpose: To measure passive rotation between C1 and C2
Method: With the patient supine, the clinician passively flexes the neck to end-range, then rotates the head to each side. The clinician notes endfeel and ROM.
Interpretation: A positive test is a 10° difference between sides[14] or visual estimate of less than 34° rotation.[39]

Assessment of Breathing Mechanics
Clinicians should assess the patient's typical breathing pattern. Breathing at rest should be primarily diaphragmatic. Some patients may rely more on accessory muscles, which may lead to problems such as scalene spasming or trigger points.[40] Patients with scoliosis may have reduced lateral costal breathing. Clinicians can place a hand(s) on the abdomen, upper chest, and lateral costal region to observe the patient's preferred breathing style. Normally, the abdomen should rise with inspiration as the diaphragm descends, but there should be little motion of the upper chest and lateral costal region. On deep inhalation, the abdomen should rise, followed by lateral and superior expansion of the lateral costal region (Fig. 17-7A) and finally superior motion of the upper chest (Fig. 17-7B). Limited rib cage expansion is a hallmark of ankylosing spondylitis.[41]

Muscle Performance
In addition to myotomal testing, the clinician should assess isometric cervical strength seated in a neutral position. Testing should include cervical flexion, extension, left and right lateral flexion, and left and right rotation. Cervical muscle strains are common, and assessment of an involved muscle or muscle group will be painful. The deep cervical flexors are key postural muscles that are frequently weak and deconditioned in patients with neck pain. The neck flexor endurance test and the cranial cervical flexion test can be used both for assessment purposes and as an exercise.

Neck Flexor Endurance Test
Purpose: To identify decreased endurance of the deep cervical flexors.[42,43]
Method: With the patient hooklying supine, the patient performs upper cervical flexion (a chin tuck) and then lower cervical flexion to lift the head 2 to 3 cm off the support surface holding the chin toward the sternoclavicular notch. Alternatively, the clinician can place the patient in the test position (Fig. 17-8).
Grading: The number of seconds the patient is able to hold the test is recorded. The ability to maintain the position for 1 minute is considered normal.

Cranial Cervical Flexion Test
Purpose: To identify decreased movement control of the deep cervical flexors. The alternate method can be used to identify decreased endurance of the deep cervical flexors.[43]
Method: With the patient hooklying supine, a pressure biofeedback unit is placed to support the patient's cervical lordosis. The unit is inflated to 20 mm Hg. While watching the pressure gauge, the patient slowly nods the head "yes" to try to increase the unit to 22 mm Hg and hold this position for 10 seconds (Fig. 17-9). The patient relaxes and the test is repeated sequentially trying to increase the pressure to 24, 26, 28, and 30 mm Hg. The test is sometimes performed using a typical blood pressure cuff.
Grading: The highest compression the patient is able to hold for 10 seconds is recorded.
Alternate Method: The test setup is similar to earlier one. However, for the endurance test, the patient first performs a maximal isometric contraction and the amount of compression is documented. The

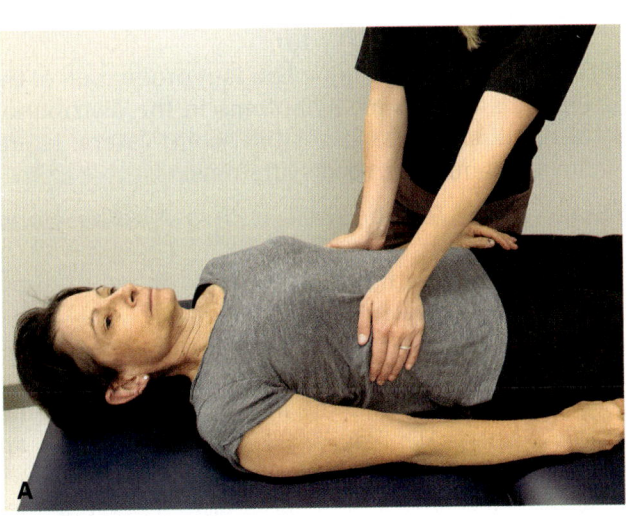
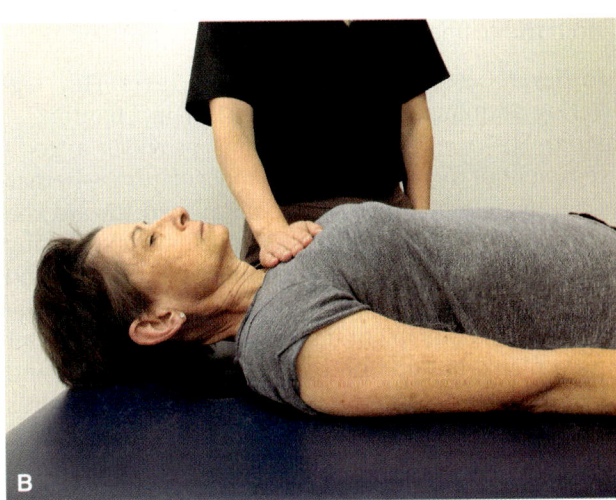

FIGURE 17-7 Assessment of lateral costal breathing (**A**) and upper chest breathing (**B**).

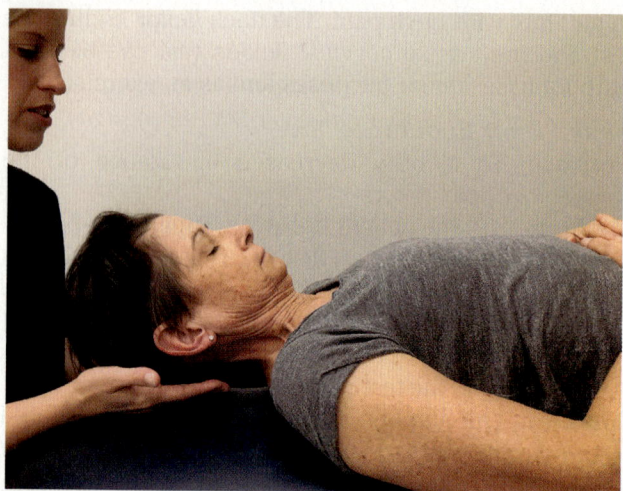

FIGURE 17-8 Neck flexor endurance test.

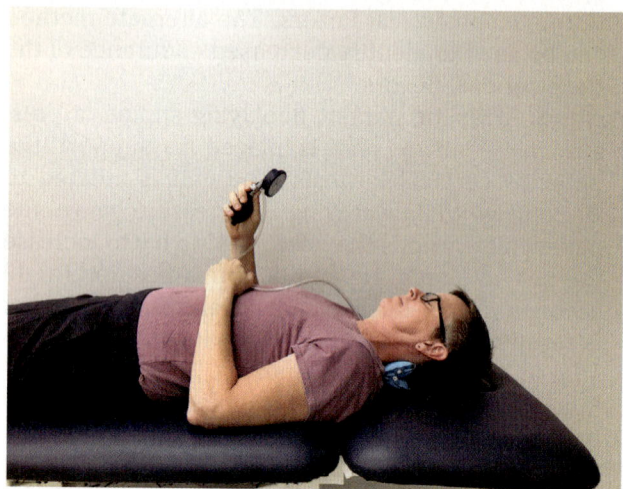

FIGURE 17-9 Cranial cervical flexion test.

patient then attempts to hold a contraction that is 60% of the maximal contraction for as long as possible. The number of seconds the patient is able to hold the test is recorded.[44]

Additional Muscle Performance Tests The leg-lowering abdominal test (see Fig. 12-7 in Chapter 12, Lumbar Spine and Sacroiliac Joint) provides a good assessment of the anterior trunk musculature, whereas the Sorenson test (see Fig. 12-8) is biased toward the posterior trunk musculature. Manual muscle testing of the trunk extensors, axiohumeral muscles, and scapulothoracic muscles is recommended. Additional core strength tests might include timed holds of a front or side plank. In addition to assessing abdominal and thoracolumbar strength, holding a front plank requires the cervical extensors and retractors to maintain a neutral head/neck posture against the pull of gravity, while a side plank better targets the cervical lateral flexors.

Muscle Length

It is common for patients with neck pain to have hypertonicity, trigger points, and/or decreased length in the upper trapezius and levator. Although not generally quantified, clinicians should assess the length of these muscles in patients with cervical pathology. The clinician should consider assessing the length of the latissimus dorsi, pectoralis major, and pectoralis minor (see Fig. 14-26, in Chapter 14, Shoulder Complex). For example, restricted latissimus dorsi length will limit functional trunk extension and overhead reaching.

Neurodynamic Testing

The **upper limb tension tests** (ULTTs) may be positive in the presence of radiculopathy (median or ulnar nerve bias) or reduced mobility of the ulnar, median, or radial nerves.[45] When performed as a means of identifying radiculopathy, it is recommended that the ulnar-biased test be performed first. If the test is negative, the clinician should perform the median nerve test. If the median nerve test is negative, the clinician should then perform the radial nerve test.[45] However, some studies find poor reliability with testing.[46] Therefore, the tests should not be used in isolation. These tests are frequently uncomfortable. Therefore, as with all tests and mobilizations, it is important to perform the test on the unaffected side first to help discriminate between discomfort and reproduction of concordant symptoms.

Upper Limb Tension Test with an Ulnar Nerve Bias
Purpose: To identify radiculopathy or reduced mobility of the ulnar nerve.[45]
Method: With the patient supine, the clinician passively moves the patient's limb through a series of positions to lengthen the ulnar nerve. The shoulder girdle is depressed, shoulder is abducted to about 100° and externally rotated, the forearm is pronated, the wrist and fingers are extended, then the elbow is slowly flexed (Fig. 17-10).
Interpretation: A positive test is reproduction of the patient's neurogenic symptoms in the distribution of the ulnar nerve. If positive, contralateral lateral flexion should increase symptoms.

Upper Limb Tension Test with a Median Nerve Bias
Purpose: To identify radiculopathy or reduced mobility of the median nerve.[43,45]
Method: With the patient supine, the clinician passively moves the patient's limb through a series of positions to lengthen the median nerve. The shoulder girdle is depressed, the wrist and fingers are extended, the forearm supinated, the shoulder is abducted to about 90° and externally rotated, then the elbow is slowly extended (Fig. 17-11). If positive,

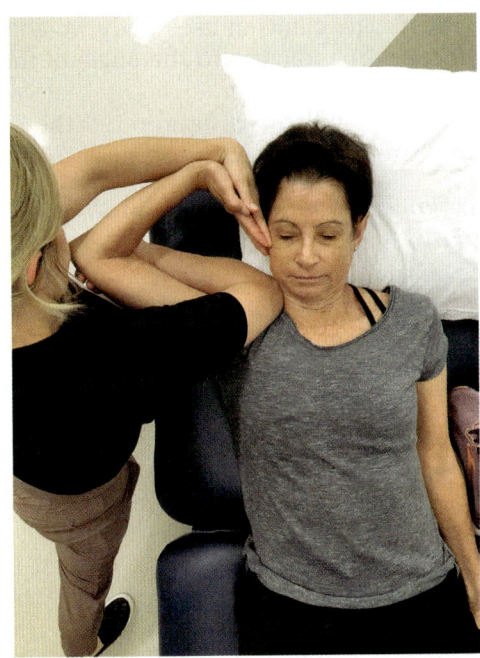

FIGURE 17-10 Upper limb tension test with an ulnar nerve bias.

positions to lengthen the radial nerve. The shoulder girdle is depressed, the shoulder is internally rotated and abducted, the elbow is extended, the forearm pronated, the fingers are flexed, then the wrist is slowly flexed (Fig. 17-12). If positive, contralateral lateral flexion should increase symptoms, whereas ipsilateral lateral flexion should decrease symptoms.

Interpretation: A positive test is reproduction of the patient's neurogenic symptoms in the distribution of the radial nerve.

Passive Accessory Intervertebral Movements

Passive accessory motion of the intervertebral joints of the cervical and upper thoracic spine can be assessed using posterior-to-anterior pressures and transverse pressures. The clinician should perform the assessment in a methodical manner, beginning either proximally at C2 and moving distally or the reverse.

Cervical Central Posteroanterior Pressure

Purpose: To assess general intervertebral joint play with an emphasis on sagittal plane motion.[47] When applying grade I and II mobilizations, this technique may be used to help decrease pain.[47] When applying grade III and IV mobilizations, this technique may be used to treat local joint hypomobility and improve cervical extension ROM.[47] For a more aggressive technique, the patient can be positioned in a greater amount of extension.

contralateral lateral flexion should increase symptoms, whereas ipsilateral lateral flexion should decrease symptoms.

Interpretation: A positive test is reproduction of the patient's neurogenic symptoms in the distribution of the median nerve.

Upper Limb Tension Test with a Radial Nerve Bias

Purpose: To identify radiculopathy or reduced mobility of the radial nerve.[43,45]

Method: With the patient supine, the clinician passively moves the patient's limb through a series of

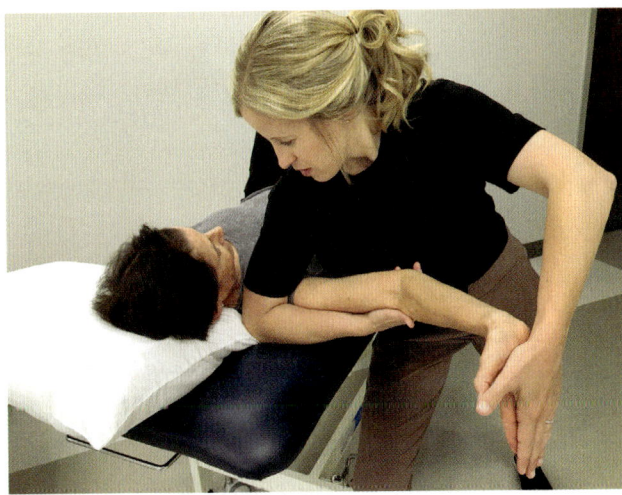

FIGURE 17-11 Upper limb tension test with a median nerve bias.

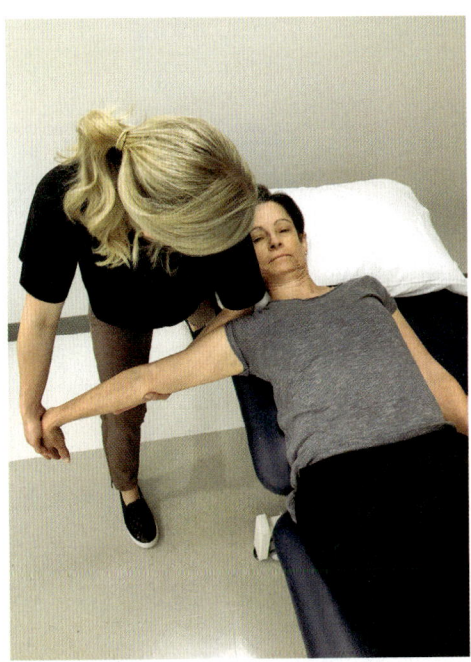

FIGURE 17-12 Upper limb tension test with a radial nerve bias.

Patient: Prone.
Clinician: The clinician stands facing the patient's feet. The thumb of the nondominant hand is placed on the spinous process of the vertebra to be mobilized. The thumb of the dominant hand (mobilizing thumb) is placed over the other thumb.
Mobilization: The clinician uses bodyweight to create a force perpendicular to the angle of the spine (Fig. 17-13).
Interpretation: The clinician should note if any symptoms are created or increased and attempt to judge the amount of motion (hypomobile, normal, or hypermobile). A positive test for instability is if symptoms are provoked or increased,[48,49] or if accessory motion is believed to be hypermobile.[50] Note that the test lacks specificity,[51] inter-rater reliability is somewhat limited,[52] and hypermobility may be asymptomatic.[53]

Thoracic Central Posteroanterior Pressure
Purpose: As with the cervical posteroanterior pressure, but with an emphasis on the thoracic spine.
Patient: Prone.
Clinician: The clinician stands at the patient's side. The clinician places the hypothenar eminence of the nondominant hand on the spinous process of the vertebra to be mobilized. The clinician's dominant hand is placed on top of the contact hand. Alternatively, for proximal thoracic mobilizations, the clinician may use the hand placement as noted for cervical spine technique for segments T1–T4.

Mobilization: The clinician uses body weight to create a force perpendicular to the angle of the spine (Fig. 17-14).
Interpretation: The test is interpreted the same as central posteroanterior pressure assessment.

Cervical Unilateral Posteroanterior Pressure
Purpose: To assess facet joint mobility with an emphasis on rotation.[47] When applying grade III and IV mobilizations, this technique may be used to treat local joint hypomobility.[47]
Patient: Prone.
Clinician: The clinician stands facing the patient's feet. The thumb of the nondominant hand is placed on the articular pillar of the vertebra to be mobilized. The thumb of the dominant hand (mobilizing thumb) is placed over the other thumb.
Mobilization: The mobilizing thumb imparts a downward force perpendicular to the angle of the spine (Fig. 17-15).
Interpretation: The test is interpreted the same as central posteroanterior pressure assessment.

Thoracic Unilateral Posteroanterior Pressure
Purpose: As with the cervical posteroanterior pressure, but with an emphasis on the thoracic spine.
Patient: Prone.
Clinician: The clinician stands at the patient's side. The clinician places the thumb of the nondominant hand on the articular pillar of the vertebra to be mobilized. The clinician's dominant hand is placed on

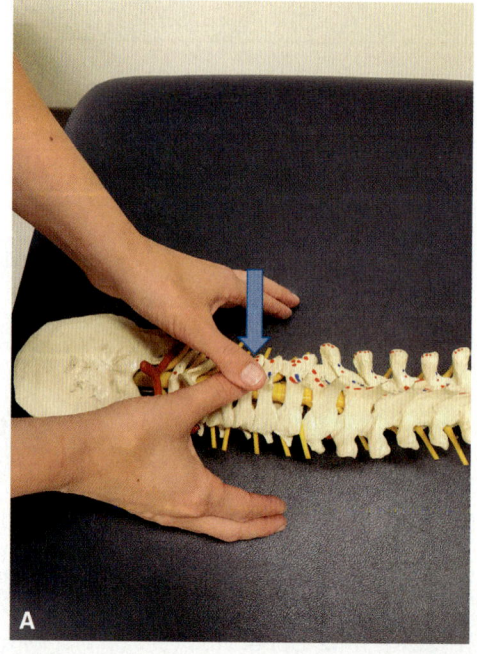 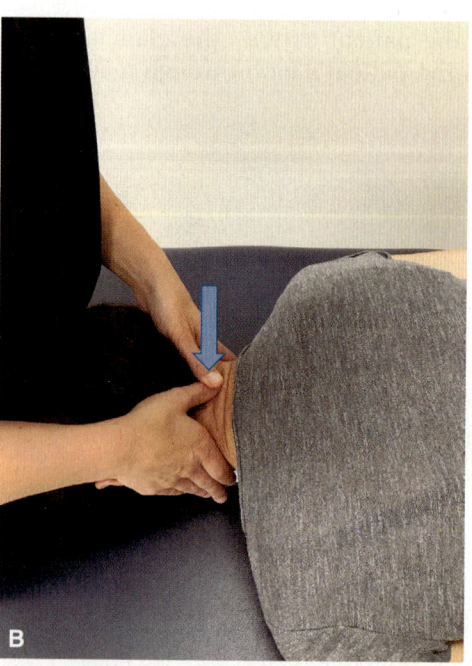

FIGURE 17-13 Cervical central posteroanterior pressure. **A.** On skeleton. **B.** On patient.

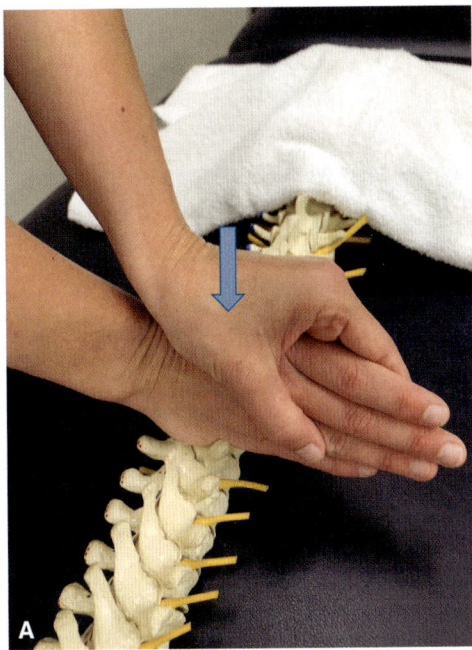
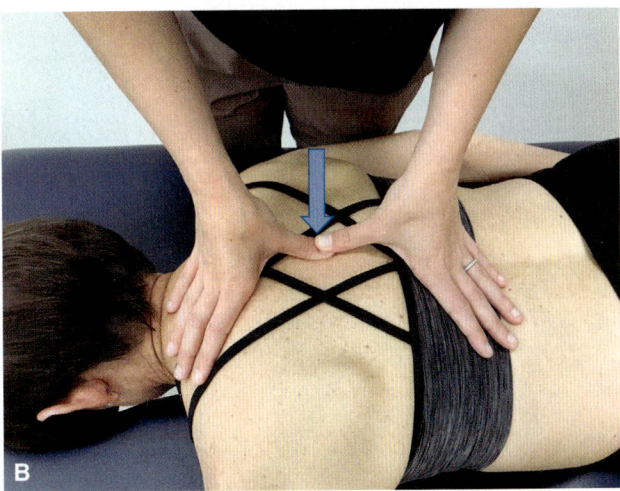

FIGURE 17-14 Thoracic central posteroanterior pressure. **A.** On skeleton. **B.** On patient using mobilizing thumb.

top of the contact hand. Alternatively, the clinician can use the hand placements used for the cervical spine technique for T1–T4 or the central thoracic posteroanterior pressures.

Mobilization: The mobilizing hand imparts a downward force perpendicular to the angle of the spine (Fig. 17-16).

Interpretation: The test is interpreted the same as central posteroanterior pressure assessment.

Cervical Transverse Pressure

Purpose: To assess facet joint mobility with an emphasis on rotation.[47] When applying grade I and II mobilizations, this technique may be used to help decrease pain.[47] When applying grade III and IV mobilizations, this technique may be used to treat local joint hypomobility.[47] For a more aggressive technique, the patient can be positioned in greater amount of cervical rotation.

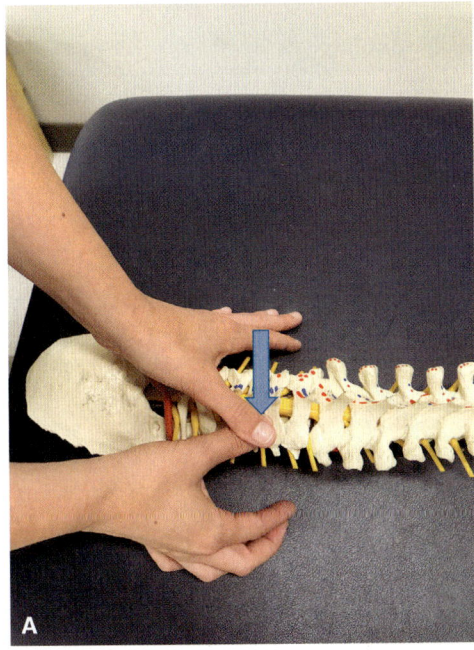
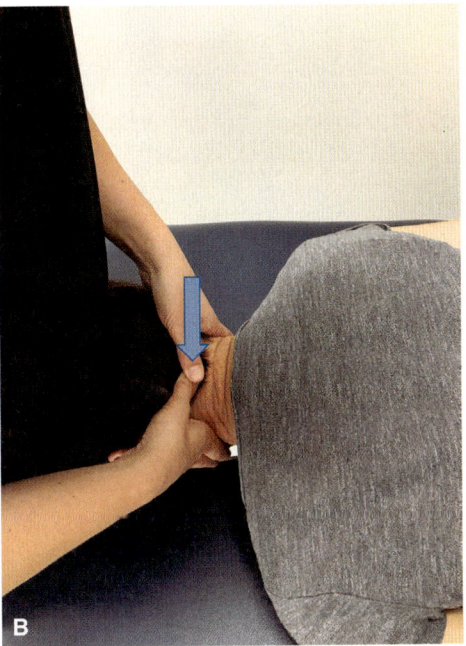

FIGURE 17-15 Cervical unilateral posteroanterior pressure. **A.** On skeleton. **B.** On patient.

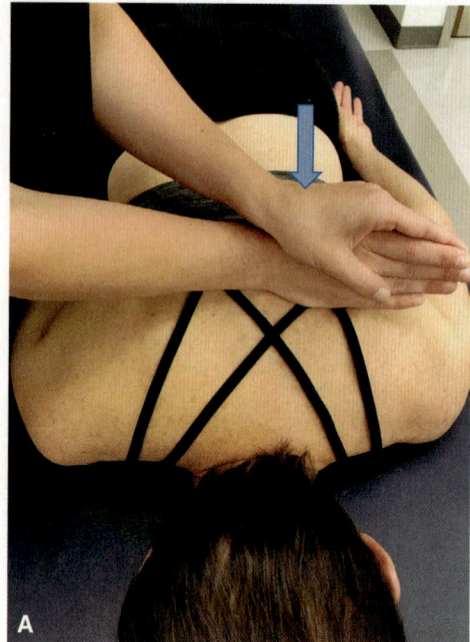
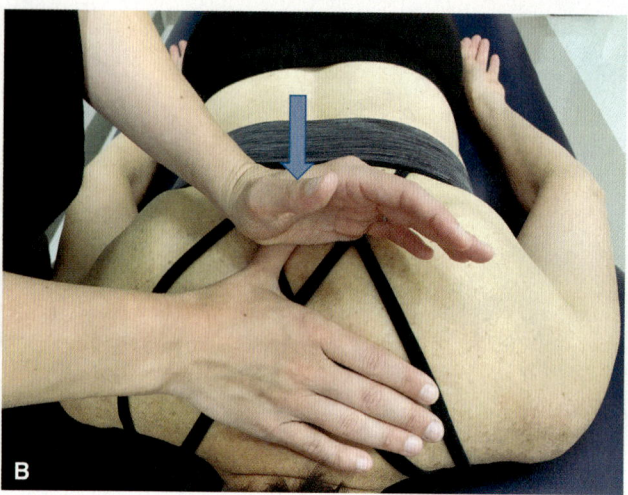

FIGURE 17-16 Thoracic unilateral posteroanterior pressure. **A.** Using hands. **B.** Using mobilizing thumb.

Patient: Prone.
Clinician: The thumb of the nondominant hand is placed lateral to the spinous process of the vertebra to be mobilized. The thumb of the dominant hand (mobilizing thumb) is placed over the other thumb.
Mobilization: The clinician imparts a transverse force to the spinous process (Fig. 17-17).
Interpretation: The clinician should note if any symptoms are created or increased and attempt to judge the amount of motion (hypomobile, normal, or hypermobile).

Thoracic Transverse Pressure

Purpose: As with the cervical transverse pressure, but with an emphasis on the thoracic spine.
Patient: Prone.
Clinician: The thumb of the nondominant hand is placed lateral to the spinous process of the vertebra

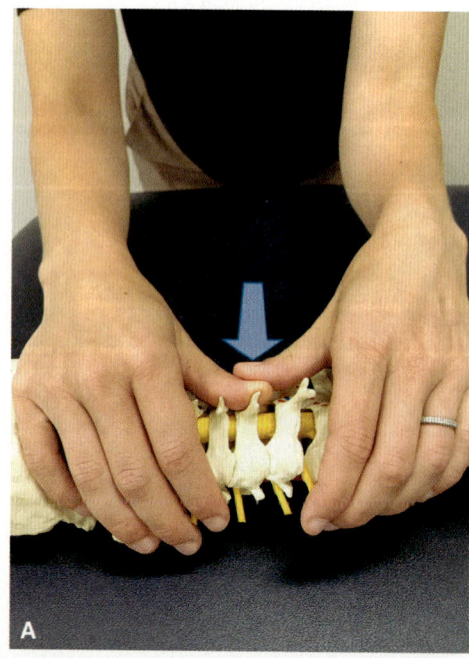
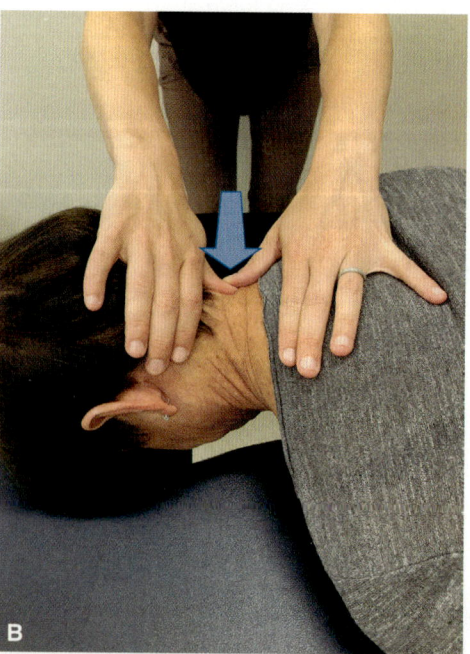

FIGURE 17-17 Cervical transverse pressure. **A.** On skeleton. **B.** On patient.

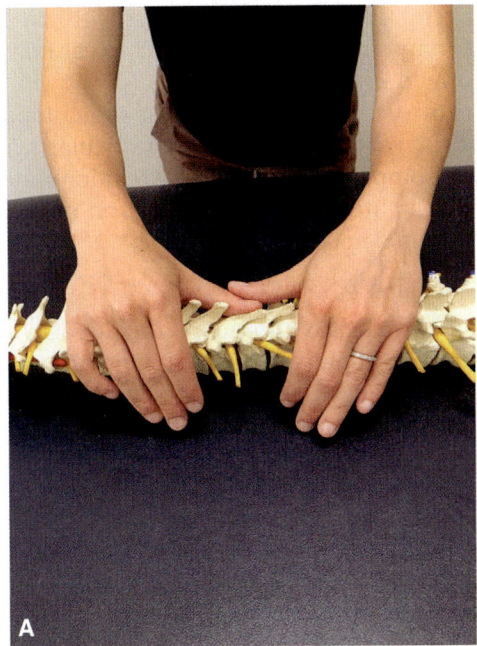

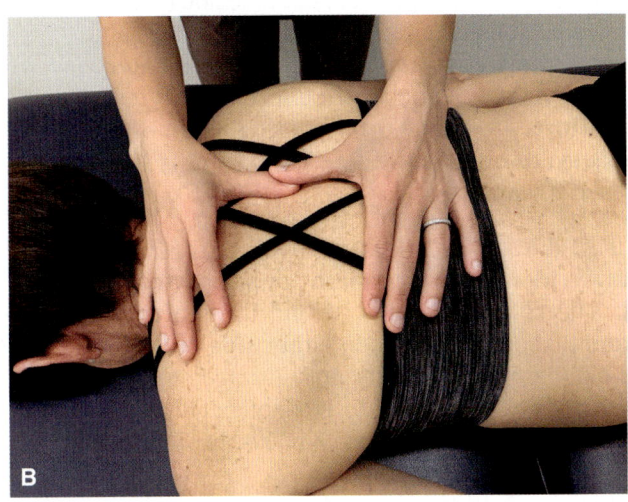

FIGURE 17-18 Thoracic transverse pressure. **A.** On skeleton. **B.** On patient.

to be mobilized. The thumb of the dominant hand (mobilizing thumb) is placed over the other thumb.
Mobilization: The clinician imparts a transverse force to the spinous process (Fig. 17-18).
Interpretation: The test is interpreted the same as cervical transverse pressure assessment.

Costovertebral Assessment Posteroanterior costovertebral joint mobility can be assessed and interpreted similar to the cervical and thoracic unilateral posteroanterior pressures. However, the clinician's point of contact is on the rib, just lateral to the costovertebral joint.

Inferior Glide of First Rib
Purpose: To assess the mobility of the first rib.
Method: With the patient seated, the clinician laterally flexes the neck toward the side to be assessed. The clinician then contacts the first rib with the 2nd metacarpophalangeal joint.
Mobilization: The clinician imparts an anterior and inferior force to the first rib (Fig. 17-19).
Interpretation: The clinician should note if any symptoms are created or increased and attempt to judge the amount of motion (hypomobile, normal, or hypermobile).

Special Tests/Provocative Testing

Clinicians should choose which special/provocative tests to perform based on the patient history and the examination to this point in order to help rule in and rule out competing differential diagnoses. Special tests for the cervical and thoracic spine include tests for

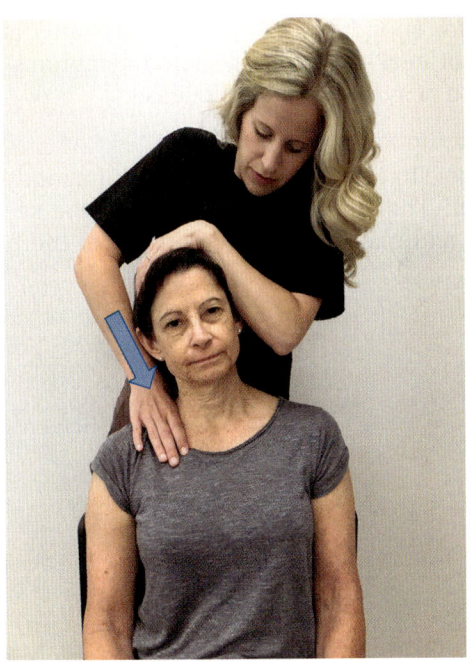

FIGURE 17-19 Inferior glide of the first rib.

radiculopathy, cervicogenic dizziness, VBI, instability, first rib position, and thoracic outlet syndrome.

Special Tests for Radiculopathy The Spurling test, cervical distraction, and cervical compression help identify the presence of cervical radiculopathy. The ULTTs may also be positive in patients with cervical radiculopathy.[45] The cervical traction and compression tests can be modified to the thoracic spine.

Spurling Test

Purpose: To identify radiculopathy or spondylosis.[46,54,55]

Method: The clinician stands behind the seated patient, placing the hands on top of the patient's head. The clinician moves the patient into lateral flexion (Fig. 17-20A) or extension and lateral flexion (Fig. 17-20B) and provides about 7 kg of axial compression. The literature supports both methods for performing this test.

Interpretation: A positive test is reproduction of the patient's symptoms on the side the patient is laterally flexed toward.

Cervical Distraction

Purpose: To identify radiculopathy or spondylosis.[54]

Method: The clinician stands behind the seated patient and places the hands on either side of the patient's skull surrounding the mastoid process. The clinician applies roughly 10 to 15 kg of axial traction by extending from the knees (Fig. 17-21). The test may also be performed in supine.

Interpretation: A positive test for radiculopathy is a reduction in radicular symptoms during traction, with a return of symptoms upon release. A positive test for spondylosis or facet arthropathy is reduction of neck pain or associated symptoms, with a return of symptoms upon release.

Cervical Compression

Purpose: To identify radiculopathy or spondylosis.[54]

Method: The clinician stands behind the seated patient and places the hands on top of the patient's skull. The clinician applies roughly 10 to 15 kg of axial compression (Fig. 17-22). The test may also be performed in supine.

Interpretation: A positive test for radiculopathy is a provocation of, or increase in, radicular symptoms during compression. A positive test for spondylosis or facet arthropathy is reproduction or increase in the patient's neck pain.

Thoracic Compression

Purpose: To identify thoracic radiculopathy.

Method: The clinician stands behind the seated patient and places the hands on the patient's shoulders. The clinician applies roughly 15 kg of axial compression (Fig. 17-23).

Interpretation: A positive test for radiculopathy is a provocation of, or increase in, radicular symptoms during compression. The test may also be painful in patients with compression fractures or spondylosis.

Thoracic Distraction

Purpose: To identify thoracic radiculopathy.

Method: The seated patient crosses arms across the chest. The clinician stands behind the patient, reaching around to hold the patient's elbows. The clinician applies roughly 15 kg of axial traction by extending from the knees (Fig. 17-24).

Interpretation: A positive test for radiculopathy is a reduction in radicular symptoms during traction. The test may also provide pain reduction for patients with compression fractures or spondylosis.

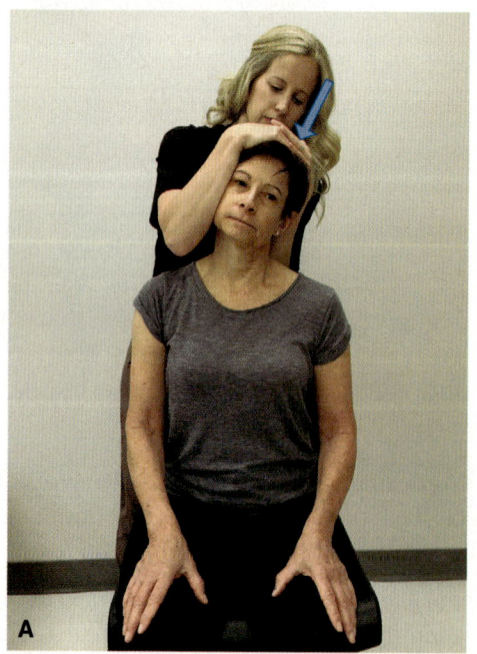 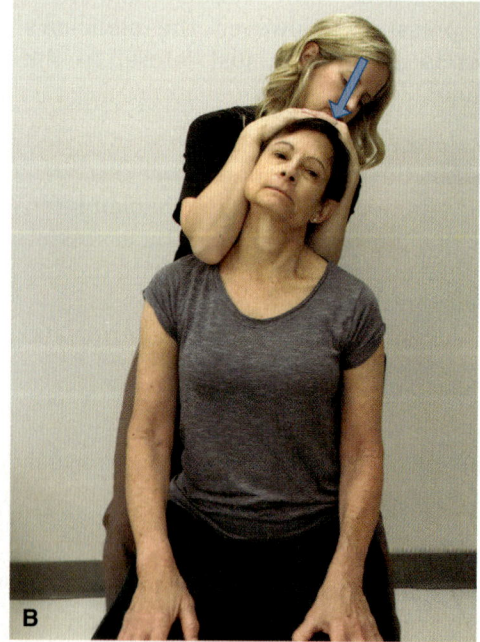

FIGURE 17-20 Spurling test. **A.** With lateral flexion. **B.** With extension and lateral flexion.

CHAPTER 17 | CERVICAL AND THORACIC SPINE 657

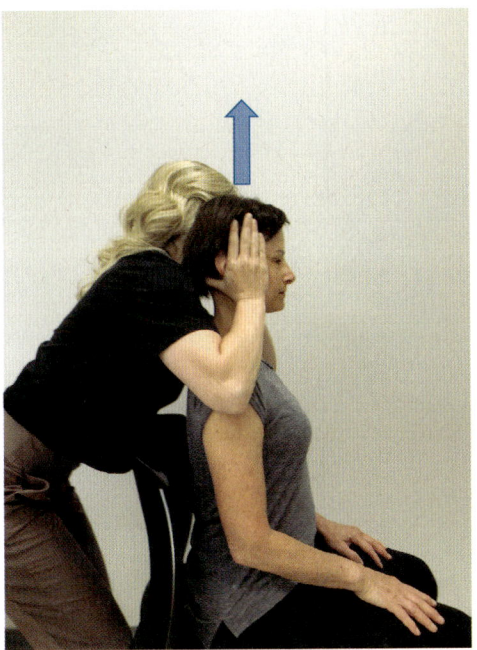

FIGURE 17-21 Cervical distraction.

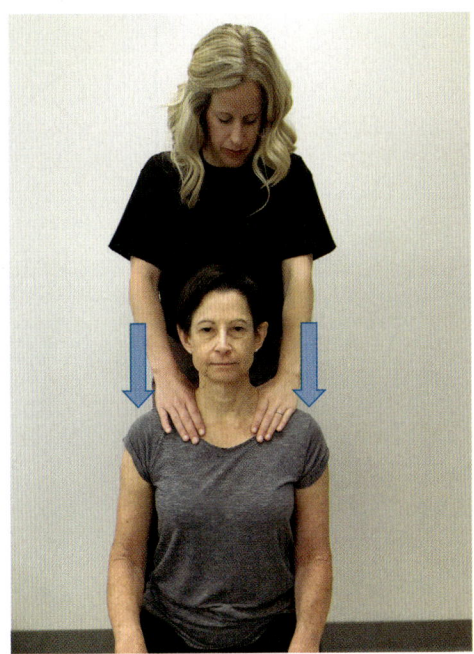

FIGURE 17-23 Thoracic compression.

Tests for Cervicogenic Dizziness There are two tests for cervicogenic dizziness: the head-neck differentiation test and the modified cervical torsion test.

Head-Neck Differentiation Test

Method: With the patient seated in a swivel chair, the clinician first rotates the chair and patient as a unit

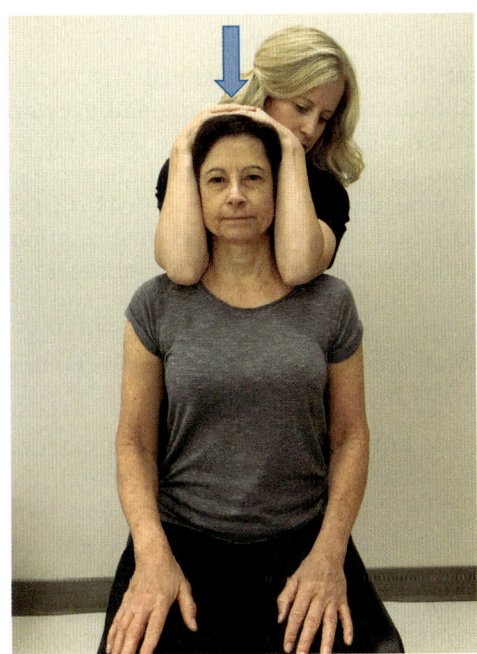

FIGURE 17-22 Cervical compression.

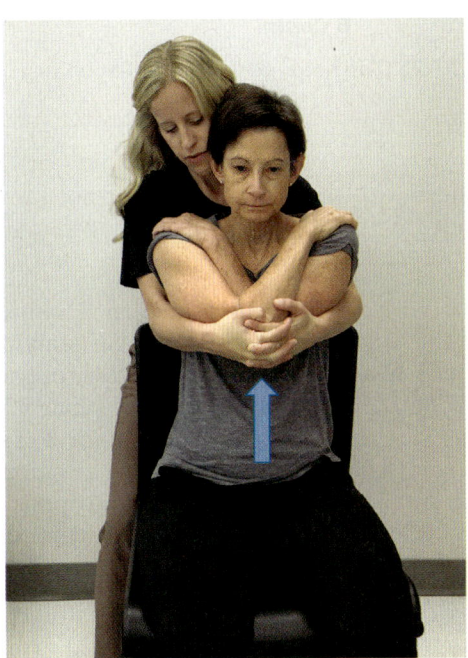

FIGURE 17-24 Thoracic distraction.

with the patient's eyes closed (Fig. 17-25A). The test is then performed with the clinician rotating the chair while asking the patient to maintain the head looking forward (torsion test, Fig. 17-25B).[17,56]

Interpretation: Dizziness created by moving en bloc indicates vestibular dysfunction. Provocation of

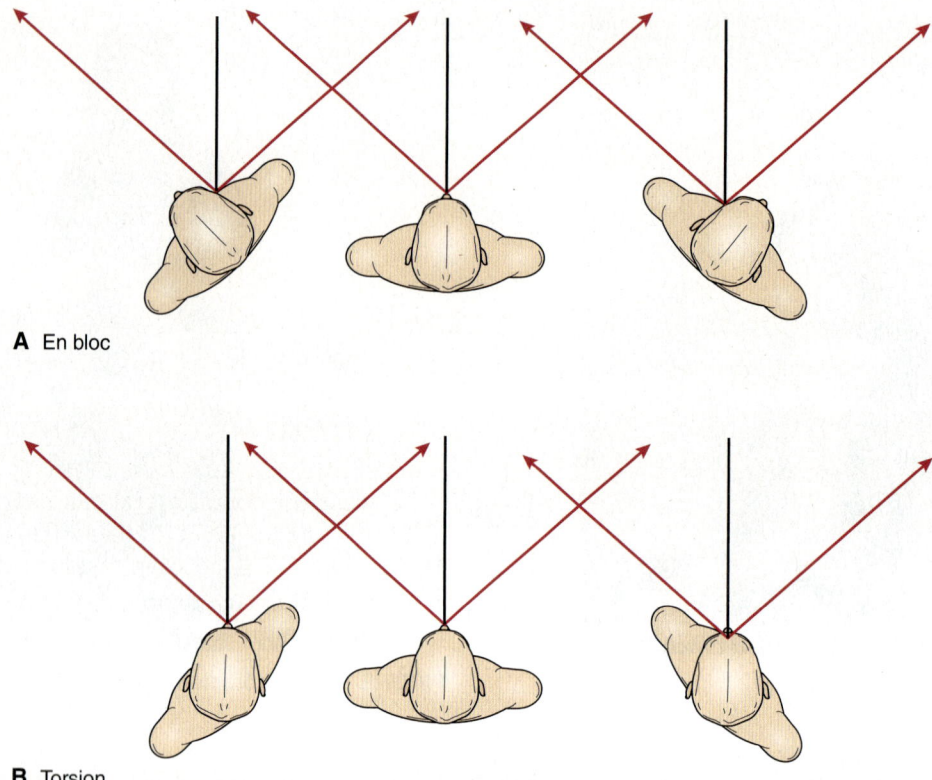

FIGURE 17-25 The head-neck differentiation test. **A.** En bloc test. **B.** Torsion test.

dizziness with the second test, but not the first, is considered a positive test for cervicogenic dizziness.

Modified Cervical Torsion Test
Method: With the patient seated in a swivel chair with the eyes closed, the clinician stabilizes the patient's head so it faces forward throughout the test. The patient then rotates the chair 45 to 90° to one side and holds the position for 30 seconds, then returns to the center starting position for 30 seconds.[56] The test is repeated to the opposite side.
Interpretation: A positive test is if symptoms are provoked in any position during testing.

Vertebrobasilar Insufficiency
Some studies found decreased vertebral and internal carotid artery flow with maximum rotation with or without extension, but this has not been consistently found.[57] Clinicians should screen for the 5D's and 3N's (Table 17-1) during a series of cervical position changes using the VBI test. A positive test is very good for ruling in VBI. However, the test has limited ability to rule out VBI. Because of the very limited sensitivity of VBI testing, clinicians should use a series of premanipulative positions before performing manipulations on the cervical spine, assessing for the 5D's and 3N's at each step. In addition, clinicians may choose to use alternate techniques, such as thoracic manipulations, rather than performing upper cervical spine manipulations when the patency of the vertebral artery is unknown.

Vertebrobasilar Insufficiency Test
Purpose: To identify potential VBI.
Method: With the patient supine and eyes open, the patient's neck is moved into the following positions and held for up to 10 seconds. Between each position, the head is returned to neutral for 10 seconds: full cervical extension, full cervical rotation to one side, full cervical rotation to the opposite side, full extension with rotation to one side, and full extension with rotation to the opposite side (Fig. 17-26).
Interpretation: A positive test is reproduction of any of the 5D's or 3N's with testing.

Cervical Instability Tests
Clinical examination of the alar and transverse ligaments has limited diagnostic accuracy.[25] A positive test warrants consultation or referral based on the individual patient situation. However, a negative test does not rule out the possibility of upper cervical instability. The clinician must take the patient history and physical examination into context. Before performing manual therapy to the upper cervical spine or cervical manipulation, the clinician should progressively stress ligaments with

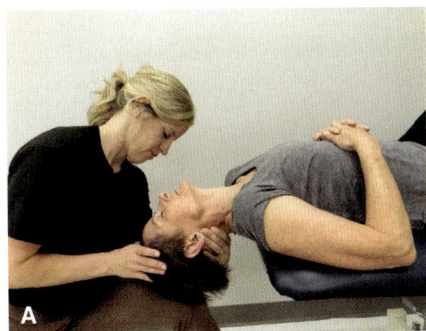 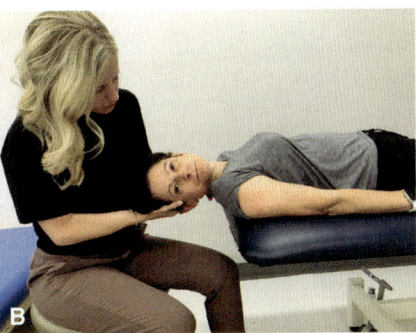 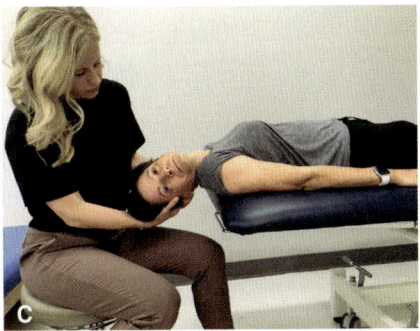

FIGURE 17-26 Progressive vertebrobasilar insufficiency testing. **A.** Extension. **B.** Rotation. **C.** Extension with rotation.

active motion, overpressure, and posterior-to-anterior pressures, ensuring no symptoms of instability are provoked.[8]

Alar Ligament Test

Purpose: To identify an incompetent alar ligament after a trauma.[17]

Method: With the patient seated, the clinician then holds the C2 spinous process with a pincer grip, while the contralateral head passively laterally flexes the patient's neck (Fig. 17-27).

Interpretation: A positive test is a lack of palpable contralateral movement of the C2 spinous process with lateral flexion.

Sharp-Purser Test

Purpose: To identify an incompetent transverse ligament.[25]

Method: With the patient seated, the neck is flexed 20 to 30° and the patient is asked about the presence of symptoms. The clinician then holds the C2 spinous process with a pincer grip to try to stabilize C2, while the contralateral hand applies a posterior force to the patient's forehead (Fig. 17-28).

Interpretation: A positive test is reduction of symptoms with the application of posterior cervical force by the clinician.

First Rib Position The cervical rotation lateral flexion test is used to identify the presence of an elevated first rib. The patient may also have a reduced or painful inferior glide of the first rib.

Cervical Rotation Lateral Flexion Test (aka Lindgren Test)

Purpose: To identify an elevated first rib.

Method: To assess the left first rib, the clinician moves patient's head to end-range right rotation, then passively laterally flexes the neck to the left (Fig. 17-29). The test is repeated on the opposite side to assess the right first rib.[43]

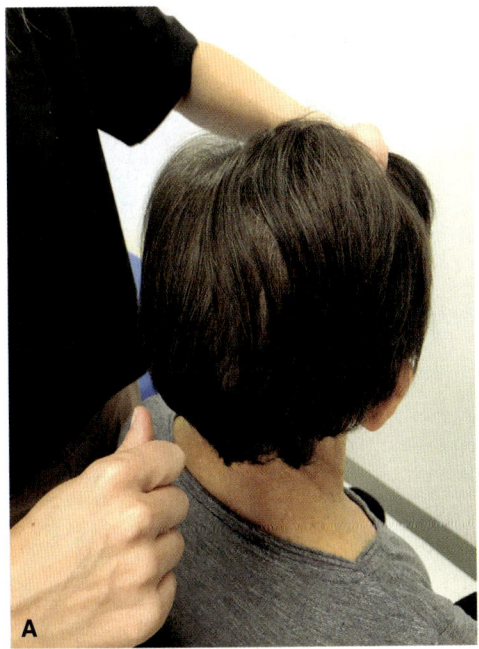 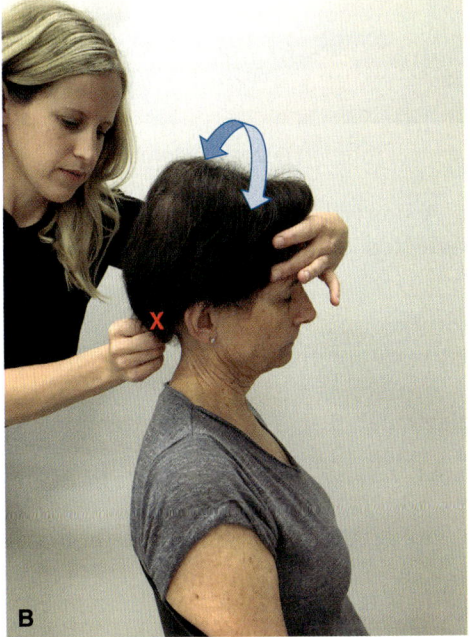

FIGURE 17-27 Alar ligament test. **A.** Pincer grip. **B.** Test.

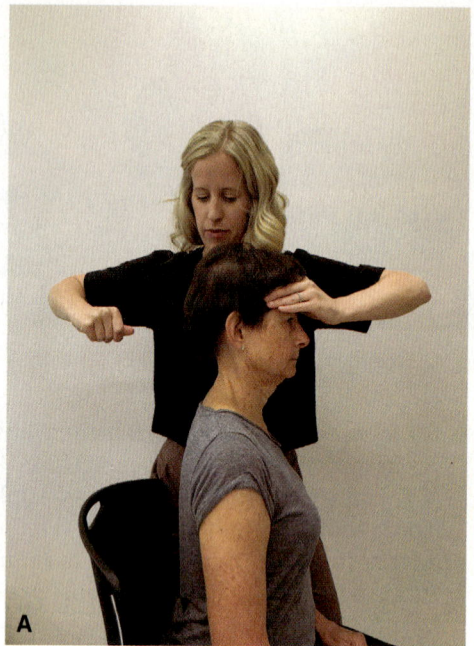
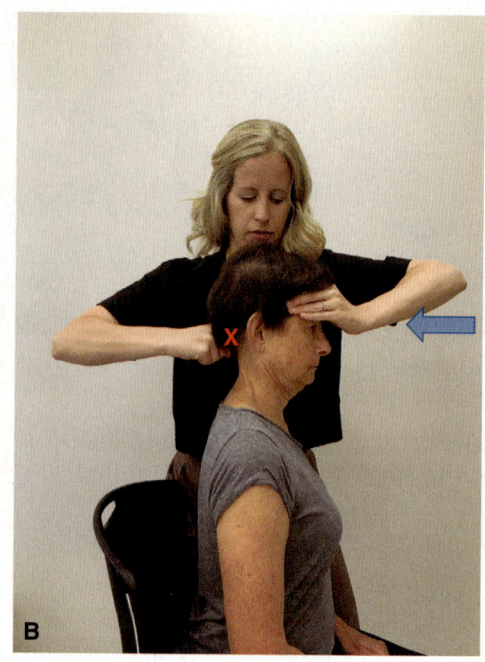

FIGURE 17-28 Sharp-Purser test. **A.** Set up. **B.** Stabilizing pincer grip to C2 with posterior force to patient's forehead.

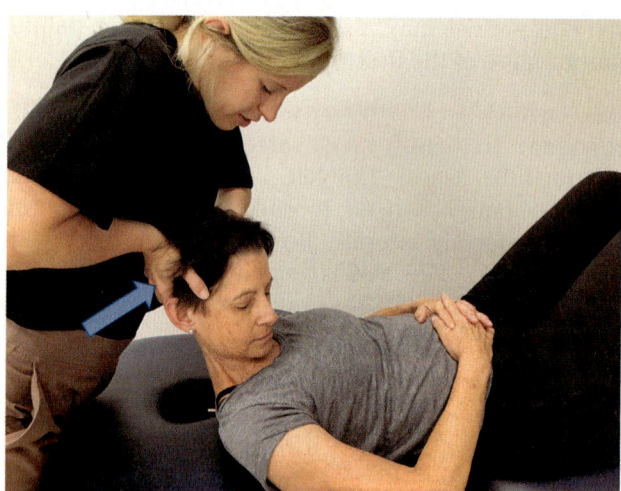

FIGURE 17-29 Cervical rotation lateral flexion test.

Interpretation: A positive test is restriction of motion on the affected side compared to the unaffected side.[58]

Special Tests for Thoracic Outlet Syndrome There are three special tests for thoracic outlet syndrome (TOS): elevated arm stress test (EAST), Adson test, and the costoclavicular test. Each test attempts to affect a different portion of the thoracic outlet.

Elevated Arm Stress Test (aka Roos Test)
Purpose: To identify TOS by reducing the thoracic outlet space

Method: The patient maintains the shoulders in 90° abduction and 90° external rotation while slowly opening and closing the hands for up to 3 minutes, while the clinician monitors the patient's radial pulse (Fig. 17-30).[59,60]

Interpretation: A positive test is production of the patient's complaint of pain or paresthesias or diminished radial pulse. These symptoms may become so noticeable that they prevent the patient from completing the test.

Adson Test
Purpose: To identify TOS by reducing the space within the scalene triangle.

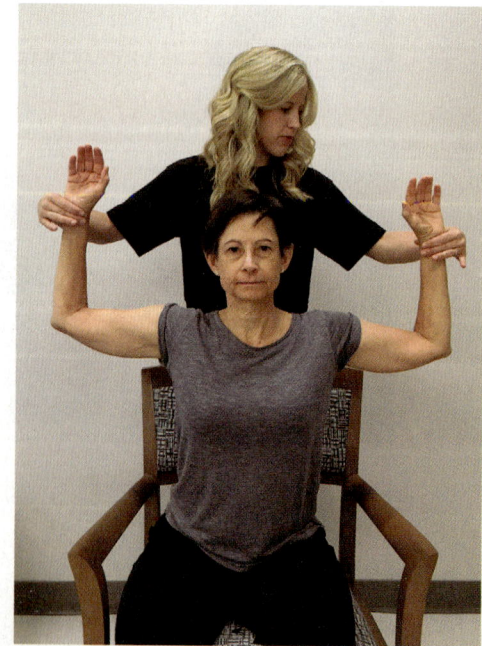

FIGURE 17-30 Elevated arm stress test.

Method: With the shoulder abducted about 30° and extended, the patient rotates toward the side being tested. While maintaining this position, the patient then inhales deeply as the clinician monitors the patient's radial pulse (Fig. 17-31).[60] Variations of this test include the addition of cervical extension[59] or rotation to the opposite side.[60]

Interpretation: A positive test is a diminished radial pulse.

Costoclavicular Test (aka Military Bracing Test)

Purpose: To identify TOS by reducing the costoclavicular space.

Method: The clinician extends the patient's shoulder and maximally retracts the scapula while palpating the radial pulse (Fig. 17-32).[60] Various modifications have been noted, including active retraction and cervical extension. Anecdotally, patients with weak scapular retractors or tight pectoral muscles are unable to reach end-range retraction actively.

Interpretation: A positive test is production of the patient's complaint of pain or paresthesias or diminished radial pulse.

PALPATION

As described in Chapter 4, Spine Osteology and Arthrology, the spinous processes of many of the cervical and most of the thoracic vertebrae are easily palpable. The root of the scapular spine and the inferior scapular angle provide a guide for the approximate location of the T3 and T7 spinous processes. The long and large lower cervical and upper thoracic vertebrae are easily palpated with the neck in flexion and thoracic spine in flexion.

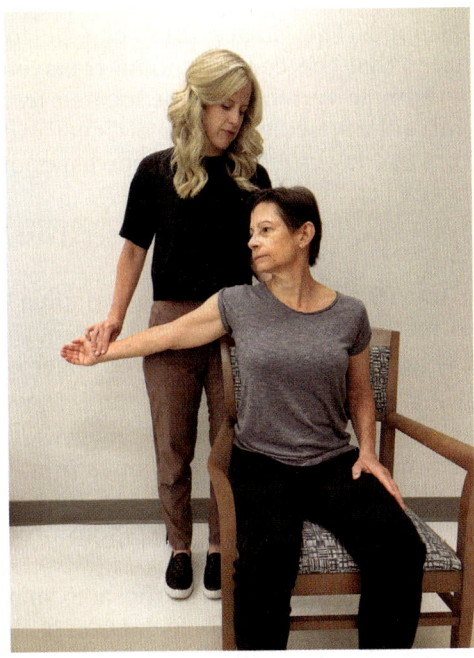

FIGURE 17-31 Adson test.

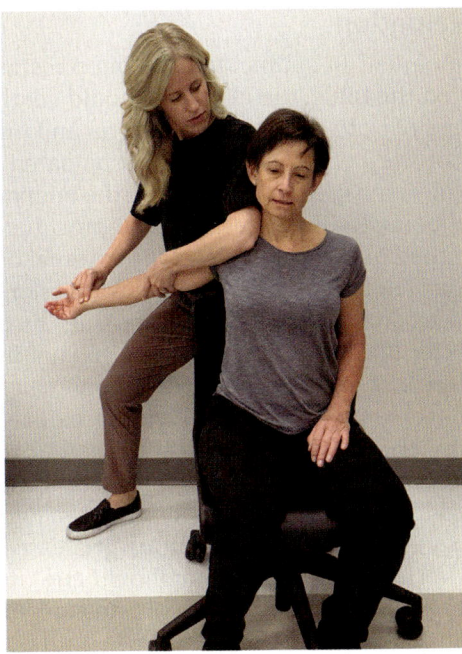

FIGURE 17-32 Costoclavicular test.

Starting Position

Palpation of the cervical and thoracic region can be conducted with the patient in sitting, standing, prone, or supine. The upright sitting or standing position allows for observation of the skin and palpation of major bony prominences. In the supine position, the weight of the head is supported, allowing greater relaxation of surrounding neck musculature and easier palpation of deeper bony prominences. The cervical and thoracic spine can also be palpated with the patient in prone. In this chapter, palpation is described for the cervical and upper thoracic spine with the patient supine and of the full thoracic spine with the patient prone.

The body position and the position of the cervical and thoracic spine should be carefully adjusted on the treatment table. In the supine position, care should be taken to adjust the head end of the table to avoid excessive neck flexion or extension.[61] For prone positioning, the patient should lie in the middle of the treatment table with the nose and face carefully positioned in the table face hole. The head end of the table should be adjusted for the desired amount of neck and thoracic flexion and extension. The patient's head should be positioned in neutral, lateral flexion, or rotation, as appropriate. The patient's arms can be in a position of comfort.

Skin Observation

The skin of the cervical and thoracic regions should be observed for blisters, scars, and discoloration. The scar from an anterior cervical disc fusion will be seen on the anterior neck.

Bony Palpation

With the patient in supine and the head resting comfortably on the table, the clinician should gently place the fingers of both hands on the lateral and posterior aspects of the neck. The occiput is palpated on the posteroinferior aspect of the skull. In the midline of the occipital bone, the external occipital protuberance, a dome-shaped bump, can be felt. The external occipital protuberance marks the center of the superior nuchal line, which can be palpated to either side. Just lateral and slightly inferior to the superior nuchal line, the mastoid processes of the temporal bone can be felt. The transverse processes of C1 vertebrae can be felt slightly anterior and inferior to the mastoid process, just posterior to the ear and the angle of the mandible (see Fig. 4-21A and B in Chapter 4, Spine Osteology and Arthrology). To palpate the spinous processes of the cervical vertebrae, the clinician should cup one hand around the side of the neck and palpate along the midline of the neck. The posterior tubercle of C1 is neither prominent nor palpable. The bifid spinous process of the C2 vertebrae can be felt in the midline of the neck, just inferior to the external occipital protuberance. The spinous processes of C3–C5 vertebrae lie deep in the neck and are not easily palpable due to the normal cervical lordosis. With the neck flexed, the long spinous processes of C6, C7, and uppermost thoracic vertebrae may be felt. The relative prominence of C7 versus T1 spinous processes varies among individuals. Owing to the long inferiorly sloping spinous processes in the thoracic spine, the tips of the thoracic spinous processes lie in a horizontal plane inferior to the corresponding vertebral body and associated transverse processes (see Fig. 4-21C in Chapter 4, Spine Osteology and Arthrology). The spinous processes of the vertebrae are normally vertically in line with each other.

The facet joints of the cervical spine feel like small domes lying deep to overlying muscle. These joints can be palpated approximately 2 to 3 cm lateral to the spinous processes. Beginning at C2, the clinician should palpate in the area of the facet joint and note any tenderness or enlargement. To confirm the vertebral level of any one cervical facet joint, the alignment can be checked against the following landmarks, as shown in Figure 17-33, the hyoid bone in line with C3 and the thyroid cartilage in line with C4 and C5.

After completion of all palpation with the patient supine, the patient can be positioned in prone for palpation of the thoracic vertebrae and associated ribs. The thoracic spinous processes can be easily palpated in the midline of the back. The thoracic vertebrae are covered by less muscle bulk than the lumbar vertebrae. The transverse process is found at the level of the accessible medial end of the associated rib that connects to the vertebra. Refer to Chapter 4, Spine

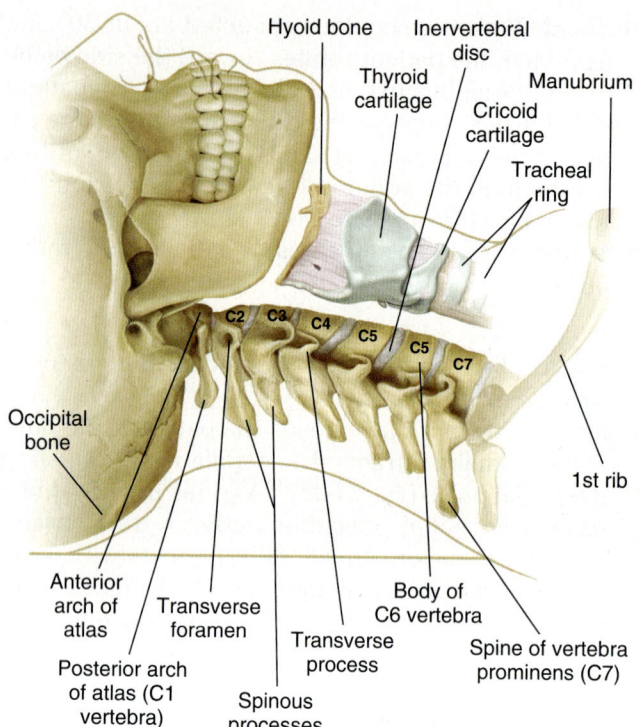

FIGURE 17-33 Cervical spine, supine position. Note major bony landmarks. (Gest TR. *Lippincott Atlas of Anatomy*. 2nd ed. Wolters Kluwer; 2020: Plate 7-13.)

Osteology and Arthrology, for rib attachments to the vertebral column. An alternative method for palpation of the thoracic transverse processes requires appreciation of the gradual increase in sloping of the thoracic spinous processes from superior to inferior until approximately T8 at which point the spinous processes are less sloped. The "finger rule" can be followed, which states that the corresponding transverse process of a thoracic vertebra can be located by moving just lateral and a specific number of finger widths superior from the lower edge of the corresponding spinous process[61] as follows:

- T1, T2 and T11, T12 spinous processes: plus one finger width
- T3, T4 and T9, T10 spinous processes: plus two finger widths
- T5–T8 spinous processes: plus three finger widths

Following the finger rule, the transverse process of T2 is located just lateral to and one finger width superior to the lower edge of the T2 spinous process. The transverse process of T9 is found two finger widths superior and just lateral to the T9 spinous process, as so forth.

The kyphotic curvature of the thoracic spine must be considered when attempting palpation of the facet joints. The facet joints can be palpated in line with the thoracic IV disc, as shown in Figure 17-34. The

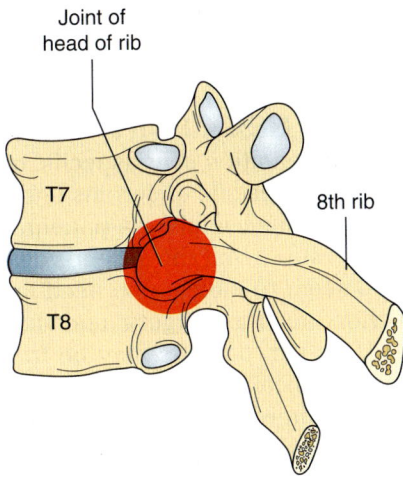

FIGURE 17-34 Relationship of thoracic spinous processes, transverse processes, and intervertebral discs. (Adapted from Oatis CA. *Kinesiology: The Mechanics and Pathomechanics of Human Movement.* 3rd ed. Wolters Kluwer; 2017: Figure 29.13.)

costotransverse joint is formed by articulation of a rib with the anterior portion of a transverse process. The transverse process and associated rib forming the costotransverse joint can be palpated just lateral to the transverse process. The tubercle of a rib can sometimes be palpated adjacent to the tip of the transverse process. The angle of the rib is the largest curvature that extends posteriorly. The superior edge of the rib is rounded, whereas the inferior edge has a sharper edge. The deep lying costovertebral joints formed by articulation of the rib with the vertebral body and IV disc are not palpable.

The articulations of the ribs with the sternum must be palpated with the patient sitting, standing, or supine. Ribs 1 through 7 articulate directly with the sternum via their costal cartilage and are called "true ribs" (Fig. 17-35). Ribs 8 through 10 connect indirectly to the ribs and are called "false ribs." Ribs 11 and 12 do not connect to the sternum and are called "floating ribs." A reliable orientation point for palpation of the anterior thoracic cage is the sternal notch that corresponds to the level of T2.

Soft-Tissue Palpation

Palpation of the neck soft tissues may be easiest to perform with the patient supine to assist with muscular relaxation. The broad proximal attachment of the superficial trapezius muscle can be palpated throughout from the external occipital protuberance along the spinous processes to T12 and along the superior nuchal line. The muscle passes along the lateral sides of the neck toward the attachment to the acromion. The upper trapezius and most superior portion of the middle trapezius can be palpated. The middle and

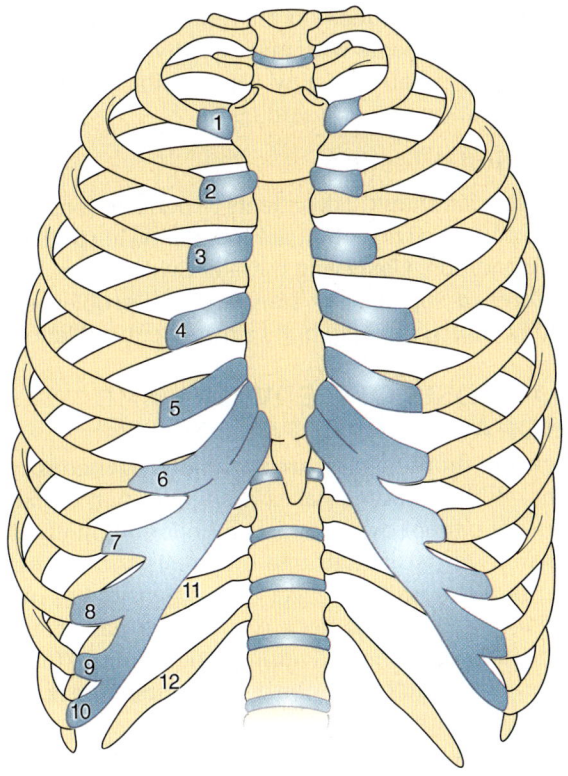

FIGURE 17-35 Sternum and ribs, anterior view. (Adapted from Oatis CA. *Kinesiology: The Mechanics and Pathomechanics of Human Movement.* 3rd ed. Wolters Kluwer; 2017: Figure 29.16.)

lower trapezius must be palpated with the patient in sitting or prone. Along the base of the skull to the mastoid processes, the trapezius and sternocleidomastoid (SCM) muscles share an attachment. The proximal and distal attachments, anterior and posterior borders, and muscle belly of the SCM muscle are superficial and easily palpable. Just posterior to the superior border of the SCM, the semispinalis capitis, splenius capitis, and levator scapulae can be palpated. The distal attachment of the levator scapulae to the superior medial portion of the scapula is easily felt beneath the trapezius.

With the patient positioned in prone, the extrinsic back muscles can be felt directly or indirectly. The trapezius and latissimus dorsi dominate the superficial posterior aspect of the back and are most easily palpated when the muscles are active. The deeper lying intrinsic muscles are not easily palpated in the thoracic region.

Gait

The clinician should perform a more global assessment of the patient's gait. Rather than considering the fine details of excessive pronation or supination, the clinician should focus on movement quality and base of support. Patients with myelopathy typically have an ataxic gait.[23] Patients may also exhibit a decrease in trunk rotation due to guarding.[62]

Functional Testing

The clinician should ask patients to perform (or simulate) some of the activities that are difficult owing to their current condition. Observing these activities, such as sleep postures or supine-to-sit transfers, and problem-solving modifications, can help build a therapeutic alliance.

DIAGNOSIS OF CERVICAL AND THORACIC SPINE PATHOLOGY

Neck and thoracic pain are both heterogeneous conditions. While in some cases a specific pathoanatomic cause of patient symptoms can be found, many times, a definitive pathoanatomic diagnosis for mechanical pain is not possible.[14] Like LBP, subgrouping or classifying patients with neck or thoracic pain may help guide interventions and improve outcomes. Most clinical practice guidelines consider grouping neck pain in terms of acuity.

- Acute pain has been present for less than 3 months.
- Chronic pain has been present for greater than 3 months.

Unlike LBP, there is some disagreement on the utility of the subacute grouping, with many guidelines collapse acute and subacute phases into one group,[10] likely because of the similarities of intervention recommendations.

The 2017 neck pain clinical practice guidelines from the American Physical Therapy Association[14] and the 2018 Royal Dutch Society for Physical Therapy[13] have adopted slightly different approaches to classifying neck pain (Table 17-6).

Using these platforms as a foundation, the following sections classify neck and thoracic pathologies using a combination of pathoanatomic and nonpathoanatomic categories recognizing that, even when an anatomic classification, such as spondylosis, is used, the true anatomic cause of symptoms may be variable or unknown.

NONSPECIFIC NECK PAIN

Perhaps, the best definition of nonspecific neck pain is neck pain without a specific or serious underlying disease. This term can be useful for a patient, as it helps the patient understand that the absence of serious pathology would seem to indicate no need for a drastic course of action, such as surgery, and that recovery is expected. However, patients may be frustrated by the inability of medical providers to find out "what is wrong." Regional interdependence and the example of forward head posture (FHP) are presented as an example of how a patient may have neck pain without a serious underlying disease/pathology.

Regional interdependence is the clinical observation that one region of the body can influence another.[63,64] Locally, fusion of two vertebrae can lead to hypermobility of the segments above and below.[65] Regionally, increased kyphosis can lead to upper cervical spine extension to allow the individual to continue to observe and interact with one's surroundings. Treatment of adjacent or regional areas may lead to symptom improvement because of the mechanical as well as centrally mediated effects. Strengthening the hip or improving dorsiflexion ROM can improve the pain of patellofemoral pain syndrome by allowing the knee to function more optimally in the sagittal plane.[66] Thoracic manipulation may reduce cervical pain through neurophysiologic effects more than creating a purely mechanical improvement in cervical motion.[64,67] In addition, pain in one region can alter muscle function in other regions.[68] For example, scapulothoracic strengthening has been shown to improve elbow pain.[69] It is thought that restoring ROM, flexibility, endurance, and strength in the thoracolumbar spine and scapular stabilizers can improve symptoms, not just in the low back but also in the thoracic and cervical regions, including nonspecific neck pain.[14]

TABLE 17-6
EXAMPLES OF CLASSIFICATIONS OF NECK PAIN

American Physical Therapy Association	Dutch Society for Physical Therapy
• Neck pain with mobility deficits • Neck pain with movement coordination impairments (including whiplash-related disorder) • Neck pain with headaches (cervicogenic headaches) • Neck pain with radiating pain (radicular pain)	• Neck pain with no signs or symptoms of major structural pathology and no or minor influence on ADLs • Neck pain with no signs or symptoms of major structural pathology but major influence on ADLs • Neck pain with no signs or symptoms of major structural pathology but presence of neurologic signs • Neck pain with signs or symptoms of major structural pathology (e.g., infection, dislocation, fracture)

ADLs, activities of daily living.

The head constitutes approximately 6% of body weight.[70] Using the concepts of regional interdependence, consider the effect suboptimal head alignment can have on the structures below. FHP is typically defined as a position of lower cervical flexion with upper cervical extension. A recent systematic review found that FHP was related to neck pain in adults.[71] Locally, FHP results in shortening of the suboccipital muscles and lengthening of the cervical extensors.[72] There is an increase in extensor muscle activity to maintain a forward gaze. The C2 nerve root and greater occipital nerve pass through the suboccipital triangle. Forward head position decreases the space within the triangle by about 19%.[72] It is thought that the combination of suboccipital shortening, increased cervical extensor activity, and/or changes in the suboccipital triangle may also be a causative factor in cervicogenic headaches (CGHs). FHP has been linked to adverse changes in the respiratory system, including decreased diaphragmatic breathing, decreased vital capacity, and increased use of accessory muscles of respiration.[70] An FHP increases the activity of mandibular elevators, which can lead to temporomandibular dysfunction.[73] Patients with an FHP have reduced proprioception,[70] which may limit their ability to self-correct to a more neutral position. FHP may also result in decreased balance.[70]

Although FHP is not a diagnosis, it appears to be a direct and indirect cause of neck pain and CGHs, while also having more remote effects on balance and posture as a whole. It is equally possible the FHP is the result of other factors. Poor vision can lead to FHP in order to adequately read a computer screen. Likewise, trunk extensor fatigue from prolonged unsupported sitting and increased kyphosis due to osteoporosis can also lead to FHP. Treatment, therefore, may include a wide variety of interventions (Fig. 17-36). Education may include reassurance that there is not an underlying serious pathology and that nonspecific neck pain is typically self-limiting. Multiple types of exercise may be helpful: postural awareness, ROM, stretching, muscular endurance exercises, strengthening, and aerobic exercise. All clinical practice guidelines recommend both education and exercise for the treatment of neck pain.[10] Manual therapy, such as joint mobilization, manipulation, and soft-tissue mobilization, although not considered to be primary interventions, are supported by lower levels of evidence and can be a useful adjunct during the plan of care of patients with nonspecific neck pain.[74,75] At this time, dry needling does not appear to provide an added benefit for patients with nonspecific neck pain[76,77] and is currently not recommended by the Canadian[11] or Dutch[13] guidelines.

There is limited information to guide clinicians in making a prognosis for patients with nontraumatic, nonspecific neck pain. Recovery will be fastest during the first 6 to 12 weeks after onset.[14] After 12 weeks, patients may still have some recovery, but improvements are likely to be slow and limited.[14]

PATHOANATOMIC CAUSES OF NECK PAIN AND CERVICAL SYNDROMES

While a pathoanatomic cause, such as cervical myelopathy, may be found for some patients with neck pain, for other patients, it may be difficult to identify a symptom generator. In some cases, such as cervical spondylosis, there may be multiple potential symptom generators. This section reviews the following classifications of neck pain: spondylosis, radiculopathy, WAD, CGH, cervicogenic dizziness, facet hypertrophy, and torticollis.

Spondylosis

Spondylosis is a more inclusive term than cervical disc degeneration or cervical arthritis as it considers all components of the spine: intervertebral disc, facet joints, and associated soft tissue. Cervical spondylosis is believed to be primarily due to age-related degeneration; however, there also appears to be an immune inflammatory component.[26] Nearly all individuals have some degree of cervical spondylosis by age 50, but like arthritis in other joints, not all are symptomatic. Changes appear to begin first in the intervertebral disc where there is a loss of disc height and reduced annular strength, leading to lateral stenosis and facet joint degeneration.[78] Myelopathy can occur in the presence of vertebral body instability. In addition, nociceptive fibers may be sensitized by inflammatory cytokines. Therefore, spondylosis may lead to radiculopathy, myelopathy, facet arthropathy, and nonspecific neck pain. The peak incidence of symptomatic spondylosis is between the ages of 40 and 60 years.[26]

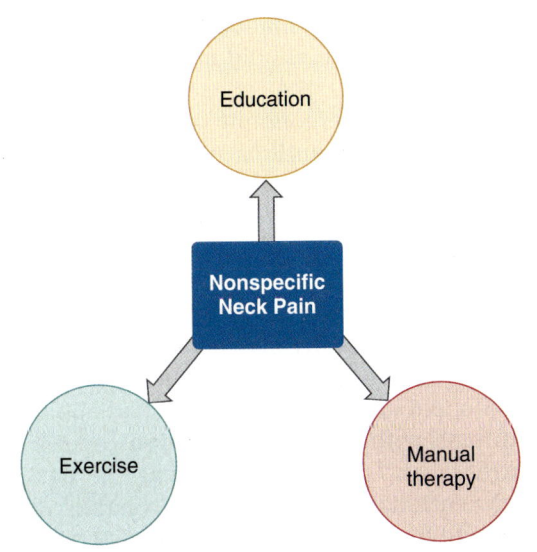

FIGURE 17-36 Nonspecific neck pain interventions.

Patients with spondylosis without radiculopathy or myelopathy typically present with a global loss of cervical motion and may have end-range pain. Cervical extension is typically painful, whereas flexion is more likely to be reported as feeling stiff. Accessory motion is typically limited and may be painful. Postural deviations and reduced cervical flexion endurance testing are common.[79] Manual traction may decrease symptoms.[26]

Conservative management with rehabilitation and analgesics is the primary treatment for cervical spondylosis. Exercises should include CROM, stretching, cervical isometrics,[79] and postural exercises[79] as needed. Joint mobilizations and manual traction may be beneficial adjuncts.[79] Self-care should include a home exercise program and may include the use of heat. A home TENS (transcutaneous electrical nerve stimulation) unit may be beneficial for patients with ongoing pain.[79]

Epidural steroid injections may provide symptom reduction for those not responding to exercise.[26] For patients with progressive neurologic decline or moderate-to-severe pain that is unresponsive to conservative management, surgery may be performed to decompress nerve roots or the spinal cord and improve spinal alignment.[26] Surgical options include cervical disc arthroplasty, fusion, and laminectomy.[80] Smoking, advanced age, diabetes, and obesity negatively impact surgical outcomes.[26]

Cervical Radiculopathy

Pathology Trauma, disc herniation, osteophytes, facet hypertrophy, spinal instability, and spondylosis may cause cervical nerve root compression, irritation, and inflammation, resulting in cervical radiculopathy.[26,44,81] The C6 and C7 nerve roots are most often affected,[81-83] with the most likely culprit being disc herniation.[6] With an incidence between 0.8 and 1.8 per 1,000,[84] cervical radiculopathy is not as common as lumbar disc herniation or lumbar radiculopathy. Although there is no gold standard for diagnosing cervical radiculopathy, most clinicians would agree that the diagnosis is best supported by identification of nerve root compression on magnetic resonance imaging (MRI) or computed tomography (CT) scan along with concordant clinical examination findings.[85,86]

History Patients with cervical radiculopathy report constant or intermittent, central, or unilateral neck pain.[27] Paresthesias or pain generally extend into the arm, forearm, or hand [14,81] and are affected by neck motion. Classically, patients with cervical radiculopathy report that arm pain is worse than neck pain.[81] Symptoms may be reduced with walking.[81] Some patients report finding some symptom relief when resting the forearm on top of the head ("shoulder abduction test"),[26] but this has low diagnostic value.[43,81] Symptoms may be worsened with certain upper extremity tasks, such as ironing, looking up, or trying to hold a phone between the ear and the shoulder.[87] Some patients report arm weakness.[87] Symptoms may gradually progress over time or may be of sudden onset. While some patients with an acute onset report a history of trauma, many report the onset during sitting, standing, or walking.[88]

Key Examination Findings Patients with cervical radiculopathy may present with the following positive findings[14,27,81,89]:

- Dermatomal paresthesia
- Myotomal weakness
- Upper extremity reflex changes
- Positive Spurling test

Paresthesias may vary from the traditional dermatomal map, differing by one level superior or inferior.[90] Symptoms are generally worsened by neck motion, and spasming may be present.[87] Manual traction or distraction may decrease symptoms.[14,26,81] Patients may have a positive ULTT.[14,81] Because there is no gold-standard test, clinicians should take into account the patient's overall clinical picture to diagnose cervical radiculopathy.[81]

Differential Diagnoses Differential diagnosis should include myelopathy, nonspecific neck pain, and peripheral nerve entrapments, such as carpal and ulnar tunnel syndromes.[89] Clinicians must also consider the possibility of a double-crush syndrome (see Chapter 15, Elbow Complex).[89]

Rehabilitation Focus and Key Points The four main treatment strategies for cervical radiculopathy are education, exercise, manual therapy, and traction (Fig. 17-37). Education should include advice to stay active, reassurance, the consequences of stress and exercise, and ergonomic advice.[91] Short-term pharmacologic interventions may be appropriate if symptoms are severe or highly irritable. Patients with chronic pain may benefit from additional information regarding pain physiology, relaxation, and coping strategies.[91]

Nearly 80% of patients with signs and symptoms of cervical radiculopathy may have a directional preference and respond to repeated movements.[12] More than 80% of patients centralized and had abolishment of symptoms with repeated extension (or retraction with extension).[92] Lateral flexion was the next most common centralizing motion.[92] A reasonable course of action would be for clinicians to use the steps outlined in Figure 17-38 to determine whether the patient has

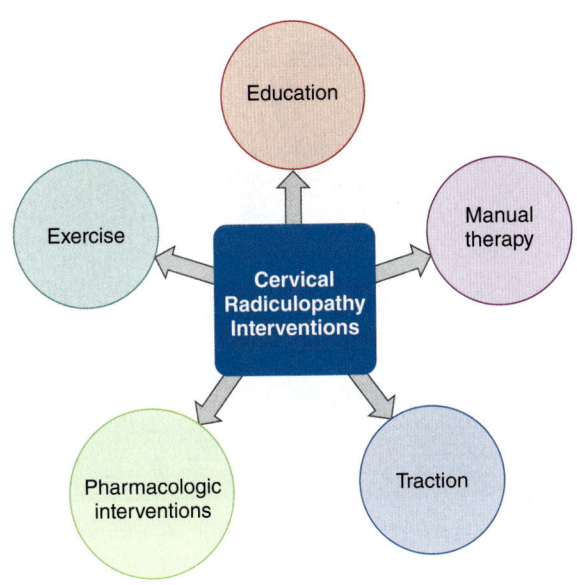

FIGURE 17-37 Cervical radiculopathy interventions.

and shown to have a 56% reduction in cervical disc herniation.[78]

Patients may also benefit from cervical stabilization exercises, including isometrics and postural exercises.[14,94] CROM exercises and stretching can be added[14,94]; however, these may not be well tolerated acutely as they may peripheralize or increase symptoms. The addition of cervical-specific exercises appears to result in quicker improvements than a more generalized strengthening and postural exercise program.[91] Aerobic exercise can assist with symptom modulation and improving general fitness.

Manual therapy can assist with symptom modulation and improving ROM.[14] Clinicians should consider cervical and thoracic joint mobilizations. In addition, thoracic manipulation may provide immediate pain reduction lasting at least 3 days and may lead to improved deep cervical flexor function.[95] Neural mobilizations in patients with cervical radiculopathy appear to improve nerve flexibility, increase neural blood flow, and may reduce neuropathic pain (Fig. 17-39).[44]

Traction decreases nerve root compression and may be used as an adjunctive intervention.[86,96] Manual traction appears to provide significant short-term reduction in pain, whereas mechanical traction may provide slightly longer pain relief.[83] Manual traction may be provided as straight distraction (Fig. 17-40) or in slight flexion and is generally held for 10 to 50 seconds, then released, and repeated. Although it is difficult to judge the amount of force provided with manual traction, about 20 lbs. (~9 kg) has been recommended. Mechanical traction is less fatiguing for the clinician, may allow for better patient relaxation, and provides more consistency. Common mechanical traction forces are in the range of 11 to 26 lbs. (5 to 12 kg) or 10% body weight.[96] Mechanical cervical traction is generally performed in supine with the neck flexed 20 to 30° for about 20 minutes, using 50 to 60 second holds with 10 to 20 seconds off.[96]

Pharmacologic interventions may be needed. Clinical practice guidelines recommend the use of topical nonsteroidal anti-inflammatory drug (NSAID) and exercise before the provision of oral NSAIDs to minimize the risk of adverse drug reactions.[86] If symptoms are not controlled, then tramadol should be considered.[86] Rarely, acute patients may benefit from the short-term use of a cervical collar to assist with symptom management.[14]

Expected Outcomes More than 90% of patients with cervical radiculopathy improve with conservative care.[97] Patients generally experience marked improvement in arm pain and neck pain and function within 6 weeks, and continued improvement occurred

a directional preference and if centralization occurs with the methodical application of cervical spine loading strategies.[86,93] Patients with evidence of centralization with repeated movements were followed by MRI

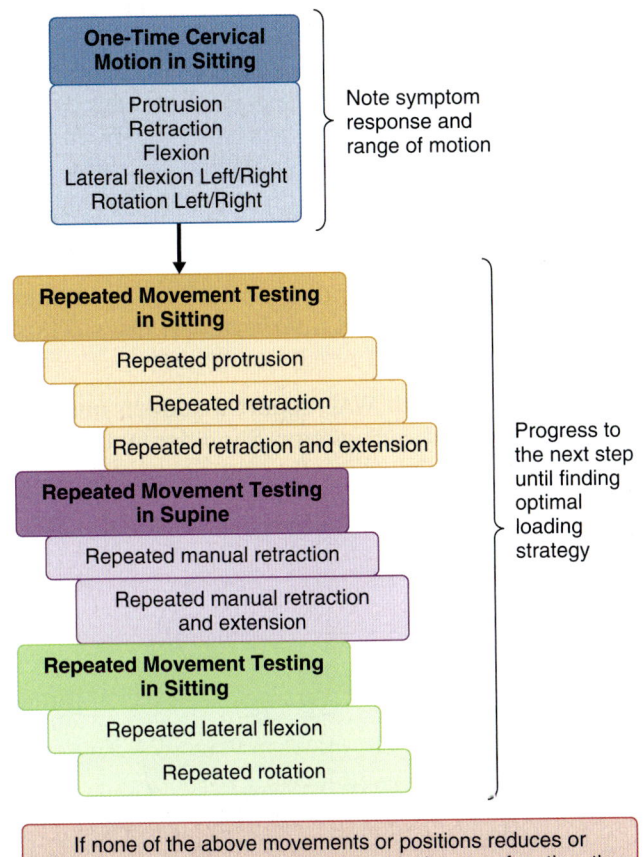

FIGURE 17-38 Cervical loading strategies.

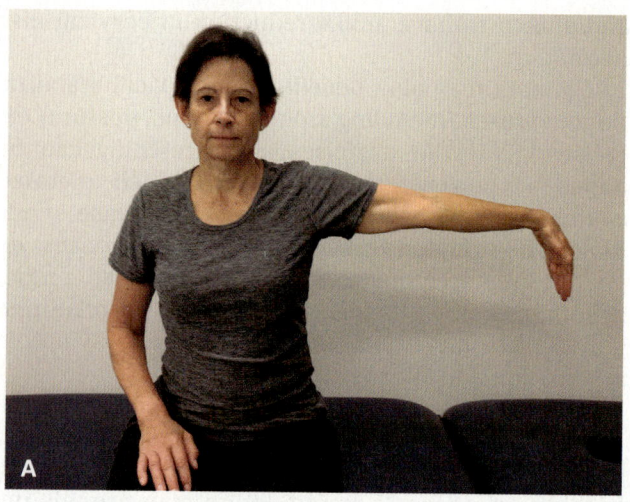
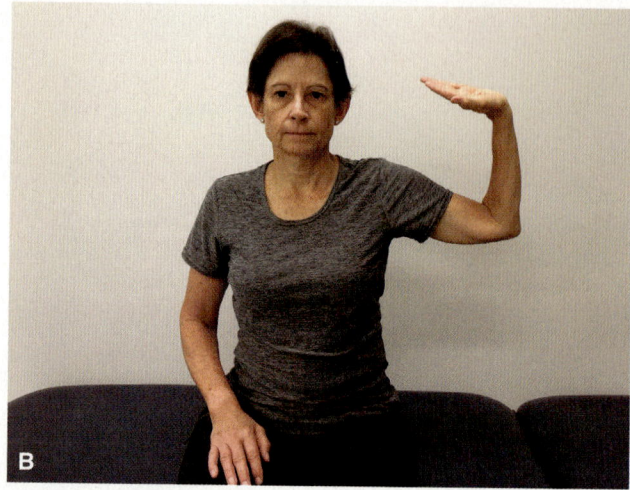

FIGURE 17-39 Upper extremity neural mobilization of the median nerve using nerve sliding technique. **A.** Elbow extension with wrist flexion. **B.** Elbow flexion with wrist extension.

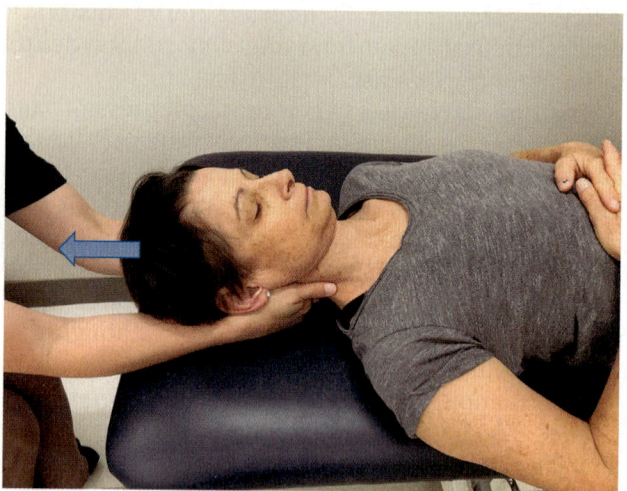

FIGURE 17-40 Manual cervical distraction in supine.

Whiplash-Associated Disorder and Neck-Coordination Deficits

Pathology WAD is a traumatic acceleration/deceleration injury of the cervical spine, most commonly from a motor vehicle accident.[10] The incidence of whiplash is 4.2 per 1,000.[104] While most individuals recover quickly from WAD, many will continue to report some degree of disability 1 year later (Fig. 17-41).[104,105] The Quebec Task Force classifies patients with WAD into grades 0–IV,[106] with grade 0 representing no complaints or signs and grade IV representing cervical fracture or dislocation. However, there is little difference in prognosis or interventions for grades 0–III.[107] Whiplash can affect numerous tissues, including muscles, ligaments, joint capsules, nerve, and intervertebral discs. Thus, patient presentation is quite heterogeneous.

History Patients with WAD report a sudden onset of painfully restricted neck motion. Shoulder motion may also be painfully limited, affecting upper extremity

over the course of a year.[97] Patients responding with centralization may fully recover in 2 to 4 weeks.[78] In addition, a recent systematic review found that exercise can reduce pain and improve function within 4 weeks.[98] Recovery is generally maintained.[83]

Surgical Interventions For those failing conservative care, epidural steroid injections may reduce symptoms.[99] Cervical fusion is the most frequent surgery performed for cervical radiculopathy[82] and results in significant clinical improvements in patient-reported outcomes.[100] Other surgical procedures, including cervical disc arthroplasty and foraminotomy with discectomy, may also be utilized.[87,101] About 80% of patients recovered within 6 weeks of surgery, with most, if not all, others recovering within 3 months.[102] Patients with a longer duration of preoperative weakness tend to have worse outcomes.[103]

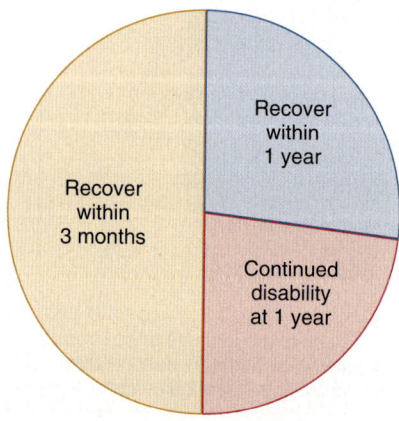

FIGURE 17-41 Recovery in whiplash-associated disorder.

function. Patients may report nausea, dizziness, headache, confusion, or concentration difficulties.

Key Examination Findings Patients with WAD typically present with decreased CROM with muscle guarding. Patients may have reduced and painful shoulder AROM. Limitations in muscle length, such as the upper trapezius, and trigger points are common. Palpation may reveal tenderness of supraspinous ligaments and/or multiple muscles within the cervical region. Cervical muscle performance testing may be painful and weak. Reduced cervical flexor endurance testing is common. If available, pressure pain threshold measurements are typically reduced locally at the neck and may be affected in widespread areas.[14]

Differential Diagnoses Differential diagnosis must include concussion and fracture, but clinicians should also consider CGH, vestibular dysfunction, VBI, and upper cervical spine instability. Multiple cervical strains and sprains are generally considered to be present with WAD.

Rehabilitation Focus and Key Points Rehabilitation should focus on education and exercise (Fig. 17-42).[74] Patients should be educated in the use of heat/ice and exercise to modulate pain, whereas collar use should be minimized.[14] Patients should be encouraged to resume normal activities as soon as possible and be reassured that symptoms are normal and do not represent serious pathology and that the natural progression for WAD for most patients is recovery within 2 to 3 months.[14,74] Both neck-specific exercises and general physical activity appear to be beneficial[108] and have no reported adverse effects.[109] Targeted exercise should address specific impairments, but general exercise may also assist with pain modulation as well as general fitness. Patients with WAD have decreased cervical proprioception.[110] This altered position sense may make it more difficult for them to attain and maintain a neutral spinal alignment, suggesting the need to include postural exercises in the plan of care. A comprehensive home exercise program should be provided.

Patients with chronic WAD should be provided with additional education regarding coping strategies such as how to reduce fear or manage activity limitations and any catastrophizing should be addressed.[74] Although evidence is limited regarding the impact of pain neuroscience education (PNE) on pain reduction and disability, PNE should be considered for patients with chronic WAD.[74] Because passive interventions have the lowest levels of evidence to support their use, they should not be first choice interventions.[74,75] However, patients with chronic WAD may benefit from manual therapy, including mobilization and manipulation of the cervical and thoracic spine, to facilitate pain modulation or improve mobility.[36,111]

Expected Outcomes It is not possible to predict WAD prognosis based on motor vehicle accident information, such as speed, direction of impact, or use of a head restraint, or even based on MRI findings.[105] Prior neck trauma,[104,107] higher initial pain (>5.5/10),[107] or anxiety may result in worse outcome.[112] There

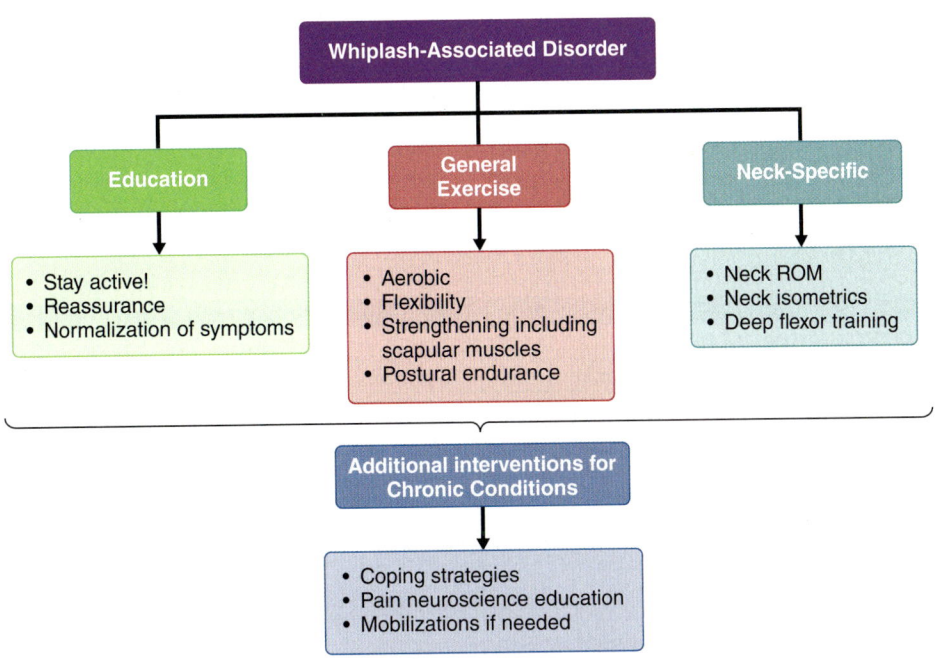

FIGURE 17-42 Interventions for whiplash-associated disorder. *ROM*, range of motion.

is conflicting evidence on the effect of preinjury psychological factors and preinjury pain, age, gender, and education level.[104,105,107] Most individuals recover quickly from WAD. However, at 1 year, many may continue to report some degree of disability.

Cervicogenic Headache

Pathology Nearly every person has experienced a headache at some point. Headaches are classified as being either primary (idiopathic) or secondary. CGHs are a form of secondary headache where symptoms appear to be the result of musculoskeletal pathology of the cervical spine. It is thought that CGHs may account for up to a quarter of all headaches.[113] Table 17-7 describes the features described by the International Headache Society that differentiate CGH from tension headaches and migraines.[114] Headache frequency is typically described as ranging from infrequent (<1 per month) to chronic (present for more than half of the month).[114]

History Patients with CGH report their headache began at the same time or after the presence of neck symptoms. Symptoms are worsened by moving the head and neck or when a certain head/neck posture is maintained for a period of time. For example, a parent may report a headache after prolonged sitting in the bleachers while watching a child play baseball. Patients should be asked about their vision and any changes in job demands/activities, such as increased time spent reading or in sustained positions.

Key Examination Findings Patients with CGH typically present with increased tone and stiffness of the suboccipital muscles.[115] This may lead to local hypomobility of passive accessory intervertebral movement (PAIVM) between the occiput and C3.[116] Global CROM is typically reduced. Most patients have a positive cervical flexion-rotation test.[116,117] Postural observation may reveal a forward head with increased thoracic kyphosis and compensatory upper cervical spine extension.[71] CGHs can be abolished with a nerve block of cervical structures.[114]

Differential Diagnoses Differential diagnosis should include other secondary sources of headache, including intracranial aneurysm, brain tumor, or central nervous system infection. In addition, clinicians should consider the effects of things like caffeine, smoking, withdrawal, and psychological distress as possible sources of a patient's headache.

Rehabilitation Focus and Key Points Rehabilitation is considered the primary treatment option for CGH.[118] The international clinical practice guideline from OPTIMa (Ontario Protocol for Traffic Injury Management) recommends exercise and education be prescribed for patients with CGH.[119] Exercise should include low-load resistance exercise for the scapular stabilizers, such as a row or prone "T" (see Fig. 14-91 in Chapter 14, Shoulder Complex). Gentle cervical isometrics and antigravity endurance holds of cervical musculature may include quadruped exercises, side plank, or increasingly longer holds of the cervical flexion endurance test. Aerobic exercise should also be integrated into the patient's program. A twice-daily home exercise program should include gentle ROM exercise progressing to stretching if needed to restore cervical motion. A recent systematic review found inconsistent benefits to the use of manual therapy in patients with CGH.[120] While another systematic review found only small, short-term reductions in pain intensity, frequency, and disability with spinal manipulation.[121] The international clinical practice guidelines recommend clinicians consider manual therapy as an adjunctive intervention to exercise for patients with CGH.[119] Clinicians should consider the addition of joint mobilization, manipulation, or soft-tissue mobilization of the neck, shoulder, and upper back region if needed.[119] Suboccipital release, either mechanically through the use of a well-placed towel roll or manually, can help reduce suboccipital tone, upper cervical spine flexion, and headaches (Fig. 17-43).

TABLE 17-7

DIFFERENTIATING COMMON HEADACHES

	Cervicogenic Headache	Tension Headache	Migraine
Headache descriptors	Unilateral headache that changes in intensity as a result of changes in cervical motion.	Mild or moderate intensity Bilateral pressure or tightening sensation	Moderate to severe intensity Unilateral throbbing aggravative by activity
Nausea/vomiting or Photophobia/phonophobia	No	No	Yes
Aura	No	No	Possible
Duration	Varied. Onset and/or resolution are coincident with cervical symptoms.	30 minutes to 1 week	4 hours to 3 days

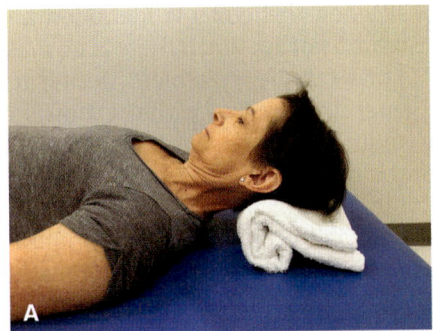 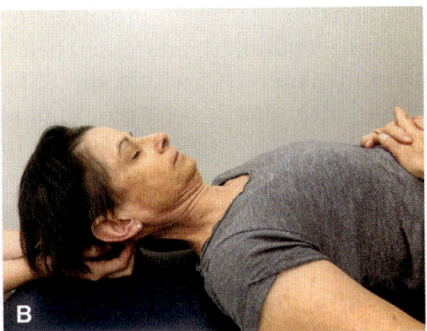 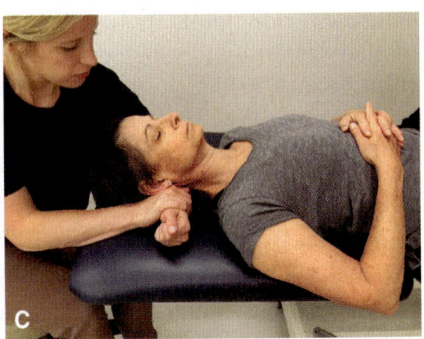

FIGURE 17-43 Suboccipital release. **A.** With small towel roll. **B.** Manually using fingertips. **C.** Manually using forearm.

Expected Outcomes Patients with CGH should expect improvements within 6 weeks.[119] For those failing to improve with these conservative interventions, single or repeated nerve blocks appear to be highly beneficial.[118,122]

Cervicogenic Dizziness

Cervicogenic dizziness is a combination of neck pathology and the sense of imbalance or unsteadiness that is provoked by head and neck motion or positioning.[110] The cause of dizziness is unclear, but may include abnormal proprioceptive input or sympathetic nervous system dysfunction. Cervicogenic dizziness is a diagnosis of exclusion.[17,123] Therefore, clinicians must rule out conditions such as vestibular dysfunction, CGH, WAD, concussion, and possible cardiovascular causes of dizziness. Cervicogenic dizziness does not produce vertigo (sense of self or environment spinning),[110] tinnitus, or an aura. Patients with cervicogenic dizziness do not have the following signs of cervical artery dysfunction: diplopia, dysphagia, dysarthria, drop attacks, nausea, or numbness around the lips. A headache may be present, but is uncommon. In contrast to other causes of dizziness listed in Table 17-8, cervicogenic dizziness symptoms last for minutes to hours.[17]

Patients with cervicogenic dizziness must have cervical pain and loss of CROM. Dizziness is brought on by cervical movement. The head-neck differentiation test and/or the modified cervical torsion test are positive for cervicogenic dizziness.[17] Patients are likely to have increased tone and tenderness of the suboccipital muscles. Central or unilateral intervertebral accessory motion testing may provoke neck symptoms or dizziness. Manual traction may reduce cervical symptoms.

Interventions for cervicogenic dizziness include manual therapy to improve cervical motion and decrease muscular tone. Upper cervical spine manipulation,[124] posterior-to-anterior pressures,[125] sustained natural apophyseal glides (SNAGS),[125] and manual traction relieve symptoms. Dry needling also appears to be effective.[126] Manual therapy should be supplemented with CROM exercises. Symptom resolution may take up to 12 weeks.[125]

Facet Arthropathy

Cervical facet arthropathy may be a degenerative lesion or a capsular restriction. Degenerative lesions are irritated by compressive or closing forces.[127] For example, a patient with right C5–C6 facet arthropathy would report right-sided posterior neck pain with cervical extension, right lateral flexion, and a right quadrant test. Symptoms would be alleviated with motions in the opposite directions (e.g., combinations of flexion, left lateral flexion, and left rotation). Unilateral posteroanterior pressures to the involved facet joint would reproduce the patient's symptoms.[17] Facet hypertrophy may progress to cervical radiculopathy.[26] Patients with facet arthropathy may have local muscle guarding. Interventions would involve CROM exercises, with an emphasis on flexion and lateral flexion to the opposite side. Deep cervical flexor endurance holds, and cervical isometrics may assist with spinal stabilization as well as modulating pain.

A capsular restriction of the facet joint would lead to restricted joint opening. A patient with a right C6–C7 facet capsular restriction would have restricted left lateral flexion and a mild restriction in left rotation and flexion. Right-sided posterolateral neck pain may be created with these movements. In addition, the clinician may notice a painful restriction in local unilateral

TABLE 17-8	
DIFFERENTIAL DIAGNOSIS OF DIZZINESS BASED ON DURATION OF SYMPTOMS	
	Duration of Dizziness
Benign paroxysmal positional vertigo (BPPV)	Seconds to minutes
Cervicogenic dizziness	Minutes to hours
Meniere disease	Intermittent bouts lasting minutes to hours
Concussion	Hours to days
Whiplash-associated disorder	Absent or days to weeks

posteroanterior joint mobility. Interventions for a capsular lesion would include stretching into flexion, lateral flexion to the opposite side, and contralateral rotation. Unilateral and transverse joint mobilizations may be beneficial.[128]

Torticollis

Torticollis is a unilateral shortening of the SCM present at birth or shortly after causing a postural deformity of ipsilateral cervical lateral flexion and contralateral rotation. The condition is the third most common congenital musculoskeletal disorder[129] and occurs more frequently after breech births, after a difficult labor, and in infants with hip dysplasia.[130] Torticollis may be the result of infant preference, caregiver preference (feeding only on/from one side), due to reduced SCM length, or due to a mass within the SCM.[131] However, differential diagnosis might also include brachial plexus injury or other neurologic injuries.[131]

The clinician should observe the infant/child for signs of pain or distress. Observe the patient's visual tracking and look for the presence of nystagmus or other visual abnormalities. The clinician should compare patient movement patterns and activities to those of a typically developing infant. The physical examination of an infant or a child with torticollis should include active and passive cervical lateral flexion and rotation in both prone and supported sitting. The clinician should palpate the SCM to identify if there is a mass as well as the general tone and elasticity of the SCM and surrounding muscles. Craniofacial asymmetries can cause torticollis by forcing an infant into a particular head posture. However, the reverse is also true. Therefore, the clinician should carefully assess for the presence of any cranial asymmetries. Given the association with hip dysplasia, hip motion should be thoroughly assessed, whereas the remaining joints should be screened for areas of hypermobility or hypomobility.

Conservative management focuses on a combination of parent education and exercise. Parents should be educated in patient positioning during sleep, waking times, and feeding that encourage symmetry. For example, prone play time may include the use of toys that encourage the infant to explore both the left and right sides. Pending the patient's response, the emphasis on passive positioning in car seats, strollers, or swings and during feeding may prioritize positioning away from the patient's preference. Parents should be taught cervical PROM for rotation and lateral flexion. A general goal would be to try to achieve 50 to 100 repetitions of each motion per day. The use of helmet therapy to assist with positioning and correction of craniofacial asymmetry with or without manual therapy may be beneficial in more severe or slowly resolving cases.[132]

Prognosis is best when torticollis is identified and addressed before 6 months of age and if there is no mass within the SCM.[131] For example, treatment during the first month of life generally resolves within 1 month of treatment but may require nearly a year of treatment if diagnosed at 6 months of age.[131] Conservative interventions are successful in 95 to 99% of cases.[130,133] Should conservative treatment fail or be delayed, botulinum injection or surgical interventions may be indicated. Surgery followed by rehabilitation is the preferred treatment plan for children older than 1 year.[129] Parents can expect full resolution within about 4 months.[129,133]

THORACIC PATHOLOGIES

This section reviews the following pathologies: compression fractures, rib/sternal fractures, scoliosis, TOS, thoracic radiculopathy, costochondritis, and slipping rib syndrome. It should be noted that the thoracic spine is often involved in LBP and neck pain. (Refer to Chapter 12, Lumbar Spine and Sacroiliac Joint, for additional information on examination and interventions of pathologies associated with lumbar spine dysfunction.)

Thoracic Compression Fractures

Pathology A vertebral compression fracture occurs when the anterior portion of the vertebral body collapses whereas the posterior vertebrae remains intact, resulting in a wedge-shaped deformity identifiable on a radiograph (Fig. 17-44). Two-thirds of compression fractures are asymptomatic and identified

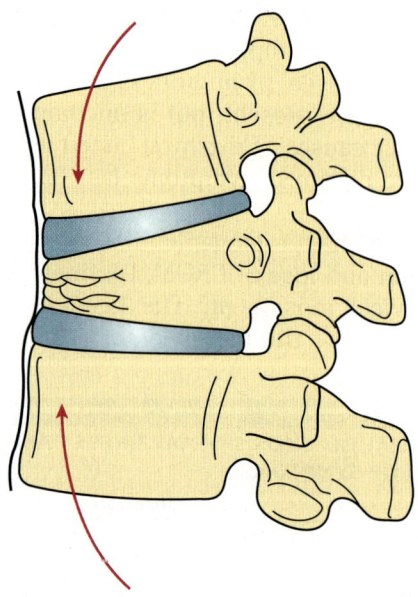

FIGURE 17-44 Schematic of a vertebral compression fracture with wedge-shaped deformity. (Adapted from Anderson MK, Barnum MG. *Foundations of Athletic Training: Prevention, Assessment, and Management.* 7th ed. Wolters Kluwer; 2022: Figure 23-20.)

incidentally during testing for other pathologies,[134,135] such as a chest x-ray for pneumonia. Ninety percent of patients with compression fractures have osteoporosis or osteopenia.[135] Compression fractures are more common in the thoracic spine due to the natural kyphotic curvature of the region. Compression fractures are twice as common in females than males, and 25% of postmenopausal women will sustain a compression fracture.[136] Compression fracture risk increases significantly with age.[137]

Risk factors for thoracic compression fractures include[135,137–140]:

- Osteoporosis or osteopenia
- Prior compression fracture
- Age over 50
- Female
- Caucasian
- Postmenopausal
- Smoker
- Low vitamin D or calcium levels
- Prolonged corticosteroid use
- Prior treatment for cancer
- Hyperparathyroidism
- Dementia
- Decreased balance
- Reduced grip strength

Patients who have had a vertebral compression fracture have a 20% increased risk of sustaining an additional fracture and a fourfold higher risk of death.[141,142] Recurrence may be due to the mechanical effects of the wedge fracture,[135] increasing stress on the vertebral bodies above and below the fracture and/or the continued presence of osteoporosis or osteopenia.[136] Patients should be asked if they have had their bone density tested (and the results) and if any treatment for osteoporosis or osteopenia has been recommended. While it is recommended that individuals diagnosed with osteoporosis or in whom an asymptomatic vertebral compression fracture is found undergo a thorough falls risk assessment,[143] this preventive step is often skipped.

History Patients with acute vertebral compression fractures generally report moderate-to-severe back pain, whereas those with chronic compression fractures generally report low levels of chronic back pain. However, as noted previously, compression fractures may also be asymptomatic. Most vertebral compression fractures are insidious or the result of minor trauma, such as sneezing, coughing, or lifting a light object. Less often, fracture is the result of a fall or motor vehicle accident.[137]

Patients with vertebral compression fractures have a mechanical presentation, with symptoms provoked with sitting, trunk flexion, and transitional movements such as rising and bed mobility.[135] Symptoms are reduced with unloading, such as lying.

Patients should be asked about a change in maximal height: a 2-cm loss of height is predictive of the presence of osteoporosis.[144] Patients with a history of cancer or who are under 50 with an insidious onset of back pain may be examined but should be simultaneously referred to rule out cancer or metastasis.[136,145] Patients should also be asked about their visual acuity and the last time they have been assessed by an eye professional, as decreased vision may increase the risk for falls.

Key Examination Findings Patient height should be measured and compared with the patient's report of maximal height. Blood pressure should be assessed, and patients should be asked about the presence of orthostatic hypotension, as hypotension increases the risk of falls.[138] Observation and posture assessment may reveal increased kyphosis. Those with more acute fractures may have muscle guarding. Patients referred with a diagnosed compression fracture should not perform trunk flexion or repeated trunk flexion because these provocative procedures are not required and increase stress on the vertebral body.

Trunk flexion in standing will increase pain complaint, whereas extension may either reduce pain or have no effect. If there is a high degree of suspicion for a compression fracture, repeated trunk flexion should not be performed as an evaluative procedure. Neurologic findings will be negative.[139] Patients may have focal tenderness over spinous processes.[146] Posteroanterior pressures will be painful and guarded. While acutely muscle performance may be limited by pain, patients with compression fractures tend to have reduced paraspinal strength and endurance.[135] Lower level exercises should be used to assess core muscle performance, such as abdominal setting, bridging, or progressive dead bug exercises (see Chapter 12, Lumbar Spine and Sacroiliac Joint). Balance should be assessed and is frequently decreased. Lower extremity strength assessment should be performed because a lack of lower extremity strength may contribute to vertebral loading, particularly during transfers.

Differential Diagnoses Differential diagnosis includes infection and cancer. Clinicians should have a high degree of suspicion for cancer in patients with a history of cancer, who have night pain, whose pain does not have a mechanical pattern, or who are under the age of 50 with insidious onset of back pain.[136,145]

Rehabilitation Focus and Key Points Conservative interventions are the mainstay of treatment for compression fractures (Fig. 17-45). Patient education

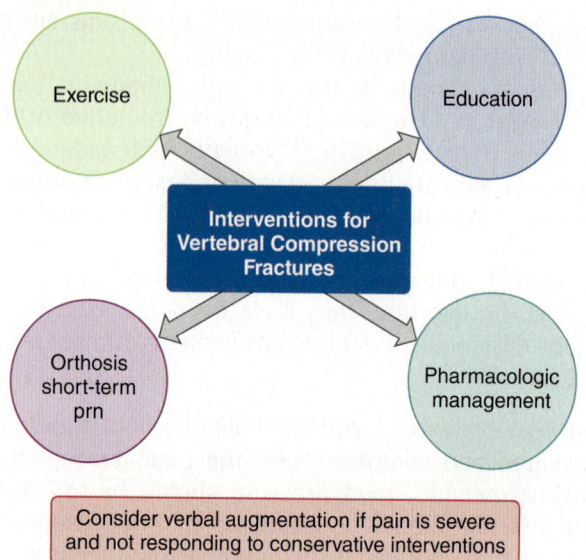

FIGURE 17-45 Interventions for vertebral compression fractures.

should include joint protection strategies, such as ways to reduce trunk flexion such as squatting rather than bending. Patients should be encouraged to be active and the importance of early mobility to prevent secondary complications of deconditioning or worsening osteoporosis.[134,136,140,147] Given the limited adherence to exercise for compression fractures, clinicians should discuss the positive benefits of exercise and its role in reducing future compression fractures.[148]

The Global Spine Care Initiative recommends postural, strengthening, stretching, and balance exercises be prescribed for patients with compression fractures.[140] Postural exercises can help reduce functional kyphosis and vertebral body compression. Prone lying and prone propping may be good positions of controlling symptoms and can be progressed to extension in lying for patients with age-related reductions in trunk extension ROM as well as help improve hip flexor length. Trunk extensor strengthening progressions can be performed in prone, standing, or quadruped based on the patient's comfort and abilities. Quadriceps and hip extensor strengthening should also be included. Balance exercises may reduce the risk of fall and future injury. Clinicians should encourage weight-bearing exercises, such as a walking program, for aerobic fitness. Patients with poor tolerance to upright activities may benefit from beginning exercise in an aquatic environment, and, if enjoyable, this can be continued long term.[135]

A thoracolumbar orthosis (see Fig. 12-35B in Chapter 12, Lumbar Spine and Sacroiliac Joint) may assist with reducing trunk flexion and decreasing paraspinal tonicity, thereby reducing vertebral body compression. Patients who have difficulty with mobility after an acute compression fracture may benefit from 4 to 6 weeks of orthotic use.[134,135,140,149]

Pharmacologic interventions can be used to reduce pain and to address bone mineral density. Nonsteroidal anti-inflammatory medications are the first line of pharmacologic pain management.[140,146,149]

Tricyclic antidepressants may be added if pain is not adequately controlled.[135] Calcium and vitamin D levels should be assessed and may be prescribed by a primary care provider as needed.[136] Bisphosphonates have been shown to increase bone mineral density in individuals with osteoporosis, with or without compression fractures, and reduce the rate of new compression fracture.[146,150]

Expected Outcomes Most patients with acute compression fractures have a gradual reduction in pain within 2 to 12 weeks.[134,151] Optimal results appear to rely on a combination of exercise and modification of daily activities to reduce trunk flexion.[152] Patients who continue to have severe pain and disability despite conservative measures may benefit from vertebral augmentation procedures, such as vertebroplasty (injection of cement into the vertebral body) or kyphoplasty (a balloon is inserted into the vertebral body to restore vertebral height followed by injection with cement).[153] Although surgical management was once thought to be extremely beneficial, it is not without complications, including infection, cement leakage, and a significant increased risk of compression fracture above and below the treated level.[135] Vertebral augmentation is now used in only about 15% of patients with compression fractures.[154]

Rib and Sternal Fractures Rib and sternal fractures are relatively rare. The four main causes of these fractures are trauma, falls, abuse, and sports. Ten percent of major trauma patients will have rib or sternal fractures.[155,156] Pulmonary complications, including pneumonia and pneumothorax, are common after rib or sternal fractures.[156] Overall mortality after rib or sternal fractures may be as high as 10%, primarily due to pulmonary complications.[155] The risk for complications after rib and sternal fractures increases with age, number of ribs fractured, and if ribs were fractured bilaterally.[155] Surgical management reduces pain, improves pulmonary function, and reduces overall complications.[157,158] A survey of patients postrib fracture revealed a high degree of fear and the perception that only time would improve function.[159] In addition, patients reported shortness of breath with activity and decreased stamina even after bony healing.[159] Rehabilitation can play a vital role immediately postinjury as well as later in recovery. Acutely, patients should be taught breathing exercises, splinting during coughing, and bed mobility.[159] Patients with high pain levels may benefit from ice, oral medication, and nerve blocks in addition to rehabilitation.[155] A progressive aerobic exercise program can assist with improving pulmonary function.[159] The patient should begin a progressive strengthening program[159]; however, shoulder exercises may begin with active-assisted ROM that incorporates breathing.

Rib fractures constitute only about 1% of all pediatric fractures.[160] Most rib fractures in children are caused by abuse, particularly for children under the age of 3 years.[161] Therefore, clinicians working with children after a rib fracture should be vigilant for other signs of abuse, including the presence of multiple fractures, repeated injuries, or reported mechanisms of injury that appear unreasonable or change over time. The child may appear withdrawn or show signs of neglect, such as inappropriate weight or poor hygiene. Any cases of suspected child abuse must be reported to the appropriate authorities immediately.

Rib and sternal fractures in sports are frequently the result of direct trauma, such as a blow to the chest in American football.[162] Sternal fractures require medical evaluation as acute cardiac arrhythmia or pneumothorax may occur.[163] Rib fractures are typically treated symptomatically with rest, ice, and analgesics. Breathing exercises should be initiated immediately. A sling may be used for 1 to 2 weeks for comfort for patients with upper rib fractures.[162] Typically, rib fractures are pain free at rest within 2 weeks. Most rib fractures in athletes are stable, allowing progressive AROM exercises to be started as soon as they are tolerated and progressed to strengthening as the athlete is able. It is recommended that athletes avoid contact/collision activities for about 6 weeks, until after bony healing takes place.[162] Most athletes return to sports in 6 to 12 weeks, although high-level athletes may return with appropriate protection and supervision after being informed of the potential risks of an early return.[162]

Sternal stress fracture may occur from repeated strong muscle contractions with or without relative energy deficiency in sport (RED-S), such as wrestling, gymnastics, golf, and weightlifting.[163,164] Stress fractures usually present with local pain that is aggravated by sport-specific activity and deep breathing. Local tenderness is common, and swelling may be present. For most patients, shoulder AROM is full.[164] Athletes with suspected stress fractures should be referred for imaging to ensure appropriate treatment. Most athletes are managed with rest, ice, and analgesics. Once asymptomatic, athletes can slowly return to sports. Healing typically requires 1 to 2 months.[164] Athletes with RED-S should be referred for nutritional or other counseling as needed.

Idiopathic Adolescent Scoliosis

Pathology Scoliosis is one of the most common orthopaedic conditions, affecting about 3% of children between the ages of 9 and 16 years.[165] Scoliosis may be congenital, neuromuscular, or idiopathic,[166] with the latter accounting for the majority of cases.[167] Scoliosis is measured using the Cobb method. The upper and lower limits of the spinal curve are identified on a frontal plane projection radiograph and a line is drawn parallel to each vertebra's endplate. The Cobb angle is the angle where these two lines cross (Fig. 17-46).[168] The diagnosis of scoliosis is given if the Cobb angle is greater than 10°.[166] Curves are generally named by the location of curvature (lumbar or thoracic) and the side of the convexity (e.g., right thoracic, left lumbar scoliosis), with the majority of cases having a primary right thoracic curve.[169] Although a radiograph only measures frontal plane angles, it is important to recognize that the scoliosis curve is three dimensional. This rotational component can be identified on three-dimensional imaging. The ribs rotate with the vertebrae such that the ribs appear more posterior on the convex side. This is identifiable using the forward bend test (aka Adam forward bend test): with the individual forward flexed, a posterior rib hump (thoracic) or lumbar bulge (lumbar) is observed on the side of the convexity. Scoliosis can

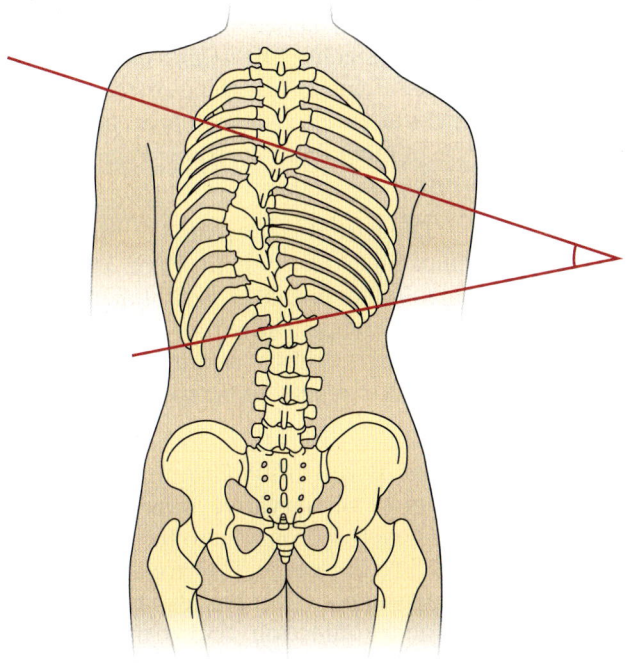

FIGURE 17-46 Cobb angle for quantifying scoliosis.

compromise pulmonary function and negatively impact psychological health due to altered cosmesis.

A 10 to 25° curve is generally considered mild.[170] Scoliosis curve progression is more likely with larger curves (>30°) and in younger, more skeletally immature patients. Curve progression is fastest during periods of rapid growth, particularly during puberty. Surgery is generally performed on individuals with larger than 40° curve.[166] Less skeletally mature individuals with smaller curves have the largest potential for early intervention.[171]

History Children and adolescents with mild scoliosis may be asymptomatic and first diagnosed during routine school physical examinations. Some individuals may be symptom free but are concerned by the cosmesis of their structural asymmetry or the poor fit of clothing. Individuals with larger curvatures may note that certain chairs or sleep positions are uncomfortable due to uneven pressure on the spine and ribcage. Patients may complain of muscular back pain that worsens as the day progresses due to the increased effort of trying to attain or maintain an upright posture.

Key Examination Findings The key findings of idiopathic adolescent scoliosis are a positive forward bend test and altered spinal alignment in standing and sitting. Trunk AROM is likely to reveal an asymmetrical loss of lateral flexion and rotation. Patients with reduced trunk extension may also have restrictions in shoulder elevation and/or latissimus dorsi length. Patients may have reduced abdominal and trunk muscle strength and endurance. Assessment of breathing patterns may reveal reduced lateral costal breathing or reduced rib expansion. Vertebral and costovertebral accessory motion may be hypomobile in some regions and hypermobile in others.

Differential Diagnoses Differential diagnosis includes neuromuscular disorders in which abnormal tone may cause spinal deformities. Spinal asymmetry may develop as a compensation for a leg length discrepancy. Although rare, rapidly developing scoliosis may be the result of a space-occupying tumor.[172]

Rehabilitation Focus and Key Points An orthosis is the most common conservative intervention for scoliosis[167] and is generally considered for individuals with larger than 25 to 29° curve.[166] Orthosis use may prevent curve progression,[173] but has also been shown to reduce pulmonary function and trunk muscle endurance.[174] While many studies recommend orthosis use for up to 23 hours per day,[175] orthoses do not need to be worn this often to be effective.[176] However, adherence to orthoses can be limited owing to brace discomfort, restrictive quality, and altered cosmesis, particularly in individuals at, or near, puberty.

Therapeutic exercise is critical for the management of scoliosis. Tissues on the concave side of the curve may become adaptively shortened without targeted stretching. Similarly, the muscles on the convex side of the curve will become elongated and weak. Postural and core stabilization exercises can help patients attain and maintain improved spinal alignment. Exercise should target rib alignment, scapular position, head-neck orientation, and breathing.[175] Endurance strengthening should include activation of local deep musculature, such as the multifidi, pelvic floor, and diaphragm, as well as global muscle stability training, such as the obliques, quadratus lumborum, and erector spinae. Patients should also be taught how to incorporate optimal spinal alignment during functional tasks. This is particularly important when weaning off of an orthosis.[175] Yoga, pilates, and tai chi have also been advocated for individuals with scoliosis.[177]

Scoliosis-specific exercises (SSEs), such as the Schroth method, Barcelona Scoliosis Physical Therapy School, and the Scientific Exercise Approach to Scoliosis, are gaining prominence in the United States and Europe.[177] SSEs focus on three-dimensional realignment of the spine including the use of breathing, corrective movements, and postural awareness and can be prescribed either in isolation or in combination with bracing. Exercises may initially require clinician manual repositioning and are progressed as able to verbal cueing and then self-correction. Exercises are progressed from positions with significant stability (supine) to more challenging positions as patient motor control and strength allows (standing or functional activities).[178] For example, a patient may sit facing a wall with rungs. The patient straddles the chair to stabilize the pelvis and then uses various hand holds to stabilize axiohumeral muscles distally. The patient is guided to move the spine more toward midline by contracting muscles to open and move the concave side of the curvature more posteriorly, while closing and moving the convex side of the curvature more anteriorly. Because most patients with scoliosis have a double curve, it takes significant practice to master the motor control necessary to perform these corrections. The exercises also must be repeated frequently to create a lasting change to patient static and dynamic alignment. Home exercises are generally performed for 15 to 45 minutes per day or 3 to 5 days per week.[176,177]

Expected Outcomes SSEs can improve or slow curvature progression, and the gains appear to be maintained throughout the patient's lifetime.[170,171]

These targeted exercises also appear to improve patient function and quality of life.[168] Best results occur when exercises are prescribed early after scoliosis diagnosis, with up to 70% of patients under the age of 10 years having significant decreases in spinal curvature and curve progression noted in only 5% of patients.[170] Patients have been shown to improve with exercise even after growth has stopped or when restarting a program if the curve has progressed over time.[167,179] Exercise is superior to orthotic use as a single intervention.[176] However, as noted previously, most studies involve some degree of bracing to be used in combination with exercise for patients with larger mild curvatures.[174]

Although promising, there is limited high-quality evidence to support the use of SSE over more general exercise.[176] Therefore, it is recommended that interventions for patients with idiopathic adolescent scoliosis include SSEs, conventional therapeutic exercise, manual therapy, and orthoses.[168] Regardless of the intervention chosen, outcomes are directly related to patient adherence.[168] Most studies note substantial improvements in spinal alignment within 4 months.[175] Continued benefits (improvement in spinal alignment or lack of curvature progression) are likely if exercise are continued.

Surgical Intervention for Idiopathic Adolescent Scoliosis Patients with significant (>40°) curvatures are treated with spinal fusion.[179] This generally involves a lengthy surgery and placement of Harrington rods on either side of the spine to realign and restrict motion of all involved spinal segments. This procedure is particularly challenging if done before the patient has stopped growing, but is the only way to truly prevent curve progression.

Adult Scoliosis

Adult scoliosis is a three-dimensional spinal deformity of at least a 10° Cobb angle[180] seen in adults over the age of 60 years.[169] Adult scoliosis may be a progression of childhood scoliosis, but more often, it is a degenerative process caused by osteoporosis and asymmetrical compression fractures.[181] Degeneration of the facet joints and intervertebral discs with resulting segmental instability likely accentuate the curvature.[169] Adult degenerative scoliosis is often accompanied by hypertrophy of the ligamentum flavum and lateral spinal stenosis.

While most cases or adult scoliosis are generally asymptomatic, patients presenting for evaluation report back and possibly leg pain that may be due to abnormal joint loading, muscular fatigue, and/or nerve root impingement. A patient's current height should be measured and compared with patient-reported maximal height. Pain of muscular origin worsens with increasing time upright or unsupported sitting, whereas stenotic pain improves with any seated position. Most compression fractures are chronic fatigue fractures and are asymptomatic; however, if acute, flexion is likely to exacerbate local bone pain due to increased vertebral body compression.

Examination should include a complete postural assessment. Hip or knee flexion contractures from osteoarthritis can create functional leg length differences that may contribute to abnormal spinal alignment. Trunk ROM is typically asymmetrically reduced with a loss of extension to be expected. A standard lower quarter neurologic screen should be performed to identify any neurologic involvement. Additional muscle performance assessments should include the gluteus maximus, gluteus medius, abdominals, and trunk extensors because these deficits can lead to functional impairments and difficulty maintaining optimal postural alignment. Gait speed may be reduced. Transfers may require increased time, upper extremity assistance, or increased hip and trunk flexion. Balance may be reduced due to age-related changes or problematic because spinal deformities may alter the normal center of gravity.

Conservative management is the first line of treatment for adult lumbar scoliosis.[182] Interventions include stretching to improve lost ROM, particularly spinal extension. More globally, stretching and manual therapy to reduce hip or knee flexion contractures is also recommended. Clinicians should compare the patient's spinal curvature in various positions. For example, a patient may present with a more flexible curvature, such that it becomes more noticeable in a weight-bearing position or with trunk muscular fatigue, or a more rigid curvature that is unaltering with position changes and attempts to manually correct alignment is met with tissue resistance. For patients with a more flexible curvature, treatment should emphasize exercise to improve and maintain spinal alignment as close to the neutral position as possible. For patients with a more rigid curvature, interventions should attempt to improve trunk endurance to prevent further deformity by countering the effect of gravity on asymmetrical spinal alignment. Weight-bearing exercise and resistance training are recommended to counteract osteoporosis and osteopenia. Balance exercises are important for this population to reduce the risk of falls. Aquatic exercise, if available, may be a useful long-term exercise mode. Aerobic exercise, such as cycling and walking, should be included in the rehabilitation plan[182] and encouraged as part of a long-term fitness program. In contrast to adolescent scoliosis, bracing does not stop curve progression and is not generally well tolerated in this population.[182]

Surgical management may be performed on individuals with a Cobb angle greater than 30° and intractable pain or disability despite rehabilitation and spinal injections.[169,182,183] However, surgery is more challenging than with adolescent scoliosis due to comorbidities like osteoporosis.[180] Surgical options include local decompression and/or fusion with or without instrumentation.[181,182] Complication rates are higher with older patients and include infection, neurologic deficits, and the need for additional surgery.[182]

Thoracic Outlet Syndrome

Pathology TOS results from compression of neurovascular structures in one of the following areas[59]:

- Scalene triangle (plexus trunks, subclavian artery)
- Costoclavicular space (plexus divisions, subclavian artery/vein)
- Subcoracoid space (plexus cords, axillary artery/vein)

Ninety to 95% of cases are neurogenic.[58,59,184] Three to 4% of cases are venous and less than 1% are arterial.[185]

TOS is more common in individuals between the ages of 20 and 50 years, with females more likely to be affected than males.[59] The condition may be congenital, traumatic, or acquired. Underlying congenital anomalies, such as the presence of a cervical rib, are usually not symptomatic until after a trauma.[58,185] Seventy prevent of cases are the result of soft-tissue restrictions, including scalene hypertrophy, muscle fibrosis after a cervical trauma, fibrous bands, the presence of an accessory muscle (scalenus minimus), or shortened pectoral muscles.[59,185] The remaining cases are the result of boney issues, including the presence of a cervical first rib, abnormal clavicle or rib fracture healing,[59,185] or dislocation of the acromioclavicular or sternoclavicular joint. Rarely, TOS is caused by obstruction from a tumor or cyst.

History Patients with TOS may report pain, paresthesias, pallor, feeling of fullness in the arm, weakness, or atrophy.[59] Most commonly, symptoms are due to lower plexus involvement (C7–T1), creating paresthesias in the medial arm, medial forearm, and ulnar two digits. Patients may also report reduced hand dexterity, lateral neck pain, or headaches, which may be severe.[58] Patients with upper plexus involvement (C5–C7) may report arm weakness as well as paresthesias in the lateral arm and radial three digits. These patients may also report symptoms spread toward the ear or a feeling of fullness within the ear.[58] There may be a history of prior neck trauma,[59] such as a motor vehicle accident. Athletes or workers in occupations requiring repetitive overhead motions may be more likely to develop symptoms due to hypertrophy or fibrosis of the pectoralis minor and scalenes.[59,186] Symptoms are typically increased or produced with static postures, such as carrying a shopping bag, walking while wearing a backpack or purse, or from a poorly fitting bra strap.[187] Symptoms may occur after exercise or activity[58] or may limit these activities. If venous involvement is present, patients will report with arm swelling and a feeling of arm heaviness or fullness with arm use.[59] Venous involvement is more commonly seen in athletes than sedentary individuals.[186]

Key Examination Findings There is no gold-standard clinical test to identify TOS. The clinician should first rule out more common pathologies, such as cervical radiculopathy or peripheral nerve entrapments. Patients may present with positive special tests, such as the costoclavicular test,[60] EAST,[58,59,185] and/or Adson.[58,59,185,186] A combination of a positive costoclavicular test and a positive EAST test increases the likelihood of TOS.[60,185] However, the absence of positive special tests does not rule out TOS.[60]

The arm of a patient with arterial TOS may be pale compared with the contralateral limb.[59,187] Blood pressure measurements should be performed bilaterally. If there is more than 20 mm Hg difference in systolic pressure, the patient should be referred for further testing.[185] Global upper extremity edema is an indicator of possible venous TOS.[59,187] If pitting edema is present however, the clinician should consider the possibility of lymphedema or deep vein thrombosis (DVT). If swelling is noted, clinicians should use the clinical prediction guideline developed by Constans et al. to determine the risk of an upper extremity DVT.[188]

The clinician should assess muscle length of the pectoralis minor and major because these may be contributing factors to patient symptoms. Many times, assessment of pectoral length or cervical lateral flexion (scalene stretching) will recreate patient symptoms.[58] Observe the resting position of the scapula and thoracic spine as well as any scapular dyskinesias as symptoms commonly are increased with overhead work.[187] Correction of scapula or thoracic positioning should be attempted to determine the effect on symptoms.[187] Muscle performance assessment should include the neck flexor endurance test, trunk extensors, as well as the lower and middle trapezius because weakness in these muscle groups may contribute to patient symptoms.

Observe the patient's breathing patterns. Patients with TOS often overuse their scalenes rather than regularly performing diaphragmatic breathing.[187] The clinician should assess the position and mobility of the first rib. Patients with TOS often have an elevated first rib and a positive cervical flexion-rotation test. An inferior glide of the first rib may be restricted and painful.[58] Palpation of the supraclavicular fossa may reproduce symptoms.[58,60] Palpation of the scalenes and pectoralis minor may reveal tenderness, trigger points, or increased tone. Patients may have positive ULTTs.[59,186]

Because symptoms may be position specific, if standard assessments have not recreated the patient's symptoms, clinicians may ask the patient to perform a symptomatic activity. For example, a baseball pitcher may have symptoms during a portion of the throwing motion. If symptoms are not provoked immediately, the position can be held for up to 3 minutes, akin to the EAST test. If symptoms are provoked, observing the ROM and flexibility required for this position may help the clinician identify impairments in range, flexibility, or strength that may need to be addressed.

Differential Diagnoses Differential diagnosis includes cervical radiculopathy,[187] carpal tunnel syndrome, ulnar tunnel syndrome, upper extremity DVT, and visceral referral from cardiac or pulmonary sources, including Pancoast tumor.[185]

Rehabilitation Focus and Key Points Symptom modulation may include rest, activity modification, and exercise. Athletes and individuals whose TOS symptoms are the result of repetitive movement are likely to benefit from at least 1 week of restricted activity.[59,185] Nonsteroidal anti-inflammatory medications may help reduce symptom irritability and local inflammation.[59,185] Patients with high irritability may benefit from periodic bouts of unweighting the shoulder girdle, such as using a pillow on top of an armrest to reduce neural tension.[187] Rehabilitation for TOS should focus on the key impairments contributing to the patient's symptoms and improving the patency of the thoracic outlet. Stretching and soft-tissue mobilization to improve muscle length and resolve trigger points of affected muscles such as the scalenes, pectoralis minor, and pectoralis major may be beneficial.[58,185] Prescribing a progressive aerobic exercise program with a goal of 30 minutes per day may assist with pain modulation.[187]

Patients with faulty breathing patterns should be taught diaphragmatic breathing. This may begin in supine with an emphasis on belly breathing while reducing upper and lateral chest motion (Fig. 17-47A). For some patient's, the clinician may need to reduce the scalenes' ability to assist with breathing by adding a large pillow under the patient's head to create active insufficiency of the scalenes (Fig. 17-47B). If needed, the clinician can then manually limit lateral costal breathing or manually facilitate diaphragmatic breathing (Fig. 17-47C). Patients with scalene hypertonicity or central sensitization may also benefit from relaxation exercises, meditation, or yoga.[187]

Inferior first rib mobilizations may help patients with an elevated first rib. Cervical and thoracic mobilizations/manipulation may be beneficial. Strengthening and movement control exercises, along with these mobility exercises, may rectify symptoms associated with scapular dyskinesia. Endurance strengthening of postural muscles may also be beneficial. Neural mobilizations have been recommended,[185,187] but there are limited data to support this intervention.

Once patients are independent with a home exercise program and no longer require manual therapy, treatment frequency may be decreased to a monthly check-in for reassessment and program modification. Patients should be encouraged to continue to be diligent with their exercise programs and postural corrections and informed that it may take up to 6 months for symptoms to fully resolve.

Expected Outcomes Approximately 70% of cases resolve with conservative management.[59] Some patients will continue to have intermittent symptoms that are position dependent. Adherence to rehabilitation, the ability to modify postures and activities, normal

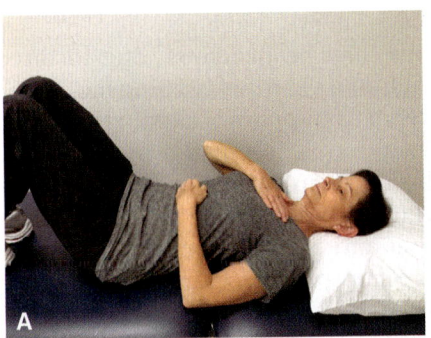
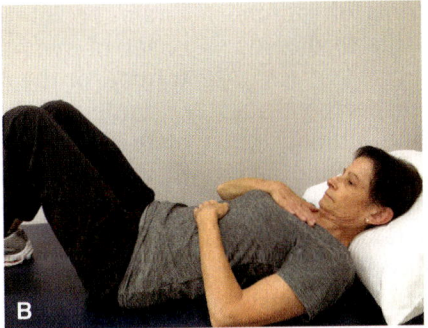
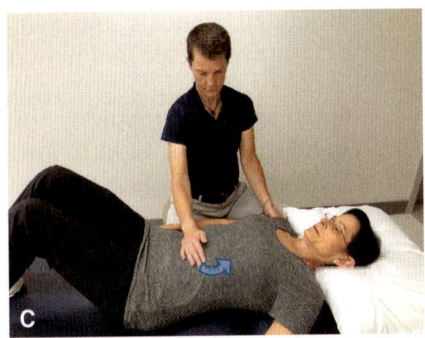

FIGURE 17-47 Diaphragmatic breathing progression. **A.** Supine with patient awareness of the rise and fall of the belly while limiting upper chest expansion. **B.** Positioning to create active insufficiency of the scalenes. **C.** Clinician facilitation of the diaphragm with a quick stretch timed at the start of inhalation.

body mass index, and nonsmoking status increase the likelihood of positive results.[58,59,185]

Surgical Management Imaging is not typically performed unless there is a suspicion of vascular involvement or the patient has failed 6 months of conservative interventions.[59] A Doppler ultrasound is a noninvasive method of determining whether there is an obstruction to arterial or venous flow.[60] Angiography is a more invasive means of identifying vascular TOS. Electrodiagnostic testing may help identify involvement of various sections of the plexus and differentiate between TOS and peripheral nerve entrapments, such as ulnar tunnel syndrome. An MRI can identify the presence of a cervical rib.

Surgical management should be considered for individuals not responding after 6 months of conservative care[185] and may include first rib excision, resection of a cervical rib, or anterior scalenectomy.[189] Fibrous bands or anatomic anomalies, such as a cervical rib, are found in almost half of the surgical patients.[185] Surgical outcomes are generally positive with a 75% success rate.[184,189] However, there are several potential surgical complications including pneumothorax or injury to portions of the plexus or the subclavian or artery or vein,[185] which warrant careful consideration and a prolonged trial of conservative care. Postoperative management should include early shoulder ROM and neural mobilizations, but strengthening should be delayed.[186]

Thoracic Radiculopathy

Thoracic radiculopathy is much less common than lumbar or cervical radiculopathy. Thoracic disc herniation accounts for less than 2% of all disc pathology and is most frequent between T8 and T11.[190] Symptoms of thoracic radiculopathy include paresthesias in a dermatomal pattern that can wrap around to the lateral and anterior chest. Radiculopathies of T1 and T2 may create upper extremity symptoms, including hand weakness or atrophy. Degenerative disc disease, trauma, and osteophyte formation can lead to lateral foraminal stenosis and symptoms of radiculopathy.[190] Rarely, symptoms may be due to discitis or a tumor.[191]

Examination and treatment of suspected thoracic radiculopathies should follow that outlined for the lumbar spine, including the use of one-time and repeated movements to try to identify a directional preference if one is present. As with lumbar spine, patients should be taught how to modify activities or positions that exacerbate symptoms with an emphasis on proper body mechanics. Neutral spine stabilization exercises can be initiated as long as peripheralization does not occur. Patients should be gradually reintroduced to functional activities involving rotation, such as golfing or tennis, to create high levels of disc stress.

Most cases of thoracic radiculopathy respond to conservative interventions.

Costochondritis

Costochondritis is inflammation of the costochondral junction or costosternal joints.[192] Patients report anterior chest pain that increases with activity or deep breathing. Onset is usually after minor activity, such as lifting, twisting, or sneezing. The condition generally presents with local tenderness of the costosternal/costochondral joints, usually unilaterally and at more than one level.[193] The 2nd through 5th costochondral junctions are most often affected.[194] Sternal or rib compression, mobilization of the costosternal joints,[194] and manually resisted breathing increase the patient's pain.[195] If swelling is present, the condition is more properly referred to as *Tietze*, but treatment and prognosis remain the same.[192] Differential diagnosis should rule out serious pathologies including those due to cardiac or pulmonary conditions as well as GERD.[193]

Costochondritis is self-limiting and generally treated with ice and short-term modification of aggravating activities.[195] Topical anesthetics can be applied if needed.[192] Because symptoms may take up at a year to resolve, patients whose symptoms are slow to resolve and significantly inhibiting function may be referred for rehabilitation.[194] A case series noted resolution of symptoms and restoration of function within five visits using an impairment-based approach with treatment directed toward improving thoracic spine and rib cage mobility.[194]

Slipping Rib Syndrome

Slipping rib syndrome is a rare, benign condition caused by hypermobility of the costal cartilages of ribs 8 through 10.[196,197] In slipping rib syndrome, the affected rib, generally rib 10, intermittently slips out of place, creating diffuse pain in the lower chest or upper abdominal region.[197] This may, in turn, lead to increased stress and hypermobility of the costovertebral ligaments, increasing the chance of recurrence.[198,199] Hypermobility may also result in intercostal muscle strain or intercostal nerve impingement.[197,200] The onset of symptoms may be insidious, due to direct trauma, or the result of a vigorous twisting motion.[197]

Patients may report a popping of slipping sensation of the inferior ribcage that is created by movement of the ribcage during deep breathing,[200] sneezing,[200] coughing,[200] bending, or athletics.[197,201] The condition is usually unilateral and is more common in females and children.[196,201] Symptoms are often vague and may appear to be abdominal in nature, requiring multiple tests to try to identify the cause of symptoms.[201] Many patients with slipping rib syndrome have concomitant psychological distress.

Palpation of the costal cartilages during respiration may reveal popping, clicking, or crepitus, and a palpable defect of the costal cartilage may be noted when compared bilaterally.[201] The hook maneuver is a clinical test to identify slipping rib syndrome. To perform the hook maneuver, the clinician curls the fingertips under the anterior costal cartilages and pulls anteriorly and superiorly. A positive test is reproduction of the patient's pain and a click.[199–201]

Slipping rib syndrome is treated with rest from provoking activities when possible, NSAIDs, ice, and physical therapy.[196,197] Rehabilitation for slipping rib syndrome is not well documented but might include short-term use of an elastic sports tape to reduce irritability, breathing exercises, and mobilization of the ribs and costovertebral joints. As irritability reduces, exercise may include quadruped trunk stabilization exercises to improve co-contraction of all trunk musculature, thoracic rotation AROM, and resisted inspiration. For athletes, progression might include resisted trunk rotation exercises beginning with small ranges.

Should conservative measures for slipping rib syndrome fail and the patient have significant disability, peripheral nerve block[197] or surgical management, including resection of a portion of the costal cartilage, may resolve symptoms.[198,200]

ADDITIONAL EXERCISES AND MANUAL THERAPY FOR THE CERVICOTHORACIC REGION

Thoracic Techniques

It can be difficult for patients to maintain near-neutral postural alignment or to change habitual movement patterns. For patients who must sit for prolonged periods of time, a prefabricated lumbar roll or a towel can help maintain the lordotic curve in chairs with insufficient lumbar support (Fig. 17-48A). Postural taping can also be used in the lumbar (Fig. 17-48B) or thoracic spine (Fig. 17-48C). When performed in an "X" pattern, the tape allows some motion in all directions but provides a tactile cue for the patient to limit slumping, flexing, or twisting. To emphasize restriction to the thoracic spine, the center of the "X" can be placed more superiorly. Unlike an orthosis, taping does not reduce trunk muscle activation and allows motion in some planes, such as extension, while discouraging motion in other directions.

Thoracic extension ROM is often limited in patients with neck or thoracic pain. Stretching into thoracic extension can include the use of the back of a chair (Fig. 17-49A), foam roller (Fig. 17-49B), or exercise ball (Fig. 17-49C) as a fulcrum. During extension, the patient can keep the elbows wide to stretch the pectorals as well.

Manual techniques may also be used to facilitate physiologic thoracic extension, such as the scoop technique (Fig. 17-50A) and a mobilization with movement (Fig. 17-50B). For the scoop technique, have the patient seated with forehead resting on folded forearms. The clinician then reaches through the patient's arms, placing fingers on the transverse processes. The clinician then applies a superior and anterior force through the fingers while simultaneously performing a scooping motion by the forearms to facilitate thoracic extension. For the mobilization with movement technique, have the patient seated with fingers crossed behind the neck with elbows close to each other. With the anterior hand, the clinician reaches under the patient's arms and grasps the patient's contralateral shoulder. The clinician's posterior hand is placed on the spinous process of the level to be emphasized. The clinician simultaneously provides an anterior and

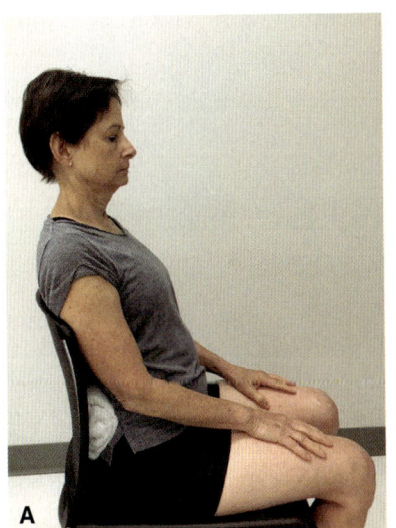
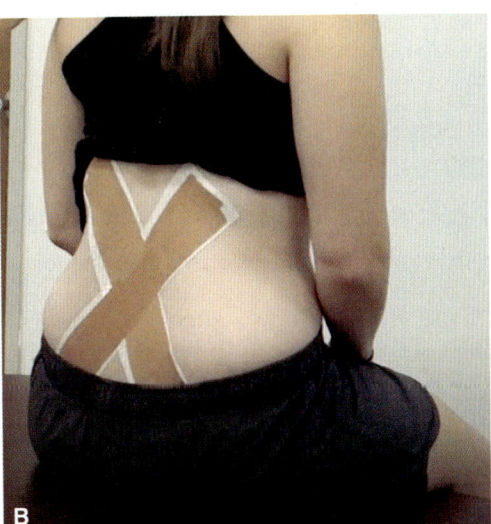
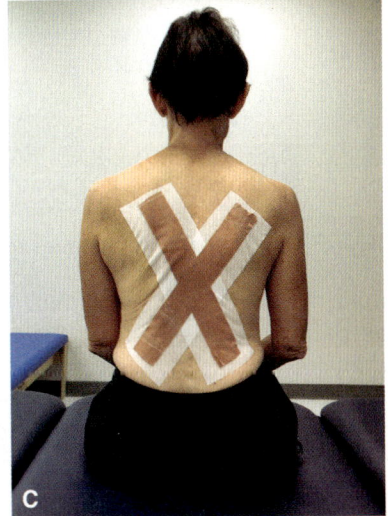

FIGURE 17-48 Methods to assist with posture correction. **A.** Lumbar roll. **B.** Postural taping for the lumbar spine. **C.** Postural taping for the thoracic spine.

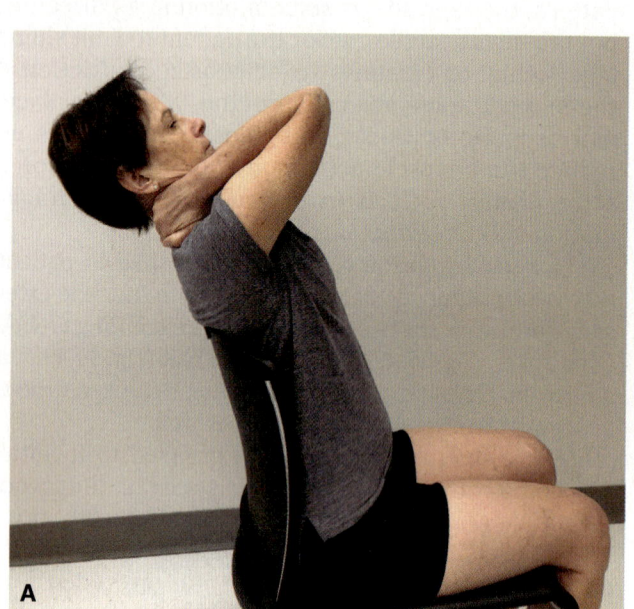
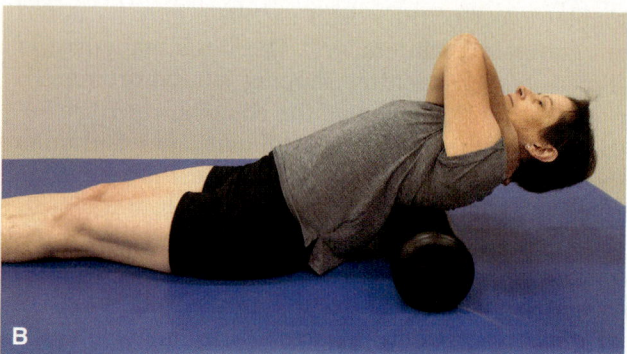
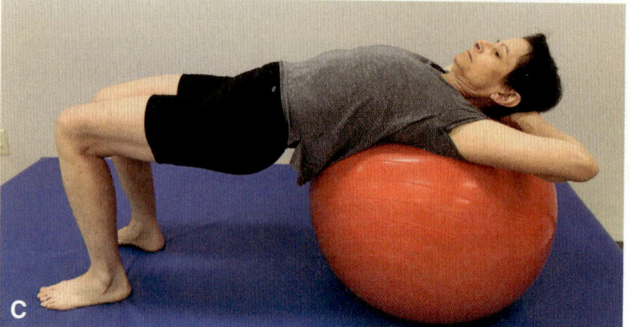

FIGURE 17-49 Stretches to increase thoracic extension. **A.** Using chair back. **B.** Using foam roller. **C.** Using exercise ball.

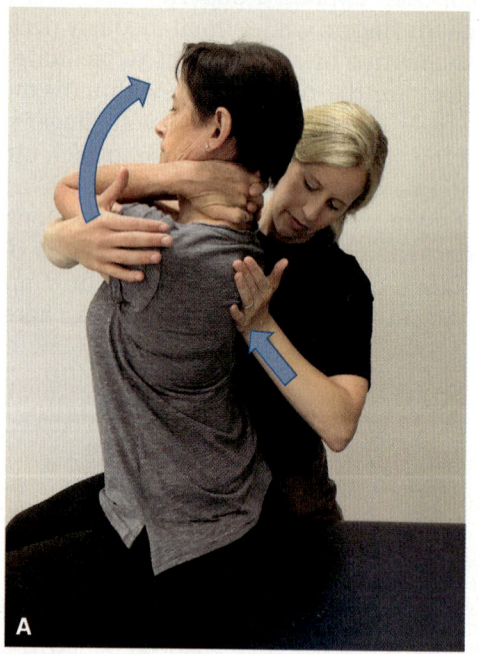
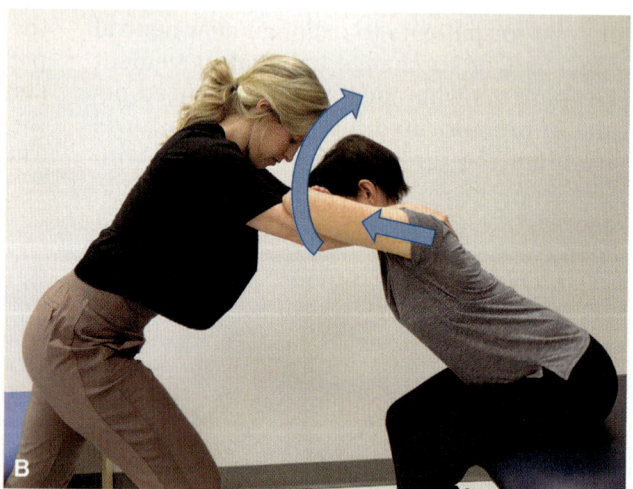

FIGURE 17-50 Manual techniques to improve thoracic extension. **A.** Mobilization with movement. **B.** Scoop technique.

superior force with the mobilizing hand while using the patient's arms to arch the patient into thoracic extension.

Thoracic rotation can be increased by performing an open book exercise (sidelying upper trunk rotation AROM) or sustaining this position as a sustained stretch (Fig. 17-51) or performing a rotational mobilization with one finger on the transverse process of the superior vertebra and another finger on the transverse process of the inferior vertebra (Fig. 17-52).

Stretching the axiohumeral muscles may be beneficial. (Chapter 14, Shoulder Complex, provides examples of ways to stretch the pectoralis major and minor.) A butterfly stretch (hands clasped behind neck with elbows relaxed out to the side) or 90/90 stretch (shoulders in 90° of abduction and 90° of external rotation)

CHAPTER 17 | CERVICAL AND THORACIC SPINE   683

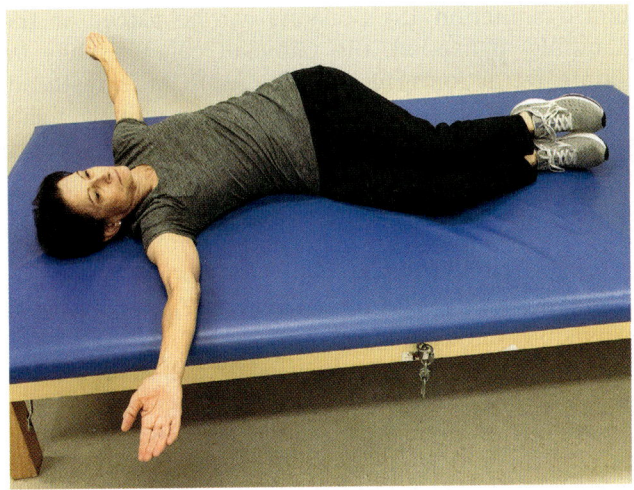

FIGURE 17-51 Open book exercise for thoracic rotation.

The following exercises in prone may help improve thoracolumbar and scapular muscular performance (Fig. 17-55): arm lift, leg lift, alternate arm and leg lift, and simultaneous bilateral arm and leg lift. For patients with limited shoulder motion or weak lower trapezii, the exercise can be modified to keep the arms at the side (Fig. 17-56). (Chapter 14, Shoulder Complex, provides additional examples of scapular muscle exercises.)

Patients with scoliosis may benefit from breathing exercises to improve posture and rib mobility. By lying on the side of the convex portion of the scoliotic curve, body weight reduces lateral costal breathing on that side. Adding abduction of the uppermost arm during inhalation helps to further expand the thoracic concavity (Fig. 17-57).

Cervical Techniques

Cervical retraction, upper cervical spine flexion, and ROM are commonly limited. Patients may utilize two fingers to glide the chin back into retraction (Fig. 17-58A). If the patient has temporomandibular

on a foam roller or towel roll placed centrally along the spine can also be beneficial (Fig. 17-53). Stretches can be held statically or performed in an on/off manner. Figure 17-54 provides an example of a manual stretch for the latissimus dorsi.

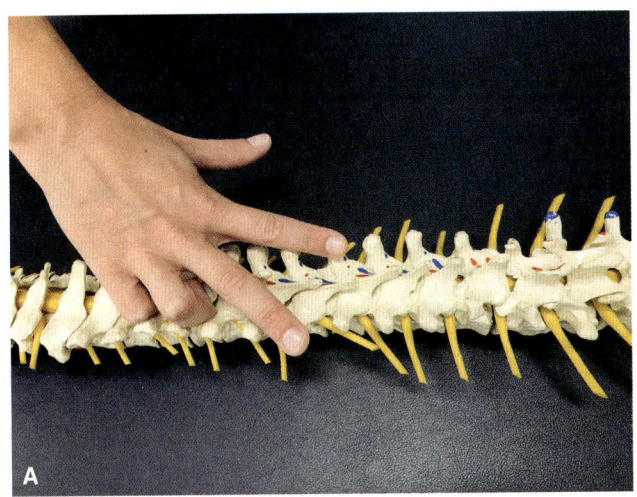
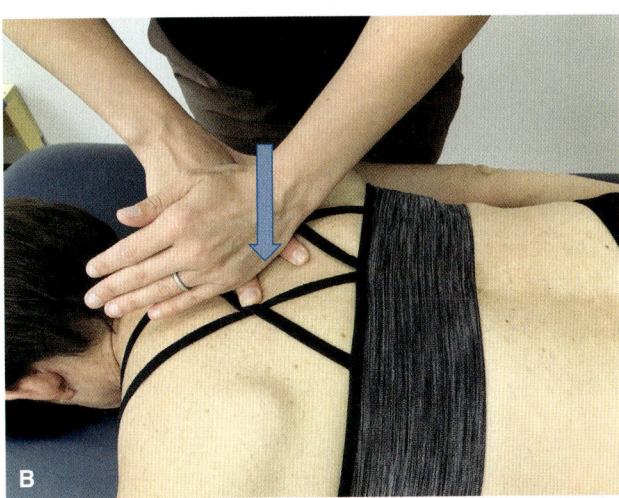

FIGURE 17-52 Mobilization to improve thoracic rotation. **A.** On skeleton. **B.** On patient.

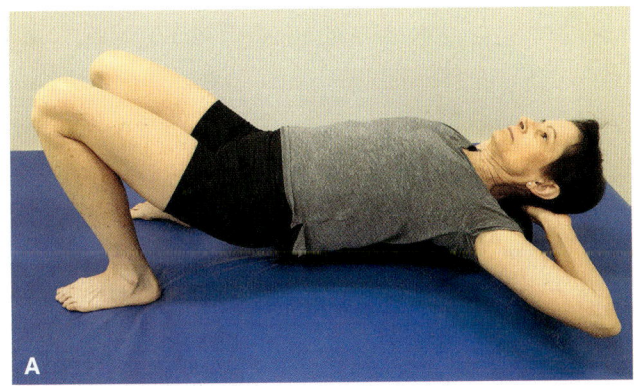
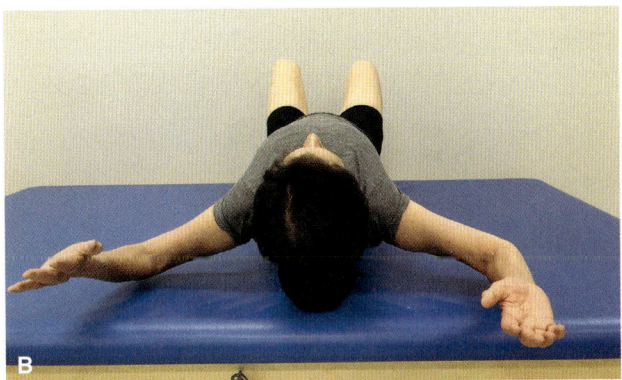

FIGURE 17-53 Pectoralis major stretches. **A.** Butterfly stretch. **B.** 90/90 stretch.

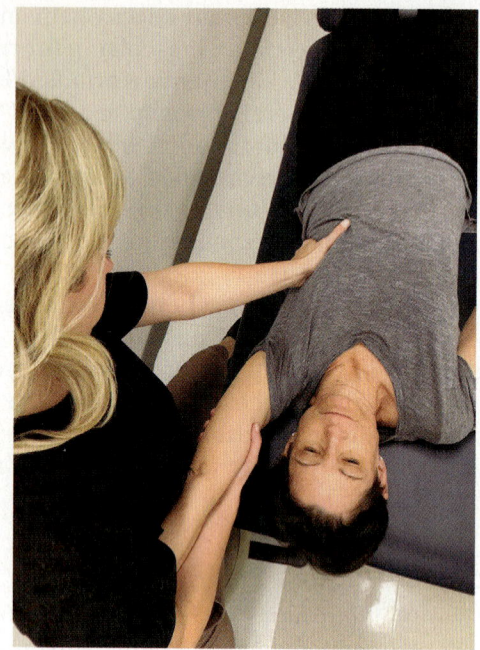

FIGURE 17-54 Latissimus dorsi stretch.

joint dysfunction, the pressure can be placed on the mandible. If needed, the clinician can manually facilitate retraction (Fig. 17-58B). As ROM is restored, the patient can perform the exercise actively, using a vertical finger placed at the sternoclavicular notch as a cue (Fig. 17-58C). Retraction can help reduce or abolish CGHs. Retraction or retraction and extension (Fig. 17-58D) may also centralize symptoms. For patients responding to unloaded positions, retraction may need to be performed in supine (Fig. 17-58E) with extension added if needed.

A towel or a strap can be used for self-mobilization. The edge of a towel or mobilization strap is placed under the articular pillar or spinous process of the vertebra to be mobilized. To facilitate rotation, the towel/strap is gently pulled horizontally across the body, creating a rotatory force (Fig. 17-59). Cervical rotation can also be manually facilitated. The clinician stabilizes C2 with the posterior hand and holds the occiput with the anterior hand. The clinician then guides the patient into rotation. The technique may be assisted

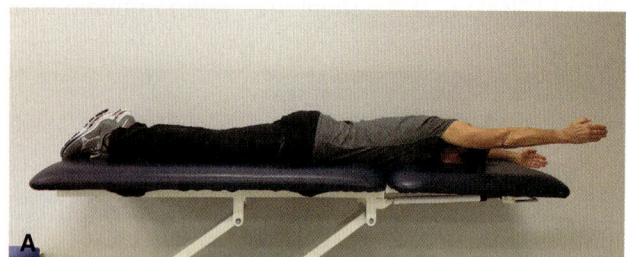
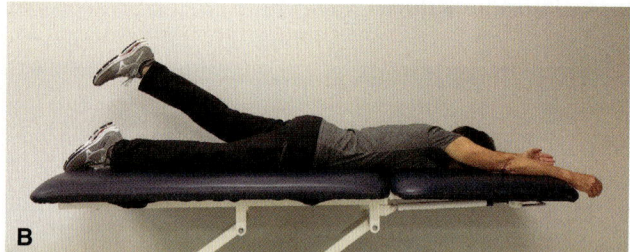
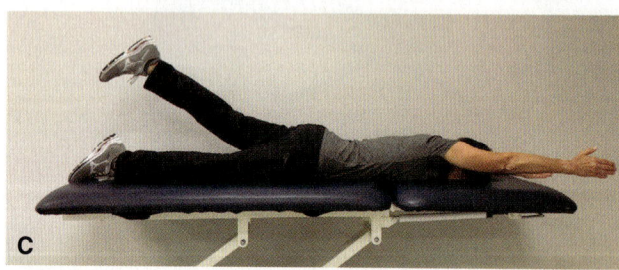
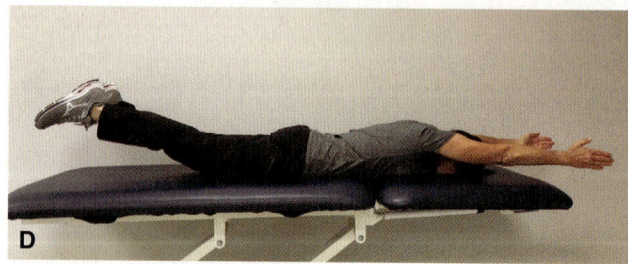

FIGURE 17-55 Thoracolumbar and scapular exercises, prone. **A.** Arm lift. **B.** Leg lift. **C.** Alternate arm/leg lift. **D.** Bilateral arm and leg lift.

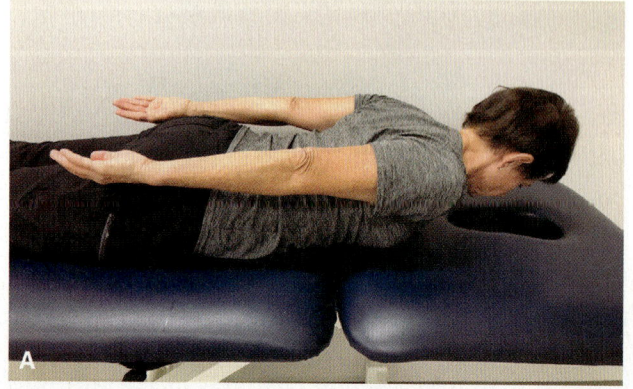
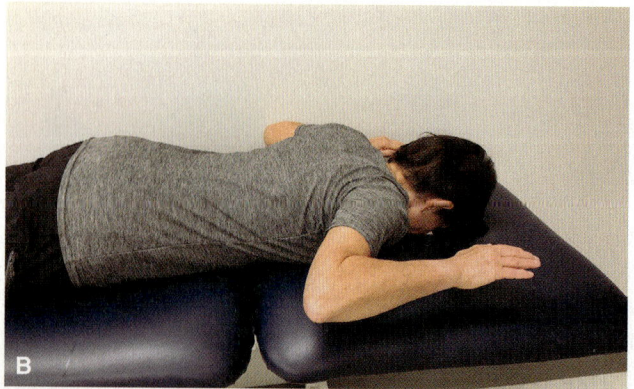

FIGURE 17-56 Prone extension and retraction **A.** Arms by side. **B.** Arms in slight abduction and external rotation.

CHAPTER 17 | CERVICAL AND THORACIC SPINE

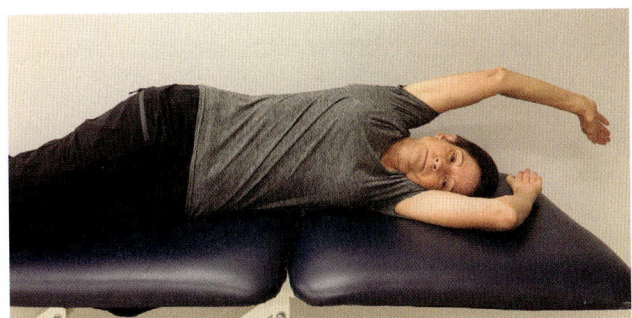

FIGURE 17-57 Facilitation of right lateral costal breathing and right rib expansion.

with the use of breathing and having the patient look toward the side of rotation.

To facilitate extension, the patient extends the head slightly, and the towel/strap is pulled along the line of the nose (Fig. 17-60). When performed at the C2 level, this movement may also help reduce the symptoms of cervicogenic dizziness.

Patients with facet arthropathy or limited lateral flexion may benefit from unilateral techniques. To perform a mobilization with movement to facilitate lateral flexion, the clinician places the mobilizing hand on the articular pillar of the segment to be mobilized, while the moving hand supports the head. The mobilizing provides an inferomedial directed force, whereas the support hand laterally flexes the patient's head toward the affected side (Fig. 17-61).

Cervical isometrics can assist with improving cervical movement control and activation (Fig 17-62). Patients can easily use two fingers to resist isometric contractions in the neutral position for the movements of upper cervical flexion (nodding motion) and lateral flexion. Retraction and extension can be awkward to use self-resistance for. Instead, these exercises can be performed against a chair with a tall back, a wall, or

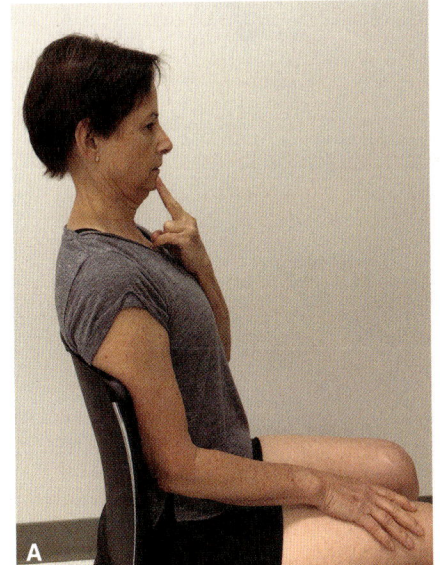
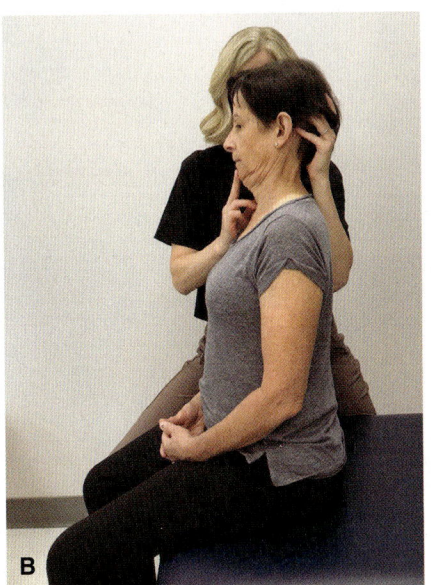
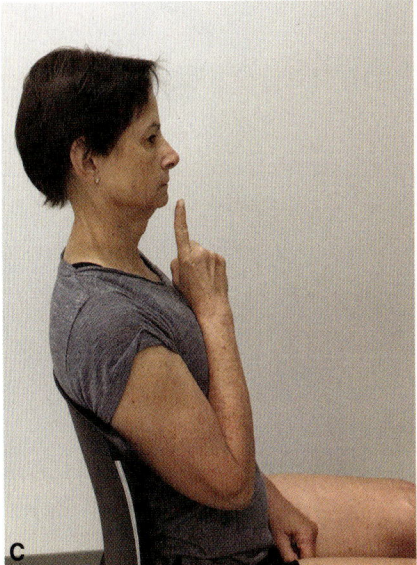
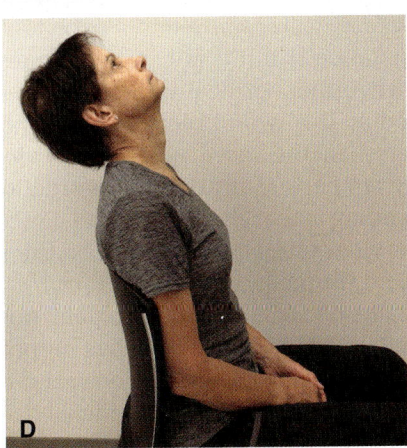
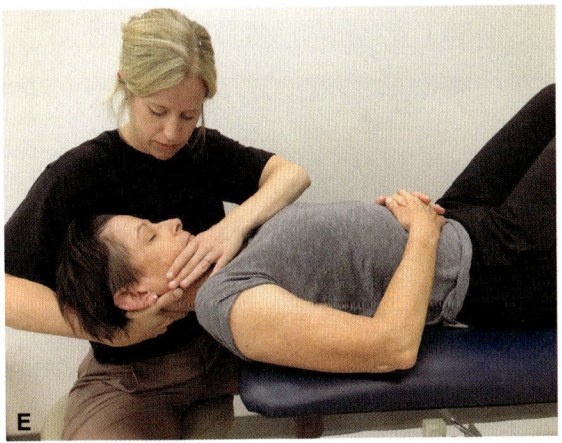

FIGURE 17-58 Cervical retraction exercises. **A.** Self-assisted. **B.** Clinician-assisted. **C.** Active. **D.** Seated retraction with extension. **E.** Supine passive retraction.

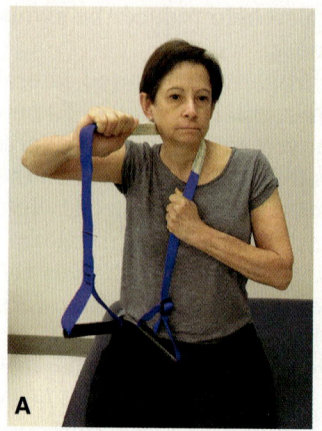 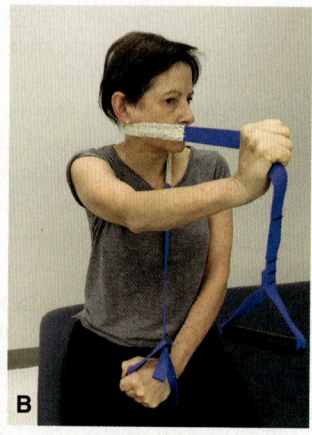 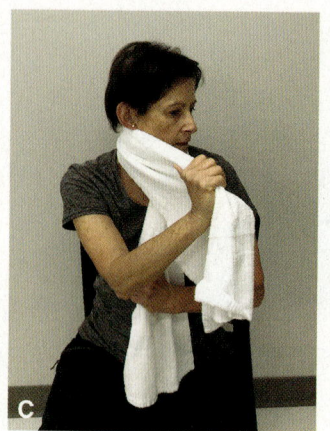 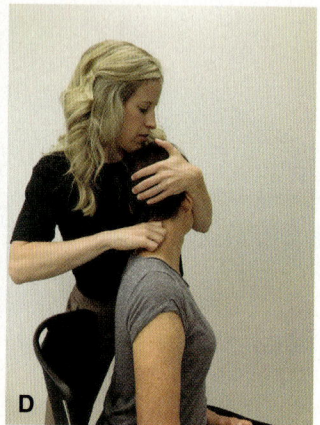

FIGURE 17-59 Self-mobilization for cervical rotation. **A.** Strap start position. **B.** Strap end position. **C.** Towel. **D.** Manual facilitation.

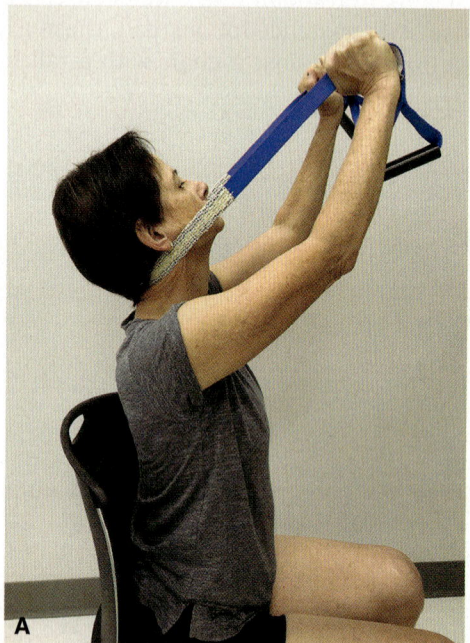 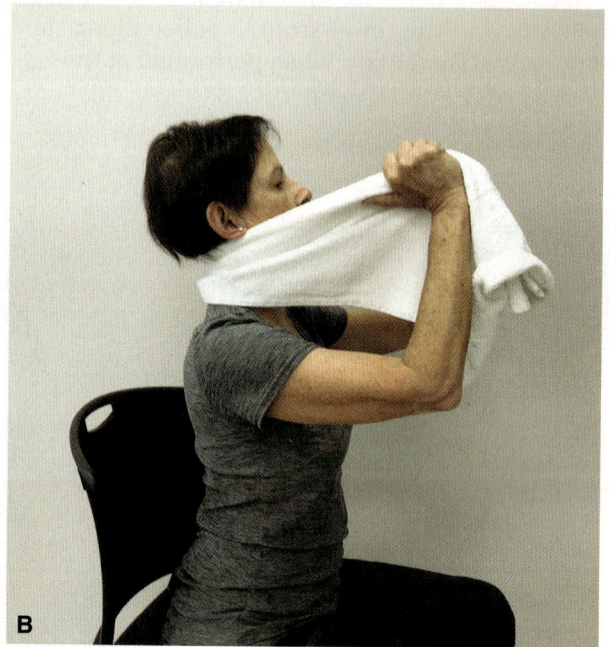

FIGURE 17-60 Self-mobilization for extension or cervicogenic dizziness. **A.** Strap. **B.** Towel.

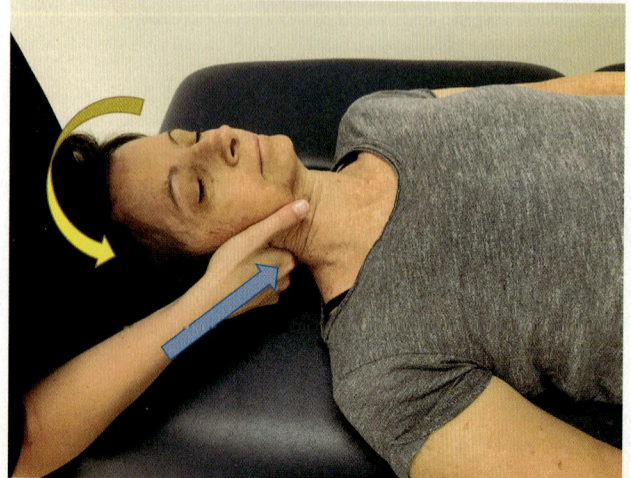

FIGURE 17-61 Mobilization with movement for cervical lateral flexion.

a resistance band. It is critical to cue patients not to perform upper cervical spine extension when trying to extend as this would recruit the suboccipital muscles rather than the more postural cervical extensors. A benefit to performing cervical retraction against a wall in standing is that the patient can concentrate not only on cervical retraction but also on the scapular retraction and thoracic extension.

Many patients with neck pain develop tightness or trigger points in the scalenes, upper trapezius, and levator scapulae. For some patients, upper trapezius stretching may need to be focused by titrating the amount of cervical rotation, flexion, and lateral flexion. Figure 17-63 provides examples of how to stretch these muscles.

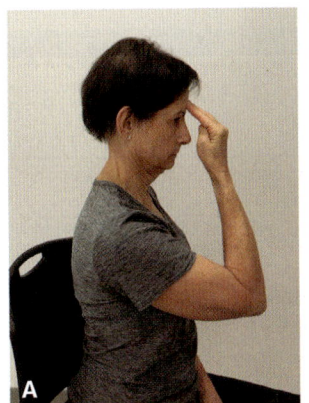 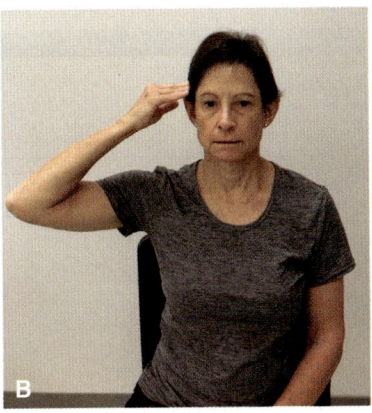 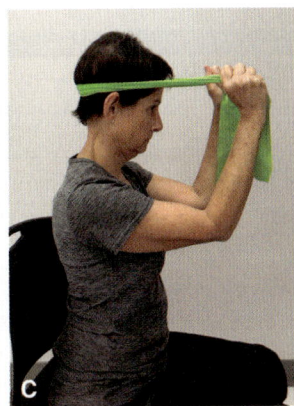 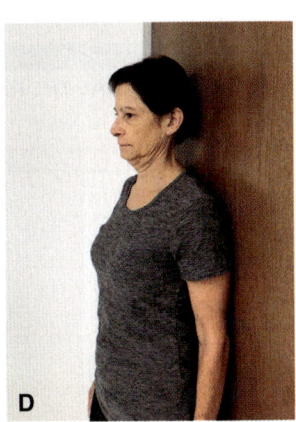

FIGURE 17-62 Cervical isometric exercises. **A.** Upper cervical flexion. **B.** Lateral flexion. **C.** Retraction against resistance band. **D.** Retraction against wall.

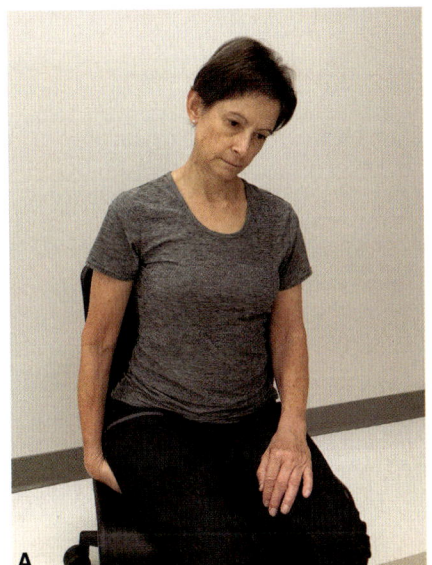 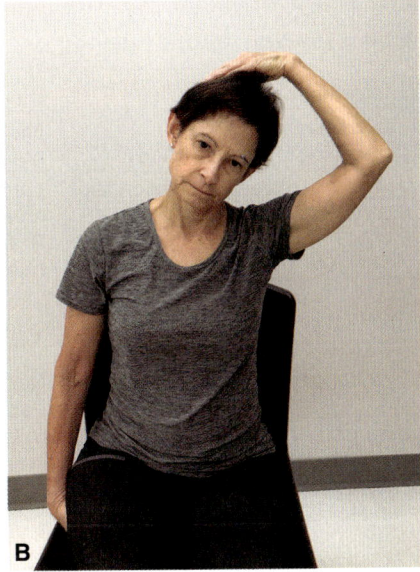 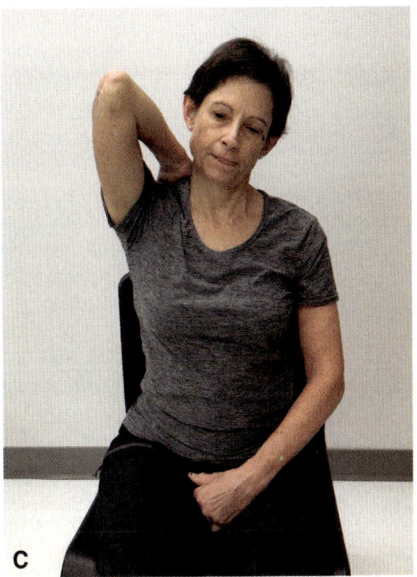

FIGURE 17-63 Stretching of the scalenes (**A**), upper trapezius (**B**), and levator scapulae (**C**).

CASE STUDY 17-1

Aiden: Patient with Upper Extremity Tingling and Numbness

Aiden is a 48-year-old jeweler who reports intermittent upper extremity tingling and numbness into her right medial upper extremity and fourth and fifth digit. Aiden reports her symptoms are noticeable while carrying things in the right upper extremity and after about 30 minutes of making jewelry. All tests begin with the uninvolved (left) side first unless otherwise noted. The physical examination of a patient with neck pathology progresses methodically to gather sufficient information to guide clinical decision-making. Table 17-9 provides an example of how an experienced clinician might organize the physical examination after performing the history and systems review.

Based on the history, there are no red flags and no signs of psychological distress. The patient's history, age, and insidious onset make the clinician consider the following diagnostic hypotheses: cervical radiculopathy, ulnar nerve entrapment, and TOS. Because radiculopathy is most common, the clinician begins with this line of investigation. When negative, the clinician moved on to performing tests for TOS and ulnar neuropathy. Although cervical distraction is one of the tests used to assist with diagnosing cervical radiculopathy, this test was not performed as the patient had no symptoms

(continued)

TABLE 17-9
SAMPLE CERVICAL-THORACIC EXAMINATION

Aiden, 48-year-old jeweler with right upper extremity paresthesias

Position	Assessments	Positive Findings
Observation	Continues from history	Forward head with upper cervical extension, protracted scapulae
Seated	T1: Interossei (A, OP, MMT) C8: Extensor pollicis longus (A, OP, MMT) C7: Wrist flexors (A, OP, MMT) C6: Wrist extensors (A, OP, MMT) C5: Deltoid (A, OP, MMT) C4: Upper trapezius (A, OP, MMT) Shoulder flexion, abduction (A, OP) Shoulder hand behind head and hand behind back (A) Dermatomes C4–T1 Peripheral nerve sensation: ulnar hand (ulnar nerve), dorsal hand (radial nerve), and palm (median nerve) Reflexes: biceps, brachioradialis, triceps patellar, Achilles Tinel: cubital tunnel, tunnel of Guyon	
Standing	Structure/posture screen Trunk AROM: flexion, extension, side glide	Mild improvement in postural deviations noted earlier
Seated neck—thoracic specific examination	Cervical ROM: protrusion, retraction, flexion, extension, lateral flexion, rotation (A, OP) Quadrant test Cervical special tests: cervical compression, Spurling Inferior glide of the first rib TOS testing: EAST, costoclavicular, Adson tests	Lateral flexion L20°/R27°, visually mild decrease in retraction Positive EAST and costoclavicular tests on right
Supine	Cervical PROM: flexion, lateral flexion, rotation, extension Neck flexion endurance test Muscle length: pectoralis minor/major Palpation: cervical soft tissue including scalenes, upper trapezius, levator scapulae, sternocleidomastoid, paraspinals, pectoralis minor ULTT Observation: breathing pattern	Neck flexion endurance test 14 seconds Pectoralis minor length: reduced B, AC joint to table 12 cm L/10 cm R Increased tone scalenes B Positive ULTT-ulnar nerve
Prone	Cervical accessory motions: central posterior-anterior pressures C2–T4 MMT: trunk raise, middle and lower trapezius Sorenson test	Prone trunk raise, B middle and lower trapezii 4/5 Sorenson test 5 seconds

A, active; *AROM*, active range of motion; *B*, bilateral; *L*, left; *MMT*, manual muscle test; *OP*, overpressure; *P*, passive; *R*, right; *TOS*, thoracic outlet syndrome; *ULTTs*, upper limb tension tests.

at the time of testing. The clinician also chose not to perform any upper cervical spine or cranial nerve assessments because the patient denied a history of trauma and had no symptoms in this region. While the ulnar nerve biased ULTT was positive, the negative tinel Test, normal sensation in the ulnar hand, and normal strength of the interossei help to rule out ulnar nerve pathology. The condition of TOS commonly involves the lower portion of the brachial plexus. Given that the ulnar nerve is derived from the inferior trunk, it is likely that the ULTT is positive due to a proximal restriction within the plexus. The clinician concluded the patient had right TOS with decreased endurance of the deep cervical flexor and trunk extensors and reduced strength of the trunk extensors and scapular stabilizers. She also had decreased length of the scalenes and pectoralis minor. Each of these impairments should be addressed within Aiden's plan of care.

CHAPTER SUMMARY

The cervical and thoracic spine is frequently a source of pain and disability. Symptoms in this region require careful attention, as the clinician must rule out referral from nearly all body systems. The clinician must not only consider pathoanatomic causes of symptoms but also recognize that nonspecific neck pain is common. It is important to identify any neural deficits and their functional implications. These must then be addressed in the plan of care. Interventions for patients with cervicothoracic dysfunction should focus on education and multiple types of exercise, but manual therapy may prove a useful adjunct.

REFERENCES

1. Hogg-Johnson S, van der Velde G, Carroll LJ, et al. The burden and determinants of neck pain in the general population: results of the bone and joint decade 2000–2010 task force on neck pain and its associated disorders. *Spine.* 2008;33(4 Suppl):S39–S51.
2. Côté P, Cassidy DJ, Carroll LJ, Kristman V. The annual incidence and course of neck pain in the general population: a population-based cohort study. *Pain.* 2004;112(3):267–273.
3. Thomas LC, Rivett DA, Attia JR, Levi C. Risk factors and clinical presentation of cervical arterial dissection: preliminary results of a prospective case-control study. *J Orthop Sports Phys Ther.* 2015;45(7):503–511.
4. Mechelli F, Preboski Z, Boissonault W. Differential diagnosis of a patient referred to physical therapy with low back pain: abdominal aortic aneurysm. *J Orthop Sports Phys Ther.* 2008;38(9):551–557.
5. Davenport D, Colaco H, Kavarthapu V. Examination of the adult spine. *Br J Hosp Med.* 2015;76(12):C182–C195.
6. Benzel EC. *The Cervical Spine.* 5th ed. Lippincott Williams & Wilkins; 2012.
7. Goodman C, Fuller K. *Pathology: Implications for the Physical Therapist.* 5th ed. Elsevier; 2021.
8. Rushton A, Rivett D, Carlesso L, Flynn T, Hing W, Kerry R. International framework for examination of the cervical region for potential of cervical arterial dysfunction prior to orthopaedic manual therapy intervention. *Man Ther.* 2014;19(3):222–228.
9. Kepler C, Anderson D. Evaluation of the cervical spine. In: Shen F, Samartzis D, Fessler R, eds. *Textbook of the Cervical Spine.* Elsevier Saunders; 2015:70–76.
10. Parikh P, Santaguida P, Macdermid J, Gross A, Eshtiaghi A. Comparison of CPG's for the diagnosis, prognosis and management of non-specific neck pain: a systematic review. *BMC Musculoskelet Disord.* 2019;20(1):81.
11. Côté P, Wong JJ, Sutton D, et al. Management of neck pain and associated disorders: a clinical practice guideline from the Ontario Protocol for Traffic Injury Management (OPTIMa) collaboration. *Eur Spine J.* 2016;25(7):2000–2022.
12. Yarznbowicz R, Wlodarski M, Dolutan J. Classification by pain pattern for patients with cervical spine radiculopathy. *J Man Manip Ther.* 2020;28(3):160–169.
13. Bier JD, Scholten-Peeters WGM, Staal JB, et al. Clinical practice guideline for physical therapy assessment and treatment in patients with nonspecific neck pain. *Phys Ther.* 2018;98(3):162–171.
14. Blanpied P, Gross A, Elliott J, et al. Neck pain: revision 2017. Clinical practice guidelines Linked to the International Classification of Functioning, Disability and Health from the Orthopaedic Section of the American Physical Therapy Association. *J Orthop Sports Phys Ther.* 2017;47(1):A1–A83.
15. Steill IG, Wells GA, Vandemheen KL, et al. The Canadian C-spine rule for radiography in alert and stable trauma patients. *JAMA.* 2001;286(15):1841–1848.
16. Michaleff ZA, Maher CG, Verhagen AP, Rebbeck T, Lin CW. Accuracy of the Canadian C-spine rule and NEXUS to screen for clinically important cervical spine injury in patients following blunt trauma: a systematic review. *CMAJ.* 2012;184(16):E867–E876.
17. Reiley AS, Vickory FM, Funderburg SE, Cesario RA, Clendaniel RA. How to diagnose cervicogenic dizziness. *Arch Physiother.* 2017;7(1):12.
18. Singh A, Tetreault L, Casey A, Laing R, Statham P, Fehlings MG. A summary of assessment tools for patients suffering from cervical spondylotic myelopathy: a systematic review on validity, reliability and responsiveness. *Eur Spine J.* 2015;24:209–228.
19. Badhiwala JH, Ahuja CS, Akbar MA, et al. Degenerative cervical myelopathy—update and future directions. *Nat Rev Neurol.* 2020;16(2):108–124.
20. Milligan J, Ryan K, Fehlings M, Bauman C. Degenerative cervical myelopathy: diagnosis and management in primary care. *Can Fam Physician.* 2019;65(9):619–624.
21. Kane SF, Abadie KV, Willson A. Degenerative cervical myelopathy: recognition and management. *Am Fam Physician.* 2020;102(12):740–750.
22. Jackson S. Cervical myelopathy in a patient referred for lower extremity symptoms. *J Orthop Sports Phys Ther.* 2017;47(7):510.
23. Nagata K, Yoshimura N, Hashizume H, et al. Physical performance decreases in the early stage of cervical myelopathy before the myelopathic signs appear: the Wakayama Spine Study. *Eur Spine J.* 2019;28(5):1217–1224.
24. McInerney S, Keil A, Jin Suh KIM. Cervical myelopathy presenting as bilateral upper extremity weakness. *J Orthop Sports Phys Ther.* 2017;47(9):691.
25. Mansfield CJ. Cervical myelopathy causing numbness and paresthesias in lower extremities: a case report identifying the cause of a false positive Sharp-Purser test. *Physiother Theory Pract.* 2019;35(4):401–408.
26. Theodore N. Degenerative cervical spondylosis. *N Engl J Med.* 2020;383(2):159–168.
27. König A, Spetzger U. *Degenerative Diseases of the Cervical Spine Therapeutic Management in the Subaxial Section.* 1st ed. Springer International Publishing; 2017.
28. Mańczak M, Gasik R. Cervical spine instability in the course of rheumatoid arthritis—imaging methods. *Reumatologia.* 2017;55(4):201–207.
29. Ali FE, Al-Bustan MA, Al-Busairi WA, Al-Mulla FA, Esbaita EY. Cervical spine abnormalities associated with Down syndrome. *Int Orthop.* 2006;30(4):284–289.
30. Hutting N, Scholten-Peeters GGM, Vijverman V, Keesenberg MDM, Verhagen AP. Diagnostic accuracy of upper cervical spine instability tests: a systematic review. *Phys Ther.* 2013;93(12):1686–1695.
31. Sullivan MJL, Bishop SR, Pivik J. The pain catastrophizing scale: development and validation. *Psychol Assess.* 1995;7(4):524–532.
32. MacDermid JC, Walton DM, Avery S, et al. Measurement properties of the neck disability index: a systematic review. *J Orthop Sports Phys Ther.* 2009;39(5):400–417.
33. Bobos P, MacDermid JC, Walton DM, Gross A, Santaguida PL. Patient-reported outcome measures used for neck disorders: an overview of systematic reviews. *J Orthop Sports Phys Ther.* 2018;48(10):775–788.

34. Favaro L, Boggs RG, Geraci J, Michael C. Conservative management of a foraminal lumbar disc herniation. *JOSPT Cases.* 2021;1(1):49–50.
35. Grijalva R, Hsu F, Wycliffe N, et al. Hoffman sign. *Spine.* 2015;40(7):475–479.
36. Snodgrass SJ, Cleland JA, Haskins R, Rivett DA. The clinical utility of cervical range of motion in diagnosis, prognosis, and evaluating the effects of manipulation: a systematic review. *Physiotherapy.* 2014;100(4):290–304.
37. Kaltenborn F. Orthopedic manual therapy for physical therapists Nordic system: OMT Kaltenborn-Evjenth concept. *J Man Manip Ther.* 1993;1(2):47–51.
38. Edmond S. *Manipulations and Mobilizations: Extremity and Spinal Techniques.* CV Mosby; 1993.
39. Hall TM, Briffa K, Hopper D, Robinson K. Comparative analysis and diagnostic accuracy of the cervical flexion-rotation test. *J Headache Pain.* 2010;11(5):391–397.
40. Simons DG, Travell JG, Simons LS. *Travell & Simons' Myofascial Pain and Dysfunction: The Trigger Point Manual (Vol 1: Upper Half of Body).* 2nd ed. Lippincott Williams & Wilkins; 1999.
41. Romagnoli I, Gigliotti F, Galarducci A, et al. Chest wall kinematics and respiratory muscle action in ankylosing spondylitis patients. *Eur Respir J.* 2004;24(3):453–460.
42. Florencio LL, de Oliveira IV, Lodovichi SS, et al. Cervical muscular endurance performance in women with and without migraine. *J Orthop Sports Phys Ther.* 2019;49(5):330–336.
43. Cleland J, Koppenhaver S, Su J. *Netter's Orthopedic Clinical Examination: An Evidence-Based Approach.* 3rd ed. Elsevier; 2015.
44. Kim DG, Chung SH, Jung HB. The effects of neural mobilization on cervical radiculopathy patients' pain, disability, ROM, and deep flexor endurance. *J Back Musculoskelet Rehabil.* 2017;30(5):951–959.
45. Apelby-Albrecht M, Andersson L, Kleiva IW, Kvåle K, Skillgate E, Josephson A. Concordance of upper limb neurodynamic tests with medical examination and magnetic resonance imaging in patients with cervical radiculopathy: a diagnostic cohort study. *J Man Manip Ther.* 2013;36(9):626–632.
46. Lemeunier N, Silva-Oolup S, Chow N, et al. Reliability and validity of clinical tests to assess the anatomical integrity of the cervical spine in adults with neck pain and its associated disorders: part 1—a systematic review from the Cervical Assessment and Diagnosis Research Evaluation (CADRE) collaboration. *Eur Spine J.* 2017;26(9):2225–2241.
47. Hengeveld E, Banks K. *Maitland's Vertebral Manipulation.* Vol 1. 8th ed. Churchill Livingstone/Elsevier; 2014.
48. Alqarni AM, Schneiders AG, Hendrick PA. Clinical tests to diagnose lumbar segmental instability: a systematic review. *J Orthop Sports Phys Ther.* 2011;41(3):130–140.
49. Abbott JH, McCane B, Herbison P, Moginie G, Chapple C, Hogarty T. Lumbar segmental instability: a criterion-related validity study of manual therapy assessment. *BMC Musculoskelet Disord.* 2005;6(1):56.
50. Seffinger MA, Najm WI, Mishra SI, et al. Reliability of spinal palpation for diagnosis of back and neck pain: a systematic review of the literature. *Spine.* 2004;29(19):E413–E425.
51. Kulig K, Landel R, Powers CM. Assessment of lumbar spine kinematics using dynamic MRI: a proposed mechanism of sagittal plane motion induced by manual posterior-to-anterior mobilization. *J Orthop Sports Phys Ther.* 2004;34(2):57–64.
52. Fritz JM, Whitman JM, Childs JD. Lumbar spine segmental mobility assessment: an examination of validity for determining intervention strategies in patients with low back pain. *Arch Phys Med Rehabil.* 2005;86(9):1745–1752.
53. Hayes MA, Howard TC, Gruel CR, Kopta JA. Roentgenographic evaluation of lumbar spine flexion-extension in asymptomatic individuals. *Spine.* 1989;14(3):327–331.
54. Thoomes EJ, van Geest S, van der Windt DA, et al. Value of physical tests in diagnosing cervical radiculopathy: a systematic review. *Spine.* 2018;18(1):179–189.
55. Shah JM, Wahezi SE, Silva K. *Spondylosis with Generalized Degenerative Disk, Uncovertebral, and Facet Pain.* Springer International Publishing; 2018:345–348.
56. Treleaven J, Joloud V, Nevo Y, Radcliffe C, Ryder M. Normative responses to clinical tests for cervicogenic dizziness: clinical cervical torsion test and head-neck differentiation test. *Phys Ther.* 2020;100(1):192–200.
57. Kranenburg HAR, Tyer R, Schmitt M, et al. Effects of head and neck positions on blood flow in the vertebral, internal carotid, and intracranial arteries: a systematic review. *J Orthop Sports Phys Ther.* 2019;49(10):688–697.
58. Kuwayama DP, Lund JR, Brantigan CO, Glebova NO. Choosing surgery for neurogenic tos: the roles of physical exam, physical therapy, and imaging. *Diagnostics (Basel).* 2017;7(2):37.
59. Li N, Dierks G, Vervaeke HE, et al. Thoracic outlet syndrome: a narrative review. *J Clin Med.* 2021;10(5):962.
60. Dessureault-Dober I, Bronchti G, Bussières A. Diagnostic accuracy of clinical tests for neurogenic and vascular thoracic outlet syndrome: a systematic review. *J Manipulative Physiol Ther.* 2018;41(9):789–799.
61. Reichert B. *Palpation Techniques. Surface Anatomy for Physical Therapists.* Thieme; 2011.
62. van Dieën JH, Reeves NP, Kawchuk G, van Dillen LR, Hodges PW. Motor control changes in low back pain: divergence in presentations and mechanisms. *J Orthop Sports Phys Ther.* 2019;49(6):370–379.
63. Sueki DG, Cleland JA, Wainner RS. A regional interdependence model of musculoskeletal dysfunction: research, mechanisms, and clinical implications. *J Man Manip Ther.* 2013;21(2):90–102.
64. McDevitt A, Young J, Mintken P, Cleland J. Regional interdependence and manual therapy directed at the thoracic spine. *J Man Manip Ther.* 2015;23(3):139–146.
65. Eck JC, Humphreys SC, Lim T-H, et al. Biomechanical study on the effect of cervical spine fusion on adjacent-level intradiscal pressure and segmental motion. *Spine.* 2002;27(22):2431–2434.
66. Willy R, Hoglund L, Barton C, et al. Patellofemoral pain: clinical practice guidelines linked to the International Classification of Functioning, Disability and Health from the Academy of Orthopaedic Physical Therapy of the American Physical Therapy Association. *J Orthop Sports Phys Ther.* 2019;49(9):CPG1–CPG95.
67. Cross KM, Kuenze C, Grindstaff T, Hertel J. Thoracic spine thrust manipulation improves pain, range of motion, and self-reported function in patients with mechanical neck pain: a systematic review. *J Orthop Sports Phys Ther.* 2011;41(9):633–642.
68. Ghamkhar L, Arab AM, Nourbakhsh MR, Kahlaee AH, Zolfaghari R. Examination of regional interdependence theory in chronic neck pain: interpretations from correlation of strength measures in cervical and pain-free regions. *Pain Med.* 2020;21(2):e182–e190.
69. Hause CJ. *Scapulothoracic Muscle Strengthening for the Management of Medial Epicondylitis.* Azusa Pacific University; 2017.
70. Szczygieł E, Fudacz N, Golec J, Golec E. The impact of the position of the head on the functioning of the human body: a systematic review. *Int J Occup Med Environ Health.* 2020;33(5):559–568.
71. Mahmoud NF, Hassan KA, Abdelmajeed SF, Moustafa IM, Silva AG. The relationship between forward head posture and neck pain: a systematic review and meta-analysis. *Curr Rev Musculoskelet Med.* 2019;12(4):562–577.

72. Patwardhan AG, Khayatzadeh S, Havey RM, et al. Cervical sagittal balance: a biomechanical perspective can help clinical practice. *Eur Spine J.* 2018;27(Suppl 1):25–38.
73. Sambataro S, Cervino G, Bocchieri S, La Bruna R, Cicciù M. TMJ dysfunctions systemic implications and postural assessments: a review of recent literature. *J Funct Morphol Kinesiol.* 2019;4(3):58.
74. Rebbeck T. The role of exercise and patient education in the noninvasive management of whiplash. *J Orthop Sports Phys Ther.* 2017;47(7):481–491.
75. Gross A, Langevin P, Burnie SJ, et al. Manipulation and mobilisation for neck pain contrasted against an inactive control or another active treatment. *Cochrane Database Syst Rev.* 2015;(9):CD004249.
76. Stieven FF, Ferreira GE, Wiebusch M, de Araújo FX, da Rosa LHT, Silva MF. Dry needling combined with guideline-based physical therapy provides no added benefit in the management of chronic neck pain: a randomized controlled trial. *J Orthop Sports Phys Ther.* 2020;50(8):447–454.
77. Gattie E, Cleland JA, Pandya J, Snodgrass S. Dry needling adds no benefit to the treatment of neck pain: a sham-controlled randomized clinical trial with 1-year follow-up. *J Orthop Sports Phys Ther.* 2020;51(1):37–45.
78. Spanos G, Zounis M, Natsika M, May S. The application of mechanical diagnosis and therapy and changes on MRI findings in a patient with cervical radiculopathy. *Man Ther.* 2013;18(6):606–610.
79. Copurgensli C, Gur G, Tunay VB. A comparison of the effects of Mulligan's mobilization and Kinesio taping on pain, range of motion, muscle strength, and neck disability in patients with cervical spondylosis: a randomized controlled study. *J Back Musculoskelet Rehabil.* 2017;30(1):51–62.
80. Zhao H, Duan LJ, Gao YS, et al. What is the superior surgical strategy for bi-level cervical spondylosis-anterior cervical disc replacement or anterior cervical decompression and fusion? A meta-analysis from 11 studies. *Medicine (Baltimore).* 2018;97(13):e0005.
81. Sleijser-Koehorst MLS, Coppieters MW, Epping R, Rooker S, Verhagen AP, Scholten-Peeters GGM. Diagnostic accuracy of patient interview items and clinical tests for cervical radiculopathy. *Physiotherapy.* 2021;111:74–82.
82. Kim HJ, Nemani VM, Piyaskulkaew C, Vargas SR, Riew KD. Cervical radiculopathy: incidence and treatment of 1,420 consecutive cases. *Asian Spine J.* 2016;10(2):231–237.
83. Romeo A, Vanti C, Boldrini V, et al. Cervical radiculopathy: effectiveness of adding traction to physical therapy—a systematic review and meta-analysis of randomized controlled trials. *Phys Ther.* 2018;98(4):231–242.
84. Park MS, Young-Su J, Seong-Hwan M, et al. Reoperation rates after surgery for degenerative cervical spine disease according to different surgical procedures: national population-based cohort study. *Spine.* 2016;41(19):1484–1492.
85. Engel G, Bender YY, Adams LC, et al. Evaluation of osseous cervical foraminal stenosis in spinal radiculopathy using susceptibility-weighted magnetic resonance imaging. *Eur Radiol.* 2019;29(4):1855–1862.
86. Kjaer P, Kongsted A, Hartvigsen J, et al. National clinical guidelines for non-surgical treatment of patients with recent onset neck pain or cervical radiculopathy. *Eur Spine J.* 2017;26(9):2242–2257.
87. Watkins RG, Watkins RG. Cervical disc herniations, radiculopathy, and myelopathy. *Clin Sports Med.* 2021;40(3):513–539.
88. Kelsey JL, Githens PB, Walter SD, et al. An epidemiological study of acute prolapsed cervical intervertebral disc. *J Bone Joint Surg Am.* 1984;66(6):907–914.
89. Tuttle J, Chutkan N. Cervical radiculopathy. In: Shen F, Samartzis D, Fessler R, eds. *Textbook for the Cervical Spine.* Elsevier Saunders; 2015:131–145.
90. McAnany SJ, Rhee JM, Baird EO, et al. Observed patterns of cervical radiculopathy: how often do they differ from a standard, "Netter diagram" distribution? *Spine J.* 2019;19(7):1137–1142.
91. Dedering Å, Peolsson A, Cleland JA, Halvorsen M, Svensson MA, Kierkegaard M. The effects of neck-specific training versus prescribed physical activity on pain and disability in patients with cervical radiculopathy: a randomized controlled trial. *Arch Phys Med Rehabil.* 2018;99(12):2447–2456.
92. Luetchford S, Declich M, Tavella R, Zaninelli D, May S. Diagnosis of cervical and thoracic musculoskeletal spinal pain receptive to mechanical movement strategies: a multicenter observational study. *J Man Manip Ther.* 2018;26(5):292–300.
93. McKenzie R, May S. *The Lumbar Spine: Mechanical Diagnosis and Therapy.* Vol 1. Spinal Publications; 2013.
94. Akkan H, Gelecek N. The effect of stabilization exercise training on pain and functional status in patients with cervical radiculopathy. *J Back Musculoskelet Rehabil.* 2018;31(2):247–252.
95. Young IA, Pozzi F, Dunning J, Linkonis R, Michener LA. Immediate and short-term effects of thoracic spine manipulation in patients with cervical radiculopathy: a randomized controlled trial. *J Orthop Sports Phys Ther.* 2019;49(5):299–309.
96. Madson TJ, Hollman JH. Cervical traction for managing neck pain: a survey of physical therapists in the United States. *J Orthop Sports Phys Ther.* 2017;47(3):200–208.
97. Beckworth WJ, Abramoff BA, Bailey IM, et al. Acute cervical radiculopathy outcomes: soft disc herniations vs osteophytes. *Pain Med.* 2021;22(3):561–566.
98. Liang L, Feng M, Cui X, et al. The effect of exercise on cervical radiculopathy: a systematic review and meta-analysis. *Medicine (Baltimore).* 2019;98(45):e17733.
99. Dillingham TR, Annaswamy TM, Plastaras CT. Evaluation of persons with suspected lumbosacral and cervical radiculopathy: electrodiagnostic assessment and implications for treatment and outcomes (part II). *Muscle Nerve.* 2020;62(4):474–484.
100. Youssef JA, Heiner AD, Montgomery JR, et al. Outcomes of posterior cervical fusion and decompression: a systematic review and meta-analysis. *Spine J.* 2019;19(10):1714–1729.
101. Sasso R, Mitchell M. Cervical disk arthoplasty. In: Shen F, Samartzis D, Fessler R, eds. *Textbook for the Cervical Spine.* Elsevier Saunders; 2015:1104–1125.
102. Mostofi K, Khouzani R. Reliability of cervical radiculopathy, its congruence between patient history and medical imaging evidence of disc herniation and its role in surgical decision. *Eur J Orthop Surg Traumatol.* 2016;26(7):805–808.
103. Kreitz T, Huang R, Beck D, Park AG, Hilibrand A. Prolonged preoperative weakness affects recovery of motor function after anterior cervical diskectomy and fusion. *J Am Acad Orthop Surg.* 2018;26(2):67–73.
104. Sterner Y, Toolanen G, Gerdle B, Hildingsson C. The incidence of whiplash trauma and the effects of different factors on recovery. *J Spinal Disord Tech.* 2003;16(2):195–199.
105. Carroll LJ, Holm LW, Hogg-Johnson S, et al. Course and prognostic factors for neck pain in whiplash-associated disorders (WAD): results of the bone and joint decade 2000–2010 task force on neck pain and its associated disorders. *Eur Spine J.* 2008;17(Suppl 1):83–92.
106. Spitzer WO, Skovron ML, Salmi LR, et al. Scientific monograph of the Quebec task force on whiplash-associated disorders: redefining "whiplash" and its management. *Spine.* 1995;20(8 Suppl):1s–73s.
107. Walton DM, Pretty J, MacDermid JC, Teasel RW. Risk factors for persistent problems following whiplash injury: results of a systematic review and meta-analysis. *J Orthop Sports Phys Ther.* 2009;39(5):334–350.

108. Ardern CL, Peterson G, Ludvigsson ML, Peolsson A. Satisfaction with the outcome of physical therapist–prescribed exercise in chronic whiplash–associated disorders: secondary analysis of a randomized clinical trial. *J Orthop Sports Phys Ther.* 2016;46(8):640–649.
109. Griffin A, Leaver A, Moloney N. General exercise does not improve long-term pain and disability in individuals with whiplash-associated disorders: a systematic review. *J Orthop Sports Phys Ther.* 2017;47(7):472–480.
110. Treleaven J, Jull G, Sterling M. Dizziness and unsteadiness following whiplash injury: characteristic features and relationship with cervical joint position error. *J Rehabil Med.* 2003;35(1):36–43.
111. Griswold D, Learman K, Kolber MJ, O'Halloran B, Cleland JA. Pragmatically applied cervical and thoracic nonthrust manipulation versus thrust manipulation for patients with mechanical neck pain: a multicenter randomized clinical trial. *J Orthop Sports Phys Ther.* 2018;48(3):137–145.
112. Sarrami P, Armstrong E, Naylor JM, Harris IA. Factors predicting outcome in whiplash injury: a systematic meta-review of prognostic factors. *J Orthop Traumatol.* 2017;18(1):9–16.
113. Pourahmadi M, Mohseni-Bandpei MA, Keshtkar A, et al. Effectiveness of dry needling for improving pain and disability in adults with tension-type, cervicogenic, or migraine headaches: protocol for a systematic review. *Chiropr Man Therap.* 2019;27:43.
114. Olesen J, Steiner T, Bendtsen L, et al. *The International Classification of Headache Disorders.* 3rd ed (iHD3). Cephalgia; 2018.
115. Park SK, Yang DJ, Kim JH, Heo JW, Uhm YH, Yoon JH. Analysis of mechanical properties of cervical muscles in patients with cervicogenic headache. *J Phys Ther Sci.* 2017;29(2):332–335.
116. Rubio-Ochoa J, Benítez-Martínez J, Lluch E, Santacruz-Zaragozá S, Gómez-Contreras P, Cook CE. Physical examination tests for screening and diagnosis of cervicogenic headache: a systematic review. *Man Ther.* 2016;21:35–40.
117. van der Meer HA, Visscher CM, Vredeveld T, Nijhuis van der Sanden MW, Hh Engelbert R, Speksnijder CM. The diagnostic accuracy of headache measurement instruments: a systematic review and meta-analysis focusing on headaches associated with musculoskeletal symptoms. *Cephalalgia.* 2019;39(10):1313–1332.
118. Barmherzig R, Kingston W. Occipital neuralgia and cervicogenic headache: diagnosis and management. *Curr Neurol Neurosci Rep.* 2019;19(5):20.
119. Côté P, Yu H, Shearer HM, et al. Non-pharmacological management of persistent headaches associated with neck pain: a clinical practice guideline from the Ontario protocol for traffic injury management (OPTIMa) collaboration. *Eur J Pain.* 2019;23(6):1051–1070.
120. Falsiroli Maistrello L, Rafanelli M, Turolla A. Manual therapy and quality of life in people with headache: systematic review and meta-analysis of randomized controlled trials. *Curr Pain Headache Rep.* 2019;23(10):78.
121. Fernandez M, Moore C, Tan J, et al. Spinal manipulation for the management of cervicogenic headache: a systematic review and meta-analysis. *Eur J Pain.* 2020;24(9):1687–1702.
122. Caponnetto V, Ornello R, Frattale I, et al. Efficacy and safety of greater occipital nerve block for the treatment of cervicogenic headache: a systematic review. *Expert Rev Neurother.* 2021;21(5):591–597.
123. Jung FC, Mathew S, Littmann AE, Macdonald CW. Clinical decision making in the management of patients with cervicogenic dizziness: a case series. *J Orthop Sports Phys Ther.* 2017;47(11):874–884.
124. Carrasco-Uribarren A, Rodríguez-Sanz J, Malo-Urriés M, et al. Short-term effects of an upper cervical spine traction-manipulation program in patients with cervicogenic dizziness: a case series study. *J Back Musculoskelet Rehabil.* 2020;33(6):961–967.
125. Reid SA, Rivett DA, Katekar MG, Callister R. Comparison of Mulligan sustained natural apophyseal glides and Maitland mobilizations for treatment of cervicogenic dizziness: a randomized controlled trial. *Phys Ther.* 2014;94(4):466–476.
126. Escaloni J, Butts R, Dunning J. The use of dry needling as a diagnostic tool and clinical treatment for cervicogenic dizziness: a narrative review & case series. *J Bodyw Mov Ther.* 2018;22(4):947–955.
127. Wilde VE, Ford JJ, McMeeken JM. Indicators of lumbar zygapophyseal joint pain: survey of an expert panel with the Delphi technique. *Phys Ther.* 2007;87(10):1348–1361.
128. Ford JJ, Slater SL, Richards MC, et al. Individualised manual therapy plus guideline-based advice vs advice alone for people with clinical features of lumbar zygapophyseal joint pain: a randomised controlled trial. *Physiotherapy.* 2019;105(1):53–64.
129. Nalawade VC. Rehabilitation in congenital muscular torticollis operated with Z-plasty: a case report. *Ind J Occup Ther.* 2020;52(2):56–60.
130. Cheng JC, Tang SP, Chen TM, Wong MW, Wong EM. The clinical presentation and outcome of treatment of congenital muscular torticollis in infants—a study of 1,086 cases. *J Pediatr Surg.* 2000;35(7):1091–1096.
131. Kaplan SL, Coulter C, Sargent B. Physical therapy management of congenital muscular torticollis: a 2018 evidence-based clinical practice guideline from the APTA Academy of Pediatric Physical Therapy. *Pediatr Phys Ther.* 2018;30(4):240–290.
132. Ellwood J, Draper-Rodi J, Carnes D. The effectiveness and safety of conservative interventions for positional plagiocephaly and congenital muscular torticollis: a synthesis of systematic reviews and guidance. *Chiropr Man Therap.* 2020;28(1):1–11.
133. Oledzka M, Suhr M. Postsurgical physical therapy management of congenital muscular torticollis. *Pediatr Phys Ther.* 2017;29(2):159–165.
134. McCarthy J, Davis AMY. Diagnosis and management of vertebral compression fractures. *Am Fam Physician.* 2016;94(1):44–50.
135. Dewar C. Diagnosis and treatment of vertebral compression fractures. *Radiol Technol.* 2015;86(3):301–323.
136. Alexandru D, So W. Evaluation and management of vertebral compression fractures. *Perm J.* 2012;16(4):46–51.
137. Takayuki T. Epidemiology of fragility fractures and fall prevention in the elderly: a systematic review of the literature. *Curr Orthop Pract.* 2017;286:580–585.
138. Piirtola M, Vahlberg T, Isoaho R, Aarnio P, Kivelä S. Predictors of fractures among the aged: a population-based study with 12-year follow-up in a Finnish municipality. *Aging Clin Exp Res.* 2008;20(3):242–252.
139. Bravo AE, Brasuell JE, Favre AW, Koenig BM, Khan AA, Beall DP. Treating vertebral compression fractures: establishing the appropriate diagnosis, preoperative considerations, treatment techniques, postoperative follow-up and general guidelines for the treatment of patients with symptomatic vertebral compression fractures. *Tech Vasc Interv Radiol.* 2020;23(4):100701.
140. Ameis A, Randhawa K, Yu H, et al. The Global Spine Care Initiative: a review of reviews and recommendations for the non-invasive management of acute osteoporotic vertebral compression fracture pain in low-and middle-income communities. *Eur Spine J.* 2018;27:861–869.

141. Ioannidis G, Papaioannou A, Hopman WM, et al. Relation between fractures and mortality: results from the Canadian Multicentre Osteoporosis Study. *CMAJ*. 2009;181(5):265–271.
142. Cauley JA, Thompson DE, Ensrud KC, Scott JC, Black D. Risk of mortality following clinical fractures. *Osteoporos Int*. 2000;11(7):556–561.
143. Fraser J. Osteoporosis: people with risk factors should undergo fracture-risk assessment. *Guidel Pract*. 2015;18(7):30–39.
144. Yeoum SG, Lee JH. Usefulness of estimated height loss for detection of osteoporosis in women. *J Korean Acad Nurs*. 2011;41(6):758–767.
145. Bhatt P, Greenberg E, Suh B. Differential diagnosis of a pathologic spine fracture. *J Orthop Sports Phys Ther*. 2018;48(7):595.
146. Slavici A, Rauschmann M, Fleege C. Conservative management of osteoporotic vertebral fractures: an update. *Eur J Trauma Emerg Surg*. 2017;43(1):19–26.
147. Svensson H, Olsson L, Hansson T, Karlsson J, Hansson-Olofsson E. The effects of person-centered or other supportive interventions in older women with osteoporotic vertebral compression fractures—a systematic review of the literature. *Osteoporos Int*. 2017;28(9):2521–2540.
148. Giangregorio LM, Gibbs JC, Templeton JA, et al. Build better bones with exercise (B3E pilot trial): results of a feasibility study of a multicenter randomized controlled trial of 12 months of home exercise in older women with vertebral fracture. *Osteoporos Int*. 2018;29(11):2545–2556.
149. Rzewuska M, Ferreira M, McLachlan AJ, Machado GC, Maher CG. The efficacy of conservative treatment of osteoporotic compression fractures on acute pain relief: a systematic review with meta-analysis. *Eur Spine J*. 2015;24(4):702–714.
150. Kaiming L, Hao G, Rui X, et al. Clinical efficacy of zoledronic acid combined with percutaneous kyphoplasty in the prevention and treatment of osteoporotic vertebral compression fracture: a systematic review and meta-analysis. *Medicine (Baltimore)*. 2021;100(13):e25215.
151. Shah LM, Jennings JW, Kirsch CFE, et al. ACR appropriateness criteria management of vertebral compression fractures. *J Am Coll Radiol*. 2018;15(11):S347–S364.
152. Li Z, Liu T, Yin P, et al. The therapeutic effects of percutaneous kyphoplasty on osteoporotic vertebral compression fractures with or without intravertebral cleft. *Int Orthop*. 2019;43(2):359–365.
153. Parreira PCS, Maher CG, Megale RZ, March L, Ferreira ML. An overview of clinical guidelines for the management of vertebral compression fracture: a systematic review. *Spine J*. 2017;17(12):1932–1938.
154. Sayari AJ, Yuzeng L, Cohen JR, et al. Trends in vertebroplasty and kyphoplasty after thoracolumbar osteoporotic fracture: a large database study from 2005 to 2012. *J Orthop*. 2015;12(4):S217–S222.
155. Coary R, Skerritt C, Carey A, Rudd S, Shipway D. New horizons in rib fracture management in the older adult. *Age Ageing*. 2020;49(2):161–167.
156. Peek J, Beks RB, Hietbrink F, et al. Complications and outcome after rib fracture fixation: a systematic review. *J Trauma Acute Care Surg*. 2020;89(2):411–418.
157. Yu K-C, Wong C-S, Kao Y, et al. Does surgery reduce the risk of complications among patients with multiple rib fractures? A meta-analysis. *Clin Orthop Relat Res*. 2019;477(1):193–205.
158. Wijffels MME, Prins JTH, Perpetua Alvino EJ, Van Lieshout EMM. Operative versus nonoperative treatment of multiple simple rib fractures: a systematic review and meta-analysis. *Injury*. 2020;51(11):2368–2378.
159. Claydon J, Maniatopoulos G, Robinson L, Fearon P. Challenges experienced during rehabilitation after traumatic multiple rib fractures: a qualitative study. *Disabil Rehabil*. 2018;40(23):2780–2789.
160. Wang H, Feng C, Liu H, et al. Epidemiologic features of traumatic fractures in children and adolescents: a 9-year retrospective study. *BioMed Res Int*. 2019;2019:1–8.
161. Kriss S, Thompson A, Bertocci G, Currie M, Martich V. Characteristics of rib fractures in young abused children. *Pediatr Radiol*. 2020;50(5):726–733.
162. Marcussen B, Negaard M, Hosey RG, Smoot MK. A case series and literature review: isolated traumatic first rib fracture in athletes. *Clin J Sport Med*. 2020;30(3):257–266.
163. Alent J, Narducci DM, Moran B, Coris E. Sternal injuries in sport: a review of the literature. *Sports Med*. 2018;48(12):2715–2724.
164. Baker J, Demertzis J, Baker JC, Demertzis JL. Manubrial stress fractures diagnosed on MRI: report of two cases and review of the literature. *Skeletal Radiol*. 2016;45(6):833–837.
165. Płaszewska M, Kotwicki T, Chwała W, Terech J, Cieśliński I. Study protocol and overview of the literature on long-term health and quality of life outcomes in patients treated in adolescence for scoliosis with therapeutic exercises. *J Back Musculoskelet Rehabil*. 2015;28(3):453–462.
166. Carroll A, Dreger M, O'Rourke P, Manal T. Adolescent spine (28.3.5). In: *The Lumbopelvic Complex: Advances in Evaluation and Treatment*. Academy of Orthopaedic Physical Therapy; 2018:1–40.
167. Fan Y, Ren Q, To MKT, Cheung JPY. Effectiveness of scoliosis-specific exercises for alleviating adolescent idiopathic scoliosis: a systematic review. *BMC Musculoskelet Disord*. 2020;21(1):1–13.
168. Burger M, Coetzee W, du Plessis LZ, et al. The effectiveness of Schroth exercises in adolescents with idiopathic scoliosis: a systematic review and meta-analysis. *S Afr J Physiother*. 2019;75(1):1–9.
169. Kim W, Porrino JA, Hood KA, Chadaz TS, Klauser AS, Taljanovic MS. Clinical evaluation, imaging, and management of adolescent idiopathic and adult degenerative scoliosis. *Curr Probl Diagn Radiol*. 2019;48(4):402–414.
170. Liu D, Yang Y, Yu X, et al. Effects of specific exercise therapy on adolescent patients with idiopathic scoliosis: a prospective controlled cohort study. *Spine*. 2020;45(15):1039–1046.
171. Zapata KA, Sucato DJ, Jo C-H. Physical therapy scoliosis-specific exercises may reduce curve progression in mild adolescent idiopathic scoliosis curves. *Pediatr Phys Ther*. 2019;31(3):280–285.
172. Sapkas G, Efstathopoulos NE, Papadakis M. Undiagnosed osteoid osteoma of the spine presenting as painful scoliosis from adolescence to adulthood: a case report. *Scoliosis*. 2009;4(1):9.
173. Negrini S, Minozzi S, Bettany-Saltikov J, et al. Braces for idiopathic scoliosis in adolescents. *Cochrane Database Syst Rev*. 2015(6):CD006850.
174. Chengfei G, Yu Z, Chunjiang F, Yan Y, Chengqi H, Mansang W. Could the clinical effectiveness be improved under the integration of orthotic intervention and scoliosis-specific exercise in managing adolescent idiopathic scoliosis? A randomized controlled trial study. *Am J Phys Med Rehabil*. 2019;98(8):642–648.
175. Yagci G, Yakut Y. Core stabilization exercises versus scoliosis-specific exercises in moderate idiopathic scoliosis treatment. *Prosthet Orthot Int*. 2019;43(3):301–308.

176. Thompson JY, Williamson EM, Williams MA, Heine PJ, Lamb SE. Effectiveness of scoliosis-specific exercises for adolescent idiopathic scoliosis compared with other non-surgical interventions: a systematic review and meta-analysis. *Physiotherapy.* 2019;105(2):214–234.
177. Marti CL, Glassman SD, Knott PT, Carreon LY, Hresko MT. Scoliosis Research Society members attitudes towards physical therapy and physiotherapeutic scoliosis specific exercises for adolescent idiopathic scoliosis. *Scoliosis.* 2015;10(1):1–7.
178. Schreiber S, Parent EC, Hill DL, Hedden DM, Moreau MJ, Southon SC. Schroth physiotherapeutic scoliosis-specific exercises for adolescent idiopathic scoliosis: how many patients require treatment to prevent one deterioration?—Results from a randomized controlled trial—"SOSORT 2017 Award Winner." *Scoliosis Spinal Disord.* 2017;12:1–8.
179. Negrini A, Negrini MG, Donzelli S, Romano M, Zaina F, Negrini S. Scoliosis-Specific exercises can reduce the progression of severe curves in adult idiopathic scoliosis: a long-term cohort study. *Scoliosis.* 2015;10(1):1–7.
180. Wong E, Altaf F, Oh LJ, Gray RJ. Adult degenerative lumbar scoliosis. *Orthopedics.* 2017;40(6):e930–e939.
181. Le Huec J, Cogniet A, Mazas S, Faundez A. Lumbar scoliosis associated with spinal stenosis in idiopathic and degenerative cases. *Eur J Orthop Surg Trauma.* 2016;26(7):705–712.
182. Diebo BG, Shah NV, Boachie-Adjei O, et al. Adult spinal deformity. *Lancet.* 2019;394(10193):160–172.
183. Peggy Guey-Chi C, Daubs MD, Berven S, et al. Surgery for degenerative lumbar scoliosis: the development of appropriateness criteria. *Spine (Phila Pa 1976).* 2016;41(10):910–918.
184. Peek J, Vos CG, Ünlü Ç, van de Pavoordt H, van den Akker PJ, de Vries JPM. Outcome of surgical treatment for thoracic outlet syndrome: systematic review and meta-analysis. *Ann Vasc Surg.* 2017;40:303–326.
185. Kuhn JE, Lebus VG, Bible JE. Thoracic outlet syndrome. *J Am Acad Orthop Surg.* 2015;23(4):222–232.
186. Ohman JW, Thompson RW. Thoracic outlet syndrome in the overhead athlete: diagnosis and treatment recommendations. *Curr Rev Musculoskelet Med.* 2020;13(4):457–471.
187. Collins E, Orpin M. Physical therapy management of neurogenic thoracic outlet syndrome. *Thorac Surg Clin.* 2021;31(1):61–69.
188. Constans J, Salmi LR, Sevestre-Pietri MA, et al. A clinical prediction score for upper extremity deep venous thrombosis. *Thromb Haemost.* 2008;99(1):202–207.
189. Yin ZG, Gong KT, Zhang JB. Outcomes of surgical management of neurogenic thoracic outlet syndrome: a systematic review and Bayesian perspective. *J Hand Surg Am.* 2019;44(5):416.e411–416.e417.
190. Wuollet A, Shahrokhn K, Hata J, Perret-Karmi D. Thoracic radiculopathy. *Crit Rev Phys Rehabil Med.* 2012;24(3):147–157.
191. Kim Y, Kim S, Oh K, Kim Y. Thoracic radiculopathy as initial symptoms of hepatocellular carcinoma: a case report. *Medicine (Baltimore).* 2018;97(27):e11635–e11635.
192. Proulx AM, Zryd TW. Costochondritis: diagnosis and treatment. *Am Fam Physician.* 2009;80(6):617–620.
193. McConaghy JR, Oza RS. Outpatient diagnosis of acute chest pain in adults. *Am Acad Fam Physician.* 2013;87(3):177–182.
194. Zaruba RA, Wilson E. Impairment based examination and treatment of costochondritis: a case series. *Int J Sports Phys Ther.* 2017;12(3):458–467.
195. Gijsbers E, Knaap SFC. Clinical presentation and chiropractic treatment of Tietze syndrome: a 34-year-old female with left-sided chest pain. *J Chiropr Med.* 2011;10(1):60–63.
196. Gress K, Charipova K, Kassem H, et al. A comprehensive review of slipping rib syndrome: treatment and management. *Psychopharmacol Bull.* 2020;50(4 Suppl 1):189–196.
197. Fares MY, Dimassi Z, Baydoun H, Musharrafieh U. Slipping rib syndrome: solving the mystery of the shooting pain. *Am J Med Sci.* 2019;357(2):168–173.
198. Bonasso PC, Petrus SN, Smith SD, Jackson RJ. Sternocostal slipping rib syndrome. *Pediatr Surg Int.* 2018;34(3):331–333.
199. Turcios NL. Slipping rib syndrome: an elusive diagnosis. *Paediatr Respir Rev.* 2017;22:44–46.
200. Mazzella A, Fournel L, Bobbio A, et al. Costal cartilage resection for the treatment of slipping rib syndrome (Cyriax syndrome) in adults. *J Thorac Dis.* 2020;12(1):10–16.
201. McMahon LE. Slipping rib syndrome: a review of evaluation, diagnosis and treatment. *Semin Pediatr Surg.* 2018;27(3):183–188.

18 | Temporomandibular Joint

Betsy Myers and June Hanks

CHAPTER OBJECTIVES
After reading this chapter, you will be able to:
1. Describe the anatomy of the joints forming the temporomandibular joint to include osteologic ligamentous, capsular, and muscular features.
2. Describe the biomechanics of the articulations of the temporomandibular joint.
3. Tailor the basic history to a patient with temporomandibular joint pathology.
4. Describe the components of the physical examination for a patient with temporomandibular joint pathology.
5. Describe the pathology, history, key examination findings, rehabilitation focus, and expected outcomes of common temporomandibular joint pathologies.
6. Hypothesize differential diagnoses of temporomandibular joint symptoms.
7. Organize the physical examination of a patient with temporomandibular joint pathology to maximize efficiency.

FUNCTIONAL ANATOMY

The temporomandibular joint (TMJ) is a modified hinge joint that permits the movements of the mandible (jaw) in the mandibular fossa of the temporal bone. The TMJ and surrounding structures (together called the *stomatognathic system*) include:

- Bones of the skull, mandible, maxilla, hyoid, clavicle, and sternum
- Dentoalveolar joints
- Teeth
- Muscles and soft tissues of the head and neck and the muscles of the cheeks, lips, and tongue
- Vascular, lymphatic, and nerve supply systems

The system works almost continuously, functioning during respiration, speech, chewing, and swallowing. Posture of the head and neck is influenced by and affects the shoulder girdle, clavicle, sternum, and scapulae. Because the center of gravity of the head lies in front of the occipital condyles, it follows that a balanced force is required to maintain an appropriate position at atlanto-occipital joint. The balance is achieved by a normal relationship and movement between the anterior and posterior neck muscles, the mandible and cranium, and the occlusion of the teeth.[1] A faulty curvature of the cervical spine is often responsible for pain, and dysfunction in the head, neck, and upper quarter[2,3] in any component of the system impacts other components. Evaluation and treatment may require an interprofessional team of physicians, dentists, therapists, and surgeons.

Osteology

Articulation between the mandible and temporal bone of the skull forms the TMJ. In fact, the bones of the TMJ do not actually articulate directly with one another, but rather with the articular disc between the mandibular fossa of the temporal bone and the condyles of the mandible. The dentoalveolar joints of the lower teeth are the components of the mandible. The upper teeth are the components of the maxilla. The maxilla articulates with the palatine bones, providing attachment for muscles of mastication, along with the hyoid, sphenoid, and zygomatic bones. For an overview of skull and mandible osteology, refer to Figure 18-1.

Mandible The mandible is the largest and strongest bone of the face,[4] serving the critical function of articulating with the two temporal bones of the skull and accommodating the lower teeth. The mandible is composed of the body and the right and left rami. The rami are oriented vertically at a near-right angle with the body. The body of the external surface of the mandible has a centrally located mental protuberance. The mental foramen, for a passage of the mental artery and nerve, is located between the mental protuberance and the mandibular angle (Fig. 18-1B). The external mandibular surface provides attachment sites for muscles of the face and neck. The internal surface of the mandible is concave side to side. The internal mandible has attachment sites for the mylohyoid, digastric, and medial pterygoid muscles (Fig. 18-2).

The superior (alveolar) border is wider posteriorly than anteriorly and consists of dentoalveolar cavities (holes) for the teeth. Most adults have 32 teeth: 8 incisors (anterior teeth on upper and lower jaw, 4 on each), 4 canine (pointed teeth just lateral to the incisors), 8 premolars (between canines and molars), and 12 molars (3 in each quadrant) (Fig. 18-3). Numbering begins at the back upper right and ends at

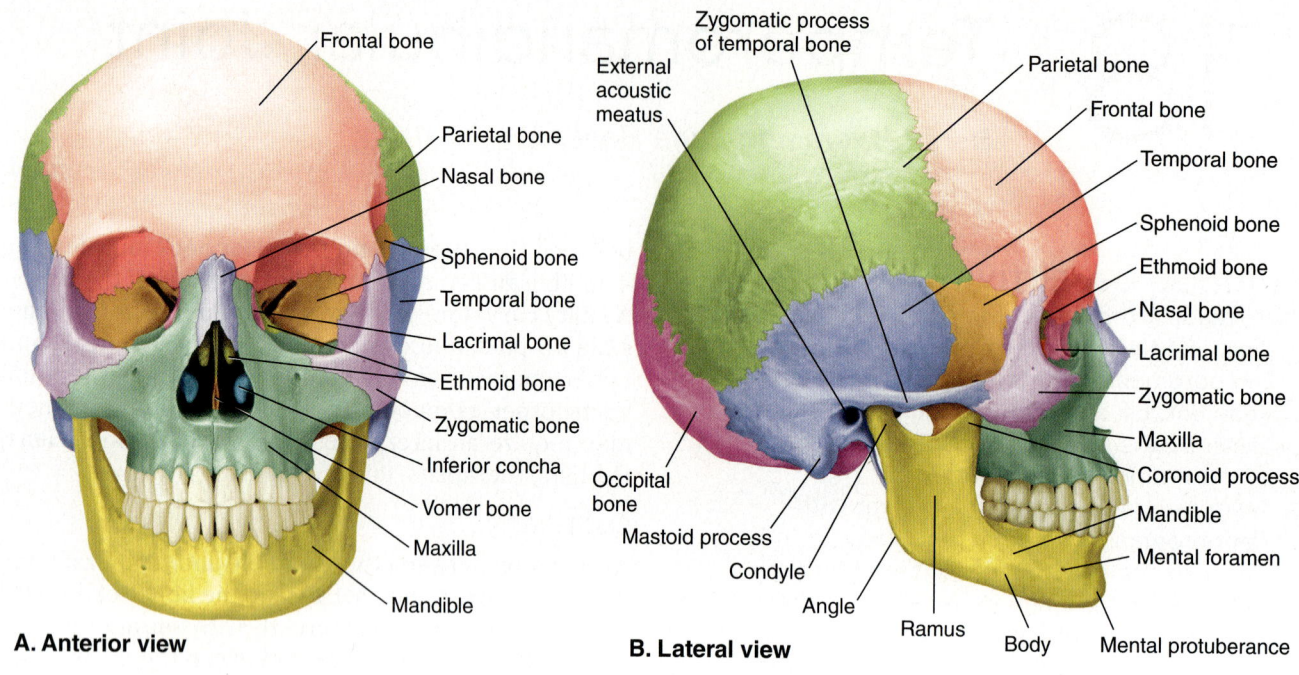

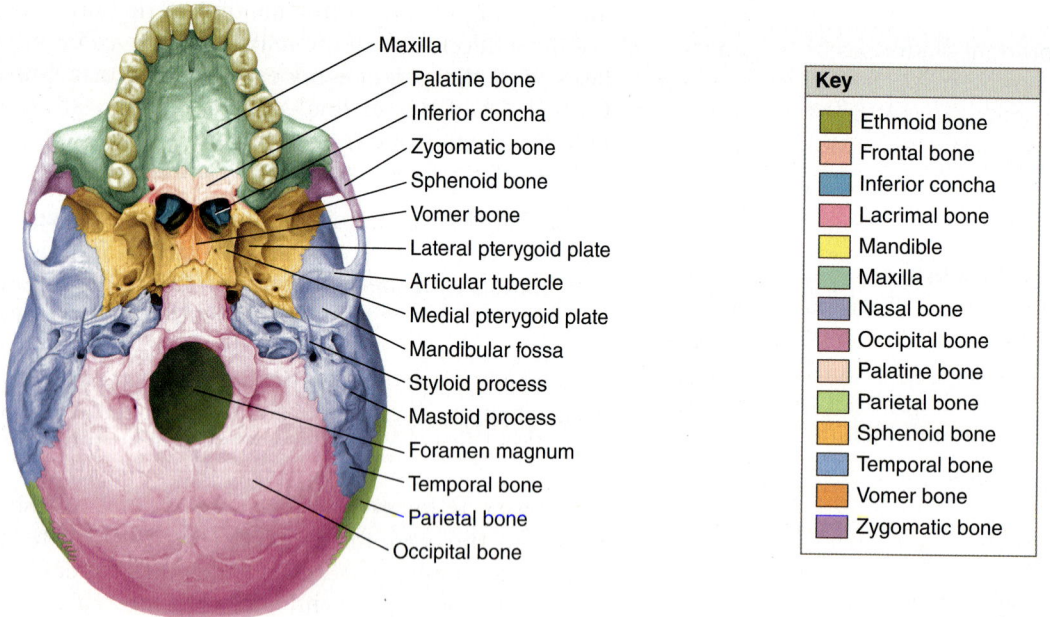

FIGURE 18-1 Skull and mandible. **A.** Anterior view. **B.** Lateral view. **C.** Inferior view. (Gest TR. *Lippincott Atlas of Anatomy.* 2nd ed. Wolters Kluwer; 2020: Plate 7-06.)

the back lower right. Normally, the upper (maxillary) teeth extend over the lower (mandibular) teeth about 1 to 2 mm.[5] Malalignments of the teeth are referred to as *malocclusions*. An overbite describes a vertical malalignment between the upper and lower teeth in which the upper front teeth excessively overlap the bottom front teeth when the back teeth are closed. In underbite, the lower teeth vertically align anterior to the upper teeth. Overjet (sometimes called *buck teeth*) describes horizontal malalignment in which the upper

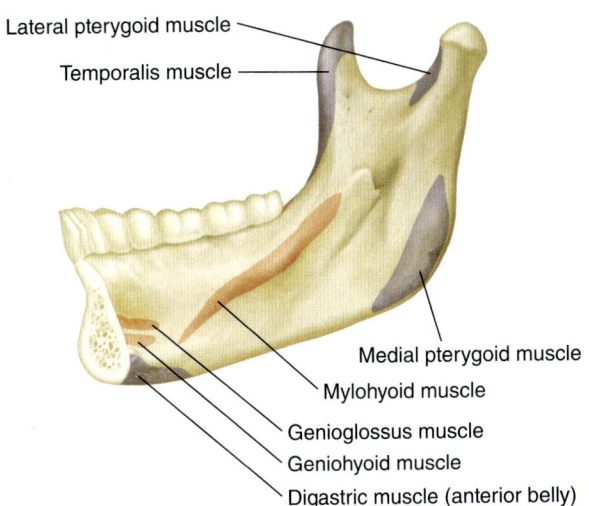

FIGURE 18-2 Mandible (cut), medial view. (Gest TR. *Lippincott Atlas of Anatomy.* 2nd ed. Wolters Kluwer; 2020: Plate 7-04.)

front teeth protrude outward toward the horizontal. Figure 18-4 depicts these malalignments.

The ramus is quadrilateral in shape and has two processes: the coronoid process and the condylar process (see Fig. 18-1B). The triangularly shaped coronoid process has an anterior convex border and posterior concave border and serves as an attachment site for the temporalis and masseter muscles. The more posteriorly located condylar process consists of the condyle and neck. The condyle is convex in shape and articulates with the articular disc. The lateral pterygoid inserts onto a depression on the anterior portion of the neck of the condyle.

Temporal Bone The temporal bone (see Fig. 18-1) forms the large, flat side and base of the skull. The outer temporal surface is smooth and slightly convex and, along with the sphenoid bone, provides attachment for the temporalis muscle. The posterior and inferior part of the temporal bone is the mastoid, which bears the prominent cone-shaped mastoid process. Anterior to the mastoid process is the long, thin styloid process. The external acoustic meatus, located just superior to the mastoid process, leads to the middle and inner ear. The zygomatic process of the temporal bone forms the posterior aspect of the zygomatic arch. Just inferior to this is the deeply concave mandibular fossa, which is divided into an anterior articular and posterior nonarticular area (Fig. 18-5). The articular portion is deeply concave. The slightly convex articular eminence limits anterior movement of the mandibular condyles. The postglenoid tubercle separates the posterior articular portion laterally from the tympanic plate.[4]

Sphenoid Bone The sphenoid bone, located anterior to and articulating with the temporal bone, is shaped like a bat or wasp with open wings. The sphenoid contributes to the hard palate of the mouth, and the inferior surface is a component of the anterior base of the skull, providing attachment for the pterygoid muscles on the medial and lateral pterygoid plates (see Fig. 18-1C). The medial pterygoid plate is located toward the midline of the skull base and ends anteriorly as the hamulus, a component of the hard palate. The pterygomandibular raphe, a fibrous band covered by membranous tissue, passes from the hamulus to the mandible and can be seen and palpated intraorally posterior and medial to the third molar. The lateral pterygoid plate provides attachment for the both the medial and lateral pterygoid muscles.

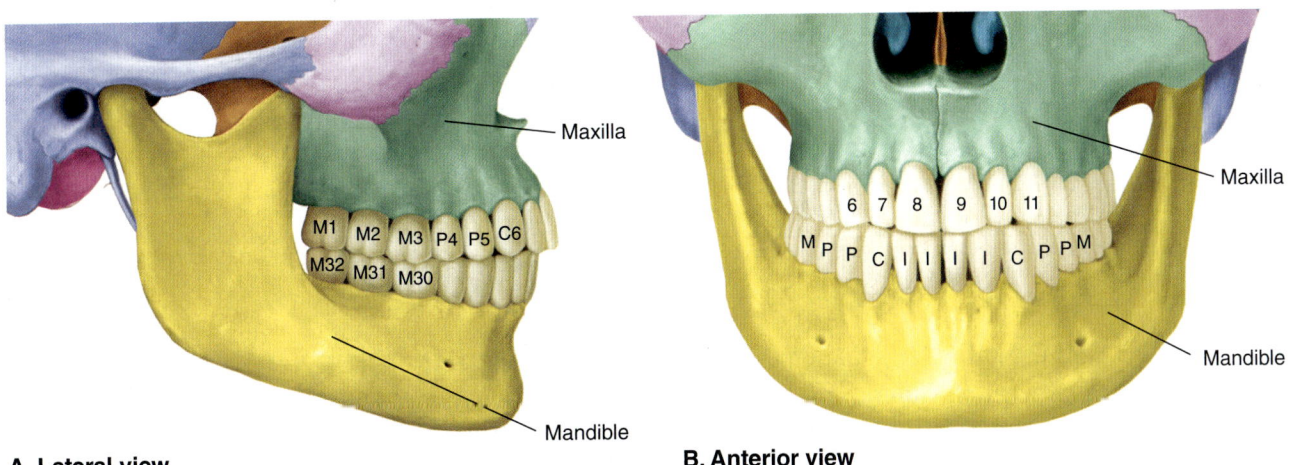

FIGURE 18-3 Teeth of the upper and lower jaw. **A.** Lateral view. **B.** Anterior view (molars not shown). Teeth are numbered for identification. *C*, canine; *I*, incisor; *M*, molar; *P*, premolar. (Gest TR. *Lippincott Atlas of Anatomy.* 2nd ed. Wolters Kluwer; 2020: Plate 7-06.)

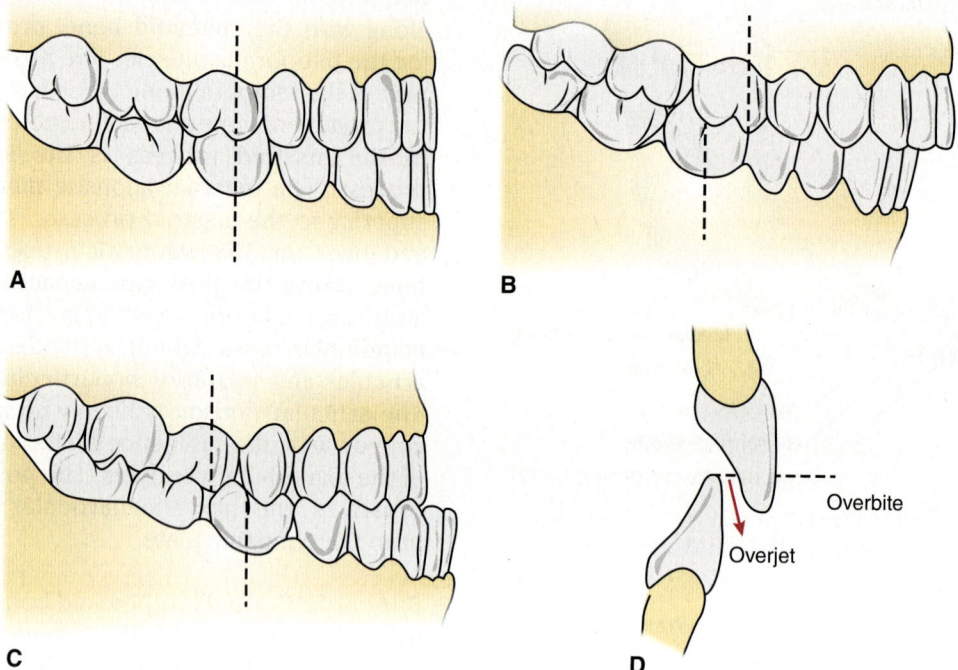

FIGURE 18-4 Malalignments of the teeth. **A.** Normal alignment. **B.** Overbite. **C.** Underbite. (A–C: Adapted from Jaffe RA. *Anesthesiologist's Manual of Surgical Procedures*. 5th ed. Wolters Kluwer Health; 2014: Figure 11.3-6.) **D.** Overbite and overjet. (Adapted from Johnson JT, Rosen CA. *Bailey's Head and Neck Surgery: Otolaryngology*. Vol 2. 5th ed. Lippincott Williams & Wilkins; 2014: Figure 135.9D.)

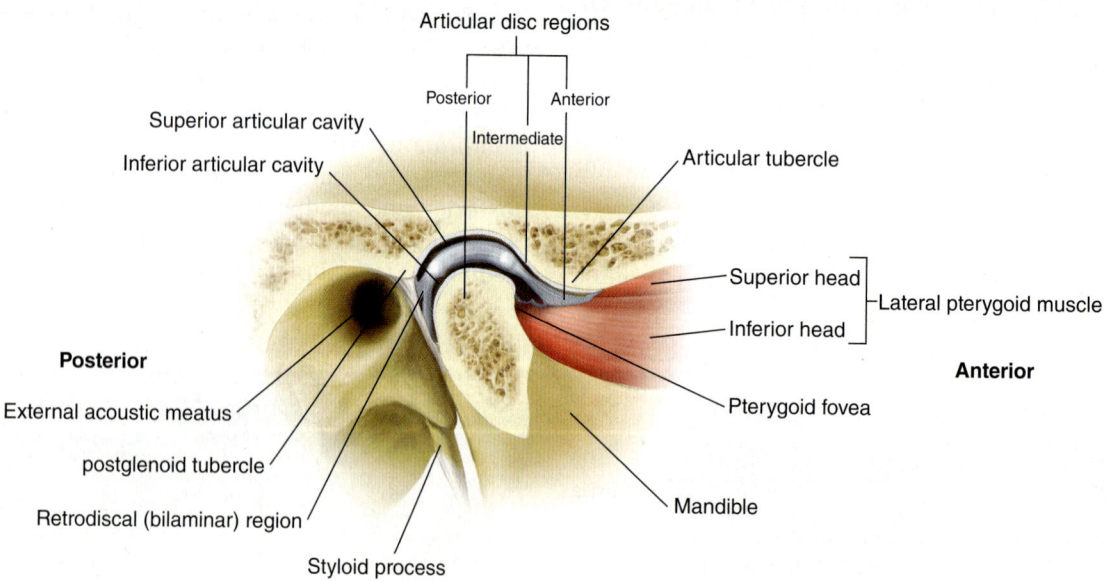

FIGURE 18.5 Temporomandibular joint, lateral view. (Gest TR. *Lippincott Atlas of Anatomy*. 2nd ed. Wolters Kluwer; 2020: Plate 7-41B.)

Hyoid Bone The U-shaped hyoid bone is located in the midline of neck between the inferior mandible and the thyroid cartilage. The hyoid does not articulate with any other bone and provides attachment for the suprahyoid and infrahyoid muscles. In the resting position, the hyoid lies just anterior to the third cervical vertebra.

JOINT STRUCTURE AND LIGAMENTS

The opposing bony surfaces of the TMJ are covered by articular cartilage. The articular surfaces are surrounded by the joint capsule that attaches superiorly to the mandibular fossa and inferiorly to the mandibular condyle. The capsule is thin and loose, particularly anteriorly in the superior cavity of the joint, but is taut posteriorly.

The articular disc (Fig. 18-5) is a biconcave fibrocartilaginous structure composed of three regions (anterior, intermediate, and posterior), separating the joint into a superior and inferior cavity.[1] The articular disc attaches:

- posteriorly to thick connective tissue with extensive neural and vascular supply
- anteriorly to the joint capsule and lateral pterygoid muscle
- medially and laterally to the sides (poles) of the condyles

With mandibular movements of protrusion and retrusion, sliding occurs between the temporal bone and the articular disc in the superior cavity. With mandibular depression and elevation, rotation and pivoting occur in the inferior cavity.[6]

The posterior attachment of the articular disc consists of loose connective tissue separated by a thin layer, forming the bilaminar retrodiscal pad located in the retrodiscal (bilaminar) region.[7] The superior lamina attaches to the postglenoid process, considered the true posterior aspect of the TMJ. The inferior lamina curves down posterior to the condyle and fuses with the capsule and condylar neck.[1] The retrodiscal pad creates a counterforce to the anterior pull of the lateral pterygoid muscle on the articular disc, for example, during yawning. The retrodiscal tissue is folded and compressed when the jaw is closed. When the jaw is opened, the condyle moves down and anteriorly, and the volume of the retrodiscal (bilaminar) region increases.[1] The rich blood and nerve supply in this retrodiscal (bilaminar) region renders the area vulnerable to inflammation with repeated or prolonged compressive forces, such as can occur with grinding and clenching of the teeth. Abnormalities in any of the structures that stabilize the articular disc can lead to disc degeneration, tearing, or perforation.[8–10]

Thickenings of the joint capsule form the lateral ligament of the TMJ, which reinforces the lateral aspect of the joint (Fig. 18-6). The joint capsule, lateral ligament, and postglenoid tubercle prevent posterior dislocation. The extrinsic ligaments are the stylomandibular ligament and sphenomandibular ligament. The stylomandibular ligament attaches to the styloid process of the temporal bone to the angle of the mandible and renders little support to the TMJ. The sphenomandibular ligament passes from the spine of the sphenoid bone to the lingula of the mandible and is a passive "swinging hinge" that bears the weight of the lower jaw, permitting protrusion, retrusion, elevation, and depression.

Movements of the Temporomandibular Joint

In the normal rest position, the mandible is maintained in position by structures and forces that support the TMJ. Resting tone in the muscles moving the TMJ is required to keep the mouth closed against gravitational forces. Movements of the TMJ are complex, occurring in multiple planes. Primary motions are mandible elevation, depression, protrusion, retrusion, and lateral shift to right and left (Fig. 18-7). The motions of chewing and grinding are combination of these motions. Depression and elevation occurs about a horizontal axis, whereas lateral deviation from side to side occurs about an anteroposterior axis. Rotation (pivoting) occurs in the lower joint cavity about the vertical axis. The movement of translation occurs in the superior joint cavity.

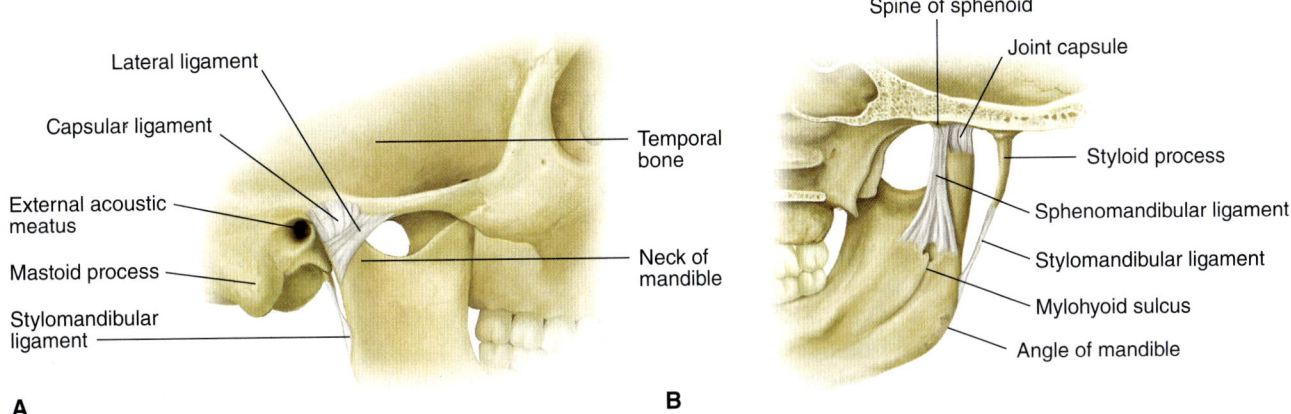

FIGURE 18-6 Joint capsule and ligaments of the temporomandibular joint. **A.** Mandible, lateral view. Lateral ligament, fibrous capsule, and stylomandibular ligament. **B.** Mandible, medial view. Sphenomandibular ligament and stylomandibular ligament. (Pansky B, Gest TR. *Lippincott's Concise Illustrated Anatomy: Head & Neck*. Vol 3. Lippincott Williams & Wilkins; 2014: Figure 2.14A & B.)

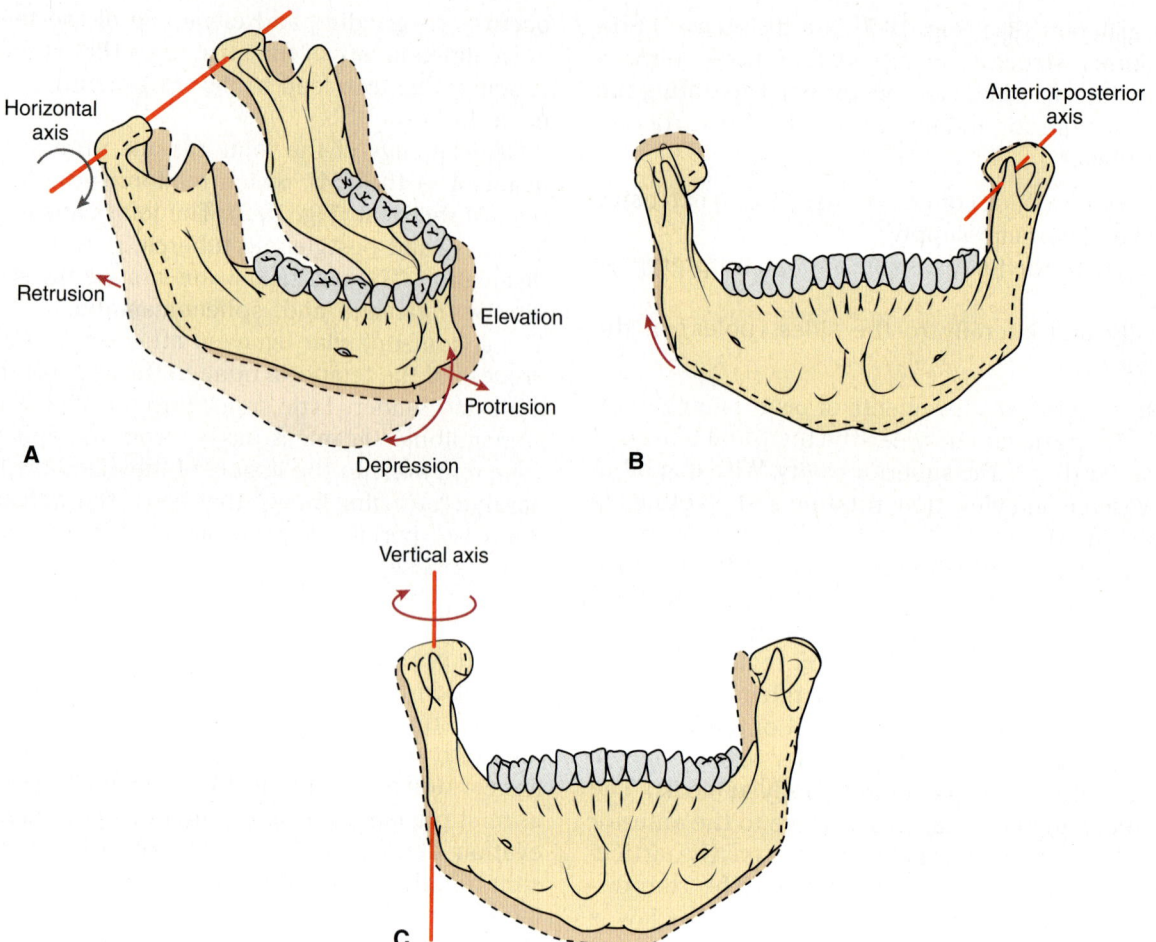

FIGURE 18-7 Movements and axes of the temporomandibular joint. **A.** Depression and elevation. **B.** Lateral deviation. **C.** Rotation (pivoting). (Adapted from Oatis, CA. *Kinesiology: The Mechanics and Pathomechanics of Human Movement.* 3rd ed. Wolters Kluwer; 2017: Figure 23.10.)

MUSCLES

The muscles acting on the mandible and TMJ are described in Table 18-1. The four primary muscles of mastication are the temporalis, masseter, lateral pterygoid, and medial pterygoid (Figs. 18-8 and 18-9). The muscles provide the majority of stabilization to the TMJ, with the ligaments playing a primary role only at end-ranges of motion. The muscles are obliquely attached relative to the TMJ joint axes such that unilateral contraction produces varied combinations of motions. For example, protrusion and deviation of the mandible to the right is produced by contraction of the right masseter muscle and left pterygoid muscles. To protrude the mandible without deviation, the right and left lateral pterygoids on each side must contract together. Similarly, the temporalis muscle acting bilaterally will elevate the mandible. Because the proximal attachment of the temporalis on the skull is lateral to the distal attachment to the mandible, unilateral contraction of the temporalis produces lateral deviation to the same side. In bilateral contraction, the angle of pull of the right and left masseter is suited for mandible elevation and protrusion, whereas the temporalis produces elevation and retrusion.[11]

The deeper mastication muscles, the lateral and medial pterygoids, are more difficult to study, leading to debate over attachments, innervation, and actions. The pterygoids are multipennate, with differing muscle fiber alignment, length, and cross-sectional area. The lateral pterygoid fibers oriented primarily in a horizontal direction and are longer in length than the medial pterygoid.[12] The lateral pterygoid has two parts, classically described as superior and inferior heads.[13,14] Some consider that the two heads have different nerve innervation patterns, with the superior head supplied by the buccal nerve and the inferior head by the mandibular trunk,[15] leading to the argument that the heads are functionally distinct.[16] Others have demonstrated two main parts with selective recruitment of various layers of the muscle during mandibular movement.[17] Others describe the lateral pterygoid as a system of fibers acting as one muscle[18] and a unique architectural arrangement dividing the muscle into oblique and horizontal planes with varying graded activity throughout

TABLE 18-1
MUSCLES ACTING ON MANDIBLE AND TMJ

Muscle	Nerve (Branches)	Proximal Attachment	Distal Attachment (to Mandible/TMJ)	Action on Mandible
Temporalis	CN V3 (deep temporal branch)	Temporal fossa	Tip and medial surface of coronoid process and anterior border of ramus	Elevation, retrusion (posterior horizontally oriented fibers)
Masseter	CN V3 (masseteric nerve)	Zygomatic bone (inferior border and medial surface of maxillary process) and zygomatic arch	Angle and lateral surface of ramus	Elevation, protrusion (limited contribution from superior fibers)
Lateral pterygoid	CN V3 (lateral pterygoid nerve)	Two heads: • Superior head: sphenoid (infratemporal surface and crest of greater wing) • Inferior head: lateral pterygoid plate (lateral surface)	• Superior head: anteromedial portion of joint capsule and articular disc • Inferior head: neck and condyloid process and pterygoid fovea (anterior fovea)	Protrusion (acting bilaterally) Contralateral lateral deviation (acting unilaterally)
Medial pterygoid	CN V3 (medial pterygoid nerve)	Two heads*: • Superficial head: maxillary tuberosity, posterior wall of the maxilla, and the pyramidal process of palatine bone • Deep head: lateral pterygoid plate (medial surface), medial pterygoid plates, pterygoid fossa	Ramus (medial surface of mandibular foramen)	Elevation and protrusion

Adapted from Moore KL, Dalley AF, Agur AMR. *Clinically Oriented Anatomy*. 8th ed. Wolters Kluwer; 2018: Table 8.11.
*El Haddioui A, Bravetti P, Gaudy J. Anatomical study of the arrangement and attachments of the human medial pterygoid muscle. *Surg Radiol Anat*. 2007;29(2):115-124; Bhojwani V, Ghabriel M, Mihailidis S, Townsend G. The human medial pterygoid muscle: attachments and distribution of muscle spindles. *Clin Anat*. 2017;30(8):1064-1071.

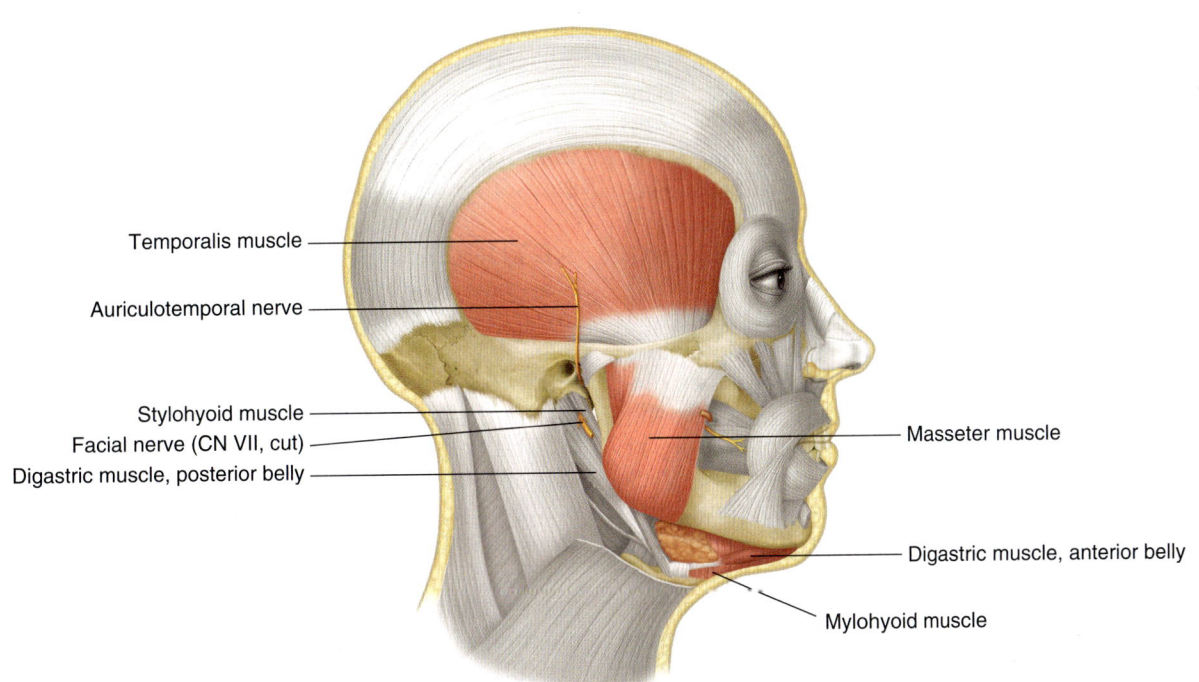

FIGURE 18.8 Muscles of mastication, superficial (temporalis and masseter), and infrahyoid muscles (digastric, mylohyoid, and stylohyoid). (Gest TR. *Lippincott Atlas of Anatomy*. 2nd ed. Wolters Kluwer; 2020: Plate 7-37.)

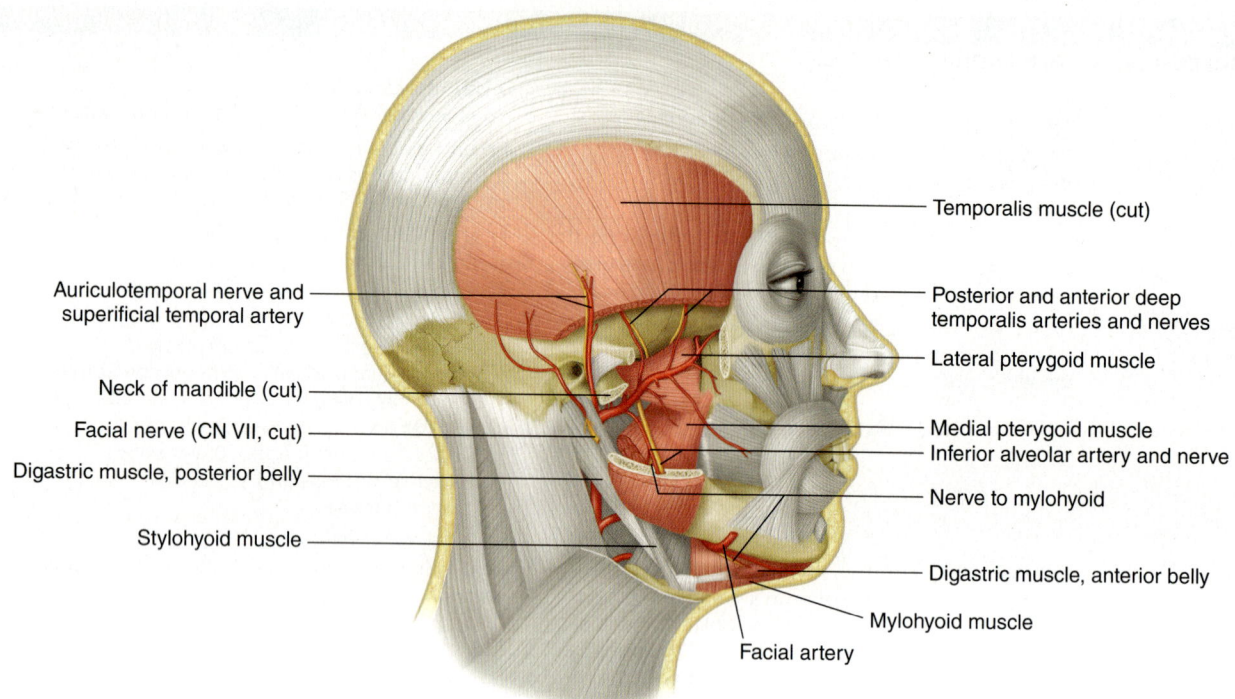

FIGURE 18.9 Muscles of mastication, deep. Portion of zygomatic arch removed with temporalis and masseter muscles cut to show lateral and medial pterygoid muscles. (Gest TR. *Lippincott Atlas of Anatomy*. 2nd ed. Wolters Kluwer; 2020: Plate 7-41A.)

the range dependent on the task demands.[17] The two lateral pterygoids must balance each other for the upper and lower teeth to properly align.

The medial pterygoid is a square-shaped muscle with superficial and deep parts. Compared to the lateral pterygoid, the medial pterygoid has shorter muscle fibers and a larger cross-sectional area, contributing to greater capacity to develop force.[12] The proximal attachments are variably described,[11,13,19–21] possibly because of significant variations among individuals. The proximal attachments of the more superficial component (head) include the tuberosity and posterior wall of the maxilla and the pyramidal process of palatine bone. The deeper component (head) attaches to the pterygoid fossa and both the medial and lateral pterygoid plates.[19,20,22] The heads join soon after formation into a single muscle that attaches distally to medial surface of the mandible, mirroring the attachment of the ipsilateral masseter to the lateral ramus of the mandible.[13] The medial pterygoid is composed of layers of aponeurotic sheets that contribute to the strength of the muscle.[19,20]

The muscles of mastication are innervated by various portions of anterior trunk of the mandibular nerve (V3), which is the third branch of the trigeminal nerve (CN V). The mandibular nerve (CN V3) branches from the main trunk in the middle cranial fossa, passes through the foramen ovale and into the infratemporal fossa where it divides to supply muscles, the skin of the cheek, anterior portion of the tongue, temporal area, and some of the suprahyoid muscles.

The suprahyoid and infrahyoid muscles act indirectly on the mandible by elevating and lowering the hyoid bone (Fig. 18-10). The suprahyoid muscles (digastric, stylohyoid, mylohyoid, and geniohyoid) depress the mandible against resistance when the infrahyoid muscles fix or depress the hyoid bone. The infrahyoid muscles are the omohyoid, sternohyoid, sternothyroid, and thyrohyoid.

ARTHROKINEMATICS

Movement of the mandible occurs in the upper and lower joint cavities. With opening of the mouth, the mandible lowers and the condyles rotate in the lower joint space, followed by translation of the articular disc in the upper joint space.[6]

The tone in the retractors and elevators of the mandibular heads holds the mandible in a retracted position when the mouth is closed and at rest, as shown in Figure 18-11A. During deep sleep, the tonic contraction relaxes and the mandible moves into a position of depression (open mouth). With wider opening of the mouth, the mandibular head and the articular disc move (translate) anteriorly with the head of the mandible positioned inferior to the articular tubercle (Fig. 18-11B). Opening and closing

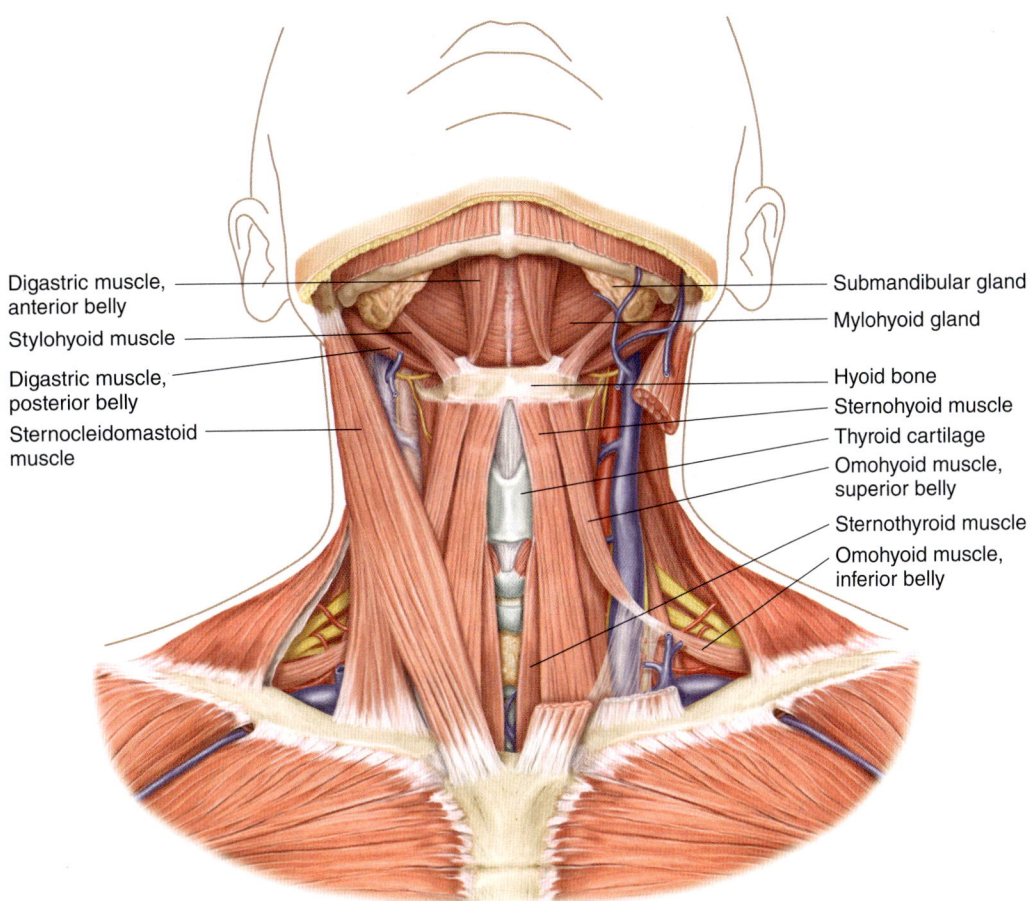

FIGURE 18.10 Suprahyoid and infrahyoid muscles. (Gest TR. *Lippincott Atlas of Anatomy*. 2nd ed. Wolters Kluwer; 2020: Plate 7-16.)

of the mandible should be in a straight line without deviation laterally and without popping or clicking at the TMJ during motion. Lowering of the mandible to a mouth-open position should allow an individual to place the width of three fingers between the teeth. Full depression of the mandible requires the mandibular heads and discs to translate and fully protrude. The mandible protrudes if translation occurs without concurrent depression of the mandible (Fig. 18.11C). With unilateral protrusion of the head and disc, the contralateral head rotates (pivots) on the inferior surface of the articular disc in the retracted position (Fig. 18-11D, E). This movement permits side-to-side chewing or grinding movements within a small range of motion (ROM).[13]

When yawning or taking a large bite, the heads of the mandible may dislocate anteriorly, passing anterior to the articular tubercles, with the mandible remaining locked and the person unable to close the mouth. Posterior dislocation is not common, due to the resistance of the lateral ligament and the presence of the postglenoid tubercle.

PALPATION

To guide palpation of the TMJ, the clinician should first identify key landmarks:

- Body, angle, ramus, and condyle of mandible
- Temporal bone
- Articular disc (palpated indirectly)
- External auditory canal

Bony Palpation

To palpate the right TMJ, the clinician can stand in front of the patient and gently place the left middle finger on the angle of the patient's mandible, with fingers 4 and 5 placed lightly on the mandible body and the index finger on the posterior portion of the mandible ramus. The index finger then slides superiorly along the external posterior surface of the mandible ramus to reach the mandible condyle, located just anterior to the external auditory canal. The index finger can be moved anterior and superior to the head of the mandible to indirectly palpate the articular disc. Palpation of the left TMJ is done in a similar manner.

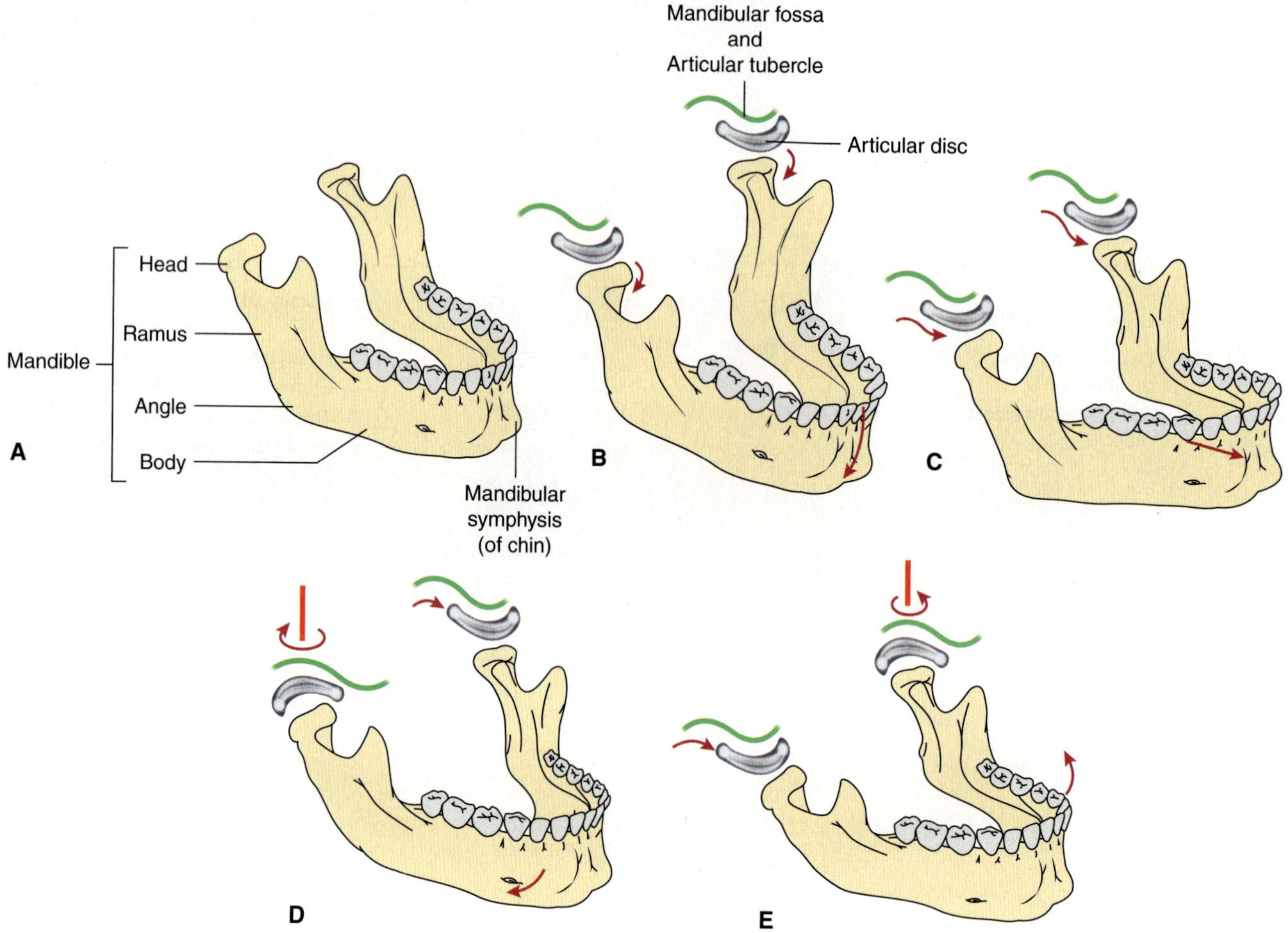

FIGURE 18-11 Movements of the mandible and articular disc. **A.** Mouth closed. **B.** Mouth open widely (mandible depressed and protruded). **C.** Mandible protruded. **D.** Mandible lateral shift to right. **E.** Mandible shift to left.

Alternately, the clinician can sit or stand at the head of a patient lying supine on the table. To palpate the right TMJ, the clinician locates the external auditory canal and tragus (thick cartilage just anterior to the external auditory canal) with the index finger and moves anteriorly about one finger width to reach the mandible condyle. The fingers 3 through 5 may rest gently on the cheek (Fig. 18.12) or along the external surface of the mandible ramus. A similar process is used to locate the TMJ on the patient's left side.

Initially, both TMJs are palpated simultaneously, to allow appreciation of differences between sides. The patient is asked to slowly open and close the mouth while the clinician palpates the movement at the TMJ. The following should be appreciated, with the start position of a closed mouth:

- Mouth opening:
  - The condyle rotates anteriorly slightly, then glides in an inferior and anteromedial direction beneath the articular tubercle (slight protrusion).
  - With wide mouth opening, the condyles rotate even farther.

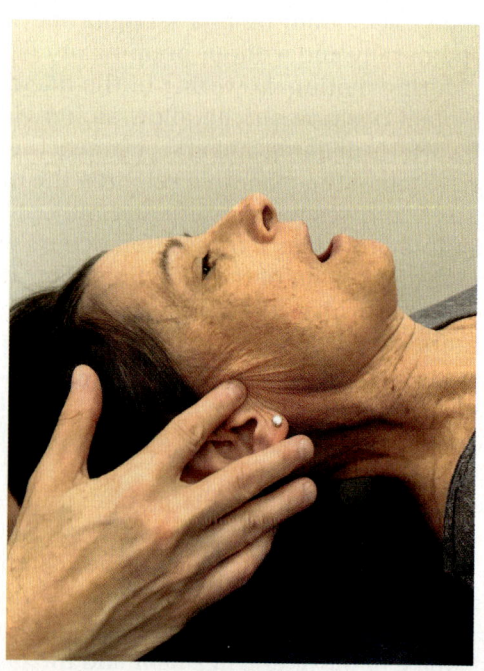

FIGURE 18.12 Palpation of the temporomandibular joint.

- Mouth closing:
  - The condyles move in reverse to return to the start position.

The condyles can be palpated in a similar manner as the patient laterally shifts the lower jaw from side to side.

Soft-Tissue Palpation

The superficial muscles of mastication, the temporalis and masseter, can be easily palpated. To palpate the temporalis muscle, the clinician places the palpating fingers on the temporalis muscle belly, just superior to the patient's ear, and gently moves the fingers toward the distal attachment on the coronoid process and ramus of the mandible (Fig. 18-13). All portions of the temporalis muscle can be palpated, except for the aspect directly deep to the posterior portion of the zygomatic arch. Palpation is facilitated by having the patient open and close the mouth.

The masseter can be palpated along its entire length from the zygomatic arch to the ramus and angle of the mandible (Fig. 18-14). The superficial and deep portions of the masseter can be palpated as the clinician places a gloved thumb on the inside of the patient's mouth by the inner cheek while the fingers are placed on the outer side of the cheek (Fig. 18-15). Asking the patient to gently press the teeth together allows the clinician to feel all aspects of the masseter.

Palpation of the medial pterygoid (see Fig. 18-9) can be combined with the intraoral palpation of the masseter. The clinician places the index or middle finger inside the patient's mouth on the medial side mandible near the angle (see Fig. 18-2) and moves the palpating finger superiorly. The hamulus of the medial pterygoid plate can be palpated on the hard palate by placing the palpating finger in the patient's mouth, posterior and medial to the third molar. The medial pterygoid can be palpated in this location as the muscle passes between attachments.

The lateral pterygoid muscle is more deeply located than the other muscles of mastication and is thus more difficult to isolate in palpation.[19,23] To palpate the lateral pterygoid intraorally, the clinician places the gloved hand inside the patient's mouth by placing with the small finger or index finger on the cheek. The patient deviates the jaw away from the side to be assessed, and the clinician palpates superiorly

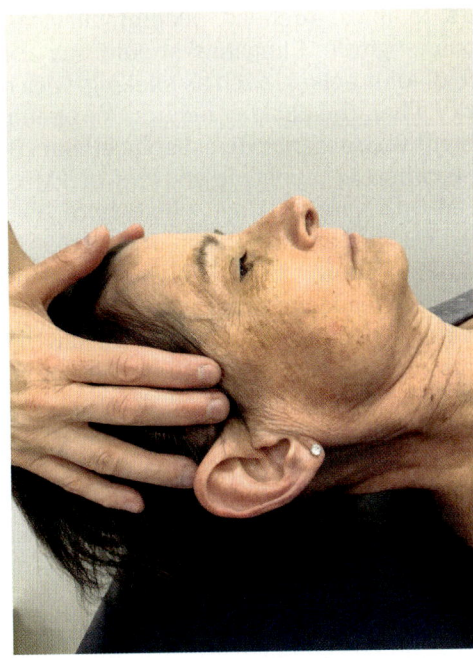

FIGURE 18.13 Palpation of the temporalis.

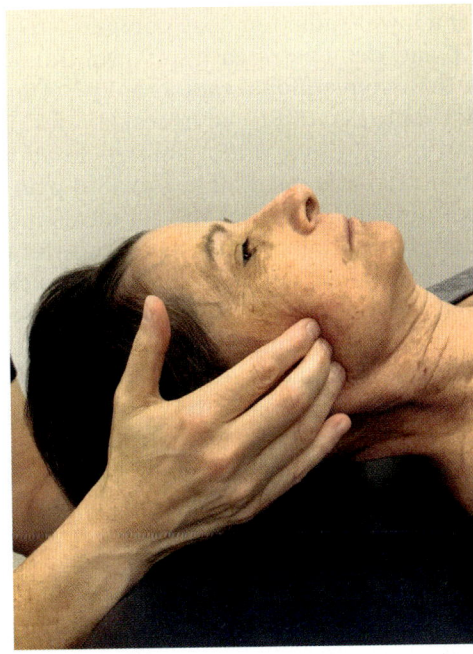

FIGURE 18.14 Palpation of the masseter (externally).

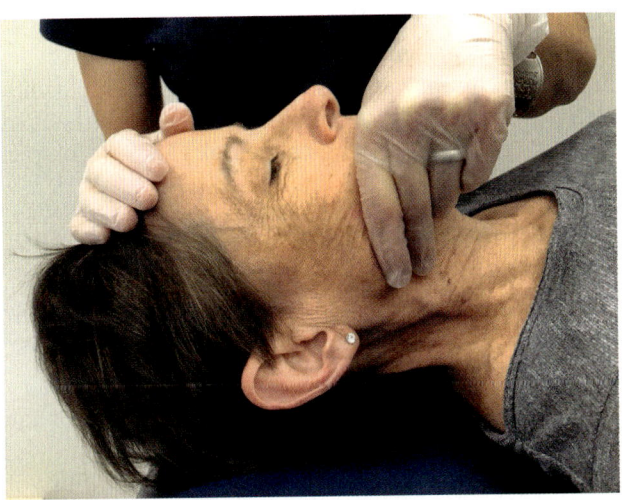

FIGURE 18.15 Palpation of the masseter (intraorally).

to the alveolar process of the maxilla to the maxillary tuberosity and continues superomedially to the lateral pterygoid plate, crossing over the superior portion of the medial pterygoid. Some consider palpation feasible, although challenging,[24] and claim ability to reliably locate trigger points and needle them consistently.[25-27] Others recommend abandoning attempts at palpation due to poor inter-tester reliability.[28] The lateral pterygoid cannot be directly palpated externally, but can be tested for strength and pain. The patient opens the mouth slightly and moves the lower jaw away from the side to be tested. The clinician applies light resistance to the movement. For example, to test the right side, the clinician would resist patient lateral deviation to the left. This test is sometimes used as a contract-relax treatment technique.[29]

INTRODUCTION TO THE EXAMINATION OF TEMPOROMANDIBULAR JOINT

The TMJ is used 1,500 to 2,000 times per day.[30] Temporomandibular dysfunction (TMD) includes musculoskeletal and neuromuscular conditions that involve the muscles of mastication, the TMJ, and associated structures.[31] It is the main source of chronic orofacial pain,[32] with a prevalence of about 13% for adults[31] and 7 to 30% for children and adolescents.[33] TMD primarily affects individuals between the ages of 20 and 40 years[34] and is more commonly seen in women[34] and smokers.[5] Several conditions are associated with TMD, including chronic headache, fibromyalgia, myofascial pain syndrome, sleep apnea, and psychiatric disorders, particularly depression or anxiety.[5] Given the multifactorial nature of TMD, an interprofessional approach, including an orthodontist, counselor, otolaryngologist, ophthalmologist, neurologist, and physical therapist, may be required for patients to attain optimal outcomes.[35]

PATIENT HISTORY: TEMPOROMANDIBULAR JOINT

The patient history assists with diagnosing or classifying a patient's condition and helps direct treatment by identifying the underlying causes of TMD and/or perpetuating factors.

Temporomandibular Dysfunction Screening Questions

The following two screening questions have proven to be reliable and valid for screening for TMD for adults[36] and adolescents.[37]

1. Do you have pain in your temple, face, jaw, or jaw joint once a week or more?
2. Do you have pain once a week or more when you open your mouth or chew?

Patients answering positively to one or both questions should be further evaluated for TMD.

Symptoms

Patients should be asked about symptom location, intensity, description, and behavior. The primary reasons patients seek treatment for TMD are limited mouth opening and pain.[34] A myogenic source of TMD can lead to bilateral or unilateral pain; however, disc dysfunction typically causes only unilateral symptoms.[38] Pain from TMD can radiate to the molar or premolar region, ears, temples, forehead, occiput, cervical region, and shoulder girdle. Clinicians should ask about the presence of joint noises, such as clicking, with motion[5] and clarify when the clicking occurs. An opening click is consistent with anterior disc displacement (DD) with reduction, whereas myogenic sources of TMD are not associated with joint clicking. A history of jaw locking helps rule in TMD[36] and is consistent with disc derangement. Patients should be asked about the presence of neck pain, headache,[39] earache, and tinnitus and whether these symptoms change with jaw motion.[40] Symptoms of TMD may fluctuate or may be intermittent. Tissue irritability should be determined to help guide the physical examination and assist with prognosis. Patients with low levels of irritability tend to improve faster and better than those with high irritability.

Trauma and Imaging

If the patient reports jaw pain and limited opening after an acute trauma, the patient should be referred for imaging, including standard or panoramic radiographs or computed tomography (CT) scan.[5] Cone-beam computed tomography (CBCT) produces high-quality images at a lower radiation dose compared to conventional CT and demonstrates less structural superimposition than conventional radiography.[41] A magnetic resonance imaging (MRI) is necessary for imaging evaluation of soft-tissue abnormalities. Routine imaging for nontraumatic onset of jaw-related pain should not be performed because an MRI (or ultrasound) may show altered morphology, such as an anterior DD,[5] on asymptomatic patients. In addition, patients can have significant improvements in motion, pain, and function, but still have abnormal morphology.[34] Nevertheless, clinicians should ask of any imaging performed and the results, even though the correlation between the clinical examination and imaging findings is poor.[34] Radiograph can demonstrate severe osteoarthritis (OA),[5] with CBCT considered the imaging technology of choice for detecting osseous changes.[42-44]

Aggravating Activities

Patients with suspected TMD should be asked about jaw-specific aggravating factors associated with jaw symptoms or headache, including chewing hard or tough food, chewing on only one side, yawning, talking, singing, kissing, and mouth opening.[5] Because sleep positions, particularly sleeping prone, can stress the TMJ, clinicians should ask if pain limits sleep or about any difficulty sleeping.

Parafunctional Behaviors

Parafunctional behaviors are movements of the jaw that are not required for normal functional demands of chewing and swallowing, speaking, and breathing.[45] Parafunctional behaviors are common in children and adults and include habits such as gum chewing, pencil chewing, and biting of the fingernails. Repetitive loading from parafunctional behaviors causes microtrauma to the TMJ and associated tissues. The Oral Behavior Checklist (Fig. 18-16) is an excellent tool to gain information regarding a variety of parafunctional behaviors that may be contributing to TMD.[46] The Oral Behavior Checklist is a 21-item questionnaire scored 0 to 4, with higher scores indicating a greater number of parafunctional behaviors.[47] Teeth clenching or teeth grinding (bruxism) may occur during the daytime when, presumably, it might be easier for the individual to use various strategies to change these behaviors, or may occur only at night, where the solution is generally a nighttime occlusal splint (aka appliance).

Past Medical History

The absence of teeth, particularly posterior teeth, is associated with TMD.[48] Therefore, clinicians should ask about prior tooth or mouth surgery and treatments for irregularities of the teeth and jaw, including the use of braces. Tooth or mouth infections can cause pain in the region of the TMJ and should be considered in patients who have had recent procedures and appropriate referrals made. Clinicians should ask about sleep dysfunction, given the link between TMD and sleep apnea and snoring. In contrast, an indirect link can be made for the association between poor vision and TMD. For example, a person who works as a data entry specialist on a computer for the majority of the workday will naturally adopt a posture of increased kyphosis, forward head, upper cervical spine extension, and mandibular depression when moving closer to the computer monitor to read information on the screen.

Psychosocial factors have been linked to TMD and can influence symptoms.[49] For example, emotional stress can create muscle hyperactivity, resulting in increased TMJ stress.[30] Clinicians should ask about stressors within the patient's life and should consider the use of a standardized psychological questionnaire, such as the Optimal Screening for Prediction of Referral and Outcome (OSPRO)—Yellow Flag Assessment.[50] As noted previously, several chronic pain conditions as well as anxiety and depression are associated with TMD. A biopsychosocial model of interventions (Chapter 19, Pain Management: A Mechanism-Centered Approach) is required to optimize treatment results in patients with chronic pain, central sensitization, and psychological distress.[51]

Outcome Measures

The Patient-Specific Function Scale (Chapter 6, Patient History) provides patients with the opportunity to note the most problematic functional activities to compare over time, regardless of pathology or body region. Although there are a number of TMJ and TMD outcome measures, there are limited data on psychometric properties.[52] The OHIP-TMD is a 20-item patient-reported outcome measure specific to patients with TMD that was adapted from a larger tool, the Oral Health Impact Profile.[53,54] The Jaw Functional Limitation Scale is a more global patient-reported outcome measure for patients with jaw symptoms.[45] Refer to Table 18-2 for details on the OHIP-TMD and Jaw Functional Limitation Scale. Other outcome measures may be appropriate based on individual patient characteristics. For example, patients with concomitant cervical dysfunction could be provided with neck-specific tools, such as the Neck Disability Index (Chapter 17, Cervical and Thoracic Spine), whereas patients with concomitant psychosocial factors that may be influencing TMJ symptoms could be provided with tools, such as the Pain Catastrophizing Scale (PCS), Tampa Scale for Kinesiophobia (TSK), or Fear Avoidance Beliefs Questionnaire (FABQ).[46]

PHYSICAL EXAMINATION: TEMPOROMANDIBULAR JOINT COMPLEX

For the TMJ, the physical examination consists of the systems review, screening examination of the cervical spine and cranial nerves,[35] and the joint-specific examination. It is common to have concomitant cervical dysfunction in patients with TMD.[55] Screening of the cervical spine and cranial nerves (see Chapter 17, Cervical and Thoracic Spine) including motor, sensory, and reflex testing should be performed as needed.[38]

A thorough description of this is found in Chapter 17, Cervical and Thoracic Spine. The clinician must rule out any potential red flags. As discussed in the history section, patients with a history of recent trauma may require imaging. Patients with abnormal cranial nerve findings or signs and symptoms of infection require referral.[5,40] Patients with widespread pain indicating a systemic condition, such as fibromyalgia, require consultation with a primary care provider or specialist.[40]

The Oral Behavior Checklist

How often do you do each of the following activities, based on the last month? If the frequency of the activity varies, choose the higher option. Please place a (✓) response for each item and do not skip any items.

	Activities During Sleep	None of the time	<1 Night /Month	1–3 Nights /Month	1–3 Nights /Week	4–7 Nights /Week
1	Clench or grind teeth when asleep, based on any information you may have	☐	☐	☐	☐	☐
2	Sleep in a position that puts pressure on the jaw (e.g., on stomach, on the side)	☐	☐	☐	☐	☐

	Activities During Waking Hours	None of the time	A little of the time	Some of the time	Most of the time	All of the time
3	Grind teeth together during waking hours	☐	☐	☐	☐	☐
4	Clench teeth together during waking hours	☐	☐	☐	☐	☐
5	Press, touch, or hold teeth together other than while eating (i.e., contact between upper and lower teeth)	☐	☐	☐	☐	☐
6	Hold, tighten, or tense muscles without clenching or bringing teeth together	☐	☐	☐	☐	☐
7	Hold or jut jaw forward or the other side	☐	☐	☐	☐	☐
8	Press tongue forcibly against teeth	☐	☐	☐	☐	☐
9	Place tongue between teeth	☐	☐	☐	☐	☐
10	Bite, chew, or play with your tongue, cheeks or lips	☐	☐	☐	☐	☐
11	Hold jaw in rigid or tense position, such as to brace or protect the jaw	☐	☐	☐	☐	☐
12	Hold between the teeth or bite objects such as hair, pipe, pencil, pens, fingers, and fingernails	☐	☐	☐	☐	☐
13	Use chewing gum	☐	☐	☐	☐	☐
14	Play musical instrument that involves use of mouth or jaw (e.g., woodwind, brass, string instruments)	☐	☐	☐	☐	☐
15	Lean with your hand on the jaw, such as cupping or resting the chin in the hand	☐	☐	☐	☐	☐
16	Chew food on one side only	☐	☐	☐	☐	☐
17	Eating between meals (i.e., food that requires chewing)	☐	☐	☐	☐	☐
18	Sustained talking (e.g., teaching, sales, customer service)	☐	☐	☐	☐	☐
19	Singing	☐	☐	☐	☐	☐
20	Yawning	☐	☐	☐	☐	☐
21	Hold telephone between your head and shoulders	☐	☐	☐	☐	☐

Copyright Ohrbach R. Available at: http://www.rdc-tmdinternational.org
Version 12May2013. No permission required to reproduce, translate, display or distribute.

FIGURE 18-16 Oral Behaviors Checklist.

Occlusion and Dentition

Observe the patient's normal jaw resting position and for clenching: when maxillary and mandibular molars are touching due to excessive contraction of the master and temporalis. The clinician should examine the patient's mouth and note the absence of any teeth. Describing teeth by number assists with discussing the patient's condition with dental professionals, such

TABLE 18-2	
COMMON OUTCOME TOOLS FOR PATIENTS WITH TEMPOROMANDIBULAR DYSFUNCTION	
Tool	Tool Basics
OHIP-TMD	• Addresses temporomandibular function specific to patients with temporomandibular dysfunction • Scoring: 0–80 • 20 items rated 0–4 with higher scores indicating worse pain/function • Seven domains: functional limitations; physical pain; psychological discomfort; physical, psychological, and social disability; and handicap • Minimum clinically important difference is about 7 points • Common diagnoses: temporomandibular dysfunction
Jaw Functional Limitation Scale	• Addresses global temporomandibular function • Scoring: 0–80 • 20 items rated 0–10 with higher scores indicating worse pain/function • Three domains: masticatory function, jaw opening, and emotional and verbal expression • Common diagnoses: jaw fracture, skeletal malocclusion, Sjögren syndrome, and temporomandibular dysfunction

as dentist and orthodontists. The absence of posterior teeth has the same effect as clenching in overloading the disc and articular surface.[35] While a prognathic (concave) or retrognathic (convex) facial profile is determined mostly by genetics, this should be documented.[35] The clinician should observe for the normal occlusion (1 to 2 mm overbite) (see Fig. 18-4).[5] Malocclusion changes the normal condyle position with jaw closure, can increase masticatory muscle activity, and is a contributing factor for TMD.[51]

The teeth should be examined for damage or excessive wear, as can occur from teeth clenching or grinding. The gums should be assessed for signs of infection. The oral cavity and tongue should be inspected. Scarring on the inside of the mouth or a scalloped appearance of the tongue is evidence of parafunctional habits in which individuals inadvertently chew on the inside of the mouth or on the tongue. Observe the patient for lip chewing.

Postural Alignment

Observe the patient for facial symmetry, jaw position at rest, and evidence of trauma. Posture dysfunction has not been shown to be consistently different between those with and without TMD[55]; however, a forward head position commonly leads to retrusion and an open jaw posture due to passive tension from the suprahyoid muscles (Fig. 18-17).[35] Therefore, the patient must actively contract the masseter and temporalis to maintain a closed mouth position. This muscular hyperactivity can lead to masticatory muscle disorders (MMDs). Increased TMJ muscle activation can also cause tooth damage.[30]

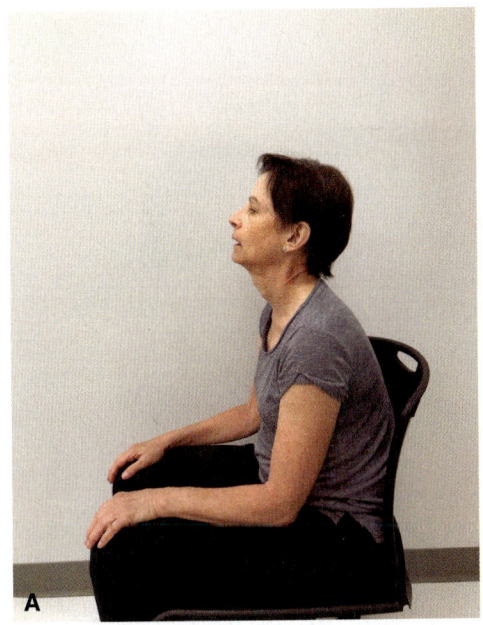
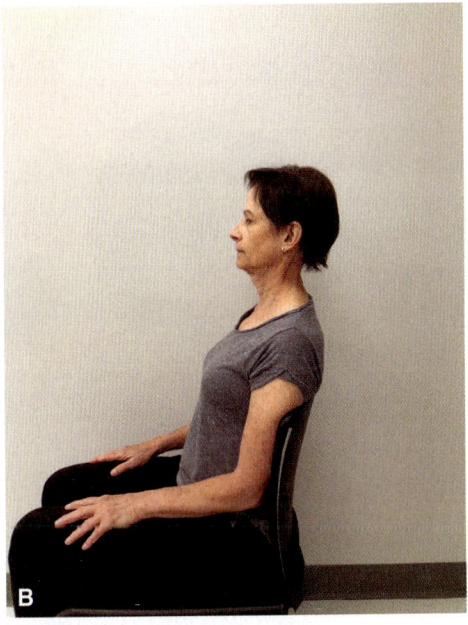

FIGURE 18-17 Relationship between posture and temporomandibular joint positioning. **A.** Slumped posture leads to open mouth positioning with retrusion. **B.** Upright posture leads to relaxed, neutral jaw positioning.

Skin and Nails

Inspect the skin and nails. Patients with parafunctional behaviors may bite their nails or cuticles.

Range of Motion

Limited active mouth opening is predictive of TMD.[49] Patients should perform active mouth opening, protrusion, and lateral deviation (Fig. 18-18). The clinician should assess TMJ movement quantity, pain provocation, and quality of active motion using normative values (Table 18-3).[56] A Therabite Range of Motion Scale, a ruler, or the end of a goniometer can be used to quantify TMJ motion (Fig. 18-19). Active mouth opening and pain-free mouth opening should be documented.[49,57] A quick test of functional mouth opening

TABLE 18-3
ACTIVE RANGE OF MOTION NORMATIVE VALUES FOR THE TEMPOROMANDIBULAR JOINT

Motion	Normative Value (mm)
Depression (mouth opening)	35–50
Occlusion (mouth closing)	Teeth approximation
Protrusion	3–7
Lateral deviation	10–15

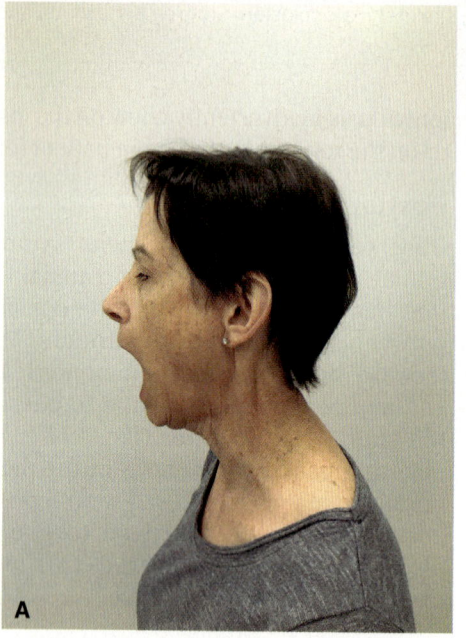
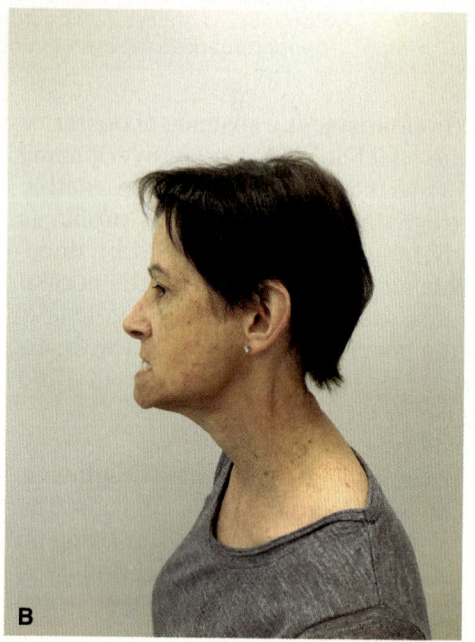
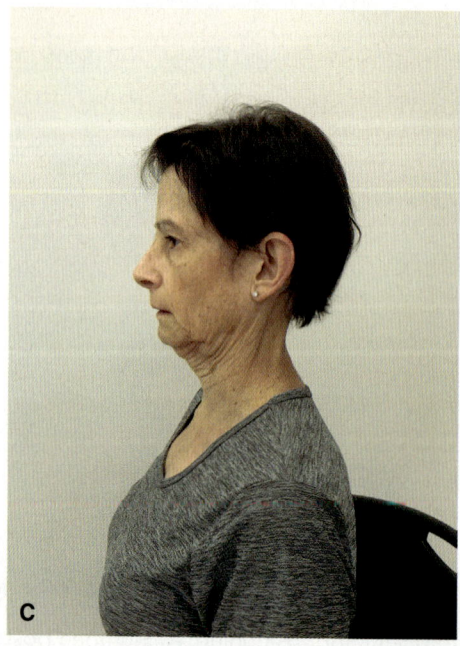
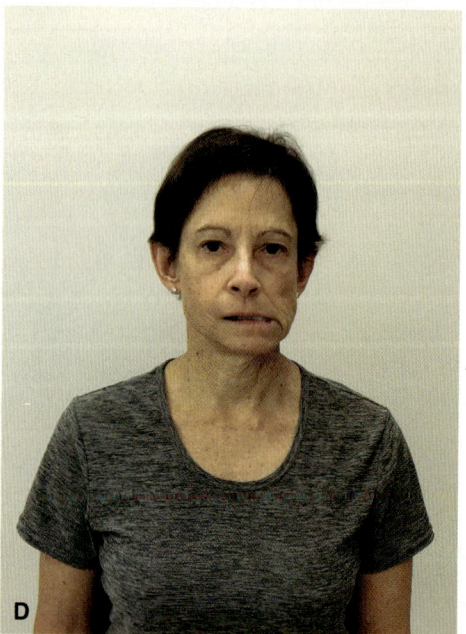

FIGURE 18-18 Temporomandibular joint active range of motion. **A.** Mouth opening. **B.** Protrusion. **C.** Retrusion. **D.** Deviation.

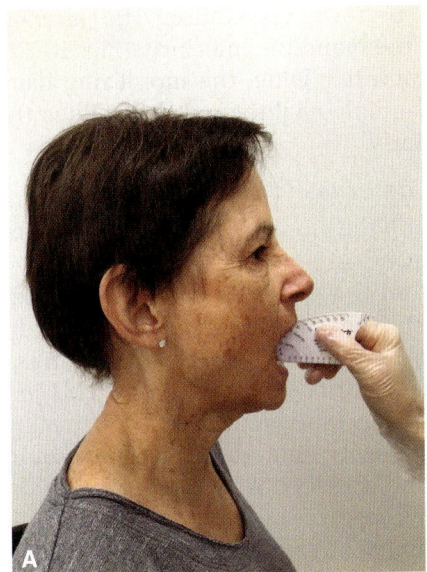 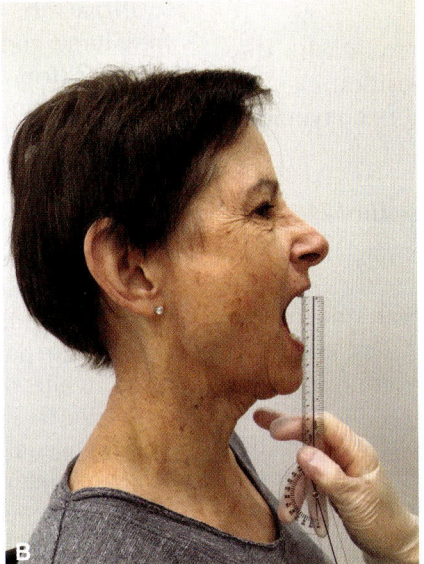 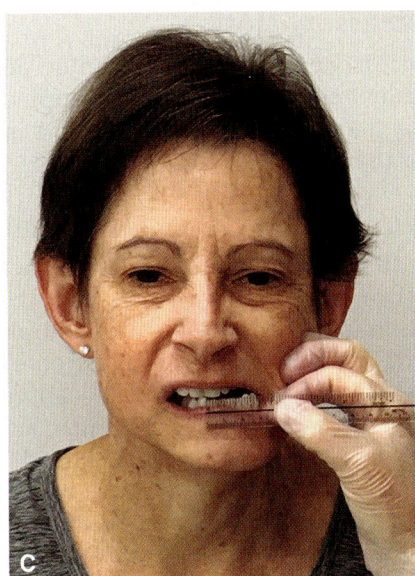

FIGURE 18-19 Quantifying active range of motion. **A.** Therabite to measure mouth opening. **B.** Goniometer to measure mouth opening. **C.** Goniometer to measure lateral deviation.

is to ask the patient to place the width of three fingers between the teeth. Mouth opening less than 30 to 35 mm is considered abnormal[5] and may be referred to as *trismus*.

The clinician should palpate anterior to the tragus during jaw motion. Clicking and popping can occur when the disc is anterior to the condylar head but then is recaptured (opening click).[5] Overpressure should be applied for symptom provocation and to determine an endfeel. A firm endfeel before normal end-range is consistent with a capsular restriction, whereas guarding may represent an internal derangement, such as a DD.[38]

Opening and closing of the mandible should be in a straight line without deflection (movement to one side or the other). Deflection during mouth opening may occur toward the affected side in cases of a capsular pattern of restriction. Movement of the jaw in an "S" pattern may indicate decreased neuromuscular control.[57]

Muscle Performance

Clinicians should perform resisted isometric testing for mandibular depression, elevation, protrusion, retrusion, and left and right lateral deviation (Table 18-4). Any symptoms during testing should be documented. Assessment of masticatory muscle performance can assist with diagnosis. For example, patients with TMD associated with MMDs will often have pain with resisted mouth closing as a result of increased masseter activation. Masticatory muscle hyperactivity is more common than muscle weakness. If masticatory muscle weakness is found with testing, it is often due to pain inhibition.[23] Because individuals with TMD have decreased bite force,[49] it may be beneficial to also measure bite force and bite endurance.

Because patients with TMD appear to have reduced cervical extensor and flexor endurance,[55] and this may contribute to poor postural alignment, clinicians should assess cervical strength and endurance in patients with TMD. In contrast, proprioceptive testing, such as accuracy of position replication or mandibular force replication, is seldom performed, because these tests do not appear to be able to distinguish between those with and without TMD[49] and these types of proprioceptive training do not improve outcomes.

TABLE 18-4

MUSCLES WORKING IN COMBINATION TO CREATE MOVEMENT OF THE MANDIBLE/TMJ

Movement	Muscles Working
Depression (mouth opening)	Bilateral lateral pterygoid and digastric muscles*
Occlusion (mouth closing)	Bilateral masseter, temporalis, and medial pterygoid muscles
Lateral deviation	Ipsilateral masseter, temporalis, contralateral pterygoid muscles
Protrusion	Bilateral pterygoids and temporalis (anterior fibers) muscles
Retrusion	Bilateral temporalis (posterior fibers), digastric, stylohyoid,* geniohyoid, and mylohyoid

*Suprahyoid muscles act in this manner when the hyoid is stabilized by the infrahyoid muscles.

Accessory Motion

Accessory motion testing can be performed with the patient seated. However, the supine position may allow the patient to relax better and is more convenient for the clinician.

Distraction and Anterior Glide of Mandible

Patient: Supine with the mouth open enough for clinician positioning.

Clinician: Standing on the contralateral side to be treated. The superior hand contacts the patient's forehead to provide stabilization, while the index finger palpated the TMJ just anterior to the tragus. The gloved mobilizing hand is placed with the thumb on the lower molars on the side to be mobilized. The index finger maintains contact with the lateral body of the mandible, whereas the remaining fingers wrap around the inferior mandible.

Mobilization: To perform distraction, the mobilizing hand glides the mandible inferiorly (Fig. 18-20). To perform an anterior glide, the mobilizing hand distracts the mandible slightly and then glides the mandible anteriorly.

Direct Lateral Glide of Mandible

Patient: Supine with the mouth open enough for clinician positioning.

Clinician: Seated on the patient's contralateral side to be mobilized. The superior (right) hand contacts the patient's forehead to provide stabilization, while the index finger palpated the TMJ just anterior to the tragus (shown on skull only to allow better visualization of technique). The gloved mobilizing (left) hand is placed with the thumb on the medial aspect of the lower molars on the side to be mobilized. The fingers wrap around the lateral mandibular ramus.

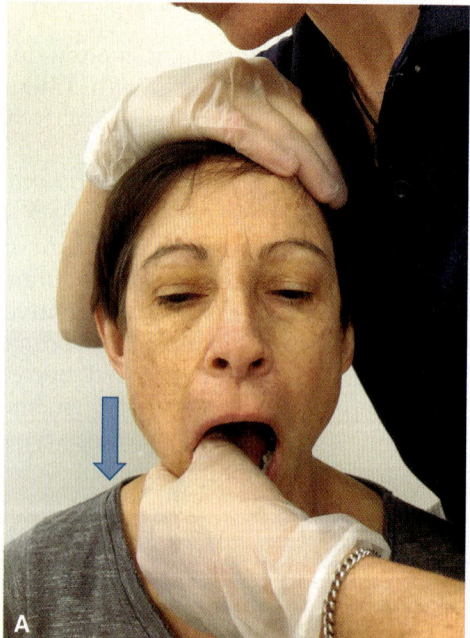
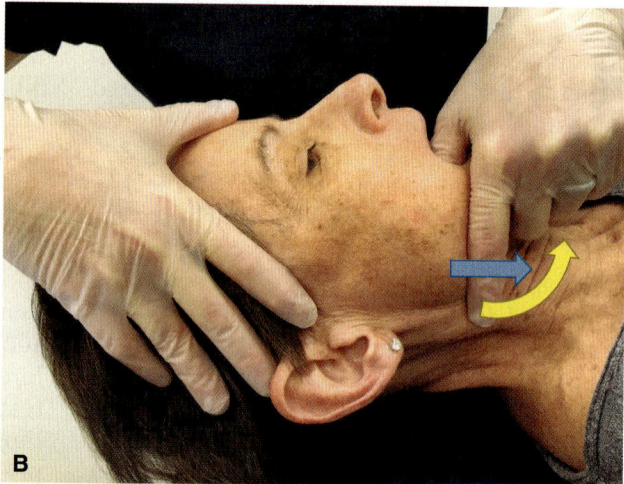
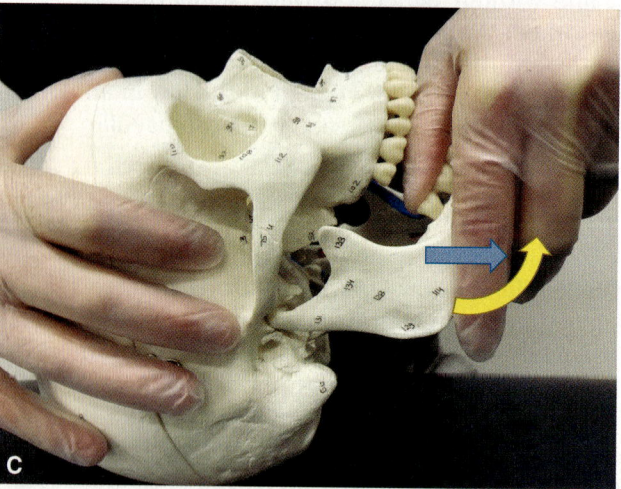

FIGURE 18-20 Distraction (*blue arrow*) and anterior glide (*curved yellow arrow*) of mandible. **A.** Seated. **B.** Supine. **C.** Performed on a skeleton.

Mobilization: The clinician creates a left or right lateral force with the mobilizing hand (Fig. 18-21).

Neurologic Testing

Light-touch sensation including the ophthalmic, maxillary, and mandibular branches of the trigeminal nerve (CN V) and the upper cervical nerves should be assessed as these can be the sources of referred pain to the TMJ region. The jaw reflex (aka the masseter reflex) further assesses trigeminal nerve function (Fig. 18-22).

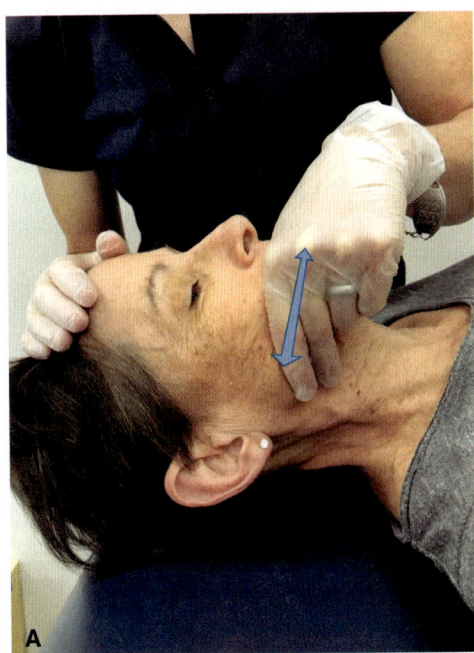

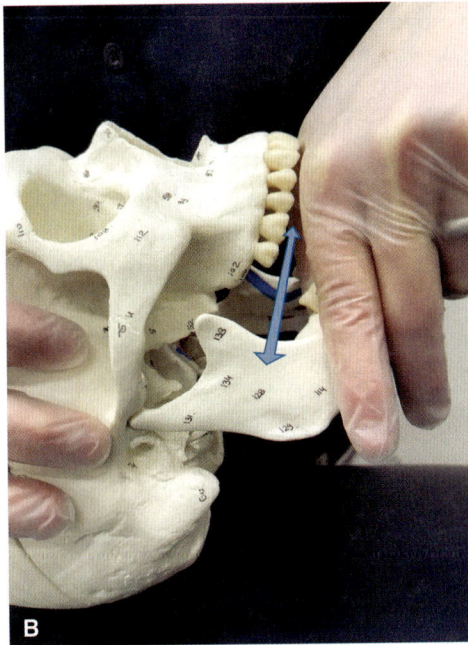

FIGURE 18-21 Direct lateral glide of mandible. **A.** On patient. **B.** On skeleton.

Palpation

Palpation should be performed as noted previously. The clinician should note the presence of any trigger points. Swelling, warmth, or erythema in the region is suggestive of infection or other medical pathology and requires immediate referral. Palpation for tenderness of the TMJ and masticatory muscles should be performed using pain pressure threshold measurements when possible (Table 18-5).[31,49] To improve reliability, the clinician should practice providing 0.5 and 1.0 kg of pressure using a strain gauge.[39] The clinician should document if this assessment reproduces the patient's familiar pain or headache.

Special Tests/Provocative Testing

Special testing for TMD is limited. The unilateral bite test and TMJ compression test are provocative tests

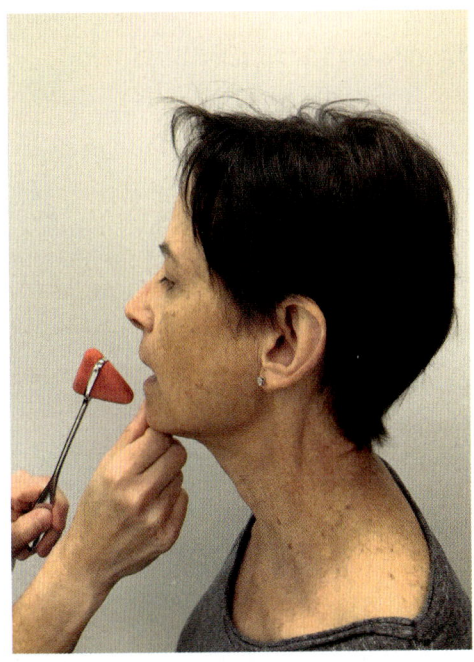

FIGURE 18-22 Jaw reflex.

TABLE 18-5	
PALPATION FOR IDENTIFYING TEMPOROMANDIBULAR DYSFUNCTION	
Location	Pressure
Lateral pole of the TMJ	0.5 kg for 2 seconds
Masseter • Origin • Body • Insertion	1 kg for 5 seconds
Temporalis • Anterior • Middle • Posterior	1 kg for 5 seconds

TMJ, temporomandibular joint.

that should be used in combination with the patient history and remaining physical examination to clarify TMD diagnoses.[38]

Unilateral Bite Test

Purpose: The unilateral bite test is sometimes called the *cotton roll test* or the *TMJ compression test*, because it was originally thought to assess only joint compressive forces. The unilateral bite test is used to assess for joint disorders or MMDs.

Method: The patient bites down on a small stack of tongue blades placed on the side of the patient's mouth (Fig. 18-23).

Interpretation: The test creates contralateral TMJ compression and ipsilateral TMJ distraction; therefore, there are multiple possible interpretations of the test (Fig. 18-24). Ipsilateral muscular pain is consistent with MMD involving the mandibular elevators, such as the masseter and temporalis.[40] Contralateral TMJ pain is associated with arthralgia due to increased joint compression.[58] A reduction in ipsilateral pain may represent ipsilateral articular pathology, such as arthralgia or DD, as the unilateral bite test unloads the ipsilateral joint. The test is also likely to be positive in the case of mandibular fracture.[38]

Temporomandibular Joint Compression Test

Purpose: The TMJ compression test involves the clinician manually loading the TMJ and related structures to identify intra-articular pathology, such as arthralgia or DD.

Method: With the patient seated, the clinician stabilizes the patient's head and neck with the posterior hand. The clinician's anterior hand provides a posterior and cranial force to the mandible (Fig. 18-25). The test can also be performed intraorally using similar hand placements to the direct lateral glide of mandible mobilization.

Interpretation: A positive test is reproduction of the patient's familiar TMJ pain with testing.[38]

Functional Testing

Functional testing of the TMJ is generally not required. However, patients who are unsure what provokes their TMJ symptoms can be asked to perform the following tasks that require significant mouth opening, increased masticatory muscle force, and/or repeated masticatory muscle action:

- Yawning
- Biting into a whole apple
- Chewing gum on one side
- Eating a bagel, Tootsie Roll, or other "chewy" food
- Biting down on a piece of hard candy

COMMON TEMPOROMANDIBULAR JOINT PATHOLOGIES

This section describes the most common TMJ pathologies a clinician is likely to see in an outpatient setting. Because many TMD interventions may be applied to

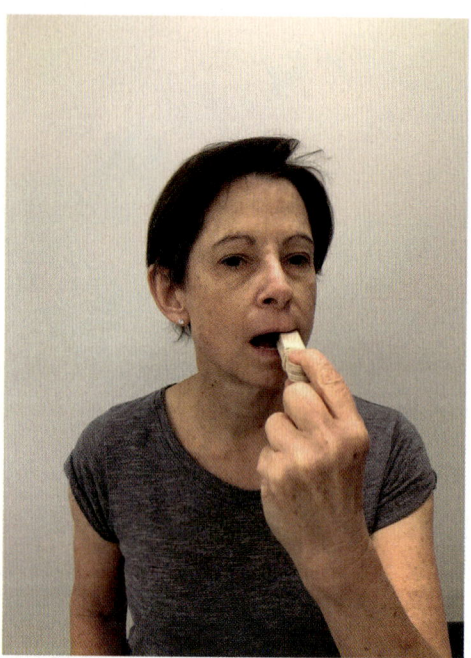

FIGURE 18-23 Unilateral bite test.

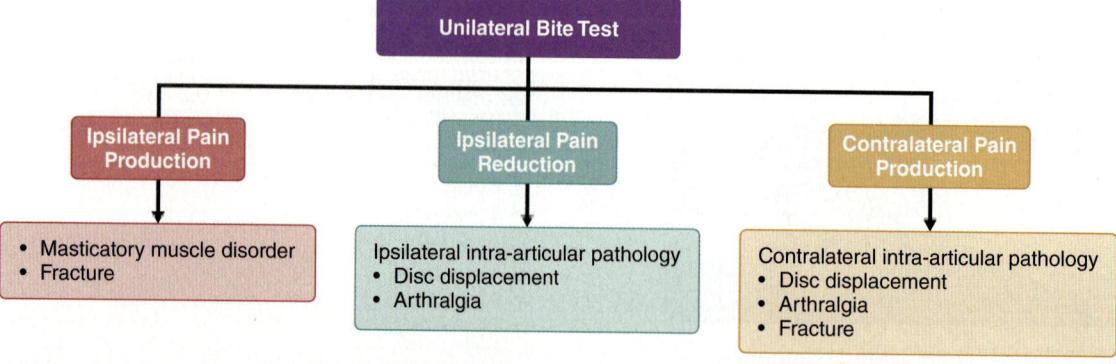

FIGURE 18-24 Unilateral bite test interpretation.

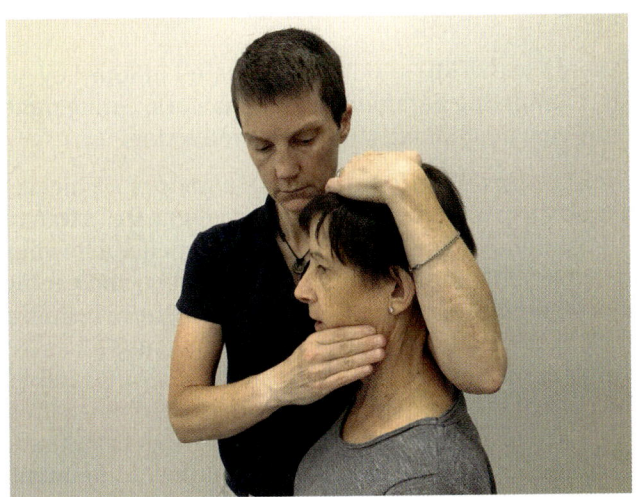

FIGURE 18-25 Temporomandibular joint compression test.

more than one condition, interventions are grouped in the following section. Classification of TMD was first done in 1992 using the research diagnostic criteria for temporomandibular disorders (RCD/TMD) classification system. The diagnostic criteria for temporomandibular disorders (DC/TMD) revised this system in 2014 with the intent of improving clinical evaluation and treatment[39] and is currently the most commonly used classification system.[31] Recently, the International Classification of Orofacial Pain (ICOP, first edition) adopted the DC/TMD criteria with only slight modification.[46] For the purposes of outpatient rehabilitation, three main diagnostic categories exist for TMD: MMDs, disc disorders, and arthralgias. Patients may fit into more than one diagnostic category.[38] In addition to the physical assessment of TMD, it is recommended that clinicians assess for psychosocial issues and pain-related disability.[40]

Masticatory Muscle Disorders

MMDs are defined by symptoms that originate from the myofascial structures of the TMJ. Patients with MMD will report that their pain is provoked by the use of the muscles of mastication, such as chewing, as well as pain with palpation of these muscles, particularly the masseter or temporalis.[46] Symptomatic trigger points are often present.[38] These patients may have limited mouth opening or the perception of difficulty opening the mouth.[31] Often, the symptoms are bilateral.[38,46] Patients with MMD have parafunctional habits, such as bruxism and clenching, and often have concomitant anxiety or stress disorders.[38]

Disc Displacements

Articular DDs occur when the articular disc is shifted or displaced relative to its normal resting position. Typically, the disc is displaced anterior and medial to the condylar head when the mouth is closed. As the mouth is opened, the disc reduces back into place on top of the condylar head, often with a palpable or audible click. This is often referred to as an *opening click*. This anterior DD with reduction is the most common TMD for adults, adolescents, and children.[31] DD is more common in females, possibly because females are more likely to have tissue laxity. Patients with this condition will report a painful popping, clicking, or snapping with jaw motion in at least one direction,[46] most commonly mouth opening. A reciprocal click, a click when the disc displaces anteriorly upon closing, may also be present.[5,38] However, disc reduction can occur without this reciprocal click.[34] Patients with DD may report intermittent limited mouth opening or, upon opening, the jaw may deflect toward the affected side during initial opening but then correct as the disc is reduced, making a "C" shape.[38,57] Patients with DD generally have unilateral symptoms and may have a positive unilateral bite test.[38]

The least common TMD is an anterior DD without reduction. Patients with anterior DD without reduction may report limited mouth opening and intermittent locking, also known as a *closed lock*, because the disc is blocking mandibular translation.[5,34,38,46] Anterior DD without reduction may be a progression of anterior DD.[59] However, this may not be the case. Some patients continue to have symptomatic anteriorly displaced discs without progression, whereas others may have anterior DDs, yet be asymptomatic.[57] Finally, some individuals with clicking and limited opening have been found to have a normal disc position.[57]

Rarely, the disc may be displaced posteriorly. This is thought to be caused by an overstretched lateral pterygoid muscle, allowing posterior DD.[60] Patients with a posterior DD may have an open lock (inability to close the mouth) or may report a closing click if the disc reduces upon closing.[60] Disc position (normal or displaced) is not directly related to the development of degenerative changes in the TMJ.[38]

Arthralgia

Temporomandibular arthralgia is degenerative joint disease of the TMJ and is seen most often in individuals over 45 years of age.[31,38] The lower joint space of the mandibular condyle and articular disc is more likely to have degeneration than the upper joint surface.[38] Patients with arthralgia have crepitus with active jaw motion and painful or limited maximal mouth opening.[46] When opening, the jaw may deflect toward the affected side due to capsular restriction.[57] Similarly, deviation to the contralateral side will be limited. Patients are likely to have a positive unilateral bite test and pain with palpation of the lateral pole of the mandibular condyle.[46] Patients with arthralgia may have limited accessory motion on the affected side. Arthralgia is evident on imaging studies. However, as with other joints, patients with positive imaging studies may not be symptomatic.[46]

Differential Diagnosis of Pain in the Region of the Temporomandibular Joint

Overall, the combination of history and physical examination is sufficient to diagnose and classify TMD without additional imaging.[31,57] Table 18-6 summarizes the typical expected key findings for patients with the three main TMDs seen within an outpatient setting. However, the clinician must consider several differential diagnoses for patients with signs and symptoms of TMD. Conditions of sinusitis,[5] recent surgery or dental procedures, infection, abscess, osteomyelitis, and temporal arteritis must be considered.[61] As noted previously, a history of trauma should raise the suspicion for fracture. Pain in the region of the TMJ may be caused by a tooth infection, cervical spine pathology, or trigeminal neuralgia.[31] Lastly, the clinician must consider chronic pain conditions and psychiatric conditions, such as anxiety and depression.[31,57]

INTERVENTIONS FOR TEMPOROMANDIBULAR DYSFUNCTION

The goals for the treatment of patients with TMD are to decrease pain, encourage muscle relaxation, re-establish normal muscle and joint activity, improve mouth opening, and improve TMJ function, such as eating.[32] Interventions for successful management may include education, exercise, manual therapy, and interprofessional collaboration (Fig. 18-26). Occasionally, the short-term use of modalities may need to be integrated into the treatment program.

Patient Education

Patients with TMD should be educated in four key areas: eliminating parafunctional behaviors, eating modifications, positioning, and stress reduction.

Eliminating Parafunctional Behaviors Clinicians should help patients identify and eliminate parafunctional behaviors, such as nail biting, pencil chewing, and jaw clenching. Gum chewing, smoking, and vaping should be discouraged. Cognitive awareness training, self-observation, and relaxation training may all assist with decreasing muscle hyperactivity. For example, the patient may be instructed in progressive relaxation exercises to be performed before bedtime or in times of stress. Creating new nail care routines to maintain healthy nails and cuticles may help curtail nail biting.

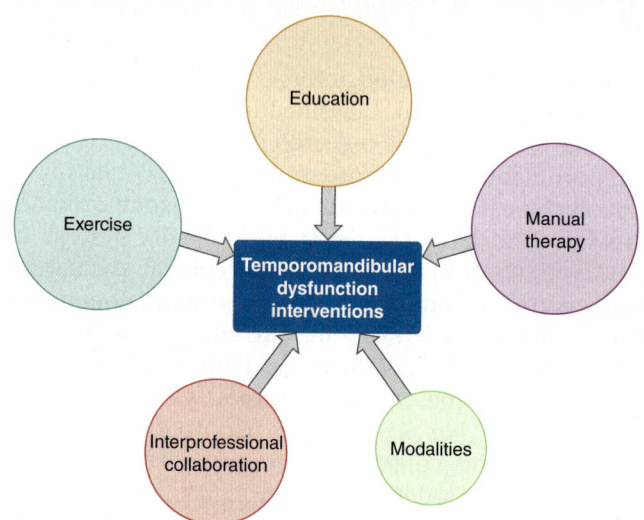

FIGURE 18-26 Temporomandibular dysfunction interventions.

TABLE 18-6			
DIFFERENTIAL DIAGNOSIS OF TEMPOROMANDIBULAR DYSFUNCTION			
Diagnosis	*Masticatory Muscle Disorders*	*Disc Displacements*	*Arthralgia*
Patient age	Between 2 and 40 years of age	Between 2 and 40 years of age	Over 45 years of age
Clicking, locking	None	Present	None
Crepitus	None	None	Present
Location	Bilateral or unilateral	Unilateral	Bilateral or unilateral
Deflection	None	Common	Possible
Deviation	None	Possible	Common
Accessory motion	Normal or guarded	Possibly limited	Decreased
Palpation	Muscles tender to palpation Trigger points possible	May have tenderness	Mandibular condyle tender to palpation May have muscular tenderness
Joint compression test	Negative	May be positive	Positive
Unilateral bite test	Increased symptoms	Decreased ipsilateral pain Increased contralateral pain	Decreased ipsilateral pain Increased contralateral pain
Cervical testing	Possible involvement	Possible involvement	Possible involvement

The clinician may encourage the patient engage in a healthy nail habit of applying hand lotion throughout the day.

Eating Modifications Patients with TMD may benefit from changing to food that is a softer consistency during periods of exacerbation.[30,62] Patients with DDs and arthralgia will benefit from avoiding full opening of the mouth.[30] Simple things like taking small bites; cutting up an apple, rather than biting into a whole one; and making slimmer sandwiches and burgers appear to be beneficial in reducing symptoms and preventing recurrence. Patients should try to limit the intake of chewy foods to decrease the workload of the masticatory muscles. Clinicians should also reinforce the importance of a healthy, balanced diet with limited use of caffeine as part of overall health.

Positioning Patients with TMD should be educated on a healthy resting jaw position: teeth slightly apart,[62] tongue gently resting against the anterior superior palate, lips closed, jaw relaxed, and breathing through the nose. A timer can be used to remind the patient to attain and maintain this rest position. Patients should be educated on the relationship between (poor) posture, TMJ position, and (increased) muscular demands. Patients should be taught to avoid extreme positioning for toothbrushing, flossing, eating, and yawning. Yawning can be modified by using the "tongue-up opening" technique in which the patient attempts to keep the tongue in contact with the anterior superior palate while yawning, thus limiting mandibular depression (Fig. 18-27).[62] Patients should try to limit yelling due to excessive mouth opening required.[62] Singing may be problematic for some individuals due to both the ROM required and the repetitive mouth movements.[62]

Patients should avoid positions that stress the TMJ. For example, students frequently sit with their head supported by their hand, leading to ipsilateral TMJ distraction and contralateral TMJ compression (Fig. 18-28). Sleeping in the prone position has a similar effect on the TMJ. Patients should be encouraged to sleep supine with a small pillow or sidelying with a soft, moldable pillow to limit prolonged TMJ stress.

Therapeutic Exercise Therapeutic exercise can help decrease TMD pain, improve mouth opening, reduce joint clicking, improve postural alignment, reduce stress, and improve function.[57,59,63] It appears that mobility exercises and performing multiple types of exercise lead to superior results.[63]

Exercises to assist with improving motion should begin with gentle warm-up exercises, such as small ROM mouth opening/closing and deviations. This should be progressed to maximal ROM opening, deviation, and protrusion.[32] Examples of exercise parameters from the literature include 10 repetitions performed six times per day.[23]

If the goal is to improve ROM, these general jaw exercises can be followed by self-assisted opening.[64] TMJ stretching can also be performed by placing two of the patient's fingers or a stack of tongue blades between the patient's front teeth for about 10 seconds

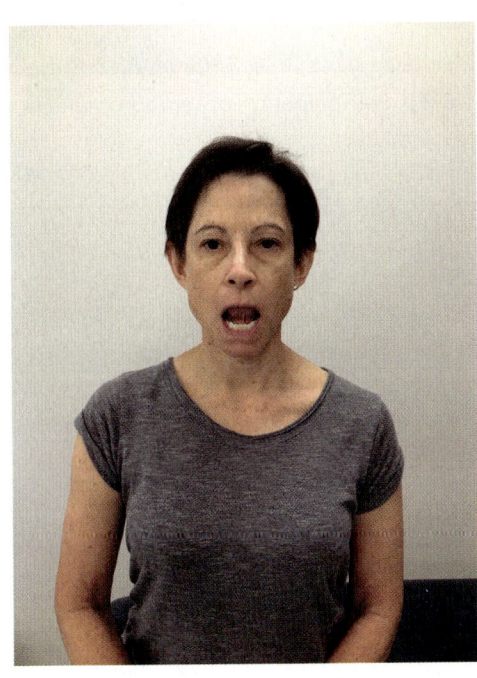

FIGURE 18-27 Tongue-up opening technique.

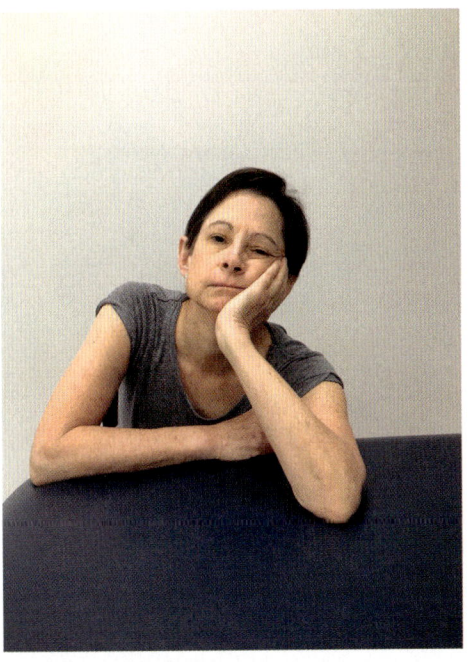

FIGURE 18-28 Poor temporomandibular joint positioning.

(Fig. 18-29). The fingers or tongue blades are removed for a rest and then repeated for about 10 repetitions. Additional tongue blades (or third finger) can be added as ROM allows. The jaw stretching can be beneficial not only for patients with arthralgia, but it is likely more beneficial for patients with limited mouth opening due to other causes, such as burns. Exercise prescription for stretching ranges from 10 to 30-second holds for 2 to 10 repetitions,[63] with more repetitions prescribed if shorter hold times are used. Typically, patients would perform 5 to 10 sets of stretching exercise.[63]

Patients with anterior DD may benefit from a series of exercises that appear to assist with patients with disc derangements, such as the following, in order:

- Open the mouth until feeling or hearing the familiar TMJ clicking sound (Fig. 18-30), then simultaneously protrude the mandible and close the mouth until the front teeth (incisors) contact each other.
- Open and close the mouth in a symptom-free range.
- Repeat the same sequence slowly for up to 3 minutes.[64]

Gentle tongue-up opening exercises may also be performed for time, with some suggesting up to 10 minutes per day.[30]

ROM exercises can be followed by gentle isometrics resisted by the clinician (Fig. 18-31). Alternatively, the patient can provide two-finger resistance to mouth opening, deviation, and protrusion.[64] Mandibular isometrics may also help with mandibular stabilization in patients with DD[65] or patients with MMDs. The patient may benefit from performing controlled mobility exercises with a mirror for feedback and focusing on moving the jaw straight forward without deviation.[30,62] When performed for neuromuscular control such as this, the following exercise parameters have proven successful: 15 to 20 repetitions, two to three times per day.[30]

Relaxation exercises such as diaphragmatic breathing where the patient breathes through the nose, yoga, or progressive relaxation exercises may improve TMJ ROM that is limited by masticatory muscle tonicity or after DD.[59] Additional exercise that might be beneficial for patients with TMD includes cervical stretching, deep neck flexor endurance training, and neuromuscular reeducation exercises for postural muscles, including the cervical, thoracic, and scapular muscles.[32,63,65]

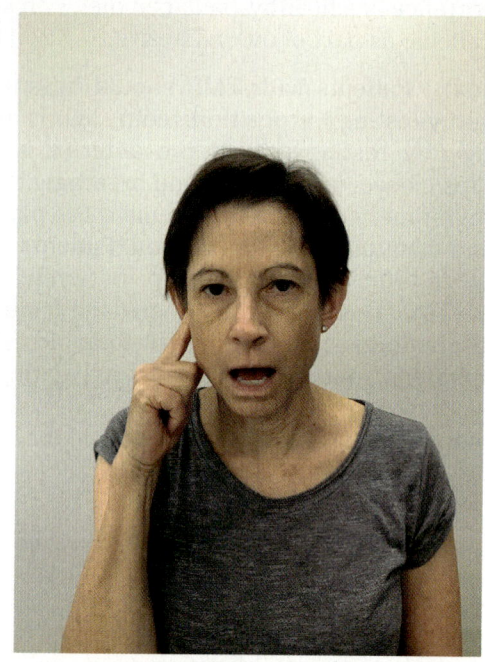

FIGURE 18-30 Self-palpation of temporomandibular joint.

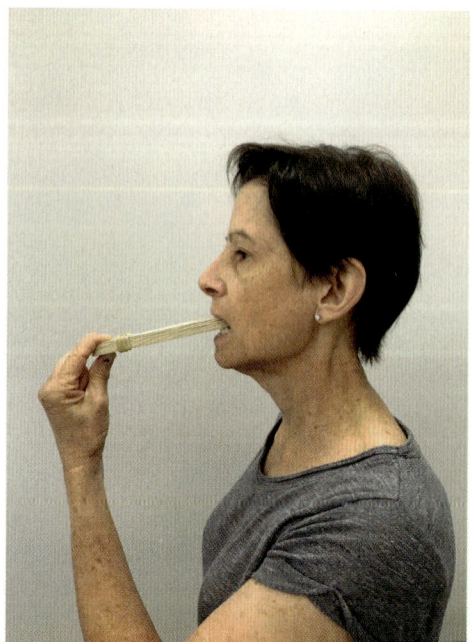

FIGURE 18-29 Use of tongue blades for jaw stretching.

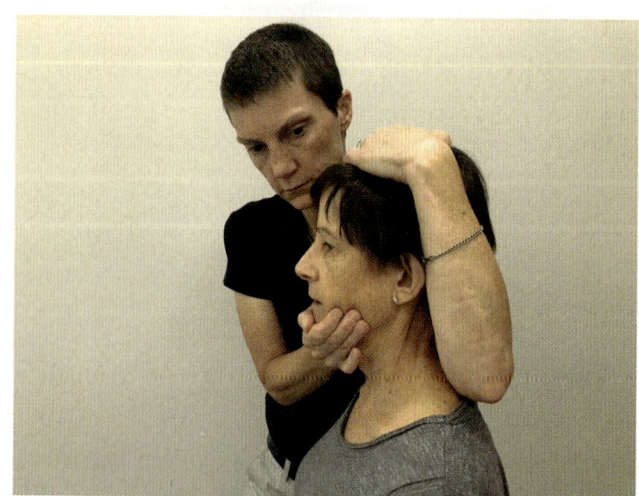

FIGURE 18-31 Clinician resisted mandibular isometric exercises.

Manual Therapy Manual therapy is a common intervention for patients with TMD.[30]

Manual therapy may have largest effect when performed on the masseter and temporalis,[23] given their ease of identification and access. Intraoral soft-tissue mobilization can be performed by the clinician to the masseter and pterygoids. The patient can also be taught individual techniques as part of a home program (Fig. 18-32). Various techniques including parallel and perpendicular strokes, effleurage, kneading, trigger point release, trigger point dry needling,[23] and muscle energy have been shown to improve motion and decrease pain.[30,66]

TMJ mobilizations may be beneficial for patients with capsular restrictions, muscle guarding, or disc derangements[38] when using the test, treat, and reassess method. The accessory motion procedures described earlier can be used to treat TMJ hypomobility, particularly when using grade III and IV mobilizations and/or performing closer to end-range. Grade I and II mobilizations performed at midrange may assist with pain modulation and muscle relaxation, thus improving overall TMJ motion. Clinicians may utilize the same hand holds as in the TMJ compression test (see Fig. 18-25) to perform an indirect medial or lateral mandibular glide.

Patient: Seated with the mouth slightly open.

Clinician: With the patient seated, the clinician stabilizes the patient's head and neck with the posterior hand. The anterior mobilizing hand holds the sides of the patient's mandible with the index thumb and index finger.

Mobilization: The clinician provides a medially or laterally directed force to the mandible with the mobilizing hand.

Patients can perform self-mobilization to target unilateral TMJ restrictions or improve lateral deviation ROM.

Patient: To mobilize the right TMJ, the patient is seated with the heel of the palm of the stabilizing (left) hand placed on the left zygomatic arch. The heel of the mobilizing (right) hand is placed on the right lateral mandibular ramus.

Mobilization: The patient creates a medial force with the mobilizing (right) hand (Fig. 18-33).

The addition of cervical manual therapy, including mobilization, manipulation, and suboccipital release, to manual therapy directed to the TMJ appears to be beneficial.[23,67] Thoracic manipulation does not appear to have additional benefit.[67] Typical manual therapy frequency is two to three times per week, but may be as infrequent as every 2 weeks.[66]

Interprofessional Collaboration

When working with patients with TMD, clinicians must consider the value of interprofessional collaboration.

A dentist or orthodontist should be consulted in the presence of altered dentition. In addition, custom-made occlusal splints are one of the most frequently

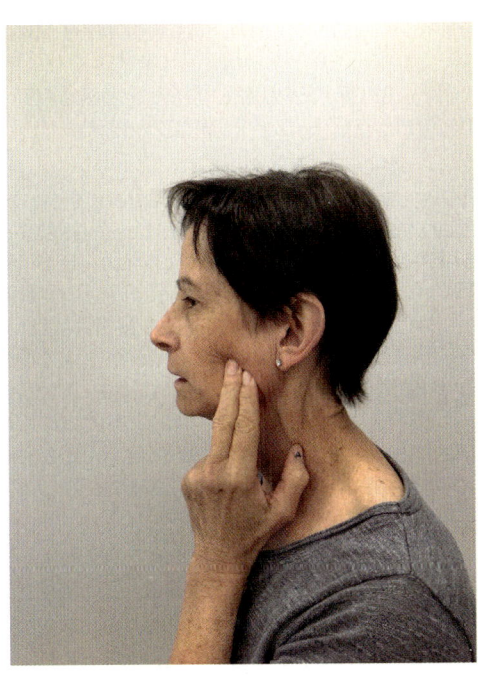

FIGURE 18-32 Patient soft-tissue mobilization of the masseter.

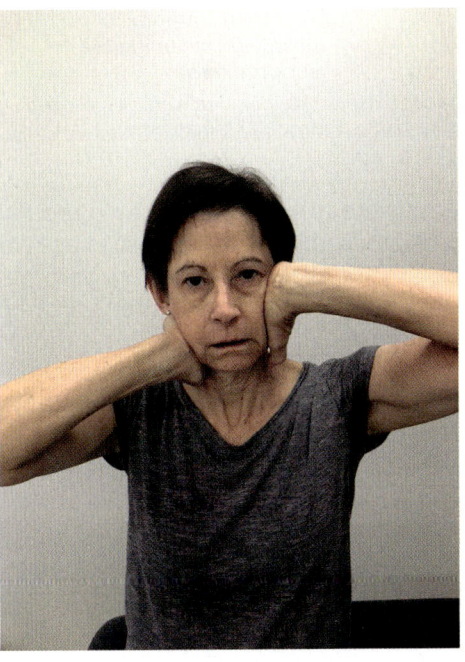

FIGURE 18-33 Self-mobilization of the right temporomandibular joint to improve mouth opening or left lateral deviation.

CASE STUDY: 18-1
Orla: Patient with Bilateral Jaw Pain

Orla is a 26-year-old nurse reporting a 6-month history of bilateral jaw pain, right greater than pain. She notes that she has difficulty opening her mouth widely, eating hard or chewy foods, and that her sleep is disrupted. She reports intermittent headaches, which she is unsure are related to her jaw pain. Orla reports she feels unsupported at work, frequently feels depressed, and has little pleasure in doing things. Her Oral Behavior Checklist score was 60/80. She denies the presence of TMJ clicking, locking, or snapping. Table 18-7 provides an example of how an experienced clinician might organize the physical examination after performing the history and systems review.

TABLE 18-7

SAMPLE TEMPOROMANDIBULAR EXAMINATION

Orla, a 26-year-old nurse with a 6-month history of bilateral jaw pain

Position	Assessments
Observation	Orla sits with a forward head with upper cervical spine extension with teeth clenched, several fingernails appear to have been chewed.
Seated	Cervical flex, ext, lat flex, rot (A, OP) Upper cervical spine flex, ext Spurling test Reflexes brachialis, biceps, triceps, jaw Dermatomes C1–T1 Myotomes C5–T1 Isometric testing cervical flex, ext, lat flex, rot Mandibular dep, elev, prot, retr, dev (A, OP) Isometric testing mandibular dep, elev, prot, retr, dev Special tests: unilateral bite test, temporomandibular compression test
Prone	Quadruped isometric hold of neutral head/neck posture MMT: middle and lower trapezius
Supine	Cervical flexion endurance test Mouth inspection TMJ accessory motion: distraction, anterior glide, lateral glide Palpation: intraoral Palpation: including the TMJ at rest and with movement, mandibular condyle, masseter, temporalis, suboccipitals

A, active; *dep*, depression; *dev*, deviation; *elev*, elevation; *ext*, extension; *flex*, flexion; *MMT*, manual muscle test; *OP*, overpressure; *prot*, protrusion; *retr*, retrusion; *TMJ*, temporomandibular joint.

Based on the history, there are no red flags, but multiple yellow flags including the patient's reports of feeling depressed, lack of interest in activities, and dissatisfaction with work. Based on the patient's age, the lack of joint clicking or locking, and the presence of parafunctional behaviors, the clinician's initial hypothesis is MMD. The patient's report of headaches and the frequent coexistence of cervical pathology with TMD, so the clinician performs a thorough screening of the cervical spine. Because the listed cervical testing was negative, the clinician deferred neural tension testing and cervical accessory motions. Next, the clinician performed a detailed examination of the TMJ, including ROM, muscle performance, and special tests. Positive examination findings included limited mouth opening but no clicking, mild limitation of lateral deviations, guarding with accessory motion assessment, the masseters were tender to palpation and contained trigger points, and the unilateral bite test produced the patient's familiar ipsilateral TMJ pain.

Before performing the supine TMJ examination procedures, the clinician assessed scapular postural muscles and cervical flexor and extensor endurance. All intraoral examination procedures are performed in sequence for maximal efficiency. Because patients are more relaxed in supine, mouth inspection, accessory motions, and palpation are performed in this position after all other information has been obtained. The clinician concluded the patient did, indeed, have MMD.

used interventions for patients with TMD. Two common devices are the Michigan bite splint and sagittal vertical extrusion device (SVED). A Michigan bite splint is used to improve condyle position, relax masticatory muscles, and prevent tooth wear.[30] An SVED is used to improve limited mouth opening, decrease pain, and improve DD.[30]

Pharmacologic interventions can be effective in assisting with pain control and muscle relaxation. Nonsteroidal anti-inflammatory medications are the first course of treatment for patients with TMD, and if not effective, a muscle relaxer may be prescribed.[5] Patients with more chronic conditions or with concomitant psychoemotional conditions may be prescribed tricyclic antidepressants, benzodiazepines, or anticonvulsants (aka gabapentin).[5]

Chronic pain is complex and multifactorial; therefore, patients with psychosocial factors contributing to their condition may benefit from the skills of a counselor, psychologist, or psychiatrist.

Modalities

Low-level laser, iontophoresis, biofeedback, and transcutaneous electrical nerve stimulation (TENS) have all been used to assist with symptom management for patients with TMD.[23,30,32] However, there is little evidence to support their use. Therefore, modalities may be best reserved as adjunctive interventions for patients with high irritability or high pain levels whose symptoms have not responded to more evidence-based rehabilitation.

EXPECTED OUTCOMES

A multifaceted approach to managing patients with TMD can lead to positive results. Patients can expect improvements in pain and increase in mouth opening ROM in 4 to 8 weeks.[30,62,64] The combination of manual therapy and exercise may be better than either alone or the use of occlusal splints or medication.[32] Patients may continue to have clicking sounds or intermittent flare-ups; therefore, patients must be educated on lifelong self-management.

Patients who fail to improve with this multifaceted approach after 6 months should be referred to an oral or maxillofacial specialist. A variety of surgical procedures may be performed on patients with TMD, including arthroscopy, condylotomy, arthrotomy, and arthroplasty.[68] Most patients are referred for a short course of therapy after surgery, including the basic exercise progression noted previously.[69]

CHAPTER SUMMARY

TMD is a relatively common condition. Because TMD is associated with several chronic pain conditions, depression, and anxiety, patient care using a biopsychosocial can be beneficial. The three primary types of TMD seen in an outpatient setting are MMDs, DDs, and arthralgia. Interventions for TMD must include education and minimizing parafunctional behaviors, therapeutic exercise, and manual therapy. A holistic approach may involve multiple health care providers to provide occlusal splints, pharmacotherapy, and counseling. Although TMD can be a chronic condition, a short course of rehabilitation is highly successful.

REFERENCE

1. Alomar X, Medrano J, Cabratosa J, et al. Anatomy of the temporomandibular joint. *Semin Ultrasound CT MR*. 2007;28(3):170–183.
2. Piancino M, Dalmasso P, Borello F, et al. Thoracic-lumbar-sacral spine sagittal alignment and cranio-mandibular morphology in adolescents. *J Electromyogr Kinesiol*. 2019;48:169–175.
3. Kim S, Lipinski L, Pujol N. Meniscal allograft transplantation with soft-tissue fixation including the anterior intermeniscal ligament. *Arthrosc Tech*. 2020;9(1):e137–e142.
4. Williams P, Warwick R, Myson M, Bannister L, eds. *Gray's Anatomy*. 37th ed. Churchill Livingstone; 1989.
5. Gauer RL, Semidey MJ. Diagnosis and treatment of temporomandibular disorders. *Am Fam Physician*. 2015;91(6):378–386.
6. Ho S. *The Temporomandibular Joint: Physical Therapy Management Using Current Evidence*; Orthopaedic Section of the American Physical Therapy Association; 2016:1–52.
7. Willard VP, Arzi B, Athanasiou K. The attachments of the temporomandibular joint disc: a biochemical and histological investigation. *Arch Oral Biol*. 2012;57(6):599–606.
8. Liu F, Steinkeler A. Epidemiology, diagnosis, and treatment of temporomandibular disorders. *Dent Clin North Am*. 2013;57(3):465–479.
9. Bernasconi G, Marchetti C, Reguzzoni M, Baciliero U. Synovia hyperplasia and calcification in the human TMJ disk: a clinical, surgical, and histologic study. *Oral Surg Oral Med Oral Pathol Oral Radiol Endod*. 1997;84(3):245–252.
10. Christo J, Bennett S, Wilkinson T, Townsend G. Discal attachments of the human temporomandibular joint. *Aust Dent J*. 2005;50(3):152–160.
11. McKinley M, O'Loughlin V, Pennefather-O'Brien E. *Human Anatomy*. 6th ed. McGraw Hill; 2021.
12. van Eijden T, Koolstra J, Brugman P. Architecture of the human pterygoid muscles. *J Dent Res*. 1995;74(8):1489–1495.
13. Moore KL, Dalley AF, Agur AMR. *Clinically Oriented Anatomy*. 8th ed. Wolters Kluwer; 2018.
14. Stöckle M, Fanghänel J, Knüttel H, Alamanos C, Behr M. The morphological variations of the lateral pterygoid muscle: a systematic review. *Ann Anat*. 2019;222:79–87.
15. Kim H, Kwak H, Hu K, et al. Topographic anatomy of the mandibular nerve branches distributed on the two heads of the lateral pterygoid. *Int J Oral Maxillofac Surg*. 2003;32(4):408–413.
16. Desmons S, Graux F, Atassi M, Libersa P, Dupas P. The lateral pterygoid muscle, a heterogeneous unit implicated in temporomandibular disorder: a literature review. *Cranio*. 2007;25(4):283–291.
17. Foucart J, Girin J, Carpentier P. Innervation of the human lateral pterygoid muscle. *Surg Radiol Anat*. 1998;20(3):185–189.
18. Murray G, Bhutada M, Peck C, Phanachet I, Sae-Lee D, Whittle T. The human lateral pterygoid muscle. *Arch Oral Biol*. 2007;52(4):377–380.

19. Bhojwani V, Ghabriel M, Mihailidis S, Townsend G. The human medial pterygoid muscle: attachments and distribution of muscle spindles. *Clin Anat.* 2017;30(8):1064–1071.
20. El Haddioui A, Bravetti P, Gaudy J. Anatomical study of the arrangement and attachments of the human medial pterygoid muscle. *Surg Radiol Anat.* 2007;29(2):115–124.
21. Oatis CA. *Kinesiology: The Mechanics and Pathomechanics of Human Movement.* 3rd ed. Wolters Kluwer; 2017.
22. Abe S, Orihara K, Kitamura S, Takizawa M, Okada M, Ide Y. Anatomical study of arrangement and attachment of the medial pterygoid muscle in Japanese men. *Bull Tokyo Dent Coll.* 1997;38(3):217–221.
23. Butts R, Dunning J, Pavkovich R, Mettille J, Mourad F. Conservative management of temporomandibular dysfunction: a literature review with implications for clinical practice guidelines (Narrative review part 2). *J Bodyw Mov Ther.* 2017;21(3):541–548.
24. Stelzenmueller W, Umstadt H, Weber D, Goenner-Oezkan V, Kopp S, Lisson J. Evidence—the intraoral palpability of the lateral pterygoid muscle—a prospective study. *Ann Anat.* 2016;206:89–95.
25. Gonzalez-Perez L, Infante-Cossio P, Granados-Nuñez M, Urresti-Lopez F, Lopez-Martos R, Ruiz-Canela-Mendez P. Deep dry needling of trigger points located in the lateral pterygoid muscle: efficacy and safety of treatment for management of myofascial pain and temporomandibular dysfunction. *Med Oral Patol Oral Cir Bucal.* 2015;20(3):e326–e333.
26. Lopez-Martos R, Gonzalez-Perez L, Ruiz-Canela-Mendez P, Urresti-Lopez F, Gutierrez-Perez J, Infante-Cossio P. Randomized, double-blind study comparing percutaneous electrolysis and dry needling for the management of temporomandibular myofascial pain. *Med Oral Patol Oral Cir Bucal.* 2018;23(4):e454–e462.
27. Gonzalez-Perez LM, Infante-Cossio P, Granados-Nuñez M, Urresti-Lopez FJ. Treatment of temporomandibular myofascial pain with deep dry needling. *Med Oral Patol Oral Cir Bucal.* 2012;17(5):e781–e785.
28. Türp J, Minagi S. Palpation of the lateral pterygoid region in TMD—where is the evidence? *J Dent.* 2001;29(7):475–483.
29. Reichert B. *Palpation Techniques. Surface Anatomy for Physical Therapists.* Thieme; 2011.
30. Wieckiewicz M, Boening K, Wiland P, Shiau Y-Y, Paradowska-Stolarz A. Reported concepts for the treatment modalities and pain management of temporomandibular disorders. *J Headache Pain.* 2015;16(1):1–12.
31. Valesan LF, Da-Cas CD, Réus JC, et al. Prevalence of temporomandibular joint disorders: a systematic review and meta-analysis. *Clin Oral Investig.* 2021;25(2):441–453.
32. Armijo-Olivo S, Pitance L, Singh V, Neto F, Thie N, Michelotti A. Effectiveness of manual therapy and therapeutic exercise for temporomandibular disorders: systematic review and meta-analysis. *Phys Ther.* 2016;96(1):9–25.
33. Christidis N, Lindström Ndanshau E, Sandberg A, Tsilingaridis G. Prevalence and treatment strategies regarding temporomandibular disorders in children and adolescents—a systematic review. *J Oral Rehabil.* 2019;46(3):291–301.
34. Muhtarogullari M, Ertan AA, Demiralp B, Canay S, Muhtaroğullari M. Correlation between clinical and magnetic resonance imaging findings in the treatment of anterior disc displacement. *Int J Prosthodont.* 2013;26(2):138–142.
35. Sambataro S, Cervino G, Bocchieri S, La Bruna R, Cicciù M. TMJ dysfunctions systemic implications and postural assessments: a review of recent literature. *J Funct Morphol Kinesiol.* 2019;4(3):58.
36. Lövgren A, Parvaneh H, Lobbezoo F, Häggman-Henrikson B, Wänman A, Visscher CM. Diagnostic accuracy of three screening questions (3Q/TMD) in relation to the DC/TMD in a specialized orofacial pain clinic. *Acta Odontol Scand.* 2018;76(6):380–386.
37. Nilsson IM, List T, Drangsholt M. The reliability and validity of self-reported temporomandibular disorder pain in adolescents. *J Orofac Pain.* 2006;20(2):138–144.
38. Shaffer SM, Brismée J-M, Sizer PS, Courtney CA. Temporomandibular disorders. Part 1: anatomy and examination/diagnosis. *J Man Manip Ther.* 2014;22(1):2–12.
39. Skeie MS, Frid P, Mustafa M, Aßmus J, Rosén A. DC/TMD examiner protocol: longitudinal evaluation on interexaminer reliability. *Pain Res Manag.* 2018:1–8.
40. Schiffman E, Ohrbach R, Truelove E, et al. Diagnostic criteria for temporomandibular disorders (DC/TMD) for clinical and research applications: recommendations of the international RDC/TMD consortium network and orofacial pain special interest group. *J Oral Facial Pain Headache.* 2014;28(1):6–27.
41. Barghan S, Tetradis S, Mallya S. Application of cone beam computed tomography for assessment of the temporomandibular joints. *Aust Dent J.* 2012;57(Suppl 1):109–118.
42. Ferrazzo KL, Osório LB, Ferrazzo VA. CT images of a severe TMJ osteoarthritis and differential diagnosis with other joint disorders. *Case Rep Dent.* 2013;2013:242685.
43. Peck CC, Goulet JP, Lobbezoo F, et al. Expanding the taxonomy of the diagnostic criteria for temporomandibular disorders. *J Oral Rehabil.* 2014;41(1):2–23.
44. Arayasantiparb R, Mitrirattanakul S, Kunasarapun P, Chutimataewin H, Netnoparat P, Sae-Heng W. Association of radiographic and clinical findings in patients with temporomandibular joints osseous alteration. *Clin Oral Investig.* 2020;24(1):221–227.
45. Ohrbach R, Markiewicz MR, McCall WD Jr. Waking-state oral parafunctional behaviors: specificity and validity as assessed by electromyography. *Eur J Oral Sci.* 2008;116(5):438–444.
46. International classification of orofacial pain, 1st edition (ICOP). *Cephalalgia.* 2020;40(2):129–221.
47. Meulen MJ, Lobbezoo F, Aartman IHA, Naeije M. Validity of the Oral Behaviours Checklist: correlations between OBC scores and intensity of facial pain. *J Oral Rehabil.* 2014;41(2):115–121.
48. Wang MQ, Xue F, He JJ, Chen JH, Chen CS, Raustia A. Missing posterior teeth and risk of temporomandibular disorders. *J Dent Res.* 2009;88(10):942–945.
49. Dinsdale A, Liang Z, Thomas L, Treleaven J. Are jaw range of motion, muscle function and proprioception impaired in adults with persistent temporomandibular disorders? A systematic review and meta-analysis. *J Oral Rehabil.* 2020;47(11):1448–1478.
50. Lentz T, Beneciuk J, Bialosky J, et al. Development of a yellow flag assessment tool for orthopaedic physical therapists: results from the optimal screening for prediction of referral and outcome (OSPRO) cohort. *J Orthop Sports Phys Ther.* 2016;46(5):327–345.
51. Skármeta NP, Pesce MC, Saldivia J, Espinoza-Mellado P, Montini F, Sotomayor C. Changes in understanding of painful temporomandibular disorders: the history of a transformation. *Quintessence Int.* 2019;50(8):662–669.
52. Mittal H, John MT, Sekulic S, Theis-Mahon N, Rener-Sitar K. Patient-reported outcome measures for adult dental patients: a systematic review. *J Evid Based Dent Pract.* 2019;19(1):53–70.
53. Durham J, Steele JG, Wassell RW, et al. Creating a patient-based condition-specific outcome measure for Temporomandibular Disorders (TMDs): Oral Health Impact Profile for TMDs (OHIP-TMDs). *J Oral Rehabil.* 2011;38(12):871–883.

54. Yule PL, Durham J, Playford H, et al. OHIP-TMDs: a patient-reported outcome measure for temporomandibular disorders. *Community Dent Oral Epidemiol.* 2015;43(5):461–470.
55. de Oliveira-Souza AIS, de OFJK, Barros M, Oliveira DA. Cervical musculoskeletal disorders in patients with temporomandibular dysfunction: a systematic review and meta-analysis. *J Bodyw Mov Ther.* 2020;24(4):84–101.
56. American Academy of Orthopaedic Surgeons. *Joint Motion: Method of Measuring and Recording.* Churchill Livingstone; 1965.
57. Connelly ST, Tartaglia GM, Silva RG. *Contemporary Management of Temporomandibular Disorders: Fundamentals and Pathway to Diagnosis.* Springer International Publishing AG; 2019.
58. Lövgren A, Visscher CM, Alstergren P, Lobbezoo F, Häggman-Henrikson B, Wänman A. The outcome of a temporomandibular joint compression test for the diagnosis of arthralgia is confounded by concurrent myalgia. *Clin Oral Investig.* 2020;24(1):97–102.
59. Chortis AG, Chorti AG, Forrester G, Georgoudis G. Therapeutic exercise in the management of anterior disc displacement of the temporomandibular joint. *Phys Ther Rev.* 2006;11(2):117–123.
60. Chossegros C, Cheynet F, Guyot L, Bellot-Samson V, Blanc JL. Posterior disk displacement of the TMJ: MRI evidence in two cases. *Cranio.* 2001;19(4):289–293.
61. Nam Y, Kim HG, Kho HS. Differential diagnosis of jaw pain using informatics technology. *J Oral Rehabil.* 2018;45(8):581–588.
62. Magesty RA, Silva MAM, Simões CASC, et al. Oral health-related quality of life in patients with disc displacement with reduction after counselling treatment versus counselling associated with jaw exercises. *J Oral Rehabil.* 2021;48(4):369–374.
63. Dickerson SM, Weaver JM, Boyson AN, et al. The effectiveness of exercise therapy for temporomandibular dysfunction: a systematic review and meta-analysis. *Clin Rehabil.* 2017;31(8):1039–1048.
64. Lindfors E, Arima T, Baad-Hansen L, et al. Jaw exercises in the treatment of temporomandibular disorders—an international modified Delphi study. *J Oral Facial Pain Headache.* 2019;33(4):389–398.
65. Cleland J, Palmer J. Effectiveness of manual physical therapy, therapeutic exercise, and patient education on bilateral disc displacement without reduction of the temporomandibular joint: a single-case design. *J Orthop Sports Phys Ther.* 2004;34(9):535–548.
66. Martins WR, Blasczyk JC, Aparecida Furlan de Oliveira M, et al. Efficacy of musculoskeletal manual approach in the treatment of temporomandibular joint disorder: a systematic review with meta-analysis. *Man Ther.* 2016;21:10–17.
67. Calixtre LB, Moreira RF, Franchini GH, Alburquerque-Sendín F, Oliveira AB. Manual therapy for the management of pain and limited range of motion in subjects with signs and symptoms of temporomandibular disorder: a systematic review of randomised controlled trials. *J Oral Rehabil.* 2015;42(11):847–861.
68. Connelly ST, Tartaglia GM, Silva RG. *Contemporary Management of Temporomandibular Disorders: Surgical Treatment.* Springer International Publishing AG; 2019.
69. Bas B, Kazan D, Kutuk N, Gurbanov V. The effect of exercise on range of movement and pain after temporomandibular joint arthrocentesis. *J Oral Maxillofac Surg.* 2018;76(6):1181–1186.

PART V

Pain Management

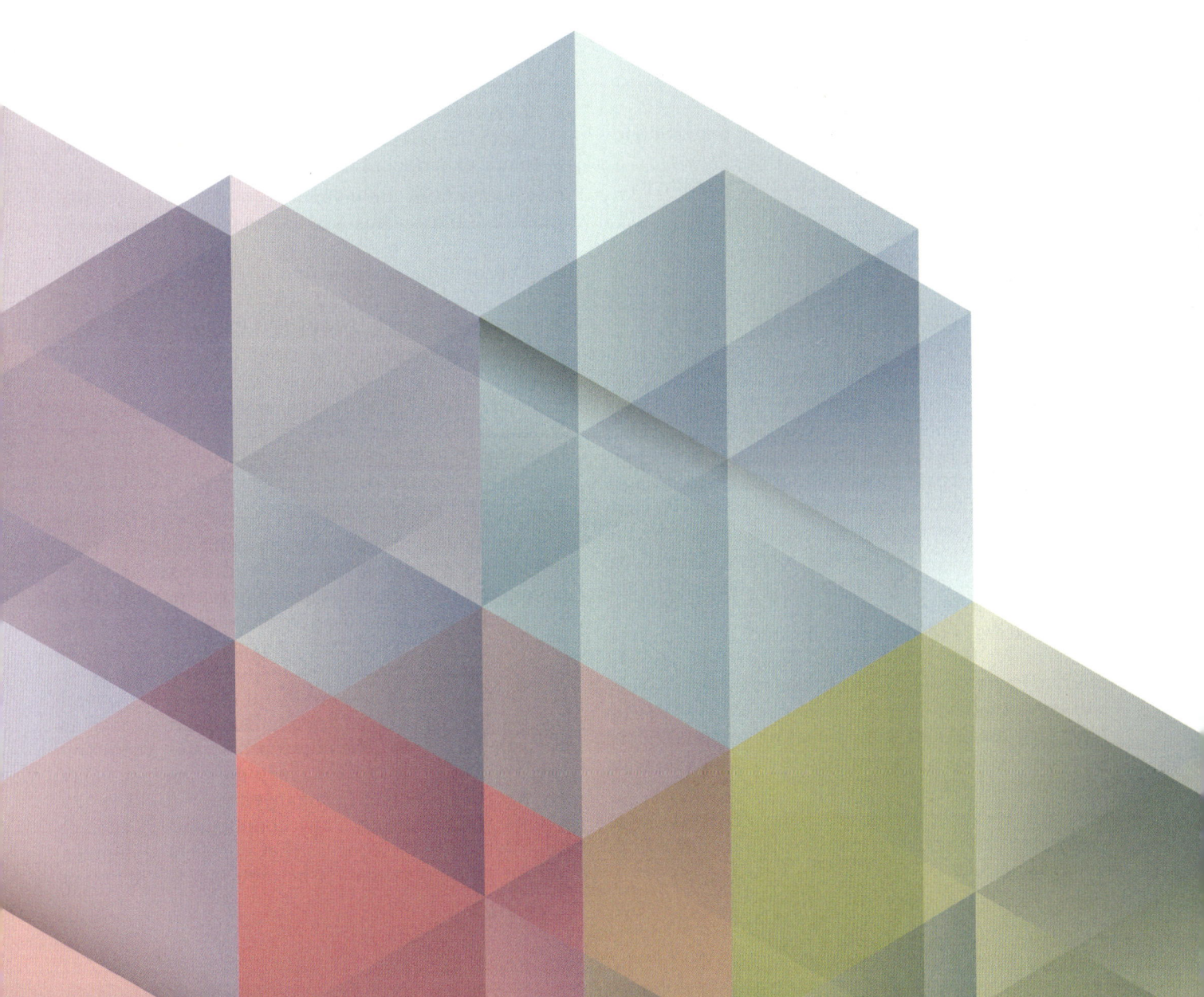

19 Pain Management: A Mechanism-Centered Approach

Craig A. Wassinger and Gisela Sole

CHAPTER OBJECTIVES
After reading this chapter, you will be able to:
1. Describe the multisystem role in the pain experience.
2. Define pain and the pain neuromatrix within the biopsychosocial model.
3. Interpret clinical history and examination findings to determine a patient's pain type.
4. Utilize validated yellow flag screening tools and pain measures as part of the patient examination process.
5. Consider the importance of patient education in promoting health literacy and self-efficacy.
6. Link commonly used therapeutic interventions (electrical modalities, manual therapy, and exercise) to different pain types.

PAIN SCIENCE DEFINITIONS AND EPIDEMIOLOGY

Pain is a common reason for seeking medical care,[1] yet the proportion of time educating health care providers on pain is quite limited.[1-3] Pain is a tremendous individual and societal burden in the United States and other countries.[4-6] Low back pain, for example, is the greatest cause of disability in the world and estimated costs in Western countries approach 2% of gross national product.[4] In the United States, the number of Americans reported to live with chronic pain has been reported as high as 116 million people at a societal cost (medical care and lost earnings) in excess of $600 billion annually.[7,8]

Recently, the International Association for the Study of Pain redefined pain as "an unpleasant sensory and emotional experience associated with, or resembling that associated with, actual or potential tissue damage."[9] This has been expanded with the following six contextual additions:

- Pain is always a personal experience that is influenced to varying degrees by biologic, psychological, and social factors.
- Pain and nociception are different phenomena. Pain cannot be inferred solely from activity in sensory neurons.
- Through their life experiences, individuals learn the concept of pain.
- A person's report of an experience as pain should be respected.
- Although pain usually serves an adaptive role, it may have adverse effects on function and social and psychological well-being.
- Verbal description is only one of several behaviors to express pain; inability to communicate does not negate the possibility that a human or a nonhuman animal experiences pain.

Key points from the definition are that pain is a real individual biopsychosocial experience in response to perceived threat. It is often protective (acute pain) but may become maladaptive (chronic pain).

ANATOMY AND PHYSIOLOGY
Anatomic structures associated with pain are primarily components of the nervous system. The four primary steps within the general pain pathway are transduction, transmission, perception, and modulation (Fig. 19-1).[10]

Peripheral Nervous System
The peripheral nervous system contributes to pain primarily via nociception. Although the terms *nociception* and *pain* are often used interchangeably, they are two distinct physiologic processes that are commonly related. Free nerves endings, or nociceptors, are peripheral nerves that respond to noxious or threatening stimuli and are found in most peripheral tissues. Noxious stimuli are commonly categorized as mechanoreceptive, chemoreceptive, and thermoreceptive. Nociceptors are usually described as thinly myelinated (A-Δ-fibers) or unmyelinated (C-fibers) afferents with relatively slow conduction velocities.[11] *Transduction* is the process that converts a stimulus into an action potential.[10] Nociception is the initiation

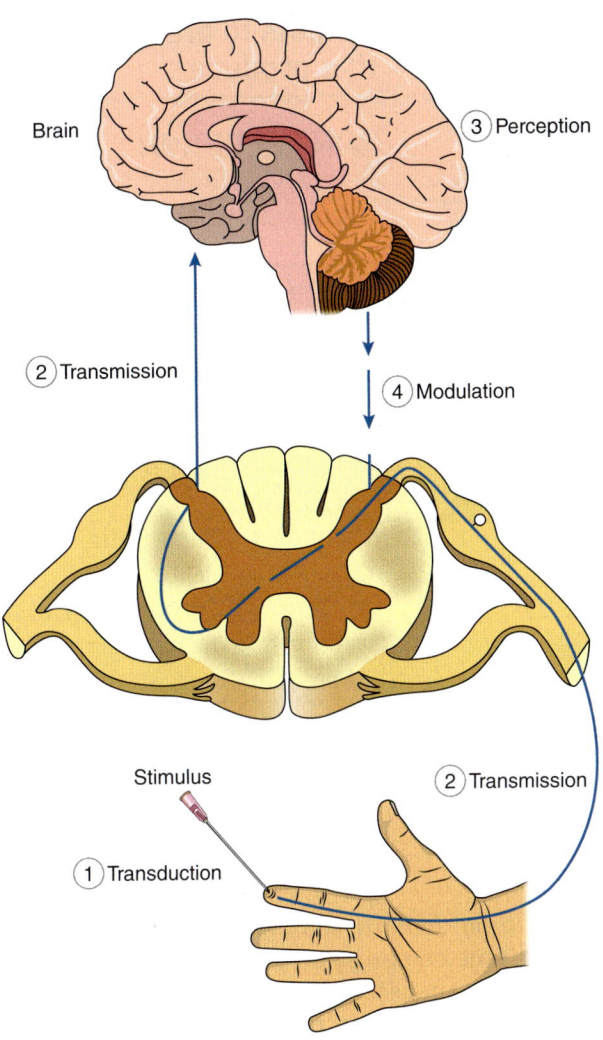

FIGURE 19-1 Steps in general pain pathway.

of a specific action potential within a free nerve ending (nociceptor) to a noxious or threatening stimulus. In the peripheral nervous system, *transmission* occurs as the propagation of the action potential from the nociceptor into the dorsal horn of the spinal cord.[10]

Central Nervous System

Transmission continues as the action potential is conveyed to the dorsal horn of the spinal cord, the afferent fibers synapse, crosses the midline, and ascends to the brain via the anterolateral system, most commonly through the spinothalamic tract.[10] As named, the spinothalamic tract terminates in the thalamus, which acts as the transmission center to higher order brain structures. Nociceptive information is then integrated with other sensory stimuli across brain structures, commonly referred to as the *pain neuromatrix*.[12] The pain neuromatrix is composed of the dorsal horn of the spinal cord and various brain structures that act to collect and interpret incoming stimuli to create a response. Key brain structures associated with the pain neuromatrix are the hippocampus, cerebellum, thalamus/hypothalamus, sensory cortices, amygdala, prefrontal cortex, cingulate cortex, and motor/premotor cortices.[12,13] *Perception* happens as the pain neuromatrix interprets the sensory, cognitive, and emotional inputs to the brain.[10]

Finally, modulation occurs in response to the incoming stimuli (threat) from within the neuromatrix. *Modulation* is the process by which primary afferent nociceptive information is upregulated or downregulated via descending information from the central nervous system.[10] This descending modulation occurs with transmission using the posterior column of the spinal cord to promote or inhibit nociceptive transmission at the interneuron within the dorsal horn.

BIOPSYCHOSOCIAL MODEL AND THE PAIN NEUROMATRIX THEORY

Pain is commonly described within a **biopsychosocial model**.[14] Pain neuromatrix theory is a psychophysiologic description of this model. Figure 19-2 portrays the pain neuromatrix model. As noted, nervous system inputs enter the body-self pain neuromatrix where they are evaluated. An individualized corresponding output is produced by the brain based on the inputs (current threats) to the individual. In addition to nervous system sensory signaling systems (nociception), additional inputs have the potential to influence the pain experience. Both cognitive- and emotion-related brain areas play a role in the interpretation of threat to the individual. The combination of these inputs (sensory, cognitive, and emotion) contributes to the evaluative process and response to threat. Importantly, the proportion of each input to the pain (body-self) neuromatrix is variable and changes over time based on personal and environmental factors. The body's response to threat is a stress response.[12,15] As such, it is also multidimensional and has implications across many bodily systems. Pain is the most commonly described output, which, by definition, has sensory and affective components. Additional outputs include changes in motor behavior, which are both voluntary and involuntary. Finally, there are changes in stress regulation, such as increases in sympathetic excitation and immune system responses to tissue damage.

An acute ankle injury can be helpful to contextualize the pain neuromatrix. In the initial musculoskeletal injury, activation of nociceptive fibers (sensory signaling systems) sends information on the location of injury to the central nervous system. This information combines with patient thoughts about the

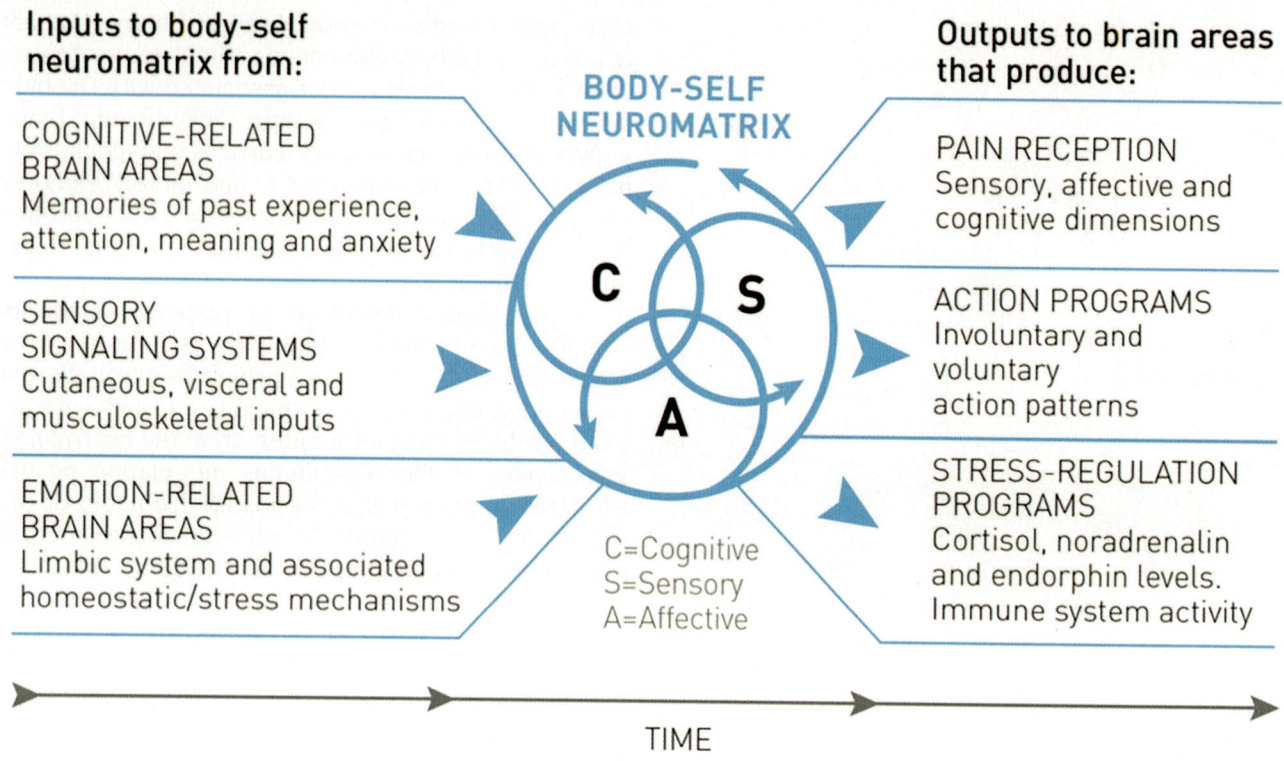

FIGURE 19-2 Pain neuromatrix model. (Melzack R. Pain and the neuromatrix in the brain. *J Dent Educ.* 2001;65: 1378-1382.)

extent of the ankle injury, details about the environment in which the injury occurs (cognitive-related brain areas), and the level of immediate and future impact (emotion-related brain areas). These inputs are continuously sampled and evaluated for threats to determine a response. A typical response could include pain in the area of injury (pain perception), local muscle guarding and decreased weight bearing (action programs), and descending modulation with localized edema (stress regulation programs). These inputs and outputs may fluctuate over time with changes in the internal and external environment of the person.

PAIN TYPES

Many attempts have been made to classify different types of pain. From a musculoskeletal rehabilitation perspective, three primary types of pain have been described: nociceptive, peripheral neuropathic, and nociplastic.[16–19]

Nociceptive Pain

Nociceptive pain specifically describes pain tied to activation of the primary afferents in response to a noxious or threatening stimulus.[17,20] Nociceptive pain arises from actual or threatened damage to non-neural tissue and is due to the activation of nociceptors.[21] Nociceptive pain is commonly linked with chemical mediators from acute tissue injury, ischemic events related to tissue compression or loading, and/or local inflammatory responses.[20] An acute acromioclavicular joint sprain that occurs in response to local ligamentous injury would be a clinical example of nociceptive pain.

Peripheral Neuropathic Pain

Peripheral **neuropathic pain** is pain that is caused by a lesion or disease of the somatosensory system.[16,22–24] Peripheral neuropathic pain is linked with altered nerve functioning and responsiveness in the peripheral nervous system and has been linked with increased neuronal excitability, abnormal impulse generation, and responsiveness to noxious stimuli (chemical, thermal, mechanical) to the peripheral nerve.[22] Median nerve compression within the carpal tunnel (carpal tunnel syndrome) is a typical clinical example of peripheral neuropathic pain.

Nociplastic Pain

Nociplastic pain describes pain that arises from altered nociception, despite no clear evidence of actual or threatened tissue damage causing the activation of peripheral nociceptors or evidence for disease or lesion of the somatosensory system causing the pain.[21] Before the term *nociplastic pain*, central sensitization was regularly used to describe this pain type. *Central sensitization* is defined as increased responsiveness of nociceptive neurons in the central nervous system to their normal or subthreshold afferent input and is a neurophysiologic phenomenon and not a pain type.[25] Thus, nociplastic pain is linked with, but not synonymous with, central sensitization. Nociplastic pain is a maladaptive nervous system dysfunction associated with altered nociceptive processing and increased responsiveness to subthreshold afferent input[19,21,26] and is chronic by definition.[21] Chronic whiplash-associated disorder and fibromyalgia would be common sample diagnoses of nociplastic pain.

The physiologic mechanisms of nociceptive, peripheral neuropathic, and nociplastic pain present differently in the clinic and, therefore, should be treated differently. Nociceptive, peripheral neuropathic, and nociplastic pain have specific clinical features, which aid clinicians in determining the most relevant pain type. Table 19-1 outlines the history findings for patients with the different types of pain. These pain types have excellent diagnostic properties *when clinicians are able to exclusively categorize* patient symptoms based on the clinical presentations listed in the table.[16–18] Patient symptoms often occur across more than one pain type and/or occur along a continuum that limits clinician's ability to precisely categorize patients by pain type. Clinically, the challenge is often determining which pain type predominates so that interventions can be appropriately aligned.

PSYCHOSOCIAL CONSIDERATIONS IN PAIN

When considering the biopsychosocial nature of pain, all aspects of the patient have the potential to impact patient presentation, treatment approaches, and outcomes.

Yellow Flag Screening

Yellow flags are commonly described as psychosocial factors that influence patient outcomes.[27] The most commonly described yellow flags relevant to musculoskeletal practice include emotional distress (anxiety and depression), fear avoidance, pain catastrophizing, self-efficacy, and patient expectation.[27–29]

Self-report tools are the accepted standard for screening and measuring yellow flags. Yellow flag screening is an abbreviated assessment process that should be used in all musculoskeletal patients to determine whether further measurement of psychosocial impairments is necessary. Several reliable and valid multidimensional yellow flag screening tools are

TABLE 19.1
CLINICAL PRESENTATION OF PAIN TYPES

Nociceptive Pain		Peripheral Neuropathic Pain		Nociplastic Pain	
Present	Absent	Present	Absent	Present	Absent
Pain localized to area of injury/dysfunction	Night pain/disturbed sleep	Pain in a dermatomal or cutaneous distribution	NA	Diffuse, nonanatomic areas of pain or tenderness on palpation	NA
Clear anatomic nature to aggravating and easing factors	Pain with other abnormal sensations	History of nerve injury, pathology, or mechanical compromise		Pain disproportionate to nature and extent of injury mechanism	
Usually intermittent and sharp with movement/mechanical provocation: may be more constant throb/ache at rest	Antalgic postures or movement patterns (e.g., constant pain)	Pain or paresthesia with mechanical/movement testing that stress neural tissue (e.g., neurodynamic tests)		Disproportionate, nonmechanical, unpredictable pain pattern in response to multiple/nonspecific aggravating or easing factors	
Associated and proportional with trauma, path process, or movement or posture				Strong association with maladaptive factors (negative emotions, poor self-efficacy, maladaptive beliefs, etc.)	

Modified from Smart KM, Blake C, Staines A, Thacker M, Doody C. Mechanisms based classifications of musculoskeletal pain: part 1 of 3: symptoms and signs of central sensitisation in patients with low back (±leg) pain. *Man Ther*. 2012;17(4):336-344.

Smart KM, Blake C, Staines A, Thacker M, Doody C. Mechanisms-based classifications of musculoskeletal pain: part 2 of 3: symptoms and signs of peripheral neuropathic pain in patients with low back (±leg) pain. *Man Ther*. 2012;17(4):345-351.

Smart KM, Blake C, Staines A, Thacker M, Doody C. Mechanisms-based classifications of musculoskeletal pain: part 3 of 3: symptoms and signs of nociceptive pain in patients with low back (±leg) pain. *Man Ther*. 2012;17(4):352-357.

available to assess psychological constructs within one questionnaire. The Örebro Musculoskeletal Pain Questionnaire[28] and the Optimal Screening for Prediction of Referral and Outcome Yellow Flag (OSPRO-YF)[30] tools are both helpful in screening for psychosocial impairments in patients with a variety of musculoskeletal disorders. The STarT Back screening tool is also used to similar effect and is specifically for patients with low back pain. Cutoff scores on these tools are predictive of poor outcomes in patients with musculoskeletal disorders and should be used as part of the evaluation process for all patients. Figure 19-3 outlines an examination pathway incorporating traditional medical condition/red flag screening with pain type and psychosocial screening.

Measurement Tools for Psychosocial Impairments

In contrast to yellow flag screening, measurement of psychosocial impairments is not necessary in all patients and should be considered when yellow flag screening indicates increased risk of psychosocial impairment or when history findings warrant further investigation (e.g., treatment for or a history of depression). Table 19-2 provides often used measurement tools for common psychosocial impairments found in clinical practice.

TABLE 19-2

COMMONLY USED PSYCHOSOCIAL MEASUREMENT TOOLS BY CONSTRUCT

Psychosocial Factor	Measurement Tool
Depression	• Personal Health Questionnaire-9 (PHQ-9) • Beck Depression Inventory I & II • Hospital Anxiety and Depression Scale (HADS)
Anxiety	• Generalized Anxiety Disorder (GAD-7) • State-Trait Anxiety Inventory (STAI) • Hospital Anxiety and Depression Scale (HADS)
Fear avoidance	• Fear Avoidance Beliefs Questionnaire (FABQ) • Tampa Scale of Kinesiophobia (TSK)
Pain catastrophizing	• Pain Catastrophizing Scale (PCS) • Coping Strategies Questionnaire (CSQ)
Self-efficacy	• Pain Self-Efficacy Questionnaire (PSEQ) • Self-Efficacy for Exercise Scale (SEES) • Arthritis Self-Efficacy Scale (ASES)
Patient expectation	• No known tools available

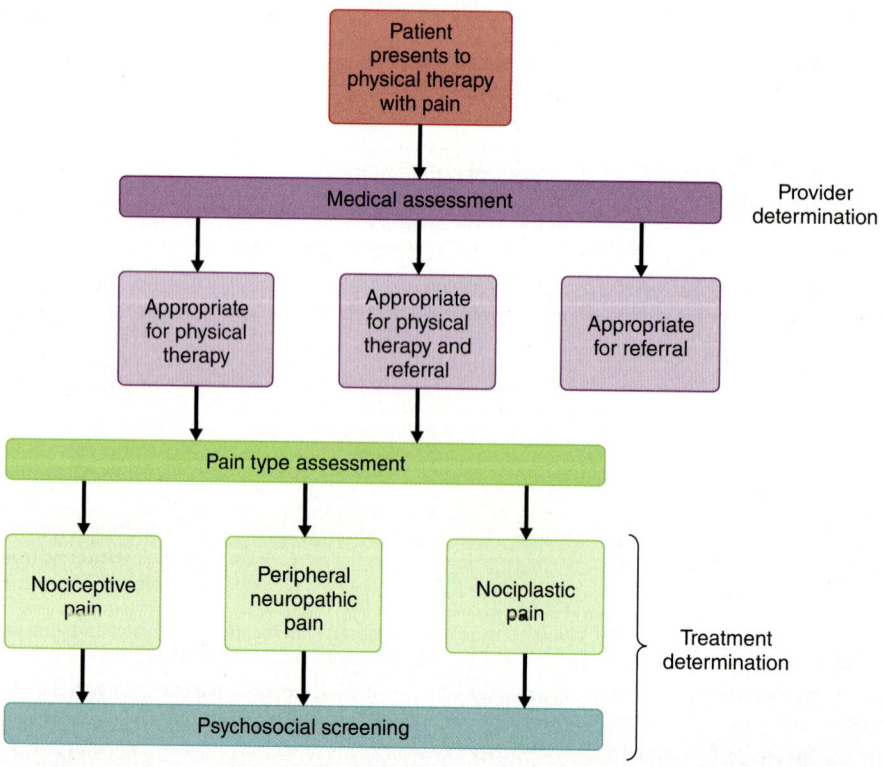

FIGURE 19-3 Proposed clinical decision-making pathway for patients in pain.

INITIAL PAIN ASSESSMENT CONSIDERATIONS

One underlying component of the assessment process should be the development of a therapeutic alliance defined as the working rapport or positive social connection between a patient and health care provider.[31] A therapeutic alliance emphasizes building rapport in order to enhance patient motivation and a sense of ownership over the treatment plan.[32] Establishing a collaborative clinician-patient therapeutic alliance with the patient and their support persons is critical to for successful rehabilitation outcomes.[33] Active listening, shared decision-making, and collaborative goal setting provide excellent opportunities to contribute to a positive therapeutic alliance (Fig. 19-4). Goals that are meaningful to the individual patient need to be defined, in addition to those that can be used as interim milestones. Goal setting should be a cooperative ongoing process, reaffirming or reestablishing these over the course of rehabilitation, if needed.[34,35]

Self-Report Scales

The Patient-Specific Functional Scale (PSFS) is a self-report functional scale that can help clinicians collaborate in goal setting. It is reliable, valid, and applicable for all body regions.[36] This scale asks patients to report their current functional score for several (commonly 3) activities as a proportion of preinjury or another baseline time period. The scale with example scores is shown in Figure 19-5.

When using the PSFS, the clinician is provided with three specific activities that the patient has self-identified as valuable and currently limited. The information from the PSFS can be used to guide both assessment and intervention strategies that are salient to the patient. Reassessment using the same tool can provide information regarding previously identified functional limitations as well as new ones that arise over the course of care. A change score 3 or above for one item or a mean change of 2/10 or above has previously been described as clinically significant.[36]

Pain Measurement and Screening

A plethora of tools are available to measure pain in a patient. The accepted clinical standard to measure pain, particularly acute pain, is patient report using some version of a 10-point scale. This can be a numeric pain rating scale (NPRS) 0 to 10 or a visual analog scale (VAS) whereby the patient indicates her or his level of pain along a 10 cm line (Fig. 19-6). VAS

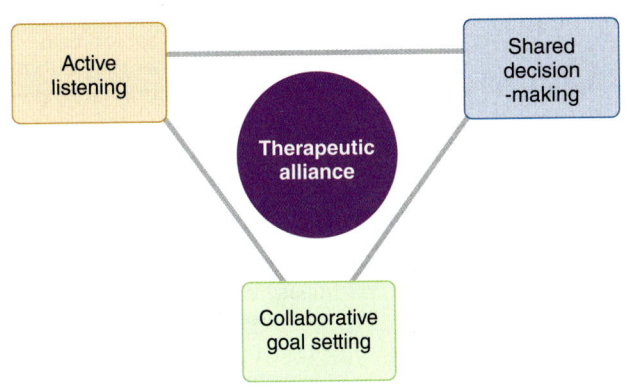

FIGURE 19-4 Clinical opportunities to promote the therapeutic alliance.

Patient-Specific Functional Scale

Directions: Choose three activities in which you are currently limited due to your injury or illness.

Determine your current ability to perform these activities using the scale below.

Patient-specific activity scoring scheme (Select one number which describes your current ability):

0   1   2   3   4   5   6   7   8   9   10

Unable to perform activity — Able to perform activity at the same level as before injury or problem

Activity	Timepoint 1	Timepoint 2	Timepoint 3	Timepoint 4	Timepoint 5
Make dinner	7				
Work full day	3				
Mow lawn	5				

FIGURE 19-5. Example of a patient-specific functional scale. (Adapted from Stratford P, Gill C, Westaway M, Binkley J. Assessing disability and change on individual patients: a report of a patient specific measure. *Physiother Can.* 1995;47(4):258-263.)

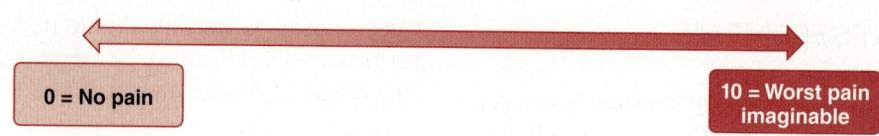

FIGURE 19-6 Visual analog scale along 10 cm line.

scores are then measured to determine the distance along the line, which is recorded as the patient's pain level. Pain measurement using the abovementioned methods is reliable and valid.[37,38] A change of 2/10 or 2 cm is commonly used to represent a clinically meaningful change in pain levels.[37–39]

Pain measurement should have two primary aims. One aim is to determine patient symptoms during a repeatable functional task. For example, if a patient's functional complaints include stair negotiation, pain should be measured *during that task* at baseline and at follow-up time periods to determine whether symptoms are changing. A second aim is to determine whether a patient's pain levels are ever 0/10 and if so during what are the conditions where this is the case. Although commonly assessed, patients' highest or worst pain level over a recent time period should be avoided as patient's pain memory has been shown to be unreliable.[40]

Several detailed self-reported pain measurement tools that may be considered for specialty pain clinics or clinical research are noted in Table 19-3 with additional supporting details.

Physical Examination Tools

Physical examination tools may also be used to objectively measure musculoskeletal pain. Pressure algometry is often used to this end, particularly for patients with chronic pain. Performance of pressure algometry involves perpendicular application of force, with an instrumented tool, to the surface of the skin that is applied slowly and with steadily increasing amounts of force. The **algometer** should be applied to the most painful site and should measure the force when the sensation *first becomes painful*, that is, the pain pressure threshold (Fig. 19-7). Force values are used to quantify regional sensitivity with increased pressure thresholds (higher force) associated with decreased sensitivity (pain) whereas decreased thresholds demonstrate the opposite. Pressure algometry has been shown to be reliable and valid. Normative values have been determined across the life span.[41,42] Clinically important differences have been described as a 15 to 25% difference from baseline.[43–45]

Patient self-report outcomes should be also used to determine pain impact on patients' function. In addition to PSFS, many other region-specific tools can be utilized for relevant patients with musculoskeletal pain. Specific examples include the Neck Disability Index, the Shoulder Pain and Disability Index, and the Lower Extremity Functional Scale.

TABLE 19-3
PAIN MEASUREMENT TOOLS

Pain Measurement Tool	Context and Use Considerations
McGill Pain Questionnaire[a]	20 questions tool that includes multiple pain categories (symptoms, affective components, evaluative components, etc.)
PEG-3[b]	Three questions screening tool to assess pain interference for **P**ain, **E**njoyment, and **G**eneral activity.
Pain DETECT Tool[c]	Seven questions tool to help determine whether the patient is experiencing peripheral neuropathic pain
Douleur Neuropathique (DN-4)[d]	Four questions (10-item) tool to help determine whether the patient is experiencing peripheral neuropathic pain
Brief Pain Inventory[e]	Nine questions tool that measures pain intensity and interference
Chronic Pain Grade Scale[f]	7-item tool used to measure pain intensity and pain-related disability in patients with chronic pain
Short-Form 36 Bodily Pain Scale (SF-36 BPS)[g]	36-item tool that measures pain intensity and interference

[a]Melzack R. The McGill Pain Questionnaire: major properties and scoring methods. *Pain.* 1975;1(3):277–299.

[b]Krebs EE, Lorenz KA, Bair MJ, et al. Development and initial validation of the PEG, a three-item scale assessing pain intensity and interference. *J Gen Intern Med.* 2009;24(6):733–738.

[c]Freynhagen R, Baron R, Gockel U, Tölle TR. Pain DETECT: a new screening questionnaire to identify neuropathic components in patients with back pain. *Curr Med Res Opin.* 2006;22(10):1911–1920.

[d]Bouhassira D, Attal N, Alchaar H, et al. Comparison of pain syndromes associated with nervous or somatic lesions and development of a new neuropathic pain diagnostic questionnaire (DN4). *Pain.* 2005;114(1–2):29–36.

[e]Cleeland C, Ryan K. Pain assessment: global use of the Brief Pain Inventory. *Ann Acad Med Singap.* 1994;23(2):129–138.

[f]Von Korff M, Ormel J, Keefe FJ, Dworkin SF. Grading the severity of chronic pain. *Pain.* 1992;50(2):133–149.

[g]Ware J, Kosinski M, Keller S. *SF-36 Physical and Mental Health Summary Scales. A User's Manual.* 2001:1994.

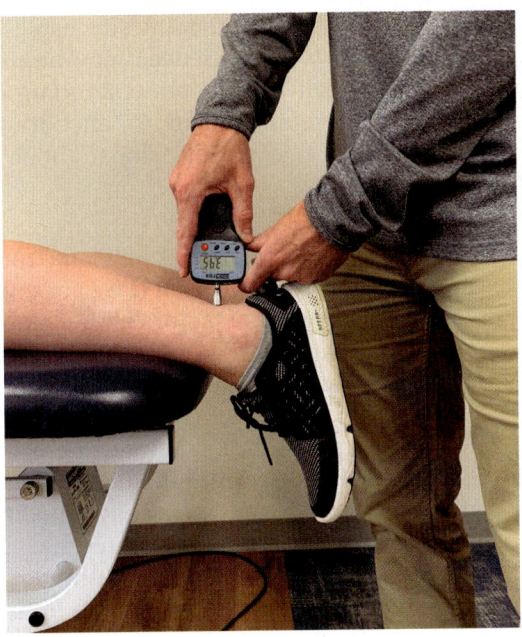

FIGURE 19-7 Pressure algometry.

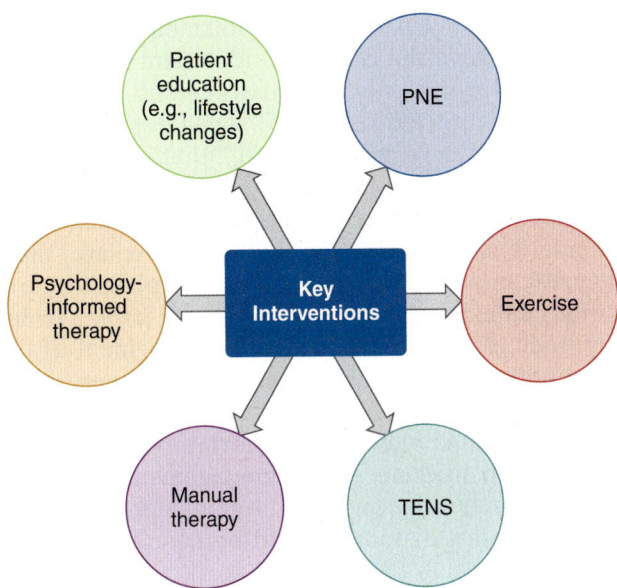

FIGURE 19-8 Key interventions. *TENS*, transcutaneous electrical nerve stimulation; *PNE*, pain neuroscience education.

Functional and Performance Assessment

Finally, patient function, performance, and other reported impairments should be measured. Numerous functional and performance tests are available to assess patients based on described functional limitations. Common examples include timed walk tests for distance (2 or 6 minutes),[25,46,47] Sit-to-Stand tests (five times or 30 seconds),[47,48] Timed Up and Go test,[49] timed functional arm and shoulder test,[50] and so on. Additional potential impairments that may be relevant to measure outcomes for patients with musculoskeletal pain include satisfaction scores with activities and rehabilitation,[51,52] sleep quality and duration,[53] daily fatigue as well as emotional and physical well-being and quality of life.[51,52]

INTERVENTIONS

Intervention selection should be based on an understanding of the patient's biologic (pain type), psychological (yellow flag), and social contributing factors to their pain and disability. These details should be integrated relevant mechanisms behind the chosen interventions. Patient education, self-management support, and exercise are considered the primary interventions for long-term rehabilitation for patients with musculoskeletal pain.[54-57] Passive interventions, such as electrophysical agents and manual therapy, can be used as adjuncts to modulate pain and promote active self-management strategies. Generic principles of these interventions (Fig. 19-8) are outlined in the subsequent section.

Patient-Specific Health Education and Self-Management Support

Patients' health literacy, expectations of treatment, as well as personal attributes, such as self-efficacy, influence treatment outcomes.[58,59] Unhelpful beliefs about pain may lead to avoidance behavior. Patients who understand their health condition are empowered to share in the decision-making process and take greater responsibility for the self-management of their condition[60]—improving health status, well-being, quality of life, and satisfaction with health care.[59,61,62] Patients with poor understanding of their condition (pain) and how to self-manage it (poor health literacy) may have poorer health outcomes, increased emergency care use, focus on passive interventions or "quick fixes," and lower use of preventive health care.[59,63,64] Lack of appropriate advice and education may lead to excessive patient dependence on the clinician, reduce self-efficacy or participation in rehabilitation, or increase fear and anxiety.

The main purpose of health education for people with musculoskeletal-related pain is to empower them to self-manage their condition, their health status, and quality of life. Using a person-centered approach, the focus should be on the patient's understanding of their pain in their context and to participate actively in collaborative decision-making through concordance in care. That is, the clinician should facilitate a deeper understanding of the reasons for decision-making and to consider their goals, preferences, beliefs, barriers, and facilitators for exercise and other lifestyle modifications.[65] A patient education focusing on cooperation between the clinician and patient (i.e., adherence to collaborative interventions versus compliance to clinician-directed activities) facilitates a partnership relationship in rehabilitation,[65] thereby contributing to and strengthening the therapeutic alliance.[66]

Educational strategies for pain self-management include basic information about immediate management of acute (nociceptive or peripheral neuropathic) pain. For nociplastic or chronic pain, a wider approach is needed, such as self-management of the pain and recurrences, when and where to seek health care, exercise and exercise prescription, and lifestyle factors, such as managing comorbidities and nutrition.[67] Sleep hygiene, stress management, and coping skills may also need to be considered.[67,68] The patient's social support should be considered, such as support within the family, at work, sports, and in the communities. Such information needs to be individualized to the person and their social support, relevant for their context.

Delivery of Patient Health Education Provision of education is an opportunity to engage with the patient and their support network. Patient education may be delivered during individual clinical sessions or in groups.[69] The education may be woven into conversations with the patients, providing "bits" of information rather than a stand-alone delivery. The patient should be encouraged to apply strategies and ways of thinking to their daily lives and to reflectively share feedback with the clinician and explore further questions. Delivery of patient health education may be supported with leaflets, audiovisual methods, websites, and Applications (Apps).[70] Face-to-face or teleconferencing sessions can be helpful.

Patient education often overlaps with psychological-informed interventions, such as using motivational interviewing to explore the patient's goals, beliefs, and abilities.[66,71] Coaching principles may be used for change of health and activity behavior.[70] Examples of psychological-informed interventions are cognitive-behavioral therapy,[72] cognitive functional therapy,[73,74] stress inoculation training,[75] and acceptance and commitment therapy.[76] These approaches have been integrated with activity- and exercise-based treatment strategies and used as part of management of persistent musculoskeletal pain,[77] shoulder pain,[78] osteoarthritis,[79] and lower back pain.[73,80,81]

Content of Patient Health Information Traditionally, patient education for musculoskeletal pain has focused mainly on the diagnosis and pathoanatomy, exercise prescription, and biomechanical-related factors (e.g., considerations of ergonomics and posture).[68,82] Biomedical diagnoses may be important to estimate prognosis and to guide referral to further investigations. Recent understanding suggests that including contemporary pain sciences may be needed to help the patient gain deeper understanding of the importance of interventions and to encourage active involvement in making decisions about their rehabilitations.

Pain Neuroscience Education Clinicians may include **pain neuroscience education** (PNE) to enhance the patients understanding of factors influencing their pain experience and appropriate self-management and self-care strategies. In essence, PNE aims to change how the patient makes sense of their pain using a positive, enabling approach.[57] Traditionally, pain was considered a "warning or marker of underlying tissue damage or disease process." Such conceptualization most likely led to the belief that chronic pain treatments should address the primary pathology. The PNE reconceptualizes pain as a "protector" or need to protect the body from harm[83] and leads the clinician and patient to place less emphasis on the "damaged structure" and harmful behaviors and more emphasis on the multifactorial dimensions of pain.

The patient's thoughts and beliefs about their pain and expectations for treatment should be established.[84] Such expectations may include their thoughts about recovery as well as value of specific interventions. For example, the clinician may explore the patient's thoughts and experiences about physical activity and exercise and their pain behavior. The yellow flag screening tools discussed previously can provide insight into potentially maladaptive patient beliefs (i.e., low expectations or pain catastrophizing). The specific PNE provided to the patient will be modified based on their beliefs, often influenced by their cultural and ethnic background. The PNE explored with the patient and their support persons may include considerations of neurophysiologic mechanisms of how the nervous system transfers messages from the periphery to the brain and how the brain interprets those messages. Those messages may be those of "danger" in addition to the direction and the space in which they move. The sensitivity of the nervous system to interpret the "danger" messages can change due to various factors, which can include comorbidities (such as type 2 diabetes) and lifestyle (sedentariness, stress, and nutrition). The clinician thus explores various dimensions with the patient, including biologic, psychological, and social factors. Such factors may be explained to the person as influencing the sensitivity of their nervous system and thereby for their pain. Specific guidelines and resources are available for patient education/PNE for patients with persistent musculoskeletal pain.[85–88]

The addition of PNE to therapy for people with chronic pain conditions may improve pain and disability in the short- and long-term outcomes for pain,[69] as well as decrease fear avoidance and pain catastrophizing.[77] PNE has been shown to be most effective for pain when combined with movement or exercise interventions compared to educational interventions alone.[77] The PNE may enhance the patient's understanding that reversing the biologic consequences of persistent pain takes time and that persevering with exercise and activity is important. The PNE has been applied to various persistent pain conditions, such as low back pain,[89] rotator cuff–related shoulder pain,[90,91] adhesive capsulitis or frozen shoulder,[92] osteoarthritis,[93] whiplash,[75] and others.[69] Adding PNE may also lead to behavioral changes, such as decreased health care utilization by people with low back pain, decreased sick leave days, and decreased health care costs, possibly reflecting improved self-efficacy.[77]

Exercise Prescription

Exercise prescription and the promotion of activity and/or movement is a core component of therapy for people with all pain types to increase their physical, cognitive, and emotional capacity.[91] The mechanisms by which movement-based interventions decrease pain is debated. Proposed mechanisms include physical, biomechanical, cardiometabolic, neurophysiologic, and psychological adaptations to increased movement and activity.[94,95] Thus, besides improving muscle strength, endurance, and aerobic capacity, exercise can reduce pain sensitivity in people with musculoskeletal pain.[96,97] Physical exercise increased functional connectivity between brain regions in healthy adults[98]; decreased pain sensitivity via descending pain modulation, as seen after aerobic exercise in athletes and others[99,100]; improved psychological impairments such as anxiety and depression[101,102]; and helped comorbid pain and health conditions, such as diabetes.[103] Given the diverse range of described mechanisms to decrease pain, it should not be surprising that systematic reviews of comparative effectiveness trials often indicate equivocal results for activity- (including graded activity) and exercise-based interventions.[104–107] Choosing an optimal or "best" exercise or therapeutic activity is currently not feasible. Therefore, the prescription of exercise should be tailored to the individual patient and consider their needs in a comprehensive biopsychosocial assessment.[57] The exercise interventions should be based on the patient's presentations, goals, and preferences, such as revealed in the PSFS. The patient should consider the selected exercises to be safe, nonthreatening, and meaningful for their lives and goals.[57] Table 19-4 outlines general aerobic and resistance exercise principles for patients with musculoskeletal pain. Exercise- and other movement-based

TABLE 19-4
GUIDING EXERCISE PRINCIPLES FOR MUSCULOSKELETAL PAIN

Aerobic Exercise

Intensity HR equivalents	• Low intensity: 40 < 55% HR_{max} • Moderate intensity: 55 < 70% HR_{max} • High intensity: 70–90% HR_{max}
Frequency	≥2 times/week; ≥6 weeks
Intensity	Low intensity (RPE 8–10) to moderate intensity (RPE 11–13); higher intensity (RPE 14–16) for goals involving more demanding work, sport or recreation where tolerated
Time	20–60 and <20 minutes with exercise intolerance. Shorter intervals can be interspersed with other exercise modalities (e.g., 3 × 7-minute walking separated by resistance exercise)
Type	Continuous and rhythmic exercises that engage major muscle groups (such as walking, jogging, swimming), but do not exacerbate symptoms
Progression	Commence RPE 8–10 grading to RPE 11–13 as tolerance increases; RPE >14 for high-intensity training Increase duration before intensity (e.g., for treadmill walking increase duration and walking speed before incline)

Resistance Exercise

Intensity 1RM equivalents	• Low intensity: 40 < 60% 1RM • Moderate intensity: 60–70% 1RM • High intensity: ≥70% 1RM
Frequency	2–3 times/week; ≥6 weeks
Intensity	Low-intensity (RPE 8–10) to moderate-intensity exercise (RPE 11–13) For more demanding work, sport or recreation consider high-intensity training (RPE 14–16)
Time	For low- to moderate-intensity exercise, 1–2 sets of 15–20 repetitions reduced/adapted for exercise intolerance. For high-intensity exercise, 1–2 sets of 8–12 repetitions
Type	Modalities that engage muscles of affected body part(s) and/or major muscle groups (weight-bearing activity, free weights, floor exercise; machines, resistance bands, motor control exercise, etc.) that do not exacerbate symptoms
Progression	Commence RPE 8–10 increasing to RPE 11–13 as tolerance and function increases; RPE >14 for higher intensity training Increase repetitions before load; commence floor exercise with short holds and higher repetitions and increase hold duration before exercise difficulty. For functional exercise, commence at a level specific to patient's presentation and increase repetitions before load

Adapted from Booth J, Moseley GL, Schiltenwolf M, Cashin A, Davies M, Hübscher M. Exercise for chronic musculoskeletal pain: a biopsychosocial approach. *Musculoskeletal Care.* 2017;15(4):413–421.

interventions, such as yoga or tai chi, are advocated for nociceptive, peripheral neuropathic, and nociplastic pain types.

Various factors influence the level of supervision and optimal intensity and dosage for exercise. Besides the patient's physical capacity, their level of fear avoidance, previous levels of activity, and self-efficacy and confidence levels may guide decision-making. Risk stratification via yellow flag screening tools (e.g., STarT Back) can also be useful. For chronic or nociplastic pain, pain should not be avoided during exercise.[108] Patients need to understand that it is safe to exercise with at levels of discomfort with which they can cope with. An "acceptable level" of pain, possibly defined on an NPRS, and a time frame for the pain to subside (e.g., within 24 hours) should be negotiated with the patient.[109] Exercises should be modified when needed, for example, with excessive or intolerable pain exacerbations. Frequent reassurance may be needed that it is safe to progressively become active, despite persisting symptoms.[57] A daily or weekly recording or diary of physical activity may help the patient identify their barriers and facilitators for such activities. Patients should be supported in a long-term maintenance program.

Electrical Modalities

Transcutaneous electrical nerve stimulation (TENS) will be used as the example modality, given the large amount of evidence evaluating its use. Recent systematic reviews indicate the evidence for TENS is often of low quality with equivocal or limited effectiveness for musculoskeletal pain conditions.[110] The cited reason is often tied to the varied parameters and application procedures across studies. The recommendations in this section are to link mechanistic basic science research with clinical application to promote best practice use of TENS in clinical practice.[111,112]

TENS has been advocated for a variety of pain types with different mechanisms of action based on patient characteristics. Conventional TENS was initially developed and described for use to gate or decrease nociceptive (C-fiber) afferents transmission within the dorsal horn of the spinal cord,[112–114] occurring via activation of large diameter (A-Δ-fibers) acting through an interneuron at the segmental level (e.g., gate theory).[113] The type described is commonly referred to as conventional or "low intensity" TENS. Conventional TENS is, therefore, beneficial for pain associated with nociception (nociceptive and nociplastic pain) when applied locally to the involved areas.[111] The setup parameters for low-intensity TENS include alternating between high (100–150 Hz) and low (0–50 Hz) frequency settings with pulse duration around 200 microseconds at an intensity that is most comfortable for the patient.

Using different application parameters, TENS has also been described to promote the release of endogenous opioids in the brain, which results in descending inhibition of nociception,[111,112,114] commonly referred to as high-intensity or "acupuncture-like" TENS. High-intensity TENS, therefore, produces a more global or systemic effect. The setup parameters for high-intensity TENS also include alternating between high (100–150 Hz) and low (0–50 Hz) frequency settings with pulse duration around 200 microseconds, yet the sensation should be "strong but tolerable." There appears to be a dose-response relationship between high-intensity TENS and analgesic effect, so encouraging the patient to routinely evaluate and increase intensity as tolerated may be considered. Owing to the different mechanism of action, high-intensity TENS may be applied at any location on the body because the response to the modality is systemic.[111,112] The varied placement of electrodes may be helpful for patients with contraindications or sensitivity to local electrode placement. Emerging evidence suggests that low-intensity TENS may also promote descending inhibition via similar mechanisms as high-intensity TENS.[111]

Beyond contraindications, clinical decision-making regarding the frequency settings on the use of TENS should also include current and past opioid medication usage. High-frequency TENS activates Δ opioid receptors, whereas low-frequency TENS activates μ opioid receptors.[115] Patients taking oral opioid medication or who are opioid tolerant are more likely to benefit from high-frequency (100–150 Hz) TENS. Oral opioids are most commonly μ opioids; thus, introducing more μ opioids in a system that has an excess already will not benefit the analgesic response.[112,116] Similarly, patients who are opioid tolerant may not exhibit any response from attempts to activate endogenous opioid release.[112,116,117]

Lastly, TENS analgesic action is primarily beneficial for evoked or movement-related pain, which is very common in musculoskeletal rehabilitation.[9,118] Thus, TENS is most appropriately used while performing painful movements or activities to decrease nociception via gating or descending mechanisms. Correspondingly, TENS is unlikely to be beneficial for resting pain or when used at rest. A sample patient vignette, Case Study 19-1, is used to apply components of TENS use and pain outcome measurement.

> ### CASE STUDY 19-1
> *Thelma: Patient with Fibromyalgia*
>
> Thelma is a 54-year-old middle school teacher with a 3-year history of fibromyalgia. Thelma is currently taking pregabalin for this condition. Her pain is variable but constant (rarely 0/10). In the past, her pain was linked with increased activity and/or work demands, yet this has been less apparent of late.
>
> **TENS considerations**: Her pain appears to be primarily nociplastic. No evidence is available that indicates a contraindication for TENS in this patient (pacemaker, skin damage, local cancer, etc.). Pad location should be at the primary site of pain if possible. Suggested device parameters include mixed frequency (2 to 125 Hz), strong but tolerable intensity, variable pulse duration from 100 to 250 microseconds. TENS should be applied when the patient is active during usual daily activities and while performing rehab activities at home or in the clinic.
>
> **Outcome measures:** Thelma's outcomes could be evaluated using a relevant functional task, such as Five Times Sit-to-Stand Test with outcomes for functional performance (time to complete) and potentially pain during the task (NPRS 0-10). Additional holistic outcomes may include sleep quality (Pittsburgh Sleep Quality Index) or quality of life (SF-36).

Manual Therapy

Manual therapy describes a broad collection of therapeutic techniques that involve skillful application of forces by the clinician to a patient with the aims of decreasing symptoms or improving other impairments, such as decreased motion.[119] The potential mechanisms behind the use of manual therapy have historically described a biomechanical process, yet these mechanisms have not been supported in research.[120,121] Current theory outlining potential mechanisms behind manual therapy offers a primarily neurophysiologic mechanism with biomechanical and psychological contributing aspects (Fig. 19-9).[52,120]

Manual therapies address pain via changes in the peripheral and central nervous system.[52] In the periphery, nociceptive chemicals (e.g., cytokines, substance P) have been shown to abate, whereas anti-nociceptive (e.g., serotonin, cannabinoids) mediators are demonstrated to increase immediately follow locally applied manual therapies.[122-126] Reported spinal cord–mediated changes with manual therapy include dorsal horn nociceptive gating with activation of proprioceptive neurons, changes in muscle and motor neuron pool activity, and hypoalgesia.[19,120,127,128] Lastly, brain-related changes have been described, which include many brain regions and connections between regions known to be linked to decreased pain responses (sensorimotor cortices, anterior cingulate cortex, insular cortex, etc.).[126,129,130] Other central nervous system–mediated changes from manual therapy are tied to shifts in autonomic nervous system function associated, which may contribute to decreased pain perception.[52,129,131] The individual responses to manual therapy are unique to each person; however, it is known that the overall effect is a transient decrease in pain that is often tied to increased function.[122,123]

Manual therapy, as a procedural intervention, will be described from an overarching perspective without detail on the specific manual therapy techniques (joint based, soft tissue, nerve focused, instrument assisted, etc.) because the described mechanisms are similar between techniques and pain outcomes have often been reported equivocal in systematic reviews.[49,132-135] The choice of technique should, therefore, depend on patient factors, such as disease or injury conditions, preferences, past experiences, and expectations, and therapist-specific details, such as skill, training, comfort, experience, and expectations. Manual interventions are advocated for both acute and chronic pain and all three pain types (nociception, peripheral neuropathic, and nociplastic).[19] Similar to TENS, manual interventions are reported to be more effective for movement, or evoked, pain compared to resting pain. Accordingly, outcomes should be focused on movement or activity as opposed to the sensory component (pain scores) alone. Additional suggested pain-related outcomes include physical and emotional functioning, global improvements (satisfaction), and the use of additional interventions for pain, such as pharmacologic use.[51]

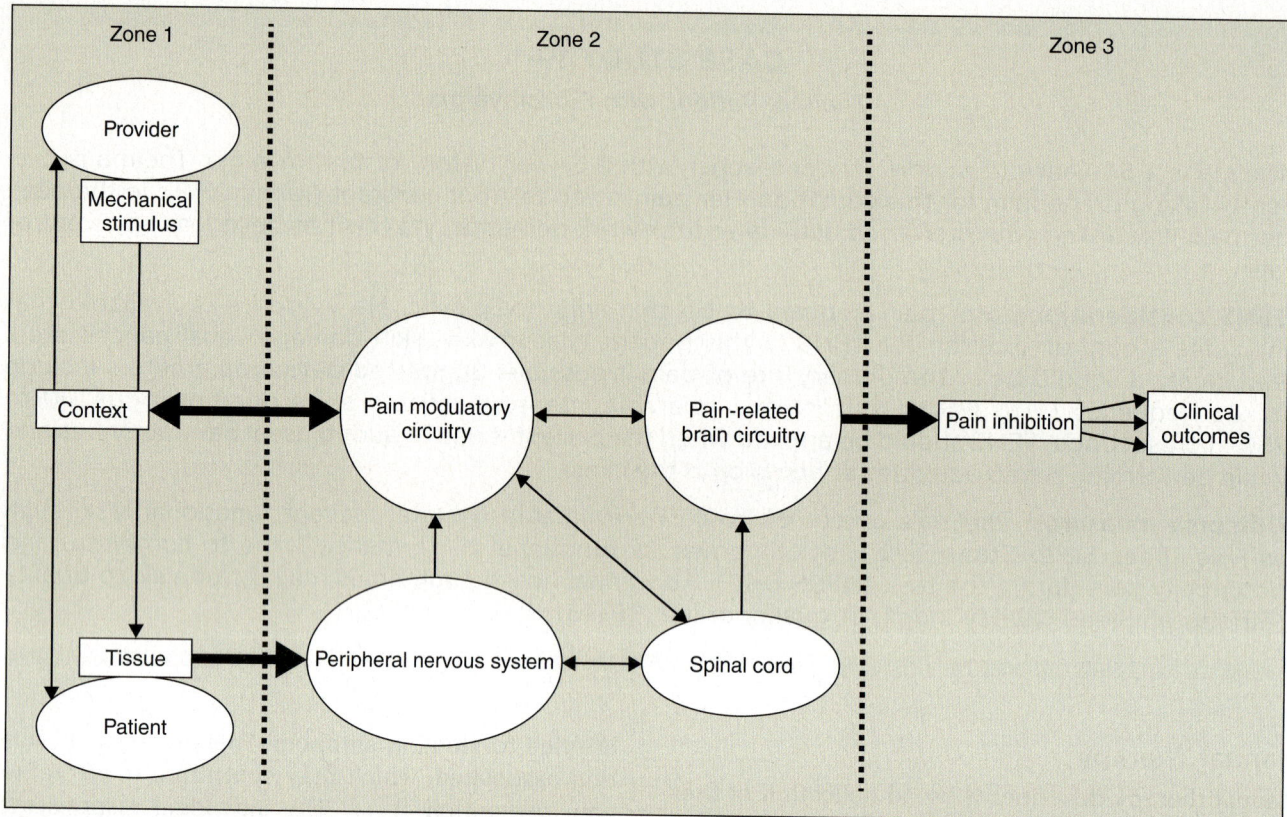

FIGURE 19-9 Mechanistic model of manual therapy. (Bialosky JE, Beneciuk JM, Bishop MD, et al. Unraveling the mechanisms of manual therapy: modeling an approach. *J Orthop Sports Phys Ther*. 2018;48(1):8–18.)

Clinical decision-making for all techniques, including manual therapies, must first consider contraindications and patient preference against manual treatment. Once these are ruled out, the type of manual intervention and sequence of interventions within a treatment session can be considered. As noted earlier, manual therapies affect multiple bodily systems, including the peripheral and central nervous system, with both local and systemic effects. Therefore, the type of manual intervention to use may be less important than other factors.[52,126] Emerging evidence links psychological components to the effectiveness of manual interventions.[52,126,136] Patient and provider beliefs, expectations, and experiences can all impact pain outcomes. The benefits from manual therapy may be enhanced by guiding patient expectations toward specific outcomes. For example, a patient with an expectation of benefit from manual therapy may have additional benefit from that treatment compared to a patient with neutral or negative expectations from the same treatment.[137] Therapists may discuss various options of manual therapy with patients to determine whether a preference exists and/or offer guidance on anticipated benefits of manual therapy to promote improved outcomes for patients.

Manual therapy should be viewed as an adjunctive treatment as opposed to a stand-alone intervention.[138] The overarching aim of manual therapies should be used to promote movement and functionally related activities or exercises that are salient to each patient. Manual therapies have been advocated, without known evidence, to be used *before* participation in active treatment activities, such as focused or general movements or exercise. Theoretically, this allows the patient to engage in exercise or other movement activities with less pain than if not preceded by manual treatments. Similarly, this may promote engagement in higher intensity activities with tolerable symptom (pain) levels.[139] Contrarily, clinicians may consider using manual therapies following all other interventions to conclude the treatment session with a pain-relieving effect. This may promote an overall positive experience of therapy via the peak-end phenomenon. A sample patient vignette, Case Study 19-2, is used to apply components of manual therapy use and pain outcome measurement.

CASE STUDY 19-2
Wilson: Patient with Post-Traumatic Knee Arthritis

Patient details: Wilson is a 46-year-old attorney with post-traumatic knee arthritis following anterior cruciate ligament repair in his early 20s. He is very active performing daily exercise and parenting his four active children. He reports knee pain and stiffness, mostly when he first gets up in the AM. Oral nonsteroidal anti-inflammatory medications are effective in treating evening pain if he has been particularly busy that day

Manual therapy considerations: Wilson's clinical details suggest nociceptive-type pain. No evidence is available, which indicates a contraindication for manual therapy in this patient (active infection, collagen disease, vascular disorders, etc.). Manual treatments may consist of joint-specific (tibiofemoral and patellofemoral glides) and soft-tissues techniques (quadriceps, peripatellar connective tissue, hamstrings, etc.) used before cycling and dynamic balance exercises in the clinic.

Outcome measures: Wilson's pain should be evaluated using a numeric pain scale (0 to 10) during his activity-based interventions (cycling and balance exercises).

CHAPTER SUMMARY

Many patients may seek therapeutic intervention for pain. Understanding pain physiology, psychosocial variables, multisystem responses, and pain types should be helpful in the examination and treatment of patients with musculoskeletal pain. Specific considerations for intervention techniques should incorporate best research evidence, intervention mechanisms, as well as clinician expertise and patient preferences within the context of shared decision-making. The focus should be on active participation of the patient and collaborative clinician-patient interactions for setting goals, decision-making, and prescription of physical activity and exercises. Patient understanding of their pain, as well as their barriers and facilitators for physical activity, is crucial for continuation of long-term activity. Long-term self-management support may be needed to enhance self-efficacy, confidence, and reassurance.

REFERENCES

1. Fishman SM, Young HM, Lucas Arwood E, et al. Core competencies for pain management: results of an interprofessional consensus summit. *Pain Med.* 2013;14(7):971–981.
2. Bement MKH, Sluka KA. The current state of physical therapy pain curricula in the United States: a faculty survey. *J Pain.* 2015;16(2):144–152.
3. Bement MKH, St Marie BJ, Nordstrom TM, et al. An interprofessional consensus of core competencies for prelicensure education in pain management: curriculum application for physical therapy. *Phys Ther.* 2014;94(4):451–465.
4. Dutmer AL, Preuper HRS, Soer R, et al. Personal and societal impact of low back pain: the Groningen spine cohort. *Spine.* 2019;44(24):E1443–E1451.
5. Hartvigsen J, Hancock MJ, Kongsted A, et al. What low back pain is and why we need to pay attention. *Lancet.* 2018;391(10137):2356–2367.
6. Buchbinder R, van Tulder M, Öberg B, et al. Low back pain: a call for action. *Lancet.* 2018;391(10137):2384–2388.
7. Simon LS. Relieving pain in America: a blueprint for transforming prevention, care, education, and research. *J Pain Palliat Care Pharmacother.* 2012;26(2):197–198.
8. Dahlhamer J, Lucas J, Zelaya C, et al. Prevalence of chronic pain and high-impact chronic pain among adults—United States, 2016. *MMWR Morb Mortal Wkly Rep.* 2018;67(36):1001–1006.
9. Raja SN, Carr DB, Cohen M, et al. The revised International Association for the Study of Pain definition of pain: concepts, challenges, and compromises. *Pain.* 2020;161(9):1976–1982.
10. Mertens P, Blond S, David R, Rigoard P. Anatomy, physiology and neurobiology of the nociception: a focus on low back pain (part A). *Neurochirurgie.* 2015;61:S22–S34.
11. Huether SE, McCance KL, Parkinson CF. *Study Guide for Understanding Pathophysiology—E-Book.* Elsevier Health Sciences; 2013.
12. Melzack R. Pain and the neuromatrix in the brain. *J Dent Educ.* 2001;65(12):1378–1382.
13. Moseley G. A pain neuromatrix approach to patients with chronic pain. *Man Ther.* 2003;8(3):130–140.
14. Engel GL. The biopsychosocial model and the education of health professionals. *Ann N Y Acad Sci.* 1978;310(1):169–181.
15. Crombez G, Eccleston C, Van Damme S, Vlaeyen JW, Karoly P. Fear-avoidance model of chronic pain: the next generation. *Clin J Pain.* 2012;28(6):475–483.
16. Smart KM, Blake C, Staines A, Thacker M, Doody C. Mechanisms-based classifications of musculoskeletal pain: part 2 of 3: symptoms and signs of peripheral neuropathic pain in patients with low back (±leg) pain. *Man Ther.* 2012;17(4):345–351.
17. Smart KM, Blake C, Staines A, Thacker M, Doody C. Mechanisms-based classifications of musculoskeletal pain: part 3 of 3: symptoms and signs of nociceptive pain in patients with low back (±leg) pain. *Man Ther.* 2012;17(4):352–357.
18. Smart KM, Blake C, Staines A, Thacker M, Doody C. Mechanisms-based classifications of musculoskeletal pain: part 1 of 3: symptoms and signs of central

sensitisation in patients with low back (±leg) pain. *Man Ther.* 2012;17(4):336–344.
19. Chimenti RL, Frey-Law LA, Sluka KA. A mechanism-based approach to physical therapist management of pain. *Phys Ther.* 2018;98(5):302–314.
20. Woolf CJ. What is this thing called pain? *J Clin Invest.* 2010;120(11):3742–3744.
21. Kosek E, Cohen M, Baron R, et al. Do we need a third mechanistic descriptor for chronic pain states? *Pain.* 2016;157(7):1382–1386.
22. Colloca L, Ludman T, Bouhassira D, et al. Neuropathic pain. *Nat Rev Dis Primers.* 2017;3(1):1–19.
23. Jensen TS, Baron R, Haanpää M, et al. A new definition of neuropathic pain. *Pain.* 2011;152(10):2204–2205.
24. Treede R-D, Jensen T, Campbell J, et al. Neuropathic pain: redefinition and a grading system for clinical and research purposes. *Neurology.* 2008;70(18):1630–1635.
25. Trouvin A-P, Perrot S. New concepts of pain. *Best Pract Res Clin Rheumatol.* 2019;33(3):101415.
26. Woolf CJ. Central sensitization: uncovering the relation between pain and plasticity. *Anesthesiology.* 2007;106(4):864–867.
27. Nicholas MK, Linton SJ, Watson PJ, Main CJ, Group DotFW. Early identification and management of psychological risk factors ("yellow flags") in patients with low back pain: a reappraisal. *Phys Ther.* 2011;91(5):737–753.
28. Linton SJ, Nicholas M, MacDonald S. Development of a short form of the Örebro Musculoskeletal Pain Screening Questionnaire. *Spine.* 2011;36(22):1891–1895.
29. Foster NE, Delitto A. Embedding psychosocial perspectives within clinical management of low back pain: integration of psychosocially informed management principles into physical therapist practice—challenges and opportunities. *Phys Ther.* 2011;91(5):790–803.
30. Lentz TA, Beneciuk JM, Bialosky JE, et al. Development of a yellow flag assessment tool for orthopaedic physical therapists: results from the optimal screening for prediction of referral and outcome (OSPRO) cohort. *J Orthop Sports Phys Ther.* 2016;46(5):327–343.
31. Crepeau EB, Garren KR. I looked to her as a guide: the therapeutic relationship in hand therapy. *Disabil Rehabil.* 2011;33(10):872–881.
32. Horvath AO, Luborsky L. The role of the therapeutic alliance in psychotherapy. *J Consult Clin Psychol.* 1993;61(4):561–573.
33. Pinto RZ, Ferreira ML, Oliveira VC, et al. Patient-centred communication is associated with positive therapeutic alliance: a systematic review. *J Physiother.* 2012;58(2):77–87.
34. Gardner T, Refshauge K, McAuley J, Goodall S, Hübscher M, Smith L. Patient led goal setting in chronic low back pain—what goals are important to the patient and are they aligned to what we measure? *Patient Educ Couns.* 2015;98(8):1035–1038.
35. Gardner T, Refshauge K, McAuley J, Goodall S, Hübscher M, Smith L. Patient-led goal setting: a pilot study investigating a promising approach for the management of chronic low back pain. *Spine.* 2016;41(18):1405–1413.
36. Stratford P, Gill C, Westaway M, Binkley J. Assessing disability and change on individual patients: a report of a patient specific measure. *Physiother Can.* 1995;47(4):258–263.
37. Hawker GA, Mian S, Kendzerska T, French M. Measures of adult pain: Visual Analog Scale for Pain (VAS pain), Numeric Rating Scale for Pain (NRS Pain), McGill Pain Questionnaire (MPQ), Short-Form McGill Pain Questionnaire (SF-MPQ), Chronic Pain Grade Scale (CPGS), Short Form-36 Bodily Pain Scale (SF-36 BPS), and Measure of Intermittent and Constant Osteoarthritis Pain (ICOAP). *Arthritis Care Res.* 2011;63(S11):S240–S252.
38. Kahl C, Cleland JA. Visual analogue scale, numeric pain rating scale and the McGill Pain Questionnaire: an overview of psychometric properties. *Phys Ther Rev.* 2005;10(2):123–128.
39. Childs JD, Piva SR, Fritz JM. Responsiveness of the numeric pain rating scale in patients with low back pain. *Spine.* 2005;30(11):1331–1334.
40. Deyo RA, Diehl AK. Measuring physical and psychosocial function in patients with low-back pain. *Spine.* 1983;8(6):635–642.
41. Fischer AA. Pressure algometry over normal muscles. Standard values, validity and reproducibility of pressure threshold. *Pain.* 1987;30(1):115–126.
42. Neziri AY, Scaramozzino P, Andersen OK, Dickenson AH, Arendt-Nielsen L, Curatolo M. Reference values of mechanical and thermal pain tests in a pain-free population. *Eur J Pain.* 2011;15(4):376–383.
43. Prushansky T, Dvir Z, Defrin-Assa R. Reproducibility indices applied to cervical pressure pain threshold measurements in healthy subjects. *Clin J Pain.* 2004;20(5):341–347.
44. Chesterton LS, Sim J, Wright CC, Foster NE. Interrater reliability of algometry in measuring pressure pain thresholds in healthy humans, using multiple raters. *Clin J Pain.* 2007;23(9):760–766.
45. Moss P, Sluka K, Wright A. The initial effects of knee joint mobilization on osteoarthritic hyperalgesia. *Man Ther.* 2007;12(2):109–118.
46. Bohannon RW, Crouch R. Minimal clinically important difference for change in 6-minute walk test distance of adults with pathology: a systematic review. *J Eval Clin Pract.* 2017;23(2):377–381.
47. Dobson F, Hinman RS, Hall M, Terwee C, Roos EM, Bennell K. Measurement properties of performance-based measures to assess physical function in hip and knee osteoarthritis: a systematic review. *Osteoarthritis Cartilage.* 2012;20(12):1548–1562.
48. Bohannon RW. Test-retest reliability of the five-repetition sit-to-stand test: a systematic review of the literature involving adults. *J Strength Cond Res.* 2011;25(11):3205–3207.
49. Desjardins-Charbonneau A, Roy J-S, Dionne CE, Frémont P, MacDermid JC, Desmeules F. The efficacy of manual therapy for rotator cuff tendinopathy: a systematic review and meta-analysis. *J Orthop Sports Phys Ther.* 2015;45(5):330–350.
50. Shah KM, Baker T, Dingle A, et al. Early development and reliability of the Timed Functional Arm and Shoulder Test. *J Orthop Sports Phys Ther.* 2017;47(6):420–431.
51. Dworkin RH, Turk DC, Farrar JT, et al. Core outcome measures for chronic pain clinical trials: IMMPACT recommendations. *Pain.* 2005;113(1):9–19.
52. Bialosky JE, Beneciuk JM, Bishop MD, et al. Unraveling the mechanisms of manual therapy: modeling an approach. *J Orthop Sports Phys Ther.* 2018;48(1):8–18.
53. Siengsukon CF, Al-Dughmi M, Stevens S. Sleep health promotion: practical information for physical therapists. *Phys Ther.* 2017;97(8):826–836.
54. Hoving C, Visser A, Mullen PD, van den Borne B. A history of patient education by health professionals in Europe and North America: from authority to shared decision making education. *Patient Educ Couns.* 2010;78(3):275–281.
55. Sassem B. *Nursing: Health Education and Improving Patient Self-Management.* Springer; 2018.

56. Vargas-Schaffer G, Cogan J. Patient therapeutic education: placing the patient at the centre of the WHO analgesic ladder. *Can Fam Phys.* 2014;60(3):235–241.
57. Booth J, Moseley GL, Schiltenwolf M, Cashin A, Davies M, Hübscher M. Exercise for chronic musculoskeletal pain: a biopsychosocial approach. *Musculoskeletal Care.* 2017;15(4):413–421.
58. Chester R, Khondoker M, Shepstone L, Lewis JS, Jerosch-Herold C. Self-efficacy and risk of persistent shoulder pain: results of a Classification and Regression Tree (CART) analysis. *Br J Sports Med.* 2019;53:825–834.
59. Wittink H, Oosterhaven J. Patient education and health literacy. *Musculoskeletal Sci Pract.* 2018;38:120–127.
60. Traeger AC, O'Hagan ET, Cashin A, McAuley JH. Reassurance for patients with non-specific conditions—a user's guide. *Braz J Phys Ther.* 2017;21(1):1–6.
61. Watson JA, Ryan CG, Cooper L, et al. Pain neuroscience education for adults with chronic musculoskeletal pain: a mixed-methods systematic review and meta-analysis. *J Pain.* 2019;20(10):1140.E1–1140.E22.
62. Trede F, Higgs J. Collaborative decision making. In: Higgs J, Jones JA, Loftus S, Christensen N, eds. *Clinical Reasoning in the Health Professions.* 3rd ed. Butterworth Heinemann; 2008:31–41.
63. Batterham RW, Hawkins M, Collins PA, Buchbinder R, Osborne RH. Health literacy: applying current concepts to improve health services and reduce health inequalities. *Public Health.* 2016;132:3–12.
64. Briggs AM, Jordan JE. The importance of health literacy in physiotherapy practice. *J Physiother.* 2010;56(3):149–151.
65. Settineri S, Frisone F, Merlo EM, Geraci D, Martino G. Compliance, adherence, concordance, empowerment, and self-management: five words to manifest a relational maladjustment in diabetes. *J Multidiscip Healthc.* 2019;12:299–314.
66. Nijs J, Wijma AJ, Willaert W, et al. Integrating motivational interviewing in pain neuroscience education for people with chronic pain: a practical guide for clinicians. *Phys Ther.* 2020;100(5):846–859.
67. Hutting N, Johnston V, Staal JB, Heerkens YF. Promoting the use of self-management strategies for people with persistent musculoskeletal disorders: the role of physical therapists. *J Orthop Sports Phys Ther.* 2019;49(4):212–215.
68. Meehan K, Wassinger C, Roy JS, Sole G. Seven key themes in physical therapy advice for patients living with subacromial shoulder pain. A scoping review. *J Orthop Sports Phys Ther.* 2020;50(6):285–293.
69. Marris D, Theophanous K, Cabezon P, Dunlap Z, Donaldson M. The impact of combining pain education strategies with physical therapy interventions for patients with chronic pain: a systematic review and meta-analysis of randomized controlled trials. *Physiother Theory Pract.* 2021;37(4):461–472.
70. Menichetti J, Graffigna G, Steinsbekk A. What are the contents of patient engagement interventions for older adults? A systematic review of randomized controlled trials. *Patient Educ Couns.* 2018;101(6):995–1005.
71. Coronado RA, Brintz CE, McKernan LC, et al. Psychologically informed physical therapy for musculoskeletal pain: current approaches, implications, and future directions from recent randomized trials. *Pain Rep.* 2020;5(5):e847.
72. Hill JC, Foster NE, Hay EM. Cognitive behavioural therapy shown to be an effective and low cost treatment for subacute and chronic low-back pain, improving pain and disability scores in a pragmatic RCT. *Evid Based Med.* 2010;15(4):118–119.
73. O'Sullivan K, Dankaerts W, O'Sullivan L, O'Sullivan PB. Cognitive functional therapy for disabling nonspecific chronic low back pain: multiple case-cohort study. *Phys Ther.* 2015;95(11):1478–1488.
74. Keeffe M, Sullivan P, Purtill H, Bargary N, Sullivan K. Cognitive functional therapy compared with a group-based exercise and education intervention for chronic low back pain: a multicentre randomised controlled trial (RCT). *Br J Sports Med.* 2020;54(13):782–789.
75. Sterling M, Smeets R, Keijzers G, Warren J, Kenardy J. Physiotherapist-delivered stress inoculation training integrated with exercise versus physiotherapy exercise alone for acute whiplash-associated disorder (StressModex): a randomised controlled trial of a combined psychological/physical intervention. *Br J Sports Med.* 2019;53(19):1240–1247.
76. Hughes LS, Clark J, Colclough JA, Dale E, McMillan D. Acceptance and commitment therapy (ACT) for chronic pain. *Clin J Pain.* 2017;33(6):552–568.
77. Louw A, Zimney K, Puentedura EJ, Diener I. The efficacy of pain neuroscience education on musculoskeletal pain: a systematic review of the literature. *Physiother Theory Pract.* 2016;32(5):332–355.
78. Louw A, Puentedura EJ, Reese D, Parker P, Miller T, Mintken PE. Immediate effects of mirror therapy in patients with shoulder pain and decreased range of motion. *Arch Phys Med Rehabil.* 2017;98(10):1941–1947.
79. Bennell KL, Nelligan RK, Rini C, et al. Effects of internet-based pain coping skills training before home exercise for individuals with hip osteoarthritis (HOPE trial): a randomised controlled trial. *Pain.* 2018;159(9):1833–1842.
80. Nielsen M, Jull G, Hodges PW. Designing an online resource for people with low back pain: health-care provider perspectives. *Aust J Prim Health.* 2016;22(2):159–166.
81. Nicholas MK, Linton SJ, Watson PJ, Main CJ. 'Decade of the Flags' Working Group. Early identification and management of psychological risk factors ("yellow flags") in patients with low back pain: a reappraisal. *Phys Ther.* 2011;91(5):737–753.
82. Ainpradub K, Sitthipornvorakul E, Janwantanakul P, van der Beek AJ. Effect of education on non-specific neck and low back pain: a meta-analysis of randomized controlled trials. *Man Ther.* 2016;22:31–41.
83. Moseley GL, Vlaeyen JWS. Beyond nociception: the imprecision hypothesis of chronic pain. *Pain.* 2015;156(1):35–38.
84. Cormier S, Lavigne GL, Choinière M, Rainville P. Expectations predict chronic pain treatment outcomes. *Pain.* 2016;157(2):329–338.
85. Butler D, Moseley L. *Explain Pain.* NOI Publishers; 2003.
86. Louw A, Puentedura E, Schmidt S, Zimney K. *Pain Neuroscience Education: Teaching People About Pain.* Orthopedic Physical Therapy Products; 2018.
87. Mosley GL, Butler DS. *Explain Pain Supercharged.* NOI; 2017.
88. Nijs J, Paul van Wilgen C, Van Oosterwijck J, van Ittersum M, Meeus M. How to explain central sensitization to patients with 'unexplained' chronic musculoskeletal pain: practice guidelines. *Man Ther.* 2011;16(5):413–418.
89. Wood L, Hendrick PA. A systematic review and meta-analysis of pain neuroscience education for chronic low back pain: short-and long-term outcomes of pain and disability. *Eur J Pain.* 2019;23(2):234–249.
90. Sole G, Macznik AK, Ribeiro DC, Jayakaran P, Wassinger CA. Perspectives of participants with rotator cuff-related pain to a neuroscience-informed pain education session: an exploratory mixed method study. *Disabil Rehabil.* 2020;42(13):1870–1879.

91. White J, Auliffe SM, Jepson M, et al. 'There is a very distinct need for education' among people with rotator cuff tendinopathy: an exploration of health professionals' attitudes. *Musculoskelet Sci Pract.* 2020;45:102103.
92. Sawyer EE, McDevitt AW, Louw A, Puentedura EJ, Mintken PE. Use of pain neuroscience education, tactile discrimination, and graded motor imagery in an individual with frozen shoulder. *J Orthop Sports Phys Ther.* 2017;48(3):174–184.
93. Nelligan RK, Hinman RS, Kasza J, Bennell KL. Effectiveness of internet-delivered education and home exercise supported by behaviour change SMS on pain and function for people with knee osteoarthritis: a randomised controlled trial protocol. *BMC Musculoskelet Disord.* 2019;20(1):342.
94. Nijs J, Lluch-Girbés E, Lundberg M, Malfliet A, Sterling M. Exercise therapy for chronic musculoskeletal pain: innovation by altering pain memories. *Man Ther.* 2015;20(1):216–220.
95. Wun A, Kollias P, Jeong H, et al. Why is exercise prescribed for people with chronic low back pain? A review of the mechanisms of benefit proposed by clinical trialists. *Musculoskelet Sci Pract.* 2020:102307.
96. Belavy DL, Van Oosterwijck J, Clarkson M, et al. Pain sensitivity is reduced by exercise training: evidence from a systematic review and meta-analysis. *Neurosci Biobehav Rev.* 2021;120:100–108.
97. de Zoete RMJ, Chen K, Sterling M. Central neurobiological effects of physical exercise in individuals with chronic musculoskeletal pain: a systematic review. *BMJ Open.* 2020;10(7):e036151.
98. Rajab AS, Crane DE, Middleton LE, Robertson AD, Hampson M, MacIntosh BJ. A single session of exercise increases connectivity in sensorimotor-related brain networks: a resting-state fMRI study in young healthy adults. *Front Hum Neurosci.* 2014;8:625.
99. Scheef L, Jankowski J, Daamen M, et al. An fMRI study on the acute effects of exercise on pain processing in trained athletes. *PAIN®.* 2012;153(8):1702–1714.
100. Naugle KM, Fillingim RB, Riley JL. A meta-analytic review of the hypoalgesic effects of exercise. *J Pain.* 2012;13(12):1139–1150.
101. Schuch FB, Vancampfort D, Richards J, Rosenbaum S, Ward PB, Stubbs B. Exercise as a treatment for depression: a meta-analysis adjusting for publication bias. *J Psychiatr Res.* 2016;77:42–51.
102. Stonerock GL, Hoffman BM, Smith PJ, Blumenthal JA. Exercise as treatment for anxiety: systematic review and analysis. *Ann Behav Med.* 2015;49(4):542–556.
103. Streckmann F, Zopf EM, Lehmann HC, et al. Exercise intervention studies in patients with peripheral neuropathy: a systematic review. *Sports Med.* 2014;44(9):1289–1304.
104. de Zoete RM, Armfield NR, McAuley JH, Chen K, Sterling M. Comparative effectiveness of physical exercise interventions for chronic non-specific neck pain: a systematic review with network meta-analysis of 40 randomised controlled trials. *Br J Sports Med.* 2021;55:730–742.
105. Oesch P, Kool J, Hagen KB, Bachmann S. Effectiveness of exercise on work disability in patients with non-acute non-specific low back pain: systematic review and meta-analysis of randomized controlled trials. *J Rehabil Med.* 2010;42(3):193–205.
106. Van Middelkoop M, Rubinstein SM, Kuijpers T, et al. A systematic review on the effectiveness of physical and rehabilitation interventions for chronic non-specific low back pain. *Eur Spine J.* 2011;20(1):19–39.
107. López-de-Uralde-Villanueva I, Munoz-Garcia D, Gil-Martinez A, et al. A systematic review and meta-analysis on the effectiveness of graded activity and graded exposure for chronic nonspecific low back pain. *Pain Med.* 2016;17(1):172–188.
108. Smith BE, Hendrick P, Smith TO, et al. Should exercises be painful in the management of chronic musculoskeletal pain? a systematic review and meta-analysis. *Br J Sports Med.* 2017;51(23):1679–1687.
109. Smith BE, Hendrick P, Bateman M, et al. Musculoskeletal pain and exercise—challenging existing paradigms and introducing new. *Br J Sports Med.* 2019;53(14):907–912.
110. Gibson W, Wand BM, Meads C, Catley MJ, O'Connell NE. Transcutaneous electrical nerve stimulation (TENS) for chronic pain-an overview of Cochrane Reviews. *Cochrane Database of Syst Rev.* 2019(4):CD011890.
111. Peng W, Tang Z, Zhang F, et al. Neurobiological mechanisms of TENS-induced analgesia. *NeuroImage.* 2019;195:396–408.
112. Vance CG, Dailey DL, Rakel BA, Sluka KA. Using TENS for pain control: the state of the evidence. *Pain Manag.* 2014;4(3):197–209.
113. Melzack R, Wall PD. Pain mechanisms: a new theory. *Science.* 1965;150(3699):971–979.
114. Sluka KA, Walsh D. Transcutaneous electrical nerve stimulation: basic science mechanisms and clinical effectiveness. *J Pain.* 2003;4(3):109–121.
115. Sluka KA, Deacon M, Stibal A, Strissel S, Terpstra A. Spinal blockade of opioid receptors prevents the analgesia produced by TENS in arthritic rats. *J Pharmacol Exp Ther.* 1999;289(2):840–846.
116. Léonard G, Cloutier C, Marchand S. Reduced analgesic effect of acupuncture-like TENS but not conventional TENS in opioid-treated patients. *J Pain.* 2011;12(2):213–221.
117. Solomon RA, Viernstein MC, Long DM. Reduction of postoperative pain and narcotic use by transcutaneous electrical nerve stimulation. *Surgery.* 1980;87(2):142–146.
118. Dailey DL, Rakel BA, Vance CG, et al. Transcutaneous electrical nerve stimulation reduces pain, fatigue and hyperalgesia while restoring central inhibition in primary fibromyalgia. *Pain.* 2013;154(11):2554–2562.
119. McCarthy CJ, Lonnemann E, Hindle J, MacDonald R, Paneris I. The physiology of manual therapy. *A Comprehensive Guide to Sports Physiology and Injury Management E-Book: An Interdisciplinary Approach.* Elsevier; 2020:121.
120. Bialosky JE, Bishop MD, Price DD, Robinson ME, George SZ. The mechanisms of manual therapy in the treatment of musculoskeletal pain: a comprehensive model. *Man Ther.* 2009;14(5):531–538.
121. Bishop MD, Torres-Cueco R, Gay CW, Lluch-Girbés E, Beneciuk JM, Bialosky JE. What effect can manual therapy have on a patient's pain experience? *Pain Manag.* 2015;5(6):455–464.
122. Sampath KK, Botnmark E, Mani R, et al. Neuroendocrine response following a thoracic spinal manipulation in healthy men. *J Orthop Sports Phys Ther.* 2017;47(9):617–627.
123. Sampath KK, Mani R, Cotter JD, Tumilty S. Measureable changes in the neuro-endocrinal mechanism following spinal manipulation. *Med Hypotheses.* 2015;85(6):819–824.
124. Degenhardt BF, Darmani NA, Johnson JC, et al. Role of osteopathic manipulative treatment in altering pain biomarkers: a pilot study. *J Am Osteopath Assoc.* 2007;107(9):387–400.
125. Vernon H, Dhami M, Howley T, Annett R. Spinal manipulation and beta-endorphin: a controlled study of the effect of a spinal manipulation on plasma beta-endorphin levels in normal males. *J Manipulative Physiol Ther.* 1986;9(2):115–123.

126. Geri T, Viceconti A, Minacci M, Testa M, Rossettini G. Manual therapy: exploiting the role of human touch. *Musculoskelet Sci Pract.* 2019;44:102044.
127. Boal RW, Gillette RG. Central neuronal plasticity, low back pain and spinal manipulative therapy. *J Manipulative Physiol Ther.* 2004;27(5):314–326.
128. Pickar JG, Wheeler JD. Response of muscle proprioceptors to spinal manipulative-like loads in the anesthetized cat. *J Manipulative Physiol Ther.* 2001;24(1):2–11.
129. Schmid A, Brunner F, Wright A, Bachmann LM. Paradigm shift in manual therapy? Evidence for a central nervous system component in the response to passive cervical joint mobilisation. *Manl Ther.* 2008;13(5):387–396.
130. Sterling M, Jull G, Wright A. Cervical mobilisation: concurrent effects on pain, sympathetic nervous system activity and motor activity. *Man Therapy.* 2001;6(2):72–81.
131. Gyer G, Michael J, Inklebarger J, Tedla JS. Spinal manipulation therapy: is it all about the brain? a current review of the neurophysiological effects of manipulation. *J Integr Med.* 2019;17(5):328–337.
132. de Luca KE, Fang SH, Ong J, Shin K-S, Woods S, Tuchin PJ. The effectiveness and safety of manual therapy on pain and disability in older persons with chronic low back pain: a systematic review. *J Manipulative Physiol Ther.* 2017;40(7):527–534.
133. Coulter ID, Crawford C, Hurwitz EL, et al. Manipulation and mobilization for treating chronic low back pain: a systematic review and meta-analysis. *Spine J.* 2018;18(5):866–879.
134. Qinguang Xu M, Bei Chen M, Yuevi Wang M, Xuezong Wang M, Dapeng Han M. The effectiveness of manual therapy for relieving pain, stiffness, and dysfunction in knee osteoarthritis: a systematic review and meta-analysis. *Pain Physician.* 2017;20(4):229–243.
135. Vincent K, Maigne J-Y, Fischhoff C, Lanlo O, Dagenais S. Systematic review of manual therapies for nonspecific neck pain. *Joint Bone Spine.* 2013;80(5):508–515.
136. Bishop MD, Bialosky JE, Penza CW, Beneciuk JM, Alappattu MJ. The influence of clinical equipoise and patient preferences on outcomes of conservative manual interventions for spinal pain: an experimental study. *J Pain Res.* 2017;10:965–972.
137. Palmlöf L, Holm L, Alfredsson L, Skillgate E. Expectations of recovery: a prognostic factor in patients with neck pain undergoing manual therapy treatment. *Eur J Pain.* 2016;20(9):1384–1391.
138. Lin I, Wiles L, Waller R, et al. What does best practice care for musculoskeletal pain look like? Eleven consistent recommendations from high-quality clinical practice guidelines: systematic review. *Br J Sports Med.* 2020;54(2):79–86.
139. Wassinger CA, Rich D, Cameron N, et al. Cervical & thoracic manipulations: acute effects upon pain pressure threshold and self-reported pain in experimentally induced shoulder pain. *Man Ther.* 2016;21:227–232.

PART VI
Applied Clinical Reasoning

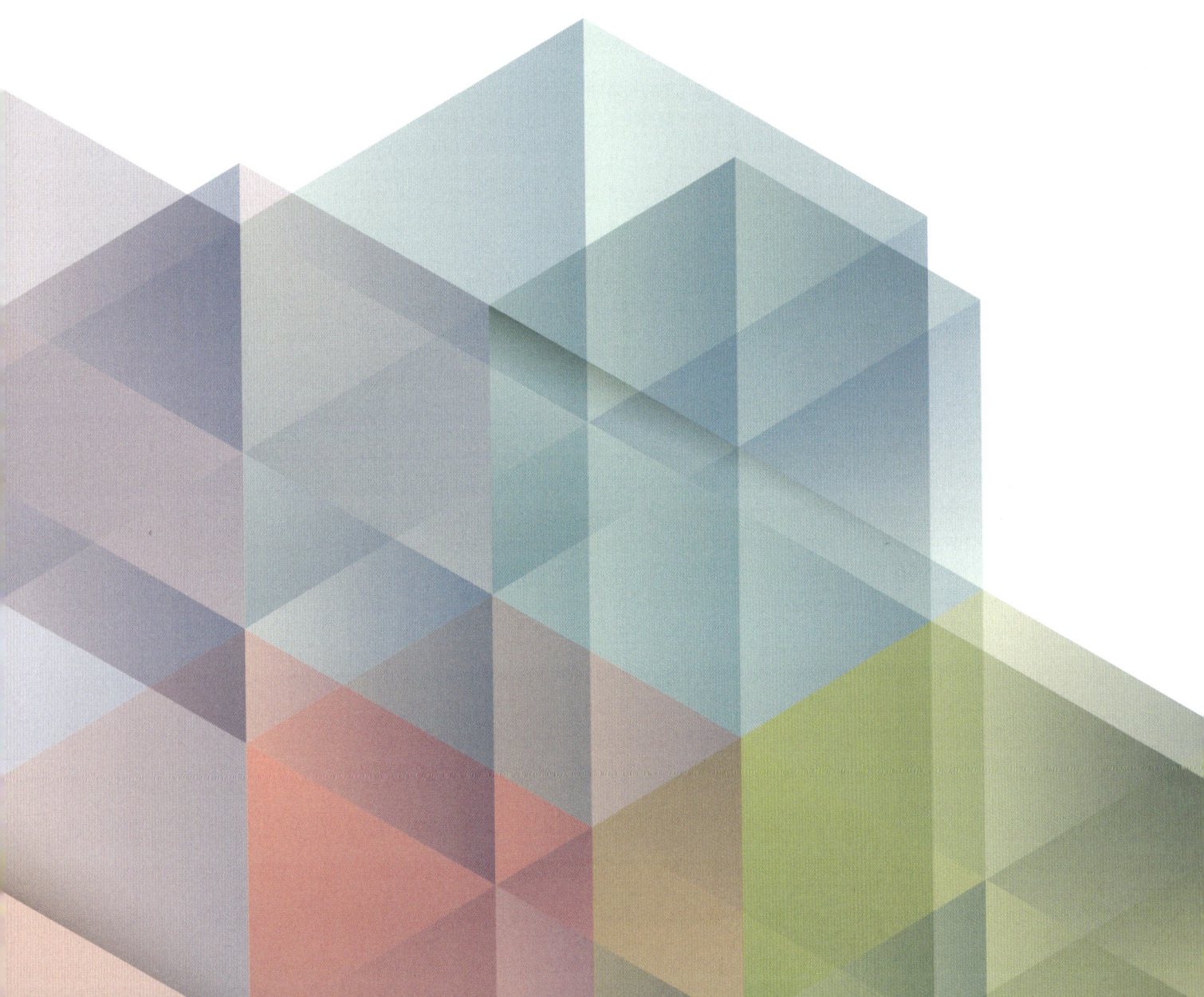

20 | Case Studies

Betsy Myers

INTRODUCTION TO CASE STUDIES

This chapter provides insights into a clinician's clinical reasoning when examining three patients. Each case contains a basic overview, patient intake forms, a history, and physical examination. An emphasis has been placed on overtly stating the clinician's thought process regarding the information provided by the patient, additional information needed, and the order and interpretation of the physical examination in order to come to a final diagnosis. Each case concludes with an overview of the recommended plan of care, with an emphasis on patient education for the session.

Case Study 20-1: McKenzie—Patient with Left Hip Pain

McKenzie is a 21-year-old volleyball player with left hip pain. Figure 20-1 contains the intake forms McKenzie completed before her clinic appointment.

History In reviewing McKenzie's intake form, the clinician notes recurrent left hip pain that began about 3 months ago. Pain is intermittent, but can be moderately severe, and is aggravated by activities such as weight training and volleyball. Symptoms are worse at the end of the day and with sitting. Overall, her hip pain is worsening. Symptom location is marked as the anterior and perhaps anterolateral left hip. This location may be consistent with a "c-sign" for intra-articular pathology but may also indicate groin pain, a stress fracture, or lumbar spine pathology.

Symptom description is consistent with a possible musculoskeletal pathology, but sharp or aching pain may also be present with pain from neurologic or visceral sources. Specifically, the clinician must consider referred pain from the lumbar spine, the gastrointestinal and genitourinary systems, and constitutional symptoms. Clarifying questions for the gastrointestinal

---

CASE STUDY 20-1
Mckenzie: Patient with Left Hip Pain

Intake Form

Name: McKenzie   Date: May 2
Age: 21   Gender: F   Race/Ethnicity: Caucasian   Preferred language: English
Reason for visit: Left hip pain
When did this start? Slowly increasing for the past 2–3 months
How did this occur? ☐ No apparent reason ☒ _____
Have you had this problem in the past? ☐ No   ☒ Yes If so, please describe (how often, how long it lasted, how resolved). Had some pain last fall during pre-season but it went away
What activities are you having difficulty performing (hobbies, sports, exercise, work): _____
Volleyball, lifting weights, squatting, sitting in class, and sometimes hard to put on shoes/socks
Describe any treatment you have tried so far to assist with this and the result (ibuprofen, ice)
Practice limited to no jumping or running — no better, ice feels good at the time
Describe any testing you have received for this and the result (x-ray, MRI, etc.):
None. Are they needed?

FIGURE 20-1 Intake form for McKenzie.

CASE STUDY 20-1 (continued)

Mark the location of your symptom(s) on the diagrams below:

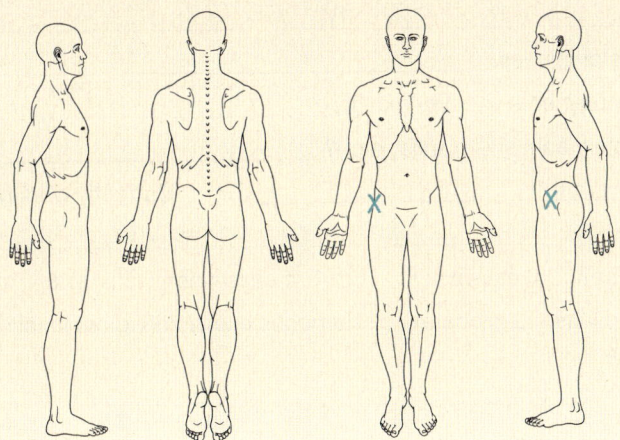

Using the following scale, 0 = No pain, 10 = Worst pain imaginable, Emergency Department necessary

What is your pain level **right now**? _1_/10

During the last 48 hours, what was your pain: **at best** _0_/10 **at worst:** _6_/10

Overall are you: ☐ getting better ☒ getting worse ☐ staying the same

Describe your symptoms: ☐ pins and needles ☐ burning ☒ aching ☒ dull
☒ sharp ☐ stabbing ☐ throbbing other: _____

What makes your symptoms **better**? ☒ activity ☐ rest ☐ morning ☐ end of day
☐ sitting ☒ walking ☒ ice ☐ heat ☐ medications: _____ Other: _____

What makes your symptoms **worse**? ☒ activity ☐ rest ☐ morning ☒ end of day
☒ sitting ☐ walking ☐ ice ☐ heat ☐ medications: _____ Other: _Weightlifting, volleyball_

Goal(s) for therapy: _Play volleyball without pain, avoid surgery_

Mark any boxes if you have a history of, or have recently experienced, the following:

☐ High blood pressure	☐ Cancer	☐ Nail changes
☐ High cholesterol	☐ Night sweats	☐ Skin changes
☐ Heart disease	☐ Night pain	☐ Vision changes
☐ Chest pain	☐ Ulcer	☐ Easy bruising
☐ Leg cramping with walking	☐ Constipation	☐ Excessive weight gain or loss
☐ Feel a heartbeat in your abdomen	☐ Incontinence	☐ Headaches
☐ Lightheadedness	☐ Abdominal pain	☐ Arthritis
☐ Diabetes	☐ Changes in menstrual pattern	☐ Muscle weakness
☐ Stroke	☐ Numbness, tingling	☐ Fatigue
☐ Epilepsy/seizures	☐ Walking or balance difficulties	☐ Morning stiffness
☒ Asthma/breathing problems	☐ Long-term steroid use	☐ Trauma (car accident or fall)

FIGURE 20-1 (continued)

> ### CASE STUDY 20-1 (continued)
>
> Are you currently pregnant? ☒ No ☐ Yes
> List prior surgeries: _Right ACL reconstruction when I was 17_
> List any other diagnoses or injuries: _____
> List any medications/supplements you are taking: _albuterol_
> List any allergies (i.e., latex, adhesives, sulfa, etc.)? _bees_
> Occupation: _college student_   Currently working? ☒ No ☐ Yes
> Recreational activities/sports: _indoor volleyball, running, lifting weights, skateboarding_
> How often do you exercise? ☐ 0 days/week ☐ 1–4 days/week ☒ 5–7 days/week
> On average, how many minutes of moderate or strenuous exercise (e.g., at least a *brisk* walk) do you engage in per week? _10 hours_
> On average, how many alcoholic drinks do you have per week: _0_
> Do you smoke? ☒ No ☐ Yes: ___packs/day, ___ yrs ☐ Former smoker: date quit ____ packs/day, __yrs,
> On average, how many hours of sleep do you get per night? _7.5_
> Does this current problem affect your sleep? ☒ No ☐ Yes
> Do you currently feel stressed? ☒ No ☐ Yes
> Do you feel down, depressed, or hopeless? ☒ No ☐ Yes
> Please note if you need any accommodations or have any preferences that may affect your therapy (i.e., religion, physical disability, etc.). _____
>
> **FIGURE 20-1** (continued)

and urogenital systems might include asking about nausea, vomiting, change of symptoms with food intake, history of urinary tract infections, painful urination, or the need to urinate more frequently. The patient should be asked specifically when her last period was and about any incidences of incontinence. Given the patient's age and the intimate nature of this discussion, the clinician may approach the topic in the following manner:

> "Many athletes with hip pain experience a small leakage of urine at times, such as during weight training or jumping activities. Is this something you have experienced?"

To investigate for possible constitutional signs and symptoms, the clinician should specifically ask McKenzie about the presence of fever, night sweats, or reduced energy levels. Although not contributory for diagnostic purposes, the clinician must review and examine the pulmonary system including finding out if McKenzie needs to have her inhaler accessible during clinic visits.

The clinician should learn more details regarding McKenzie's right anterior cruciate ligament (ACL) reconstruction. For example, was the ACL injury noncontact or contact related? What are McKenzie's perceptions of her right knee function? Does she have any pain in her right knee? Does she consider her right leg to be her "bad" leg, potentially leading to greater left lower extremity forces with volleyball-related activities and squatting?

Activity both improves and worsens McKenzie's symptoms and requires follow-up questions. Interestingly, McKenzie notes a hobby of running, but this was not listed as an aggravating activity. This requires confirmation as running is a high load on the hip that would likely be painful in the case of a stress fracture. Conversely, the hip is in a relatively neutral or extended position, which is less likely to be problematic for a patient with femoroacetabular impingement syndrome (FAIS). The clinician must clarify McKenzie's position in volleyball, her handedness, and explore if there is a specific skill in volleyball or weight training that is problematic (e.g., jumping or asymmetrical lifting). Pain with sitting is common with lumbar disc pathology, but can occur with hip dysfunction as well. The clinician may ask if sitting is immediately painful, painful after a while, or if the type of chair (e.g., amount of lumbar support or the degree of hip flexion/chair height) influences her symptoms.

The clinician should get a sense of the irritability of McKenzie's symptoms. She has noted both sharp pain and dull, aching pain. For example, the clinician should try to understand if these symptoms occur together or does sharp pain transition into a dull ache over the course of the day or practice or is the sharp pain intermittent with certain movements but the dull aching sensation something that occurs at the end of the day. The clinician should gain an understanding of McKenzie's perception of what is wrong with her hip now as well as in the past. This is particularly important because McKenzie noted on her intake form that one of her goals for treatment was to avoid surgery. Given her prior knee surgery and her recurrence of hip pain, McKenzie may believe that surgery is the only true solution to this athletic injury or perhaps she has a teammate with hip pain who required surgery. If McKenzie's response appears to indicate psychological distress, the clinician may want to have her complete the Fear Avoidance Beliefs Questionnaire (FABQ) or the Tampa Scale for Kinesiophobia (TSK) and/or refer McKenzie to a mental health professional. To learn more about her hip-specific complaints, the clinician could ask McKenzie to complete the Harris Hip Score or Modified Harris Hip Score.

Based on the history, the clinician has initial hypotheses of pain referred from the lumbar spine, labral pathology, FAIS, groin pain, and stress fracture. To clarify symptoms that are more consistent with lumbar pathology, the clinician asks about paresthesias, symptoms in other locations, and a history of back pain. To help rule in/out labral pathology, the clinician specifically asks about the presence of clicking, catching, or locking and the impact of twisting activities, such as getting in/out of the car. McKenzie denied pain in other locations and has never had back pain. She reports her sharp pain is more of a sharp pinching pain with deep squatting, performing digs when playing the back row in volleyball, and sitting upright. If these activities are performed repeatedly, her hip will constantly ache, but the sharp, pinching will still occur intermittently with those activities.

TABLE 20-1

MCKENZIE: A 21-YEAR-OLD VOLLEYBALL PLAYER WITH LEFT HIP PAIN

Position	Assessments	Positive Findings
Observation	Continues from history	
Seated	Great toe ext/L5 (A, OP, MMT) Ankle dorsiflexion/L4 (A, OP, MMT) Ankle plantarflexion (A) Knee ext/L3 (A, OP, MMT) Hip ER (A, OP, MMT) Hip IR (A, OP, MMT) Hip flexion/L1,2 (A, OP, MMT) Dermatomes L1–S2 Reflexes: Achilles, patellar Special test: fulcrum test	MMT hip ER 4B PROM L hip IR 25°*
Standing	Structure/posture screen including leg length and rotational changes such as femoral torsion and resting foot posture Trunk AROM flex, ext, side glide Trunk quadrant test	
Supine	Knee PROM: flex, ext Hip PROM: flex, rot, abd, add Muscle length: gastrocnemius, hamstring, Thomas test	PROM L hip flex 100°* bony endfeel, L IR* capsular endfeel Muscle length: Thomas test hip flexed 30° with the knee flexed 90°, hip extended 10° with the knee extended.
Left sidelying	MMT: R hip abd, L hip add	R hip abd 4
Prone	Hip PROM: ext, IR Special test: Craig test MMT: hip ER, hamstring (S1,2), gluteus maximus, trunk ext Functional test: prone plank	PROM: hip ext R15° capsular endfeel/L 10° capsular endfeel MMT hip ER 3+B, glue max 4 B Functional test: prone plank with cues, fatigued at 30"
Right sidelying	MMT: L hip abd, R hip add	L hip abd 4
Supine	Palpation: anterior hip including hip flexors, hip adductors, inguinal ligament, abdominals MMT: leg-lowering abdominal test Special tests: FABER, FADIR, scour	MMT: leg lower 3+ Special tests: positive FADIR, pain with scour at end-ranges of flex but no increase in pain with compression

(continued)

TABLE 20-1 (continued)
MCKENZIE: A 21-YEAR-OLD VOLLEYBALL PLAYER WITH LEFT HIP PAIN

Position	Assessments	Positive Findings
Standing	Footwear inspection Gait Single leg balance: eyes open (and observe for Trendelenburg sign), eyes closed MMT: plantarflexion Functional testing: squat, single leg squat, jump, volleyball approach jump, dig	Single leg stance eyes open R15 seconds/L20 seconds, eyes closed 3 seconds B Functional tests: • Squat >90° hip flexion,* gluteus dominant pattern with an excessive anterior pelvic tilt • Single leg squat with increased valgus R > L, poor balance, and anterior pelvic tilt • Dig positioning "uncomfortable," pain with increased hip flex range of motion

*Reproduction of patient's symptoms.
A, active; AROM, active range of motion; ER, external rotation; Ext, extension; IR, internal rotation; L, left; MMT, manual muscle test; OP, overpressure; P, passive range of motion, PROM, passive range of motion; R, right.

Physical Examination Based on the history, there are no red flags for the clinician to consider. The physical examination begins with the systems review. Heart rate, blood pressure, oxygen saturation, and respiratory rate are taken. The patient's height and weight are measured. All findings were considered normal. Table 20-1 provides the sample flow of the remainder of the physical examination by an experienced clinician. All tests begin with the uninvolved right side unless otherwise noted. Any positive findings are listed in the right-hand column.

The seated examination begins by performing a lower quarter neurologic screen to identify potential lumbar spine involvement. This is followed by standard position testing of hip rotation range of motion (ROM) and strength. The standing examination first includes a global look at structure/posture followed by trunk active range of motion (AROM) and the quadrant test to finish clearing the lumbar spine. Before performing higher level functional tasks in the standing position, the clinician examines the patient in lying. The knee is cleared by performing passive range of motion (PROM). The clinician then assesses hip PROM and muscle length of key lower extremity muscle groups. Note that this clinician chose not to assess hip joint mobility, but another clinician may have chosen to perform this assessment. In McKenzie's case, the clinician may have made this decision for several reasons. First, hip instability was not considered a potential differential diagnosis. Second, it is difficult for patients to relax with hip accessory motion testing. Third, the result of the assessment (normal versus hypomobile) does not change the differential diagnosis.

With McKenzie in sidelying, the clinician assesses hip abductor and adductor strength. The clinician could have assessed the patient's ability to perform a side plank at this time, but deferred this. Note that left sidelying is used for manual muscle testing (MMT) of the right (top) gluteus medius, whereas a left side plank assesses the right (lower) gluteus medius. Because the clinician noted poor strength of the uninvolved right gluteus medius first, it was decided that the side plank on the involved side would likely be poor. However, the clinician may well assess a side plank later on or use a unilateral or bilateral side plank as a strengthening exercise if appropriate.

Prone assessments included checking for femoral torsion, given the asymmetrical hip rotation noted in sitting. In addition, because patients with FAIS may have increased hip rotation ROM when assessed in neutral hip flexion, the amount of rotation achieved in the standard position is compared with that noted in the standard position. This was indeed the case for McKenzie. Lastly, the clinician assessed hip external rotation (ER) strength with the hip in neutral as an indicator of hip abductor function for running or landing from a jump, which occurs in a more extended position than the traditional seated MMT.

The clinician then proceeded to perform tests that were most likely to be provocative: FADIR, FABER, and scour. Location-specific palpation was also performed after referred pain from the lumbar spine was ruled out. Core strength was assessed functionally with a plank but also with the traditional leg-lowering abdominal MMT. The clinician would have performed knee-specific testing, including ligamentous stability and meniscal pathology, if McKenzie noted any knee-specific complaints. Lastly, the clinician returned the patient to standing and progressed from gait assessment to the highest level of functional tests for the session, choosing items that the patient noted difficulty with (squat) as well as volleyball-specific tasks. The clinician could have examined hop testing as well. However, the functional tests chosen provided a rich picture of the patient's functional abilities.

The clinician concluded that McKenzie had FAIS, specifically limiting hip flexion but also hip internal rotation. Her condition is exacerbated by poor hip and abdominal strength, decreased neuromuscular control of the hip/pelvis, and reduced balance. Lumbar pathology was ruled out by lack of provocation with trunk AROM and quadrant testing, along with a normal lower quarter neurologic screen and symptom reproduction with hip-specific testing. While a positive fulcrum test rules in a stress fracture, a negative test cannot rule out a stress fracture. The clinician believed a stress fracture is improbable given lack of pain with high-load activities such as playing front row in volleyball and running in combination with finding no significant changes to her training and a normal body mass index. Groin pain was ruled out by symptom-free hip flex/adduction and abdominal testing.

The clinician discussed the examination findings with McKenzie, including explaining the pathology of FAIS. The clinician educated McKenzie in activity modification, including limited squat depth, particularly when lifting weights. Because there appears to be a slight inflammatory component to McKenzie's symptoms, she was instructed to ice her hip after practice and when the hip is sore, providing specifics regarding ice location, time, and method. The clinician obtained McKenzie's permission to discuss her case with her volleyball athletic trainer and/or coach to ensure coordination of care. The clinician emphasized the impairments that might be contributing to her condition and related how improving these impairments might not only improve her hip symptoms, but potentially reduce the risk of another noncontact ACL injury or other lower extremity injury. The clinician presented rehabilitation options, including hip and core strengthening, balance and neuromuscular control exercises, and hip flexor stretching. Also, the clinician noted that once her symptoms were less irritable, hip joint mobilizations and stretching into hip flexion and internal rotation would be attempted to try to gain ROM, particularly hip flexion, as this was functionally limiting her sitting and volleyball digs. To address McKenzie's concern regarding a potential need for imaging, the clinician noted that a radiograph might confirm the diagnosis of FAIS, but that bony changes (such as cam and pincer lesions) are frequently asymptomatic. In addition, the clinician noted that most patients are able to resume symptom-free athletic participation in less than 3 months of appropriate rehabilitation and that only a small percentage of patients with FAIS require surgery.

Case Study 20-2: Dekohta—Patient with Right Buttock Pain

Dekohta is a 31-year-old male with right buttock pain. Figure 20-2 contains the intake forms Dekohta completed before his clinic appointment.

CASE STUDY 20-2
Dekohta: Patient with Right Buttock Pain
Intake Form

Name: Dekohta   Date: April 5
Age: 31   Gender: M   Race/Ethnicity: Native American   Preferred language: English
Reason for visit: Glute/hamstring pain
When did this start? 2 weeks ago
How did this occur? ☐ No apparent reason   ☐ When performing a deadlift
Have you had this problem in the past? ☒No   ☐Yes If so, please describe (how often, how long it lasted, how resolved).
What activities are you having difficulty performing (hobbies, sports, exercise, work):
Cannot perform my normal weight lifting or running, sore with sitting a long time
Describe any treatment you have tried so far to assist with this and the result (ibuprofen, ice)
Stretching my glute and hamstring have not helped
Describe any testing you have received for this and the result (x ray, MRI, etc.):
None

FIGURE 20-2 Intake form for Dekohta.

(continued)

CASE STUDY 20-2 (continued)

Mark the location of your symptom(s) on the diagrams below:

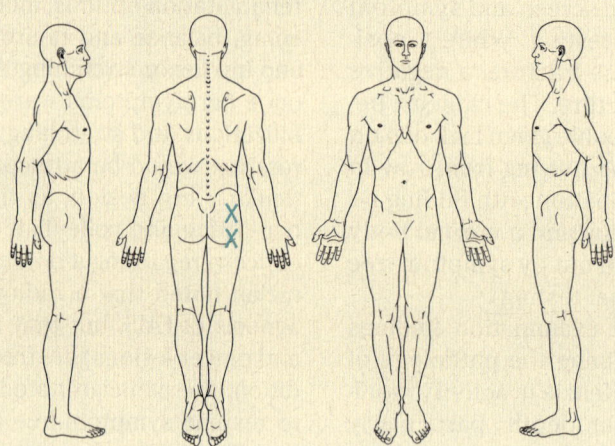

Using the following scale, 0 = No pain, 10 = Worst pain imaginable, Emergency Department necessary
what is your pain level **right now**? __1__/10
During the last 48 hours, what was your pain: at best __1__/10 at worst: __5__/10
Overall are you: ☐ getting better ☐ getting worse ☒ staying the same
Describe your symptoms: ☒ pins and needles   ☐ burning   ☒ aching   ☒ dull
   ☐ sharp ☐ stabbing   ☐ throbbing   other: _____
What makes your symptoms **better**? ☒ activity ☐ rest ☒ morning ☐ end of day
   ☐ sitting ☒ walking   ☐ ice ☐ heat ☐ medications: _____ Other: _Lying down_
What makes your symptoms **worse**? ☒ activity ☐ rest ☐ morning ☒ end of day
   ☒ sitting ☐ walking   ☐ ice ☐ heat ☐ medications: _____ Other: _Weightlifting, running, putting on socks_

Goal(s) for therapy: _Learn what is wrong and return to normal activities without pain_

Mark any boxes if you have a history of, or have recently experienced, the following:

☐ High blood pressure	☐ Cancer	☐ Nail changes
☐ High cholesterol	☐ Night sweats	☐ Skin changes
☐ Heart disease	☐ Night pain	☐ Vision changes
☐ Chest pain	☐ Ulcer	☐ Easy bruising
☐ Leg cramping with walking	☐ Constipation	☒ Excessive weight gain or loss
☐ Feel a heartbeat in your abdomen	☐ Incontinence	☐ Headaches
☐ Lightheadedness	☐ Abdominal pain	☐ Arthritis
☐ Diabetes	☐ Changes in menstrual pattern	☒ Muscle weakness
☐ Stroke	☒ Numbness, tingling	☐ Fatigue
☐ Epilepsy/seizures	☐ Walking or balance difficulties	☒ Morning stiffness
☐ Asthma/breathing problems	☐ Long-term steroid use	☐ Trauma (car accident or fall)

FIGURE 20-2 (continued)

> **CASE STUDY 20-2 (continued)**
>
> Are you currently pregnant? ☒ No ☐ Yes
> List prior surgeries: _Hernia surgery when I was 2 months old_
> List any other diagnoses or injuries: _____
> List any medications/supplements you are taking: _B vitamins_
> List any allergies (i.e., latex, adhesives, sulfa, etc.)? _____
> Occupation: _Actuary/statistician_   Currently working? ☐ No ☒ Yes
> Recreational activities/sports: _Weight train, trail running, fishing_
> How often do you exercise? ☐ 0 days/week   ☒ 1–4 days/week   ☐ 5–7 days/week
> On average, how many minutes of moderate or strenuous exercise (e.g., at least a *brisk* walk) do you engage in per week? _150_
> On average, how many alcoholic drinks do you have per week: _0_
> Do you smoke? ☒ No ☐ Yes: ___packs/day, ___ yrs ☐ Former smoker: date quit _____ packs/day, __ yrs,
> On average, how many hours of sleep do you get per night? _6_
>   Does this current problem affect your sleep? ☐ No ☒ Yes
> Do you currently feel stressed? ☒ No ☐ Yes
> Do you feel down, depressed, or hopeless? ☒ No ☐ Yes
> Please note if you need any accommodations or have any preferences that may affect your therapy (i.e., religion, physical disability, etc.). _____
>
> **FIGURE 20-2** (*continued*)

History In reviewing Dekohta's form, the clinician notes a 2-week history of what he describes as right "glute/hamstring" pain (marking the right buttock on the body diagram) that began while performing a deadlift. Symptoms are constant, ranging in intensity from mild to moderate, and have not changed much since onset. Symptoms are described as pins and needles, aching, and dull. Musculoskeletal symptoms are commonly described as dull and aching or sore and hurting. It would not be unusual to have an onset of musculoskeletal pain, such as a strain from heavy lifting as described by Dekohta. The lack of improvement over 2 weeks is somewhat suspicious, but may represent inadequate load reduction and activity modification that is delaying healing. The clinician must consider that pins and needles are more commonly the result of neurogenic involvement and that aching pain may also represent referral from visceral sources.

The clinician should obtain additional details regarding the onset of symptoms, including information such as:

- How much the patient was attempting to deadlift
- How many repetitions were performed
- How this load compares to his usual weight training routine
- When in the workout this occurred
- Whether he could he continue the workout
- Whether he could stand upright and walk normally after the workout

The clinician will need to clarify the region of symptoms both currently and since onset. For example, Dekohta should be specifically asked about the presence of back pain during this episode; symptoms in the right thigh, calf, or foot; and left buttock or leg symptoms. In addition, the clinician should ask if Dekohta has a history of back pain, hamstring strains, or hip problems. Dekohta reports attempts at stretching the "glute and hamstring" did not help. It would be useful to learn more about what was tried by having the patient demonstrate these stretches, describe the stretching parameters used, and note any changes with the stretches. It is possible that aggressive stretching of an acutely strained muscle is preventing normal tissue healing.

The pattern of symptoms increasing with weight training, running, sitting, and putting on socks (flexing) and reducing while lying down would seem to indicate that Dekohta's symptoms are affected by disc loading. The clinician should clarify the impact of his current condition on function, such as how long he can sit before symptoms increase and specifically what weight training or running he is currently able to perform.

The clinician should explore Dekohta's notations of excessive weight change, weakness, sleeping difficulties, and stiffness. These are constitutional symptoms that may indicate a systemic pathology. The clinician should ask how Dekohta's weight has changed and over what period of time. In addition, the clinician must determine whether the muscle weakness is specific to deadlifting due to right buttock pain, or if the other lower extremity or other regions are also affected. Difficulty sleeping is not uncommon with an acute injury, but night pain that prevents an individual from returning to sleep is worrisome. The clinician should ask if Dekohta normally gets only 6 hours of sleep per night or if his sleep pattern is limited by his current complaint. In addition, the clinician should ask if Dekohta is able to find a position that is comfortable and, if woken due to pain, whether he is able to go back to sleep. Morning stiffness might be expected as a somewhat normal complaint after an acute injury but, if more global, may represent a systemic inflammatory condition. The clinician should continue to explore potential constitutional symptoms by asking Dekohta if he has had a fever or is feeling generally well, with the exception of his chief complaint of right buttock symptoms. It would be helpful to clarify why Dekohta is taking the Vitamin B supplements and ensure that he is not taking any other medications or supplements. The key result of this line of questioning was that Dekohta has been trying to lose weight in an attempt to obtain a normal body mass index and had experienced a planned loss of 10 pounds over the course of 4 weeks via diet and exercise.

Given the location of Dekohta's symptoms, the clinician should also review the cardiopulmonary, gastrointestinal, and genitourinary systems. Dekohta's buttock symptoms are lower than would be expected with an abdominal aortic aneurysm, and he does not appear to have any of the more common comorbidities, such as smoking or hypertension. However, the clinician should inquire about the presence of a throbbing pain, and if present follow this up with palpation of the abdominal aorta in addition to the planned assessment of blood pressure. Dekohta has not noted taking any medication for this condition, such as an anti-inflammatory drug. An acute injury may respond positively to an anti-inflammatory drug, but it is possible that he tried an anti-inflammatory medication and stopped because of the lack of response, a side effect to the medication, or an unreported ulcer. Therefore, the clinician should ask specifically if Dekohta has tried anti-inflammatory medications and the result, as well as determine whether his symptoms are affected by food intake. To explore the potential referral from the genitourinary system, the clinician should enquire about bladder function, sexual dysfunction, and saddle anesthesia. The patient's remote history of hernia surgery may indicate a weak abdominal wall and requires the clinician to assess for a possible hernia during the physical examination. Although there do not appear to be any signs of psychological distress based on the intake form, the clinician should be observant for this throughout the history and examination.

Based on the history and negative findings from queries into non-neuromusculoskeletal systems, the clinician has initial hypotheses of nonspecific low back pain (LBP), disc pathology, deep gluteal syndrome, or muscle strain (gluteal, hip rotator, or hamstring). However, the clinician must still consider the possibility of a hernia causing referred pain.

TABLE 20-2
DEKOHTA: A 31-YEAR-OLD ACTUARY/STATISTICIAN WITH RIGHT BUTTOCK PAIN

Position	Assessments	Positive Findings
Observation	Continues from history	
Seated	L5: great toe extension (A, OP, MMT) L4: ankle dorsiflexion (A, OP, MMT) L3: knee extension (A, OP, MMT) L1/2: hip flexion (A, OP, MMT) Hip external rotation (A, OP, MMT) Hip internal rotation (A, OP, MMT) Dermatomes L1–S2 Reflexes: patellar, Achilles, Babinski, biceps, brachioradialis, triceps	
Standing	Structure/posture screen Gait Single leg balance Standing PF (S1,2) MMT Baseline trunk AROM flexion, extension, side glide Repeated trunk flexion x 5 Repeated trunk extension x 10	Mild decrease in lordosis Baseline symptoms: R buttock pain Baseline trunk flex fingertips to mid-shin, extension mildly decreased, both increased buttock symptoms, no worse Repeated trunk flexion produced R LBP and increased buttock symptoms, worse Repeated trunk extension increased back and buttock symptoms, no worse

TABLE 20-2 (continued)
DEKOHTA: A 31-YEAR-OLD ACTUARY/STATISTICIAN WITH RIGHT BUTTOCK PAIN

Position	Assessments	Positive Findings
Supine	Muscle length: gastrocnemius Hip PROM: flexion, abduction Hip: scour, FADIR, FABER SLR (also assesses hamstring length) Trunk flexion in lying Repeated trunk flexion in lying x 10	Baseline supine symptoms: R buttock and R LBP, reduced from standing Trunk flexion in lying increased back symptoms, no worse
Prone	Hip extension (P) MMT: gluteus maximus, HS (S1,2) Prone prop Repeated extension in lying x 10 x 3 Palpation: gluteals, hamstrings, lumbar paraspinals Posterior-to-anterior pressures: central and unilateral L5–L1	Baseline supine symptoms: R buttock and R LBP, same as supine Extension in lying: • Set 1: abolished back pain, reduced buttock pain, better • Set 2: reduced buttock pain, increased extension ROM, better • Set 3: no effect Palpation: increased tone of right hip external rotators Posterior-to-anterior pressures of L5 produced right low back pain, no worse
Supine	Palpation: inguinal region Abdominal drawing in maneuver Leg-lowering abdominal test	Leg-lowering abdominal test 4, produced buttock pain, no worse

A, active; *L*, left; *LBP*, low back pain; *MMT*, manual muscle test; *OP*, overpressure; *P*, passive; *PF*, plantarflexion; *R*, right; *SLR*, straight leg raise.

Physical Examination The physical examination should begin with the systems review. Heart rate, blood pressure, oxygen saturation, and respiratory rate were taken. The patient's height and weight were measured. The clinician should observe skin integrity, scarring, ecchymosis, and edema. All findings were considered normal. Table 20-2 provides the flow of the remainder of the physical examination by an experienced clinician. All tests begin with the uninvolved left side unless otherwise noted. Any positive findings are listed in the right-hand column.

The seated examination begins with a lower quarter neurologic screen to identify potential lumbar spine involvement and assessment of hip rotation ROM and strength. Because Dekohta has reported paresthesias leading to suspicions of neurologic involvement, the clinician chose to perform upper extremity reflexes as a point of comparison. Despite a negative seated examination, the clinician cannot rule out lumbar spine involvement without assessing trunk AROM. Therefore, the clinician moves on to the standing examination, beginning first with a gross appreciation of Dekohta's structure and posture, followed by a logical progression of assessing balance on one limb before repeated unilateral plantarflexion. While it may seem that the clinician assessed the S1,2 myotome twice, this choice was intentional. Hamstring strength was assessed due to symptoms reported in the region of the hamstring, whereas plantarflexion strength was considered important, given Dekohta's hobbies of weight lifting and running.

Despite not having back pain initially, careful attention to symptom location and intensity allowed the clinician to recognize Dekohta's symptoms changed as a result of repeated trunk motion. Repeated trunk flexion worsened symptoms (creating LBP and worsening buttock symptoms), whereas repeated trunk extension transiently increased both back and buttock symptoms. Given the lack of directional preference in a loaded (standing) position in the sagittal plane, the clinician proceeded to the lying examination. The lack of symptom provocation with seated hip rotation testing combined with the increase in symptoms with trunk AROM helped narrow the clinician's diagnostic hypotheses to the lumbar spine. Therefore, the supine examination began with clearing the hip before returning to methodically loading the trunk in lying. Given Dekohta's report of increased pain with sitting and standing trunk flexion worsening symptoms, it was unlikely that unloaded flexion in supine would be the patient's directional preference. However, the clinician recalled that lying down improved his symptoms and wanted to take a logical, meticulous approach and try this loading strategy, carefully noting a new baseline for symptoms with each position change. The prone examination revealed Dekohta's directional preference for unloaded trunk extension. The clinician performed posteroanterior joint mobilizations to see if these might further reduce symptoms. However, another clinician may have chosen to skip this assessment, given the patient's positive response to repeated extension in lying.

The clinician completed the physical examination by assessing for a possible hernia, given the patient's past medical history and report of heavy lifting. This was chosen, despite having found a directional preference, to ensure a holistic approach to patient care. Because a hernia was considered improbable, this was not investigated immediately. If the clinician had a higher degree of suspicion that the patient's symptoms were caused by a hernia, this would have been performed at the start of the physical examination. The Thomas test was not performed, given the clinician's observation of normal ROM with gluteus maximus testing (hip extension with the knee flexed 90°). The clinician chose to defer hip abductor strength assessment, given the ease of which symptoms were changed based on loading. The clinician could also have deferred leg-lowering abdominal testing but took a cautious approach, first trying an abdominal drawing in maneuver before the actual MMT. The clinician recalled that the vast majority of patients with a directional preference, even those with unilateral symptoms, respond to repeated movements in the sagittal plane. The decision to meticulously follow a strategic loading process of exhausting the sagittal plane before exploring other planes proved beneficial.

As a result of the history and physical examination, the clinician concluded that Dekohta had nonspecific LBP that centralized with unloaded trunk extension. He also appeared to have suboptimal core strength, although this was not thoroughly investigated, given how easily his symptoms changed based on trunk loading. The clinician informed Dekohta of the examination findings and related that most patients with a directional preference typically recover with about a month of rehabilitation. The clinician emphasized the need to try to avoid or limit trunk loading (weight training through the trunk and trunk flexion activities) short term to allow tissue healing. The clinician reviewed methods to reduce trunk loading while at work, including the use of a chair with lumbar support, the use of a standing desk, and frequent changes of position. The clinician explained the concepts of centralization and peripheralization as guiding principles for home exercise and activity modification at this time. A home program of repeated extension in lying was prescribed to be performed in sequential sets of 10 repetitions, until symptoms were not further improved, with repetition of this sequence 3 to 5 times a day. An abdominal exercise program could have been prescribed but was deferred to minimize the chance of symptom aggravation, given the production of buttock pain with abdominal strength testing. The plan of care included assessment hip abductor strength, trunk extensor strength, and trunk extensor endurance strength. Once symptoms have resolved, the clinician planned to observe Dekohta performing his weight training, including a deadlift, beginning at a low intensity.

Case Study 20-3: Jamal—Patient with Bilateral Shoulder Pain

Jamal is a 39-year-old handyperson with bilateral shoulder pain. Figure 20-3 contains the intake forms Jamal completed before his clinic appointment.

CASE STUDY 20-3
Jamal: Patient with Bilateral Shoulder Pain

Intake Form

Name: Jamal   Date: Aug 8
Age: 39   Gender: M   Race/Ethnicity: African American   Preferred language: English
Reason for visit: L > R shoulder pain
When did this start? 5 weeks ago
How did this occur? ☒ No apparent reason   ☐ When performing a deadlift
Have you had this problem in the past? ☒ No   ☐ Yes   If so, please describe (how often, how long it lasted, how resolved).
What activities are you having difficulty performing (hobbies, sports, exercise, work): Reaching overhead, lifting overhead, dry walling, washing back
Describe any treatment you have tried so far to assist with this and the result (ibuprofen, ice): ibuprofen
Describe any testing you have received for this and the result (x-ray, MRI, etc.): None

FIGURE 20-3 Intake form for Jamal.

CASE STUDY 20-3 (continued)

Mark the location of your symptom(s) on the diagrams below:

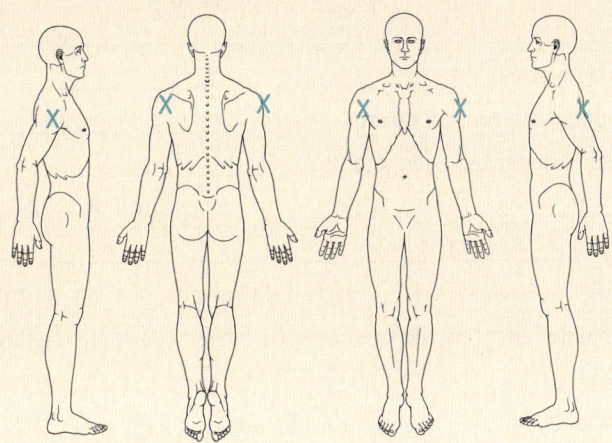

Using the following scale, 0 = No pain, 10 = Worst pain imaginable, Emergency Department necessary

what is your pain level **right now**? __2__/10

During the last 48 hours, what was your pain: **at best** __0__/10 **at worst:** __7__/10

Overall are you: ☐ getting better ☒ getting worse ☐ staying the same

Describe your symptoms: ☐ pins and needles ☐ burning ☒ aching ☒ dull
☐ sharp ☐ stabbing ☐ throbbing other: _____

What makes your symptoms **better**? ☐ activity ☐ rest ☐ morning ☐ end of day
☐ sitting ☐ walking ☐ ice ☐ heat ☒ medications: _ibuprofen_ Other: _____

What makes your symptoms **worse**? ☒ activity ☐ rest ☐ morning ☒ end of day
☐ sitting ☐ walking ☐ ice ☐ heat ☐ medications: _____ Other: _My job_

Goal(s) for therapy: _Work without pain_

Mark any boxes if you have a history of, or have recently experienced, the following:

☒ High blood pressure	☐ Cancer	☐ Nail changes
☒ High cholesterol	☐ Night sweats	☐ Skin changes
☐ Heart disease	☐ Night pain	☐ Vision changes
☐ Chest pain	☐ Ulcer	☐ Easy bruising
☐ Leg cramping with walking	☐ Constipation	☐ Excessive weight gain or loss
☐ Feel a heartbeat in your abdomen	☐ Incontinence	☐ Headaches
☐ Lightheadedness	☐ Abdominal pain	☐ Arthritis
☐ Diabetes	☐ Changes in menstrual pattern	☐ Muscle weakness
☐ Stroke	☐ Numbness, tingling	☐ Fatigue
☐ Epilepsy/seizures	☐ Walking or balance difficulties	☐ Morning stiffness
☐ Asthma/breathing problems	☐ Long-term steroid use	☐ Trauma (car accident or fall)

FIGURE 20-3 (continued)

> **CASE STUDY 20-3 (continued)**
>
> Are you currently pregnant? ☒ No ☐ Yes
> List prior surgeries: <u>Tonsils, right knee meniscus surgery</u>
> List any other diagnoses or injuries: _____
> List any medications/supplements you are taking: <u>Hydrochlorothiazide, simvastatin</u>
> List any allergies (i.e., latex, adhesives, sulfa, etc.)? _____
> Occupation: <u>Handyperson</u>   Currently working? ☐ No ☒ Yes
> Recreational activities/sports: <u>Race car driving</u>
> How often do you exercise? ☐ 0 days/week ☒ 1–4 days/week ☐ 5–7 days/week
> On average, how many minutes of moderate or strenuous exercise (e.g., at least a *brisk* walk) do you engage in per week? <u>60</u>
> On average, how many alcoholic drinks do you have per week: <u>5</u>
> Do you smoke? ☒ No ☐ Yes: ___packs/day, ___ yrs ☒ Former smoker: date quit <u>3yrs, 2</u>packs/day, <u>11</u>yrs,
> On average, how many hours of sleep do you get per night? <u>6</u>
> Does this current problem affect your sleep? ☐ No ☒ Yes
> Do you currently feel stressed? ☐ No ☒ Yes
> Do you feel down, depressed, or hopeless? ☒ No ☐ Yes
> Please note if you need any accommodations or have any preferences that may affect your therapy (i.e., religion, physical disability, etc.). _____
>
> **FIGURE 20-3** (*continued*)

History In reviewing Jamal's intake form, the clinician notes intermittent moderate left more than right shoulder pain of insidious onset 5 weeks ago. Symptoms are a dull, aching sensation and increase with overhead and hand behind the back activities. Symptoms are increased with activity, as the day goes on, and while working. Jamal reports symptoms are worsening. The patient has a history of hypertension and hypercholesterolemia, for which he takes medications, and a distant history of smoking. There is no prior history of shoulder pain, but Jamal had a prior right knee surgery.

The response to anti-inflammatory medications, symptoms worsening with high-demand shoulder activities, and symptom description appear consistent with a mechanical shoulder problem. However, based on Jamal's history and location of symptoms, the clinician should ask clarifying questions that address the cardiovascular, pulmonary, gastrointestinal, and urogenital systems as well as constitutional factors and a psychological screening. For example, cardiac-related symptoms might also be increased with overhead activities; however, cardiac symptoms are unlikely to be created with reaching behind the back. The clinician should enquire about the patient's medications, ensuring he is taking the prescribed dosage regularly. Because the lungs are a possible source of shoulder pain and Jamal has a history of smoking, the pulmonary system requires further investigation. The clinician should congratulate Jamal on smoking cessation and ask what made him decide to stop smoking. For example, it would be good for the clinician to know if Jamal stopped smoking after being told he was developing emphysema or if it was for some other reason. Clarifying questions are warranted, such as asking about chest pain, shortness of breath, fatigue, the presence of a cough, and if shoulder symptoms come on with activities that stress the heart but not the shoulders, such as walking, running, or biking. Although some of these questions were on the intake form, clarification that these items are in fact negative is important.

Clarifying questions for the gastrointestinal and urogenital systems might include asking about nausea, vomiting, change of symptoms with food intake, history of urinary tract infections, painful urination, or the need to urinate more frequently. Constitutional symptoms such as fatigue have been covered already, but the clinician may ask about the presence of fever or if Jamal has had any recent illnesses. The clinician should learn more about Jamal's knee surgery, such as when the surgery occurred and how the knee is functioning now. Lack of normal knee function may require compensation from other areas, and, if his knee surgery was recent, sepsis should be considered.

Jamal has two potential yellow flags: he notes he is currently feeling stressed and that his job makes his symptoms worse. While it is reasonable that the physical demands of being a handyperson might increase shoulder pain, and that the worsening of symptoms may make Jamal stressed due to fear he may not be able to continue working, it is possible that he is exhibiting pain-associated psychological distress, fear avoidance behavior, or abnormal coping behaviors. It is also possible that the stress Jamal has noted is unrelated to his current shoulder complaint. The clinician might begin with the following inquiries:

- "I see that your shoulder pain is aggravated by work. I know you do some drywalling, but the job of a handyperson is quite varied. Can you guide me through the activities of a typical workday so I can better understand the specifics of your job?"
- "Have there been any changes in your job demands in the past 2 months?"
- "You have noted on your intake form that you feel stressed. Can you tell me more about that?"

Jamal reports that his passion is restoring old homes requiring fine craftsmanship. He reports that normally, his boss is able to find this type of work for him, but for the past 2 months, his crew has been working solely on building a new subdivision. Therefore, his job demands have changed to primarily drywalling with some painting, performed mostly at or above shoulder height.

Jamal's symptoms are exacerbated by overhead work, requiring a position of sustained cervical extension as well as shoulder elevation. The clinician must clarify the location and type of symptoms, specifically asking about the presence of neck pain or headache, tingling or numbness, and forearm, hand, or lower extremity symptoms. Cervical extension may aggravate cervical stenosis, a posterior disc herniation, or myelopathy, causing bilateral shoulder pain. The clinician must learn the patient's hand dominance and more about the left versus the right shoulder symptoms. For example, did both shoulder symptoms begin at the same time? Are the symptoms similar in each shoulder? Is one shoulder worse than the other? While the patient has not noted stiffness, weakness, clicking, catching, locking, or a feeling of instability, the clinician should ask if Jamal is experiencing these shoulder-specific problems to help rule in/out competing diagnoses, such as adhesive capsulitis, osteoarthritis, ruptured tendon, labral pathology, and instability. The clinician should learn about the patient's exercise habits and the effect of exercise on shoulder symptoms. The patient's hobby of race car driving is somewhat unique. The clinician should learn if the patient has a history of any race-related injuries or accidents.

The clinician should choose at least one outcome measure for the patient to complete. Assuming the history does not reveal neck-related symptoms, the Disabilities of Arm, Shoulder, and Hand (DASH) questionnaire would be appropriate. Pending the patient's response to yellow flag inquiry, the clinician may want to have Jamal complete the FABQ or the TSK.

Based on the history, the clinician has initial hypotheses of pain referred from the cervical region, rotator cuff tendinopathy, scapular dyskinesia, and subacromial impingement syndrome (SIS). Glenohumeral osteoarthritis, although more common in individuals over the age of 65, is also possible, given the patient's highly physical job demands and recreational hobby of car racing. Adhesive capsulitis is considered less likely, given Jamal reports the ability to perform overhead work and reach behind the back. Instability and labral pathology are considered improbable based on the patient's response to shoulder-specific symptoms. However, the clinician must still consider referred pain from non-musculoskeletal sources.

Physical Examination Based on the history, there are no red flags for the clinician to consider. The physical examination should begin with the systems review. The clinician should learn Jamal's learning style and observe his affect and engagement throughout the session. Heart rate, blood pressure, oxygen saturation, and respiratory rate were taken. The patient's height and weight were measured. The clinician should observe skin integrity, scarring, nail status, and edema. Observation of gross coordinated movements should be performed, given the low potential for myelopathy. All findings were considered normal.

TABLE 20-3
JAMAL: A 39-YEAR-OLD HANDYPERSON WITH BILATERAL SHOULDER PAIN

Position	Assessments	Positive Findings
Observation	Continues from history	
Seated	Cervical flex, ext, lat flex, rot (A, OP) Spurling test Reflexes brachialis, biceps, triceps Dermatomes C4–T1 Finger add (A, MMT) Thumb ext (A, MMT) Elbow flex, ext (A, P, MMT) Upper trapezius MMT Shoulder ER arms at side, flex, ext, scaption, abd (A, OP, MMT) Scapular assistance and retraction tests Shoulder combined hand behind neck and behind back reach (A) MMT: ER and IR with arms at sides MMT: shoulder flex, ext, abd Special tests: supraspinatus test, ER lag test, Neer impingement test, Hawkins-Kennedy test, horizontal adduction test Palpation: including long head of biceps, subacromial region, anterior and posterior shoulder, upper trapezius, levator scapulae, and posterior rotator cuff	Shoulder AROM: Flex L155/R150 Scap L160/R155 Painful arc on the R Hand behind the back to L T10/R T12* MMT: shoulder abduction L4/R4* Special tests: positive R Neer impingement, B Hawkins-Kennedy, and L horizontal adduction tests Palpation: increased tone upper trapezii, trigger points in right infraspinatus, tender B supraspinatus humeral attachment region
Supine	PROM: shoulder flex, scap, IR, ER MMT: serratus anterior Glenohumeral accessory motion: anterior, posterior, inferior Muscle length: pectoralis minor/major	Shoulder PROM: Flex L158/R155* Scap L162/R160* IR L 60/R50* Glenohumeral accessory motion reduced B posteriorly and inferiorly
Prone	MMT: ER, IR, rhomboid, middle trapezius, lower trapezius, trunk extensors Plank hold Sorenson test	MMT: ER 4 B, lower trap 3 + B, trunk extensors 3 Sorenson test 10 seconds
Standing	Functional test: mock drywall work, lifting, lifting 5 and 10# dumbbell overhead	Decreased thoracic extension Pain with higher levels of elevation B
Seated	Thoracic ext, rot (AROM, OP)	Reduced kyphosis reversal, reduced ROM

*Reproduction of patient's symptoms.
A, active; abd, abduction; AROM, active range of motion; ER, external rotation; Ext, extension; flex, flexion; IR, internal rotation; L, left; lat flex, lateral flexion; MMT, manual muscle test; OP, overpressure; P, passive range of motion, PROM, passive range of motion; R, right; ROM, range of motion; rot, rotation; scap, scaption.

Table 20-3 provides the sample flow of the remainder of the physical examination by an experienced clinician. All tests begin with the less involved left side unless otherwise noted. Any positive findings are listed in the right-hand column.

The seated examination begins with clearing the cervical spine and elbow (active motion with overpressure and MMT) of potential involvement. To clear the cervical spine, the clinician performs a cervical screen of AROM with overpressure and Spurling test. Upper extremity myotomes, dermatomes, and reflexes are then performed. The clinician chose to use elbow flexion and extension for testing the C6 and C7 myotome rather than the wrist flexors and extensors. This choice was made because assessment of the elbow was required, given the elbow joint is the joint distal to the glenohumeral joint and, therefore, is also part of the clearing examination for the shoulder, whereas the wrist musculature is not. To finish clearing the elbow, the clinician also performs overpressure to elbow flexion and extension. This is followed by a gross appreciation of shoulder AROM viewed from both the front and behind to observe the quantity and quality of motion, including any abnormal scapulohumeral rhythm or scapular dyskinesia.

The seated examination rules out the cervical spine, rotator cuff rupture, adhesive capsulitis, and scapular dyskinesia. Positive findings are consistent with SIS, rotator cuff tendinopathy, and glenohumeral arthritis. The lack of crepitus and normal ER ROM helps to rule out glenohumeral arthritis. Reduced glenohumeral joint accessory motions and painful end-ranges are consistent with SIS. The prone examination findings of decreased posterior cuff strength along with impaired trunk extensor strength and endurance provide additional possible causative factors for SIS. The clinician's observation of reduced functional thoracic spine extension leads to additional testing of thoracic spine extension and rotation ROM and an additional causative factor for Jamal's symptoms.

The clinician concluded that Jamal had SIS exacerbated by reduced thoracic spine extension motion, reduced glenohumeral accessory motion, reduced posterior cuff and thoracic muscle performance, and a significant change in job demands. The clinician discussed the examination findings with Jamal, including the lack of serious pathology (no rotator cuff tear, no cervical involvement, and no referral from non-musculoskeletal systems). The clinician reiterated the inflammatory component to Jamal's symptoms by noting both how the anti-inflammatory medication ibuprofen helped relieve his symptoms and how his symptoms were less intense when not performing impinging tasks. The clinician discussed the positive anti-inflammatory effects of icing his shoulder routinely, especially after work, in addition to the potential adverse effects of prolonged ibuprofen use. Jamal was instructed in activity modifications to reduce impingement, including using a ladder more often, alternating work tasks between high and low levels, and asking his supervisor about the ability to limit overhead work for at least the following week. The clinician presented rehabilitation options, including stretching, strengthening, and joint mobilizations to the shoulder and thoracic spine, and noted that most patients with SIS report a resolution of symptoms within 8 weeks of starting interventions.

CHAPTER SUMMARY

There are many possible approaches to each patient interaction. The three cases included in this chapter provided examples of integration of information gathered on the patient intake forms, patient history, and physical examination to determine possible and probable causative factors to the patient symptoms. The logical progression of questioning and the physical examination with minimal positional changes are provided. The reader is encouraged to review the detailed information presented in this test to further explore potential functional tests and outcome measures.

APPENDIX A
GLOSSARY

Accessory motion arthrokinematic motions occurring at articular surfaces, also known as joint play.

Algometer device used to identify the pressure and/or force eliciting a pressure-pain threshold.

Apoptosis cellular death in which cell actively destroys itself.

Arthrokinematic motion movement between adjacent articular surfaces, such as gliding.

Articular cartilage smooth, low-friction tissue located at the ends of bones in synovial joints.

Avascular necrosis (aka osteonecrosis) death of bone tissue due to lack of blood supply.

Bankart lesion detachment of the anteroinferior portion of the glenoid labrum that occurs with anterior humeral dislocation.

Biceps tenodesis surgical release of the long head of the biceps from the glenoid with reattachment on the humerus.

Biceps tenotomy surgical release of the long head of the biceps without reattachment.

Biopsychosocial model of pain approach to understanding pain that describes the interaction between genetic makeup (biology), mental health and behavior (psychology), and social and cultural contexts.

Capsular pattern of restriction pattern of loss of motion at a joint that indicates restriction of the entire capsule due to effusion or fibrosis.

Cauda equina syndrome a serious collection of symptoms caused by damage to the terminal portion of the spinal cord.

Centralization phenomenon in which distal symptoms related to the spine are reduced or move proximal/toward the midline as a result of movement.

Clearing examination limited examination of the joints proximal and distal to the suspected area of pathology.

Clonus a stretch reflex that is exaggerated, rhythmic, and oscillating suggestive of an upper motor neuron lesion.

Close-packed position the position of a joint in which the capsule and ligaments are taut and there is maximal joint congruency.

Complex regional pain syndrome (CRPS) broad term describing excess and prolonged pain and inflammation that follows an injury to an arm or leg, previously known as reflex sympathetic dystrophy (RSD). CRPS has acute (recent, short-term) and chronic (lasting >6 months) forms.

Conjunct rotation obligatory motion that occurs at the joint surface that is not under voluntary control.

Constitutional symptoms nonspecific cluster of signs and symptoms that signal possible systemic disease process or pathology.

Convex-concave pattern of movement describes the roll and glide pattern that occurs with movement.

Cyriax testing (aka isometric testing in a midrange position) designed to assess the status of the muscle-tendon unit along with its innervation.

Derangement spinal disorder in which symptoms centralize (or peripheralize) as a result of changes in spinal loading.

Dermatome area of skin that is innervated primarily by one spinal nerve root.

Directional preference direction of mechanical loading that reduces, centralizes, and/or abolishes patient symptoms.

Double-crush injury when a nerve is compressed at more than one point, less compression is required to adversely affect nerve function.

Effusion intra-articular swelling.

Elastic cartilage tissue found in external ear and epiglottis that has higher amounts of elastin to provide strength and elasticity.

Endfeel the quality of resistance to movement the examiner feels at the end point of movement; may be normal or abnormal.

Entrapment (aka entrapment neuropathy) compression of a peripheral nerve.

Fibrocartilage strong tissue consisting of type I and type II collagen fibers in intervertebral discs and articular cartilage.

Force couple a system in which the force of one muscle (the primary agonist) works with the antagonist muscle producing a resultant movement.

Glenohumeral internal rotation deficit (GIRD) at least a 20° loss of glenohumeral internal rotation compared with the contralateral side.

Hemarthrosis bleeding within a joint, commonly occurs with intra-articular fracture and anterior cruciate ligament rupture.

Herniated nucleus pulposus migration of the disc nucleus against sensitive neural tissue.

Hill-Sach lesion osseous deformity of the posterosuperior humeral head from impacting the anterior glenoid during an anterior glenohumeral dislocation.

Instability subjective complaint of discomfort or lack of function due to excessive arthrokinematic translation.

Instant center of rotation (aka instantaneous center of rotation) the point around which motion takes place at a particular moment in time.

Irritability the ability of a tissue to handle stress, how easily symptoms are provoked. Once provoked, how intense symptoms are and how long it takes to return to baseline. Rated as none, low, moderate, or high.

Isometric testing in a midrange position (aka Cyriax testing) designed to assess the status of the muscle-tendon unit along with its innervation.

Jendrassik maneuver method used to reinforce an absent or diminished reflex.

Joint mobilization passive movement of the articular surface used to assess joint mobility, promote pain relief, or increase motion.

Laxity increased joint mobility as assessed with joint mobility testing or special tests.

Loose-packed position *see* open-packed position

Lower quarter neurologic screen cluster of tests designed to identify damage to a spinal nerve; includes trunk active range of motion, myotome, dermatome, reflex testing of the lower quarter.

Myelopathy compression of the spinal cord.

Myotome a muscle that is primarily innervated by one spinal nerve root.

Neurodynamic tests assessments of nerve tension by lengthening the tissue (e.g., straight leg raise and upper limb tension test).

Neurogenic claudication symptoms of tingling, numbness, and/or pain due to compression of spinal nerves.

Neuropathic pain pain caused by inflammation, irritation, or neural tissue compression. Associated with damage to the neurons in the body, following an infection or injury to the area, either of which will result in messages of pain being sent to the central nervous system.

Nociceptive pain pain from physical damage or potential damage to the body tissue without damage to the nerve itself. Includes radicular pain (occurs when nerve roots are irritated); somatic pain (occurs when pain receptors in tissues are activated) and visceral pain.

Nociplastic pain describes a category of pain arising primarily from alterations of neural processing with no known tissue damage.

Noncapsular pattern of restriction loss of motion at a joint that does not follow a predictable pattern, most commonly caused by intra-articular mechanical block or extra-articular lesion.

Open-packed position (aka loose-packed position) the position of a joint in which there is the greatest amount of slack in the capsule and ligaments and the least amount of articular congruency.

Osteochondritis dissecans (OCD) a joint disorder involving the articular surface and subchondral bone occurring most often in children and adolescents that is thought to be caused by lack of blood supply.

Osteokinematic motion rotary movement of a bony segment that occurs during physiologic motion such as knee flexion.

Pain Neuroscience Education (PNE) approach to pain intervention that aims to change patient perception of pain using a positive, enabling approach that emphasizes the multifactorial dimensions of pain.

Painful arc increased pain or pain in the range of 70 to 120° of shoulder elevation.

Panner disease painful elbow disorder in children due to changes in the surface of the capitellum.

Passive accessory intervertebral movement (aka PAIVM) mobilization technique that produces movement of a mobile vertebral segment without the active participation of muscles related to the movement.

Peripheralization phenomenon in which distal symptoms related to the spine are increased or move distally/away from the midline as a result of movement.

Plexopathy pathology involving a nerve or nerves within a plexus.

Provocation test type of special test designed to create or increase a patient's familiar symptoms.

Quarter screen regional examination that includes observation; gross assessment of structure and posture; assessment of motion, muscle length, and strength; and functional testing.

Radiculopathy pathology involving a spinal nerve root.

Red flags signs and symptoms that might indicate the presence of serious or nonmusculoskeletal pathology for which referral is required, should not be used in isolation.

Review of systems part of the history in which the clinician screens relevant body systems.

SLAP lesion *see* superior labrum anterior to posterior

Slipped capital femoral epiphysis (aka SCFE) disorder of adolescents in which the growth plate of the femoral head moves ("slips") with respect to the rest of the femur. The head of the femur stays in the cup of the hip joint, whereas the rest of the femur is shifted downward and backward off the femoral neck.

Special tests clinical procedures thought to assess specific anatomic structures or pathologic processes.

Spondylolisthesis pathologic slippage of one vertebral body on another.

Spondylolysis fracture of the pars interarticularis.

Spondylosis (aka cervical spondylosis) all-encompassing term for degenerative changes to the cervical spine.

Stability description of clinical course of a patient's condition: improving, staying the same, worsening.

Subtalar joint neutral theoretical concept that there is a neutral position of the subtalar joint where the joint is neither pronated nor supinated.

Superior labrum anterior to posterior injury to the superior labrum anterior to posterior to the long head of the biceps attachment on the glenoid.

Systems review limited examination of key body systems.

Tendinopathy broad term for pathology of a tendon, may be inflammatory, degenerative, or both.

Tenosynovitis inflammation of the synovial sheath surrounding a tendon.

Upper limb tension test (aka brachial plexus tension test, Elvey test, or ULTT) test to stress neurologic structures in the upper limb by placing the upper limb joints into specific position to stress components of the major nerves.

Upper quarter neurologic screen cluster of tests designed to identify damage to a spinal nerve; includes cervical active range of motion, myotome, dermatome, reflex testing of the upper quarter.

Vertebrobasilar insufficiency condition characterized by poor blood flow to the posterior portion of the brain due to blockage of vertebral arteries.

Yellow flags signs or symptoms that indicate the potential for pain-associated psychological distress and fear-avoidance beliefs.

APPENDIX B
OSTEOKINEMATIC AND ARTHROKINEMATIC MOTIONS

TABLE B-1
LOWER EXTREMITY OSTEOKINEMATIC AND ARTHROKINEMATIC MOTIONS

Joint	Motion	Normative Value (Degrees)	Arthrokinematic Glide to Restore Motion*	Open-Packed Position
Hip	Flexion	0–120	Inferior glide of femur	30° flexion, 30° abduction, and slight lateral rotation
	Extension	0–30	Anterior glide of femur	
	Abduction	0–45	Inferior glide of femur	
	Adduction	0–30	Lateral distraction of femur	
	Internal rotation	0–45	Posterior glide of femur	
	External rotation	0–45	Anterior glide of femur	
	Global motion	NA	Lateral distraction or inferior glide of femur	
Tibiofemoral	Flexion	0–135	Posterior glide of tibia, to a lesser extent internal rotation of tibia	25° flexion
	Extension	0 to up to 10	Anterior glide of tibia, to a lesser extent external rotation of tibia	
	Global motion	NA	Long-axis distraction	
Patellofemoral	Flexion	0–135	Inferior glide of patella	Full extension
	Extension	0 to up to 10	Superior glide of patella	
Talocrural	Dorsiflexion	0–20	Posterior glide of talus	Mid-inversion/eversion and 10° plantar flexion
	Plantarflexion	0–50	Anterior glide of talus	
	Inversion	0–35	NA	
	Eversion	0–15	NA	
	Global motion	NA	Talocrural distraction	
Rearfoot	Inversion	5	Lateral glide of calcaneus	Midway between extremes of range of motion with 10° plantar flexion
	Eversion	5	Medial glide of calcaneus	
	Global motion	NA	Subtalar distraction	
Great toe MTP	Extension	0–70	Dorsal glide of proximal phalanx	0–10° extension
	Flexion	0–45	Plantar glide of proximal phalanx	
	Global motion	NA	Distraction of proximal phalanx	
Lesser toe MTP	Extension	0–40	Dorsal glide of proximal phalanx	0–10° extension
	Flexion	0–40	Plantar glide of proximal phalanx	
	Global motion	NA	Distraction of proximal phalanx	
Great toe IP	Extension	0	Dorsal glide of distal phalanx	Slight flexion
	Flexion	0–90	Plantar glide of distal phalanx	
	Global motion	NA	Distraction of distal phalanx	
Lesser toe PIP	Extension	0	Dorsal glide of middle phalanx	Slight flexion
	Flexion	35	Plantar glide of middle phalanx	
	Global motion	NA	Distraction of middle phalanx	
Lesser toe DIP	Extension	0	Dorsal glide of distal phalanx	Slight flexion
	Flexion	60	Plantar glide of distal phalanx	
	Global motion	NA	Distraction of distal phalanx	

*Based on concave-convex rule in the open kinetic chain, requires clinical decision-making. (See Chapter 11 for hip; Chapter 10 for tibiofemoral and patellofemoral; and Chapter 9 for the remainder of the text discussed in the table.)

DIP, distal interphalangeal; *IP*, interphalangeal; *MTP*, metatarsophalangeal; *PIP*, proximal interphalangeal.

TABLE B-2
UPPER EXTREMITY OSTEOKINEMATIC AND ARTHROKINEMATIC MOTIONS

Joint	Motion	Normative Value (Degrees)	Arthrokinematic Glide to Restore Motion*	Open-Packed Position
Glenohumeral	Flexion	0–180 (shoulder girdle)	Inferior glide of humerus	30° flexion, 30° abduction, and slight lateral rotation
	Extension	0–60	Anterior glide of humerus	
	Abduction	0–180 (shoulder girdle)	Inferior glide of humerus	
	External rotation	0–90	Anterior glide of humerus	
	Internal rotation	0–70	Posterior glide of humerus	
	Horizontal abduction	0–45	Anterior glide of humerus	
	Horizontal adduction	0–135	Posterior glide of humerus	
	Global motion	NA	Lateral distraction of humerus	
Elbow	Flexion	0–150	Humeroulnar distraction, ventral radiohumeral glide	25° flexion
	Extension	0	Humeroulnar medial/lateral tilt, dorsal radiohumeral glide	
Forearm	Supination	0 to about 80–90	Proximal RU ventral glide, Distal RU dorsal glide	Proximal RU: 70° flexion and 35° supination
	Pronation	0 to about 80–90	Proximal RU dorsal glide, Distal RU ventral (or palmar) glide	Distal RU: 10° supination
Elbow/forearm	Global motion	NA	Humeroulnar and humeroradial distraction	
Wrist†	Flexion	0–80	Dorsal glide of distal segment	Radiocarpal joint: neutral with slight ulnar deviation
	Extension	0–70	Palmar glide of distal segment	
	Radial deviation	0–20	Ulnar glide of distal segment	Midcarpal joint: Neutral with slight flexion and ulnar deviation
	Ulnar deviation	0–30	Radial glide of distal segment	
	Global motion	NA	Distraction of distal segment	
Finger MCP	Flexion	0–90	Palmar glide of proximal phalanx	Slight flexion
	Extension	0–45	Dorsal glide of proximal phalanx	
	Global motion	NA	Distraction of proximal phalanx	
Finger PIP	Flexion	0–100	Palmar glide of proximal phalanx	10° flexion
	Extension	0	Dorsal glide of proximal phalanx	
	Global motion	NA	Distraction of proximal phalanx	
Finger DIP	Flexion	0–90	Palmar glide of distal phalanx	30° flexion
	Extension	0	Dorsal glide of distal phalanx	
	Global motion	NA	Distraction of distal phalanx	
Thumb CMC	Flexion	0–15	Ulnar glide of 1st metacarpal	Midway between flexion/extension and between abduction/adduction
	Extension	0–20	Radial glide of 1st metacarpal	
	Abduction	0–70	Dorsal glide of 1st metacarpal	
	Adduction	0	Palmar glide of 1st metacarpal	
	Global motion	NA	Distraction of 1st metacarpal	
Thumb MCP	Flexion	0–50	Palmar glide of proximal phalanx	Slight flexion
	Extension	0	Dorsal glide of proximal phalanx	
	Global motion	NA	Distraction of distal phalanx	
Thumb IP	Flexion	0–80	Palmar glide of distal phalanx	10° flexion
	Extension	0–30	Dorsal glide of distal phalanx	
	Global motion	NA	Distraction of proximal phalanx	

*Based on concave-convex rule in the open kinetic chain, requires clinical decision-making. (See Chapter 14 for glenohumeral joint; Chapter 15 for elbow, forearm, and elbow/forearm joints; and Chapter 16 for the remaining joints discussed in the table.)
†Includes radiocarpal and midcarpal joints.
CMC, carpometacarpal; DIP, distal interphalangeal; IP, Interphalangeal; MCP, metacarpophalangeal; PIP, proximal interphalangeal; RU, radioulnar.

APPENDIX C
PERIPHERAL AND SEGMENTAL NERVE INNERVATION

TABLE C-1
LOWER EXTREMITY PERIPHERAL AND SEGMENTAL INNERVATION

Muscles	Peripheral Nerve	Nerve Root	Myotome	Plexus
Iliopsoas	Femoral	L1–L3	L1–L2	Lumbar
Pectineus	Femoral	L2–L3		Lumbar
Sartorius	Femoral	L2–L3		Lumbar
Quadriceps femoris	Femoral	L2–L4	L3	Lumbar
Gracilis	Obturator	L2–L3		Lumbar
Adductor brevis	Obturator	L2–L4		Lumbar
Adductor longus	Obturator	L2–L4		Lumbar
Adductor magnus	Obturator, tibial	L2–L4		Lumbar
Obturator externus	Obturator	L3–L4		Lumbar
Tensor facia latae	Superior gluteal	L4–L5		Sacral
Gluteus maximus	Inferior gluteal	L5–S2		Sacral
Gluteus medius	Superior gluteal	L5–S1		Sacral
Gluteus minimus	Superior gluteal	L5–S1		Sacral
Tibialis anterior	Deep fibular	L4–L5	L4	Sacral
Extensor digitorum longus	Deep fibular	L5–S1		Sacral
Extensor hallucis longus	Deep fibular	L5–S1	L5	Sacral
Extensor digitorum brevis	Deep fibular	S1–S2		Sacral
Gemellus superior	Nerve to obturator internus	L5–S1		Sacral
Obturator internus	Nerve to obturator internus	L5–S1		Sacral
Gemellus inferior	Nerve to quadratus femoris	L5–S1		Sacral
Quadratus femoris	Nerve to quadratus femoris	L5–S1		Sacral
Piriformis	Nerve to piriformis	L5–S2		Sacral
Semimembranosus	Tibial	L5–S1	S1, S2	Sacral
Semitendinosus	Tibial	L5–S1	S1, S2	Sacral
Biceps femoris	Tibia (long head), common fibular	L5–S2		Sacral
Fibularis	Superficial fibular	L5–S1	S1, S2	Sacral
Tibialis posterior	Tibial	L4–L5		Sacral
Gastrocnemius	Tibial	S1–S2	S1, S2	Sacral
Soleus	Tibial	S1–S2		

Genitofemoral nerve:
Femoral branch
Genital branch (with ilioinguinal nerve)
Lateral femoral cutaneous nerve
Cutaneous branches of obturator nerve
Anterior cutaneous branches of femoral nerve
Lateral sural cutaneous nerve
Saphenous nerve
Superficial fibular nerve
Sural nerve
Deep fibular nerve
Lateral plantar nerve
Medial plantar nerve

Anterior

APPENDIX C | PERIPHERAL AND SEGMENTAL NERVE INNERVATION

TABLE C-1 (continued)
LOWER EXTREMITY PERIPHERAL AND SEGMENTAL INNERVATION

Muscles	Peripheral Nerve	Nerve Root	Myotome	Plexus
Flexor digitorum longus	Tibial	S2–S3		Sacral
Flexor hallucis longus	Tibial	S2–S3		Sacral
Small muscles of foot	Lateral plantar	S1–S2		Sacral
Flexor digitorum brevis	Medial plantar	S2–S3		Sacral
Flexor hallucis brevis	Medial plantar	S2–S3		Sacral
Perineal and sphincters	Pudendal	S2–S4		Sacral

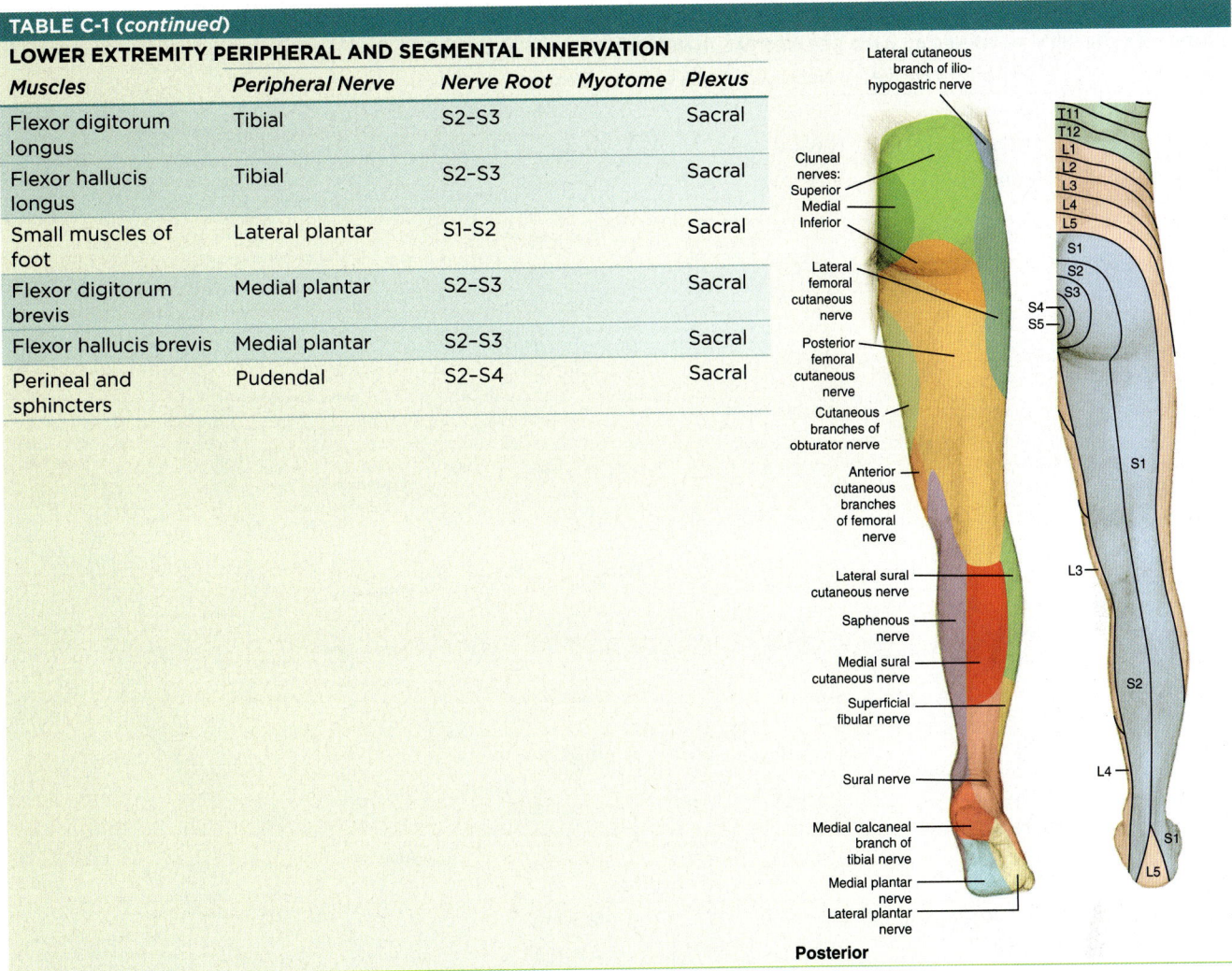

TABLE C-2
UPPER EXTREMITY PERIPHERAL AND SEGMENTAL INNERVATION

Muscle	Peripheral Nerve	Nerve Root	Myotome	Plexus
Sternocleidomastoid	Accessory	CN XI		Cranial
Trapezius	Accessory	CN XI		Cranial
Cervical muscles	Cervical	C1–C4	Flexors: C1–C3 Lateral flexors: C2–C4	Cervical
Diaphragm	Phrenic	C3–C5		Cervical, brachial
Scalenes	Ventral rami of C3–8	C3–C8		Cervical, brachial
Levator scapulae	Dorsal scapular	C5 (C3–C4)		Cervical, brachial
Rhomboids	Dorsal scapular nerve	C4–C5		Cervical, brachial
Infraspinatus	Suprascapular	C4–C6		Cervical, brachial
Supraspinatus	Suprascapular	C4–C6		Cervical, brachial
Teres minor	Axillary	C4–C6		Cervical, brachial
Deltoid	Axillary	C5–C6	C5	Brachial
Biceps brachii	Musculocutaneous	C5–C6	C6	Brachial
Brachialis	Musculocutaneous	C5–C6		Brachial
Coracobrachialis	Musculocutaneous	C5–C7		Brachial
Subscapularis	Subscapular	C5–C7		Cervical, brachial

(continued)

TABLE C-2 (continued)
UPPER EXTREMITY PERIPHERAL AND SEGMENTAL INNERVATION

Muscle	Peripheral Nerve	Nerve Root	Myotome	Plexus
Teres major	Subscapular	C6–C7		Cervical, brachial
Latissimus dorsi	Thoracodorsal	C6–C8		Brachial
Triceps brachii and anconeus	Radial	C6–C8	C7	Brachial
Anconeus	Radial	C7–T1		Brachial
Brachioradialis	Radial	C5–C7		Brachial
Extensor carpi radialis longus	Radial	C5–C8	C6	Brachial
Extensor carpi radialis brevis	Posterior interosseous	C6–C8	C6	Brachial
Supinator	Posterior interosseous	C5–C6		Brachial
Abductor pollicis longus	Posterior interosseous	C7–C8		Brachial
Extensor carpi ulnaris	Posterior interosseous	C7–C8	C6	Brachial
Extensor digiti minimi	Posterior interosseous	C7–C8		Brachial
Extensor digitorum	Posterior interosseous	C7–C8		Brachial
Extensor indicis	Posterior interosseous	C7–C8		Brachial
Extensor pollicis brevis	Posterior interosseous	C7–C8		Brachial
Extensor pollicis longus	Posterior interosseous	C7–C8	C8	Brachial
Flexor carpi radialis	Median	C6–C7	C7	Brachial
Pronator teres	Median	C6–C7		Brachial
Flexor digitorum superficialis	Median	C7–T1		Brachial
Abductor pollicis brevis	Median	C8–T1		Brachial
Flexor digitorum profundus	Median, Ulnar	C8–T1		Brachial
Flexor pollicis brevis	Median	C8–T1		Brachial
Flexor pollicis longus	Median	C8–T1		Brachial
Lumbricals (the two lateral)	Median	C8–T1		Brachial
Opponens pollicis	Median	C8–T1		Brachial
Flexor carpi ulnaris	Ulnar	C7–C8	C7	Brachial
Palmaris longus	Ulnar	C8–T1		Brachial
Lumbricales (the two medial)	Ulnar	C8–T1		Brachial
Abductor digiti minimi	Ulnar	C8–T1		Brachial
Adductor pollicis	Ulnar	C8–T1		Brachial
Flexor digiti minimi brevis	Ulnar	C8–T1		Brachial
Interossei	Ulnar	C8–T1	T1	Brachial
Opponens digiti minimi	Ulnar	C8–T1		Brachial

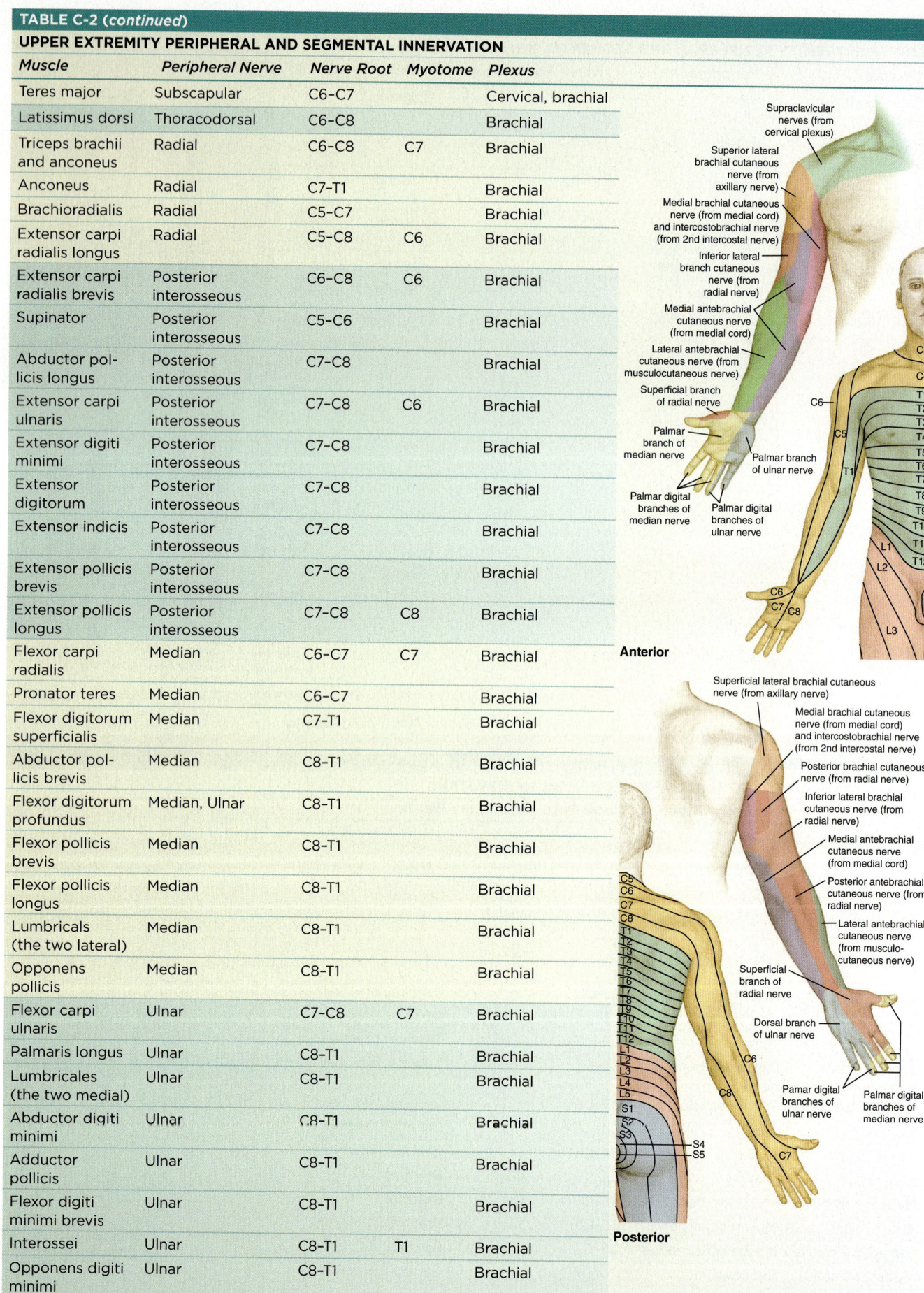

INDEX

Page numbers in *italics* denote figures; those followed by a t denote tables.

A

AAA (*see* Abdominal aortic aneurysm)
Abdominal aortic aneurysm (AAA), 375
Abdominal muscles, 82, *83–84*
Abduction, 39
   and adduction, 198
   hyperextension-external rotation test, 349, *349*
   inferior humeral glide, 497–498, *498*
Abnormal response, 158, 162
AC joint separations (*see* Acromioclavicular joint, separation)
AC shear test (*see* Acromioclavicular joint, compression test)
Accessory bones, 189, *190*, *191*
Accessory joint movement, 43 (*see also* Arthrokinematic movement)
Accessory motion, 43
   hip joint, 346–347, *346*
   knee joint, 281–282, *282*
   physical examination, 161–163, *162*, 163–164t
   wrist and hand complex, 603–606, 603t, *604–606*, 605t
ACDF (*see* Anterior cervical discectomy with fusion)
Acetabulum, hip joint, 330, *331*
Achilles tendinopathy
   differential diagnoses, 239
   expected outcomes, 240
   history, 239
   key examination findings, 239, *240*
   pathology, 239
   rehabilitation focus and key points, 239–240, 240t
Achilles tendon, 21
   pathology tests, 221
      arc sign, 221
      Royal London Hospital test, 221
      Thompson test, 221
   rupture, 240–241
      postoperative rehabilitation, 241
      surgical outcomes, 241
ACL (*see* Anterior cruciate ligament)
Acromioclavicular (AC) joint
   compression test, 464, *465*
   and ligaments, *440*, 441–442
   separation, 474–476, 475t
Acromioclavicular degenerative joint disease, 476
Acromion, 437
Activation/movement control–biased tests, 385
Active compression test (*see* O'Brien active compression test)
Active piriformis test, 390, *390*
Active range of motion (AROM), 150, 383
   interpretation of symptoms, 154
   quality, 150
   quantity, 150
   signs and symptoms, 150–151
Acute lumbar strains, 413–414
Acute tendon rupture, 599
Adduction, 39
Adductor test, 348, *348*
Adhesive capsulitis, 478–481, *479*, *479–481*
Adson test, 660–661, *661*
Adult scoliosis, 677–678
Aerobic exercise, 409
Aggravating activities, 706–707
Aggrecan, 8t, 9
Alar ligament test, 659
Alcohol abuse, 128
Alcoholism, 128
Algometer, 732, *733*
ALL (*see* Anterior longitudinal ligament)
α-chains (*see* Polypeptide chains)
Anatomical snuffbox, 592, *592*
Ankle
   impingement, 238–239, *239*
   injury, acute, 727–728
   sprain
      differential diagnoses, 236
      expected outcomes, 236t, 237
      history, 236
      key examination findings, 236, 236t, *237*
      pathology, 234–236
      rehabilitation after lateral ankle surgery, 238
      rehabilitation focus and key points, 236–237, *238*
      surgical interventions, 238
      surgical outcomes, 238
Ankle and foot
   accessory motion, 214
      distal tibiofibular joint mobilization, 214–215, *215*
      intermetatarsal joint mobility, 216–217, *217*
      interphalangeal joint mobilizations, 217–218, *218*
      intertarsal joint mobility, 216, *217*
      metatarsophalangeal joint mobility, 217, *218*
      proximal tibiofibular joint, 214, *215*
      subtalar joint mobilizations, 215–216, *217*
      talocrural joint mobilization, 215, *216*
   achilles pathology tests, 221
      arc sign, 221
      Royal London Hospital test, 221
      Thompson test, 221
   ankle pathologies (*see specific types*)
   case study, 250
   distal tibial alignment, 210–211, *211*
   examination, introduction to, 204
   first ray position and mobility, 210
   foot pathologies (*see specific types*)
   footwear and gait, 223, 223t
   fractures
      differential diagnoses, 234
      expected outcomes, 234
      history, 233
      key examination findings, 233–234
      pathology, 233
      rehabilitation focus and key points, 234, *234*, *235*
   functional testing, 223, *224*
   hypermobility tests, 222
      navicular drop test, 222, *222*
      windlass test, 222, *222*
   joint, 204–205, 206t
   muscle length, 213, *213*
   muscle performance, 213, *214*
   neurodynamic testing, 214
   palpation, 222–223
   paresthesias tests
      dorsal and plantar tinel test, 219
      metatarsal compression test, 218, *219*
      mulder sign, 218–219
      thumb index finger squeeze test, 218, *219*
   physical examination, 205–207, *207*, 207t
   range of motion, *212*, 212–213, 212t
   reflexes, 214
   sensory tests, 214
   skin and nails, 211–212
   sprains and instability tests, 219
      anterior drawer test, 219, *220*
      external rotation stress test, 220, *221*
      fibular translation test, 220–221
      forced dorsiflexion test, 219–220, *220*
      lateral talar tilt test, 220, *221*
      medial talar tilt test, 219, *220*
      syndesmotic squeeze test, 220, *221*
   structure, 207
      bony structure and alignment, 207–209, *208*, 208t
      forefoot varus and valgus, 210, *211*
      subtalar joint neutral, 209–210, *209*, *210*
Ankle–foot complex biomechanics
   ankle complex, 198–199
      midtarsal joint, 200–203, *202*
      subtalar joint, 200, *201*
      talocrural joint, 199–200, *199*, *200*

771

Ankle–foot complex biomechanics (*continued*)
  ankle–foot motions terminology, 198
  distal intertarsal joints, 203
  intermetatarsal joints, 203
  interphalangeal joints, 203
  metatarsophalangeal joints, 203
  structural relationships, 197–198
  tarsometatarsal joints, 203
Annulus fibrosis, 55–57
Anterior and lateral neck muscles, 88–90, 89t
Anterior ankle impingement, 238
Anterior atlanto-occipital membrane, 71
Anterior cervical discectomy with fusion (ACDF), 100
Anterior cruciate ligament (ACL), 12, *13*, 260, 263–264, *263*
  injuries
    conservative management *versus* prehabilitation, 294–295, *294*, *295*, 295t
    expected outcomes, 299, *299*
    history, 294
    pathology, 293–294, *293*
    post–anterior cruciate ligament rupture evaluation, 294
    postoperative rehabilitation focus and key points, 296–299, 297–298t, *298*
    prevention, 299–300, *300*
    reconstruction surgery, 295–296, 297t
  reconstruction, 748
Anterior drawer test, 219, *220*
Anterior glide
  clavicle on sternum, 464
  humerus, 462, *462*
Anterior longitudinal ligament (ALL), 66, 66t
Anterior scapular slide test (*see* Anterior slide test)
Anterior slide test, 473
Anterior superior iliac spine (ASIS), 334, 338
Anterior talofibular (ATF) ligament, 193
  sprain, 154
Anterior/posterior pelvic tilt, 339
Antibiotics, 127
Apophysitis, 310
Apoptosis, 20
Appendicular skeleton, 48
Apprehension test, 287, *287*, 470, *470*
Aquatic therapy, 292
Arc sign, 221
Arches of hand, 570–571, *570*
Arm-trunk, 446
Arthralgia, 715–716
Arthritis (*see specific entries*)
Arthritis Self-Efficacy Scale (ASES), 730t
Arthrofibrosis, 309
Arthrokinematic movement, 39–40, 40t, *41*, 42
  elbow, 526–527
    humeroradial joint, 526, *527*
    humeroulnar joint, 526, *526*
    proximal radioulnar joint, 526–527, *527*
  hip, 339
  hypomobility, 44
  knee joint, 272, *272*
  by region, 93–96, *93–96*
  spinal, 92, *93*, 766–767
  temporomandibular joint, 702–703, *704*
Arthrology
  joint motion, 38–39
    accessory movements, 43
    arthrokinematics, 39–40, 40t, *41*
    close-packed position, 42–43
    conjunct rotation, 40–41
    convex-concave pattern of movement, 42, *42*
    instant center of rotation, 41–42, *41*
    open-packed position, 43
    osteokinematics, 39, *39*
  joint motion assessment, 43–44
    hypermobility and hypomobility, 44
    joint mobilization, 44–47, *46*, 46t
  synovial joints, 36–37, *36*
    differentiation of joint receptors, 37t
    joint surface shape, 38, 38t, *39*
    neurology, 37–38
    nutrition and lubrication, 38
Articular cartilage, 9–10, 10t, 36, 168
  healing, 24
  injuries, 23–24, 293
  knee joint, 293
  treatment, 24
Articular disc, *698*, 699, *704*
  disc displacements, 715
Articular surface, 187
ASES (*see* Arthritis Self-Efficacy Scale)
ASIS (*see* Anterior superior iliac spine)
Assistive device, walking with, 113
ATF ligament (*see* Anterior talofibular (ATF) ligament)
Athletic taping, 633, *634*
Atlas, 69–70, *69*
Auricular surfaces, 73
Avulsion, 17
Axial rotation, *56*, 268
Axial skeleton, 48
Axiohumeral muscles, 448t, 452
Axis, 69–70, *69*
Axon, 29–30
  terminal, 30

B

Babinski reflex test, 158
Back/lower extremity pathology, 341
Balance assessments, 113–114, 113t, *114*, 317
Balance exercises, 409
Balance training, 237
Ballottement test
  knee, 283, *284*
  wrist and hand complex, 607, *608*
Bankart lesion, 490
BAPS (*see* Biomechanical ankle platform system)
Beck Depression Inventory I & II, 730t
Belly press test, 467–468
Berg Balance Scale, 113t, 597
Biceps brachii, 447t, *449*, 451
Biceps load I and II tests, 472, *473*
Biceps pathology, 495, 495t
Biceps rupture, distal, 552
Biceps tenodesis, 494
Biceps tenotomy, 494
Bicipital groove, 437
Big picture assessment, 178, *179*, 429
Bilateral jaw pain, 720
Bilateral shoulder flexion, 500, *500*
Biomechanical ankle platform system (BAPS), 248
Biomechanics, intervertebral disc, 55–56, *55–56*
Biopsychosocial model, 727–728, *728*
Bone, 10–12, *11*, *12*, *13*, 168
  collar, 11
  healing, 26–28, *27*
  injury, 25–26, *26*, 26t
  matrix, 13, *13*
  nonsurgical and surgical immobilization options for, 28
  postsurgical complications, 28, *29*
  stress injuries, 231–233
  treatment, 28, *28*, 29t
Bony palpation (*see specific entries*)
Bony processes, 53
Bony remodelling, 11–12, *13*
Bony structure and alignment, wrist and hand complex, 600, *600*
Boutonniere deformity, 620
Brachial plexus, 62
Brief Pain Inventory, 732t
British Athletics Muscle Injury Classification, 24
Brostrom method, 238
Buck teeth, 696
Bursae, 169
  hip joint, 330, *331*
Bursitis, 311
Burst fracture, 51, *51*
Buttock
  case study, 751–756
  pain, 751–756

C

C-sign, 746
C1 vertebra (*see* atlas)
C2 vertebra (*see* axis)
Cadence, 107, 109
Caffeine, 128
CAIT (*see* Cumberland Ankle Instability Tool)
Calcaneocuboid joint, 193–194
Calcaneofibular ligament (CFL), 188, 193
Calcaneus, 187–189, *188*
Calcified matrix, *13*
Canadian C-spine rule, *644*
Capitate, 569
Capsular pattern of restriction, 151–152
Capsule fibers, 332
Cardiac-related medications, screening for, 127
Cardiovascular and pulmonary systems, 375–376
  review of systems, 455
Carpal compression test, 610, *610*
Carpal glides, isolated, 605, *605*, 605t
Carpal tunnel, 592, *592*

Carpal tunnel syndrome (CTS), 597, 628–629, *629*
Carpals, 566, *567*, 568–570, *569*
Carpometacarpal (CMC) joints, 575, *576*
Carpometacarpal grind test, 606
Cartilage, 9–10, 10t (*see also specific types*)
Case studies
   Dekohta (buttock pain), 751–756
      history, 753–754
      intake form, *751–753*
      physical examination, 754–755t, 755–756
   Jamal (bilateral shoulder pain), 756–761
      history, 758–759
      intake form, *756–758*
      physical examination, 759–761, 760t
   McKenzie (hip pain), 746–751
      history, 746–749
      intake form, *746–748*
      physical examination, 749–750t, 750–751
Cauda equina syndrome, 376
CBCT (*see* Cone-beam computed tomography)
CDH (*see* Cervical disc herniation)
Cell body, 30
Cells, 3–4, *4*, 4t
Central nervous system (CNS), 29
   anatomy and physiology, 727
Central posteroanterior pressure, 387, *388*
Central sensitization, 728–729
Central slip test, 609, *609*
Central stenosis, 101
Cerebrospinal fluid (CSF), 64
Cervical and thoracic spine
   case study, 687–688
   cervical radiculopathy, 666–668
   cervicogenic dizziness, 671, 671t
   cervicogenic headache, 670–671, 670t, *671*
   description of, 641
   diagnosis of, 664
   exercises and manual therapy, 681–687, *681–687*
      cervical techniques, 683–687, *683–687*
      thoracic techniques, 681–683, *681–683*
   facet arthropathy, 671–672
   frontal plane movement, 94–95
   horizontal plane movement, 94, *94*
   nonspecific neck pain, 664–665
   palpation, 661–664
      bony palpation, 662–663
      functional testing, 664
      gait, 663–664
      skin observation, 661
      soft-tissue palpation, 663
      starting position, 661
   pathoanatomic causes, 665–672
   patient history
      brain aneurysm or mass lesion, 644
      cancer, 645–646
      cervical myelopathy, 644–645, 646t
      chief complaint, 642–643
      fracture, 644
      general medical information, 642
      infection, 646
      lifestyle and occupation, 642
      location and intensity of symptoms, 643
      neck pathology, history of, 642
      onset, 643
      outcome measures, 646, 646t
      red flag screening, 644–646
      review of systems, 641–642
      symptom behavior, 643–644
      symptom quality, 643
      upper cervical spine instability, 645
      vertebrobasilar insufficiency, 644
   physical examination
      Adson test, 660–661, *661*
      alar ligament test, 659
      breathing mechanics, assessment of, 649
      cervical central posteroanterior pressure, 651–652
      cervical compression, 656
      cervical distraction, 656
      cervical instability tests, 658–659
      cervical transverse pressure, 653–654
      cervicogenic dizziness, tests for, 657–658
      costovertebral assessment, 655
      head-neck differentiation test, 657–658, *658*
      inferior glide of first rib, 655
      Lindgren test, 659–660, *660*
      Military Bracing test, 661, *661*
      modified cervical torsion test, 658
      muscle length, 650
      muscle performance, 649
      neurodynamic testing, 650–651
      neurologic examination, 647
      observation, 646–647
      passive accessory motion, intervertebral joints, 651–655
      radiculopathy, special tests for, 655–656
      range of motion, 648–649
      Roos test, 660
      sharp-purser test, 659, *660*
      special/provocative tests, 655–661
      spurling test, 656
      structure and posture, 647–648
      thoracic central posteroanterior pressure, 652
      thoracic compression, 656
      thoracic distraction, 656–657
      thoracic transverse pressure, 654–655, *655*
      thoracic unilateral posteroanterior pressure, 652–653, *653*
      vertebrobasilar insufficiency test, 658–659
   sagittal plane movement, 93–94, *93*
   spondylosis, 665–666
   thoracic pathologies, 672–681
      adult scoliosis, 677–678
      costochondritis, 680
      idiopathic adolescent scoliosis, 675–677
      slipping rib syndrome, 680–681
      thoracic compression fractures, 672–675, *674*
      thoracic outlet syndrome, 678–680
      thoracic radiculopathy, 680
   torticollis, 672
   whiplash-associated disorder and neck- coordination deficits, 668–670
Cervical compression, 656
Cervical disc herniation (CDH), 97, 99–100
Cervical distraction, 656
Cervical instability tests, 658–659
Cervical myelopathy, 644–645, 646t
Cervical radiculopathy, 666–668
Cervical screen, 430
Cervical spine fracture, 149
Cervical transverse pressure, 653–654
Cervical vertebrae, 53t, *54*
   characteristics of, 69–71, *69–70*
   ligaments of, 71
   middle and lower, 70–71, *70*
   upper, 69–70, *69–70*
Cervicogenic dizziness, 671, 671t
   tests for, 657–658
Cervicogenic headache, 670–671, 670t, *671*
Chair push-up test, elbow and, 538, *538*
Check-rein ligament, 577
Chondroitin sulfate, 7t, 9
Chronic Exertional Compartment Syndrome, 245
Chronic Pain Grade Scale, 732t
CKCUEST (*see* Closed kinetic chain upper extremity stability test)
Clancy impingement test (*see* Horizontal adduction test)
Claudication, 205
Clavicle, 436–437, *436*
Claw toes, 208
Clearing examination, 149
Clicking, 150–151
Clinician-generated joint mobilizations, 496–498, *497–499*
Clonus, 158, 161
Close-packed position, 163
   hip, 338
   joint, 42–43
   spine, 60
Closed-chain movement, 340
Closed kinetic chain upper extremity stability test (CKCUEST), 502, *503*
Closed lock, 715
Closed wound healing, 20–21
CMC joints (*see* Carpometacarpal (CMC) joints)
CNS (*see* Central nervous system)
Coccyx, 74
Codman's exercise, 479, *479*
Collagen fibers, 4–6
   assembly of, *5*
   types of, 6, *6*, 7t
Collar bone (*see* Clavicle)
Collaterals, 30
Colles fracture, 572, *574*, 626, *627*
Combined plane shoulder motion testing, 459–460, *460*
Combined Task Force (CTF), 98
Compact bone, 10–11, *11*
Complex regional pain syndrome (CRPS), 629–630, 629t, *630*
Component movement (*see* Arthrokinematic movement)
Comprehensive examination, 146

Compression forces on tissues, 16, *16*
Compression fracture, 51, *51*
Computed tomography (CT), 75, 136, *137*, 706
Cone-beam computed tomography (CBCT), 706
Conjunct rotation, 40–41
Connective tissue, 2–3
  components
    cells, 3–4, *4*, 4t
    fibers, 4–6, *5–6*, 7t
    ground substance of extracellular matrix, 6–9, 7t, *8*, 8t, 9t
  composition, *2*, 3t
  location, and function of, 3t
  proper and specific, *3*
  response of, *16*
  specific structures
    bone, 10–12, *11*, *12*, *13*
    cartilage, 9–10, 10t
    fascia, 14
    ligaments, 12, *13*
    tendons, 12–13, *14*
Connective tissue proper, 2
Constant-length phenomenon, 154
Constitutional symptoms, 142, 376, 456
Continuous passive motion (CPM) machines, 309
Contractile lesions, special tests for, 465–468
Contractile tissue, special tests for, 347
  adductor test, 348, *348*
  resisted external derotation test, 347, *348*
  trendelenburg test, 347, *348*
Conventional/"low-intensity" TENS, 736
Convex-concave pattern of movement, 42, *42*
Coping Strategies Questionnaire (CSQ), 730t
Coracobrachialis, 447t, *449*, *451*
Core strength testing, 183
Corner stretch, 487, *487*
Corticosteroids, 127–128
Costochondritis, 680
Costovertebral assessment, 655
COSTS + Function and Goals, 129, *129*
Cotton roll test (*see* Unilateral bite test)
Cozen test, elbow and, 536, *537*
CPM machines (*see* Continuous passive motion (CPM) machines)
Crank test, 472, *472*
Crepitus, 150
  during movements, 459
Cross body test (*see* Horizontal adduction test)
CRPS (*see* Complex regional pain syndrome)
CSF (*see* Cerebrospinal fluid)
CSQ (*see* Coping Strategies Questionnaire)
CT (*see* Computed tomography)
CTS (*see* Carpal tunnel syndrome)
Cuboid, 189
  whip manipulation, 247–248, *248*
Cubonavicular joint, 194
Cumberland Ankle Instability Tool (CAIT), 206t

Cuneiforms, 189
Cushioned shoe, 116
Custom foot orthotics, 117–118
Cyriax, 146
  testing, 155, 158t

D

DDD (*see* Degenerative disc disease)
DDs (*see* Disc displacements)
De Quervain syndrome, 624, 624t
Decorin, 8t, 9
Deep extensors of wrist, *582*
Deep flexors of wrist, *585*
Deep gluteal syndrome (DGS), 378, 389
  active piriformis test, 390, *390*
  differential diagnoses, 415
  expected outcomes, 415
  history, 414
  key examination findings, 414–415
  pathology, 414, *415*
  rehabilitation and key points, 415
  seated piriformis stretch, 390, *390*
Deep layer medial collateral ligament (dMCL), 263
Deep vein thrombosis (DVT), 458
Degenerative disc disease (DDD), 96–97, *97*, 407–408
Degenerative joint disease (DJD), 239, 275
Deltoid, 447t, *449*
Demifacets, 72, *72*
Dendrite, 29
Dense connective tissue, 2–3
Derangement, 379
Dermatan sulfate, 7t
Dermatome screen, 169, 180, 430–431, *431*
DGI (*see* Dynamic Gait Index)
DGS (*see* Deep gluteal syndrome)
Diffuse ecchymosis, 211
Digastric muscle, *701*, *702*, *703*
Digital stress test, 608
DIP joint (*see* Distal interphalangeal joint)
Direct lateral glide of mandible, 712–713, *713*
Directional preference, 379
Disabilities of Arm, Shoulder, and Hand (DASH) questionnaire, 598, 759
Disc bulge, 98
Disc displacements (DDs), 715
Distal interphalangeal (DIP) joint, 570
Distal intertarsal joints, 203
Distal radioulnar dorsal glide, elbow and, 535, *535*
Distal radioulnar joint (DRUJ), 571, *571*
Distal radius, 566
  fractures, 626–627, *627*
Distal tibial alignment, 210–211, *211*
Distal tibiofibular joint, 191
  mobilization, 214–215, *215*
Distraction and anterior glide of mandible, 712, *712*
Distraction forces on tissues, 16, *16*
DJD (*see* Degenerative joint disease)
dMCL (*see* Deep layer medial collateral ligament)
Dorsal and plantar tinel test, 219
Dorsal finger injuries, 620

Dorsal radiocarpal and midcarpal glides, 604, *604*
Dorsal radiohumeral glide, elbow and, 534
Double support, 107
Douleur Neuropathique (DN-4), 732t
Drop arm test, 465, *466*
DRUJ (*see* Distal radioulnar joint)
Dupuytren contracture, 621
Dural root sheath, 64
DVT (*see* Deep vein thrombosis)
Dynamic Gait Index (DGI), 113, 113t

E

Early active motion protocol, 623
Eating modifications, temporomandibular dysfunction, 717
ECM (*see* Extracellular matrix)
Edema management, 627
Effusion, 165
  tests, 283
    ballottement test, 283, *284*
    modified stroke test, 283, *284*
Ehlers-Danlos syndrome, 490
Elastic cartilage, 9, 10t
Elastic fibers, 6
"Elastohydrodynamic" lubrication, 38
Elbow complex
  anatomy
    carrying angle, 516
    joint capsule, 518
    joints, 515, *516*
    ligaments, 516–518, 517t, *518*
    movement, 522, *522*, 523t
    muscles, 522–525, *524*
    neurovascular, 518–522, *518–521*
    osteology, 513–515, *514–515*
    stability, 525–526
  arthrokinematics
    humeroradial joint, 526, *527*
    humeroulnar joint, 526, *526*
    proximal radioulnar joint, 526–527, *527*
  case study, 560
  differential diagnosis, 554, *554*, 554t
    medial elbow symptoms, 555t
  examination of, 528–529
  mobilization treatment techniques, 554–555
    humeroulnar distraction mobilization, 554, *555*
    posterior radiohumeral mobilization, 554, *555*
    radioulnar spreading, 555, *556*
  palpation, 527–528, *528*
  pathologies, 540–553
    biceps rupture, distal, 552
    dislocation, 544
    fractures, 548, 549t
    internal derangement, 553
    lateral epicondylalgia, 540–543, *540–543*
    medial apophysitis, 553
    medial epicondylalgia, 543–544, *544*
    median nerve, compression neuropathies of, 551, 552t
    nerve compression, 549–552, *550*

olecranon bursitis, 553
osteoarthritis, 547–548
osteochondritis dissecans, 553
Panner disease, 553
posterolateral rotatory instability, 546–547
radial nerve, compression neuropathies of, 551–552
stress fractures, 548–549
triceps rupture, distal, 552–553
valgus instability, 544–546
patient history, 529–530
chief complaint, 529
location of symptoms, 529
onset, 529
outcome measures, 529–530, 530t
personal factors, 529
review of systems, 529
physical examination, 530–540
accessory motion, 533–535
chair push-up test, 538, *538*
Cozen test, 536, *537*
distal radioulnar dorsal glide, 535, *535*
dorsal radiohumeral glide, 534
elbow flexion test, 538–539, *539*
elbow instability, special tests for, 536–538
epicondylalgia, special tests for, 536, *537*
functional testing, 540
humeroradial distraction, 534, *534*
humeroradial pathology, special test for, 538
Maudsley test, 536, *537*
Mill test, 536
muscle length, 531, 532t
muscle performance, 532, 532t
neurodynamic testing, 533
palpation, 540
pronator compression test, 539, *539*
proximal radioulnar dorsal glide, 534, *535*
proximal radioulnar ventral glide, 534, *535*
push-up test, 538
radiocapitellar compression test, 538, *539*
range of motion, 531, 531t
reflexes, 533
sensory tests, 532–533
skin, 531
special tests for peripheral nerve pathology, 538–540
special/provocative tests, 535–540, *536*
structure, 531
tear drop pinch test, 539–540, *539*
valgus stress test, 536, *537*
varus stress test, 537–538, *538*
ventral radiohumeral glide, 534, *535*
therapeutic exercises, 556–559, *556–559*
Elbow flexion test, 538–539, *539*
Elbow instability, special tests for, 536–538
Electrical modalities, 736
Electrodiagnostic testing, 139
Electromyography (EMG), 139
Elongation of tissue, 17

End feel, 153–154
Endocrine system, 376
Endoneurium, 30
Endotenon, 13
Entheses, 262
Entrapment, 169
Epicondylalgia, special tests for, 536, *537*
Epithelial tissue, 2
Ethylene-vinyl acetate (EVA), 114
Evolute, 267
Excursion, 161
Exercise prescription, 735–736, 735t
Exercises and manual therapy (*see also specific techniques*)
cervical and thoracic spine, 681–687, *681–687*
cervical techniques, 683–687, *683–687*
Extension, 39
Extensor expansion, 590–591
Extensor retinaculum, 590–591, *590–591*
Extensor tendon disruption, 619–621, 619t, *619–620*
External rotation, 368
lag test, 466, *466*
stress test, 220, *221*
Extracapsular ligaments, 36
Extracellular matrix (ECM), 2
ground substance of, 6–9, 7t, *8*, 8t, 9t
Extrinsic back muscles, 77, 77t, *78*

F

FAAM (*see* Foot and ankle ability measure)
FABER test, 348–349, *349*, 361, 750
FABQ (*see* Fear Avoidance Beliefs Questionnaire)
Facet joints
arthropathy, 671–672
differential diagnoses, 412
expected outcomes, 412–413
history, 412
key examination findings, 412, 412t
pathology, 412
rehabilitation focus and key points, 412
test/quadrant test, 389, *389*
close- and open-packed position, 60
innervation, 60
intervertebral disc height and, 60
and movement, 58–60, *58*
regional orientation, 58–59, *59*
sliding at, *93*
FADI (*see* Foot and ankle disability index)
FADIR test, 350, *350*, 750
FAIS (*see* Femoroacetabular impingement syndrome)
False ribs, 663
Fascia, 14
Fascicles, 31
Fatigue testing, 156
FDP (*see* Flexor digitorum profundus)
FDS (*see* Flexor digitorum superficialis)
Fear Avoidance Beliefs Questionnaire (FABQ), 380, 707, 730t, 749, 759
Feiss line, 208, *208*
Femoral neck torsion, angle of, 330, 332, *332*
Femoral torsion, 344, *344*

Femoroacetabular impingement syndrome (FAIS), 746–751
differential diagnoses, 357
expected outcomes, 358
history, 357
key examination findings, 357
pathology, 356–357, *357*
rehabilitation after surgery, 358
rehabilitation focus and key points, 357–358
Femur
hip joint, 330, *331*
knee joint, 260, *261*
FFI (*see* Foot function index)
Fibers, 4–6, *5–6*, 7t, 30
Fibril-associated collagens, 6, 7t
Fibril-forming collagens, 6, 7t
Fibrocartilage, 9, 10t
Fibromyalgia, 737
Fibronectin, 9, 9t
Fibrosis, 168
Fibula, 185–186
knee joint, 262
Fibular (lateral) collateral ligament, 12, *13*
Fibular translation test, 220–221
Fibularis strain, 154
Finger flexor repair, rehabilitation after, 622–624, *622*, *624*
Finger osteoarthritis, 617–619, *618*
Finkelstein test, 609, *609*, 624t
First carpometacarpal arthroplasty, 617
First carpometacarpal joint osteoarthritis, 615–617, *615–617*
FITT (*see* Frequency, intensity, time, and type)
Fitzgerald test, 350–351, *351*
Flexion, 39
inferior humeral glide, 496–497, *498*
prone humeral distraction, 498, *499*
sidelying shoulder, 500, *500*
Flexion-extension rotation, 267
Flexor digitorum profundus (FDP), 591
Flexor digitorum superficialis (FDS), 591
Flexor pollicis longus tenosynovitis, 614–615
Flexor rotators, 268
Flexor tendon sheaths, 591, *591*
Floating ribs, 663
Foam tubing, 618, *618*
FOOSH injury, 597
Foot and ankle ability measure (FAAM), 206t
Foot and ankle disability index (FADI), 206t
Foot arches, 203–204
Foot function index (FFI), 206t
Foot orthotics, 117
custom, 117–118
functions, 117
heel lifts, 118
prefabricated, 117
wedges, 118
Footwear, 114
components, 114–115, *115*, 115t
fitting, 115–116, *116*, 116t
functions, 114
recommendations, 116–117, 117t
running shoes, 116, *116*
types, 114

Force couples of shoulder, 452–453, *452–453*
Forced dorsiflexion test, 219–220, *220*
Forces, 340, *341*
Forefoot bones
   metatarsals, 189, *190*
   phalanges, 189
   sesamoids, 189
Fovea sign, 610, *610*
Fracture, 26–27, 626–628, *627* (see also Bones)
   distal radius fractures, 626–627, *627*
   elbow, 548, 549t
   hand fractures, 628
   hip
      pathology, 355, *355*
      postoperative course, 356, *356*
   lumbar, 413
   management, 233
   potential postsurgical complications with management, *29*
   scaphoid fracture, 627–628
   types, *26*, 26t
   types of surgery for fixation, 29t
Frequency, intensity, time, and type (FITT), 128
Friction forces on tissues, 16, *16*
Froment sign, 610, *611*
Frontal plane analysis, 111
Frozen shoulder (see Adhesive capsulitis)
Fulcrum test, 351, *351*
Full can test (see Supraspinatus test)
Functional ankle instability, 235
Functional Reach Test, 113, *114*
Functional testing, 156, 166, 223, *224* (see also specific entries)
   knee joint, 289–290, *289–291*
   lower quarter screen, 181
   lumbar spine and sacroiliac joint, 393
   wrist and hand complex, 611–613, *612*, 613t
Funnel approach, 124

G

Gaenslen test, 390, *391*
GAGs (see Glycosaminoglycans)
Gait, 107
   abnormalities, 111–112, 112t
   age impact on, 112
   analysis, methods of, 110–111, *111*
   assistive devices and, 113
   characteristics, 109–110
   cycle, 107
   distance terminology, 107–109
   foot orthotics, impact of, 117
      custom, 117–118
      functions, 117
      heel lifts, 118
      prefabricated, 117
      wedges, 118
   footwear, impact of, 114
      components, 114–115, *115*, 115t
      fitting, 115–116, *116*, 116t
      functions, 114
      recommendations, 116–117, 117t
      running shoes, 116, *116*
      types, 114
   gait cycle, phases of, 107, *108*, 108t
   knee joint, 289
   lumbar spine and sacroiliac joint, 393
   muscle activity during, 110, *110*
   speed, 408
   standardized assessments, 113–114, 113t, *114*
   temporal terminology, 107–109, *108*, *109*
   training, 355
Gamekeeper's thumb, 613
Gastrointestinal system, 376
   review of systems, 455
General medical information, 126–128, 127t
Generalized Anxiety Disorder (GAD-7), 730t
Geniohyoid, 702
Genitourinary systems, 376
Genu recurvatum, 266
GH joint (see Glenohumeral joint)
GIRD (see Glenohumeral internal rotation deficit)
Glenohumeral (GH) joint
   arthrokinematics, 446
   dynamic stabilization of, 444–445
   instability, *490*, 490–493, 490t, 492–493t
   and ligaments, 443–446, 445t
   osteoarthritis, 477
   osteokinematics, 445–446, 445t, *446*
   static stabilization of, 443–444, 443t, *444*, 445t
Glenohumeral internal rotation deficit (GIRD), 459, *459*
Glenoid fossa, 443, *444*
Glenoid labrum, 443, *444*
Glide, 40, 161, *162*
Gluteal muscles, 84, 88
Gluteus maximus, 279
Glycocalyx, 30
Glycoproteins, 2
   multiadhesive, 9, 9t
Glycosaminoglycans (GAGs), 2, 6–9, 7t
Golfer's elbow, 543
Grades, 44
Great toe, 195
Greater trochanteric pain syndrome (GTPS)
   differential diagnoses, 361
   expected outcomes, 361
   history, 360
   key examination findings, 360–361
   pathology, 360
   rehabilitation focus and key points, 361
Grind test, 288, *288*
Groin pain, 342, 361–362, *361*, 362t
Ground substance, 2
   extracellular matrix, 6–9, 7t, *8*, 8t, 9t
GTPS (see Greater trochanteric pain syndrome)

H

H-taping, 633, *634*
HADS (see Hospital Anxiety and Depression Scale)
Hallux rigidus, 227, *227*
Hallux valgus
   differential diagnoses, 225
   history, 225
   key examination findings, 225
   pathology, 224, *225*
   physical therapy outcomes, 226
   rehabilitation
      focus, 225–226, *226*
      after surgery, 226–227
Hamate, 569
Hamstrings (HSs), 338
Hand (see also Wrist and hand complex)
   fractures, 628
   tool dexterity test, 613t
Handheld dynamometry, 461, *461*
Hard callus formation, 27
Harris Hip Score, 749
Haversian canals, 10
Hawkins-Kennedy impingement test, 469, *469*
Head, arms, and trunk (HAT), 330, 340
Head-neck differentiation test, 657–658, *658*
Healing
   articular cartilage, 23–24
   bone, 26–28, *26–29*, 26–27t, 29t
   factors affecting healing, 21, *21*
   inflammatory phase, 18–20, *20*
   ligament, 23
   muscle, 24–25, *25*
   nerve/neuron, 29–33, *30–31*, 32t
   tendon, 21–22
Health habits, 128–129, 128t
Heel lifts, 118
Hemarthrosis, 275
Hematoma formation phase, 27
Heparan sulfate, 7t, 9
Heparin, 7t
Herniated disc (see Herniated nucleus pulposus)
Herniated nucleus pulposus (HNP), 97, *98*, 404–405
   differential diagnoses, 405
   expected outcomes, 405–406, *406*
   history, 405
   key examination findings, 405
   and nerve root involvement, classification of, 98–99, *99*, 99t
   rehabilitation focus and key points, 405, *406*
   treatment for, 100
High-intensity/"acupuncturelike" TENS, 736
Hip
   additional joint mobilization treatment techniques, 363–367, *365–367*
   additional therapeutic exercises, 367–369, *367–369*
   biomechanics
      arthrokinematics, 339
      closed-chain movement, 340
      forces, 340, *341*
      motion, 339–340
      osteokinematics, 338–339
      stability, 338
   case, 369
   case study, 746–751
   differential diagnosis, 363, *364*, 365t
   examination, introduction to, 341
   flexion, 368
   fracture, 355, 369–370
   functional anatomy, 330

angle of femoral neck torsion, 330, 332, *332*
angle of inclination, 330, *332*
joint capsule, 332–333
ligaments, 332–333, *334–335*
muscles, 333–334, *336–337*, 338t
osteology, 330, *331*
palpation, 334, 337
instability
    differential diagnoses, 359–360
    expected outcomes, 360
    history, 359
    key examination findings, 359
    pathology, 358–359, *359*
    rehabilitation focus and key points, 360
    surgical options, 360
pain, 746–751
patient history, 341
    back/lower extremity pathology, 341
    chief complaint, 342
    location of symptoms, 342
    onset mechanism, 342
    patient-specific function scale, 342, 343t
    review of systems, 341–342
physical examination, 342–343
    accessory motion, 346–347, *346*
    femoral torsion, 344, *344*
    functional testing, 352–353, 352t
    gait, 351
    leg length discrepancy, 343, *344*
    muscle length, 345, 345t
    muscle performance, 345
    neurodynamic testing, 345
    palpation, 351
    pathologies (*see specific types*)
    range of motion, 345, 345t
    reflexes, 345
    sensory tests, 345
    skin, 345
    special tests/provocative testing, 347–351, *348–351*
    structure, 344
    tibia and femur length, 344, *344*
strength testing, 416
Hip abductor strength, 367
Hip-spine syndrome, 404
Hoffmann test, 161
Horizontal adduction test, 469, *469*
Horizontal pull, 474
Hornblower test, 466lower *467*
Hospital Anxiety and Depression Scale (HADS), 730t
HS tendinopathy (*see* Proximal hamstring tendinopathy)
"Hug-a-tree" exercise, 501, *502*
Humeroradial distraction, elbow and, 534, *534*
Hyaluronan, 7t, 8, 9
Hyoid bone, 698
Hyperesthesia, 392
Hypermobility
    and hypomobility, 44
    tests, 222
        navicular drop test, 222, *222*
        windlass test, 222, *222*

Hyperpronation, 208
Hypomobile joints, 161, 162
Hypomobility, 44

I

ICR (*see* Instant center of rotation)
Idiopathic adolescent scoliosis, 675–677
IGHL (*see* Inferior glenohumeral ligament)
Iliofemoral ligament, 332
Iliotibial band pathology, special test for, 288
    noble compression test, 288, *288*
Iliotibial band syndrome (ITB) syndrome, 309–310
Inclination, angle of, 330, *332*
Inferior glenohumeral ligament (IGHL), 444
Inferior glide
    acromion on clavicle, 464
    clavicle on acromion, 463, *463*
    clavicle on sternum, 464, *464*
    humerus, 462, *463*
        in abduction, 497–498, *498*
        in flexion, 496–497, *498*
Inflammatory phase of tissue healing, 18–20, 19t, *20*
Infrahyoid muscle, 702, *703*
Infrapatellar fat pad, 265
Infraspinatus, 447t, *449*
    positioning, 454, *454*
Instability tests, 388
    prone instability test, 389, *389*
Instability/labral pathology, 470–474
Instant center of rotation (ICR), 41–42, *41*, 446
Intercarpal joints, 573–575, *574–575*
Interdigital/morton neuroma
    differential diagnoses, 229
    expected outcomes, 229
    history, 228
    key examination findings, 228–229
    pathology, 228
    rehabilitation focus and key points, 229
Interfibrillar component (*see* Ground substance)
Intermediate flexors of wrist, 584
Intermediate layer of intrinsic back muscles, 77, *79*
Intermetacarpal joint mobilization, 605, *606*
Intermetatarsal joints, 203
    mobility, 216–217, *217*
Intermittent shoulder pain, 502–503
Internal rotation lag test, 467
International Classification of Diseases (ICD-10) codes, 167
International Functioning, Disability, and Health (ICF) classification, 167
Interneurons, 29
Interphalangeal (IP) joints, 195, 203, 577
    mobilizations, 217–218, *218*, 606
Interprofessional collaboration, 719, 721
Intersection syndrome, 624, 624t
Interspinous ligament, 66–67, 66t
Intertarsal joints, 194
    mobility, 216, *217*
Intertransverse ligament, 66, 66t
Interventions, pain, *733*
    electrical modalities, 736

exercise prescription, 735–736, 735t
manual therapy, 737–738, *738*
patient-specific health education and self-management support, 733–735
Intervertebral disc (IVDs), 48
    biomechanics, 55–56, *55–56*
    height, facet joint and, 60
    lumbar, pressure, *57*
    nutrition, 56–58
    pathology, 57–58, *98*
Intervertebral joints, movement of, 81t
Intra-articular fibrocartilage, 168
Intra-articular pathology tests, 350
    FADIR test, 350, *350*
    Fitzgerald test, 350–351, *351*
    fulcrum test, 351, *351*
    scour test, 350, *350*
Intra-articular swelling, 165
Intracapsular ligaments, 36
Intramembranous ossification, 10
Intrinsic back muscles, 77–79, 77t, *79–80*
(*see also specific muscles*)
Intrinsic strengthening, putty for, *633*
Inversion/eversion, 198
Inverted double V system, 578, *578*
Investing fascia, 14
Ipsilateral coupling, 90, *92*
Irritability, 133, 134t
Ischiofemoral ligament, 332–333
Isokinetic assessment, 461, *461*
Isokinetic testing, 158
Isometric testing, 155, 158t
IVDs (*see* Intervertebral disc)

J

Jaw Functional Limitation Scale, 707, 709t
Jaw reflex, 713, *713*
Jebsen hand function test, 613t
Jendrassik maneuver, 158
Jensen's classification system, 98
Joint capsule, 36, 168–169, 332–333
Joint mobilization, 44–47, *46*, 46t, 240 (*see also specific entries*)
    clinician-generated, 496–498, *497–499*
    elbow, 554–555
        humeroulnar distraction mobilization, 554, *555*
        posterior radiohumeral mobilization, 554, *555*
        radioulnar spreading, 555, *556*
    general guidelines for, 45–46, *46*
    grades of mobilization, 46, *46*
    indications and contraindications for, 45
    patient-generated, 498–499, *499*
    technique, 46–47, 46t
Joint of Luschka (*see* Uncovertebral joint)
Joint protection strategies, 633, *633–634*
Joint receptors, 37, 37t
Joint surface shape, 38, 38t, *39*
Joints (*see also specific joints*)
    elbow, 515, *516*
    hypomobility, 161, 212
    mobility, 161
    motion, 38–39
        accessory movements, 43
        arthrokinematics, 39–40, 40t, *41*

Joints (continued)
    close-packed position, 42–43
    conjunct rotation, 40–41
    convex-concave pattern of movement, 42, *42*
    instant center of rotation, 41–42, *41*
    open-packed position, 43
    osteokinematics, 39, *39*
  motion assessment, 43–44
    hypermobility and hypomobility, 44
    joint mobilization, 44–47, *46*, 46t
  shoulder complex, 438–440, *438–439*
    acromioclavicular joint and ligaments, *440*, 441–442
    glenohumeral joint and ligaments, 443–446, 443t, *444*, 445t, *446*
    scapulohumeral rhythm, 446–447
    scapulothoracic joint, 442–443, *442*
    sternoclavicular joint and ligaments, 440–441, *440–441*
    subacromial space, 443, *443*
  synovial joints, 36–37, *36*
    differentiation of joint receptors, 37t
    joint surface shape, 38, *39*
    neurology, 37–38
    nutrition and lubrication, 38
    stability of, 36
    traditional anatomical classification of, 38t
  temporomandibular joint, 698–699, *699*
  wrist and hand complex
    carpometacarpal joints, 575, *576*
    distal radioulnar joint, 571, *571*
    interphalangeal joints, 577
    metacarpophalangeal joints, 575–577, *576–577*
    midcarpal and intercarpal joints, 573–575, *574–575*
    radiocarpal joint, 571–573, *572–574*
Joints osteology, 185, *186*
  accessory bones, 189, *190*
  distal tibiofibular joint, 191
  forefoot bones
    metatarsals, 189
    phalanges, 189
    sesamoids, 189
  great toe, proximal phalangeal joint of, 195
  interphalangeal joints, 195
  intertarsal joints, 194
  leg bones
    fibula, 185–186
    tibia, 185
  metatarsophalangeal joints, 195
  midfoot bones, 189
    cuboid, 189
    cuneiforms, 189
    navicular, 189
  midtarsal joint, 193
    calcaneocuboid joint, 193–194
    talonavicular joint, 193, *194*
  plantar aponeurosis, 195, *196*
  proximal tibiofibular joint, 191
  rearfoot bones
    calcaneus, 187–189, *188*
    talus, 186–187, *188*
  relationships and palpation by region
    dorsal aspect, 196–197
    lateral aspect, 197
    medial aspect, 195–196
    plantar aspect, 197
    posterior aspect, 197
  subtalar joint, 193
  tarsal coalitions, 189, *190*
  tarsometatarsal joints, 194–195
Jumper's knee, 302

K

Kallikrein, 18
Keratan sulfate, 7t, 9
Key pinch, 602
Keystone, 569
Kidney/ureteral stones, 376
Kinetic chain, 428
Kirschner wire, 627
Knee, 109–110
  arthrokinematic movements of, *41*
  biomechanics, 265, *266*
    alignment, 266–267, *267*
    osteokinematics, 267–268, *267*
  bursae, 265, *265*, 266t
  case study, 319–320
  collateral ligaments, 263
    lateral collateral ligament, 263
    medial collateral ligament, 263
  cruciate ligaments, 263
    anterior cruciate ligament, 263–264, *263*
    posterior cruciate ligament, *263*, 264
  differential diagnosis, 311, *312–313*, 313t
  examination, introduction to, 274
  history, 274–275, 276t
  joint capsule and synovium, 265
  joint mobilization techniques, 311–316, *313–316*
  menisci and associated ligaments, 262–263, *262*
  muscles, 268, *269–271*
  osteology
    femur, 260, *261*
    fibula, 262
    patella, 261, *261*
    tibia, 260–261, *261*
  other knee ligaments, *264*, 264–265, 264t
  palpation, 271–272
    arthrokinematics, 272, *272*
    patellofemoral joint, 272–274, *273*
  pathologies (*see specific types*)
  physical examination, 275, 277t
    accessory motion, 281–282, 282t
    functional testing, 289–290, *289–291*
    gait, 289
    muscle length, 278, 278t, *279*
    muscle performance, 278–280, *280–281*, 280t
    neurodynamic testing, 280–281
    palpation, 289
    range of motion, 277–278, 277t
    reflexes, 280
    sensory tests, 280
    skin and soft tissue, 277
    special tests/provocative testing, 283–288, *283–288*
    structure, 277
  post-traumatic knee arthritis, 739
  therapeutic exercises, 316–318, *316–318*
Kyphosis, 49, *50*

L

Labral pathology, 493–495, *493*
Lachman test, 285, *285*
Laminin, 9, 9t
Lateral ankle sprain, 171–172
Lateral collateral ligament (LCL), 263
  injuries, 301–302
Lateral distraction of humerus, 462, *463*
Lateral flexion, *56*
Lateral humeral distraction with belt, 498, *498*
Lateral pelvic tilt, 339
Lateral pterygoid, 700–702, 701t, 705–706
Lateral stenosis, 101
Lateral talar tilt test, 220, *221*
Latissimus dorsi, 448t
Laxity, 490
LDH (*see* Lumbar disc herniation)
LEFS (*see* Lower extremity function scale)
Leg bones
  fibula, 185–186
  tibia, 185
Leg length discrepancy, 343, *344*
Leg-lowering abdominal test, 385
Legg-Calvé-Perthes disease, 363
Levator ani, 82
Levator scapulae, 448t
Lift-off test, 467, *467*
Ligament reconstruction and tendon interposition (LRTI), 617
Ligaments, 12, *13* (*see also specific entries*)
  acromioclavicular joint and, *440*, 441–442
  cervical vertebrae, 71, *71*
  characteristics of, 69–71, *69–70*
  elbow, 516–518, 517t, *518*
  glenohumeral joint and, 443–446, 443t, *444*, 445t, *446*
  hand, 579, 579t
  healing, 23
  hip joint, 332–333, *334–335*
  injury, 23
  knee joint, 284–285
    lachman test, 285, *285*
    posterior drawer test, 285–286, *286*
    quadriceps active drawer test, 286
    valgus stress tests, 286–287, *287*
  physical examination, 169
  spine osteology
    stabilizing sacroiliac joint, 75t, *76*
  sternoclavicular joint and, 440–441, *440–441*
  treatment to promote healing, 23
  wrist, 577–578, *578*
    extrinsic ligaments, 578t
    intrinsic ligaments, 578t
Ligamentum flavum ligament, 66, 66t
Ligamentum nuchae (*see* Nuchal ligament)
Limb posture and use, wrist and hand complex, 600
Limb symmetry index (LSI), 298
Lindgren test, 659–660, *660*
Little Leaguer elbow, 553

Load-and-shift test, 471, *471*
Local strengthening, 237
Localized swelling, 165
Location-specific palpation, 750
Log roll test, 349, *349*
Long-axis distraction, 161
Loose connective tissue, 2–3
Lordosis, 49, *50*
Low back pain, 726
  associated with centralization, 396
    differential diagnoses, 397
    expected outcomes, 399
    history, 396–397
    key examination findings, 397, *397*
    rehabilitation focus and key points, 397–399
  associated with mobility deficits, 394
    differential diagnoses, 395
    expected outcomes, 396
    history, 394
    key examination findings, 394–395, *395*
    rehabilitation focus and key points, 395–396, *396*
Lower extremity function scale (LEFS), 206t, 275
Lower extremity peripheral and segmental nerve innervation, 768–769t
Lower quarter neurologic screen (LQNS), 179, *180*
  dermatome screen, 180
  myotome screen, 180
  reflex screen, 180, 180t
  trunk screen, 180
Lower quarter screen (LQS), 428
  case, 182–183
  components, 177, *177*
    functional testing, 181
    integument, 181
    lower extremity motion, 180–181, 181t
    lower quarter neurologic screen, 179–180
    muscle length and strength, 180–181, 181t
    observation, 177–178
    structure and posture, 178–179, *178*, 179t
    vasculature, 181
  general rules for, 177
  purpose of, 176–177
LQNS (*see* Lower quarter neurologic screen)
LQS (*see* Lower quarter screen)
LRTI (*see* Ligament reconstruction and tendon interposition)
LSI (*see* Limb symmetry index)
Lubrication, 38
Lumbar (L3) vertebra, 53t, *54*
Lumbar disc herniation (LDH), 97, 100
Lumbar plexus, *62*
Lumbar spine and sacroiliac joint
  case, 419–420
  diagnosis, 393–394
  examination, introduction to, 375
  front plane movement, 96
  functional testing, 393
  gait, 393
  horizontal plane movement, 96, *96*
  nonspecific low back pain
    associated with centralization, 396–397, *397–399*, 398t
    associated with mobility deficits, 394–396, *395–396*
    expected outcomes, 396
    muscle activation and movement control deficits, 399–404, *400–404*, 400t
  palpation, 391
    bony palpation, 392, *392*
    skin observation and, 391–392
    soft-tissue palpation, 392–393, *393*
    starting position, 391
  passive accessory intervertebral movements, 387
    central posteroanterior pressure, 387, *388*
    transverse pressure, 388, *389*
    unilateral posteroanterior pressure, 387–388, *388*
  pathoanatomic classifications, 404
    acute lumbar strains, 413–414
    deep gluteal syndrome, 414–415, *415*
    degenerative disc disease, 407–408
    facet joint arthropathy, 412–413, 412t
    herniated nucleus pulposus, 404–406, *406*
    hip-spine syndrome, 404
    lumbar and pelvic fractures, 413
    myofascial pain syndrome, 414
    pelvic floor muscle dysfunction, 406–407, 407t
    sacroiliac joint dysfunction, 415–419, 416–417t, *418*
    spondylolisthesis, 411
    spondylolysis and stress reactions, 411–412
    stenosis, 408–410, 409t, *410*, 411t
  patient history
    back pathology, 377–378
    chief complaint, 378
    general medical information, 377
    lifestyle and occupation, 377
    location and intensity of symptoms, 378–379, *378*
    neck pathology, 377
    onset, 378
    outcome measures, 380, 380t
    patient demographics, 377
    symptom behavior, 379, 379t
    symptom quality, 379
    tracking symptoms, 379–380, *380*
  physical examination, 381
    hip range of motion, 384–385
    muscle length, 385
    muscle performance, 384–385
    neurodynamic testing, 385–387, *387*
    neurologic examination, 381, *382*
    observation, 381
    structure and posture, 382, *382*
    trunk muscle performance, 385, 385t, *386*
    trunk range of motion, 383–384, 383t, *384*
  review systems, 375
    cardiovascular and pulmonary systems, 375–376
    constitutional symptoms, 376
    endocrine system, 376
    gastrointestinal and genitourinary systems, 376
    psychiatric system, 376
  sagittal plane movement, 95–96
  special tests/provocative testing, 388–390, *389–391*
Lumbar vertebrae, 72–73, *73*
Lunate, 568, 625, 626t

M

Magnetic resonance imaging (MRI), 136, 138, *138*, 706
  spinal stenosis, 101, *101*
Major deep layer of intrinsic back muscles, 78, *80*
Mallet finger, 599, *599*
  deformity, 600
Malocclusions, 696
Manchester short splint, 623
Mandible, 695–697, *696–698*
  direct lateral glide of, 712–713, *713*
  distraction and anterior glide of, 712, *712*
  movements of, *704*
Mandibular angle, 695, *696*
Manipulation, 44
Manual muscle testing (MMT)
  case studies, 750, 756, 760
  knee, 278
  physical examination, 155
  wrist and hand complex, 602
Manual therapy
  general guidelines, 45–46, *46*
  lumbar spine and sacroiliac joint, 396, 403, 405, 408
  pain management, 737–738, *738*
  temporomandibular dysfunction, 719, *720*
  wrist and hand complex, 616, *616*
Manubrium, *436*
Marfan syndrome, 490
Masseter, 700–702, *701*, 701t
  palpation of, 705, *705*
  reflex (*see* Jaw reflex)
Mastication muscles, 700–702, *701–702*
Masticatory muscle disorders (MMDs), 715
Maudsley test, elbow and, 536, *537*
McGill Pain Questionnaire, 732t
MCL (*see* Medial collateral ligament)
McMurray test, 284, *285*
MCP joints (*see* Metacarpophalangeal joints)
MDI (*see* Multidirectional shoulder instability)
MDT (*see* Mechanical diagnosis and therapy)
Mechanical diagnosis and therapy (MDT), 379
Mechanistic model of manual therapy, *738*
Medial collateral ligament (MCL), 153, 263
  injuries, 300
Medial compartment, 306
Medial patellar tilt test, 288, *288*
Medial pterygoid, 700–702, 701t, 705
Medial talar tilt test, 219, *220*

Medial tibial stress syndrome (MTSS)
  differential diagnoses, 244
  expected outcomes, 244
  history, 244
  key examination findings, 244
  pathology, 244
  rehabilitation focus and key points, 244
  surgical interventions, 244
Median nerve, 592, *593*
Medical tests, 129
Medication, 126–127
  reconciliation, 377
Meniscal injuries
  differential diagnoses, 292
  expected outcomes, 292
  history, 291
  key examination findings, 291–292
  pathology, 290, 292t
  rehabilitation after surgery, 292–293
  rehabilitation focus and key points, 292
Meniscal pathology, 284
  McMurray test, 284, *285*
  Thessaly test, 284, *284*
Meniscal repairs, 293
Menisci, 262–263, *262*
Metacarpals, *567, 570*
Metacarpophalangeal (MCP) joints, 575–577, *576–577*
  flexion, *620*
  mobilization, 605, *606*
Metatarsal compression test, 218, *219*
Metatarsalgia
  differential diagnoses, 227–228
  expected outcomes, 228
  history, 227
  key examination findings, 227
  pathology, 227
  rehabilitation focus and key points, 228, *228*
Metatarsals, 189
Metatarsophalangeal (MTP) joint, 109, 115, 203
  mobility, 217, *218*
MFPS (*see* Myofascial pain syndrome)
Michigan bite splint, 721
Michigan State University (MSU) classification, 99
Midcarpal and intercarpal joints, 573–575, *574–575*
Midcarpal instability, 625
Midcarpal shift test, 607–608, *608*
Midfoot bones, *187*
  cuboid, 189
  cuneiforms, 189
  navicular, 189
Midtarsal joint, 193–194, *194*, 200–203, *202*
Military bracing test, 661, *661*
Mill test, elbow and, 536
Minnesota rate of manipulation test, 613t
Minor deep layer of intrinsic back muscles, 79, *80*
MMDs (*see* Masticatory muscle disorders)
MMT (*see* Manual muscle testing)
Modalities, 721
Modified Carter Wilkinson scale, 151
Modified Duran protocol, 623
Modified Harris Hip Score, 749

Modified sleeper stretch, 499, *499*
Modified stroke test, 283, *284*
Modulation, 726–727, *727*
Motion analysis, 109
Motion control shoe, 116
Motor (efferent) neuron, 29
Movement system impairment, 400
MRI (*see* Magnetic resonance imaging)
MTP (*see* Metatarsophalangeal joint)
MTSS (*see* Medial tibial stress syndrome)
Mulder sign, 218–219
Multiadhesive glycoproteins, 9, 9t
Multiangle isometric quadriceps test, 287–288
Multidirectional shoulder instability (MDI), 490
Muscle, 579
  elbow, 522–525, *524*
  hand
    dissection, *586–588*
    intrinsic muscles, 586t
  healing, 25, *25*
  hip joint, 333–334, 336–337, 338t
  injury, 24
  physical examination, 169
  shoulder complex
    axiohumeral muscles, 448t, 452
    force couples of the shoulder, 452–453, *452–453*
    scapulohumeral muscles, 447–451, 447t, *449–451*
    scapulothoracic motions and muscle working as prime movers, 448t
    scapulothoracic muscles, 448t, 451–452
  spine osteology, 75, 81t
    anterior and lateral neck muscles, 88–90, 89t
    extrinsic back muscles, 77, 77t, *78*
    intrinsic back muscles, 77–79, 77t, *79–80*
    stabilizing muscles, 80–88, 81t–82t, *82–87*
    suboccipital muscles, 88, *88*
  temporomandibular joint, 700–702, *701–703*, 701t
  tissue, 2
  treatment, 25
  wrist
    deep extensors of, *582*
    deep flexors of, *585*
    extrinsic muscles of, 579–580, 579–580t
    intermediate flexors of, *584*
    superficial extensors of, *581*
    superficial flexors of, *583*
Muscle activation and movement control deficits, 399–401, *400*, 400t
  differential diagnoses, 402
  expected outcomes, 403
  history, 401
  key examination findings, 401–402, *401–402*
  rehabilitation focus and key points, 402–403, *402–404*
Muscle activity, 110, *110*
Muscle length (*see specific entries*)

Muscle performance, 345 (*see also specific entries*)
  joint-specific examination, 155, 155t
    cyriax testing, 155, 158t
    fatigue testing, 156
    functional testing, 156
    isokinetic testing, 158
    manual muscle testing, 155
    myotomal testing, 155, 156–157t
    sensory tests, 158, *159*
  testing, 487
Muscle strength, 180–181, 181t
Musculoskeletal system, 148
  disorders, 146
  pain, guiding exercise principles for, 735t
  pathology, 125
Myelopathy, 101
Mylohyoid muscle, *701, 702, 703*
Myofascial pain syndrome (MFPS), 414
Myotomal testing, 155, 156–157t
Myotome screen, 180, 430, 430t

N

Navicular, 189
Navicular drop test, 222, *222*
NCS (*see* Nerve condition study)
Neck Disability Index, 707
Neer impingement test, 469, *469*
Nerve compression, 549–552, *550*
Nerve condition study (NCS), 139
Nerve root involvement, disc herniation and, 98–99
Nerve/neuron, 29–31, *30–31*
  anatomy of, *30*
  healing, 31–32
  injury, 31, 32t
  innervation, peripheral and segmental, 768–770t
  pathology, special tests for, 610–611
  treatment, 32–33
  wrist and hand complex, *596*
    median nerve, 592, *593*
    radial nerve, 592, *595*
    ulnar nerve, 592, *594*
Nervous tissue, 2
Neural structures, movement and impact on, 90
Neurodynamic testing, 214, 345 (*see also specific entries*)
  knee joint, 280–281
  lumbar spine and sacroiliac joint, 385
    prone knee flexion, 386
    slump test, 386–387, *387*
    straight leg raise, 385–386
  wrist and hand complex, 603
Neurologic testing (*see specific entries*)
Neuromuscular electrical stimulation (NMES), 292, 309
Neuromuscular systems, 148
Neuropathic pain, 728, 729t
Nitroglycerin, 127
NMES (*see* Neuromuscular electrical stimulation)
Noble compression test, 288, *288*
Nociceptive pain, 726, 728, 729t
Nociplastic pain, 728–729, 729t

Noncapsular pattern of restriction, 152–153
Nonspecific low back pain (LBP), 751–756
Nonsteroidal anti-inflammatory drugs (NSAIDs), 376, 377
Non–weight-bearing subtalar joint neutral, 209
NPRS (*see* Numeric pain rating scale)
NSAIDs (*see* Nonsteroidal anti-inflammatory drugs)
Nuchal ligament, 66t, 68
Nucleus pulposus, 55
Numeric pain rating scale (NPRS), 731
Nutrition, 38
    intervertebral disc, 56–58

O

OA (*see* Osteoarthritis)
O'Brien active compression test, 473
Older adults
    exaggerated kyphosis, 51, *51*
Olecranon bursitis, 553
Open-packed (or loose-packed) position
    joint, 43
    spine, 60
Open packed position, 161
Open reduction and internal fixation (ORIF), 626
Open wound healing, 20–21
Opening click, 715
Optimal Screening for Prediction of Referral and Outcome (OSPRO), 141, 707
Optimal Screening for Prediction of Referral and Outcome Yellow Flag (OSPRO-YF), 730
Optimal test battery, 299
Oral Behavior Checklist, 707, *708*
Oral Health Impact Profile for TMDs (OHIP-TMDs), 707, 709t
Orebro Musculoskeletal Pain Questionnaire, 730
ORIF (*see* Open reduction and internal fixation)
Osborne ligament, 522
OSPRO (*see* Optimal Screening for Prediction of Referral and Outcome)
OSPRO-YF (*see* Optimal Screening for Prediction of Referral and Outcome Yellow Flag)
Ossification, 10
Osteoarthritis (OA)
    differential diagnoses, 353
    elbow, 547–548
    expected outcomes, 353
    finger, 617–619, *618*
    first carpometacarpal joint, 615–617, *615–617*
    glenohumeral, 477
    history, 353
    key examination findings, 353
    knee
        differential diagnoses, 307, 307t
        expected outcomes, 308
        history, 306
        key examination findings, 306–307
        pathology, 306
        rehabilitation focus and key points, 307–308, 307–308t
    pathology, 352–353
    rehabilitation focus and key points, 353
    special tests for, 606
Osteoblasts, 11–12, *13*
Osteochondritis dissecans, 553
Osteoid, 12, *13*
Osteokinematic (or physiologic) hypomobility, 44
Osteokinematic movement, 44
    by region, 93–96, *93–96*
    spine osteology, 92, *92*, 92t, 766–767
Osteokinematics, 39, *39*
    hip joint, 338–339
Osteopontin, 9, 9t
Ottawa Ankle Rules, 205–206, *207*
Ottawa Knee Rules, 275, 277t

P

Pain, 726
    anatomy and physiology
        central nervous system, 727
        peripheral nervous system, 726–727
    biopsychosocial model and pain neuromatrix theory, 727–728, *728*
    general pathway, steps in, 727
    initial assessment considerations, *731*
        functional and performance assessment, 733
        pain measurement and screening, 731–732, *732*, 732t
        physical examination tools, 732, *733*
        self-report scales, 731, *731*
    interventions, *733*
        electrical modalities, 736
        exercise prescription, 735–736, 735t
        manual therapy, 737–738, *738*
        patient-specific health education and self-management support, 733–735
    psychosocial considerations in measurement tools for psychosocial impairments, 730, 730t
        yellow flag screening, 729–730, *730*
    science definitions and epidemiology, 726
    sensation, 158
    types, 729t
        nociceptive pain, 728, 729t
        nociplastic pain, 728–729, 729t
        peripheral neuropathic pain, 728, 729t
Pain Catastrophizing Scale (PCS), 380, 707, 730t
Pain DETECT Tool, 732t
Pain neuromatrix, 727
    theory, 727–728, *728*
Pain neuroscience education (PNE), 734–735
Pain Self-Efficacy Questionnaire (PSEQ), 730t
Painful arc, 459, *459*
    movement, 150
Painful joints, 162
Palmar aponeurosis, *586–587*
    and flexor tendon sheaths, 591, *591*
Palmar glide of scaphoid, 631–632, *632*
Palmar ligaments, *578*
Palmar pinch, 602
Palmar radiocarpal glide
    and midcarpal glides, 604, *604*
    with movement, 631, *632*
Palpation, 222–223 (*see also specific entries*)
    cervical and thoracic spine, 661–664
        bony palpation, 662–663
        functional testing, 664
    elbow, 527–528, *528*
    hip joint, 334, 337, 351
    knee joint, 289
    lumbar spine and sacroiliac joint, 391
        bony palpation, 392, *392*
        skin observation and, 391–392
        soft-tissue palpation, 392–393, *393*
        starting position, 391
    physical examination, 164–166, 165t
    shoulder complex, 474
        bony palpation, 453–454
        soft-tissue palpation, 454–455, *454*
    special considerations with, 611
    spine, 90, *91*
    temporomandibular joint
        bony palpation, 703–705, *704*
        soft-tissue palpation, 705–706, *705*
    wrist and hand complex
        bony palpation, 596–597
        soft-tissue palpation, 597
Pancoast tumor, 125
Panner disease, 553
Paper grip test, 213
Parafunctional behaviors, 707, *708*
    eliminating, 716–717
Paresthesias, 214
    tests
        dorsal and plantar tinel test, 219
        metatarsal compression test, 218, *219*
        mulder sign, 218–219
        thumb index finger squeeze test, 218, *219*
Passive accessory motions, 161
Passive overpressure, 43
Passive range of motion (PROM), 151, 383
    end feel, 153–154
    interpretation of symptoms, 154
    quantity, 151–153
    signs and symptoms, 153
Patella, 261, *261*
Patellar fracture, 303
Patellar instability
    differential diagnoses, 304
    expected outcomes, 304
    key examination findings, 304
    pathology, 303–304
    rehabilitation focus and key points, 304
Patellar tendinopathy, 261
    differential diagnoses, 302
    expected outcomes, 303
    history, 302
    key examination findings, 302
    pathology, 302
    rehabilitation focus and key points, 302, *303*, 303t
Patellofemoral joint, 272–273
    alignment, 273, *273*
    kinematics, 273–274
    mobilization, 281–282, *282*

Patellofemoral pain syndrome (PFPS), 146
  differential diagnoses, 305–306
  expected outcomes, 306
  history, 304–305
  key examination findings, 305, *305*
  pathology, 304, *305*
  rehabilitation focus and key points, 306
Patellofemoral pathology, special test for knee joint, 287
    apprehension test, 287, *287*
    grind test, 288, *288*
    medial patellar tilt test, 288, *288*
    multiangle isometric quadriceps test, 287–288
Pathoanatomic diagnosis, 166
Patient education, 716–719, *717–719*
Patient-generated joint mobilizations, 498–499, *499*
Patient history, 122–125 (*see also specific entries*)
  advantages, 142, 144
  general demographics, 125–126, *127*
  health history, 126
    general medical information, 126–128, 127t
    health habits, 128–129, 128t
    medical tests, 129
  intake form, *123–124*
  key elements, *123*
  review of systems, 141–144, *142*, 142t, *143*
  symptom investigation, 129
    chief complaint, 129–130
    function, 140–141, *140–141*
    goals, 141
    onset, 130–131, *130*
    stability, 139–140, *140*
    symptoms, 131–133, *131–132*, 132t
    treatment and testing, 133–139, *134–139*, 135t
Patient-Specific Functional Scale (PSFS), 140, *140*, 342, 343t, 707, 731, *731*
Patient-specific health education, pain, 733–734
  content of information, 734
  delivery of, 734
  pain neuroscience education, 734–735
Patient-Specific Outcome Tool, 275, 598
Pattern recognition, 125
PCL (*see* Posterior cruciate ligament)
PCS (*see* Pain Catastrophizing Scale)
Pectoralis major, 448t
Pectoralis minor
  length assessment, 460, *460*
  manual stretching of, 487, *488*
PEG-3, 732t
Pelvic diaphragm, 82
Pelvic floor muscle (PFM), 82–83, *85–87*
  dysfunction, 406–407, 407t
Pelvic fractures, 413
Pelvic rotation, 339–340
Perception, 726–727, *727*
Perdue pegboard test, 613t
Performance-Oriented Mobility Assessment (POMA), 113, 113t
Perichondrium, 10
Perineurium, 31

Periosteum, 10
Peripheral nervous system (PNS), 29, *31*
  anatomy and physiology, 726–727
  injury grading system, 32t
Peripheral neuropathic pain, 728, 729t
Peripheralization, 379
Peritendinitis, 22
Personal Health Questionnaire-9 (PHQ-9), 730t
PFasc, 229
Pfirrmann classification system, 99
PFM (*see* Pelvic floor muscle)
PFPS (*see* Patellofemoral pain syndrome)
PGs (*see* Proteoglycans)
Phalanges, 189, *567*, 570
Phalen test, 610, *610*
PHQ-9 (*see* Personal Health Questionnaire-9)
Physical examination (*see also specific entries*)
  case, 171–172
  clearing examination, 149
  clinical decision-making, 166–168
    articular cartilage, 168
    bone, 168
    bursae, 169
    intra-articular fibrocartilage, 168
    joint capsule, 168–169
    ligaments, 169
    muscle, 169
    nerves, 169–170
    tendons, 169
  components of, 147, *147*
  integrated approach to treatment, 170–171
  introduction to, 146–148
  joint-specific examination, 149–150
    accessory motions, 161–163, *162*, *163–164*t
    functional testing, 166
    gait, 166
    mobility, 166
    muscle length, 154–155
    muscle performance, 155–158, 155t
    neurodynamic tests, 161
    palpation, 164–166, 165t
    range of motion, 150–155, *151–152*, 153t, 154t
    reflexes, 158, 161, 161t
    special tests, 163
    structure, 150
    transfers, 166
  plan of care, 170
  prognosis, 170
  purposes of, 146
  quarter screen, 149
  systems review, 148–149
Piano key sign, 465, 607, *608*
PIIS (*see* Posterior inferior iliac spine)
Pinch assessment, 602, *602*
PIP joint (*see* Proximal interphalangeal joint)
Piriformis syndrome (*see* Deep gluteal syndrome)
Pittsburgh Knee Rules, 275, 277t
Plain film radiography, 135
Plane of scapula, 438, *438*

Plank, 487, *487*
Plantar aponeurosis, 195, *196*
Plantar fasciopathy
  differential diagnoses, 230
  expected outcomes, 231
  history, 230
  key examination findings, 230
  pathology, 229–230
  rehabilitation focus and key points, 230–231
  surgical interventions, *231–233*
Plantar flexion/dorsiflexion, 198
Plexopathies, 169
Plica syndrome, 310
Plicae, 265
PLL (*see* Posterior longitudinal ligament)
Plyometric functional tests, 223
Plyometrics, 298
PNE (*see* Pain neuroscience education)
PNS (*see* Peripheral nervous system)
Polypeptide chains, 4
Polyurethane (PU), 114
POMA (*see* Performance-Oriented Mobility Assessment)
Popeye deformity, 495
Popliteal cyst, 277
Positioning, temporomandibular dysfunction, 717, *717*
Post-traumatic knee arthritis, 739
Posterior apprehension test, 471, *472*
Posterior atlanto-occipital membrane, 71
Posterior capsule, 499, *499*
Posterior cruciate ligament (PCL), 12, *13*, *263*, 264
  injuries, 300–301, *301*
Posterior drawer test, 285–286, *286*
Posterior glide
  clavicle on sternum, 464
  humerus, 462, *462*
Posterior inferior iliac spine (PIIS), 392
Posterior longitudinal ligament (PLL), 66, 66t
Posterior superior iliac spine (PSIS), 75, 90, 334, 378
Posterior talofibular (PTF) ligament, 186, 187, 193
Posterior thigh thrust, 390
Postoperative physical therapy, 309
Posture and temporomandibular joint positioning, 709, *709*
Power grips, 611, *612*
Precision grip, 611–612, *612*
Precision handling, 612–613
Prefabricated foot orthotics, 117
Prefabricated wrist orthosis, 633, *633*
Preoperative rehabilitation, 309
Press test, 609
Pressure algometry, 732, *733*
Primary intention, 21
Primary tissue injury, 18, *18*
Progressive tendon loading, 240
Proliferative phase of tissue healing, 19t, 20
PROM (*see* Passive range of motion)
Pronated foot/supinated foot, 198
Pronation/supination, 198
Prone ball catch, 501, *501*
Prone external rotation, 501, *501*

Prone humeral distraction in flexion, 498, *499*
Prone instability test, 349–350, *350*, 389, *389*
Prone knee flexion, 386
Prone "T" exercise, 501, *501*
Prone "Y" exercise, 501, *501*
Proteoglycans (PGs), 2, 6–9, 8t
Provocation tests, 163
Proximal femoral shaft, 330
Proximal hamstring (HS) tendinopathy
    differential diagnoses, 362
    expected outcomes, 362
    history, 362
    key examination findings, 362
    pathology, 362
    rehabilitation focus and key points, 362, *363*
Proximal humerus, 437, *437*
    with major bony landmarks, *438*
Proximal interphalangeal (PIP) joint, 570
Proximal radioulnar joint (PRUJ), 571
Proximal tibiofibular joint, 191, 214, *215*
PRUJ (*see* Proximal radioulnar joint)
PSEQ (*see* Pain Self-Efficacy Questionnaire)
PSFS (*see* Patient-Specific Functional Scale)
PSIS (*see* Posterior superior iliac spine)
Psychiatric system, 376
Psychosocial impairments
    measurement tools for, 730, 730t
PTF ligament (*see* Posterior talofibular ligament)
PU (*see* Polyurethane)
Push-up test, elbow and, 538
Pyramid of Progressive Force, 623

Q

Quadrant test, 389, *389*
Quadriceps active drawer test, 286
Quadriceps contusion, 310–311, *311*
Quadriceps/Q angle, 274
Quarter screen, 149
Quick-DASH, 598

R

Radial bursa, 614
Radial nerve, 592, *595*
Radial radiocarpal and midcarpal glides, 604–605
Radial wrist pain, 624–625, 624t
Radiculopathy, 169, special tests for, 655–656
Radiocapitellar compression test, elbow and, 538, *539*
Radiocarpal and midcarpal distraction, 604
Radiocarpal joint, 571–573, *572–574*
Radiographs, 135, 135t
Radionuclide bone scan, 138–139, *139*
Radius and ulna, 566, *567–569*
Rancho Los Amigos Gait Assessment Form, 111, *111*
Range of motion (ROM), 150 (*see also specific entries*)
    active range of motion (AROM), 150
        interpretation of symptoms, 154
        quality, 150
        quantity, 150
        signs and symptoms, 150–151
    elbow and, 531, 531t
    hip joint, stability tests, 348
        abduction-hyperextension-external rotation test, 349, *349*
        FABER test, 348–349, *349*
        log roll test, 349, *349*
        prone hip instability test, 349–350, *350*
    knee joint, 267, 277–278, 277t
    lumbar spine and sacroiliac joint, 384–385
    passive range of motion (PROM), 151
        end feel, 153–154
        interpretation of symptoms, 154
        quantity, 151–153
        signs and symptoms, 153
Rearfoot bones
    calcaneus, 187–189, *188*
    talus, 186–187, *188*
Rearfoot varus, 210
Red flags, 141
    screening, 644–646
Reflexes (*see also specific entries*)
    arc, *32*
    elbow and, 533
    hip joint, 345
    knee joint, 280
    physical examination, 158, 161, 161t
    screen, 180, 180t, 431, 432t
    wrist and hand complex, 603
Relative motion orthosis, *620*
Relocation test, 470, *471*
Remodeling phase, 27
    tissue healing, 18, 19t
Resisted external derotation test, 347, *348*
Reticular fibers, 6
Reticulin (*see* Reticular fibers)
Retrocalcaneal bursitis, 241
Reverse total shoulder arthroplasty (rTSA), 477
Review of systems, 455–456
    cardiovascular and pulmonary systems, 455
    constitutional symptoms, 456
    gastrointestinal system, 455
    patient history, 141–144, *142*, 142t, *143*
    physical examination, 148–149
    urogenital system, 455
Rheumatoid arthritis, 572, *573*
Rhomboid major, 448t
Rhomboid minor, 448t
Right anterior knee pain, 319–320
Roos test, 660
Rotation, 39
Rotator cuff muscles, 447–448, *449* (*see also specific muscles*)
Rotator cuff pathology, 481–485, 482t, 483–485, 484t
Royal London Hospital test, 221
rTSA (*see* Reverse total shoulder arthroplasty)
Running shoes, 116, *116*
Rupture, 17
    extensor tendon, 619, *619*

S

Sacral plexus, *62*
Sacroiliac compression, 390
Sacroiliac dysfunction, 390
    Gaenslen test, 390, *391*
    posterior thigh thrust, 390
    sacroiliac (anterior) gap, 390
    sacroiliac compression, 390
Sacroiliac gap, 390
Sacroiliac joint (SIJ), 73, *74–75*
    dysfunction
        differential diagnoses, 416
        expected outcomes, 418
        history, 416
        key examination findings, 416
        pathology, 415–416
        rehabilitation focus and key points, 416–418, 416–417t, *418*
    ligaments stabilizing, 75t, *76*
    as part of pelvic basin with osteologic landmarks, *74*
Sacrotuberous ligament, 393
Sacrum, 73, *73*
Sagittal vertical extrusion device (SVED), 721
Scaphoid, 568, 625, 626t
    compression test, 599, *599*
    fracture, 149, 627–628
    palmar glide of, 631–632, *632*
    shift test, 606–607, *607*
Scapholunate advanced collapse, 626
Scapula, *436*, 437, *438*
    movements of, 438–440, *439*
    plane of, 438, *438*
    resting position on the thorax, *439*
Scapular assistance test, 468, *468*
Scapular distraction, 496, *497*
Scapular dyskinesia, 468, 485–488, *486–488*
    causes of, 489
    corner stretch, 487, *487*
    plank, 487, *487*
Scapular mobilization, 463, *463*
Scapular retraction test, 468, *468*
Scapulohumeral muscles, 447–451, 447t, *449–451*
Scapulohumeral rhythm, 446–447
Scapulothoracic joint, 442–443, *442*
Scapulothoracic motions and muscle working as prime movers, 448t
Scapulothoracic muscles, 448t, 451–452
SCFE (*see* Slipped capital femoral epiphysis)
Scoliosis, *50*, 51, *51*
Scotty dog, 51
Scour, 750
    test, 350, *350*
Screening
    for cardiac-related medications, 127
    for hip fracture, 342–343
    for musculoskeletal system, 148
    neuromuscular system, 148–149
Screw-home mechanism, 41
Seated piriformis stretch, 390, *390*
Secondary tissue injury, 18
Seddon Classification System, 31
SEES (*see* Self-Efficacy for Exercise Scale)

INDEX

Self-Efficacy for Exercise Scale (SEES), 730t
Self-management support, pain, 733–735
Self-mobilization for carpal tunnel syndrome, 628, *629*
Self-palpation of temporomandibular joint, 718, *718*
Self-report scales, 731, *731*
Self-report tools, 729–730 (*see also specific tools*)
Sensory (afferent) neuron, 29
Sensory tests, 158, *159*, 214 (*see also specific entries*)
  hand, 602, *603*
  hip joint, 345
  knee joint, 280
Serratus anterior, 448t
Sesamoids, 189
SGHL (*see* Superior GH ligament)
Sharp-purser test, 659, *660*
Shear forces on tissues, 16, *16*
Sheet-forming and anchoring collagens, 6, 7t
Shock-absorbing footwear, 307
Short-Form 36 Bodily Pain Scale (SF-36 BPS), 732t
Shoulder blade (*see* Scapula)
Shoulder complex
  additional joint mobilization techniques
    clinician-generated joint mobilizations, 496–498, *497–499*
    patient-generated joint mobilizations, 498–499, *499*
  additional therapeutic exercises, 499–502, *499–502*
  arthroplasty, 477–478, *477*
  bilateral, pain, 756–761
  case study, 502–503, 756–761
  differential diagnosis, 495, *496–497*, 496t
  elevation, 446
  examination of, 455
  functional anatomy, 435–436, *435*
    osteology, 436–437, *436–438*
  girdle, 435, *435*
  joints, 438–440, *438–439*
    acromioclavicular joint and ligaments, *440*, 441–442
    glenohumeral joint and ligaments, 443–446, 443t, *444*, 445t, *446*
    scapulohumeral rhythm, 446–447
    scapulothoracic joint, 442–443, *442*
    sternoclavicular joint and ligaments, 440–441, *440–441*
    subacromial space, 443, *443*
  muscles
    axiohumeral muscles, 448t, 452
    force couples of the shoulder, 452–453, *452–453*
    scapulohumeral muscles, 447–451, 447t, *449–451*
    scapulothoracic motions and muscle working as prime movers, 448t
    scapulothoracic muscles, 448t, 451–452
  palpation
    bony palpation, 453–454
    soft-tissue palpation, 454–455, *454*
  pathologies, 456
    acromioclavicular degenerative joint disease, 476
    acromioclavicular joint separation, 474–476, 475t
    adhesive capsulitis, 478–481, *479–481*, 479t
    biceps pathology, 495, 495t
    glenohumeral instability, *490*, 490–493, 490t, 492–493t
    glenohumeral osteoarthritis, 477
    labral pathology, 493–495, *493*
    rotator cuff pathology, 481–485, 482t, *483–485*, 484t
    scapular dyskinesia, 485–488, *486–488*
    shoulder arthroplasty, 477–478, *477*
    sternoclavicular joint pathology, 476–477
    subacromial impingement syndrome, 488–489
    suprascapular neuropathy, 495
  patient history
    chief complaint, 457
    location of symptoms, 456
    neck pathology, 456
    onset, 456
    outcome measures, 457–458, 457t
    patient characteristics, 456
    review of systems, 455–456
    shoulder pathology, 456
    symptom behavior, 457
  physical examination
    accessory motion, 461–464, *462–464*
    functional testing, 474, *474*
    muscle length, 460, *460*, 460t
    muscle performance, 461, *461*
    neurodynamic testing, 461
    palpation, 474
    range of motion, 459–460, 459t, *459–460*
    reflexes, 461
    sensory tests, 461
    skin, 458–459
    special tests/provocative testing, 464–474, *465–474*
    structure, 458, 459t
Sidelying horizontal adduction, 499, *499*
Sidelying shoulder flexion, 500, *500*
SIJ (*see* Sacroiliac joint)
SIS (*see* Subacromial impingement syndrome)
Sit-to-stand tests, 733
Six-minute walk test, 113t, 408
Skier's thumb, 613
Skin, 164–165 (*see also specific entries*)
  mobility, 165
  moisture and texture, 165
  observation, 164
  swelling, 165, 165t
  temperature, 165
SLAC wrist (*see* Scapholunate advanced collapse)
SLAP lesions (*see* Superior labrum anterior and posterior lesions)
Sleep, 128
Sleep disturbances, 128
Slide, 39–40
Slip-lasted construction design, 114
Slipped capital femoral epiphysis (SCFE), 342, 363
Slipping rib syndrome, 680–681
Slump test, 386–387, *387*
sMCL (*see* Superficial medial collateral ligament)
Smith fracture, 572, *574*, 626, *627*
Soft callus formation, 27
Soft tissue
  impingement, 238
  palpation, 392–393, *393*, 454–455, *454*
    temporomandibular joint, 705–706, *705*
    wrist and hand complex, 597
  wrist and hand complex, 600–601
Somatic sensory neurons, 29
Specialized connective tissue, 3
Speed test, 473, *473*
Sphenoid bone, 697
Spinal cord, *61*
  and vertebral column, 65
Spinal coupling, 90, *92*
Spinal dural sac, 64
Spinal ganglia, *61*
Spinal nerve, 60–64
  exit from vertebral column, 61t
  formation of, *60*
  plexuses formed by anterior rami of, 62–63
Spinal stenosis, 100–101, *101*
Spine extension, *56*
Spine flexion, *56*
Spine osteology, 48–49
  facet joints
    close- and open-packed position, 60
    innervation, 60
    intervertebral disc height and, 60
    and movement, 58–60, *58*
    regional orientation, 58–59, *59*
  intervertebral disc
    biomechanics, 55–56, *55–56*
    nutrition, 56–58
  kinematics
    arthrokinematic movement, 92, *93*
    movement and impact on neural structures, 90
    osteokinematic and arthrokinematic movement by region, 93–96, *93–96*
    osteokinematic movement, 92, *92*, 92t
    spinal coupling, 90, *92*
  muscles, 75, 77t, 78–80, 81t
    anterior and lateral neck muscles, 88–90, 89t
    extrinsic back muscles, 77
    intrinsic back muscles, 77–79
    stabilizing muscles, 80–88, 81–82t, *82–87*
    suboccipital muscles, 88, *88*
  palpation, 90, *91*
  regional characteristics for vertebrae, ligaments, and discs, 68–69, *68*
    cervical vertebrae and ligaments, 69–71, *69–70*
    coccyx, 74
    ligaments of cervical vertebrae, 71, *71*
    lumbar vertebrae, 72–73, *73*
    sacrum, 73, *73*
    thoracic vertebrae, 71–72, *72*

sacroiliac joint, 74–75, *74*, 75t, *76*
spinal cord segment and spinal nerve, 60–64
    exit from vertebral column, 61t
    formation of, *60*
    plexuses formed by anterior rami of, *62–63*
spinal ganglia, *61*
vertebral canal
    contents of, 64, *65*
vertebral column (*see* Vertebral column)
Splinting, 620, *620*
Spondylolisthesis, 51
    differential diagnoses, 411
    expected outcomes, 411
    history, 411
    key examination findings, 411
    pathology, 411, 411t
    rehabilitation focus and key points, 411
    surgical interventions, 411
Spondylolysis/stress reactions, 51, 412–413
Spondylosis, 642, 665–666
Sprains and instability tests, 219
    anterior drawer test, 219, *220*
    external rotation stress test, 220, *221*
    fibular translation test, 220–221
    forced dorsiflexion test, 219–220, *220*
    lateral talar tilt test, 220, *221*
    medial talar tilt test, 219, *220*
    syndesmotic squeeze test, 220, *221*
Spurling test, 656, 760
Stabilizing muscles, 80–82, *82*
    abdominal muscles, 82, *83–84*
    gluteal muscles, 84–86, 88
    pelvic floor muscles, 82–83, *85–87*
    trunk, 81–82t
STAI (*see* State-Trait Anxiety Inventory)
Stance phase, 107
STarT Back Screening Tool, 380, 730
State-Trait Anxiety Inventory (STAI), 730t
Stenosing tenosynovitis (*see* Trigger finger)
Stenosis, lumbar
    differential diagnoses, 409
    expected outcomes, 410
    history, 408
    key examination findings, 408–409, 409t
    pathology, 408
    rehabilitation focus and key points, 409–410, *410*
    surgical interventions, 410
Step length, 107
Step width, 107
Sternoclavicular (SC) joint
    and ligaments, 440–441, *440–441*
    pathology, 476–477
Stomatognathic system, 695
Straight leg raise test, 385–386
Strength-biased tests, 385
Stress
    to annular fibers, *57*
    fractures, elbow, 548–549
    on intervertebral disc, 55–56
    on layers of annulus fibrosis, 56
    on tissue, 15–16, *15–17*
Stretching, 240
Stride length, 107, 109
Strobel-lasted construction design, 114

Structural assessment, 179
Structural relationships, 197–198
Stylohyoid muscle, *701*, 702, *703*
Subacromial bursa, 443, *443*
Subacromial impingement, 468–469
Subacromial impingement syndrome (SIS), 488–489, 756–761
Subacromial space, 443, *443*
Suboccipital muscles, 88, *88*
Subscapularis, 447t, *449*
    release, 480, *481*
Subtalar joint, 193, 200, *201*
    mobilizations, 215–216, *217*, 247, *248*
    neutral, 209–210, *209, 210*
Sulcus test, 471, *472*
Superficial extensors of wrist, *581*
Superficial flexors of wrist, *583*
Superficial layer of intrinsic back muscles, 77, *79*
Superior (alveolar) border, 695
Superior GH ligament (SGHL), 444
Superior glide of clavicle on sternum, 464
Superior labrum anterior and posterior (SLAP) lesions, 493–495
Suprahyoid muscle, 702, *703*
Suprapatellar bursa, 265
Suprascapular neuropathy, 495
Supraspinatus, 447t, *449*
    positioning, 454, *454*
Supraspinatus test, 465
Supraspinous ligament, 66t, 67–68
SVED (*see* Sagittal vertical extrusion device)
Swan-neck deformity, 622
Swing phase, 107
Symptoms
    associated symptoms, 133
    constancy, 133
    irritability, 133, 134t
    location, 131–132, *132*
    modifying factors, 133
    quality of, 132–133, 132t
    severity, 133, 133t
    24-hour pattern, 133
Syndecan, 8t, 9
Syndesmotic squeeze test, 220, *221*
Synovial fluid, 36, 38
Synovial inflammation, 168
Synovial joints, 36–37, *36*
    differentiation of joint receptors, 37t
    joint surface shape, 38, 38t, *39*
    neurology, 37–38
    nutrition and lubrication, 38
    stability of, 36
    traditional anatomical classification of, 38t
Synovium, 265

T

T1 vertebra, 72
T12 vertebra, 72
Tailor bunions, 208
Talocrural joint, 199–200, *199, 200*
    mobilization, 215, *216*
Talonavicular joint, 193, *194*
Talus, 186–187, *188*

Tampa Scale for Kinesiophobia (TSK), 296, 380, 707, 730t, 749, 759
Taping, 237
Tarsal coalitions, 189, 190, 191
Tarsal Tunnel Syndrome (TTS), 243–244
Tarsometatarsal joints, 194–195, 203
    rotation of, 248, *249*
TDH (*see* Thoracic disc herniation)
Tear drop pinch test, 539–540, *539*
Teeth
    examination of, 709
    malalignments of, *698*
    upper and lower jaw, 695, *697*
Temporal bone, 697, *697–698*
Temporalis, 700–702, *701*, 701t
    palpation of, 705, *705*
Temporomandibular dysfunction (TMD)
    interventions for, 716
        interprofessional collaboration, 719, 721
        modalities, 721
        patient education, 716–719, *717–719*
        screening questions, 706
Temporomandibular joint (TMJ)
    arthrokinematics, 702–703, *704*
    case study, 720
    examination of, 706
    expected outcomes, 721
    functional anatomy, 695–698, *696–698*
    interventions for temporomandibular dysfunction, 716
        interprofessional collaboration, 719, 721
        modalities, 721
        patient education, 716–719, *717–719*
    joint structure and ligaments, 698–699, *699*
    movements of, 699, *700*
    muscles, 700–702, *701–703*, 701t
    osteology, 695–698, *696–698*
    palpation
        bony palpation, 703–705, *704*
        soft-tissue palpation, 705–706, *705*
    pathologies, 714–715
        arthralgia, 715–716
        differential diagnosis of pain, 716, 716t
        disc displacements, 715
        masticatory muscle disorders, 715
    patient history
        aggravating activities, 706–707
        past medical history, 707
        outcome measures, 707, 709t
        parafunctional behaviors, 707, *708*
        symptoms, 706
        temporomandibular dysfunction screening questions, 706
        trauma and imaging, 706
    physical examination, 707
        accessory motion, 712–713, *712–713*
        functional testing, 714
        muscle performance, 711, 711t
        neurologic testing, 713, *713*
        occlusion and dentition, 708–709
        palpation, 713, 713t
        postural alignment, 709, *709*
        range of motion, 710–711, 710t, *710–711*
        skin and nails, 710
        special tests/provocative testing, 713–714, *714–715*

Temporomandibular joint compression test, 714, *715*
Tenascin, 9, 9t
Tendinitis, 22
Tendinopathy, 22, 169
Tendinosis, 22
Tendon, 12–13, *14*
    gliding, 623–624, *624*
    injury, 21–22
    treatment to promote healing, 22
Tenosynovitis, 169
TENS (*see* Transcutaneous electrical nerve stimulation)
Tension forces on tissues, 16–17, *16*
Teres major, 447t, *449*
Teres minor, 447t, *449*
TFC (*see* Triangular fibrocartilage)
TFCC (*see* Triangular fibrocartilage complex)
THA (*see* Total hip arthroplasty)
Thenar eminence, 597
Therapeutic alliance, 731, *731*
Therapeutic exercises, 248, *250*
    additional, 499–502, *499–502*
    temporomandibular dysfunction, 717–718, *718*
Thessaly test, 284, *284*
Thompson test, 221
Thoracic (T6) vertebra, 53t, *54*
Thoracic compression, 656
    fractures, 672–675, *674*
Thoracic disc herniation (TDH), 100
Thoracic distraction, 656–657
Thoracic outlet syndrome, 678–680
Thoracic radiculopathy, 680
Thoracic spine
    frontal plane movement, 95
    horizontal plane movement, 95
    sagittal plane movement, 95
Thoracic transverse pressure, 654–655, *655*
Thoracic unilateral posteroanterior pressure, 652–653, *653*
Thoracic vertebrae, 71–72, *72*
Three-jaw chuck, 602
Thrust technique, 46
Thumb
    ball rolling exercise, 616, *617*
    carpometacarpal joint mobilization, 606, *606*
    index finger squeeze test, 218, *219*
    spica taping, 633
Tibial (medial) collateral ligament, 12, *13*
Tibial plateau, 260
Tibialis posterior dysfunction (TPD)
    differential diagnoses, 243
    expected outcomes, 243
    history, 242
    key examination findings, 242–243
    pathology, 241–242, 241–242t
    rehabilitation focus and key points, 243, *243*
Tibiofemoral joint mobilization, 281, *282*, 311, 313, *313*
Tilt of distal radius, 566, *568*
Timed Up and Go (TUG) test, 113t, 733
Tinel test, 624t
Tip-to-tip pinch, 602

Tissues (*see also specific tissues*)
    behavior, 15–16, *15–16*
        composition, 17
        properties, 17, *17*
    fatigue, 131
    healing, *19*, 19t
        abnormalities in wound healing, 21
        closed and open wound healing, 20–21
        factors affecting healing, 21, *21*
        inflammatory phase, 18–20, *20*
    injury, 17–18
        primary tissue injury, 18, *18*
        secondary tissue injury, 18
    irritability, 133, 479–480, 479t
    various loading modes to, *16*
TKA (*see* Total knee arthroplasty)
TMD (*see* Temporomandibular dysfunction)
TMJ (*see* Temporomandibular joint)
Tongue blades for jaw stretching, 717–718, *718*
Tongue-up opening technique, 717, *717*
Torticollis, 672
Total hip arthroplasty (THA), 353–355, 354t
Total knee arthroplasty (TKA), 308–309
Total shoulder arthroplasty (TSA), 477–478, *477*
TPD (*see* Tibialis posterior dysfunction)
TrAb (*see* Transversus abdominis)
Trabeculae, 10
Traction/distraction, 161
Tracts, 31
Transcutaneous electrical nerve stimulation (TENS), 736
Transduction, 726–727, *727*
Transient or wandering cells, 3
Translation, 39
Transmembrane collagen, 6, 7t
Transmission, 726–727, *727*
Transverse pressure, 388, *389*
Transversus abdominis (TrAb), 82, 399
Trapezium, 570
Trapezoid, 570
Trauma and imaging, 706
Trendelenburg gait, 385
Trendelenburg test, 347, *348*, 416
Triangular fibrocartilage (TFC), 566, *568*
Triangular fibrocartilage complex (TFCC), 566, 571, *571*
    dorsal components, 572
    grind test, 609, *609*
    injury, 625
    palmar components, 572
    pathology, special tests for, 609–610
    ulnar components, 572
Triceps rupture, distal, 552–553
Trigger finger, 621–622, *622*
Trigger points, 414
Triquetrum, 568, 625, 626t
Trismus, 711
Tropocollagen, 4
True ribs, 663
Trunk muscle performance, 385
    activation/movement control–biased tests, 385, 385t, *386*
    strength-biased tests, 385
Trunk screen, 180

TSA (*see* Total shoulder arthroplasty)
TSK (*see* Tampa Scale for Kinesiophobia)
TTS (*see* Tarsal Tunnel Syndrome)
TUG test (*see* Timed Up and Go test)

U

UCL (*see* Ulnar collateral ligament)
Ulna, radius and, 566, *567–569*
Ulnar and radial collateral stress test, 608, *608*
Ulnar collateral ligament (UCL), 613–614, *613*
Ulnar drift of metacarpals, 617, *618*
Ulnar nerve, 592, *594*
    compression at tunnel of Guyon, 629
    paralysis, 600, *600*
Ulnar radiocarpal and midcarpal glides, 604, *605*
Ultrasound imaging, 139, *139*
Uncovertebral joint, 70
Unilateral bite test, 714, *714*
Unilateral posteroanterior pressure, 387–388, *388*
Upper extremity peripheral and segmental nerve innervation, 769–770t
Upper quarter neurologic screen (UQNS), 428, 430–431, *430*, *431*, 431t
Upper quarter screen (UQS)
    case, 432–433
    components, 428–429, *429*
        functional testing, 432
        integument, 432
        observation, 429
        structure and posture, 429–430, 429t
        upper extremity motion and strength, 431–432, 432t
        upper quarter neurologic screen, 430–431, *430*, *431*, 431t
        vasculature, 432
    general rules, 428
    purpose of, 428
UQNS (*see* Upper quarter neurologic screen)
UQS (*see* Upper quarter screen)
Urinary incontinence, 376
Urogenital system, 455

V

Valgus, 198
    collapse, 293
    instability, elbow, 544–546
    stress test, 286–287, *287*, 536, *537*
Van Rijn's classification, 99
Varus stress test, 537–538, *538*
VAS (*see* Visual analog scale)
Vascular testing, 603
VBI (*see* Vertebrobasilar insufficiency)
Ventral radiohumeral glide, 534, *535*
Versican, 8t, 9
Vertebra prominens, 71
Vertebrae, typical, 52–55, *53–55*
    comparisons by region, 53t
    components of, 53
Vertebral arch, 53
Vertebral body, 53
Vertebral canal, contents of, 64, *65*

Vertebral column, 48–49, *48*, 61
  curvatures
    during maturation, *49*
    normal alignment and, 50–52, *50–52*
    normal curvatures of, *49*
  ligaments of, 64, 66–68, 66t, *67*
  movement of, 64
  osteokinematic movement of, *92*
  pathologies of
    cervical disc herniation, 99–100
    classification of herniated nucleus pulposus and nerve root involvement, 98–99, *99*, 99t
    degenerative disc disease, 96–97, *97*
    herniated nucleus pulposus (*see* Herniated nucleus pulposus)
    lumbar disc herniation, 100
    spinal stenosis, 100–101, *101*
    thoracic disc herniation, 100
  role of, 49
  spinal nerve exit from, 61t
  in thoracic spine, *72*
  typical vertebrae, 52–55, *53–55*, 53t
Vertebrobasilar insufficiency (VBI), 644
  test, 658–659
Victorian Institute of Sports Assessment-Achilles (VISA-A), 206t
Visual analog scale (VAS), 731–732

W

"W" exercise, 500, *500*
Walking speed, 107–109, 112
Wall angels, 500, *500*
Wartenberg syndrome, 624, 624t
Watson test (*see* Scaphoid, shift test)
Wedge fracture (*see* Compression fracture)
Wedges, 118
Whiplash-associated disorder and neck-coordination deficits, 668–670
Windlass test, 222, *222*
Wolff law, 15, *15*
Wound healing (*see also* Healing)
  abnormalities, 21
  closed and open, 20–21
Wrist and hand complex
  additional joint mobilization treatment techniques, 630
    palmar glide of scaphoid, 631–632, *632*
    palmar radiocarpal glide with movement, 631, *632*
  case study, 635
  differential diagnosis, 630, 630t, *631*
  examination of, 597
  functional anatomy, 566
  joints of
    carpometacarpal joints, 575, *576*
    distal radioulnar joint, 571, *571*
    interphalangeal joints, 577
    metacarpophalangeal joints, 575–577, *576–577*
    midcarpal and intercarpal joints, 573–575, *574–575*
    radiocarpal joint, 571–573, *572–574*
  ligaments of
    hand, 579, 579t
    wrist, 577–578, *578*, 578t
  muscles of, 579–588, 589t
  nerves supplying, *596*
    median nerve, 592, *593*
    radial nerve, 592, *595*
    ulnar nerve, 592, *594*
  osteology
    arches, 570–571, *570*
    carpals, 566, *567*, 568–570, *569*
    distal end of radius and ulna, 566, *567–569*
    metacarpals, *567*, 570
    phalanges, *567*, 570
  palpation
    bony palpation, 596–597
    soft-tissue palpation, 597
  pathologies
    carpal tunnel syndrome, 628–629, *629*
    complex regional pain syndrome, 629–630, 629t, *630*
    dupuytren contracture, 621
    extensor tendon disruption, 619–621, 619t, *619–620*
    finger osteoarthritis, 617–619, *618*
    first carpometacarpal arthroplasty, 617
    first carpometacarpal joint osteoarthritis, 615–617, *615–617*
    flexor pollicis longus tenosynovitis, 614–615
    fracture, 626–628, *627*
    radial wrist pain, 624–625, 624t
    rehabilitation after finger flexor repair, 622–624, *622, 624*
    swan-neck deformity, 622
    triangular fibrocartilage complex injury, 625
    trigger finger, 621–622, *622*
    ulnar collateral ligament injuries, 613–614, *613*
    ulnar nerve compression at tunnel of guyon, 629
    wrist instability, 625–626, 626t
  patient history
    chief complaint, 598
    hand dominance, 597
    mechanism of onset, 597
    occupation and recreational activities, 597
    outcome measures, 598, 598t
    prior history, 598
  physical examination, 598–600, *599*
    accessory motion, 603–606, 603t, *604–606*, 605t
    functional testing, 611–613, *612*, 613t
    muscle length, 602
    muscle performance, 602, *602*
    neurodynamic testing, 603
    range of motion, *601*, 601–602, 601t
    reflexes, 603
    sensory tests, 602, *603*
    skin and nails, 601
    special considerations with palpation, 611
    special tests/provocative testing, 606–610, *607–611*
    structure and posture, 600–601, *600*
    vascular testing, 603
  specific anatomic regions of
    anatomical snuffbox, 592, *592*
    carpal tunnel, 592, *592*
    extensor retinaculum and expansion, 590–591, *590–591*
    palmar aponeurosis and flexor tendon sheaths, 591, *591*
  therapeutic interventions
    interventions for range of motion, 632
    interventions for strengthening, 632–633, *633*
    joint protection strategies, 633, *633–634*
Wrist instability, 625–626, 626t

Y

Y-shaped arcuate ligament, 265
Yellow Flag Assessment, 707
Yellow flags, 142
  screening, 729–730, *730*
Yergason test, *474*

Z

Zona orbicularis, 333
Zygapophyseal joints (*see* Facet joints)